Clinical
Diagnosis of
Mental Disorders
A Handbook

Clinical Diagnosis of Mental Disorders
A Handbook

Edited by
Benjamin B. Wolman

Plenum Press · New York and London

Library of Congress Cataloging in Publication Data

Main entry under title:

Clinical diagnosis of mental disorders.

Includes bibliographies and index.
1. Mental illness – Diagnosis. 2. Psychological tests. 3. Diagnosis, Differential. I.
Wolman, Benjamin B. [DNLM: 1. Mental disorders – Diagnosis. WM141 C641]
RC469.C58   616.8′9′075   78-14969
ISBN 0-306-31141-0

© 1978 Plenum Press, New York
A Division of Plenum Publishing Corporation
227 West 17th Street, New York, N.Y. 10011

Printed in the United States of America

Contributors

Joel Allison, Ph.D.
Department of Psychology
Yale University
New Haven, Connecticut 06520

Andrea Alper
Doctoral Program in Clinical Psychology
Long Island University
Brooklyn, New York 11201

Leopold Bellak, M.D.
Department of Psychiatry
Albert Einstein College of Medicine
Bronx, New York 10461

Thomas J. Boll, Ph.D.
Division of Child and Adolescent Psychiatry
University of Virginia Medical Center
Charlottesville, Virginia 22901

James N. Butcher, Ph.D.
Psychology Department
University of Minnesota
Minneapolis, Minnesota 55455

Beth Clark
Doctoral Program in Clinical Psychology
Long Island University
Brooklyn, New York 11201

Jennifer Cole, Ph.D.
Department of Psychology
University of Michigan
Ann Arbor, Michigan 48104

Steve DeBerry
Doctoral Program in Clinical Psychology
Long Island University
Brooklyn, New York 11201

Deborah Lee Doller, Ph.D.
Department of Psychology
Arizona State University
Tempe, Arizona 85281

John E. Exner, Jr., Ph.D.
Doctoral Program in Clinical Psychology
Long Island University
Brooklyn, New York 11201

Cynthia Fielding
Doctoral Program in Clinical Psychology
Florida Institute of Technology
Melbourne, Florida 32901

Leonard D. Goodstein, Ph.D.
Department of Psychology
Arizona State University
Tempe, Arizona 85281

John R. Graham, Ph.D.
Department of Psychology
Kent State University
Kent; Ohio 44240

Emanuel F. Hammer, Ph.D.
Faculty, National Psychological Association
    of Psychoanalysis
381 West End Avenue
New York, New York 10024

David L. Hayes, Ph.D.
Department of Psychology
Michigan State University
East Lansing, Michigan 48824

Wayne H. Holtzman, Ph.D.
Hogg Foundation for Mental Health
The University of Texas at Austin
Austin, Texas 78712

vi

CONTRIBUTORS

Max L. Hutt, Ph.D.
21 Regent Drive
Ann Arbor, Michigan 48104

Etta Karp, Ph.D.
Mental Retardation Institute
New York Medical College
New York, New York 10035

Chase Patterson Kimball, M.D.
Department of Psychiatry
University of Chicago
Chicago, Illinois 60637

Joseph D. Matarazzo, Ph.D.
Department of Medical Psychology
University of Oregon School of Medicine
Portland, Oregon 97201

Martin Mayman, Ph.D.
Department of Psychology
University of Michigan
Ann Arbor, Michigan 48109

Harold Michal-Smith, Ph.D.
Mental Retardation Institute
New York Medical College
New York, New York 10035

Murry Morgenstern, Ph.D.
Mental Retardation Institute
New York Medical College
New York, New York 10035

Jum C. Nunnally, Ph.D.
Department of Psychology
Vanderbilt University
Nashville, Tennessee 37203

Patricia L. Owen, Ph.D.
Psychology Department
University of Minnesota
Minneapolis, Minnesota 55455

Fred J. Pesetsky, Ph.D.
1905 Grovedale
Jackson, Michigan 49203

Vladimir Pishkin, Ph.D.
Veterans Administration Hospital
Oklahoma City, Oklahoma 73104

Albert I. Rabin, Ph.D.
Department of Psychology
Michigan State University
East Lansing, Michigan 48824

Morris I. Stein, Ph.D.
Department of Psychology
New York University
New York, New York 10003

Frederick C. Thorne, M.D., Ph.D.
Clinical Psychology Publishing Co., Inc.
Brandon, Vermont 05733

Edwin E. Wagner, Ph.D.
Department of Psychology
University of Akron
Akron, Ohio 44325

Robert I. Watson, Jr., Ph.D.
Institute of Advanced Psychological Studies
Adelphi University
Garden City, New York 11530

Harold Wilensky, Ph.D.
Psychological Center
City University of New York
New York, New York 10031

Benjamin B. Wolman, Ph.D.
International Encyclopedia of Psychiatry,
    Psychology, Psychoanalysis, & Neurology
10 West 66th Street
New York, New York 10023

Joseph Zubin, M.D.
New York Psychiatric Institute
New York, New York 10032

Preface

For centuries the "treatment" of mentally disturbed individuals was quite simple. They were accused of collusion with evil spirits, hunted, and persecuted. The last "witch" was killed as late as 1782 in Switzerland.

Mentally disturbed people did not fare much better even when the witchhunting days were gone. John Christian Reil gave the following description of mental patients at the crossroads of the fifteenth and sixteenth centuries:

> We incarcerate these miserable creatures as if they were criminals in abandoned jails, near to the lairs of owls in barren canyons beyond the city gates, or in damp dungeons of prisons, where never a pitying look of a humanitarian penetrates; and we let them, in chains, rot in their own excrement. Their fetters have eaten off the flesh of their bones, and their emaciated pale faces look expectantly toward the graves which will end their misery and cover up our shamefulness. (1803)

The great reforms introduced by Philippe Pinel at Bicêtre in 1793 augured the beginning of a new approach. Pinel ascribed the "sick role," and called for compassion and help. One does not need to know much about those he wants to hurt, but one must know a lot in order to help. Pinel's reform was followed by a rapid development in research of causes, symptoms, and remedies of mental disorders.

There are two main prerequisites for planning a treatment strategy. Before starting any therapeutic procedure, be it chemical or physical, or one of the numerous psychotherapeutic techniques, the therapist must decide what bothers the patient, and, resultingly, how to treat him. Only irresponsible quacks and ignoramuses treat without knowing what kind of a condition they are treating, and blindly apply their meager knowledge or guesswork.

Responsible therapy starts with diagnosing the patient's condition. In the dark Middle Ages all kinds of headaches were often "treated" by bloodletting, which was sometimes fatal. Mental patients were "treated" by exorcism and flogging.

Contemporary professionals in any of the healing arts, be it general medicine, dentistry, or treatment of mental disorders, must know before they act. The knowledge of the condition of the patients is called diagnosis. The clinician's decision on how to treat the patient must be determined by his knowledge of the patient's condition, and the method of treatment must be based on thorough diagnostic study of every single case.

vii

The number of men, women, and children in the United States who suffer a variety of mental disorders is more than 20 million, and every year about 3 million people seek professional help. Mental health professionals, psychiatrists, clinical psychologists, psychiatric social workers, and psychiatric nurses try their best to cure or at least to alleviate the sufferings of their patients, and apply a variety of chemical, physical, and psychological methods of treatment.

The aim of this volume is to acquaint them with the much-needed knowledge of diagnostic tools. It is divided into two parts. The first part describes in detail the various diagnostic techniques, and the second part dwells on the problems of differential diagnosis.

In organizing and editing this volume, I was greatly encouraged by the most efficient cooperation of all the authors, and I was guided by the wise suggestions of the members of the Editorial Board. Mr. Seymour Weingarten, formerly the Executive Editor of Plenum Publishing Corporation, has offered most cordial assistance.

BENJAMIN B. WOLMAN

Contents

Part I: Diagnostic Techniques

Part II: Differential Diagnosis

I
Diagnostic Techniques

1

Research in
Clinical Diagnosis

JOSEPH ZUBIN

1. Introduction

By its very nature, the process of clinical diagnosis simulates a research process since it involves the testing of a variety of plausible hypotheses before a final decision is reached. Thus, in a sense, every clinical diagnosis is a research undertaking. Despite this, formal research into clinical diagnosis is of relatively recent vintage. It has two aspects: research into the decision-making process—leading to a diagnosis and research into the results of this process—the diagnosis itself. While the decision-making process itself is now being investigated experimentally, we shall limit ourselves to research in diagnosis itself with special reference to its improvement.

Clinical diagnosis in the mental disorders has a long past, reaching back nearly 34 centuries to the ancient Hindu scriptures (*Caraka Samhita*, 1949), but its history is rather brief, dating back only to Pinel and Esquirol at the beginning of the nineteenth century, who were among the first systematizers in psychopathology. Research in clinical diagnosis was hardly begun before the last quarter of the nineteenth century, after Kraepelin's systematic nosology took hold.

A historical survey of the development of research in clinical diagnosis will have to be left to historians. Here we will be concerned primarily with the current status and future of research into clinical diagnosis.

Perhaps the most apt characterization of the continued search for improvement in diagnosis was made by Heinrich Kluver (personal communication), who wrote:

> I guess something has to be done in re the diagnostic discrepancies, etc. you speak of. As things are, attempts are still made, as [A.] Hoche in Freiburg once expressed it, "To clear turbid solutions by pouring them continually from one glass to the other."

2. Interest in Diagnosis

For a long time, clinical diagnosis was in the doldrums; because no effective therapies were available, it was a mere academic exercise, even when the diagnosis was

JOSEPH ZUBIN • New York Psychiatric Institute, New York, New York 10032.

undisputed. The first breakthrough came with the discovery of the cause of general paresis, which enabled the clinician to appeal to an objective criterion, the Wassermann test, to validate the results of his clinical interviews, observations, and history of the patient. A similar breakthrough occurred subsequently when the cause of pellagra with psychosis was discovered. These advances are hardly remembered as achievements of psychopathology today because the disorders are rare and are no longer regarded as part of psychopathology. Similar notable discoveries in etiology were made in the field of mental retardation, and, although quite a number of inborn errors of metabolism and other genetic abnormalities have been discovered, the proportion of mentally retarded conditions for which the etiology is known is still very small. In the etiology of the mental disorders, especially in the functional disorders, little if any dramatic progress has been made, although the research efforts have been prodigious. We are still abysmally ignorant. Despite the conquest of general paresis, pellagra with psychosis, and several mental defect disorders, interest in diagnosis remained at a low ebb until the advent of the somatotherapies in the 1930s and 1940s. Since these therapies seemed to be most suitable for only certain types of patients, interest in diagnosis was rekindled, but choice of treatment, important as it is, is only one of the purposes of diagnosis. The ideal diagnostic nomenclature should maximize the communicative utility of the diagnostic label, optimize its prognostic potential and its explanatory powers in relation to etiology, and, of course, optimize choice of treatment. To attain this ideal is the goal of research in clinical diagnosis.

3. Defining Mental Health

The first set of problems that one faces in entering this field is the absence of defining boundaries between mental health and mental disorder and, within the vague boundaries of the mental disorders, the nebulous distinctions between the various disorders. The response to this chaotic condition has varied from Szasz's (1961) denial of the existence of mental disorders to the attempts of men like Leonhard (1936, 1959) to subdivide the disorders into minute subgroupings. Leonhard makes meticulous distinctions within diagnostic categories based on hypothetical brain dysfunctions. Szasz, on the other hand, claims that mental disorders are based on arbitrary distinctions between essentially normal but nonconforming individuals made by a psychiatric establishment bent on preserving its status and powers. Apparently, some clinicians and researchers can live with the fluid boundaries like fish in the ocean, while others, rather like groundhogs, require more specific boundaries.

Perhaps the most important concept requiring definition is mental health itself. No one would quarrel about the diagnosis of a severely chronic schizophrenic whose condition is of long duration, even though the etiology of this disorder would involve considerable controversy. But the vast majority of those seeking relief from mental disorder and those affected with it but who have not accepted the patient role do not fall into this extreme category. How can one arrive at a definition of mental health and mental disorder which though not ironclad can nevertheless be useful, or do we not need such definitions? Could we not hide behind the definition adopted by some practitioners that mental disorders are defined by the types of individuals whom mental health professionals serve? This, indeed, is the definition suggested by Linder (1965).

It is true that even in a more basic science like biology definitions of such fundamental terms as "species" remain open-ended (J. Huxley, 1940). Nevertheless, it is important to define the field of interest even though the boundaries remain vague. If we accept the notion that man is bombarded continually by environmental challenges emanating from the ecological niche which he occupies (physical, social, and cultural parameters of the niche) and that his health depends on his capacity to maintain his homeostasis in the face of these challenges, then "health" can be defined as the degree to which he maintains his dynamic balance and "illness" is its opposite.

4. Taxonomic Problems

The taxonomic problem of classifying the types of illnesses which can arise from the exogenous and endogenous challenges that face man's adjustment is quite complicated. Simple description is not enough, since similar topographical descriptions can arise from a variety of causes. We need to dig deeper under the surface into the etiology of the disorders. Just as simple description of animals is not sufficient for a good taxonomy unless the developmental and evolutionary aspects of the animal's structure and behavior are uncovered, so in the case of the mental disorders the sources of the maldevelopment must be understood for a complete classification. Unfortunately, we know very little about the etiology of most mental disorders, and, furthermore, once the etiology becomes known, the disorder is lost to psychopathology, as was the case with general paresis, pellagra with psychosis, and various types of mental retardation. But what can one do when facing the disorders of unknown origin? One solution is to limit oneself to description alone, but, as was pointed out previously, this is not enough. A better solution is to develop "as if" etiologies in the form of scientific models of etiology. This has been done elsewhere (Zubin, 1972), and the most useful models now dominating research are (1) ecological, (2) developmental, (3) learning, (4) genetic, (5) internal environmental, and (6) neurophysiological. Each of these models is so broad in scope that entire schools of psychopathology can pass through its portals without touching. Furthermore, none of them works in isolation. In order to provide for interaction between them, a super-model or second-order model has been suggested, viz. vulnerability (Zubin, 1976). This model stipulates that when a stressor of sufficient magnitude impinges on a person, a crisis develops which, depending on the degree of vulnerability of the person, either is dissipated so that the individual can return to his precrisis status or, if the person is sufficiently vulnerable, develops into an episode of disorder. It further postulates that the disorder is time limited and that when the stressful situation is overcome the individual will return to his preepisode status (Zubin, 1976). The causes of this vulnerability are to be sought in the six etiological models described earlier, and each of these models can provide markers to identify the vulnerable individuals. (Zubin & Spring, 1977).

Why is it so difficult to deal with diagnosis in psychopathology? Psychopathologists tend to look up to their colleagues in the field of the physical disorders as being more advanced in their nosology. The advantages that physical bases provide for classification are obvious. But how systematic is the classification of so-called physical (nonmental) disorders? To begin with, the first classification systems were merely based on individual symptoms or signs. The development of the concept of a syndrome as a concatenation of symptoms and signs is due to Sydenham in the seventeenth century.

Then, as science and medicine advanced, the classification of disorders followed the new discoveries. When anatomy yielded its secrets through dissection, morbid anatomy became the basis for classification; then followed cellular pathology in the wake of the microscope, and bacterial infection following the work of Koch and Pasteur; and thus the concept of disease entities each produced by a single etiological agent was born. Since then, electrophoresis, chromosome analysis, and electron microscopy have provided new criteria for classification based on biophysical structures, genes, and molecules. Ironically, the new techniques did not make a clean sweep of the status quo in nosology, but, like the English language, absorbed all the new invaders and produced a crazy quilt of classification embodying both the old and the new. Thus there are still diseases based on symptoms, syndromes of symptoms, morphological and physiological anomalies, morbid anatomy and physiology, bacterial or other exogenous agents, biochemical defects, genetic abnormalities, ultrastructural abnormalities, and so on and on. Any attempt at finding a unifying concept in current nosology is doomed to failure because of the congeries of methods used in classification. In the field of psychopathology, the nomenclature could be simpler since we deal primarily only with symptoms and signs and their combination into syndromes. Had the various DSM's and their progenitors limited themselves to description alone, diagnosis might have indeed been simpler. However, various admixtures of description and presumed etiology tended to be the basis for diagnosis in the past. It is one of the advantages of the newly proposed DSM III that putative etiology is kept out of the diagnosis. However, here too the advances made in genetics, biochemistry, and biophysics are beginning to have their effect, although because we have not yet found the etiology of any of the mental disorders we must depend on behavioral syndromes. But the behavior of the patient is determined not only by his mental disorder but also by his underlying premorbid personality, and it is this mixture which he presents at the time of admission. If we could separate the behavior due to the mental disorder from the behavior due to his premorbid personality and to their interaction, we could recognize the focal disorder in isolation from its surround and probably find this factor characteristic of all similarly afflicted patients. What we perceive, however, is not the effect of the *focal disorder* alone, but the effect of the illness, which reflects the premorbid personality and the focal disorder and their interaction. This is why no two schizophrenics are alike—their focal disorder may be the same but their illness is different. The relation between premorbid personality and psychopathology is still moot and involves such thorny issues as the distinction between "trait" and "state."

Elsewhere (Zubin, 1965) I have examined the relationship between premorbid personality and psychopathology and have pointed out that logically they might be related in one of three ways: (1) As identical—as Freud might have viewed them. (2) As independent—as Kraepelin might have thought. Or (3) as interacting—as Adolf Meyer might have thought. But it might be valuable to adopt the assumption of independence or the null hypothesis and study premorbid personality as an independent variable or set of variables. In fact, studies in Lund, Sweden, have found that the premorbid personality does not relate to occurrence of mental disorder, but does color it once it appears. Consequently, we must begin a determined effort to study premorbid personality if we are to clarify diagnosis.

Turning now to the current scene, what has research in clinical diagnosis accomplished?

If we accept the dictum of the philosophy of scientific taxonomy following Alexander Wolf (1929) regarding the need for mutually exclusive and exhaustive categories based on the most important characteristics of the thing concerned (the disorder) and on the actual relations between them and accept the importance of having "natural" rather than "artificial" classification systems, then our progress in attaining our goals has been but little. We have, however, made some progress. In the first place, when the unreliability of the clinical interview method became apparent as a result of investigations of the interview after World War I, attempts were made to develop self-rating inventories and scales to be filled out by the patient and checklists and rating scales to be filled out by the interviewer. The self-reporting instruments have the advantage of eliminating interviewer bias and interpretation by putting the onus on the individual's response rather than on the response of the interviewer to the patient's behavior. That this strategy does not guarantee a better result is, of course, quite obvious. The self-reporting inventories have generally not been found to be so useful for the classification of inpatients, although they have been found quite useful in minor disorders, primarily in dealing with student populations and in surveys of the general population.

5. Diagnostic Techniques

It is interesting to note that in a recent study Dohrenwend and his colleagues found that the common denominator in such self-reports seems to be related more to Jerome Frank's (1973) demoralization factor than to psychopathology.

The checklists and rating scales used by interviewers were not provided with standardized methods for obtaining the information and therefore were not always comparable from patient to patient. To obtain a more systematic method for the collection of the information, the clinical interview itself was brought under control by providing a systematic structured format for it. The first step was to standardize the usual mental status examination (Mental Status Schedule, Spitzer, Burdock, & Hardesty, 1964). The questions to be asked of the patient were specified in a proper sequence and directions for coding the responses were laid down. The mental status schedule, which had been the psychiatrist's mainstay, was converted into this kind of systematic structured interview in our laboratory, yielding high reliability in scoring of items, as well as considerable validity. This technique underwent a series of modifications based on experience gained in the various studies conducted under the aegis of the Biometric Research Unit of the New York State Department of Mental Hygiene (Zubin, 1972). We worked with three types of interviews: (1) a nonprobing Structured Clinical Interview (SCI) by Burdock and Hardesty (1968), (2) a medium-probing Mental Status Schedule (MSS) by Spitzer et al. (1964) and the Psychiatric Status Schedule (PSS) by Spitzer, Endicott, Fleiss, and Cohen (1970), and (3) a deep-probing Present State Examination (PSE) by Wing, Birley, Cooper, Graham, and Isaacs (1967). These interviewing methods have demonstrated their value in two major studies—the US-UK Diagnostic Project (Cooper, Kendell, Gurland, Sharpe, Copeland, & Simon, 1972) and the WHO Pilot Study in Schizophrenia (World Health Organization, 1973). The US-UK project was initiated to determine why the national statistics show such disproportionate frequency of affective disorders in the United Kingdom and of schizophrenia in the United States. When the newly developed systematic structured interviews (Gurland, cited in Zubin, Salzinger,

Fleiss et al., 1975) were applied to samples of patients admitted to hospitals in the two countries, the cross-national differences turned out to reflect different diagnostic practices of psychiatrists rather than differing characteristics of patients in the two countries. Whereas the US-UK project limited itself to two cultures but investigated the entire panoply of mental disorders, the WHO study limited itself to one disorder but investigated its incidence, form, and course in nine different cultures. This investigation found specific syndromes of schizophrenia ubiquitously distributed in developing and in advanced cultures from Ibadan, Nigeria, to Washington, D.C.

Other advances in descriptive psychopathology have been (1) the use of computers that simulate the clinician's decision processes and arrive at a diagnosis (Spitzer & Endicott, cited in Zubin et al., 1975; Wing, Cooper, & Sartorius, 1974), (2) the provision of mathematical methods for clustering individuals with shared psychopathological characteristics into more homogeneous subgroups (Fleiss & Zubin, 1969; Wing & Nixon, 1975), and (3) the development of behavior analytic descriptions of patient characteristics (Kanfer & Saslow, 1969; Salzinger, cited in Zubin et al., 1975). Rather than emphasizing the presence of symptoms per se, behavior analytic description relates deviant behavior to environmental contingencies that initiate and sustain it. Description is therefore focused on aspects of the individual and his environment that are of immediate relevance to behavior modification therapy.

A dispassionate view of where we stand in descriptive psychopathology today leads to the conclusion that we have made considerable progress and perhaps gone as far as we can go but that this is still not far enough. Through the use of systematic structured interviews and operational criteria for selecting a diagnosis a high degree of agreement on diagnosis can be attained. We can now objectively describe the characteristics of patients we deal with so that replication of basic research and treatment findings on similar patients is possible. Moreover, we can demonstrate that individuals suffering from such syndromes of psychopathology as schizophrenia can be found in parts of the world that differ widely in cultural and ecological conditions.

However, we cannot presuppose that reliable description of a syndrome implies valid understanding of its underlying cause. We need to do more than describe, since description never cured anyone, nor did it by itself reveal etiology. Although treatment can often not await a thorough knowledge of etiology, the discovery of an effective cure for any disorder is less likely to result from chance than from an understanding of factors that cause the disorder. As in the classification of organisms, in which taxonomy looks to common origins of descent, so in the classification of disorders we look for common causes producing the disorder. But how can progress be made when with but few exceptions we are abysmally ignorant of the causes of mental disorder and even more poignantly ignorant of the efficacy of the treatment? When faced with such ignorance, one can only contemplate possible or "as if" causes, formulate them into parsimonious scientific models, and proceed to test the hypotheses they generate (Zubin & Spring, 1977).

We have already indicated the types of scientific models which can help establish a more basic aspect of the etiology of the mental disorders.

What needs to be done further? We cannot be satisfied with reliability alone—we must also ask whether our judgments are valid. Here is where we flap our wings in a vacuum at present. How can we improve validity?

6. The Problem of Validity

Of the four types of validity—predictive, construct, concurrent, and content—we will deal only with the first two, predictive and construct validity, since concurrent validity is really a type of reliability and content validity refers to whether the measure covers adequately the entire area under investigation.

6.1. Predictive Validity

Outcome and course of the disorder provide criteria for the predictive validity of the diagnosis. Thus, if the diagnosis of affective disorder leads to a more rapid release than for schizophrenics, this can be taken as a vindication of the diagnosis since this is the outcome we would expect.

6.2. Construct Validity

What else do we expect patients in a given category to have in common besides similarity in outcome?

These expectations have been embodied in a set of scientific models for etiology and have been described earlier in two groups: field theory models, consisting of the ecological developmental and learning theory models, and molecular or biological models, consisting of genetic, internal environmental, and neurophysiological models.

Accepting the genetic model, we would expect that diagnostic system to be most valid which showed the highest transmission rate of schizophrenia in relation to consanguinity. As a matter of fact, a test of the American and British diagnostic systems as well as a Swedish one—Essen-Möller's—was made in Gottesman and Shield's (1972) twin study, and the highest transmission rate was found in Essen-Möller's system.

Accepting the ecological model, we would, for example, expect to find the highest rates of schizophrenia in individuals occupying the deprived, isolated, and oppressed ecological niches in our cities—and this indeed turns out to be the case.

Accepting the developmental model, we would, for example, expect the highest rates among those who according to Sullivan never had a chum, i.e., had deviant friendship patterns in their adolescence.

Accepting the learning theory model, we would expect that families with deviant rearing patterns would give rise to more psychopathology.

Accepting the internal environment model, we would expect to find biochemical indicators such as monoamine oxidase differentials in schizophrenics and their relatives.

Accepting the neurophysiological model, we would expect to find deviant patterns in the processing of information input reflecting deviation in attention and arousal. These hypotheses have been tested by such techniques as reaction time, sensory integration, pupillography, skin conductance, and evoked potentials.

Each of these scientific models would require some modification of our diagnostic procedures in order to provide data for the construct validity of the diagnosis. Thus the genetic model would require more careful interviewing methods of blood relatives to determine family incidence of mental disorder. The ecological model would require a more careful examination of the ecological niche the person occupied, stressing not only the generally accepted parameters such as socioeconomic status and crowding but also the more subtle aspects of available opportunities for growth, privacy, etc. The developmental model would place more emphasis on premorbid history, and the learning theory model would require more careful surveys of family structure. The internal environmental model would require a careful survey of body chemistry and metabolism along the lines dictated by recent findings, while the neurophysiological model would require the application of the specific laboratory techniques found to be differential between patients and normals as well as between patient groups (Sutton, 1973).

7. Problems in Research in Diagnosis

In addition to the problems presented in the general overview described thus far, there are certain specific problems in research in diagnosis which require further investigation.

7.1. Determination of "Casedness"

Much of the research in diagnosis has dealt with individuals who come willingly or are brought for help and hence may be considered, with rare exceptions, as probably being mentally ill. The function of the examiner in such instances is to determine the particular type of disorder that is present. Rarely does he have to decide whether the individual is a "case" or not. In community surveys, the very opposite situation holds. The number of cases is relatively rare, but the decision whether a given individual represents a case or not must be made very frequently. We have made considerable progress in differential diagnosis in the studies of patients, but have made little if any progress in determining casedness. This is where more research is needed, especially longitudinal studies, in which preliminary indications of casedness can be followed up. More indirect approaches such as the findings of markers which do not indicate currently present psychopathology but characterize individuals who may later develop a disorder are needed (Zubin & Spring, 1977; Zubin & Gurland, 1977).

7.2. Dimensionality vs. Typology in the Distribution of Mental Disorders

If two categories of patients are to be differentiated, some discontinuity must exist which separates them into two distinct groups. Since there is no single characteristic which identifies a given disorder (excepting general paresis and a few other disorders for which a single cause has been found), we must look at a pattern or syndrome of characteristics or dimensions as a basis for classification. If we consider the distribution of groups of individuals along the dimensions of a given syndrome, we might consider the following possibilities. Limiting ourselves to three dimensions for the sake of clarity, although the argument could be extended to n dimensions, the population may be distributed normally or symmetrically over the three dimensions, so that there are no troughs or valleys of rarity in the three-dimensional surface. In that case, it would be difficult to find natural boundaries for separating the total population into subgroups. On the other hand, if troughs exist, so that clusters of individuals can be found between pairs of troughs, it would be easy to identify these clusters into subgroups. However, even if there are no natural cleavages in the dimensions, there might be certain boundaries such as arise in hypertension which are recognized as separating different types of individuals, even if there are no points of rarity or cleavage in the three-dimensional space. Last, there may be certain qualitative characteristics that separate groups such as combinations of hallucinations and delusions. Which of these possibilities now characterize the distribution of the mentally ill is difficult to determine, but unless we can find boundaries between groups our definitions of disorder categories will remain nebulous. The problem becomes even more complicated because the boundaries may reflect the patient's behavior, the behavior of the examiner in evaluating the patient's behavior, or the norms imposed by society.

The advent of the drug era has brought a search for subtypes of the various diagnostic categories which have similar responses to specific drugs. This has opened up a demand for clustering technique which would identify the individuals belonging to the various homogeneous subtypes by means of their common profiles. The frequent failure to replicate such findings has resulted in the conclusion that blind empirical searches for such subtypes without any underlying testable hypotheses constituted a vain attempt at lifting oneself by his own bootstraps. Fleiss and Zubin (1969) have pointed out that we need better mathematical models for typology before wasting our time in uncharted courses.

Futhermore, the differences between the dimensional approach and the typological approach are often vitiated by the factor analytic approach used in determining the dimensions, since this approach makes assumptions which nullify typological assumptions. For example, typology thrives on nonlinear relationships between variables and on discontinous nonnormal distributions, the very assumptions that factor analysis contradicts. Consequently, it is foolhardy to expect to find types when the assumptions they are based on are not compatible with the techniques used to find the types.

There is another point of view, however, which would indicate that the conflict between dimensionality and typology is ephemeral. It can be best illustrated by an incident during a prior conference on diagnosis (Katz, Cole, & Barton, 1967). The same question had been raised then, over 10 years ago, and the discussion had lasted until late in the evening. I couldn't fall asleep that night, and, waking at 4 a.m., I turned on the TV only to discover that I had tuned into the *Farmer's Hour* and was listening to a lecture on pomology—how to tell good from bad apples. Apparently, the earlier method was to have an apple knocker tap the apple with his knuckles to determine whether it had too much core and whether it was immature. Today, the reporter indicated, the method consists of conveying the apples on a conveyor belt under two sets of monochromatic lights. The amount of light absorbed is read off a dial which automatically determines the fate of the apple. Apparently, the typology of the apple knocker has been converted to a dimensional measure for classifying the apples. Upon further thought, I concluded that actually this dimensionality is probably the reflection of the genetic makeup of the apple seed—again a typological classification into good and bad genes. But genes accomplish their work by secreting certain biochemical substances (amino acids) in smaller or larger quantities. Again, the typological genetic classification has been altered to a continuous dimensionality. And so on. . . . Apparently the state of the art determines whether typology or dimensionality is to be preferred for classification, and there is no essential difference between the two.

Futhermore, mathematical techniques can probably be developed for converting a typological classification into a dimensional one and vice versa.

Currently, the battle between typology and dimensionality is seesawing with no definitive superiority by either approach. Thus the dimensional approach which has been championed by factor analysts like Eysenck on psychometric grounds has received some support from an unexpected quarter in the form of the spectrum concept of schizophrenia promulgated by Kety, Rosenthal, Wender, and Schulsinger (1968). On the other hand, investigators of depression have found markers which support the typological approach in differentiating unipolar from bipolar depressions (Fieve & Dunner, 1974).

7.3. Operational Criteria

Because of the absence of objective criteria for classification based on either behavioral or psychophysiological markers, dependence must be placed on the phenomenological approach through interviewing. Nevertheless, although the phenomenological data are not easy to classify, certain combinations can be established as guides which will render the classification procedure more objective. To accomplish this end, specific definitions are required for the common terms used in psychopathology, such as "anxiety," "depression," and "depersonalization." Specific criteria can be prescribed that must be present before a decision regarding the presence or absence of a given phenomenon can be accepted. Similarly, in codifying the individual symptoms into a syndrome, specific criteria can be prescribed before the syndrome is regarded as present. Kraepelin had originally focused on the course of the illness as a primary criterion in separating dementia praecox from manic-depressive psychosis, but, following Bleuler's reformulation of the problem, more primacy was given to symptomatology. This second tradition has been further developed by Schneider (1959), Langfeldt (1939), the Biometrics Research Unit (Gurland, cited in Zubin et al., 1975; Spitzer & Endicott, cited in Zubin et al., 1975), the WHO Pilot Study of Schizophrenia (World Health Organization, 1973), and cognate groups. These groups have specified the psychopathological characteristics of schizophrenic behavior along the well-known dimensions of perceptual dysfunction, speech disorder, delusions, hallucinations, affective and cognitive dysfunction, and so on. However, these classic symptoms do not in themselves indicate a particular diagnosis, since they tend to be manifested by a diverse and heterogeneous group of patients. To reduce this heterogeneity and yet save the symptom or syndrome approach, Feighner, Robins, Guze, Woodruff, Winokur, and Munoz (1972) and subsequently Spitzer and Endicott (cited in Zubin et al., 1975) have proposed operational definitions of schizophrenia and the other mental disorders for the new *Diagnostic and Statistical Manual* (DSM III) of the American Psychiatric Association. Each disorder is operationally defined by explicit criteria. These criteria take the form of sets of characteristics, a specified number of which must be presented before a given diagnosis is warranted. Because the specific psychopathological features associated with each official DSM III diagnosis can now be explicated, the reliability of diagnostic decisions can be enhanced (Spitzer & Endicott, cited in Zubin et al., 1975) and the heterogeneity that characterized the DSM III diagnostic categories can be greatly reduced (Zubin & Spring, 1977).

8. Conclusion

Research in clinical diagnosis in modern times was forced on psychopathology by the advent of the somatotherapies in the 1930s and 1940s, when it became obvious that the various somatotherapies did not affect all patients similarly. The greater need for classification was even more accentuated by the drug therapies, and better diagnoses and assessment became a necessity. The ideal diagnosis should maximize the communication value of the diagnostic label, optimize its prognostic potential and its explanatory power, and provide a basis for the best therapeutic choice.

To attain this ideal goal, mere description was not enough. First, description leads to characterization of the illness rather than the disorder itself. By "illness" is meant the interaction between the focal disorder and the premorbid personality and the ecological niche the person occupies. That is why individuals who suffer from the same focal disorder do not always seem alike. Despite these difficulties, considerable success has been attained in providing systematic interviewing techniques and operational criteria for describing the disorders.

Second, we need to dig deeper than the surface description and deal with the etiology of the disorder. Since we do not have any knowledge of the etiology of most mental disorders, we have to resort to the stratagem of inventing scientific models of etiology and testing them against observation and in this way attempt to establish the validity of the diagnoses. Six scientific models have been described: (1) ecological, (2) developmental, (3) learning, (4) genetic, (5) internal environmental, and (6) neurophysiological. Each of these can provide hypotheses for testing predictive and construct validity. A second-order model which may prove to be a common denominator running through all the models is provided by the vulnerability model, which regards the patient as a vulnerable individual who when subjected to sufficient stress and strain will develop an episode. But this episode is time limited; only his vulnerability persists after the episode ends. The goal of preventive intervention is to prevent future episodes from developing in the vulnerable. To this end, two types of markers must be found: (1) those that identify the vulnerable individual and (2) those that identify the beginnings and ends of episodes. When these are discovered, the diagnosis of the mental disorders will become clearer and the tremendous affliction which they bring society will be reduced.

9. References

Burdock, E. I., & Hardesty, A. S. *Structured clinical interview.* New York: Springer, 1968.

The Caraka Samhita. Jamnagar, India: Shree Gulab-Kuniverba Ayurvedic Library, 1949.

Cooper, J. E., Kendell, R. E., Gurland, B. J., Sharpe, L., Copeland, J. R. M., & Simon, R. J. *Psychiatric diagnosis in New York and London: A comparative study of mental hospital admissions* (Maudsley Monograph No. 20). London: Oxford University Press, 1972.

Feighner, J. P., Robins, E., Guze, S. B., Woodruff, R. A., Winokur, G., & Munoz, R. Diagnostic criteria for use in psychiatric research. *Archives of General Psychiatry,* 1972, *26,* 57–63.

Fieve, R. R., & Dunner, D. L. Unipolar and bipolar affective states. *The nature and treatment of depression.* In F. F. Flach, & S. C. Draghi (Eds.), New York: Wiley, 1974.

Fleiss, J. L., & Zubin, J. On the methods and theory of clustering. *Multivariate Behavioral Research,* 1969, *4,* 235–250.

Frank, J. D. *Persuasion and healing.* Baltimore: Johns Hopkins Press, 1973 (originally published 1961).

Gottesman, I. L., & Shields, J. *Schizophrenia and genetics.* New York: Academic Press, 1972.

Huxley, J. S. Introductory: Towards the new systematics. In J. S. Huxley (Ed.), *The new systematics.* Oxford: Clarendon Press, 1940.

Kanfer, F. H., & Saslow, G. Behavioral diagnosis. In C. M. Franks (Ed.), *Behavior therapy: Appraisal and status.* New York: McGraw-Hill, 1969.

Katz, M. M., Cole, J. L., & Barton, W. E. *The role and methodology of classification in psychiatry and psychopathology.* Chevy Chase, Md.: U.S. Department of Health, Education, and Welfare, 1967.

Kety, S. S., Rosenthal, D., Wender, P. H., & Schulsinger, K. The types and prevalence of mental illness in the biological and adoptive families of adopted schizophrenics. In D. Rosenthal & S. S. Kety (Eds.), *The transmission of schizophrenia.* Elmsford, N.Y., Pergamon Press, 1968.

Langfeldt, G. *The schizophreniform states.* Copenhagen: Munksgaard, 1939.

Leonhard, K. *Die Defect schizophrenen krankheits Bilder.* Leipzig: Thieme, 1936.

Leonhard, K. *Aufteilung der endogenen Psychose,* (2nd ed.). Berline, 1959.

Linder, R. Diagnosis: description or prescription? A case study in the psychology of diagnosis. *Perceptual and Motor Skills,* 1965, *20,* 1081–1092.

Schneider, K. [*Clinical psychopathology*] (M. W. Hamilton, trans.). New York: Grune & Stratton, 1959.

Spitzer, R. L., Burdock, E. I., & Hardesty, A. S. *Mental Status schedule.* New York: Biometrics Research Unit, New York State Psychiatric Institute, 1964.

Spitzer, R. L., Endicott, J., Fleiss, J. L., & Cohen, J. The psychiatric status schedule, *Archives of General Psychiatry,* 1970, *23,* 41–55.

Szasz, T. *The myth of mental illness.* New York: Hoeber-Harper, 1961.

Sutton, S. Fact and artifact in the psychology of schizophrenia. In M. Hammer, K. Salzinger, & S. Sutton (Eds.), *Psychopathology: Contributions from the social, behavioral, and biological sciences.* New York: Wiley, 1973.

Wing, J., & Nixon, J. Discriminating symptoms in schizophrenia. *Archives of General Psychiatry,* 1975, *32,* 853–859.

Wing, J. K., Birley, J. L. T., Cooper, J. E., Graham, P., & Isaacs, A. D. Reliability of a procedure for measuring and classifying present psychiatric state. *British Journal of Psychiatry, 113,* 1967; 499.

Wing, J. K., Cooper, J. E., & Sartorius, N. *The measurement and classification of psychiatric symptoms.* Cambridge: Cambridge University Press, 1974.

Wolf, A. Classification. *Encyclopaedia Britannica* (14th ed., vol. 5). London: The Encyclopaedia Britannica Co., 1929, p. 777. Quoted in M. Shepherd. Definition, classification and nomenclature: A clinical overview. In Kemali et al. (Eds.), *Schizophrenia today.* London: Pergamon Press, 1976.

World Health Organization. *Report of the international pilot study of schizophrenia,* Vol. 1. Geneva: WHO, 1973.

Zubin, J. The program of the biometrics research unit. Reprinted from *The Psychiatric Quarterly,* 1972, *46* (*3*), 439–448.

Zubin, J. Psychopathology and the social sciences. In O. Klineberg & R. Christie (Eds.), *Perspectives in social psychology.* New York: Holt, Rinehart and Winston, 1965.

Zubin, J. Scientific models for psychopathology in the '70s. *Seminars in Psychiatry,* 1972, *4,* 283–196.

Zubin, J. Role of vulnerability in the etiology of schizophrenic episodes. In L. J. West & D. E. Flinn (Eds.), *Treatment of schizophrenia: Progress and prospects.* New York: Grune & Stratton, 1976, pp. 5–43.

Zubin, J., & Gurland, B. J. The United States–United Kingdom project on diagnosis of the mental disorders. In L. L. Adler (Ed.), *Issues in cross-cultural research.* New York: New York Academy of Sciences, 1977, pp. 676–686.

Zubin, J., & Spring, B. Vulnerability—A new view of schizophrenia. *Journal of Abnormal Psychology,* 1977, *86,* 103–126.

Zubin, J., Salzinger, K., Fleiss, J. et al. Biometric approach to psychopathology: Abnormal and clinical psychology–statistical, epidemiological, and diagnostic approaches. *Annual Review of Psychology,* 1975, *26,* 671.

2

Classification and Diagnosis of Mental Disorders

BENJAMIN B. WOLMAN

1. Introduction

The purpose of classification of mental disorders is to facilitate diagnosis. To diagnose means to discern, to find out to what extent a particular disease, disorder, or dysfunction differs from other diseases, disorders, or dysfunctions, and what it has in common with similar ones. Every single case is unique, that is, an *idiophenomenon,* because it is a disease or a disorder of a particular person at a particular period of time. However, if it shares certain characteristics with other cases, these common characteristics permit putting them together into categories or classes and form general *nomothetic* conclusions.

"Classification" is the name of such a process of grouping together objects or events or concepts on the basis of at least one common trait or characteristic. One can choose any criterion or any common element. Thus one could divide all cases of mental or behavior disorders (I am using these terms interchangeably) into male and female, children and adults, hospitalized and ambulatory, rich and poor, urban and rural, and so on, depending on the vantage point of the classifying person. A hospital administrator who assigns rooms to patients can be concerned with their age and sex or with their level of income and the kind of insurance they have. A sociologist or anthropologist who studies mental disorders is interested in ecological factors, class, race, religion, ethnic background, family dynamics, and so on. There are innumerable ways of classification: one could divide mental patients into those who are married or who are single; those on medication, those only in psychotherapy, or those receiving both; those who are correctly diagnosed or misdiagnosed; those receiving or not receiving treatment; and so on.

It is not easy to dismiss any of the above classificatory systems. The question is which to choose.

Are there any objective criteria?

BENJAMIN B. WOLMAN • 10 West 66th Street, New York, New York 10023.

2. Logical Principles

BENJAMIN B.
WOLMAN

Classification is a procedure in formal logic. It means grouping together objects, bodies, attributes, or concepts. It is a selective procedure, for the proverbial cake could be cut in more than one way. For instance, it is perfectly logical to classify one's students according to age, sex, religion, race, ethnic origin, and so on. One can divide them into those who wear glasses and those who don't, into those whose marks are above or below the average, or into those who play tennis and those who don't. Each of these classifications serves a definite purpose (Hempel, 1961; Nagel, 1961).

Small wonder that there have been innumerable classificatory systems of mental disorders. The earliest systems go far back in human history, when some hallucinating individuals were believed to be God-inspired saints and prophets, while most disturbed people were persecuted as possessed by Satan and practicing witchcraft.

No classificatory system, as such, is better or more essential than another. A real estate broker classifies his acquaintances into those who buy and those who take up his time without buying; but a neighbor who is a bridge player classifies the same people as nonplayers, beginners, good players, and masters of bridge.

Scientific classification enables the formation of general concepts, for when objects or events are put together into a class or category on the basis of at least one common denominator it becomes possible to make generalizations. These generalizations, often called "empirical laws," enable science to move away from idiophenomena and to operate and communicate; e.g., a proposition "John Doe is a schizophrenic" is meaningless unless the class of schizophrenia has been clearly defined.

There are two rules in regard to scientific classification: economy and usefulness. A classification is economical when (1) no object within a given system of classification belongs to more than one class and (2) every object belongs to a certain class. For example, if we divide tables in a storage room according to height and classify those below 3 feet as low and those above 4 feet as tall, we have left out some tables. If we classify as low those that are below 4 feet and as tall those that are above 3 feet, those between 3 and 4 feet belong to both classes and our classification is uneconomical.

The economical classification of biological species divides them into plants and animals, and animals into vertebrates and invertebrates, enabling the biologists to make general and truthful statements pertaining to each class.

Classification of mental disorders based merely on symptomatology is usually uneconomical. Consider autistic patterns of behavior, typical not only of schizophrenic children but also of children after encephalitis or anoxia (Wolman, 1970). Hallucinations may accompany a great many disorders. So do depressions, anxieties, phobias, homosexual impulses, psychosomatic disorders, addictions, antisocial behavior, etc. Most of these symptoms accompany more than one type of mental disorder.

Viewing from a purely logical point of view, the classificatory system of the American Psychiatric Association published in 1968, the DSM II, is an exercise in logical error. The *Diagnostic and Statistical Manual, DSM II,* divides all mental disorder into organic and nonorganic. This is a perfectly logical division and, naturally, *tertium non datur;* it excludes a third category, which is neither organic nor inorganic. However, mental deficiency was assigned to this never never possible place in DSM II!

Moreover, every clinician knows that psychosomatic or psychophysiological phenomena are associated with certain mental disorders. They are, by definiton, psycho—somatic, and they do not form a separate clinical entity outside the neuroses, psychoses, and so on. The DSM II does, however, assign them as a clinical category separated from any other mental disorder.

The DSM II follows the traditional subdivision of schizophrenia, and it adds the category of "schizoaffective" disorder, sort of a hybrid between schizophrenia and the manic-depressive psychosis.

3. Clinical Diagnosis

As stated above, there are two main requirements for an adequate classificatory system: economy and usefulness. The first requirement is quite obvious, but there is no consensus of opinion concerning clinical usefulness.

Certainly all clinicians would agree that diagnosis is the ultimate purpose of classification of behavior disorders. However, this agreement borders on tautology. Nosology is the science of classification of diseases; classification is a systematic arranging of objects or ideas in classes; and diagnosis means discerning, or distinguishing, that is, finding out the specific traits or characteristics that enable the clinician to put a particular disease or disorder into a class of similar cases.

In other words, when a clinician studies a case of a disease or a disorder and arrives at a conclusion concerning the particular nature of the case, his further decisions as what to do about it are greatly facilitated if it is possible to relate the particular case to a class or category of similar cases. An adequate classificatory system enables the clinician to reason, for example, as follows: "Mr. A. cannot go to sleep unless he touches the alarm clock innumerable times. He brushes his teeth always in the same manner, four times up and four times down. He feels miserable when he is unable to have his lunch at 12:15," and so on. His sex, age, and occupation are coincidental to diagnosis, but the above overt symptoms permit diagnosis of his case as an obsessive-neurosis provided that all other cases with similar symptoms have been put together in the same class. Thus an adequate classificatory system is a necessary prerequisite for a clinical diagnosis and for a resulting treatment strategy.

Imagine a clinician who does not have any classificatory system. Suppose he noticed certain symptoms, such as running nose, but he was unable to relate them to any of the nosological categories. What kind of treatment should he apply? In medieval times headaches were often treated by blood letting, which could have been fatal for some patients. Some mentally disturbed individuals were treated by exorcism, cold packs, flogging, and so on, irrespective of the nature of their disorder.

Wolman's *Dictionary of Behavioral Science* (1973b, p. 99) defines *diagnosis* as "identification of diseases, handicaps, and disorders on the basis of observed symptoms; diagnosis is classification on the basis of observed characteristics."

A correct assessment of distinct features (symptoms) common to a certain class or group of disorders is the mainstay of clinical diagnosis, and an adequate classificatory system should facilitate diagnostic procedures.

4. Symptomological Considerations

Psychologists and psychiatrists have pointed to four clinically significant criteria for classification of mental disorders: symptomatology, etiology, prognosis, and treatment. These are not identical, and are not even similar terms. Early students of mental disorders classified mental disorders on the sole basis of apparent manifestations of the patient's behavior. The first great reformer of treatment methods, P. Pinel, divided the mentally sick patients into melancholic, manic with delirium, manic without delirium and dementive (Alexander & Seleznick, 1977). These four categories corresponded to what one could see on the wards. Some patients were passive, sad, and despondent, and they were naturally classified as melancholic. The hyperactive, elated patients were divided into delirious and nondelirious. The mental defectives or dementives formed a separate category.

Soon Pinel's system came under criticism, especially as clinicians noticed that the very same melancholics become manic and vice versa. The condition was described by Kahlbaum as cyclic disorder, and after E. Kraepelin's sixth edition of his *Lehrbuch* (1899), has become a standard category of manic-depressive psychosis.

The ninth edition of Kraepelin's *Lehrbuch* (1927) consists of two volumes of 2425 pages. Kraepelin's systems followed the model of other medical specialties, and delved into the etiology, symptomatology, prognosis, and incidence of each disorder. Although Kraepelin offered a detailed description of every clinical entity, his system has linked symptomatology with other aspects of mental disorders, and especially prognosis (to be discussed later on).

Since Kraepelin's time, psychiatrists and psychologists have argued about the value of symptomatology vs. other diagnostic criteria. Freud's system, to be discussed later on, strongly leans toward etiology. Presently, there is a strong tendency to get away from inferrable and not always proven etiological data toward symptomatology.

Advocates of behavior modification methods suggest that diagnostic procedures should be limited to the assessment of observable symptoms. Overt behavior is identified with the disorder, and the clinician should amass all the information concerning the visible symptoms and their reinforcement contingencies (Ferster, 1966; Kanfer & Saslow, 1969; Ullman & Krasner, 1969; and many others).

A different approach but one also stressing overt behavior has been introduced by Albee (1969), Bower (1966), Phillips (1968), Scheff and Scheff (1966), and others. The common denominator of all these authors is their suggestion to relate behavior disorders to the patient's level of social competence and adequacy and ability for observable successful adjustment.

Foulds (1969) introduced the postulate of the existence of one "personal illness" that encompasses all clinical manifestations of maladaptation, and he distinguished between symptoms and traits. According to Foulds, the person's impaired ability to engage in social relationships is the core of all disorders. Foulds distinguished four clinical conditions—personality disorder, neurosis, integrated psychosis, and non-integrated psychosis—viewed in a downward order of declining social adjustment.

Phillips (1968) introduced a bidimentional classificatory system based on (1) social direction of the symptoms and (2) their mode of expression. He distinguished three social dominance patterns—turning against oneself, against others, and away from others—and four modes of expression—thought, affection, somatization, and action.

In 1974 the American Psychiatric Association had appointed a task force on Nomenclature and Statistics to prepare a third edition of the *Diagnostic and Statistical Manual of Mental Disorders* (DSM). The first edition of this Manual (DSM III) was published in 1952, and the second (DSM II) in 1968; the third (DSM III) is in press, but its outline was published in 1977 by Pinsker and Spitzer in B. B. Wolman's

International Encyclopedia of Psychiatry, Psychology, Psychoanalysis, and Neurology (Vol. 3, pp. 160–164).

19

CLASSIFICATION
AND DIAGNOSIS OF
MENTAL DISORDERS

The DSM III emphasizes observable data. "When DSM I was published, etiology was emphasized. It is apparent now that much of what was in 1952 thought to be etiology must now be regarded as speculation. The empirical emphasis of DSM III is not intended to detract from psychodynamic psychiatry but emphasize the distinction between observation and inference. . . . Diagnosis should be based upon what is observed and known" (Pinsker and Spitzer, 1977, p. 161).

While there is a good reason for moving away from unproven speculations toward observable facts, one can raise valid objections against using symptomatology as the sole criterion for classification of mental disorders. For one thing, there is no general agreement concerning the choice of the symptoms for classificatory purposes. For example, Edwards (1972) compared American and British psychiatric diagnoses of schizophrenia and discovered far-reaching differences in the choice of symptoms. For instance, 68.7% of American psychiatrists believe that distortion in perception, and especially hallucinations, are indicative of schizophrenia, while only 25.6% of British psychiatrists believe that hallucinations are a most important symptom of this disorder.

Moreover, symptoms can be misleading. Consider physical health and disease. High temperature, coughing, nasal discharge, diarrhea, local swelling, weight loss, and so on could signal a variety of mild, moderate, and severe physical illnesses. Depression, impotence, aggressiveness, psychosomatic symptoms, delusions, and hallucinations could be associated with a host of different organic and psychogenic mental disorders. Some symptoms may be coincidental to a particular mental disorder. They might be related to the patient's religious or political beliefs, cultural background, socioeconomic status, and so on, and not necessarily to the individual's particular mental disorder.

Zubin (1967), in an analysis of problems related to the classification of behavior disorders, stressed the question of continuity vs. discontinuity in the behavioral patterns of the patients. Discontinuous patterns could be coincidental to a particular disorder, although they could be easily noticeable and even striking.

Apparently, a classificatory system based solely on overt symptoms leaves too many questions unanswered, and the main question is what is indeed the essential element of a particular type of disorder?

5. Etiological Considerations

Kraepelin (1927) distinguished between endogenous and exogenous mental diseases. He believed that, e.g., epilepsy and schizophrenia are caused by internal changes in the brain, while delirium tremens is caused by alcohol, which is an external factor. The DSM II (1968) was primarily guided by etiological considerations, albeit not too consistently. For example, the division of disorders into organic and nonorganic is clearly etiological.

Freud's classificatory system was par excellence etiological. Initially, Freud divided all mental disorders into "actual neuroses" caused by organic factors and "psychoneuroses" caused by psychological factors. Freud linked the origin of psychoneuroses to fixation at or regression to infantile developmental phases as shown in Table 1 (quoted after Fenichel, 1945, p. 101).

Table 1. Freud and Abraham's Timetable

Stages of libidinal organization	Stages in development of object love	Dominant point of fixation
1. Early oral (sucking) stage	Autoeroticism (no object, preambivalent)	Certain types of schizophrenia (stupor)
2. Late oral-sadistic (cannibalistic) stage	Narcissism: total incorporation of the object	Manic-depressive disorders (addiction, morbid impulses)
3. Early anal-sadistic stage	Partial love with incorporation	Paranoia, certain pregenital conversion neuroses
4. Late anal-sadistic stage	Partial love	Compulsion neurosis, other pregenital conversion neuroses
5. Early genital (phallic) stage	Object love, limited by the predominant castration complex	Hysteria
6. Final genital stage	Love (postambivalent)	Normality

Within the Freudian frame of reference, Glover (1968) suggested a new classification system related to two factors: (1) the Freud-Abraham stage of psychosexual fixation or regression (Table 1) and (2) the predominance of a particular defense mechanism of introjection and projection. Bour (1966) applied both Freudian and Adlerian systems to diagnosis and emphasized three sets of characteristics: (1) the changes in aggressive and sexual drives, (2) the psychosexual developmental stage, and (3) the dominant psychodynamic mechanisms typical in a particular disorder.

Kendall (1968) in Great Britain and Angst (1966) in Switzerland have introduced etiology to classification of depressive disorders. Kendall distinguished between endogenous and reactive depression. Angst related the unipolar depression from the bipolar manic-depressive disorder to premorbid history.

Kantor and Herron (1966), Cancro and Sugarman (1968, 1969), Goldstein, Held, and Cromwell (1968), and many others suggested a division of schizophrenic syndromes into process and reactive, based on a "bad" or "good" premorbid story.

An all-inclusive classificatory system closely related to etiological factor was introduced by Thorne (1967).

While etiological factors continue to play a highly significant role in diagnosis and classification of mental disorders, one must point to two main difficulties with classification based on etiology. First, several etiological data are controversial. For instance, some authors maintain that schizophrenia is inherited, while others maintain that it is acquired. The second difficulty is related to the particular nature of causal relations in psychology, for there is no evidence that the same causes always produce the same effects or that a certain effect is always a result of a certain cause (Wolman, 1965b and c).

Consider children's thumbsucking. Is thumbsucking always produced by the same cause? Investigators have revealed several possibilities: (1) Some children suck when the holes in the nipple are too small; apparently, they get tired and give the bottle up, but suck their thumbs because they are hungry. (2) When sucking the breast of an affectionate mother, sucking becomes a pleasurable experience; children suck their thumbs any time they are upset, as if seeking the soothing pleasure of sucking. (3) Children who did not suck in childhood or were weaned too early suck their thumbs as if trying to recapture the missed gratification.

Clinical observations (Wolman, 1964) yielded a rainbow variety of reactions. Some patients react to frustration with aggression or regression; others become very depressed. A schizophrenic patient, defeated in her efforts to set fire to the hospital, reacted with obvious relief. As she explained later, she realized that "she was not as dangerous as she has thought, if one stupid doctor and one moronic attendant could overwhelm her." For a while she screamed "We are outnumbered," but later she felt happy that finally someone "did not take her nonsense." Apparently her reaction to frustration was ambivalent and included both protest and relief.

Pavlov's dog suffered a "nervous breakdown" when he was exposed to conflicting stimuli in an ellipse approaching a circle. Would a man suffer a nervous breakdown if he could not distinguish between his girlfriend and her twin sister? Would he not find some way out?

Psychological propositions are exasperatingly varied. Physicists can remove air from a tube in order to find out whether bodies fall with the same speed in a vacuum. Humans do not fit into evacuated tubes; moreover, their behavior is guided by a variety of reasons. Men marry for a variety of rational and irrational reasons; so also do they love, hate, come together, and part. Simple and uniform generalizations do not do justice to the complexity of human behavior.

6. Prognostic Considerations

Every practitioner in any one of the healing professions is naturally concerned with prognosis. One classificatory system went so far as to link it to the anticipated outcome. According to Zilboorg and Henry,

> The most distinguishing point of the Kraepelinian system was the prognostic attitude, closely connected with diagnosis. The Hippocratic principles of prognosis thus entered into psychiatry under a very singular guise. One diagnosed by prognosis, as it were, and if the prognosis proved ultimately correct, the diagnosis was considered correct. This was a departure from a vital and sound principle of general medicine. One cannot say that because a disease ends in a certain definite way it is a certain definite disease. Kraepelin himself was apparently unaware of this singular deviation from medical principles and did not forsee that the fatalism with which it was imbued weakened even further the rather unstable and never too strong rational therapeutic interest with regard to mental diseases. There is no doubt that it was not Kraepelin's intention to diminish the therapeutic efforts or to keep them only within the limits of the aging tradition of hospital management and humanitarian tolerance. But the therapeutic efforts were to become based on the complacent, expectant attitude that if the disease is a manic-depressive psychosis the patient will get well, and if it is a dementia praecox the patient will deteriorate—or, in the most turgid language of psychiatric formalism, if it is a manic-depressive psychosis "the prognosis is good for the attack," and if it is a dementia praecox the prognosis is unfavorable. (Zilboorg & Henry, 1941, p. 456)

The distinction between *reactive* (good premorbid) and *process* (poor premorbid) types of schizophrenia (Cancro & Sugarman, 1969; Kantor & Herron, 1966; and others) gave rise to a certain degree of optimism in predictability and prognosis. Goldstein et al. (1968) discovered that most reactive schizophrenics develop paranoid symptoms while process schizophrenics have a 50:50 chance of becoming paranoid.

Prognostic studies conducted by Hunt (1951) at the Great Lakes Naval Training Center showed that psychiatric interviews had some predictive validity, but they failed in predicting successful behavior of psychiatrically healthy men. In other words, whenever psychiatrists dealt with clearly disturbed individuals, their diagnosis had a considerable prognostic value, but in cases of mild difficulties their diagnosis led to no significant prognostically valid results.

Several researchers have arrived at similar negative conclusions. Holt and Luborsky (1958) studied psychiatric residents and pointed to the difficulty in predicting their future professional success. Fisher, Epstein, and Harris (1967) faced similar difficulties in trying to predict the performance of Peace Corps volunteers.

I believe that the very nature of human behavior renders clinical predictions exceedingly difficult if not totally impossible. Human beings do not act in a vacuum, and their behavior almost always represents a psychosocial field. Every observer, no matter how objective, influences the observed. In physics, under Einstein's influence, there has been a growing awareness of the fact that any observer-observed situation represents a field. Wrote Jeans: "Every observation involves a passage of a complete quantum from the observed object to the observing subject, and a complete quantum constitutes a not negligible coupling between the observer and the observed. We can no longer make a sharp division between the two. . . . Complete objectivity can only be regained by treating observer and observed as parts of a single system" (Jeans, 1958, p. 143).

The difference in the choice of vantage point can lead to far-reaching differences in the results of observation. Compare, for instance, Freud's and Sullivan's ideas concerning schizophrenia. The reclining position of the neurotic patient and the sparse communication from the mostly silent psychoanalyst facilitated transference phenomena. Freud, the keen observer, noticed them and made them the cornerstone of his therapeutic method. However, when a psychotic patient was asked to recline with a psychoanalyst sitting behind his couch and watching him, a different reaction took place. Silence was probably perceived as rejection, and the invisible analyst became a threatening figure. The patient withdrew even more into his shell, and, if he did communicate, he would not dare to communicate his true feelings. Such a behavior gave the impression of narcissistic withdrawal and lack of transference feelings toward the psychoanalyst.

Sullivan worked in a hospital where patients were moving back and forth and were acting out their feelings. He saw patients in interpersonal relations, and, being a keen observer, he did not fail to notice the socially induced changes in their behavior. The here-and-now interaction became the clue to the understanding of the psychotic patient. Most probably what has been observed in participant observation was not the patient as an isolated entity but the patient in interaction with the therapist, that is a *psychosocial field*.

One must therefore conclude that the present status of a mental patient is but one of many determinants of his future behavior. How he will act in the future will be greatly influenced by his interaction with several other people (among them the therapist), and it is, therefore, rather unpredictable (Wolman, 1964, 1966a).

7. Therapeutic Considerations

The study of mental or behavioral disorders (I am using these two terms interchangeably) is an empirical science. Like all other empirical sciences, psychopathology describes factual data and puts them into classes or categories.

There are no other rules for this generalization procedure except formal-logical principles (Nagel, 1961).

However, the empirical psychopathological science serves as a basis for the applied sciences which deal with the treatment of mental disorders. These applied sciences or praxiologies (Wolman, 1965b, 1973c) prescribe actions directed toward a certain goal. For example, education, which is one of the praxiologies, sets goals and develops means leading toward the attainment of the educational goals. Clinical psychology and psychiatry as praxiologies aim at curing behavior disorders and develop physical, chemical, and psychological methods which should enable practitioners to attain the therapeutic goals.

In choosing a motto of my *Handbook of Clinical Psychology* (1965a), I paraphrased Auguste Comte's famous dictum, *"Savoir pour prevoir"* (to know in order to predict), and suggested that the motto of clinical psychology should be *"Savoir pour aider autrui"* (to know in order to help others).

Helping a disturbed person to become not disturbed or at least less disturbed is the main goal of psychiatry and clinical psychology. The empirical science of psychopathology is the very foundation for the praxiological science of treatment. It is a two way street, for adequate therapy is based on empirical knowledge of mental disorder, and the empirical study of mental disorders must not overlook its main application. In short, a therapy which is not based on scientific psychopathology is quackery, but an empirical research in psychopathology which is not related to therapy goes nowhere and could be useless, for it may deal with insignificant and irrelevant issues.

It seems therefore that therapy should be the choice vantage point for any classificatory system. This decision raises several relevant questions concerning the aims, method, and overall therapeutic philosophy (Wolman, 1973c, 1976). What is, indeed, the goal of treatment of mental disorders?

Other praxiologies have it much easier. Consider education. Educational praxiology has a given, built-in, *immanent* goal which is determined by the biological process of growth and maturation. The immanent goal of all educational systems, whether John Dewey's or J. F. Herbart's, whether American or Soviet, is to help and guide children in the natural process of becoming mature adults. However, since the concepts of maturing and adulthood greatly depend on cultural settings and social philosophies, the educational praxiology must determine *transcendent* goals appropriate for each society and culture.

It seems that the concept of mental health should serve as the immanent goal of all treatment methods, but it is one of the highly controversial issues in current research (Albee, 1969; Bower, 1966; Gurland, 1977; Jahoda, 1958; Phillips, 1968; Laing, 1967; Strupp, 1972; Szasz, 1961; Wolman, 1973a). Moreover, there is very little evidence concerning the efficacy of the various therapeutic systems (Eysenck, 1961; Strupp, 1972).

During World War II, Stockings (1945) suggested that military psychiatrists should diagnose schizophrenic patients on the basis of their reaction to methods of treatment. Those schizophrenics who reacted favorably to IST (insulin shock treatment) were labeled as "dysglycotics," and those who responded to ECT (electric shock treatment) were named "dysoxics." However, such a system was open to severe criticism for lack of clear evidence concerning the efficacy of the various treatment methods, and it could not last for long becuase the advent of new methods would have rendered it obsolete. Moreover, it seems that many contemporary therapeutic strategies are little, if at all, related to diagnostic evaluations (Kreitman, Sainsbury, Morrissey, Towers, & Scrivener, 1961).

The fact is that therapeutic techniques based on various schools of thought claim similar results. One can substantially reduce depression by the use of ECT, lithium bicarbonate, and several other antidepressants, and by highly diversified psychotherapeutic methods such as classic psychoanalysis, existential analysis, nondirective therapy, and so on and so on. Quite often there is no adequate scientific explanation as to why certain methods produce certain results while other methods fail.

Small wonder that many therapists are given to diagnostic apathy and, in extreme cases, to diagnostic nihilism. Many clinicians apply one and the same method to whatever case they deal with. In some cases their accidental approach may work, but in many other cases such a hit-and-miss method may prove counterproductive and even harmful.

Some clinicians go even further and reject the very idea of classification. Laing (1967) maintains that diagnostic categories are dehumanizing and self-fulfilling prophesies. For example, schizophrenics behave in a peculiar way because they are treated as schizophrenics. No less extreme ideas have been expressed by Szasz (1961, 1969), who maintains that psychiatric classification is merely a strategy of personal constraint.

Unfortunately, all these ideas fail to solve the problem under consideration. Deprived of any classification, psychiatrists and clinical psychologists would have to view every case as a totally new and unique occurrence, a true idiophenomenon that defies any generalization. Unable to generalize and draw general conclusions, would clinicians be able to learn anything and profit from their experience? There would be no other way but to start from scratch every time they see a new patient!

8. The Problem of Generalizations

Disappointment in the existing diagnostic systems was voiced by several authors (Albee, 1969; Phillips, 1968; Szasz, 1961; Sarbin, 1967; Scheff and Scheff, 1966; Wolman, 1973c). The main criticism has been leveled against the term "mental disease." Many authors have stressed the fact that disturbed and disorganized behavior is itself maladjustment, and there is no need to relate it to a medical model. As Phillips and Draguns (1971) summarized, at present the importance is accorded to the person's interaction with his environment and adjustment, rather than to a hypothetical disease entity.

There are, however, considerable differences among the advocates of the nonmedical approach. Some authors prefer to deal with overt behavior only (Ferster, 1966; Ullman and Krasner, 1969), while others include also unconscious elements of human behavior (Wolman, 1965a, 1967, 1973a). Furthermore, some authors emphasize flux and change in behavior (Albee, 1969; and many others), while other authors seek more stable elements (Grinker, 1969; Zubin, 1967).

More than 10 years ago, Zubin (1967) pointed to the chaotic state in this area. One of the main difficulties is related to the specific nature of psychological data and the apparent need for caution in generalization and classifications. For instance, such general categories as ascendance-submissiveness, masculine-feminine traits, introvert-extravert, domineering parents or children, "strong" mother and "weak" father, overprotection, overindulgence, and dependence-independence may miss the point entirely. A manic-depressive is both ascendant and submissive, depending on mood; he is often aggressive to others and self-defeating to himself. He may be self-sacrificing and overselfish, oversentimental and overbrutal. A schizophrenic may oscillate between overdependence and independence syndromes; he may fear a fly and run into a lion's den; he may worry about hurting the feelings of the person whom he murders; parents of schizophrenics are overprotective and overindulgent.

Physical scientists have an easier job. Their electrons, energy, loads, temperatures, sizes, and locomotions seem to behave in a more reasonable way than humans do. Hence the rules of logic and mathematics are applicable to the study of the physical world.

Humans who study humans are exposed to several disadvantageous conditions. Their objectivity can be questioned; their power to set the conditions of observations is so great as to raise suspicion; their subjects are irrational; and scientific observation or experimentation may easily become a two-way process, in which both observer and observed participate.

The observer's methods and tools are an important variable in the subject's performance. He sets the conditions under which the observation will take place and determines what actually will be performed. The detached position of the psychoanalyst whose armchair was outside the patient's field of vision was probably causing further withdrawal in schizophrenic patients, and led Freud to believe that schizophrenia was a narcissistic nontransference disorder (Freud, 1935). Fenichel, Federn, Sullivan, Hill, Fromm-Reichmann, Wolman, and others, who took a participant attitude, reversed Freud's notion on transference in schizophrenia.

This does not mean that every case of mental disorder is a unique, unrepeatable phenomenon which renders impossible any generalization and classification. Actually, everything and everybody is an idiophenomenon, but on the basis of a single common trait sciences can group any number of idiophenomena and draw generalizations (Wolman, 1960a, 1971, 1972a). For instance, no oak tree is identical with any other oak tree, because every single oak tree has something specific and unique, at least because no two oak trees can grow in exactly the same place. However, all oak trees have at least one common trait which permits us to put all of them together into one class and draw general conclusions. When a botanist or a gardener "diagnoses" a tree as being an oak, he does not prescribe its future development as an oak, nor does he constrain the developmental process, notwithstanding Szasz's and Laing's stern warnings.

9. Causal-Etiological Approach

All these considerations inevitably lead one to abandon, at least temporarily, the idea of classification based on a single factor, be it symptomatology, etiology, or therapeutic goals and methods. The only possible way out of this perplexing situation is to base the classificatory system on a combination of several factors. Etiological data seem to be exceedingly valuable provided that the knowledge of causes will allow the therapist to predict the symptoms and serve as an adequate basis for the selection of an appropriate treatment method, and of the increasingly important issue of prevention.

At this point, one must caution against an oversimplistic assumption that the removal of causes will necessarily obliterate the results. A careless campfire can start a huge forest fire, but extinguishing the campfire will not put an end to the forest fire.

In diagnostic procedures, one could apply Tolman's (1932) formula of independent variables, intervening variables, and dependent variables. Assuming that etiological factors, whatever they are, are the independent variable, the clinician, armed with the knowledge of intervening variables, should be able to predict the symptoms, that is, the dependent variables. Or with a knowledge of symptoms (the dependent variable) and the intervening variables, he should be able to explain (to "predict" in reverse time order) what caused the symptoms. For instance, if a patient fears open spaces (agoraphobia), the clinician applies his knowledge of an appropriate conceptual system that could serve as intervening variable (Wolman, 1960a). By the same token, when the clinician finds the underlying etiology, he should be able to predict that his patient will fear open spaces.

I am using this method in my psychotherapeutic practice which I call "interactional psychoanalytic psychotherapy" (Wolman, 1965c, 1967, 1976). Accepting a modified psychoanalytic model (to be explained later on) as the intervening variable, I have pursued diagnostic interviews either starting from etiological data leading to anticipatory hypothesis of symptoms or starting from symptoms and hypothetically deducing their causes.

A classificatory system should include etiology and symptomatology, or, as Marchais (1966) suggested, should be based on all three factors: etiology, symptomatology, and indications for treatment.

An adequate classificatory system must relate the therapeutic goal to relevant etiological and prognostic factors. This suggestion hinges on accepting the causal principle in psychology and its application both to past events, i.e., etiology, the study of causes, and to the future outcomes, anticipated by prognostic studies.

The causal principle has been questioned by theoretical physicists and philosophers of science, and Einstein's fourth dimension undermined the concept of temporal sequence that underlies causality. Moreover, the causal hypothesis in physics smacks of anthropomorphism, for it sounds as if, e.g., the clouds have produced the rain, or the heat has made bodies to increase their size.

Neither of these two problems exists in psychology. Human life has a clearly time-determined beginning and end, and temporal sequences are self-evident. And to deny the fact that human actions produce certain results would smack of reimorphism (Wolman, 1971, 1972a).

10. Defining Mental Health

The first step is to seek an objective definition of mental health. As mentioned above, there have been several efforts to define mental disorders by relating them to mental health (Alexander & Seleznick, 1966; Blashfield, 1976; Fisher et al., 1967; Hunt, 1950; Jahoda, 1958; Grinker, 1969; Helzer, Robins, Woodruff, Reich, & Wish, 1977; Menninger, Mayman, & Pruyser, 1963; Kanfer and Saslow, 1969; Woodruff, Goodwin, & Guxe, 1974; and many others).

Jahoda (1958) suggested that the main difference between mental disturbances and normality are clearly defined deficiencies in (1) awareness, acceptance, and correctness of self-concept; (2) continued growth and self-actualization; (3) integration and unity of personality; (4) autonomy and self-reliance; (5) perception of reality and social sensitivity; and (6) mastery of the environment and adequacy in meeting the demands of life. According to Jahoda, deficiencies in these traits are signs of abnormality.

27

CLASSIFICATION
AND DIAGNOSIS OF
MENTAL DISORDERS

11. Mental Health and Survival

It might be useful to compare mental health to physical health without necessarily accepting the medical model. "Health" and "disease" are not opposite terms, and both describe the level of physical adjustment of a living organism. Life and death are two opposite states of an organism. When a physician diagnoses an individual as being in good health, he means that this individual has a good chance for survival and for an adequate use of his organism. A person diagnosed as very ill is in lethal danger. The main measure of severity of a physical disease is the estimated distance from mortal danger. Severity of symptoms is not always the best indicator of the severity of a disease; a bleeding nose or diarrhea may be more spectacular than the initial stages of cancer, yet cancer is more severe because it carries a much higher probability of death. When a lethal danger is improbable, the disease is considered less severe; when the probability is high, the disease is considered severe. Health and disease are degrees or measures on the continuum of life and death. When the heart and lungs of an individual are healthy, they facilitate an optimum of life; when the structure or function of these organs is inadequate, they are abnormal, i.e., sick. Death is the final point of physical abnormality, the dead end of life. Not all diseases lead to death; some of them incapacitate the individual, reduce his vitality, and prevent the use of his potentialities.

Despite the diversity of opinions, practically all clinicians agree that mental health and mental disorder are not opposites. Moreover, analogous to physical health, mental health is an indicator of one's chances for survival. Mental disorders are not diseases of a specific organ, and they do not lead to death. However, mental disorders impair adjustment. They reduce one's ability to cope with stress, they affect one's emotional life, they impair one's perception of reality. Severe mental disorders incapacitate the individual and turn him into a helpless creature who could not survive unless taken care of. The dead end of physical illness is death; the dead end of mental disorder is the inability to live.

One can point to empirical criteria for determination of mental health and mental disorder. These criteria should enable us to determine observable degrees of normality and abnormality. The four criteria are (1) optimal success, (2) emotional balance, (3) cognitive functions, and (4) social adjustment (Wolman, 1965a, 1967, 1973a).

12. Optimal Success

All living organisms resist destruction and adjust to their environment. The actions of all organisms are directed toward the protection of their individual lives and procreation of the species.

The apparent common denominator of human motivation is the struggle for survival, for self-realization, for success and satisfaction. Normal individuals use their resources in this struggle; in most cases, their achievements are proportional to their innate and acquired potentialities and to environmental factors. This is, however, not the case with mentally disturbed individuals. Their accomplishments usually fall short of what could be reasonably expected. They either give up, defeat themselves, or try to destroy themselves. The inability to use one's mental and physical resources is one of the outstanding signs of mental disorder.

13. Emotional Balance

Cannon, Pavlov, Freud, Goldstein, and others introduced similar principles, calling them "homeostasis," "equilibrium," "constancy," or "equipotentiality," respectively. Although these terms are not identical, they all convey the idea that whenever an organism is exposed to a stimulation that disturbs its equilibrium, the behavior of the organism aims at the restoration of the initial state.

All human beings react to life situations with joy and sorrow, pleasure and pain, elation and depression. The normal or healthy individuals react to stimuli in an appropriate, proportionate, controllable, and adjustive manner.

Normally, we react with pleasure and joy to situations in which we are successful and with grief to failure. There are, however, people who react with sorrow and regret to success and seem to enjoy defeat. Their emotional reaction is inappropriate. Some of these people bring misery on themselves. Others cannot find satisfaction in success; they are unable to appreciate what they have and constantly look for "greener pastures," but no pasture is green enough and no success brings gratification. Disturbed people are often their own worst enemies, defying their own efforts, avoiding pleasure, and seeking pain. In some extreme cases of schizophrenia, to be discussed later, the normal pain-pleasure reaction is reversed or even nonexistent.

Normal emotional reaction is proportionate to the stimulus. If a man who is mentally balanced and emotionally healthy loses money, his reaction will be proportionate to the magnitude of the loss and to the ensuing financial hardship. If the loss is small, his worry will be mild and of short duration. A less well-balanced individual will react differently. Some disturbed individuals cannot take frustration, and despair whenever they meet hardships or suffer a loss. Disturbed individuals are inclined to see doom in the face of a mild frustration. Some individuals accuse themselves of being misfits and recall their past major and minor troubles; some blame others.

A well-balanced individual will do whatever is possible to regain a loss and prevent the recurrence of losses in the future, recognizing that self-accusations or accusations of others cannot restore a lost object or person. Disturbed individuals tend to perpetuate their depressed or aggressive moods instead of trying to compensate for past losses and to prevent future misfortunes. Their emotional balance cannot be easily restored, and the depressed or agitated anxiety states are likely to occur again and again. The failure in coping with hardships often leads to increasing irritability, and each new frustration adds to the difficulty in restoring emotional balance. Apparently, mental disorder is a dynamic process with a distinct tendency for deterioration. In psychosis, the ability to face frustration and to act in a constructive fashion may be lost altogether. The slightest frustration may throw the individual off and cause uncontrollable emotional outbursts. Some psychotics are in a state of perpetual fury, continuous panic, or unbearable tension and depression.

The criterion of emotional balance can therefore be applied toward the distinction of the severity of a disorder. Emotionally balanced individuals are "normal"; those who are poorly balanced are less normal; serious emotional dysbalance indicates severe mental disorder.

14. Perception

The third criterion of mental health relates to the soundness of the cognitive functions. In order to survive, one must perceive things as they are. An erroneous perception, an oversight of danger, or an inability to distinguish wish from truth may jeopardize one's life. A realistic perception of the outer world and of one's life increases one's chance for survival and helps in optimal adjustment.

In most mental disorders, the individual's perception of himself and of others is disturbed. This may not be due to a physiological or anatomical deficiency in the sensory organs as is true in the case of sight or hearing impairments, nor be due to a lack of ability to perceive, compare, and reason as in mental deficiency. In mental disorder, the mental apparatus is, in most cases, fully or partly preserved, but it seems that the individual is unable to use his mental capacities and cannot perceive himself or other people correctly.

Freud called the ability to see things as they are "reality testing." The neonate, said Freud (1938/1949, p. 42), is unable to distinguish inner stimuli from stimuli coming from the outside world. Me and not-me are not clearly separated. Gradually, by checking their perceptions and manipulating the perceived objects, infants learn to test reality, that is, to distinguish between inner and outer stimuli, between their own feelings and the external world, between wish and truth.

Sullivan (1953) suggested another distinction. He believed that the earliest stage of thinking in human life is the "prototaxic" mode, that is, a state of unconscious, diffused, and indistinguishable experiences. In the next stage, the "parataxic," the individual perceives the world as a series of experiences in a nonlogical order; he looks upon himself as if he were the center of the universe. In the third stage, the "syntaxic," the individual develops the ability to check his perceptions against the perceptions of others, and validates them through the consensus of the group. This consensual validation is actually one of the methods by which reality can be tested.

Everyone may occasionally err in perception, but, as a rule, we are capable of reality testing and of correcting our errors. In mentally disturbed individuals, this ability is impaired or nonexistent, and the more they are disturbed, the poorer is their perception of reality.

Most neurotics either have an exaggerated notion of their own status and importance or underestimate their resources and status. Feelings of omnipotence and inadequacy are frequent symptoms of mental disorder, for how people feel and think about themselves is an area in which wish and reality can be badly confused.

The situation may become quite serious when the individual's picture of the outside world becomes distorted. When an individual misconstrues or misinterprets what he perceives, it is delusion. For example, when a person flees from a policeman who simply wants to check his driver's license, in fear that the policeman will arrest him for a noncommitted crime, or when he ascribes hostile feelings to his friends who are loyal and trustworthy, his reality testing is practically nonexistent. This distortion of perception is called delusion. Hallucination is perceiving things that do not exist at all; that is, perception without external stimulation, such as seeing ghosts or hearing voices. A hallucinating patient is unable to distinguish his inner fears, wishes, and dreams from the outer world and its events. His ability for reality testing is lost, and no reasoning or explanations can restore it. In sleep, there is no reality testing; in dreams, we experience our own wishes and fears as if they were true, objective facts.

The question of cultural influences must be raised in connection with the problem of perception of reality. In various cultures, myth and truth have often been confused, and dreams have been often taken for reality. "With us a person would be neurotic or psychotic who talked by the hour with his deceased grandfather, whereas such communication with ancestors is a recognized pattern in some Indian tribes," wrote Horney (1937, p. 15).

When everyone else accepts delusion, it is rather difficult for an individual to perform reality testing. Thus when the belief in ghosts, voices, spirits, and witches is a well-entrenched cultural feature, everyone experiences this culturally determined delusion, and it is not easy to perform reality testing. The doubts one may have cannot be consensually validated, because the delusion is generally accepted as reality. But even at that time, an individual who believes that he himself has turned into a stone, or who believes that his genuine friends hate him, is mentally disturbed. Thus reality testing is an important criterion of mental disorder within the cultural limitations.

15. Social Adjustment

Each social group has its share of constructive, life-preserving, cooperating factors, as well as its share of disruptive, destructive, and antisocial forces. However, a society in which mutual respect, consideration, and cooperation prevail certainly has better chances for survival than a society in which the norm is "cutthroat competition" and hate of all against all. The latter society will be constantly in the throes of internal struggle and will probably end in the mutual annihilation of its members, if it is not destroyed by outside enemies who exploit its inner dissension.

No society can afford the free play of hostile and disruptive forces; these forces must be checked to the point where they do not threaten the survival of the group. There is great diversity in the codes with which societies regulate the display of hostility. The Judeo-Christian civilization believes in the sanctity of all human life; some societies limit their "thou shalt not kill" to members of their own group only; and even the most primitive societies do not tolerate unchecked intragroup hatred and belligerence.

Normal individuals are capable of living on friendly terms with their group. They are capable of cooperating with others and of entering into social relations based on mutual respect, agreement, and responsibility. They are capable of accepting and honoring commitments to other people. They may disagree with others without becoming disagreeable, and they can understand that others may disagree with them. They may fight in self-defense in a manner approved by their cultural group. Thus the fourth and last criterion of mental health is social adjustment, which hinges on four patterns of social interaction: the hostile, instrumental, mutual, and vectorial. Mature individuals relate in a self-controlled hostile way in self-defense; they are instrumental in their breadwinning functions; they are mutual in friendship, social love, and marriage; they are vectorial toward their children and toward whoever needs their help (Wolman, 1956, 1958, 1960b).

Some individuals are more instrumental, or more mutual, or more vectorial in behavior patterns. Mature behavior is not perfect behavior; it is rational and balanced, corresponding to Freud's model of id-ego-superego, with the rational ego keeping a reasonable balance among the animalistic demands of the id, the moralistic commandments of the superego, and the realistic pursuit of practical goals.

Mentally disturbed individuals are usually socially maladjusted and as a rule find it difficult to relate to others. They may overdo or underdo in their instrumental, mutual, or vectorial attitudes. Often, believing other people to be hostile, they fear and distrust others, shy away from them, and withdraw into seclusion. Sometimes they hate people, and at the same time fear their own hostile impulses. In severe cases, the hostility breaks through; in a catatonic fury, a mental patient may attack everything and everybody. The severity of social maladjustment usually corresponds to the severity of mental disorder, although this is not a simple relationship. The interactional patterns and interindividual relations of an individual offer valuable diagnostic cues.

Social adjustment must not be confused with conformity. Were these two identical, all ethnic, religious, and political minorities would be considered maladjusted; every inventor, every creative writer, every political reformer, and every pioneer of social, religious, or scientific progress could be branded as emotionally unhealthy. Social adjustment is the ability for a peaceful and friendly interaction with other individuals, while conformity means unconditional acceptance of certain social norms and mores. Social adjustment does not exclude an individual's differences of opinion with someone else, but implies the ability to cope with these differences in a friendly and realistic manner, rather than becoming anxious and hostile. It is quite possible that the conformists rather than the nonconformists are maladjusted. Most probably, insecure and immature individuals are afraid to be different and cannot tolerate differences of opinion.

16.   Irrational Behavior or Mental Disease?

Rational behavior is geared toward survival. However, rationality and irrationality do not qualify as health and disease, respectively. A diseased organism can be a victim of morbid genes, faulty metabolism, infection, poisoning, or traumatic events. These terms are not applicable to nonorganic mental disorders. Mentally unhealthy people are, to some extent, victims of whatever factors have caused their disorder, but they are not merely passive, bedridden, helpless victims. Mental disorder is irrational behavior, whether it involves erroneous perception, exaggerated emotionality, or avoidance of one's friends. Schizophrenics, for instance, display all three of these symptoms. Schizophrenia is not a disease of the brain or vasomotor system; schizophrenia is the total person; it is an irrational way of handling one's life. Symptoms in mental disorder are hardly coincidental; they usually serve a purpose; that is, they usually represent a search for something or an escape from something. They are morbid, irrational ways of coping or rather failing to cope with life.

The sick role is a passive role; one succumbs to pneumonia, typhoid fever, smallpox, thrombosis, or fracture of bones. One does not succumb in the same way to obsessive-compulsive neurosis, sexual frigidity, severe depression, or schizophrenia.

Health and sickness are states of an organism. Good health means good chances for survival, while poor health and disease point to a danger to life. No one is perfectly healthy, nor is anyone absolutely normal mentally. Mental normality and abnormality are a matter of degree. The more realistic one's perceptions, the more balanced one's emotionality, and the more satisfactory one's interaction with other people, the more one is normal; less well-balanced people are disturbed. There are degrees and levels of mental health just as there is a continuum of physical health.

17. Methodological Considerations

BENJAMIN B.
WOLMAN

One cannot analyze behavior disorders in a vacuum outside the context of behavioral science. Psychopathology is a branch of psychology and abnormal behavior is a certain type of behavior, just as a rotten apple is still an apple. With this in mind, one must relate psychopathological concepts to a certain theoretical model in psychology.

Models are neither true nor false. They are merely methods of presentation which do or do not facilitate (1) communication and (2) further research. Some models are more general, more flexible than others; some models have a greater heuristic value than the others. For instance, Jung's personality model (Wolman, 1978) is rather cumbersome. Hull's model (Wolman, 1960a) is clear and streamlined, but it covers only certain aspects of human behavior.

Freud's conceptual system offers distinct advantages in its consistency and clarity, and enables us to relate etiological data to theoretical models (Wolman, 1977). As such, it has stimulated further research which is branching off into distinct diagnosis systems such as those of Glover (1968), Bour (1966), and Wolman (1973a).

Clinical practice needs descriptive and easily ascertainable concepts and models. Clinicians work with people, and such terms as "weak ego," "libido," and "repression" are not empirical terms and they fail to describe what patients think, feel, and do.

Quite naturally, clinicians seek terms related to what they can see. The St. Louis research is a good example of the efforts to cast diagnostic criteria in terms of overt behavior (Helzer et al., 1977; Murphy, Woodruff, Herjanic, & Fischer, 1974; Woodruff et al., 1974). The work of Eysenck (1961), Kanfer and Saslow (1969), and Ferster (1966) follows a similar line, and the DSM III is coated in terms of observable data (Pinsker & Spitzer, 1977; Spitzer, Endicott, & Robins, 1975).

It seems, however, that going to extreme in the direction of symptomatology, as DSM III does, may put psychopathology back to a pre-Kraepelin era and deny the important developments in etiology and concept formation.

For instance, Freud's topographic theory, which distinguishes three "mental layers" of conscious, preconscious, and unconscious, enables researchers and clinicians to go beyond the observable data and include inferrable data in a methodologically adequate manner. Empirical propositions in psychology and psychopathology describe (1) observable events, such as "the patient broke several dishes," (2) introspectively observable data, such as "the patient believed a 'voice' told him to break the dishes," and (3) inferrable data, such as "the patient is unable to distinguish between outer, sensorily perceived stimuli and stimuli that came from within."

Freud's dynamic theory introduced the concepts of emotional energy (libido), the activating, releasing force (eros), and the investing or charging of energy in objects (cathexis), thus permitting some sort of an estimate of emotional balance between self-and-object cathexis which represents normality, and a dysbalance which indicates a disorganized personality and disturbed behavior.

Freud introduced a personality model, called the structural theory, composed of the id, ego, and superego. The inherited instinctual forces of love (eros) and hate (thanatos) are seated in the id, the "boiling cauldron" of all human impulses. The id follows blindly the principle of immediate gratification of needs, regardless of consequences (the "pleasure principle"). The newborn child's personality is composed of the id only, but as the child grows a shell develops and turns into the protective and controlling part of the personality, called ego. The id is entirely unconscious and wholly irrational in its pursuit of immediate gratification; the ego is an outgrowth of the id. It pursues pleasure, but not at all costs. Acting as guardian of the system, the ego's main task is survival under optimal conditions. The ego controls the unconscious impulses and guides the entire behavior toward an optimal adjustment to life.

Standing at the extreme opposite of that instinctual reservoir represented by the id is the superego. The superego develops as a result of introjection of parental images and an identification with their "do's" and "don'ts." The superego represents one's guilty conscience and the internalized voices of parents, teachers, and other authority figures whose moral standards the individual has accepted.

The ego of well-adjusted individuals exercises control over the organism. It satisfies the animalistic demands of the id, but it does so in a way that does not invite adverse repercussions. The ego also takes into consideration the moralistic demands of the superego, provided that they are not too exaggerated. The ego keeps a reasonable balance between the conflicting demands of the id and the superego, and acts in a realistic fashion, anticipating the consequences of its actions.

A weak ego is a sign of mental disorder. A state of anxiety arises when the ego is pressured by the id or the superego. Mental symptoms result from the morbid efforts of the ego to retain its control against undue inner pressures. As long as the ego is still in charge of the entire system, the disorder is mild and called neurosis. A psychosis begins to develop when the ego fails to control the system, and a flood of unconscious impulses originating in the id or the superego sweeps over the conscious state.

18. Wolman's Nosological System

Wolman (1965a, 1966a, 1966b, 1970, 1973a) has attempted to build a bridge between Freud's theoretical system and observable behavior. Interpersonal relations seemed to offer the best choice, for human interaction is not only an observable but also an indicator of highly relevant adjustment processes. Freud's personality model requires some modification in regard to social relations. The term "cathexis" is merely a logical construct that enables us to distinguish between various types of object relations. Freud's studies dealt with the cathecting individual and omitted the cathected object. Sociologically oriented neoanalysts such as Horney and Sullivan were concerned with this issue. Instead of Freudian love, sexual or aim-inhibited, Horney introduced protection and safety; instead of Freud's active cathexis of libido or need to love, she emphasized the need to be loved. Sullivan went even further in his theory of interpersonal relations; he tied personality directly to interpersonal relations. Without using the term "cathexis," he emphasized empathy, describing it as a kind of "emotional contagion or communion" between the child and parental figures. Freud dealt with the individual who cathects his libido in the object; Wolman suggested including also the cathected object in the study. This enables one to use the important contributions made by the neoanalytic schools without abandoning Freudian personality theory.

This new concept of "interindividual cathexis" is merely a logical construct and has been introduced because of its methodological flexibility and usefulness. Thus, in instrumental relationships, the individual's aim is to receive libido cathexes from others; in mutual relationships, the individual aims at receiving libido cathexes as well as at giving them to those from whom he aims to receive; and, in vectorial relationships, the individual aims to object-cathect, to give to others. A well-balanced individual is capable of functioning in all three types of relationships. His libido is reasonably balanced in interindividual relationships and is properly divided between intercathexes and intracathexes. A dysbalance in interindividual cathexes, caused by interaction between the individual and his environment, inevitably leads to a dysbalance in intraindividual cathexes. In other words, improper social relations must cause personality disorder.

Another modification of Freud's theory of personality has been suggested (Wolman, 1960a) and pertains to the destructive instincts and the theory of death. Freud suggested the theory of thanatos as the death instinct, the opposite of eros, or the life instinct, which serves to protect life. How can this supposed death instinct protect death? No living organism uses instinctual energy to die or to increase or to protect death, nor is it true "that the final aim of the destructive instinct is to reduce living things to an inorganic state" (Freud, 1938/1949, p. 20). Certain organic processes continue after the organism as a whole dies, and no living organism turns with death into a rock.

Starting with Charles Darwin and continuing with T. Huxley, I. P. Pavlov, T. Schjeldrupp-Ebbe, and recently K. Lorentz, biologists pointed to the use of physical force for self-defense as the general law of nature. Lorentz believes that hate is a more general and fundamental pattern than love and that hostility is the primary pattern in the animal kingdom; it is the main drive in the struggle for survival. When man is hungry or hurt or when his energies are low, the available energy is predominantly destructive, and he can be easily provoked to violence. The hostile drive, called "ares," serves life, too. Its emotional energy, called "destrudo," can be cathected analogously to libido.

Through the developmental stages of life, there is a gradual modification in the intercathexes and intracathexes of libido, usually combined with destrudo. Oral love is a fusion of object libido with an obvious predominance of destrudo. In the anal stage, in "tenderness," object cathexis of libido becomes stronger. At the phallic stage, in possessive-protective love, there is an additional gain of libido over destrudo. In well-adjusted adults, destrudo is partially sublimated, partially aim-inhibited, and partially adequately repressed. Destrudo is primitive and archaic, and there are no developmental stages analogous to those of libido, for there cannot be any progress in destrudo. Destrudo takes over when libido fails. In emergencies, in states of severe deprivation, starvation, lack of sleep, exhaustion, and pain, destrudo takes over. When love cannot help, hate is called in.

Destrudo is the controlling power of the organism only in a state of serious regression. In normal states, it is partially fused with libido and partially sublimated, but it never has pure, uncontrolled, savage liberty. An unbound, bursting-out destrudo is symptomatic of severe mental disorder.

The modification of Freud's personality model permits classification of mental disorders according to their type and the degree of their severity. The type of disorder could be ascertained by applying the concept of balanced cathexes to normal and abnormal behavior. A normal person balances his libido (friendly) and destrudo (hostile) impulses and cathects (invests, charges) them partly in oneself and partly in others. When one's libido is excessively self-cathected, the individual is narcissistic; he loves himself and no one else, he is an exploitative psychopath or sociopath (I use these terms interchangeably, but I prefer the latter one). If an individual's libido is excessively cathected in others, especially parental figures, he will develop compulsive behavior and/or, eventually, a full-blown schizophrenia. If an individual's moods swing from one extreme to another, from extreme libido self-cathexis toward excessive libido-object cathexis, he is probably hysteric and, if he deteriorates, he will end up as a manic-depressive psychotic.

Sociopaths hate whoever refuses to be used and exploited by them; schizophrenics fear their own hostility; and the manic-depressives hate those who don't love them and hate themselves for not being loved.

The Freudian concept of cathexes has been translated by Wolman (1965b, 1966a, 1967, 1970, 1973a) into observable interactional categories. When an individual relates in a hostile (H) manner to others, his destrudo is object-cathected. If an individual's libido is self-cathected and he expects others to take care of his needs and wishes, his attitude to others is narcissistic-hyperinstrumental, because he perceives others as tools to be used. He is basically hostile to other people.

If his libido has been excessively hypercathected, especially in parents or parental substitutes, his self-cathexis has been impoverished. Too much of libido has been given away, in a hypervectorial manner. He cares for others too much, and resents his resentment of giving too much without receiving. He tries to overcontrol his destrudo out of fear of hurting those he loves so much.

The third clinical type exhibits dysbalance in his social relations and distribution of libido and destrudo cathexes. He swings from object- to self-cathexis, from love to hate. He loves too much and expects too much in return, and hates others and self for his inevitable frustrations. His social, mutual relations are disturbed and he is called therefore dysmutual.

Based on a modified Freudian view of personality and the four criteria for mental health presented above, Wolman sees three basic types of "sociogenic" mental disorders. The hyperinstrumental type is highly instrumental in any situation and in regard to all people, always asking for something for nothing and showing no consideration for his fellow man. This type of disturbed person corresponds to what has usually been called the "psychopath" or the "sociopath" and has usually been the rejected child. The hypervectorial type is always ready to give, to protect, and to sacrifice himself. In childhood, this type was not able to act as a child but was forced into a role of protector of his protectors (i.e., the guardian of his inadequate parents). This type covers all that is described under the name "schizophrenic" and related conditions. The third type is the dysmutual type who is characterized by cyclic moods of extreme reaction, corresponding to what has been called "manic-depressive." These individuals at one time overdo in their love for others as the hypervectorial do, and at another time they feel no love for lovers and are as selfish as the hyperinstrumentals are. Typically, their childhoods were characterized by rejection and inattention except at times of extreme stress (e.g., when sick or injured), when they were showered with excessive amounts of attention and overprotection.

Within each type, Wolman describes five levels of disorder moving from neurosis to complete collapse of personality structure (see Table 2). These levels are said to function on a continuum, but Wolman points out that not every mentally disturbed individual must go through all or any levels of deterioration:

All mental disorders represent a continuum of deterioration. When rocks fall down, some roll one level down and come to a stop; some roll down step by step; some skip a step; some roll down all the way through. The fact that some rocks roll only one step down and some skip steps does not contradict the fact that there are five distinct steps on the slope.

These five steps are empirically observable phenomena. What has been added here is the *link* between them, the idea of *continuity* in mental processes, counterposed to a rigid and untrue assumption voiced by some workers that a neurotic cannot go psychotic. (Wolman, 1965a, p. 1135)

19. Emphasis on Etiology

Wolman's classificatory system is one of the possible systems that meet the requirement for economy and usefulness, because it combines symptomatology, etiology, and prognosis, enabling the clinicians to make diagnostic judgments and plan appropriate treatment strategies.

The emphasis on etiology offers certain significant advantages because it helps to distinguish the distinct roots of similar symptoms. Consider depression. Depression as a symptom is a cluster of feelings of angry helplessness, despair, and dependence. It is a catchall, almost as broad as high temperature in physical illness. Even more so, because perfectly balanced and well-adjusted individuals can get depressed when they are physically wounded, or when they have lost their jobs or have lost someone dear to them. Such an exogenous depression is not a sign of maladjustment provided that it is appropriate, that is, caused by a real harm or loss, proportionate to what happened, reasonably controllable, and leading to adjustive actions.

Endogenous depressions are usually pathological, but they may have a variety of causes, and lead to a host of different behaviorial patterns. In a vast majority of cases, the causes of depression determine its course. For instance, in schizophrenia (Wolman, 1966a, 1970), depression is very deep and can go on forever except for periods of the so-called spontaneous recovery. In manic-depressive disorder, depression reaches a certain low point which may lead to self-termination (more about depression later on). Obviously, psychotherapy with schizophrenics differs from psychotherapy with manic-depressives (Wolman, 1973a, 1976; Krauss and Krauss, 1977a).

Table 2. Classification of Psychogenic Mental Disorders

	Narcissistic—hyperinstrumental type (I)	Depressive—dysmutual type (M)	Schizohypervectorial type (V)
Neurotic level	Hyperinstrumental (narcissistic neuroses)	Dysmutual neurosis (dissociations, hysterias, and depressions)	Hypervectorial neurosis (obsessional, phobic, and neurasthenic neuroses)
Character neurotic level	Hyperinstrumental character neurosis (narcissistic character)	Dysmutual character neurosis (depressive and hysteric character)	Hypervectorial character neurosis (schizoid and obsessional character)
Latent psychotic level	Latent hyperinstrumental (psychopathic narcissism bordering on psychosis)	Latent dysmutual psychosis (borderline depressive psychosis)	Latent vectoriasis praecox (borderline and latent schizophrenia)
Manifest psychotic level	Hyperinstrumental psychosis (psychotic psychopathy and moral insanity)	Dysmutual psychosis (manifest depressive psychosis)	Vectoriasis praecox (manifest schizophrenia)
Dementia level	Collapse of personality structure		

A similar reasoning could be applied to a great many symptoms. The meaning of a symptom and the best way of coping with it depend on its etiology. This rule applies to practically all psychosomatic symptoms. On several occasions, I treated patients with psychosomatic skin troubles, heart disturbances, and gastrointestinal diseases. The first step was to send them for a thorough medical examination, and refuse to work with them until I had received from the physician or hospital totally negative results. Having received this green light, I had to find what was the unconscious purpose, the primary or secondary gain, in a particular symptom.

This teleological question is actually an etiological one. Why did a particular patient develop a particular symptom depending on what bothered him and what he wished to avoid or to gain?

Such an approach also facilitates preventive action. While the immediate task of clinicians is to seek remedies for existing ills, their moral obligation to society goes beyond that of a repairman. Armed with the knowledge of causes and results, they must actively participate in developing programs for the prevention of mental disorders (Wolman, 1972b).

20. Nature vs. Nurture

Mental disorders are either inherited, acquired, or caused by a combination of both. If they are inherited, they are transmitted through the genes. Those mental disorders which are not inherited are acquired through interaction with either the physical or the social environment. Thus mental disorders can be divided into three large categories related to their origins. Those that originate in the organism through heredity or through interaction with the physical environment (injuries, poisons, and so on) are "somatogenic" (*soma* means "body"). The inherited disorders are "genosomatogenic," because they are caused by genes. The physically acquired mental disorders are "ecosomatogenic," because they are caused by interaction with the environment, the ecos. All other disorders stem from faulty interindividual relations, i.e., they are psychosocial, but since the interaction with the social environment is the cause of morbid conditioning and cathexis, we shall call these disorders sociogenic or sociopsychogenic.

21. Early Childhood Experiences and Clinical Patterns

Interaction with one's social environment is synchronic with birth. The neonate faces parents and/or other adults whose attitudes exercise a tremendous impact on his development. As a rule, the earlier the infant is exposed to a noxious interaction, the greater is the damage to his personality.

One can distinguish three main parent-child interactional patterns that adversely affect the child's mental health. Some parents reject their child, some expect too much from him and overdemand, and some shift from acceptance to rejection and vice versa.

Some parents do not demand love from their children, nor do they offer any love to them. The child growing up in this kind of environment feels lonely and rejected, and perceives the world as a place where one either exploits others or is exploited by them. Rejected children soon learn to take advantage of other people's weaknesses, assuming that everyone else does the same. Viewing the world as a jungle serves as a justification for their own extreme selfishness. They regard their exploitative and hostile behavior as the self-preservatory response of an innocent creature facing a hostile world.

Clinical observations indicate three prototypical settings which are conducive to fostering such selfish, hyperinstrumental, hypernarcissistic personality types: institutions, underprivileged homes, and wealthy homes. The institutional environment, where anonymous counselors deal with anonymous "cases" in a cold, uninvolved, matter-of-fact way, distributing so many cups of milk and so many penalties for violation of the institutional discipline, is most likely to produce secondary narcissism (A. Freud, 1967).

Many hyperinstrumentals are underprivileged children who have been reared in an atmosphere of constant bickering, and were rejected by parents who resented the burden of taking care of their offspring. Members of underprivileged families often create an atmosphere where the jungle ethic prevails and the entire world seems to be populated by enemies.

In the third category are children of well-to-do families where the parents have characteristically substituted money for affection and nurturance. The child of such a background has no one to emulate or to identify with and is forced to live a hollow, selfish existence of unfulfilled wishes.

These narcissistic, hyperinstrumental children, when they deteriorate, typically become psychopaths. Milder cases of hyperinstrumentals are selfish and hostile people who feel that others are hostile. They are sensitive to their own suffering and deprivations, but have no empathy or sympathy for anyone else. In more severe cases, there is a total lack of moral restraint, consideration, and compassion for one's fellow man, and often a tendency to defy the law while proclaiming and believing in one's own innocence. The hyperinstrumentals, who are exploitative and generally oral-cannibalistic, operate on the principle that weak enemies and neutrals have to be destroyed and friends are to be used. The destrudo of hyperinstrumentals is highly mobilized and ready to strike against the outer world (object directed). A hyperinstrumental, perceiving himself as an innocent, poor, hungry animal, sees people as enemies: either he will devour them or they will devour him. Highly aggressive, the narcissistic hyperinstrumental type is actually a coward, brutal and cruel to those who fear him but obedient and subservient to those he fears. In the milder, neurotic cases, he appears as a selfish, frightened individual. In more severe cases, he is cruel when deteriorated. The most severe cases are described in terms of psychotic psychopathy, called by Prichard (1835) "moral insanity."

At the other extreme are parents who love their children but expect too much love in return. Insecure parents demand that the child love them and elicit in the child a premature emotional involvement. These immature and insecure people invite a reversal in social roles. They act as if they were the children who need to be loved, and demand the kind of love and affection from the child that would more properly be expected to come from their own parents. In such families, the parents' attitude toward the child is instrumental, and the child is forced too early into a costly, loving, vectorial attitude toward his parents. The child, in effect, is robbed of his childhood and must prematurely become an adult. His parents, disappointed in one another, expect him to compensate for all the love and affection they failed to obtain from each other. Moreover, the child is not allowed to express his dissatisfaction, discomfort, and dissent, nor is he permitted to act out childhood tantrums. In short, a child exposed to immature, overdemanding, and instrumental parents is expected to become a model child who renounces his own desires to please his parents. The child is forced into an extreme and too early hypervectorial attitude.

This parent-child interaction forces the child to worry about his truly or allegedly weak, sick, or dying parents. The child is forced to become a "model child," a protector of his protectors (Wolman, 1966a, 1970). The model child may try, at the devastating cost of impoverishment of his own emotional resources, to overcontrol his impulses. However, as soon as the emotional resources of love (the libido) have been overspent, the emotional energy of hate (the destrudo) takes over. Overspent love turns to hatred for oneself and others. The "fallen angel" soon becomes a hateful devil who is no longer able to control his hostile impulses. He hates himself for hating others, and is afraid of love that becomes overdemanding and threatening. The extreme result is schizophrenia. Typically, schizophrenics are individuals who as small children were forced to worry about their parents. Throughout their lives they feel compelled to strive for perfection and are unreasonably harsh on themselves. They appear to treat life as an obligation to be honored, as a ritual to be followed, or as a mission to be fulfilled, showing unlimited sympathy for those who suffer. Their love tends to be excessively loyal, often to the point of a domineering and despotic overprotectiveness. The loss of controls results in a full-blown schizophrenic episode, driven by uncontrollable hatred (Bellak & Loeb, 1969; Hill, 1955; Jackson, 1960; Wolman, 1966a, 1970, 1973a).

The depressive states of all kinds and levels have given rise to a good deal of controversy in psychiatric and psychological literature. Obviously not all depressed moods are pathological. One of the main criteria of mental health suggested by Wolman is emotional balance:

> All living organisms act in accordance with the law of homeostasis. This law states that whenever the human organism is exposed to stimulation which disturbs its equilibrium, a reaction takes place that is aimed at the restoration of the initial equilibrium. This principle applies to all functions of the organism, including emotional life. Human beings respond with pleasure and pain, joy and sorrow, elation and depression to situations in which they find themselves. The normal or mentally healthy individual reacts emotionally to stimuli in proportion to their magnitude (stronger reaction to the stronger stimuli and weaker reaction to the weaker stimuli) so that the best possible adjustment and restoration of emotional balance result. Thus, the emotionally balanced individual acts in a rational manner that enhances his chances for successful living; he reacts to stress in an adjustive manner. The reaction of the mentally sick or emotionally unbalanced individual may be exaggerated and out of proportion to the stimulus. Some individuals are in the throes of despair whenever they meet hardships or suffer a loss. Even when the loss is negligible and can be easily replaced, the disturbed individual is carried away by his emotions and acts in an irrational manner that certainly will not make matters better. One may expect a deterioration in this individual's ability to cope with hardships. Gradually increasing irritability and growing difficulty in restoring the emotional balance bear witness to an aggravation of the mental disorder. Emotionally balanced individuals are 'normal'; those who are poorly balanced are less normal. Severe emotional dysbalance is one of the indicators of the severity of the disorder. (Wolman, 1965a, p. 1128)

Wolman (1966b, 1973a) has suggested a solution to the problem of unipolarity or bipolarity. He has distinguished four clinical syndromes of the depressive psychosis, which he calls manifest dysmutual psychosis (Krauss and Krauss, 1977a). The dysmutual psychosis is basically a state of depression, but when the patient's ego surrenders to the superego these merge in a state of blissful elation or mania. The second syndrome is paranoia. When the failing ego externalizes superego pressure, it perceives the outer world as a rejecting and punishing mother who will eventually be forced to accept her suffering child. This is basically the dynamics of paranoia. The third syndrome is agitated depression. It starts wherever the ego is crushed between the cruel superego and savage id. There are no elated moods, no escape mechanisms, no respite from the unbearable depression. Suicidal danger is very high in this syndrome. The last syndrome is simple deterioration, when both the ego and the superego are defeated by the id.

The manic syndrome does not bring genuine joy and happiness. It is an escape, a desperate reaction to an unbearable feeling of depression. The dynamics of this syndrome represent the surrender of the ego to the superego. When the pressure of the superego becomes unbearable, the ego renounces further resistance and turns away from reality as if refusing to deal with it. In a manic mood, the self-righteous superego determines what is true and false: thus manic patients may express dogmatic and self-assured opinions about matters they have not considered heretofore. They become omniscient sages and judges who know everything and have the final say on all problems.

The manic mood may be precipitated by a severe blow to one's self-esteem, a loss of a close relative or friend, or the loss of status or property. In reaction to these events, the dysmutual hates those who have let him down, and he blames even those who were thoughtless enough to desert him by death. This hate is then taken up by his superego and turned on the self.

Introjection of the image of the rejecting or deceased parent, most often the one of the opposite sex, is typical for the dysmutual disorders. This introjected "love object" functions in a manner analogous to that of the rejecting parent; it is hostile and cruel, but only up to a certain point. The despairing ego tries to reach this point by accepting defeat, by magnifying it, and by making life look more horrible than it is. Then it turns to the superego as if to say, "See how miserable I am! You are right, I deserve to be punished. So beat me, but love me."

In some but not all cases of dysmutual psychosis, the superego accepts the surrender. When the ego gives up in despair, the superego accepts the defeat, embracing the wounded ego as would the bad mother who suddenly felt sorry for her suffering infant.

Once the dysmutual turns self-hate into self-pity, his mood changes radically. The ego, loved by the superego, is full of love and friendship. A manic patient becomes everyone's friend: thus a married woman in a manic state invited strange men she met on the street to share her bed; a manic man offered help and distributed money to whomever he met.

The ego that surrendered its prerogatives to the superego does not exercise proper jurisdiction over emotion and motility. The superego is self-righteous; so are the words and deeds of a manic, who believes that his wishes cannot be questioned and his whims are the law.

In elation there is no delay, no reality principle, no planning or caution. Whatever the manic feels like doing, he will do immediately, here and now. If he is sexually aroused, he may proposition the first girl he meets and become furious if she turns him down. If he is highly aroused he is likely to rape her. He cannot take the slightest frustration.

The manic-depressive wants to be absorbed by his mother. His delusions and hallucinations have to do with martyrdom, with being lost and found, with being

Cinderella saved by a good fairy or a slave led by a Messiah toward the lost paradise. A typical fantasy is of a disaster that will force mother to love them.

Schizophrenics wish to be God or Messiah. Since their parents have been weak and unreliable individuals, they must fill the void by becoming the omnipotent, omniscient, benevolent, or destructive God-Father, who saves, protects, or punishes his parents. Thus, whereas the schizophrenic rescues, the manic-depressive wants to be rescued. In the manic phase, he can be joined with the powerful parents and thereby acquire omnipotence and immortality.

However, even in a manic mood there is an underlying fear of losing the newly regained paradise. Manic patients avoid facing real issues out of a fear that the sharp pin of reality may prick the balloon of their blissful illusion. Thus no real planning or practical steps are taken for fear that the implementation of an idea may bring hardships and disappointment.

Not all dysmutual psychotics are capable of manic denial. In some cases, there is no escape from the assaults of the superego. The patient may feel happier if he has had the opportunity to outshine others and bask in the glory of his achievements, but since no human being can always be victorious and constantly admired by others, the short-lived moods of good feeling yield to severe depression.

One psychotic reaction to depression is full-blown paranoia. A way of defending against the self-directed destrudo (i.e., hate of the superego toward the ego) is to project the hate, as if saying, "I do not hate myself, but *they* hate me."

This projective-paranoid mechanism may be used by the ego on many occasions. It takes place whenever the ego is attacked by the superego and the ego is no longer capable of engaging in adequate reality testing.

In schizophrenia, when the ego is exposed to intolerable accusations from the superego, it develops paranoid accusations. In psychopathic disorders, when the patient's aggressiveness evokes hostile reactions, the patient denies that he was ever hostile; he believes himself to be an innocent sheep surrounded by a pack of wolves.

In dysmutual disorders, projections become systematized, reproducing the Cinderella story of a persecuted child finally rewarded for his sweetness and goodness. Every paranoid is a martyr, persecuted by a bad mother (stepmother) who is expected to become a good godmother.

When one feels painfully rejected, he may deny the rejection and pretend that he is greatly loved, or he may come to believe that he is a victim of a conspiracy. In either case, he employs the mechanism of projection. In the first case, he projects his love for the rejecting love object; in the second, he projects his hatred for the love object, whom he hates for turning down his love. Dysmutual patients tend to exaggerate and advertise their feelings. They often take signs of friendliness or even simple kindness as evidence of great love, and proceed to fall in love accordingly. Sometimes they are carried away by their own wishful thinking and imagine that other people are madly in love with them. A repeated pattern of this nature can assume the proportions of paranoia.

22. Continuum Hypothesis

The distinction between neurosis and psychosis has been another difficult issue. Pinsker and Spitzer (1977, p. 162) report that in DSM III "psychoses" and "neuroses" are not used as principles of classification:

"Psychotic" is used as an adjective to describe certain aspects of severity of illness. "Neurosis" is referred to as a speculative etiologic concept.

   The concept of "the psychoses" as a group of conditions seems rooted in the mental hospital, at a time when no one was identified as a mentally ill person unless psychotic. But if the term "psychotic" describes a certain degree of impairment of reality testing, disruption of thinking process, disorganization of behavior, or inability to function, the disorder (or disorders) which causes the psychotic impairment must have been present in mild form before the psychotic level of impairment was reached. Further clinicians do not usually classify their patients as "psychotic" as a precursor to determining whether or not the exact diagnosis is organic brain syndrome, mood disorder or schizophrenia, the historical subdivision of the psychoses (ICDA, 1968).

   Some psychiatrists diagnose schizophrenia in patients who have never been psychotic; others insist that psychosis at some time during the course of illness is essential before the diagnosis can be made. Yet even with this more stringent approach, the schizophrenic patient is not psychotic at all times. It is inconsistent to describe a patient as suffering from a psychosis, while acknowledging that he is not psychotic. (Pinsker and Spitzer, 1977, p. 162)

Wolman's system assumes a continuum; neurosis and psychosis are levels of disorder and not separate clinical entities:

My assumption is that the normal personality is a balanced personality. Once an imbalance in cathexes starts, the ego, in accordance with Freud's "constancy principle" and its main task of protection of the organism, tries to counteract the maladjustive processes. The struggle of the ego against pressures from within creates profound feelings of anxiety with a great variety of ego-protective symptoms. Although the nature of the symptoms depends on the nature of threat or damage and is specific in each of the three types of disorder, the common denominator for this level of all three types is anxiety and ego-protective symptoms. As long as the ego is capable of asserting itself using a galaxy of defense mechanisms, it is *neurosis*. It can be a hyperinstrumental neurosis, a dysmutual neurosis, or a hypervectorial neurosis; they are different *types* of neurosis, but they are the same, first level of mental disorder.

   When the ego so-to-say comes to terms with the neurotic symptoms and the neurotic symptoms or attitudes become "included in the ego" or "blended into personality" (Fenichel, 1945, p. 463ff.), then neurosis becomes "character neurosis" or "character disorder," or "personality disorder." These three names describe the same category, the same second level of mental disorder.

   Sometimes the defenses are inadequate and a neurosis or a character neurosis may turn into a latent or manifest psychosis. A neurosis does not have to become first character neurosis and then a latent psychosis and later on a manifest psychosis. Character neurosis serves as a "protective armor" (Reich, 1945), a rigid set of ego-protective symptoms that prevents further deterioration into psychosis, but sometimes even armor may break. Yet, in some cases, in spite of a severe psychotic deterioration the individual still is not manifestly psychotic. He somehow continues functioning on a slim margin of ego controls; a mild noxious stimulus may throw him into a manifest psychosis. As long as his ego keeps on going and a contact with reality is preserved, it is *latent* and not a manifest psychosis.

   The main difference between neurosis and psychosis lies in the strength of the ego. As long as the ego controls the id and preserves the contact with reality, it is neurosis. Psychosis is a neurosis that failed; it is a defeat of the ego that lost the contact with reality and a victory of the id. (Wolman, 1966b, pp. 57–58)

23. Conclusions

   Apparently, there is more than one way to classify mental disorders, and several classificatory systems meet the formal logical requirement of economy. The question of their usefulness is still unresolved, but pure symptomatology offers little if any guidance in planning therapeutic and preventive strategies. An adequate classificatory system must therefore incorporate several factors, delve into etiology, and link conceptual systems with observable symptoms.

Albee, G. W. Emerging concepts of mental illness and models of treatment: The psychological point of view. *American Journal of Psychiatry*, 1969, *125*, 870–876.

Alexander, F. G., & Seleznick, S. T. *The history of psychiatry*. New York: Harper & Row, 1977.

American Psychiatric Association. *Diagnostic and statistical manual of mental disorders. DSM II*. Washington, D.C.: Author, 1968.

Angst, J. *Zur Ätiologie und Nosologie endogener depressiver Psychosen*. Berlin: Springer, 1966.

Bellak, L., & Loeb, L. (Eds.). *The schizophrenic syndrome*. New York: Grune & Stratton, 1969.

Blashfield, R. K., & Draguns, J. G. Evaluative criteria for psychiatric classification. *Journal of Abnormal Psychology*, 1976, *85*, 140–150.

Bour, P. Proposition concrète en matière de nosologie psychiatrique. *Annales Medicopsychologiques*, 1966, *2*, 508–511.

Bower, E. M. Mental health, social competence and the war on poverty. *American Journal of Orthopsychiatry*, 1966, *36*, 652–654.

Cancro, R., & Sugarman, A. A. Classification and outcome in process-reactive schizophrenia. *Comprehensive Psychiatry*, 1968, *9*, 227–232.

Cancro, R., & Sugarman, A. A. Psychological differentiation and process-reactive schizophrenia. *Journal of Abnormal Psychology*, 1969, *74*, 415–419.

Edwards, G. Diagnosis of schizophrenia: An Anglo-American comparison. *British Journal of Psychiatry*, 1972, *120*, 385–390.

Eysenck, H. J. (Ed.). *Handbook of abnormal psychology: An experimental approach*. New York: Basic Books, 1961.

Fenichel, O. *The psychoanalytic theory of neurosis*. New York: Norton, 1945.

Ferster, C. B. Classification of behavior psychology. In L. Krasner & L. P. Ullman (Eds.), *Research in behavior modification*. New York: Holt, Rinehart and Winston, 1966.

Fisher, J., Epstein, L. J., & Harris, M. R. Validity of the psychiatric interview. *Archives of General Psychiatry*, 1967, *17*, 744–750.

Foulds, G. A. *Personality and personal illness*. London: Tavistock, 1969.

Freud, A. Comments. In H. Witmer (Ed.), *On rearing infants and young children in institutions*. Washington: Children's Bureau, 1967, *1*, 49–55.

Freud, S. *An outline of psychoanalysis*. New York: Norton, 1949. (Originally published in 1938.)

Glover, E. *Birth of the ego*. New York: International Universities Press, 1968.

Goldstein, M. J., Held, J. M., & Cromwell, R. Premorbid adjustment and paranoid-nonparanoid status in schizophrenia. *Psychological Bulletin*, 1968, *70*, 382–385.

Grinker, R. W. Emerging comcepts of mental illness and models of treatment: The medical point of view. *American Journal of Psychiatry*, 1969, *125*, 865–879.

Gurland, B. Classification, nosology, and taxonomy of mental disorders. In B. B. Wolman (Ed.), *International encyclopedia of psychiatry, psychology, psychoanalysis, & neurology*. New York: Van Nostrand/Aesculapius, 1977, Vol. 3, pp. 156–160.

Helzer, J. E., Robins, L. N., Woodruff, R. A., Jr., Reich T., & Wish, E. D. Reliability of psychiatric diagnosis. I. A methodological review. *Archives of General Psychiatry*, 1977, *34*, 129–133.

Hempel, C. G. Introduction to problems of taxonomy. In J. Zubin (Ed.), *Field studies in the mental disorders*. New York: Grune & Stratton, 1961, pp. 3–22.

Hill, L. B. *Psychotherapeutic intervention in schizophrenia*. Chicago: University of Chicago Press, 1955.

Holt, R. R., & Luborsky, L. *Personality patterns of psychiatrists*. New York: Basic Books, 1958.

Horney, K. *The neurotic personality of our time*. New York: Norton, 1937.

Hunt, H. F. Clinical methods: Psychodiagnostics. *Annual Review of Psychology*, 1950, *1*, 207–220.

Hunt, W. A. An investigation of naval neuropsychiatric screening procedures. In H. Guetzkow (Ed.), *Groups, leadership, and men*. Pittsburgh, Pa.: Carnegie Press, 1951, pp. 245–256.

Jackson, D. (Ed.). *The etiology of schizophrenia*. New York: Basic Books, 1960.

Jahoda, M. *Current concepts of mental health*. New York: Basic Books, 1958.

Jarvis, E. *Insanity and idiocy in Massachusetts: Report of the Commission on Lunacy*. Cambridge, Mass.: Harvard University Press, 1855.

Jeans, J. *Physics and philosophy*. Ann Arbor, Mich.: University of Michigan Press, 1958.

Kanfer, F. H., & Saslow, G. Behavior diagnosis. In C. W. Franks (Ed.), *Behavior therapy: Appraisal and status*. New York: McGraw-Hill, 1969, pp. 417–444.

Kantor, R., & Herron, W. G. *Reactive and process schizophrenia*. Palo Alto, Calif.: Science and Behavior Books, 1966.

Kendall, R. E. *The classification of depressive illness.* London: Oxford University Press, 1968.

Krauss, H. H., & Krauss, B. J. Manic-depressive disorder: Wolman's view. In B. B. Wolman (Ed.), *International encyclopedia of psychiatry, psychology, psychoanalysis, & neurology.* New York: Van Nostrand/Aesculapius, 1977, Vol. 6, pp. 487–488. (a)

Krauss, H. H., & Krauss, B. J. Nosology: Wolman's system. In B. B. Wolman (Ed.), *International encyclopedia of psychiatry, psychology, psychoanalysis, & neurology.* New York: Van Nostrand/Aesculapius, 1977, Vol. 8, pp. 86–88. (b)

Kreitman, N., Sainsbury, P., Morrissey, J., Towers, J., & Scrivener, J. The reliability of psychiatric diagnosis. *Journal of Mental Science,* 1961, *107,* 887–908.

Laing, R. D. *The politics of experience.* New York: Ballantine, 1967.

Lorr, M. Classification of the behavior disorders. *Annual Review of Psychology,* 1961, *12,* 195–216.

Marchais, P. De quelques principes pour l'établissement d'une nosologie en psychiatrie. *Annales Medico-psychologiques,* 1966, *2,* 512–522.

Meehl, P. The cognitive activity of the clinician. *American Psychologist,* 1960, *15,* 19–27.

Menninger, K., Mayman, M., & Pruyser, P. *The vital balance: The life process in mental health and illness.* New York: Viking, 1963.

Murphy, G. E., Woodruff, R. A., Jr., Herjanic, M., & Fischer, J. R. Validity of the diagnosis of primary affective disorder: A prospective study with a five-year follow-up. *Archives of General Psychiatry,* 1974, *30,* 751–756.

Nagel, E. *The structure of science.* New York: Harcourt, Brace, 1961.

Phillips, L. *Human adaptation and its failures.* New York: Academic, 1968.

Phillips, L. & Draguns, J. G. Classification of the behavior disorders. *Annual Review of Psychology,* 1971, *22,* 447–482.

Pinsker, H., & Spitzer, R. Classification of mental disorders, DSM-III. In B. B. Wolman (Ed.), *International encyclopedia of psychiatry, psychology, psychoanalysis, & neurology.* New York: Van Nostrand/Aesculapius, 1977, Vol. 3, pp. 160–164.

Prichard, J. C. *Treatise on insanity.* London: Gilbert & Piper, 1835.

Reich, W. *Character analysis.* New York: Orgone Institute, 1945.

Sarbin, T. R. On the futility of the proposition that some people be labelled "mentally ill." *Journal of Consulting Psychology,* 1967, *31,* 447–453.

Scheff, T. J., & Scheff, T. I. *Being mentally ill: A sociological theory.* Chicago: Aldine, 1966.

Spitzer, R. L., Endicott, J., & Robins, E. Clinical criteria for psychiatric diagnosis and DSM-III. *American Journal of Psychiatry,* 1975, *132,* 1187–1192.

Stockings, G. T. Schizophrenia in military psychiatric practice. *Journal of Mental Science,* 1945, *91,* 110–112.

Strupp, H. H. Ferment in psychoanalysis and psychotherapy. In B. B. Wolman (Ed.), *Success and failure in psychoanalysis and psychotherapy.* New York: Macmillan, 1972, pp. 71–103.

Sullivan, H. *The interpersonal theory of psychiatry.* New York: Norton, 1953.

Szasz, T. *The myth of mental illness.* New York: Harper & Row, 1961.

Szasz, T. (Ed.). *Ideology and insanity.* New York: Doubleday, 1969.

Thorne, F. C. *Integrative psychology.* Branden, Vt.: Clinical Psychology, 1967.

Tolman, E. C. *Purposive behavior in animals and men.* New York: Appleton-Century-Crofts, 1932.

Ullman, L. P., & Krasner, L. *A psychological approach to abnormal behavior.* Englewood Cliffs, N.J.: Prentice-Hall, 1969.

Wolman, B. B. Leadership and group dynamics. *Journal of Social Psychology,* 1956, *43,* 11–25.

Wolman, B. B. Explorations in latent schizophrenia. *American Journal of Psychotherapy,* 1957, *11,* 560–588.

Wolman, B. B. Instrumental, mutual acceptance and vectorial groups. *Acta Sociologica,* 1958, *3,* 19–27.

Wolman, B. B. *Contemporary theories and systems in psychology.* New York: Harper, 1960. (a)

Wolman, B. B. Impact of failure on group cohesiveness. *Journal of Social Psychology,* 1960, *51,* 409–418. (b)

Wolman, B. B. The fathers of schizophrenic patients. *Acta Psychotherapeutica,* 1961, *9,* 193–210.

Wolman, B. B. Non-participant observation on a closed ward. *Acta Psychotherapeutica,* 1964, *12,* 61–71.

Wolman, B. B. Mental health and mental disorders. In B. B. Wolman (Ed.), *Handbook of clinical psychology.* New York: McGraw-Hill, 1965, pp. 1119–1139. (a)

Wolman, B. B. Schizophrenia and related disorders. In B. B. Wolman (Ed.), *Handbook of clinical psychology.* New York: McGraw-Hill, 1965, pp. 976–1029. (b)

Wolman, B. B. Toward a science of psychological science. In B. B. Wolman and E. Nagel (Eds.), *Scientific psychology.* New York: Basic Books, 1965, pp. 3–23. (c)

Wolman, B. B. Family dynamics and schizophrenia. *Journal of Health and Human Behavior,* 1965, *6,* 163–169. (d)

Wolman, B. B. *Vectoriasis praecox or the group of schizophrenias.* Springfield, Ill.: Thomas, 1966. (a)

Wolman, B. B. Dr. Jekyll and Mr. Hyde: A new theory of the manic depressive disorder. *New York Academy of Sciences,* 1966, *28,* 1020–1032. (b)

Wolman, B. B. (Ed.) *Psychoanalytic techniques.* New York: Basic Books, 1967.

Wolman, B. B. *Children without childhood: A study of childhood schizophrenia.* New York: Grune & Stratton, 1970.

Wolman, B. B. Does psychology need its own philosophy of science? *American Psychologist,* 1971, *26,* 877–886.

Wolman, B. B. (Ed.) *Child psychoanalysis.* New York: Van Nostrand Reinhold, 1972.

Wolman, B. B. *Call no man normal.* New York: International Universities Press, 1973. (a)

Wolman, B. B. *Dictionary of behavioral science.* New York: Van Nostrand Reinhold, 1973. (b)

Wolman, B. B. Concerning psychology and the philosophy of science. In B. B. Wolman (Ed.), *Handbook of general psychology.* Englewood Cliffs, N.J.: Prentice-Hall, 1973. (c)

Wolman, B. B. (Ed.) *The therapist's handbook.* New York: Van Nostrand Reinhold, 1976.

Wolman, B. B. Psychoanalysis as science. In B. B. Wolman (Ed.), *International encyclopedia of psychiatry, psychology, psychoanalysis, & neurology.* New York: Van Nostrand/Aesculapius, 1977, Vol. 9, pp. 149–157.

Wolman, B. B. *Psychoanalysis as a scientific system.* In press.

Woodruff, R. A., Jr., Goodwin, D. W., & Guxe, S. B. *Psychiatric diagnosis.* New York: Oxford University Press, 1974.

World Health Organization. *International classification of diseases (ICD-8).* Geneva: Author, 1975.

Zilboorg, G., & Henry, G. W. *A history of medical psychology.* New York: Norton, 1941.

Zubin, J. Classification of the behavior disorders. *Annual Review of Psychology,* 1967, *18,* 373–406.

3

The Interview: Its Reliability and Validity in Psychiatric Diagnosis

JOSEPH D. MATARAZZO

1. History of the Interview

The interview is probably as old as the human race. It quite likely traces its roots to the first conversation in which either Adam or Eve interrogated the other or one of their children regarding some alleged transgression. It differs from the more common, spontaneous, everyday communicative encounter in that the interview is a deliberately initiated conversation wherein two persons, and more recently more than two, engage in verbal and nonverbal communication toward the end of gathering information which will help one or both of the parties better reach a goal. This goal or destination for which the interview serves as a data-gathering instrument is occasionally clearly defined by one or both parties, but, for the experienced as well as novice interviewer, such a goal even today is unfortunately more often than not still too ill-defined and inadequately stipulated.

Humanity's earliest written records reveal that since antiquity the interview by any of a variety of names has been used professionally in succession by ancient gods, priests and priestesses, philosophers, physicians, members of the clergy, and attorneys. In the nineteenth century, it became a standard tool of newspaper reporters and, in the twentieth century, a necessary tool used by numerous other professional persons. More specifically, the Oxford dictionary indicates that the word *interview* first appeared in print as such in 1514 to designate "a meeting of persons face to face, especially for the purpose of formal conference on some point." In 1548, it was used to mean "to have a personal meeting with [each other]" and "to meet together in per-

JOSEPH D. MATARAZZO • Department of Medical Psychology, University of Oregon School of Medicine, Portland, Oregon 97201.

son." And, in 1869, its meaning was extended to include "to have an interview with [a person]; specifically, to talk with so as to elicit statements for publication." Also in 1869, as indicated above, the term "interviewer" appeared in print to designate "one who interviews; specifically, a journalist who interviews a person [an interviewee] with the object of obtaining information for publication."

A concomitant of the acceleration of the industrial revolution which was taking place throughout much of the world during the twentieth century was the emergence of a variety of new professionals: clinical psychologists, psychiatrists, economists, social workers, sociologists, anthropologists, professional nurses, detectives, business executives, salesmen, television reportorial interviewers, and talk show interviewers, pollsters, motivation researchers, public opinion takers, college and other educational guidance specialists, vocational rehabilitation and other types of counselors, bank personnel who specialize in loans, department store and finance company interviewers, welfare caseworkers, employment agency specialists, thought-reform interrogators, and, most recently, paraprofessional counselors of all types, to name but a few of the different types of individuals using the interview as a major data-gathering communicative tool in their work. In aggregate, these various newly recruited professionals and paraprofessional persons have given rise to a vast new industry, the communications professions.

2. Sociological Interviews

In a brief review of the history of the interview from the perspective of sociology, Riesman and Benney (1956) outline its development from the diplomatic encounters between heads of state during the post-Renaissance period; through its introduction by Horace Greeley as a technique useful to newspaper men; through its use by Mayhew, Booth, LePlay, and Quetelet in understanding the working classes of a newly developing industrial society and, concurrently, its use by Freud in his then developing psychoanalytic method; and finally to its use by twentieth-century social scientists such as Roethlisberger and Dickson, Lazarsfeld, Merton, and others. Commenting on the twentieth-century developments in uses of the interview, Riesman and Benney wrote:

> In social research, market research, industry, social work, and therapy interviewing has become in fifty years a major white-collar industry—one of those communications professions which represents the shift of whole cadres into tertiary areas. (p. 3)

Elsewhere in their paper, Riesman and Benney include such pithy comments as these:

> Interviewing itself is a middle-class profession, in pursuit of middle-class concerns. (p. 12)

> We do know that the interview is taking on something of the nature of a *rite de passage* as one moves from one institution to another, from school to army to job to other jobs and finally to the gerontological social worker. (p. 15)

They also cite a 1952 book by Kephart in which he reports that over half the current labor force either changes jobs or takes new employment annually and that all but a few of what they numbered a labor force of 30 million individuals find that "an interview is the major factor in their new placement." As a matter of fact, Bellows and Estep (1954) estimated that 150 million selection interviews were taking place annually in the United States alone during that same time. With the advent during the 1960s and 1970s of legislation which effectively bars the use by American industry of tests and other objective psychological assessment instruments in personnel hiring, the interview is in the United States today the major, if not exclusive tool in such hiring. Inasmuch as the use of psychological testing in industry was not as far advanced in other parts of the world as it was in the United States at the time of this recent legislation, one may conclude that the interview is today the tool of choice in industry throughout all industrialized countries of the world. Recalling also that millions of interviews are conducted yearly by mental health specialists in the United States alone, if one were to add up, worldwide, all the interviews conducted by specialists from all the communications professions in 1 year, it is conceivable that the sum would exceed hundreds of millions, if not billions. In view of these astronomical numbers and the related professional man-hours and monies of investment that they represent, it may be surprising for the reader to learn how little, relatively speaking, is known even by professionals about the historical facts, the present status, or even the reliability and validity of the interview—whether used in the mental health or one of the other professions enumerated above.

3. Diagnostic Interviews

Before examining the empirical research information available on the interview as a data-gathering instrument, it is important for the purposes of this chapter to point out that in medicine, psychology, and psychiatry, and probably to an extent greater than that in any of the other communications professions, data from the interview cannot be separated from inferences concurrently made from behavioral and related observations of the individual being interviewed. Detectives, reporters, and other interviewers make mental note of shifts in gaze and in posture, facial flushes, hesitations, circumlocutions, non sequiturs, delusional content, and similar nonverbal or nonlexical communications, but, to date, only in the mental health professions have attempts been made to systematically use such cues as integral parts of a diagnostic appraisal. The history of the use of such verbal and nonverbal observational cues in early forms of the "mental status" examination as a basis for classification, nosology, and diagnosis is intimately intertwined with the history of medicine, psychiatry, and psychology dating back to the earliest records of the human race. The reader interested in an excellent historical review of the actual nosological system in use for psychiatric classification and diagnosis in each era from the period 2600 B.C., through Hippocrates and Plato of the classic Greek period (fifth and fourth centuries B.C.), through early Christianity, the Dark Ages, the Renaissance, through the great writers of sixteenth-, seventeenth-, and eighteenth-century medicine, and, finally, into the nineteenth and twentieth centuries will find this history in rich and detailed text in Zilboorg (1941) and in neat but comprehensive outline in the appendix of the book by Menninger, Mayman, and Pruyser (1963). Included in the outline provided by the latter are the specific diagnostic classifications used by each of the well-known and lesser giants, including Hippocrates, Plato, Galen, Avicena, Saint Thomas Aquinas, Paracelsus, Sydenham, Linneaus, Kant, Pinel, Rush, Esquirol, Maynert, Wernicke, Kraepelin, Bleuler, Freud, Meyer, Southard, and William Menninger (whose work in World War II gave birth to the American Psychiatric Association's 1952 *Diagnostic and Statistical Manual of Mental Disorders* DSM I, and to the revised second edition, DSM II, published in 1968). Other chapters in the present volume concern themselves with the complex issues involved in the earlier and current diagnostic systems for classifying the mental disorders. In the present chapter, we shall deal with these diagnostic categories only from the perspective of the clinician's major diagnostic tool, the interview.

4. Freud and the Dynamic Interview

Our treatment of the interview in this chapter likewise perforce must cut across the subject matter of the psychodynamics involved in personality theories in addition to the just described, relatively more static product called diagnosis. Concurrent with their interest in classifying the psychiatric disorders, the same historical figures listed above also concerned themselves with human nature, the essence of human-ness, and, in particular, ways of characterizing and describing the individual dif-ferences which help define each individual both as a member of a larger class and as a unique entity. The insights of Socrates, Plato, Saint Thomas, and other early phil-osophers, theologians, physicians, psychologists, and novelists who from the dawn of time also offered rich, and, in some cases, surprisingly modern psychodynamic personality theories ring as true today as they did many centuries ago. The purposes of the present chapter do not permit a review of such theories, although Durant (1939), Ehrenwald (1976), Ellenberger (1970), and Zilboorg (1941) are a few of the many writers who have catalogued and offered comment on that specific tributary in the history of the interview.

Despite the contributions of Socrates and these earlier and modern theorists, the contributions to clinical interviewing of one figure, Sigmund Freud, are probably without parallel. During the late nineteenth century, when most of the psychiatry of the Western world was under the influence of Emil Kraepelin's static nosological and descriptive psychiatry which classified all patients into one of only several dozen types, Sigmund Freud developed a variant of the doctor-patient interview called the free association method which permitted him insights and glimpses into the "repres-sed" and "unconscious" memories and basic human impulses which make each hu-man unique. As a result, a new era in the history of ideas, one which has lasted al-most a century to date, was born. It is of interest that medicine and psychiatry were slower to accept the insights into the individual, and human nature more generally, which Freud felt were being made possible by this new type of interview interaction, than were anthropology, literature, and psychology. Actually, it was the psychologist G. Stanley Hall who, at Clark University in 1909, gave Freud his first academic hear-ing, and William James, J. J. Putnam, and Morton Prince who did so much to pop-ularize and otherwise disseminate Freud's views. Historians record that it was not until psychiatry began in about 1920 to divorce itself as an appendage of neurology that it too accepted the psychodynamic discoveries, observations, and theories of Freud (Menninger et al., 1963, pp. 61–62, 467).

A description of the development of Freud's use of the interview in psycho-therapy, including some of the historical antecedents of his approach, has recently been reported elsewhere (Matarazzo, 1979). Here one need only state that Freud's innovations in interview technique were intimately related to his psychotherapeutic technique, which, in turn, was a direct outgrowth of his theory of infantile sexuality and later adult personality development. The details of these are too well known to repeat here. Suffice it to say that Freud's clinical interview-derived insights led him (1) to reverse the preoccupation of philosophers, physicians, and scientists with the conscious aspects of human behavior and focus their interest instead on what he called the powerful "unconscious" elements, especially as these were revealed in dreams, free associations, slips of speech, etc.; (2) to introduce such new concepts as the id, ego, and superego for describing psychic structure; (3) to focus attention on the ubiquitous role of anxiety in human behavior and man's employment of a variety of defense mechanisms (repression, projection, rationalization, reaction formation, etc.) for coping with it; and finally (4) to explain how all this knowledge could be used by the interviewer as psychoanalytic interview therapy proceeded and as such predictable interview stages as transference, resistance, and others unfolded.

Freud's interviewing technique was designed to help the patient explore his unconscious and conscious personality to an extent which would permit what Wolberg (1954, p. 8) and others have called a "reconstruction" of his basic personality. The objectives of Freud's insight therapy with reconstructive goals thus were (1) insight into unconscious conflicts, with efforts to achieve extensive alterations of basic character structure, and (2) the expansion of personality growth, with development of new adaptive potentialities. The psychoanalytic interviewing techniques are designed expressly to accomplish these hoped-for goals.

As suggested earlier, until almost the middle of the twentieth century, and quite likely because of the highly idiosyncratic and grossly unreliable psychodynamic syndromes which Freud used as his psychiatric diagnoses (Stoller, 1977), standard textbooks of psychiatry made little mention of Freud or his psychodynamic interview method. Rather, these modern textbooks focused primarily on descriptive psychiatric diagnosis and, in the few conditions where this was known, included some statements about etiology (e.g., paresis and other organic conditions) and treatment (e.g., ECT in the depressions). The closest these pre-1950 psychiatry textbook authors came to mentioning the interview was in a discussion of how to take a psychiatric history or how to perform a mental status examination. Nevertheless, influenced by the parallel developments in Freudian psychoanalysis, dynamic psychiatry, and clinical psychology, a few psychiatrists began to integrate the insights derived from these new developments into regular psychiatric and clinical psychological (in contrast to classical psychoanalytic) interview practice.

One of the interview techniques based on a modified psychoanalytic theory is Wolman's (1965, 1973) sociodiagnostic interview. Wolman endeavors to build bridges between Freud's conceptual system and observable behavior. His main emphasis is on interactional patterns (he calls his version of psychoanalysis "interactional psychoanalysis"), in the belief that the vast majority of behavior disorders are caused by morbid intrafamilial interaction.

In his experimental studies in social psychology, summarized by London (1977), Wolman distinguished three types of social relations. When individuals enter social relationships with the aim of having their needs taken care of, their attitude is instrumental; when their aim is to give and to take, it is mutual; when their aim is to give, it is vectorial.

Studies of the family's pathogenic role, especially in schizophrenia, led Wolman (1965) to the conclusion that most behavior disorders are caused by mismanagement of men (children) by men (adults). Wolman introduced a tripartite classificatory system. According to this system, people totally rejected in childhood develop narcissistic-instrumental disorders (sociopathic type); children exposed to overdemanding and blaming parents are forced into hypervectorialism (schizotype); and, finally, children exposed to an emotional seesaw of rejection interrupted by occasional outbursts of affection develop dysmutual disorders (depressive types).

Wolman (1973) also suggested five levels of deterioration applicable to all three clinical types: (1) neurosis, (2) character neurosis, (3) latent psychosis, (4) manifest psychosis, and, finally, (5) dementive state.

Wolman's sociodiagnostic interview (1965) is geared to discovery of salient interactional patterns in childhood regarded as main diagnostic clues. Thus, for instance, he expects sociopaths (narcissistic-hyperinstrumentals) to be highly critical of their parents, while the schizotype, on any level of deterioration, would feel guilty of his hostility and speak kindly and sympathetically of his parents. Other leading clinical psychologists and psychiatrists writing during the 1940s, 1950s, and 1960s suggested still other improvements on Freud's theoretical views, and these new ideas, too, began to become integrated into clinical practice.

Along with the millions of employment interviews conducted in the United States annually, individuals in the several mental health professions quite likely conduct in this country alone between 100,000 and 200,000 such psychotherapy interviews daily. They no doubt carry out during the same day many thousands of diagnostic interviews on these and other patients—patients referred to them by the courts, other professional colleagues, or former patients, or self-referred patients. It is on these diagnostic interviews that considerable empirical research and controversial findings have been published during the past four decades. In fact, attacks on the utility of the interview as a data-gathering tool have come as much from critics who question the reliability and validity of the diagnosis reached on the basis of such limited interview data as from critics who question the reliability and validity of the effects of the professional activity carried on longitudinally across many interview sessions called psychotherapy. We turn next to an examination of the complex issues involved in determining the reliability and the validity of the diagnosis reached by mental health professionals who use the interview for classifying their patients by use of any of the nosological systems for such diagnosis now extant.

5. Reliability of Psychiatric Diagnosis

The word *diagnosis* is derived from the Greek preposition *dia* (apart) and *gnosis* (to perceive or to know). Thus to know the nature of something requires at the same time distinguishing it from others. Ancient Egyptian and Sumerian records of 4500 years ago include scattered references which reveal that as far back as 2600 B.C. writers of that era could describe with modern-sounding precision the two clinical syndromes which we today call melancholia and hysteria. One thousand years later, in the famous Ebers papyrus (1500 B.C.), one finds excellent descriptions of two other still currently recognized clinical conditions, alcoholism and senile deterioration. One of the earliest systematized psychiatric classification schemes was contributed a thousand years later by Hippocrates, who, working in the fourth century B.C., divided all mental illnesses into the following diagnostic categories: (1) phrenitis, (2) mania, (3) melancholia, (4) epilepsy, (5) hysteria, and (6) scythian disease, or what we today call "transvestism." As cited above, Menninger et al. (1963, pp. 449–489), in a clearly presented and extensive outline, trace the changes next introduced in such "psychiatric" diagnoses from the time of Plato through the Dark Ages and Renaissance, through Kraepelin, and then up to the present. A reader following this history cannot help but be impressed with the observation that, despite the mixture from ancient times through the eighteenth century of demonology and science in the attempts by a succession of writers to describe the etiology of such psychiatric conditions, most of the actual classifications themselves (namely psychosis, epilepsy, alcoholism, senility, hysteria and other neuroses, and mental retardation) and the descriptions of their clinical features have changed little during the last 2500 years. The promulgation of specific subcategories (e.g., schizophrenia vs. manic-depressive types of psychoses) within these global general categories has, however, varied considerably from one era to another, despite the lack of much change in these larger, more global diagnostic classifications (e.g., psychosis).

Notwithstanding the fact that global classifications of insanity were consistently recognized throughout all epochs, psychiatry and clinical psychology were too young and thus could not participate in the explosions in data gathering and empiricism in scientific knowledge which took place during the sixteenth, seventeenth, eighteenth, and nineteenth centuries in physics, biology, chemistry, and the related older sciences. A beginning empiricism did not come to the mental health sciences until five decades ago, not until the first few hundred clinical psychologists and psychiatrists entered the field and began to give definition to their respective, newly developing professions. As their increasing numbers made it possible, a few stalwarts began to seek empirical evidence that the human judgment called diagnosis was a reliable (stable and reproducible) datum. The requirement that one should check the accuracy across another examiner (or oneself at a later time) of one's specific diagnostic classification of a mentally ill person most likely was perceived throughout each successive era in the long history which predated the modern era of empiricism in psychiatric diagnosis. Nevertheless, from man's earliest recorded times there no doubt were recognized pathognomonic features of mental illness that one could almost take for granted as signs of severe mental derangement, and thus all observers would agree on this global diagnosis. The convulsive symptom of epilepsy probably was one such universally recognized datum, as no doubt also was hallucination a classic datum indicating the presence of psychosis or similarly grave mental derangement. Writing on the latter subject in the year 1790, Immanual Kant, then professor at the University of Königsberg, included the following passage in his treatise on the classification of mental illness:

> The only feature common to all mental disorders is the loss of common sense (*sensus communis*), and the compensatory development of a unique sense (*sensus privatus*) of reasoning, e.g., a person sees in broad daylight on his table, a light shining which another person, standing nearby, does not see; or one hears a voice which no one else hears. For it is a subjectively necessary indicator of the correctness of our overall judgments, and hence of the soundness of our minds, that we compare our judgment with the judgment of others; that we do not isolate ourselves with our own judgment but, on the contrary, act with our private judgment as if the matter were being judged publicly. (Kant, 1964, p. 19)

It probably would be a fair guess that in the early history of modern clinical psychiatry and psychology few clinicians would not agree at first blush that a person who saw a light shining on a table which others did not see, or heard a voice which no one else heard, was hallucinating and, in the absence of data that the individual was a mystic, an alcoholic, or a drug addict, or had a brain tumor, conclude that such a person was psychotic. Furthermore, such experienced clinicians quite likely would have believed as a matter of faith that if any two of them independently interviewed this patient, they no doubt would get the same history of hallucination and, with such history, each reach the same diagnosis. That is, their interrater agreement on the diagnosis of psychosis would be perfect, or near perfect, in this and similar patients.

However, in the absence of empirical evidence it was equally likely that, despite demonstrable similarity in their professional training and their avowed allegiance to the same diagnostic classification system such as the American Psychiatric Association's current one, two experienced clinicians interviewing the same patient might disagree and, empirically, reveal little interrater agreement or reliability. Concerned about this potential disagreement between clinicians, especially those working in state hospitals where such diagnosis was mandatory, Kempf over 50 years ago sounded the following warning:

> If each important institution can be induced to give, sealed, to a central committee, its actual working system for classifying cases as dementia praecox, manic-depressive, paranoia, hysteria, and neurasthenia, illustrated by cases, the differences would probably be so varied that the whole system would have to be abandoned because the faithful assumption that symptoms are similarly applied and evaluated throughout psychiatry would be brutally discredited. (Kempf, 1920)

Some 30 years later, Roe, in commenting on research by clinical psychologists at midcentury, echoed a similar concern about the unreliability of psychiatric diagnosis:

> On the other hand, clinicians have managed to take time for research, as witness the papers coming out in such numbers on the use of various psychological devices for making psychiatric diagnoses. I suggest that much of this research is not only a waste of time and a perpetuation of errors, but is actually preventing advance in the field. There are many reasons why this is true, but one of the most potent is that it involves clinging to a classification which has long since been outlived. I submit that using techniques which are not too precisely validated, if they are validated at all, to place patients in psychiatric categories, the inadequacy of which is admitted by all concerned, is a treadmill procedure guaranteed to keep us moving in circles. (Roe, 1949, p. 38)

On the other side, Kahn and Cannell wrote:

> The interview must be considered to be a measurement device which is fallible and which is subject to substantial errors and biases. All this does not suggest, however, that the interview should be discarded. . . . [We] need to learn more about the sources of bias and to develop methods for eliminating them. (Kahn & Cannell, 1957, p. 179)

In this section we shall examine the utility of the interview in making psychiatric diagnoses. Until only a decade ago, the number of research workers who found diagnostic judgments based on psychiatric interviews unreliable outnumbered those who reported studies showing that they were reliable. Early investigators who believed interviewer-based psychiatric diagnosis to be unreliable were Ash (1949), Boisen (1938), Eysenck (1959), Masserman and Carmichael (1938), Mehlman (1952), Pasamanick, Dinitz, and Lefton (1959), and Scott (1958). Arrayed against them were these early defenders of the reliability of interview-based psychiatric diagnosis: Hunt, Wittson, and Hunt (1953), Foulds (1955), Schmidt and Fonda (1956), Seeman (1953), Kreitman, Sainsbury, Morrissey, Towers, and Scrivener (1961), Beck (1962), Wilson and Meyer (1962), and Sandifer, Pettus, and Quade (1964). In addition, several early authors have contributed excellent theoretical and review articles in this general area: Beck (1962), Caveny, Wittson, Hunt, and Herrmann (1955), Eysenck (1961), and Zigler and Phillips (1961). These last papers did much to clarify the pertinent issues in the reliable-unreliable debate. Rotter (1954, pp. 250–257) actually outlined steps for improving the reliability of interview-derived judgments.

In the past decade, considerable sophistication has been introduced into reliability research of this type. However, before considering this new research, it will prove instructive in regard to the purposes of this chapter to review the pre-1965 studies on both sides of the interrater reliability debate.

6. Early Studies Showing the Unreliability of Psychiatric Diagnosis

One of the first studies on the reliability of psychiatric diagnosis was reported by Masserman and Carmichael (1938). On the basis of a follow-up of 100 psychiatric patients, a year after discharge from a mental hospital, these authors reported that in 40% of the cases the original diagnoses required "major revision" a year later. However, how much this change in psychiatric diagnosis 1 year later was a function of the unreliability of the original diagnosis or of the unreliability of the second diagnosis, or both, and how much it was a function of actual changes in the patient's clinical status during the 1-year interval, if at all, cannot be assessed from the Masserman and Carmichael data. (The 1974 Murphy, Woodruff, Herjanic, and Fischer study of stability of diagnosis over time which is reviewed in the last pages of the present chapter is a highly sophisticated current reexamination of this same problem.)

A study which involved several diagnoses arrived at simultaneously, although reasonably independently, was reported by Ash (1949). In his study, 52 white males were evaluated in a government-related clinic in a joint interview by two or three psychiatrists who worked full time in this clinic. Typically, one of the psychiatrists conducted a physical examination of each man and then called his colleague(s) in for the psychiatric interview. The psychiatric interview was jointly conducted, each psychiatrist asking whatever questions he wished. However, each psychiatrist recorded his diagnosis independently. Specific diagnoses were not discussed.

Ash presented his results for pair combinations of the three psychiatrists for varying combinations (N's of 38–46) of the 52 cases and jointly for all three raters for the 35 out of 52 patients who were seen simultaneously by all three psychiatrists. An earlier, pre-1952 version of the official nomenclature of the American Psychiatric Association (1952) was used for their diagnostic judgments. This involved five major categories (mental deficiency, psychosis, psychopathic personality, neurosis, and "normal range" but with "predominant personality characteristic") and some 60 specific diagnostic subcategories. Because this study is quoted so often as evidence of the unreliability of psychiatric diagnosis, the results of the agreement levels among the three psychiatrists in the 35 cases examined by all three in simultaneous conference are shown in Table 1. It can be seen that the agreement for all three psychiatrists for the major category diagnosis was 45.7% while for specific subcategory diagnosis it was only 20%. (As might be expected, two out of the three of these psychiatrists, in different combinations of two, showed agreement levels higher than these: 51.4% and 48.6%, respectively.)

The present writer pointed out in an earlier review of this reliability vs. unreliability literature (Matarazzo, 1965) that, in essence, these results show that three psychiatrists could agree completely in 45.7% of the cases for five broad categories (where chance expectation would be 1 in 5, or 20%, if the base rates of the five conditions were known and equal—which they certainly are not) and in 20% of the cases

Table 1. Agreement in Diagnoses among Three Psychiatrists (35 cases)[a]

Type of agreement	Three psychiatrists agree	Two out of three agree	None agree	Total
Major category				
Percent	45.7	51.4	2.9	100.0
N	(16)	(18)	(1)	35
Specific diagnosis				
Percent	20.0	48.6	31.4	100.0
N	(7)	(17)	(11)	35

[a] Adapted from Ash (1949).

in specific categories (where chance expectation would be 1 in 60, or 1.7% if the base rates again were known and equal). However, it was pointed out by the present writer that with an N as small as 35, such considerations appeared overly refined even if the base rates could be determined.

Ash clearly pointed out the limitations of his study imposed by this small N. He also pointed out the possible limitations imposed by the joint conference method and the fact that his 60 (and seemingly only 55 specific) subcategories did not utilize the entire APA diagnostic system. However, what neither Ash nor other reviewers of his study seem to have concerned themselves with is that 104 (75%) out of 139 diagnoses made on the 52 cases by the three psychiatrists were diagnoses of "normal range"; i.e., 75% of Ash's diagnoses were reasonably "normal" with a "predominant personality characteristic" (see Ash, 1949, p. 273, Table 1). This latter included such specific subcategories as aggressive type; unethical, egocentric, and selfish type; shiftless, lazy, uninhibited, dull, adynamic type; nomadic type; and balanced personality. It was not surprising to this writer to find that three psychiatrists agreed no more than is shown in Table 1 when so many of their cases (75%) were not frank psychiatric ones. Actually, one can be impressed that they agreed as well as they did on what is essentially a study of the reliability of judgment of personality characteristics of a predominantly normal group of 35 men. It quite likely is because he handled this large normal group differently that Zubin (1967, p. 382) reports in Ash's study agreement levels for two out of three psychiatrists of 64% and 38%, where we have in Table 1 (and also in 1965) report agreement levels of 51.4% and 48.6% for the major and specific categories, respectively.

Although not utilizing two independent clinicians each examining the same patient, the study by Mehlman (1952) did utilize a large sample of Toledo State Hospital patients ($N = 4016$). His hypothesis was that since assignment of patients to a ward psychiatrist was random, then if psychiatric diagnosis were reliable, the *relative frequencies* of patients in different diagnostic categories would not differ from one admitting psychiatrist to another. Mehlman broke down his data by sex and showed that 16 different psychiatrists on the female services and nine psychiatrists on the male services did in fact differ among themselves in the frequency with which they utilized (1) an organic vs. a psychogenic diagnosis and (2) a manic-depressive vs. a schizophrenic diagnosis. He did not report means, standard deviations, or other data, limiting his results simply to the significance levels of the χ^2 values for each of these pair dichotomies.

A similar "relative frequency" study was conducted by Pasamanick et al. (1959) and led them to caution that "psychiatric diagnosis is at present so unreliable as to merit very serious question when classifying, treating and studying patient behavior and outcome" (p. 127). Their study also used only a very indirect method of assessing reliability (relative frequency of six different diagnostic categories assigned to patients on three female wards of the Columbus Psychiatric Institute and Hospital) and thus, while important, is not a conclusive investigation of the reliability of psychiatric diagnosis. As a matter of fact, a subsequent relative frequency study by Wilson and Meyer (1962), reporting the diagnostic consistency in a psychiatric liaison service at The Johns Hopkins Hospital, revealed the incidence of almost identical percentages for various diagnostic categories in samples from two consecutive years—a finding in direct contrast to those of the two studies just reviewed. Whether the positive, albeit also indirect, findings of Wilson and Meyer were due to differences in (1) patient population, (2) psychiatrists, (3) hospital settings, (4) the temporal interval, or a host of other factors could not be evaluated from these published reports. The study by Boisen (1938), also a relative frequency investigation, revealed that the percentage of patients with the same diagnosis was markedly different in three states (Illinois, Massachusetts, and New York), thus implicating still other potential factors in the unreliability findings.

Other early writers who questioned the reliability of psychiatric diagnosis were Eysenck (1952, pp. 33–34), Roe (1949, p. 38), and Scott (1958, p. 32). In the characteristic tough-minded manner with which he has served as a critic of other things psychological, Eysenck, after reviewing the studies of Ash and several others, had this to say: "We may then regard it as agreed that psychiatric diagnosis is of doubtful validity and low reliability." Eysenck continued that since the use, by psychologists, of psychological testing techniques leads to no further improvement in the reliability of diagnosis, "then it is small wonder that so many psychologists have eschewed the Kraepelinian straightjacket in order to indulge in Freudian manic spells which give them at least the illusion of usefulness" (1952, pp. 33–34).

7. Early Studies Showing the Reliability of Psychiatric Diagnosis

One of the most vigorous research groups to study the psychiatric interview was that of Hunt and Wittson and their associates. During hostilities and for the period of a decade following World War II, this group, which worked together in wartime Navy neuropsychiatric screening from 1941 to 1945, published a number of studies and theoretical articles on the reliability and validity of psychiatric diagnosis. References to this work will be found in Hunt (1955) and in many volumes of the *Journal of Clinical Psychology* from 1955 on. Whereas the Hunt and Wittson studies of the 1940s and early 1950s were on the reliability and validity of psychiatric diagnosis (and related military selection procedures), the later program of research of Hunt and his other colleagues was designed around the important premise that psychiatric diagnosis is merely one example of a more general psychological process—clinical judgment—and that the latter human act has much in common with psychophysical and other judgments.

Although only one of the studies of this research group (Hunt et al., 1953) was directed exclusively to the question of the reliability of psychiatric diagnosis, a number of their validity studies also bore on the reliability problem—possibly even more than this one reliability study itself. We shall review these validity studies later in this chapter. Here we will review the 1953 reliability study. In the Hunt et al. (1953) study, these investigators concerned themselves with "the reliability or consistency of diagnosis, or more specifically with the question of agreement between psychiatrists in a diagnostic situation" (p. 53). However, they were careful to point out two important assumptions: (1) that by the "reliability of diagnosis" is meant whether the same diagnosis will be rendered on a repeat examination by the same or some other psychiatrist, and (2) that diagnosis is essentially a process of taxonomic categorization with prediction as its function (p. 55). Their many subsequent (predictive) validity reports which we review later thus should be understood as intimately related to the reliability question, and validity and reliability should not be clearly distinguished.

The Hunt et al. (1953) study examined the reliability or consistency of the psychiatric diagnoses in a group of 794 naval enlisted men (examined in the psychiatric unit at a naval precommissioning installation) who were found to be unsuitable for service and who were transferred to a naval hospital for medical survey with the neutral, nonbiasing designation "diagnosis unknown, observation." However, a diagnosis had been made of each man and was included in his record and held at the precommissioning station.

Table 2 shows the amount of agreement between the psychiatric diagnoses made on each man in the two installations. The authors point out that, inasmuch as the primary function of a naval neuropsychiatric department is the implicit prediction of unsuitability for military service, their first measure of reliability concerned the number of men considered unsuitable by both psychiatric staffs. The remarkably high agreement (93.7%) on this category is not invalidated by such relevant considerations as the fact that, in receiving the recruit, the hospital unit thereby recognized that the precommissioning station felt something was wrong with him. The personal, administrative, theoretical orientation, and other considerations whereby disagreements among different clinicians abound are too well known to deserve elaboration.

The data on 681 of the 794 men (113 could not be fitted into the three broad categories) were next examined for agreement in the two examining units across three broad or major diagnostic categories (including psychosis, psychoneurosis, and personality disorder, as in Ash's 1949 study), and all 794 men were studied for agreement in specific diagnosis (32 subcategories). The reliability values (54.1% and 32.6%, respectively) also shown in Table 2 are not as high as for the unsuitable-for-service diagnosis.

Commenting on the high agreement (93.7%) on the unsuitability diagnosis and

Table 2. Diagnostic Agreement between Precommissioning Station and Naval Hospital[a]

	Precommissioning station (number of cases)	Hospital (number of cases)	Agreement (%)
Unsuitable for service	794	744	93.7
Agreement within major categories	681	369	54.1
Agreement on specific diagnosis	794	259	32.6

[a]Adapted from Hunt et al. (1953, p. 59).

the low agreement (32.6%) on the specific diagnosis, the authors raised the validity question when they pointed out that (in the 1940s) it was of little practical difference in care, treatment, or social implications whether a man was classified as "psychoneurotic: anxiety" or "emotionally unstable." In any event, the study by Hunt et al. is not the best test of the reliability of psychiatric diagnosis since, like Ash's study, it used (young) men who were sufficiently within the normal range to have been accepted for military service before being identified at the precommissioning station. This type of study needed repetition with psychiatric hospital patients, even though the Hunt et al. findings are of considerable interest in that they utilized two different clinicians (as Ash did), each seeing the same individual, and not the indirect relative frequency approach.

Although Hunt et al. cautioned that their results "may be influenced by factors specific to the naval situation and that broad generalizations to civilian practice are dangerous, if justified at all" (p. 60), the similarity of their results to those of Ash was striking (54.1% vs. 45.7% and 32.6% vs. 20.0%, for broad and specific categories respectively).

However, unlike Ash, who interpreted his results solely in a reliability framework, Hunt and Wittson and their co-workers, as we shall see later in this chapter, published a series of follow-up studies which demonstrated the validity and thus, indirectly, the reliability of their psychiatric diagnoses (broad and specific categories as well as the very reliable category of unsuitability for military service).

It was not long after Hunt and Wittson had reported their evidence for the very high reliability of their "unsuitability for service" diagnosis that Schmidt and Fonda (1956) published a study in which, utilizing a format similar to that used by Ash, they reported good evidence for the reliability of their major psychiatric categories. Schmidt and Fonda conducted their study at Connecticut's Norwich State Hospital and utilized 426 patients each interviewed by one of eight psychiatric residents and next independently interviewed by one of three board-certified staff psychiatrists. Each of the two interviewers used 40 specific diagnostic categories from DSM I published in 1952 by the American Psychiatric Association. Additionally, these 40 specific diagnostic classifications were further grouped into three superordinate or major categories: organic, psychotic, and character(ological disorder). As shown in Table 3, Schmidt and Fonda found that the independent interrater agreement on these three major categories between resident and senior psychiatrists across the 426 patients was as follows: organic, 92% (178 out of 193); psychotic, 80%; and character disorder, 71%. When averaged across all three of these major categories to produce one summarizing value for the reliability of global diagnosis, the agreement

Table 3. Major Category Agreement: Resident with Chief Psychiatrist[a]

Resident	Chief psychiatrist			
	Organic	Psychotic	Character	Number
Organic	(178)	12	12	202
Psychotic	12	(128)	9	149
Character	3	21	(51)	75
N	193	161	72	(426)

[a] Adapted from Schmidt and Fonda (1956).

**Table 4. Percentage Agreement on Psychiatric Diagnoses Obtained by
Two Independent Psychiatrists**

	Ash	Schmidt and Fonda	Kreitman et al.	Beck et al.	Sandifer et al.
	(1949)	(1956)	(1961)	(1962)	(1964)
Number of patients	35	426	90	153	91
Agreement in major category	51	84	78	70	—
Agreement in specific diagnosis	48	55	63	54	57

reached 84%. When analyzed further for the average reliability of diagnosis for 11 specific subtypes within these three global groups, the interrater agreement was found to be 55%. Thus, whereas this last figure (55%) agreed with Ash's figure of 48.6% for the specific classification, the Schmidt and Fonda finding of 84% agreement was considerably higher than the 51.4% reported by Ash in our Table 1 for the major category (two psychiatrists).

During the next decade, three additional reliability studies were published, and each reported percentage agreements closer to those of the Schmidt and Fonda study than to those of the Ash study. These studies were reported by Kreitman et al. (1961), Beck, Ward, Mendelson, Mock, and Erbaugh (1962), and Sandifer et al. (1964), and the results of these three studies are summarized in our Table 4 along with those of Ash and of Schmidt and Fonda.

After reviewing the interrater reliability studies conducted through 1964 and summarized here in our Table 4, Zubin offered the following conclusions:

> The findings indicate "that the degree of overall agreement between different observers with regard to specific diagnoses is too low for individual diagnosis. The overall agreement on general categories of diagnosis, although somewhat higher, still leaves much to be desired. The evidence for low agreement across specific diagnostic categories is all the more surprising since, for the most part, the observers in any one study were usually quite similar in orientation, training and background. (Zubin, 1967, p. 383)

In reviewing this same research up through 1965, the present writer (Matarazzo, 1965) was a bit more optimistic. Over a decade later, he is even more optimistic. Given the fact that empirical research was still in its infancy in psychiatry and clinical psychology, the results in Table 4 reveal, first, that there was by 1964 a fair degree of interrater reliability across two interviewers or raters for the more global or major psychiatric classifications. Second, it is also obvious that this reliability drops a bit when the judgments within a major category are made more specific and less global, although the reader who has worked in a state hospital or other mental health facility will quite likely still be impressed by the degree of agreement shown in these earliest studies even within specific categories. In any event, the reader interested in a lucid and most convincing set of hypotheses about the types of personal and highly idiosyncratic factors which led to the relatively low reliabilities of psychiatric diagnosis in the era before 1965 will find these in the in-depth studies of the proclivities of individual mental health diagnosticians carried out by Raines and Rohrer (1955, 1960).

8. The Problem of Base Rates

In his review of the literature on the reliability of such psychiatric diagnosis over a decade ago, this writer (Matarazzo, 1965) was struck by the fact that the studies summarized in Table 4 had not concerned themselves with a serious potential methodological flaw, namely the issue of base rates. That is, the assessments of the degree of interrater agreement shown in Table 4 had neglected to take into account the frequency with which any particular specific diagnosis did or did not occur in a population or sample of patients. This problem was mentioned in the writer's 1965 review in his discussion of the data in Table 1 from Ash's study. It also was highlighted in a study of clinical diagnosis by Hunt, Schwartz, and Walker (1964). However, it will be given more prominence in the present chapter because, even a decade or two after this potential methodological flaw was cited, only a few investigators and textbook writers have given it the attention it deserves. H. F. Hunt (1950), in an early annual review chapter, was one of the first to highlight the importance of the problem of base rates. Subsequently, the New York State Psychiatric Institute (Columbia University) team of Cohen (1960), Spitzer, Cohen, Fleiss, and Endicott (1967), and Fleiss (1971) elaborated further on the issue of base rates and developed statistical procedures (the kappa statistic) for handling a number of other problems involved in such interrater research, including how to control for the percentage of agreement two independent diagnosticians should reach on the basis of chance alone. During the past decade, Spitzer, Fleiss, Cohen, and their colleagues in New York and Woodruff, Robins, Guze, and their colleagues at the Washington University School of Medicine in St. Louis each have used the kappa statistic and related sophisticated methodology and thereby, as will be shown in a later section, have improved considerably the quality of research on the reliability and validity of psychiatric diagnosis. Formulas for kappa (K) and weighted kappa (K_w) have been published, and hypothetical examples have been furnished by both groups. The formula for K is as follows:

$$K = \frac{p_o - p_c}{1 - p_c}$$

where p_o is the observed proportion of agreement and p_c is the agreement expected by chance alone. The hypothetical data in our Table 5 cited by Helzer, Robins, Taibleson, Woodruff, Reich, and Wish (1977) of the St. Louis group illustrate the use of kappa. In this hypothetical study of the reliability of the psychiatric diagnosis of schizophrenia, two clinicians independently examine the same 100 patients and give each patient one of two diagnoses: "schizophrenia" or "not schizophrenia." From these judgments, there are three possibilities regarding diagnostic agreement: (1) both clinicians agree on schizophrenia, (2) both agree on not schizophrenia, and (3) they disagree. The last category can be broken down further into those patients for whom the first examiner diagnosed schizophrenia whereas the second did not, and for whom the second examiner diagnosed schizophrenia whereas the first did not, thus making the four possible combinations shown in Table 5.

All the data needed to compute kappa are given in Table 5. The proportion of observed agreement (p_o) is based on the total number of interviews (all 200) rather

Table 5. Hypothetical Values for Agreement by Two Randomly Selected Clinicians for the Diagnosis of Schizophrenia

	First examiner	Second examiner	Number of patients involved	Number of interviews involved
Both clinicians diagnose schizophrenia in the same patient	20	20	20	40
Both clinicians diagnose not schizophrenia in the same patient	72	72	72	144
First clinician diagnoses schizophrenia; second clinician says not	6	0	6	12
Second clinician diagnoses schizophrenia; first clinician says not	0	2	2	4
		Total	100	200

than on the total number of patients (100). Table 5 shows that the frequency with which both clinicians are in full agreement is 20 + 72, or 92 patients. Thus p_o is 20 + 72 divided by 100, or .92. The proportion of agreement (frequency) based on chance alone (p_c) in this sample of 200 interviews is 48 patients. It is based on the number of times or frequency that a diagnosis (in this case of schizophrenia) is made by either examiner in their 200 interviews. Thus there are 40 (20 + 20) such instances in the first row, 6 instances in the third row, and 2 instances in the fourth row. That is, a positive diagnosis (the diagnosis of schizophrenia) is given 48 times out of 200 interviews, yielding a proportion of 48 divided by 200, or .24. The proportion of times the diagnosis of not schizophrenia is given in this sample of patients likewise is 152 out of 200 interviews, yielding a proportion of .76. That is, if the two examiners do not even see the patients at all, but instead routinely merely assign each one the diagnosis of schizophrenia, they will be correct in 24 of the patients out of 100. Likewise, if they each diagnose each of the 100 patients as not schizophrenic even without seeing one of them, they will have correctly identified 76 of them merely because there are that many in the sample to begin with. The proportion p_c in the formula is designed to offer a correction for such chance "hits" and is computed in our example as $p_c = (48 \div 200)^2 + (152 \div 200)^2 = (.24)^2 + (.76)^2$, or .64. The values of .92 and .64, when entered in the formula for kappa given above, yield $K = (.92 - .64) \div (1 - .64)$, or $K = .28 \div .36$, for a final value of $K = .78$. Thus the reliability of psychiatric diagnosis of our two clinicians in Table 5, with appropriate statistical correction and control, is .78.

Kappa has been applied in several actual clinical studies during the past decade, and we shall examine these studies and results shortly. Additionally, in an important methodological contribution, Spitzer and Fleiss (1974) reanalyzed the data in each of the studies summarized here in our Table 4, substituting kappa as the statistic in each instance. Not surprisingly, inasmuch as they now controlled for chance agreement in each study, they found the levels of agreement to be considerably lower than those shown in our Table 4. However, before we review the use of kappa in subsequently studied new samples of patients, we must first examine another methodological issue, namely the necessary stipulation that before two clinicians go about testing the reliability of their diagnostic classification they must first agree on what it actually is that they will be examining for in their patients. In other words, how objectively specifiable are each of the supposedly distinct psychiatric diagnoses found in DSM II, or in any of the other currently extant classificatory systems?

63

THE INTERVIEW:
ITS RELIABILITY
AND VALIDITY IN
PSYCHIATRIC
DIAGNOSIS

9. The Era of Operational Definitions in Psychiatric Diagnoses

During the days when the present writer was a young faculty member at the Washington University School of Medicine from 1950 to 1955, Robins and Guze and their colleagues already had identified the fact that the problem of low interrater reliability in psychiatric diagnosis arose out of the inability of two examiners to write down and therefore agree in advance what symptoms or other behaviors had to be present before a specific diagnosis of, for example, schizophrenia, hysteria, manic-depressive psychosis, or alcoholism would be made. Clearly a diagnosis or other classification can be no better than the classifier's knowledge and understanding of the conditions or other observations he or she is classifying. In the statement made by Immanuel Kant 200 years ago and quoted earlier in this chapter, he implied that most persons would agree that an individual who experienced hallucination was mentally ill. Beyond this quite likely universally agreed-on observation involving this most global and grossest classification or discrimination imaginable (mentally ill vs. not mentally ill), the data summarized here in Tables 1 through 4 make quite clear that broadly educated and highly trained mental health professionals agree less and less, one with the other, as the categories and classifications of the behavior disorders they must discriminate become progressively more specific.

Professionals of comparable experience disagree on the particulars required for any given diagnosis not only from one hospital to another but also often with each other in the same institution (see Table 3), where, it might have been assumed, there would be a fairly high level of agreement as to definition of various disorders. The reader will not be surprised to learn, therefore, that a condition such as schizophrenia is diagnosed differently by psychiatrists in Great Britain from the way it is diagnosed by their American counterparts. Edwards (1972) presents a comparative listing of the actual symptoms reported by experts as necessary for the diagnosis of schizophrenia in the two countries. Thus, for example, 68.7% of the American psychiatrists participating in the survey checked that hallucinations are of primary importance in the diagnosis of schizophrenia, as against only 25.6% of the British psychiatrists who agree with them on the relative importance of this behavioral symptom.

It was disagreement and problems of this type, evident even in the staff of a single psychiatric hospital or facility, that demanded that some common yardstick or measuring instrument be devised if future research were to be improved. The St. Louis group thus set about patiently and painstakingly during the 1950s, 1960s, and 1970s to develop a structured interview by use of which they standardized the method for eliciting data from each patient and, next, classified the products of this interview into explicit clinical criteria for each of 16 psychiatric disorders. Their explicit criteria for individual diagnostic classifications (such as hysteria, alcoholism, depression, schizophrenia) were published in a series of individual papers, and the whole was then integrated and reproduced in a single article by Feighner, Robins, Guze, Woodruff, Winokur, and Munez (1972) and later, for easy reference and accessibility, in a book by Woodruff, Goodwin, and Guze (1974). To provide the reader with an example of their approach, their operational definition of the symptoms which an interviewer must elicit or observe before making the diagnosis of depression was given as follows:

Depression: the following three requirements *must* be met:

1. *Dysphoric mood* characterized by symptoms such as the following: depressed, sad, despondent, hopeless, feeling "down in the dumps," irritable, fearful, worried, or discouraged.

2. *At least 5 of the following 8 criteria:* (a) Poor appetite or weight loss of 2 pounds a week or 10 pounds or more a year when not dieting. (b) Difficulty in sleeping, including insomnia or hypersomnia. (c) Loss of energy; namely fatiguability, tiredness. (d) Agitation or retardation. (e) Loss of interest in usual activities, or decrease in sexual drive. (f) Feelings of self-reproach or guilt (either may be delusional). (g) Complaints of or actually diminished ability to think or concentrate, such as slow thinking or mixed-up thoughts. (h) Recurrent thoughts of death or suicide, including thoughts of wishing to be dead. (Note: If only 4 of these 8 criteria are found, diagnose as "probable depression" rather than "depression.")

3. *A psychiatric illness lasting at least one month with no preexisting conditions* such as schizophrenia, anxiety neurosis, phobic neurosis, obsessive, compulsive neurosis, hysteria, alcoholism, drug dependency, antisocial personality, homosexuality and other sexual deviations, mental retardation, or organic brain syndrome.
(General Note: Patients with life-threatening or incapacitating medical illness preceding and paralleling the depression do not receive the diagnosis of primary depression.)

Each of the many psychiatric conditions contained in DSM II is not as clearly defined by Woodruff et al. as is depression above. Yet a large enough number of the important psychiatric conditions (16 plus an all-important residual category called "undiagnosed psychiatric illness") are such that, with the additional research data contained in the separate chapters of their book devoted to each condition, it is now possible for other investigators to begin to use the definitions of the St. Louis group (and, as will be described below, those provided by the New York State Psychiatric and St. Louis collaborative team of Spitzer, Endicott, and Robins and colleagues) and thereby markedly enhance research by removing the critical barrier of disagreement in the definition of what was being classified which has impeded prior research on the reliability of psychiatric diagnosis. The potential gain from the use of their operationally explicit criteria is sufficiently obvious that this approach has been incorporated into DSM III, which the American Psychiatric Association has indicated will go into effect in 1979 (Spitzer, Sheehy, & Endicott, 1977).

In a collaborative study involving the St. Louis and the New York State Psychiatric Institute groups, and with funding from the National Institute of Mental Health, Spitzer, Endicott, and Robins (1975) expanded and modified the 1972 Feighner et al. criteria for a selected group of 23 functional psychiatric disorders, and demonstrated that the use of these 23 operational definitions increased rater-to-rater reliability considerably. These definitions are a further refinement of those in the Woodruff et al. (1974) version.

The structured interview which has been developed by this St. Louis group to reliably elicit the presence or absence of the requisite behavioral criteria for each of their operationally defined diagnoses begins with asking about name, age, and a few demographic items and is followed by an open-ended question covering the present illness. It next proceeds to a standardized list of 150 items covering current or past psychiatric symptoms, prior hospitalizations, family history, and a mental status examination. Reports indicate that the whole interview can be accomplished in 30–90 min, with a mean length of 60 min. Individual items are asked in a fixed sequence, but the actual phrasing of most questions is left to the interviewer, who also decides whether, when, and how to elicit more information on ambiguous responses. The operational definitions provided for each of the interview items reduce such ambiguity considerably. In the St. Louis (and New York State Psychiatric Institute) classificatory scheme, a patient can be given more than one diagnosis (i.e., a primary one and one or more secondary ones), and frequently is.

10. 1977 Reliability Studies Using Operational Definitions and Kappa   **65**

THE INTERVIEW:
ITS RELIABILITY
AND VALIDITY IN
PSYCHIATRIC
DIAGNOSIS

10.1. St. Louis Group

When we were commenting earlier in this chapter on the methodological flaw involving base rates and chance inherent in the studies summarized in our own Table 4, we indicated that Spitzer and Fleiss (1974) reanalyzed the data from the individual studies shown in Table 4 by applying the kappa statistic correction to them. They also tabulated many more specific diagnoses than we show in our Table 4. Spitzer and Fleiss then computed an average kappa across the studies. Their conclusion from these reanalyzed data was that

> There are no diagnostic categories for which reliability is uniformly high. Reliability appears to be only satisfactory for three categories: Mental deficiency, organic brain syndrome (but not its subtypes), and alcoholism. The level of reliability is no better than fair for psychosis and schizophrenia and is poor for the remaining categories. (Spitzer & Fleiss, 1974, p. 344)

A test of the utility of the explicit and operational criteria offered by the St. Louis group to improve diagnostic reliability was recently published by that group (Helzer, Clayton, Pambakian, Reich, Woodruff, & Reveley, 1977) and the results were compared by them to those published earlier (and partly summarized in our Table 4) which also were subsequently reanalyzed by Spitzer and Fleiss using kappa.

Helzer et al. utilized three psychiatrists: a first-year resident, a junior medical school staff psychiatrist, and a senior faculty psychiatrist. Each of 101 new patients admitted to the psychiatric service of the medical school in St. Louis was interviewed twice, once within 24 hr of admission by one of the three psychiatrists and again, independently, by a second psychiatrist about 24 hr later. Each psychiatrist saw about an equal number of patients, and each interviewer came first or second about equally. The results are reported in our Table 6.

The frequency of diagnosis shown in the first column is based on the 202 interviews (101 patients seen twice). Thus, acknowledging multiple diagnoses (the aver-

Table 6. Diagnostic Frequency and Interrater Concordance[a]

Diagnosis	Frequency of diagnosis (%)	Overall agreement (%)	Specific agreement (%)	Kappa ($N = 101$)	Kappa ($N = 71$)	From Spitzer and Fleiss (1974)
Depression	81	86	84	.55	.70	.41
Mania	13	96	73	.82	.93	.33
Anxiety neurosis	35	89	73	.76	.84	.45
Schizophrenia	5	96	43	.58	.66	.57
Antisocial personality	15	95	72	.81	.85	.53
Alcoholism	35	88	71	.74	.73	.71
Drug dependence	15	96	76	.84	.85	—
Hysteria (female subjects only)	18	88	68	.72	.72	—
Obsessional illness	7	97	67	.78	.79	—
Homosexuality	3	99	75	.85	.79	—
Organic brain syndrome	6	92	20	.29	.36	.77
Undiagnosed psychiatric illness	18	76	20	.19	—	—
Average concordance	—	92	62	.66	.75	—

[a]Adapted from Helzer, Clayton, Pambakian, Reich, Woodruff, and Reveley (1977).

age per patient was 2.5) in the 202 interviews conducted by a series of two interviewers, a diagnosis of current or past depression was made 164 times, or 81% of the total. Because an average of 2.5 diagnoses was made per patient, this figure does not mean that 81% of the 101 patients were diagnosed as having primary affective disorder, depressed type. That is, inasmuch as diagnoses were nonpreemptive in this study, any given patient might (and some in fact did) have another psychiatric illness clearly antecedent to depression. The first row in Table 6 merely catalogues the percent of the 202 interviews which included depression as one of the diagnoses among the 2.5 generated per each of the 202 such interviews. After depression, anxiety and alcoholism (each with 35%) were the next most frequently assigned diagnoses as shown in the first column of Table 6.

The second and third columns of Table 6 show percentage of overall agreement (the raw percentage of agreement in individual cases by the two interviewers) and specific agreement (the percentage of agreement after excluding the 18% undiagnosable cases shown in the second from the bottom row). The fourth column presents the test-retest reliability (kappa) for the 101 patients across the two interviewers for each diagnostic category.

Inasmuch as the St. Louis group believes the classification "undiagnosed psychiatric illness" is an operationally defined category which must be used at this early stage of knowledge, they encourage its use whenever a clinician is unsure of the diagnosis. As shown in the second from the bottom row of our Table 6, the two interviewers used this category in 18% of the 202 interviews. The authors recomputed kappa for their data excluding these patients, and the values of kappa for the 71 patients for whom both interviewers gave a positive diagnosis are shown in the second from last column of Table 6.

Whether one examines the values of kappa for specific diagnosis on all 101 patients or the values of kappa only on the smaller sample of 71 patients, the values show strikingly higher interrater reliability for specific psychiatric diagnosis than published heretofore (see the results of earlier research in our Table 4). In fact, even when these earlier results in our Table 4 are corrected and kappa is applied, as was done by Spitzer and Fleiss for six of the earlier reliability studies (and reproduced here in the last column of our Table 6), the kappa values obtained by the St. Louis group were found in direct comparison by them (see the fifth and sixth columns in Table 6) to be markedly higher in all categories except organic brain syndrome. (Helzer, Clayton, Pambakian, Reich, Woodruff, & Reveley explain that this surprisingly low value for organic brain syndrome resulted in their study because there were too few such organic patients, namely only 6% of the interviews, and also because their operational criteria for this category are less well defined).

10.2. NIMH Collaborative Research Program

Investigators working in the same general area but located in different settings not infrequently pool their talents and produce a product that neither could have produced alone. With support from an NIMH grant to study the psychobiology of depression, Spitzer and Endicott and their colleagues at the New York State Psychiatric Institute were able to join forces in furthering research on the reliability and validity of psychiatric diagnosis with Robins in St. Louis, as well as with colleagues at the Harvard and Iowa medical schools. Together, these collaborators have produced two important research and clinical tools: (1) a manual of *Research Diagnostic Criteria* consisting of explicit, relatively easy to utilize operational definitions of 25 psychiatric disorders, many of which may become part of DSM III (Spitzer, Endicott, & Robins, 1977), and (2) a standardized interview schedule for eliciting the history and related present status and clinical information needed for determining in which of these 25 categories a given patient should be classified (Endicott & Spitzer, 1977). This collaborative team of investigators utilized new inpatients from their four settings and applied their recently developed research tools in what may be three of the best-designed studies to date on the reliability of psychiatric diagnosis. Two of the three studies involved joint interviews whereby one rater conducted the interview and the other merely observed, with each giving an independent diagnosis. The third study utilized two different and independent interviewers and a test-retest interval which ranged from 1 day to 1 week for different patients. The results of these three reliability studies are shown in Table 7. Inasmuch as this collaborative team could begin with and then improve on the operational definitions and the structured interview utilized in St. Louis by Helzer, Clayton, Pambakian, Reich, Woodruff, and Reveley (1977), the resulting even higher reliability values from their three studies shown in our Table 7 relative to Table 6 may not be too surprising.

Table 7.   Kappa Coefficients of Agreement for Major Diagnostic Categories Using the Research Diagnostic Criteria (RDC)[a]

	Joint interviews		Test-retest (N = 60)
	Study A (N = 68)	Study B (N = 150)	
Present episode			
Schizophrenia	.80	—	.65
Schizoaffective disorder, manic type	—	—	.79
Schizoaffective disorder, depressed type	.86	.85	.73
Manic disorder	.82	.98	.82
Major depressive disorder	.88	.90	.90
Minor depressive disorder	—	.81	—
Alcoholism	.86	.97	1.00
Drug abuse	.76	.95	.92
Lifetime			
Schizophrenia	.75	.91	.73
Schizoaffective disorder, manic type	—	—	—
Schizoaffective disorder, depressed type	.94	.87	.70
Manic disorder	.89	.93	.77
Hypomanic disorder	.85	—	.56
Major depressive disorder	.97	.91	.71
Minor depressive disorder	—	.68	—
Alcoholism	.88	.98	.95
Drug abuse	.89	1.00	.73
Obsessive compulsive disorder	—	1.00	—
Briquet's disorder	.79	.95	—
Labile personality	—	—	.70
Bipolar I	.93	.95	.40
Bipolar II	.79	.85	—
Recurrent unipolar	.81	.83	.80
Intermittent depressive disorder	—	.85	.57

[a]Adapted from Spitzer, Endicott, and Robins (1977).

The test-retest correlations for specific psychiatric diagnoses shown in the whole of Table 7 and in the second from the last column in Table 6 reach levels which traditionally have characterized the best psychometric tests currently extant and widely utilized in clinical practice and research, namely the Wechsler Intelligence Scales, the Minnesota Multiphasic Personality Index, and similar instruments. These same 1977 correlations for specific diagnoses reported in Table 7 also are at or above the relatively high levels of reliability reached for very global diagnostic categories in the earlier (1940–1965) period of reliability research already reviewed in this chapter. If investigators in other settings can demonstrate the same degree of reliability across independent clinicians for the diagnostic categories which have been painstakingly operationally defined by the collaborative project group and the St. Louis group, a major chapter will have been turned in the history of psychiatric diagnosis. Helzer, Clayton, Pambakian, Reich, Woodruff, and Reveley acknowledge that two elements of their research design may have increased their values of kappa shown in Table 6: (1) that they permitted an average of 2.5 diagnoses per interview and also (2) that the results they obtained by use of the structured interview were reviewed by a research faculty member to see if the interviewer had failed to record a datum that, in fact, had come out in the interview. If future research reveals that these two factors did increase the values of kappa, then we will have identified two operationally specifiable factors that have impeded prior research and that must be studied in greater detail in the future. The results in Table 7, however, seem to have resulted as much from the use of very explicit operational definitions as from factors comparable to these two from the St. Louis study.

11. Reliability of Diagnosis in Medicine

Reviewers have for too long bemoaned the low reliabilities typically obtained in research on psychiatric diagnosis. The implication in such critical reviews was that the reliability of diagnosis was higher in other branches of medicine than it was in psychiatry and clinical psychology. In their same article, Helzer, Clayton, Pambakian, Reich, Woodruff, and Reveley (1977) cite a review of the literature by Koran (1975a, 1975b) of published test-retest studies from the medical literature which reveal that this is not so. We shall here cite only three of the many studies reviewed by Koran.

In the first of these studies that Koran reviewed, Acheson (1960) reported a study in which a physician read 53 electrocardiogram tracings and reread them a year later. He used three classifications for comparison: the tracings were read both times as (1) normal, (2) questionably abnormal, or (3) abnormal. The value of kappa was reported by Koran to be .70.

In the second study reviewed, Norden, Phillips, Levy, and Kass (1970) calculated the level of agreement for the presence or absence of chronic pyelonephritis found through intravenous pyelograms. As a test of interrater agreement, two radiologists made independent interpretations of the same X-ray films. Koran's reanalysis of the data using kappa indicated that the value of the kappa obtained was .28 if "undecided" films were included and .43 if they were excluded.

The third study was reported by Felson, Morgan, Bristol, Tendergrass, Dessen, Linton, and Regen (1973) and involved the reliability of an X-ray diagnosis of pneumoconiosis in coal miners. The study involved a comparison of the diagnosis of this disease in 14,520 films which were read by one of seven staff radiologists and independently by one of 24 radiologists, with the physicians in both these groups each having had considerable experience in pneumoconiosis interpretation. The results revealed a kappa value for the sets of pairs of radiologists of .47, a result that Felson et al. considered unacceptably low reliability.

The interested reader will find a number of other related studies from the medical literature in Koran's review. Helzer, Clayton, Pambakian, Reich, Woodruff, and Reveley (1977) consider that their results summarized in our Table 6 offer good evidence for reliability when evaluated against previous studies of psychiatric diagnosis and also against the reliability of medical diagnosis represented in these three and other studies reviewed by Koran. The present writer agrees with these authors and hopes that in future research on the reliability of psychiatric diagnosis other investigators will be stimulated to use the explicit criteria and operational definitions published by the St. Louis group.

12. The Use of Computers in Psychiatric Diagnosis

The use of explicit, objectively specifiable criteria in arriving at differential diagnoses also makes possible the use of computers to ease the burden of reaching such differential judgments in the face of mounds of clinical data on a single patient. The New York State Psychiatric Institute group was quick to see this potential and began to write programs for logical decision tree branching and related decision making which could be fed into a modern, high-speed computer. Their product was DIAGNO and its subsequent revisions, DIAGNO II and DIAGNO III, a computer-based diagnostic model which has written into it the signs and symptoms of 79 different psychiatric diagnoses found in the diagnostic manual (DSM II) of the American Psychiatric Association. To improve the efficiency of DSM II, the New York group believes that they and others should provide DIAGNO with objective definitions for each psychiatric diagnosis similar to the operational definitions developed by the St. Louis group. The New York group also is experimenting with diagnostic models based on discriminant function and on a Bayesian probability classification as alternatives to DSM II.

In a number of studies published to date, the New York group has compared the degree (reliability) of agreement in differential diagnosis of information both fed to DIAGNO and elicited by an experienced psychiatrist (or an experienced therapist), and the results show beginning promise for such computer-derived differential diagnoses (Melrose, Stroebel, & Glueck, 1970; Fleiss, Spitzer, Cohen, & Endicott, 1972; Spitzer, Endicott, Cohen, & Fleiss, 1974; Spitzer & Endicott, 1974). Differential diagnosis by computer as against clinician for specific psychiatric dysfunctions actually reached the phenomenally high level of agreement of 65 out of 100 cases in one of their recent studies (Spitzer & Endicott, 1974). Continuation of this line of research can only help to produce heuristically useful information which will improve the reliability and, ultimately, the validity of differential psychiatric diagnosis—not only for broad, global categories but clearly also for the more highly discrete, specific conditions which clinicians long have wished to describe and thus better treat. There are, however, serious problems related to the reliable clinical use of computers for differential diagnosis, and their application currently seems far from imminent (Spitzer et al., 1974; Endicott & Spitzer, 1977).

We must now move on to a problem, one artfully addressed in a recent paper by Blashfield and Draguns (1976), which is equal in importance to that of reliability, namely the validity of a given psychiatric diagnosis. Any clinician or investigator could promulgate a criterion that is highly reliable in the sense that independent interviewers could be shown to achieve 100% agreement in its use. For example, one could postulate that the color of one's hair is a pathognomonic sign of schizophrenia, namely assert that all patients with red hair will be given the diagnosis of schizophrenia, that such redheads will be given no other diagnosis but schizophrenia, and that the label schizophrenia will be given to no other patient but to those with red hair. It is obvious that the specific diagnosis of schizophrenia so defined should achieve a test-retest correlation of 1.00 across independent clinician examiners. The question now is: having established reliability, how good (valid) is the product? Put differently, the demonstration of high reliability is merely a prior condition for embarking on the clinician's and investigator's true purpose—the development and demonstration of a valid method of prediction, treatment, and control. One can have high reliability without validity, but validity cannot be other than poor without the demonstration of a universally acceptable high level of reliability in the description and identification of the class of phenomena under investigation. However, in order to provide a proper perspective for consideration of this important issue of validity, it is necessary to review the function of psychiatric diagnosis. This is because consideration of the issue of "validity" without prior consideration of the question of "validity for what purpose or end" is a meaningless exercise.

13. Psychiatric Diagnosis: Its Functions and Purposes

The purposes and power of classification have been recognized since ancient times. The act of classification, based on accurate and reliable description and implying the possibility of prediction for the future, is basic to all science. It also is basic to every other aspect of living, for without classification we would not discriminate days and nights, the seasons, edible vs. inedible foods, and a myriad of other categories and classifications which we take for granted but which make survival possible.

Diagnosis in clinical practice essentially is no more and no less than the process of introducing order into one's observations, with an attendant increase in meaningfulness and ultimately control. Clinical diagnosis is the first cousin of taxonomy in biology, chemistry, and physics and involves merely the labeling of an object or a phenomenon in order to indicate its inclusion in a class of similar objects or phenomena. Placing an object or a phenomenon in a certain class is a labor-saving device that makes it possible to infer on the basis of this class membership the possession of certain class characteristics without the necessity of laboriously having to demonstrate each and every one of them a priori. Thus classifications owe their existence to an economizing principle of the human intellect. A new classification, such as the description of a new clinical syndrome, can be very fruitful if it helps put old observations in a new light and generates new questions for better treatment, prevention, control, or future research. But, as we have seen in the above sections on reliability, no classification can be any better than the classifier's knowledge and understanding of the observations he or she is classifying.

Diagnosis is not in and of itself tied to any particular set of categories, clinical descriptions, or other operational definitions. For example, the interested clinician or researcher could find today any one of the three following diagnostic systems (or others) suitable to his or her purposes: (1) the highly reliable-appearing structured interview and attendant diagnostic classifications developed by the St. Louis group and detailed in Woodruff et al. (1974) and shown in our Table 6, (2) the equally promising standardized interview schedule called the Present State Examination (PSE) for the more reliable diagnosis of schizophrenia which is being tried out concurrently to test its universality in nine countries under the auspices of the World Health Organization (Carpenter, Strauss, & Bartko, 1973), and (3) the heuristically equally promising Boston City Hospital Behavior Checklist for the diagnosis of psychopathology developed by Nathan and his colleagues from systems analysis principles (Martorano & Nathan, 1972; Martorano & Nathan, 1978). Once having demonstrated that a single category or total system of classification (diagnosis) based on one of these three methods (or others) is reliable, one may next proceed to test its validity. Before doing so, however, one must first be clear as to what end one has in mind against which to test the validity of one's diagnostic classifications. Writing from the perspective of an applied clinical neuropsychiatric unit which had served the Navy in World War II, Caveny et al. (1955) were aware of this need when they pointed out that, although the specific functions of psychiatric diagnosis are infinite, four of these functions of diagnosis appear to be critical: (1) administrative, (2) therapeutic, (3) research, and (4) prevention.

The administrative function of psychiatric diagnosis involves its use in such important administrative acts and decisions as recordkeeping and reporting and related epidemiological uses, selecting the type of ward suited for custodial care, deciding whether to admit or reject someone for service in the military, or, if already in, whether to offer or not offer a course of treatment, deciding whether to indict a prisoner as the first step in entry into the formal criminal and legal system or to bypass this system by the a priori acceptance of the defense of mental illness with referral of the individual to a hospital instead, and so on. One might extend this administrative function to include communicative aspects in that a universally accepted diagnostic classification scheme permits individuals in different settings to use a common language when communicating about any class of psychiatric patient.

The function of diagnosis in psychiatric or psychological treatment is well known. With the advances in scientific knowledge of the past several decades, a diagnosis of "primary depression" or "acute schizophrenic episode" or "fear of elevators" immediately narrows down considerably for most of today's clinicians the options for the treatment of choice for each of these conditions. As the science of mental and behavioral therapy, including its powerful pharmacological and behavioral variants, proceeds to full development, diagnosis and therapy of choice in many instances will be synonymous. Even within the constraints imposed by today's still relatively limited knowledge of which treatment is best for which specific condition, reliable diagnosis permits chronicling the natural history of different psychological and psychiatric disabilities, thus ensuring more reliable judgments of prognosis based purely on this knowledge of typical course of the disease or behavioral condition alone.

The function of diagnosis in research also is well known. Even with their obvious limitations, the classificatory schemes of Kraepelin, or of DSM I, were better than no scheme at all, as witness the results in our Table 4. Although these schemes are not as heuristically or clinically powerful as the results which a more reliable classificatory system such as the one underlying the results in our Table 7 makes possible, the total absence of even a rudimentary classification scheme would negate the possibility that future research could ever lead to further knowledge and ultimately to better treatment. The three research programs identified earlier in the present section are representative of the role reliable diagnosis plays in good research, and vice versa.

The fourth and ultimately most important function of diagnosis is prevention or control. It is not enough that reliable diagnosis might lead to efficient and effective therapy and treatment on purely clinical, pragmatic, or ad hoc grounds, without an understanding of the condition itself. Reliable diagnosis also will enhance the search for commonalities across classes and other abstractions not inherent or immediately apparent in one type of class alone. As the reports at the end of this chapter of the studies by Wender (1977), Winokur (1977), and Van Praag (1977), and others will substantiate, these searches for commonalities may lead potentially to discovery of new knowledge about the condition merely from knowledge of its membership in a broader class and, it is hoped, make it possible more effectively to either completely eradicate the condition, immunize people against it, treat them better for it, contain it, or otherwise bring it under control. It is thus clear that reliable diagnosis is merely the first step in the never-ending search for exemplars, correlates, and other indices of validity which one day will permit the full-scale prevention or control of psychiatric and behavioral disability.

With these introductory statements we shall now examine the state of our knowledge concerning the validity of psychiatric diagnosis based solely on the clinical interview. We shall confine our discussion to two types of validity, concurrent and predictive validity, because, unlike the area of psychological test validation, in the area of psychiatric and behavioral diagnosis the issues of content validity and face validity are of limited importance, and a sufficient data base knowledge on which to establish beginning construct validity may not be available in the foreseeable future.

14. Predictive Validity

14.1. World War II U.S. Navy Studies

Although often overlooked by most reviewers of the literature on the validity of psychiatric diagnosis, the studies carried out by Hunt and Wittson and their colleagues in a U.S. Navy neuropsychiatric unit in World War II are classic examples of the type of sophistication, and also the resources, required for good validity research. In one such validity study (Hunt, 1951; Raines, Wittson, Hunt, & Herrmann, 1954), these investigators reasoned that if psychiatric diagnostic screening procedures of recruits at the precommissioning training center (boot camp) were efficacious in reducing subsequent psychiatric attrition during later service among the same groups screened, then the amount of subsequent attrition should be in inverse ratio to the number eliminated during training. That is, the more men discharged for psychiatric reasons during training, the less psychiatric attrition would be expected among the remaining same group of men during subsequent military service.

Fortunately, the peculiar conditions necessary for testing their hypothesis existed in the U.S. Navy during the first part of 1943. At one recruit base, Sampson, the commanding officer was not sympathetic to psychiatric screening, and relatively few discharges were permitted. At Great Lakes, the commanding officer allowed the psychiatric unit to discharge as many men as it saw fit. At Newport, where the investigators worked, the commanding officer asked the psychiatric unit to hold the discharge rate to roughly 4%. According to Hunt et al., in 1943 the three naval training stations were operating under conditions where the quality of the recruit populations, the professional competence of the staff engaged in psychiatric screening, and the actual psychiatric examination procedures in use were all roughly comparable.

To check their hypothesis, Hunt et al., knowing the earlier discharge rates for each station, after the war, obtained the records of a sample of approximately 1300 men seen in each of the recruit centers during the same month in 1943 in order to see what the discharge rate was for these same men in the 2½ years of subsequent naval service. To cross-validate their findings, they repeated the procedure for samples for each of three additional months.

The results, shown in Table 8, are clear-cut: the higher the screening center's rate of diagnosing unsuitability for service, the lower the subsequent psychiatric attrition rate in the same group sample; the lower this training discharge rate (as at Sampson), the higher the subsequent rate of breakdown in this same group under the later military conditions. As mentioned earlier, Hunt et al. also point out that careful inspection of these results indicates that there may be a curve of diminishing returns, since as more men are discharged, there is less and less return in lowered attrition rate. Thus, in April 1943, Great Lakes discharged almost twice as many men as Newport (4.5% vs. 2.6%), but its attrition rate was diminished by only one-sixth. Hunt et al. suggest that one may ask whether, beyond an optimal point, the slight improvement in subsequent discharge rate is worth the large man-

Table 8. Psychiatric (Unsuitability-for-Service) Discharge Rate during Training and Subsequent Psychiatric Attrition during Service[a]

Training center	Number of recruits screened	Percent discharged during training	Percent discharged subsequently
January 1943			
Great Lakes	1310	4.4	2.6
Newport	1255	5.0	3.7
Sampson	1350	0.7	4.1
April 1943			
Great Lakes	1525	4.5	1.5
Newport	1173	2.6	1.8
Sampson	2823	0.7	3.0
June 1943			
Great Lakes	1347	5.9	3.2
Newport	1294	4.2	3.0
Sampson	1284	0.7	3.7
July 1943			
Great Lakes	1350	5.2	3.3
Newport	1310	3.0	3.6
Sampson	1354	1.3	5.0

[a] Adapted from Hunt (1951).

power loss entailed by the doubled number of training center discharges—a social, economic, and ethical question not answerable by scientists alone.

In commenting on the results shown in Table 8 and the related validity studies of his group, Hunt carefully reminds us of a fact pertinent here, i.e., that in studying the reliability and validity of psychiatric diagnosis, one need not always be bound by the superficially enticing concept of reliability and validity of diagnosis for single individuals, taken one at a time across a total sample, as, for example, in the studies by Ash (1949), Masserman and Carmichael (1938), and others. Hunt writes:

> The fulfillment of [the clinician's] predictions is often influenced by complex and uncontrolled environmental factors. There are many areas, and many types of behavior, that are not amenable to prediction at present, and some may never be. It must be stressed that the predictions made in psychiatric selection are essentially group predictions rather than individual predictions, since the question of prediction in the individual instance raises many confusing philosophical and mathematical issues in the use of probability data in the clinical sciences. In psychiatric selection we are not making a prediction concerning the future behavior of each and every individual passing through the selection process, but rather making a prediction concerning the total behavior of the group to which the individual belongs on our continuum. We do not hope to be right in each and every individual prediction, but rather to have a high proportion of successes in any group or series of predictions. (Hunt, 1955, pp. 201–202)

Thus it was appropriate to raise a question, as we did in the last section, pertinent to the several studies showing lack of reliability of psychiatric diagnosis, namely the question of reliability for what. As Zigler and Phillips (1961) make clear, and as Caveny et al. (1955), Hunt et al. (1953), and Blashfield and Draguns (1976) have elaborated, the function of psychiatric diagnosis is not a unitary one. Studies on the predictive validity of such diagnosis must keep these various purposes in mind.

Hunt and his co-workers published numerous additional "historicoexperimental" validity studies, only several of which will be reviewed here. In a study conducted in 1944 (Wittson & Hunt, 1951), 944 cases of naval personnel were sent for interview because of suspected psychiatric symptoms (picked up by enlisted men conducting vocational aptitude placement exams). On the basis of merely a very brief psychiatric interview, these cases were diagnosed and placed into three classes: (1) mild symptoms, treatment not indicated; (2) moderate symptoms, shore duty (but not sea duty) indicated; and (3) severe symptoms, hospitalization indicated. Years later, the subsequent naval careers of 932 of these 944 men were studied for the 1-year period after this mild-moderate-severe diagnosis was made, and the psychiatric discharge rates during that 1-year period were determined. The results, presented in Table 9, show a remarkable clarity. The subsequent rate of psychiatric discharge

Table 9. Incidence of Subsequent Neuropsychiatric Discharges among Men Interviewed and Diagnosed as to Severity of Psychiatric Condition (1944 sample)[a]

Diagnosis	Total number	Subsequent NP discharge	
		Number	Percent
Mild	527	34	6.5
Moderate	367	74	20.2
Severe	38	34	89.7

[a]Adapted from Wittson and Hunt (1951).

(often accomplished far from the scene of the original diagnosis and independent of it) paralleled the original prediction (differential diagnosis); i.e., mild, moderate, and severe ratings had subsequent discharge rates of 6.5%, 20.2%, and 89.7% respectively. The normal attrition rate for discharges among unselected Navy men during this same period was 1.6%, a figure one-tenth as large as the figure of 15.6% which obtained for the total group of 932 men shown in Table 9.

The authors did not carry out a check on the reliability of their three-category diagnostic classification. However, as pointed out by us in the last section, good validity implies good reliability. That is, although the results shown in Table 9 clearly establish the validity of the original diagnostic classificatory process, as Hunt and Wittson interpreted their results, the results also establish, ipso facto, the practical reliability of the original crude three-group psychiatric diagnostic system. That is, in the absence of methodological flaws in the research design, to the extent that the three-category differential diagnosis worked (predicted) as well as it did in this study, the diagnostic classificatory scheme must have been of sufficient reliability to merit serious further attention and use. Or, put another way, had the test-retest reliability for the "suitable-for-service" vs. "not-suitable-for-service" dichotomy implied by the three classifications shown in Table 9 been only of the order of, for example, .50–.80, this fact would have to be interpreted within the context of the validity results shown in the same table. Granted that the results shown in Table 9 might have been even more striking if the three-category diagnostic scheme shown in this table had better than, for example, a .50–.80 kappa test-retest reliability across two psychiatrists, the demonstrated validity results attest to not inconsiderable reliability for the original diagnostic classifications. However, despite this relatively low hypothetical reliability, the validity results shown in Table 9 cannot be discarded. In most instances, if not all, reliability cannot be divorced from validity. However, few students of the reliability of psychiatric diagnosis have been fortunate enough to be part of a long-range program of research which would make possible such a test of reliability through its validity correlates. Pasamanick et al. (1959, p. 130) provide some such validity data in their table showing the results (validity) of ECT, drugs, and psychotherapy for different diagnostic categories (reliability). We shall consider some modern studies of this type in the next section.

In a study (Hunt et al., 1952) related to the one shown in Table 9, these investigators determined the subsequent psychiatric discharge rates of three groups of men in whom the initial diagnosis varied as to degree of "certainty" and "severity" as determined by who conducted the psychiatric examination and by the time, energy, and number of professional personnel required to arrive at the diagnosis. The three diagnostic groups used were as follows: (1) undiagnosed—despite the presence of some indication of psychiatric difficulty the clinician concerned was unable to attach a definite diagnostic label; (2) diagnosed—indications of a psychiatric difficulty were present, and a definite psychiatric diagnosis could be made; and (3) board hearing recommended—diagnosed cases, each of which was felt to possibly indicate unfitness for further military service and which were consequently referred by the psychiatrist to the next higher authority, the aptitude board, for final decision, but each of which nevertheless resulted in assignment to military duty by the board after careful consideration. The subjects in the diagnosed and undiagnosed groups also were sent to duty, this diagnosis notwithstanding. As a futher control group against which to check their hypothesis of differential subsequent psychiatric discharge rates in these three groups, Hunt et al. included a group of false positives, i.e., men referred to the observation ward for psychiatric examination but judged by the examining clinician to be "normal," or free from any positive symptomatology. The study was cross-validated in samples from 2 successive years. Some 20 clinicians were involved in the study. The original diagnosis was evaluated against a criterion of psychiatric discharge by the end of the war (December 31, 1945).

The results shown in Table 10 also are strikingly clear. As the confidence level or definiteness of severity of condition of the initial diagnosis increased from none (no NP), through least, moderate, and highest, the subsequent psychiatric discharge rate likewise increased in stepwise fashion. There seems little doubt that this additional "experiment of nature" by these authors adds to the confidence one can have in the reliability, as well as the validity, of the process of psychiatric diagnosis involved in the four classes of judgments shown in Table 10.

In additional studies, Hunt and his co-workers cited evidence to show that despite the lower test-retest correlations found by them and others for such specific diagnoses as schizoid personality, psychopath, and alcoholic, the validity correlates of these diagnoses as determined by subsequent military history of each man showed remarkable power for them. For example, men diagnosed as psychopaths subsequently showed a higher incidence of disciplinary infractions and fewer hospitalizations, while neurotics showed the reverse, etc. They also cited evidence to show that individuals diagnosed as "low intelligence," "low intelligence plus psychiatric symptoms" (but both groups were still sent to duty), or "normal" controls, all three being evaluated as groups, had markedly contrasting subsequent differential discharge rates for psychiatric, medical, and disciplinary reasons. References to these and numerous other validity studies can be found in Hunt (1955).

The results from this program of research on the validity of psychiatric diagnosis in the military situation were impressive. Nevertheless, the results required follow-up and attempt at cross-validation by others. Cross-validation on other samples was especially necessary in view of the provocative publication by Sharp (1950), a front-line army psychiatrist with the 99th Division, who, because of a shortage of manpower, took 395 mild neuropsychiatrically diagnosed soldiers into the Battle of the Bulge and found that, during 50 days of the battle, only 45 of the 395 were unable to function due to psychiatric or medical reasons. Although 50 days may be too short a test of predictive validity, such a report required more attempts at cross-validation of the Hunt et al. findings.

Table 10. Incidence of Subsequent Neuropsychiatric Discharge among Groups Differing in Definiteness of Initial Diagnosis[a]

Confidence level of initial diagnosis	1942		1943		1944	
	N	Percent	N	Percent	N	Percent
Highest (board)	42	21.4	1	0.0	31	32.3
Moderate (diagnosed)	126	15.9	126	15.9	93	29.0
Least (undiagnosed)	126	8.7	126	8.7	93	14.0
Control (no NP)	42	0.0	42	4.8	31	0.0

[a] Adapted from Hunt et al. (1952).

14.2. Post-World War II Peacetime Studies

77

THE INTERVIEW:
ITS RELIABILITY
AND VALIDITY IN
PSYCHIATRIC
DIAGNOSIS

The results demonstrating a fair degree of predictive validity reproduced in our Tables 8, 9, and 10 were collected by Hunt et al. under the peculiar conditions, manpower stresses, strains, and related problems which obtained in a military service during wartime. Accordingly, Hunt, Herrmann, and Noble (1957) attempted to cross-validate their wartime findings by studying a large group of new recruits who had commenced training at the Great Lakes Naval Training Center in the year 1952, a period when the Navy no longer was involved in meeting manpower requirements for a global war. Upon his arrival at the Training Center, each recruit was given a brief psychiatric screening interview as a part of his entering physical examination. Upon completion of the interview, the interviewer rated each recruit in one of four categories. Recruits judged to be free of psychiatric defect and fully qualified for duty were given a rating of 1. Those giving evidence of mild, transient, or mildly severe dysfunction were assigned a 2 rating; and those found to show evidence of a more moderate, chronic dysfunction were assigned a 3 rating. Those recruits found unsuitable for service were discharged under the less urgent manpower needs of 1952, thereby, unfortunately, obviating follow-up of their subsequent military career.

Table 11 presents the follow-up results with a sample of 2406 recruits. As is shown, of the subsample of 617 recruits found to have no psychiatric condition, follow-up after a period of 3 years revealed that fewer than 1% (.81) had received a discharge for psychiatric reasons, 2.43% for a medical reason, and 1.64% for bad conduct. As the total in the last column shows, the total discharge rate for all three of these reasons combined was 4.88% for this group having no psychiatric defect.

The next two rows show a progressive increase in total subsequent attrition: 8.73% for recruits given a rating of 2 for a mild psychiatric defect at entry and 11.24% for those judged to be more moderately disturbed and given a higher rating of 3. These 1952–1955 results cross-validate the Hunt et al. wartime studies for 1942, 1943, and 1944 and, once again, are good evidence for the predictive validity of the brief neuropsychiatric interview of the psychiatric team members who conducted that part of the initial physical examination.

Hunt et al. offered two important observations regarding their study of this 1952 sample. First, they called attention to the inability of categories 2 and 3 to predict differentially the subsequent psychiatric attrition in the ranks of these recruits.

Table 11. Incidence of Subsequent Neuropsychiatric Discharges among Men Interviewed and Diagnosed as to Severity of Psychiatric Condition (1952 sample)[a]

Boot camp psychiatric diagnosis	Total number	Reason for and percent discharged during next 3 years of duty			
		Psychiatric	Medical	Bad conduct	Total
1. No defect	617	.81	2.43	1.64	4.88
2. Mild defect	1273	2.99	2.99	2.75	8.73
3. Moderate defect	516	2.71	3.88	4.65	11.24

[a]Adapted from Hunt, Herrmann, and Noble (1957).

As a matter of fact, as the second column of Table 11 shows, the subsequent discharge rate for psychiatric reasons (2.71%) of the recruits in the most disabled category (category 3) was less than the discharge rate (2.99%) for category 2, a reversal of the prediction. Hunt et al. interpret this finding as suggesting that their interviewers could not make such a fine discrimination as that required by a rating of 3 vs. 2. On the other hand, examination in Table 11 of the subsequent rates of attrition for these two groups for medical reasons or bad conduct, plus the total column, strongly suggests to the present reviewer that such fine discriminations and valid predictions were, in fact, being made. All that the interviewers failed to do was to predict differentially among categories 1, 2, and 3 the specific reason for the subsequent discharge, attaining quite well this differential prediction in two areas (medical and bad conduct types of discharges) and less well for psychiatric reasons, per se.

The second observation offered by Hunt et al. was that their psychiatric interviewers could not reliably differentiate within another subset of data which they also collected but which are not shown in our Table 11. Thus, in this other part of their study, they tried to predict from an interview with each man the subsequent discharge rates of two subsamples of such young men who had volunteered for special duty (e.g., submarine service). Of 655 such healthy volunteers so screened by them in 1952, a total of 531 were judged qualified as a result of this special brief psychiatric interview and 124 were judged not qualified. Subsequent discharges for these two subgroups of otherwise healthy recruits showed that the "qualified" group had a higher level of discharge (2.82%) than found in the group judged not qualified (2.42%). Cross-validation of this last finding in samples drawn in 1953 and in 1954 again showed inability of the interviewer to make this judgment of differential success within such a group of healthy volunteers. What these findings indicate is that there obviously is a limit to the capacity of such brief psychiatric interviews for success in studies of predictive validity. That the Navy then stopped using such a special but still brief psychiatric interview for selecting men for hazardous duty is not surprising. The Hunt et al. results appeared to be clear evidence that such fine discriminations within what were two subgroups of psychiatrically healthy men were not possible. Nevertheless, these 1952 data shown in our Table 11 served as an excellent cross-validation a decade later of the predictive validity so clearly evident in our Tables 8, 9, and 10.

Another decade after this 1952 sample was studied, Plag and Arthur (1965), from the United States Navy Neuropsychiatric Research Unit at San Diego, carried out still another cross-validation study. Their populations included recruits who commenced their boot camp training in May, August, and November of 1960 and in February of 1961. By 1960, these Navy researchers had developed a standardized 195-item personal and psychological screening questionnaire which was filled out by each recruit at the time of his initial medical examination. This completed questionnaire served as the basis for the brief psychiatric interview which typically came at the end of this medical examination. It was still standard practice in the Navy in 1960 to use the product of these initial psychiatric screening interviews to refer those recruits who seemed to need further study for a hearing by an aptitude board, one comparable to that mentioned in our Table 10, for determination of neuropsychiatric fitness to remain in the Navy.

Plag and Arthur reported that of 3616 new recruits in the 1960–1961 samples under study, a total of 216, or about 6%, were judged by the aptitude board unsuitable to continue in the service. As a test of the predictive validity of the Navy's 1960–1961 psychiatric screening activity, a total of 134 of these 216 enlisted men were purposely graduated into the fleet from recruit training. Checks of the characteristics of these 134 men revealed that they were representative of the total 216. In addition, Plag and Arthur paired each of these 134 psychiatrically diagnosed recruits with 134 matched controls taken from the remaining pool of 3400 recruits already found to be suitable for service, and compared the subsequent military history of both groups two years later.

The results are shown in Table 12. As can be seen in the second column, 27.6% of those who were judged "unsuitable" for service in recruit training but nevertheless allowed to commence a career as naval enlisted men had been discharged on follow-up 2 years later. In the healthier control group judged "suitable" for service, the attrition rate was 14.2%. Plag and Arthur interpret these 2-year follow-up results as evidence of the predictive validity of naval neuropsychiatric screening. However, they also were impressed by the fact that, within the group of 134 recruits who would have been discharged based on their individual screening and psychiatric interview, there nevertheless were 97 men (72.4%) who were still on active duty 2 years later as against the 37 men (27.6%) who had been dropped as unsuitable. Thus to have discharged all 134 in the recruit phase (that is, the full 6% designated as unsuitable by the aptitude board in boot camp) would have lost to the service the 97 men who survived on active duty 2 years later.

From their study of the subsequent military histories of the two subsets (the matched healthy controls vs. the psychiatrically diagnosed group), Plag and Arthur derived some valuable insights into why, for example, some of the men who were diagnosed unsuitable in boot camp did adjust and thus succeed 2 years later (e.g., the naval experience offers an environment for further maturation for some young men). Nevertheless, the authors were concerned about the cost-benefit ratio of such psychiatric interviewing and indicated that "although the system of psychiatric screening currently utilized has statistical validity, its practical value is limited. The utility of the procedure, however, is dependent upon administrative considerations which are beyond the scope of this report" (p. 540).

As our earlier discussion of the present Table 8 identifies, it is just these "administrative considerations" which led Hunt et al. to point out that in psychiatric interview screening "There may be a curve of diminishing returns, since as more men are discharged, there is less and less return in attrition rate." The 6% discharge among Plag and Arthur's total naval sample of recruits in the 1960–1961 period is higher

Table 12. Incidence of Subsequent Neuropsychiatric Discharges among Men Diagnosed in Boot Camp as Unsuitable for Service by Use of a Screening Questionnaire and Psychiatric Evaluation[a]

Boot camp psychiatric diagnosis	Total number	Percent subsequently discharged after differing numbers of years of service	
		2 years	4 years
Unsuitable for service	134	27.6	46.5
Suitable for service	134	14.2	27.6

[a] Results from Plag and Arthur (1965), Plag and Goffman (1966), and Brown (1971).

even than the highest similar discharge level for all recruits attained in 1943 and reproduced in our Table 8. That this 1960–1961 Plag and Arthur control group sample is atypical can be surmised from the fact that approximately 4% of all World War II military recruits were subsequently discharged because of psychiatric or behavioral unsuitability (Ginzberg, Anderson, Ginsberg, & Herma, 1959, pp. 34–36, p. 61). From the results shown in our earlier Table 8, one may agree with the implication in Hunt's data that administrative curtailment of a rate of discharge above about 3%, while seemingly unfeeling, might have been cost-effective in his study and also in the Plag and Arthur study, given the otherwise good predictive validity of such psychiatric interviews as is shown in our Tables 8 and 12.

From another perspective, one may take the opposite tack and argue that for some situations, and admitting that the total cost of achieving it may be very high, even a 1% improvement in the success of psychiatric and psychological interviewing would be cost effective. An example that comes to mind is in the selection of astronauts who one day will be responsible for piloting spaceships which will cost billions of dollars to deploy and sustain in space. If a future predictive validity study in the selection of such astronauts showed that the gain from the use of a psychiatric interview with such potential astronauts was only 1%, even cost-conscious administrators might feel it had been worth the gain in this unusual instance. Likewise, as a second example, clinicians working in the prisons who one day, relative to a control group of match controls, accurately identify even one more deranged individual from a sample of individuals known to pose a potential threat to a world leader also will be judged to have proven the worth of such psychiatric interviewing in the minds of many persons. Predictive validity can generate results in statistical terms, as evidenced in the data in the tables in this chapter. However, educated minds will have to interpret these data, with the full understanding that different interpreters may reach diametrically opposed conclusions.

Despite the absence of any discussion in relation to the data in Table 12 by Plag and Arthur as to why their sample of recruits judged to be normal and "suitable for service" yielded the subsequent unusually high attrition rate of 14.2% (compared to the attrition rate of only 1.6% for the comparably "normal" group discussed in relation to our Table 9), their 2-year-data in Table 12 offer good evidence for predictive validity. The data are even more convincing if, as is done in the last column of Table 12, one adds the data from a subsequent report by Navy Captain Earl Brown in a discussion of another paper (see p. 152, *American Journal of Psychiatry*, 1971, Vol. 128) and from a report by Plag and Goffman (1966) that the two groups of recruits in this first follow-up Plag and Arthur report (1965), when followed-up for 2 more years, showed a differential attrition rate of 46.5% vs. 27.6% at the end of 4 years of naval duty. To anyone familiar with military rates of discharge, these last data appear to be impressive indeed even without a knowledge of the actual attrition rate for the rest of the Navy during 1960–1961. It certainly could not have been anywhere near the almost 50% value of 46.5% shown in Table 12 for the psychiatrically "unsuited for service" group. In any event, the almost 20% greater attrition (46.5% vs. 27.6%) after 4 years relative to the control group's admittedly relatively high value is impressive evidence for the predictive validity of a brief psychiatric process involving a screening interview.

14.3. A United States Army Study

Comparable data from the United States Army which just as clearly raise the question of the cost effectiveness of neuropsychiatric screening were published by Egan, Jackson, and Eanes (1951). They followed the Army careers of 2054 men who had previously been rejected by the Army for neuropsychiatric reasons but who later were in fact inducted during 1942–1946. Follow-up showed that 18% of these once-rejected inductees were given subsequent neuropsychiatric discharges, and 82% performed satisfactorily during their subsequent years of Army service. This compared to a rate of 6% neuropsychiatric discharge vs. 94% of enlisted personnel who served satisfactorily in the whole United States Army during that same period; that is, the former rejectees had a threefold greater discharge rate from Army military duty than did regular inductees (18% vs. 6%).

Thus this Egan et al. World War II study yielded results comparable to those of Hunt and Wittson et al. and also comparable to those of the Plag and Arthur study. All three gave evidence of predictive validity for their psychiatric screening. Nevertheless, like the Navy studies, Egan's Army study showed a remarkable 82% success rate for the men who would have been rejected outright. Only administrators with the responsibility for the overall success of such missions and the public to whom they report, are the ones who ultimately must judge whether or not weeding out 18% of such individuals who ultimately would fail was worth the cost of also weeding out 82% who would not. Research on the predictive validity of the interview, or any other assessment device, in industry as well as the military essentially boils down to each person with the authority to continue or discontinue such assessment finding his or her own answer to this last question to the satisfaction of that subset of society to which he or she is ultimately responsible.

14.4. Illiteracy in 1951 and 1972

In another study from the Navy group, almost three decades ago Hunt and Wittson (1951) reported on a 1951 sample of 940 naval recruits and a second 1951 sample of 473 naval recruits who (1) were found on screening during their initial boot camp medical examination to be illiterate, (2) were given special remedial literacy training by the Navy, and (3) were sent to duty rather than being discharged. Hunt and Wittson found that the rate of discharge during the subsequent 12 months of duty for ineptitude, other neuropsychiatric reasons, and bad conduct was 18.8% and 18.1% respectively, in the two samples. Inasmuch as the discharge rate for the Navy as a whole during 1951 was about 5.1% these values indicate a threefold increase in the probability of subsequent discharge among illiterates who received special literacy training.

Fifteen years later, during 1967–1972, Hoiberg, Hysham, and Berry (1974) carried out a cross-validation predictive validity study of this earlier Hunt and Wittson study. The Hoiberg et al. cross-validation sample of 1518 naval recruits given remedial literacy training showed a 1-year follow-up discharge rate of 18.0% (a figure comparable to that of Hunt and Wittson) as against a comparable 1-year attrition rate during the same period of only 1.7% in a control group sample of 1520 literate naval recruits matched for scores on the Armed Forces Qualification Test (AFQT). Although "ineptitude" accounted for the bulk of the reasons for attrition in each of the three Navy samples (1951, 1951, and 1967–1972), the attrition due exclusively to "other neuropsychiatric reasons" in these three samples was 3.0%, 3.4%, and 5.5% respectively. These rates of attrition are considerably higher than the 1.0% found in the control group used by Hoiberg et al. in their 1967–1972 study.

It thus would appear that a datum that is easily obtained either by psychiatric history or by a simple objective test, namely illiteracy, has considerable predictive validity for subsequent failure due to neuropsychiatric factors.

14.5. Some Classic Studies Which Yielded Negative Results

The studies reviewed in the last several sections above all present good evidence for the predictive validity of the psychiatric interview as a screening tool in the military situation. However, in the period following World War II some now classic studies were published which reported a failure to find evidence of predictive validity for clinical judgments involving specific personality characteristics. These studies reported the failure of neuropsychiatric assessment in (1) selection for the wartime clandestine strategic services (OSS Assessment Staff, 1948), (2) the prediction of success as a pilot (Holtzman and Sells, 1954), (3) the prediction of success in psychiatric residency training (Holt & Luborsky, 1958) and also in clinical psychology training and later professional work (Kelly & Fiske, 1951; Kelly Goldberg, 1959), (4) the prediction of success for officer candidates in the United States Marine Corps (Wilkins et al., 1955), and finally (5) the prediction of success in the Peace Corps (Fisher, Epstein, & Harris, 1967).

These classic studies are by now sufficiently well known that they need not be reviewed here other than to state that the psychological and psychiatric judgments and discriminations made by the clinicians in these studies were very fine discriminations within groups of essentially very healthy subjects. Not one of these classic studies involved what Cronbach and Gleser (1965) identify as "broad-band" categorizations such as the global classification of "suitability" vs. "unsuitability" utilized in the Hunt et al. studies. As was described in relation to Tables 8, 9, 10, 11, and 12, those predictive studies pitted interview-derived judgments made on a sample of psychiatrically unfit recruits against similar judgments of a sample that was fit. These just-listed classic studies which produced no evidence of predictive validity took samples comparable to this fit group and searched for the predictive validity of considerably finer gradations within it. The results showed such finer clinical judgments to have little predictive validity. It long has been recognized that when the most unfit are removed from a predictive validity study the possibility of a successful study is reduced considerably. The successful Navy and Army predictive studies reviewed above did not suffer from this well-known restriction-of-range problem. The interested reader will find the role of this problem described in the recent cross-validation by Kandler, Plutchik, Conte, and Siegel (1975) of the lack of predictive validity in determining the level of success during training of psychiatric residents first reported by Holt and Luborsky (1958). Kandler et al. quite appropriately point out that it is unreasonable to expect an interview of 1 or 2 hr duration to predict the 3-year level of follow-up success of 17 highly able psychiatric residents who were chosen from a pool of 99 such applicants. Had there been a subsample of neuropsychiatrically unsuitable residents included among those 17 selected and allowed to continue, results not unlike those of Hunt et al. reviewed above might have been forthcoming.

14.6. The Failure of Differential Diagnosis in the Legal Arena

Anyone who reads the daily newspapers has known for a long time that experts from the mental health professions frequently disagree one with another on their psychiatric diagnoses when they testify as expert witnesses in court trials. Almost without fail the expert called by the defense offers the opinion that the accused is legally insane. This testimony is followed by that of an expert with similarly impressive credentials who is called by the prosecution and who offers the opinion that the accused is legally sane. The practical effect of such disagreement is to nullify completely, in the minds of the jury and the public, the opinion of either expert. After numerous replays of such public displays of lack of reliability of psychiatric diagnosis, lay persons, jurists, and attorneys have come to expect it and are, in fact, visibly surprised when such experts from opposing sides agree. Disagreement is what is expected, and both sides and the public today routinely place little credence on such testimony in this area of psychiatric diagnosis.

Much less known, however, have been the costs in human terms of the lack of reliability and validity of psychiatric diagnosis in other areas of the legal system: specifically, the incarceration often for a lifetime of individuals either in a state hospital or in a prison following psychiatric testimony which has been accepted by the court that the accused is criminally insane. In such cases, typically when a heinous assault or crime has been committed and reports of it are given daily front-page coverage, psychiatrists on both sides usually are in agreement that the accused is insane and thus should be removed from society lest the criminal act be repeated. In the past, society's interest in such deranged individuals dissipated quickly following the sensational trial, and, once incarcerated, they were forgotten by all but their keepers. Large states such as New York and California have housed untold numbers of such individuals, keeping them incarcerated in state hospitals long after their prison terms expired. The prediction of mental health specialists based on psychiatric interview that an individual is dangerous and constitutes a threat to society remained for the most part surprisingly unchallenged. Recently, however, Ennis and Litwack (1974) and Ziskin (1975, 1977) have reviewed the literature which shows the lack of reliability of the psychiatric diagnosis that a person is criminally dangerous and point out the human costs to untold thousands of persons of such unreliable and invalid diagnostic predictions. Among many other topics covered, each review highlights the now famous 1966 precedent-setting Supreme Court decision which was handed down in the Baxstrom vs. Herold case. The Supreme Court held that those alleged criminally insane individuals remaining in the New York State Department of Corrections hospitals after their prison terms had expired must be released immediately by the corrections department and committed to a state hospital under due process in the civil courts. Affected were 967 patients who had been incarcerated in maximum-security hospitals following determination by psychiatrists that they were mentally ill and too dangerous for release or even for transfer to civil hospitals. Overnight these 967 patients were released from the criminal justice system and committed by civil court order to other state hospitals.

In effect, this court decision was an experiment of nature not unlike the Navy studies in World War II reported by Hunt and his colleagues in which recruits psychiatrically diagnosed as unsuitable for service were nevertheless permitted into naval service. Follow-up 1 year later of the 967 criminally insane and dangerous patients who were transferred to civil hospitals revealed that (1) 147 of them had been discharged to the community and (2) 702 presented no special problems to the hospital staff or to other patients. Only 7 of the original 967 were found to be so difficult to manage or dangerous that they had to be recommitted to a Department of Corrections hospital.

A second follow-up 4 years later of the original 967 patients revealed that (1) 281 of them (27%) were living successfully in the community, (2) only 9 of the 967 had been convicted of a crime (only 2 of the 9 for a felony), and (3) a total of only 29 (3%) of the 967 were incarcerated in a correctional facility or hospital for the criminally insane.

One of the reviewers of these results commented as follows:

> In statistical terms, Operation Baxstrom tells us that psychiatric predictions are incredibly inaccurate. In human terms, it tells us that but for a Supreme Court decision, nearly 1,000 human beings would have lived much of their lives behind bars, without grounds privileges, without home visits, without even the limited amenities available to civil patients, all because a few psychiatrists, in their considered opinion, thought they were dangerous and no one asked for proof. (Ennis & Litwack, 1974, p. 713)

Ennis and Litwack also review a later study, one believed to be the most extensive study to date in the prediction of dangerousness in criminal offenders. In this study a team of five mental health experts, including two or more psychiatrists, was asked to conduct an unusually thorough clinical examination of a group of individuals who previously had been convicted of serious assaultive crimes (often sexual in nature) and to predict which ones again would commit assaultive crimes if released. Despite this psychiatric prediction of dangerousness in each instance, the court released 49 such individuals following a hearing. Follow-up 5 years later showed that 65% of these 49 had not been found to have committed another violent crime. Ennis and Litwack (1974) add: "In other words, two thirds of those released despite predictions of dangerousness by the professional team did not in fact turn out to be dangerous" (p. 713).

No reader can be other than impressed by the human costs associated with this false-positive prediction in cases of the two-thirds of individuals who were erroneously diagnosed. What Ennis and Litwack underplay in the statement just quoted is that the diagnosis and prediction were surprisingly accurate in 35% of the cases.

Neither scientists nor reviewers of the literature can answer the critical issue which is involved here, namely what costs society is willing to pay for what benefits. This issue of a cost-benefit ratio was addressed earlier in this chapter in relation to the data summarized in Table 12. Only a total society, or each individual community within it, after listening to the arguments of proponents of civil liberties, jurists, penologists, moralists, religious leaders, and mental health professionals, among many other individuals, can decide whether it wishes to wrongly continue to incarcerate two out of every three once-convicted felons because of such psychiatric predictions in order to protect itself from the one-third who, these last base rates indicate, will be the ones who will repeat the criminal assault. The issue is as thorny as is the debate about pornography. There simply are questions which experts are no better equipped to answer than are other citizens, and thus each community must reach its own consensus. Whether psychiatric or psychological diagnosis of dangerous-ness, with its recognized degree of invalidity, is better than no such opinion because of the human costs of overprediction is, at this stage of our knowledge, best left to the courts to decide in each and every individual case. To take an extreme example, one such court may choose to incarcerate indefinitely an individual who savagely and wantonly murders one or a dozen strangers, whereas another court hearing the same testimony about the same individual may decide that prison for a fixed term is ap-propriate. Ziskin (1977 supplement) presents evidence that more and more courts are aware of the other than good validity of such psychiatric predictions and are deciding in favor of defendants instead of the prosecution in such instances. As the art and science of psychiatric diagnosis become even more refined, as bit by bit certainly ap-pears to be the case from the studies so far reviewed in this chapter, the courts and society more generally will have better information on which to base their answers to these questions; questions which expose our moral fabric as a people. When dealing with millions of military recruits during total mobilization in wartime, an increase in predictive validity as to who later will become a psychiatric casualty of, say, 10% or 20% or 30% (see Tables 9 and 10), will help identify correctly hundreds of thousands of such potential future neuropsychiatric casualties. This predictive gain is accom-plished at the cost of erroneously similarly diagnosing many hundreds of thousands of false positives who, experience has shown, will not break down psychiatrically. Such false positives have apparently been a cost society was willing to pay during war-time. Society must now take a close look at predictions of dangerousness, and related diagnoses, within its civilian sectors and determine what price, if any at all, it is willing to pay for even one false-positive diagnosis, let alone a total of 60–95% of all such diagnoses within the legal arena. As mentioned above, scientists can collect such data; society itself must make the value judgment in each individual instance.

14.7. Stability Over Time of Diagnosis of Primary Affective Disorder

The several reviews of the predictive validity of the psychiatric interview in the military situation cited earlier were included in the present chapter because they were prospective studies and as such still are the best such validity studies available. Nevertheless, the fact that they dealt with what Cronbach and Gleser (1965) call a broad-band diagnostic classification—namely psychiatrically "suited" for military duty vs. "unsuited"—was both the strength and the weakness of these military studies. It was a strength because it overcame the problems associated with the low reliabil-ity of the specific diagnoses (see our Table 4) for the reason that by the use of such a rubric as "unsuitable" one lumped together into one global, undifferentiated diag-nosis all the potential reasons why a person was judged inadequate and thus pre-dictably would fail. This lumping together into one broad category removed the problem of discriminating or specifying more finely which type of psychiatric dis-ability was present while it also retained the potential that, if any one of many po-tential problems was present, the opportunity to demonstrate predictive validity for such a condition was enhanced.

The weakness of using general classifications such as "psychiatrically suitable" or "psychiatrically unsuitable" when dealing with everyday psychiatric and behav-ioral conditions in the civilian setting is that they are too general for differential pre-dictions which require different dispositions based on finer differential diagnosis.

With the advent during the 1950s and 1960s of new drugs which are potentially differentially effective for different types of psychiatric and behavioral disabilities, and the seemingly similar potential of biofeedback and the new behavior therapies developed in the 1960s and 1970s, more opportunities than ever before are being presented to the mental health professions to both better treat these conditions and carry out more sophisticated studies of the predictive validity of differential diagnosis.

As described in Sections 9 and 10, Robins, Guze, Winokur, Goodwin, Woodruff, Murphy, and their colleagues at the Washington University School of Medicine in St. Louis have been actively attempting to provide more objective and standardized operational definitions (differential diagnostic criteria) of a number of the most common psychiatric and behavioral dysfunctions. The first successes of that enterprise corresponded with the just-mentioned developments which showed promise for differential pharmacological and behavioral treatment. Not surprisingly, then, the St. Louis group mounted a series of studies which used the follow-up procedure as a criterion measure against which to assess the predictive validity (in the sense of stability of the disorder) of their initial differential diagnosis (predictor). This group has adopted the "disease model" or "natural history model of disease" first proposed by the seventeenth-century London physician Thomas Sydenham as their general model for studying the predictive validity of their objectively standardized, operationally defined, differential psychiatric diagnostic classifications. Sydenham's model employs inductive logic and proved itself immensely fruitful in medical diagnosis during the past three centuries. His model had three requirements which must be met in establishing a disease or disorder as a discrete entity: (1) description of the disease in question (inclusion criteria); (2) delimitation of the disease in question from similar diseases already described (exclusion criteria); (3) follow-up studies, establishing that the disease either goes away or remains the same disease, i.e., does not turn into something else (outcome criteria). To these, the St. Louis group added two more: (4) laboratory findings (as independent measures of etiology and pathogenesis) and (5) family studies showing clustering of the disease (as independent evidence of etiology).

A guiding premise underlying the research of this St. Louis group has been that the validity of differential clinical diagnosis in psychiatry and clinical psychology will remain a matter of faith until systematic programs of research have shown such discrete diagnoses to be stable over time, i.e., not changing into other diseases or dysfunctions. Furthermore, the search for objective and more reliable neuro-biochemical, behavioral, and psychophysiological indices of such stable disorders must be preceded by reliable classification by clinical criteria of homogeneous groups of patients in each clinical classification.

As one test of predictive validity within the natural history model, Murphy, Woodruff, Herjanic, and Fisher (1974) studied prospectively, in a 5-year follow-up design, the natural history of 43 patients given a specific diagnosis of primary affective disorder by use of their published objective criteria. (See this operational definition in Section 9 of this chapter.) The same two diagnosticians (G.E.M. and R.A.W.) diagnosed the patients both initially and at follow-up, using published diagnostic criteria previously agreed on. Different interviewers did the follow-up interviews, and they were blind to the earlier diagnosis and kept that way by being forbidden to inquire about the nature of the complaints and treatment on the index admission. They took only an interval history of the intervening 5 years. In rediagnosing the patients, the authors too were blind to the previous diagnosis and had only the interval history and current clinical picture to work from. (The question of whether a diagnostician might recall after 4 years a diagnosis previously given was answered when one of the authors tested his recall and performed much worse than chance; G. E. Murphy, personal communication.) To some readers this might appear to be but another study in interrater reliability of specific diagnosis. However, following Sydenham's model, Murphy et al. (p. 754) in an important contribution point out that patient reliability (stability of the patient's condition over time) is quite different from either (1) stability of a single diagnostician's test-retest classification or (2) agreement in diagnosis between two independent raters on the same day. If psychiatric conditions are so fickle that any given patient's dysfunction fluctuates haphazardly, changing over time from one discrete diagnostic classification to another highly dissimilar one, studies of reliability of the judgments of clinicians are doomed to failure from the outset. If, on the other hand, a condition such as depression or affective disorder could be shown to be stable over a 5-year period, confidence in the objective criteria used in both its original and its follow-up diagnosis would be enhanced.

In the study here being reviewed, Murphy et al. (1974) found that the second diagnosis independently agreed with the first diagnosis of primary affective disorder given 5 years earlier for 37 out of the 43 patients, i.e., in 86%. It is important to point out that these 43 patients were part of a larger sample of 115 psychiatric patients of whom 82 were reinterviewed after 5 years and that both initially and at follow-up the diagnosticians were asked to classify each patient into one of 19 possible differential psychiatric classifications (e.g., schizophrenia, alcoholism, hysteria, and anxiety neurosis, in addition to primary affective disorder). This 86% agreement is a level of reliability (and predictive validity in the investigator's purposes) for specific diagnosis well beyond that previously reported by other groups (see the present Table 4), although about at the same level as the 84% agreement for depression previously reported by this group and here summarized earlier in the third column of our Table 6.

What this finding means is that use of the operational definition of primary affective disorder (and other psychiatric disorders) promulgated by this group can yield a homogenous cluster of patients who are highly similar on specified criteria, thus facilitating to a considerable extent the probability that further research will not be in vain due to the poor reliability (validity) of the original diagnosis.

As a matter of fact, some additional predictive validity studies of this type as might come to the mind of the reader were carried out by this St. Louis group. These also have dealt with the variables of prognosis over time and stability of the condition over time. For example, Robins and Guze (1970) used the five natural history criteria described earlier in the present section as background for a heuristically useful review of the literature designed to better refine their operationally defined criteria for the diagnosis of schizophrenia. In particular, their review of the published literature on the natural history or course of schizophrenia (however defined subjectively by each investigator) revealed that groups of such samples of patients from throughout the world further divided themselves, over time, into two subgroups: (1) those with a good prognosis (remission from schizophrenia) and (2) those with a poor prognosis (schizophrenia still present). The authors' literature review, plus their own ongoing clinical study, revealed that there is at least one objective criterion that can reliably distinguish between these two postulated subgroups of patients with schizophrenia, namely the psychiatric history of first-degree relatives. Specifically, by use of their own operationally defined criteria for the diagnosis of schizophrenia, they discerned that (1) good-prognosis patients with schizophrenia have a predominance of affective disorder among their psychiatrically ill first-degree relatives, whereas, in contrast, (2) poor-prognosis patients have a predominance of schizophrenia among their first-degree relatives. They concluded furthermore that apparent "schizophrenia" with a good prognosis, what they later reclassified as "schizophreniform illness" (Woodruff, Goodwin, & Guze, 1974, p. 32) is not a mild form of schizophrenia but is, rather, a different disorder altogether. In their view, only poor-prognosis schizophrenia (what others have called chronic, process, or true schizophrenia) should be diagnosed by Bleuler's earlier term, "schizophrenia."

The reader interested in the gains achieved in diagnostic definition by the discovery of such objective criteria will find the chapter on schizophrenia (as well as the other conditions) in the recent Woodruff et al. book (1974) interesting reading.

Stability over time as a variable which enters into differential diagnosis was studied by this same group in primary affective disorder as reviewed above, and also in a series of papers on a sample of patients who did not fit any of the inclusive and exclusive criteria for their other diagnoses and who thus by their criteria are given the positive diagnosis of "undiagnosible."

15. Concurrent Validity

15.1. Adoption Studies in Schizophrenia

It long has been recognized worldwide that the diagnosis schizophrenia is a heterogeneous grab bag which means somewhat different things to each clinician who uses it. Wender (1977) summarizes four different uses of the term *schizophrenia:* (1) process, chronic, or true schizophrenia (Kraepelin's well-described dementia praecox); (2) reactive or acute schizophrenia (used in the United States to designate a schizophrenic condition with a rapid onset, usually in relation to identifiable stress, in individuals with a good premorbid personality adjustment and with good therapeutic prognosis); (3) pseudoneurotic, borderline, or ambulatory schizophrenia (used in the United States, each with its own clinical features); and (4) schizoid or schizothyme (used by Bleuler and Kallman to describe neurotic psychopathology less severe than the psychotic condition of chronic or acute schizophrenia).

Beginning with these four loosely defined but nevertheless relatively homogeneous and clinically seemingly disparate diagnostic classifications of what he and others would later call the "schizophrenic spectrum" of disorders, Wender posed an important question, one open to empirical study: namely do these four diagnostic groups cluster together genetically within an individual family or do they differentiate themselves into genetic transmissions which are discrete for one or more of the four conditions? To get around the thorny nurture vs. nature methodological problem within such family transmission, Wender utilized the strategy of studying adopted vs. biological relatives of schizophrenic patients. Beginning with a total of 5500 adoptees, Wender identified 17 with a diagnosis of chronic schizophrenia, 7 with acute schizophrenia, and 9 with borderline schizophrenia. He identified 33 adoptees as his control group, one carefully matched adoptee with each of these 33 patients in his schizophrenic index group. He next searched for the prevalence of chronic, acute, and borderline schizophrenics, as well as individuals who could be diagnosed as schizoid, in the families of these index and control patients. In time, such painstaking analyses led him to postulate the existence of a schizophrenic spectrum. He recently summarized the results of his adoption studies as follows:

> [These adoption studies] have documented a genetic contribution to the chronic and borderline schizophrenias; they have shown that the borderline schizophrenias are related to the chronic schizophrenias; and they have, in addition, provided some evidence that the acute schizophrenias and the schizoid states may also be related to the "true" schizophrenias. The data are stronger for the borderline schizophrenias and schizoid states; therefore, before the membership of the latter in the schizophrenic spectrum is seconded, additional confirmatory data are needed. Finally, these studies have not only documented the existence of a relationship between borderline schizophrenia(s) and chronic schizophrenia but have, by a logical bootstrap operation, helped us to define the characteristics of the borderline schizophrenias. This should be of considerable value in its own right, for only by breaking down this confusing group of disorders into relatively homogeneous groups can we hope to obtain meaningful data in regard to their natural history, pathogenesis, diagnosis, and response to treatment. (Wender, 1977, pp. 126–127)

It is obvious from this brief summary statement that the use of reasonably clear operational definitions of four homogeneous subgroupings within the global schizophrenia rubric combined with the methodology of using adoptees has helped refine even further each of these four initial subgroupings. It is the further use of bootstrap operations of the type utilized by Wender that will bring even greater clarity (reliability and validity) to the diagnosis of schizophrenia and other mental disorders. We turn next to the studies in Iowa of Winokur, one of the early members of the St. Louis group, on the affective disorders as a second example of the use of family history in the better delineation of a specific in contrast to a global psychiatric diagnosis.

15.2. Genetic Studies in the Affective Disorders

Winokur (1977) has recently reviewed his investigations during the past two decades of genetic transmission in the study of the affective disorders. He acknowledges that the vast bulk of published data in psychiatric diagnosis is concerned with (1) the clinical description of the syndrome and (2) the course of the disorder. And although he points out that (3) response to differential treatment is still in its infancy as a new diagnostic tool, he believes that the most efficient way to make a diagnosis ultimately is by (4) the use of signs, symptoms, and behaviors that are pathognomonic for each psychiatric disorder. Unfortunately, few pathognomonic psychiatric or behavioral indicators which are observable in a patient have been discerned to date. As a result, Winokur and others have turned their search to pathognomonic indicators which might be discerned in the family history.

Specifically, Winokur (1) identified a group of patients with a homogeneous clinical picture and outcome, (2) further separated these patients into subgroups on the basis of specific variables (e.g., age at onset, sex, special clinical features), and (3) next searched for specific genetic-familial configurations of psychiatric disorders in these subgroups. As an alternative methodology, he occasionally began with step 3 and worked backward through steps 2 and 1. In one early study he and his colleagues began with 426 patients who by clinical criteria manifested an affective disorder. These 426 patients were next further subdivided into two groups: (1) those who had a two-generation history (parent and proband or parent and child) of affective disorder and (2) those with no other family history of psychiatric disorder. The results of this family study showed that those patients who had a two-generation history of affective disorder had a highly significant excess of admissions for mania, but, equally interesting, their family histories showed no difference in prior admissions for depression. Thus, starting with a difference in apparent familial transmission (two-generation vs. one-generation), Winokur and his colleagues discovered the presence of a previously unsuspected additional clinical finding, namely that mania is significantly more likely to be found in a family where there are two generations of affectively disordered individuals than in a family where no other psychiatric disorder is present. Inasmuch as the syndrome of depression, in contrast to mania, does not differ in terms of familial transmission, Winokur postulated that there are at least two reliably and validly distinct types of affective disorder: (1) manic-depressive disorder and (2) depressive disorder. That is, that as suggested above by Wender about schizophrenia, depression also covers a broad spectrum of distinct but related disorders. Winokur points out that, in studies concurrent in time with his own, Angst in Zurich and Perris in Sweden started with patients with both mania and depression and compared them to patients showing only depression and came up with a similar finding. Perris utilized the diagnosis of "bipolar" for those patients with mania and depression and the diagnosis of "unipolar" for those patients with depression alone.

These early findings of apparent differential genetic transmission in the different affective disorders helped launch still additional studies during the past decade, specifically, neurochemical and electrophysiological studies of the affective disorders as well as studies utilizing a variety of demographic variables. Space does not permit a full review of these studies here, although the following recent summary statement by Winokur suggests the methodology used and the general nature of the studies conducted by his group and other investigators:

It is clear that depression disease is more likely seen in early onset patients. To use a definition of depression spectrum disease which encompasses these points is unwieldly. Further . . . one may note that the depressed relatives of the early onset patients are equally likely to have a late onset (before and after 40). There is a logical problem in using the age of onset as a defining factor. An early onset female could well be used as a depression spectrum disease proband; however, if her relative had an illness after 40, one would question the validity of this break. In fact, this late onset relative could be used as a pure depression disease proband. For these reasons, we have been concerned with a reasonable and workable definition of depression spectrum disease. As a significant qualitative and quantitative difference seems to be the presence or absence of alcoholism in a family, *we have defined depression spectrum disease as an illness in any patient who had a rigorously diagnosed depression and has an alcoholic or antisocial member in the first-degree relative group*. Certainly, from the family studies, the presence of alcoholism or antisocial personality in a first-degree relative would be associated with being an early onset female depressive but this would not be an invariable finding. There would be too much overlap with other types of patients. Thus, the definition of depression spectrum disease is dependent on the familial disease pattern as well as the clinical picture in the proband. (Winokur, 1977, p. 146)

To this Winokur then added the following recapitulation:

Through the use of genetic variables, it has been possible to separate bipolar from unipolar affective disorder . . . Using a similar methodology, it has been possible to delineate two types of unipolar disorders—depression spectrum disease and pure depressive disease. An initial workup using a linkage methodology has suggested that these two unipolar illnesses are in fact distinct entities. Should the findings be replicated, we will be able to say that three types of affective disorders have been discovered, where in the past only one was presumed to have existed. (Winokur, 1977, p. 150)

15.3. Biochemical and Other Pathophysiological Studies

Throughout this chapter we stressed that differential psychiatric classification and diagnosis have been based in the past primarily on (1) the clinical symptomatology and related features, (2) etiology (as in paresis or Korsakoff syndrome), and (3) the natural history or course of the disorder. Advances in the study of the neurobiology of mental and behavioral disorders since 1958 have added heuristically and clinically provocative new findings on which to erect a fourth and potentially even more reliable and valid diagnostic definition for some of these disorders, namely the unique and operationally specifiable and clinically demonstrable biochemical and pathophysiological indicators which are associated with them.

Van Praag (1977) reviews the history of these biomedical discoveries in depression, albeit, interestingly, he uses terminology for this disorder which differs from that of Winokur and his co-workers. He begins with the parallel facts that concurrent with, but independent of, the introduction of antidepressant drugs as a therapy for depressions in 1958 two different types of compounds with such an antidepressant effect were discovered. These were (1) tricyclic antidepressants (prototype imipramine, Tofranil) and monamine oxidase (MAO) inhibitors (prototype iproniazid, Marsilid). Although these tricyclic antidepressants and MAO inhibitors are chemically unrelated, they show two important similarities: (1) clinically they each exert a beneficial therapeutic effect on depression (especially "vital" or "endogenous" depression) and (2) biochemically they each behave as monoamine agonists in the brain, albeit via different mechanisms.

Van Praag then reviews a large number of biomedical studies carried out during the past 20 years in this broad field, including studies on metabolism, related chemical research, postmortem research, pharmacological research, and therapeutics. This review leads him to offer the following general conclusions:

> I believe that the above discussed relations between monoamine metabolism and treatment results with compounds which influence monoamine lend support to two concepts—the concept that disorders of central monoamine metabolism can play a role in the pathogenesis of "vital" (endogenous) depressions, and the concept that the group of "vital" depressions is a heterogeneous one in biochemical terms. At least two types of "vital" depression exist; 5-hydroxytryptamine (serotonin) deficiency plays a role in the pathogenesis of one, while noradrenaline deficiency is important in the pathogenesis of the other. Both of these types of depression are indistinguishable in psychopathological terms.
>
> Patients of the first group seem to respond best to antidepressants with a strong ability to potentiate 5-hydroxytryptamine (serotonin) and less to noradrenaline-potentiating compounds, while the reverse applies to the noradrenaline-deficient patient. The cerebrospinal fluid supplies no reliable information on the presence or absence of a central noradrenaline deficiency; . . . renal 3-methoxy-4-hydroxyphenylglycol excretion is more instructive in this respect. . . . It was already known that renal 3-methoxy-4-hydroxyphenylglycol and cerebrospinal fluid show poor correlation. A possible explanation is that 3-methoxy-4-hydroxyphenylglycol in the lumbar cerebrospinal fluid is chiefly of spinal, not of cerebral origin. (Van Praag, 1977, pp. 177–179).

These quotations from Van Praag, and the ones from Winokur and Wender included in the immediately preceding section, provide the reader with insight into the directions of the investigative steps that have been taken during the past decade to produce the considerable improvement in the reliability of the specific diagnoses which occurred between the time of the studies shown in our Tables 6 and 7 and the time of earlier studies shown in our Table 4. The recent statements of Spitzer, Sheehy, and Endicott (1977), the form of an earlier definition for affective disorder which we included earlier in Section 9 of this chapter, the Research Diagnostic Criteria (RDC) of Spitzer, Endicott, and Robins (1977), and the standardized Diagnostic Interview of Endicott and Spitzer (1977) suggest that the soon-to-be-introduced DSM III will contain operational definitions of specific diagnostic classifications which potentially may utilize family history and otherwise may approximate in detail the operational specificity suggested in the quotations from Wender and from Winokur. These new features no doubt will make DSM III a more useful document than is DSM II. That other problems may appear also is clear, and we turn next to one of these.

16. DSM III: An Increase in Reliability, Validity, and Also Interprofessional Conflict

Throughout this chapter, reference has been made to the earlier DSM I, the current DSM II, and the forthcoming DSM III. Although each of these diagnostic classificatory systems was a product of the work of successive committees of the American Psychiatric Association, the research on the reliability and validity of diagnosis of the products of these systems, which we reviewed in detail throughout this chapter, was carried out by scientists with allegiance to no single professional guild. That is, the scientists and clinicians who have used these diagnostic systems have been clinical psychologists and other social behavioral scientists as well as psychiatrists. A criticism recently was forthrightly sounded by Schacht and Nathan (1977) that the developers of DSM III are not being allowed to do their work guided solely by scientific criteria but instead are injecting into DSM III self-serving, partisan elements which reflect exclusively a medical model for all the psychiatric and behavioral dysfunctions and which thus can help only the guild of psychiatry in the economic arena of clinical practice. Nathan has served as a member of a three-person committee of the American Psychological Association which had liaison with the DSM III committee of the American Psychiatric Association and thus has observed firsthand the types of political issues which can cloud the development of a new and otherwise heuristically important scientific system. Following their cataloguing of the positive contributions of DSM III, Schacht and Nathan provide the reader with a glimpse of how a large number of mental health clinicians and scientists will regard DSM III with other than enthusiasm:

> To imply, as [do the developers of DSM-III], that DSM-III was influenced only by professional concerns rather than professional territorialism suggests to us an exceptional lack of candor. . . .
>
> In our judgment, DSM-III has the potential to be very bad for psychologists, despite the real and potential advances in scope, diagnostic reliability, and diagnostic logic it represents. . . . It is entirely possible, for example, that promulgation of DSM-III as an official action of the American Psychiatric Association will carry sufficient weight to call it to the attention of insurers and legislators who will see in it quasi-official recognition of the primacy of physicians in the diagnosis and treatment of the disorders categorized by DSM-III.

Perusal of the references which end this chapter will reveal that the scientists who have brought the study of the reliability and validity of psychiatric and behavioral diagnosis to the threshhold of scientific respectability (1) have come from a number of different professions and (2) have published their operational definitions and their reliability and validity correlates and exemplars in scientific journals which have allegiance to society and not to a single guild. As a member of the scientific community, the present writer is proud of the scientists who have contributed to these advances and whose works he reviewed here. Much of what will be DSM III already is published in the open literature and has been reviewed in the present chapter. It would be embarrassing for all of us if DSM III or the companion documents which other guilds purportedly are attempting to develop in competition with DSM III were published in other than the open scientific literature. The race in the open field of science has been and continues to be exhilarating and rewarding enough for each of us. Having shown that psychiatric and behavioral diagnoses have adequate reliability and beginning validity, those of us who are interested next can launch the series of programmatic studies which will be needed to begin to unravel the question of which of these conditions are exclusively medical or behavioral, or a combination of both.

17. References

Acheson, R. M. Observer error and variation in the interpretation of electrocardiograms in an epidemiological study of coronary heart disease. *British Journal of Preventive and Social Medicine*, 1960, *14*, 99–122.

American Psychiatric Association. *Diagnostic and statistical manual, mental disorders, first edition.* Washington, D.C., 1952.

Ash, P. The reliability of psychiatric diagnosis. *Journal of Abnormal and Social Psychology*, 1949, *44*, 272–277.

Beck, A. T. Reliability of psychiatric diagnoses: A critique of systematic studies. *American Journal of Psychiatry*, 1962, *119*, 210–216.

Beck, A. T., Ward, C. H., Mendelson, M., Mock, J. E., & Erbaugh, J. K. Reliability of psychiatric diagnoses. II. A study of consistency of clinical judgments and ratings. *American Journal of Psychiatry*, 1962, *119*, 351–357.

Bellows, R. M., & Estep, M. F. *Employment psychology: The interview.* New York: Rinehart, 1954.

Benney, M., Riesman, D., & Star, S. A. Age and sex in the interview. *American Journal of Sociology*, 1956, *62*, 143–152.

Blashfield, R. K., & Draguns, J. G. Evaluative criteria for psychiatric classification. *Journal of Abnormal Psychology*, 1976, *85*, 140–150.

Boisen, A. Types of dementia praecox: A study in psychiatric classification. *Psychiatry*, 1938, *1*, 233–236.

Carpenter, W. T., Jr., Strauss, J. S., & Bartko, J. J. Flexible system for the diagnosis of schizophrenia: Report from the WHO International Pilot Study of Schizophrenia. *Science*, 1973, *182*, 1275–1278.

Caveny, E. L., Wittson, C. L., Hunt, W. A., & Herrmann, R. S. Psychiatric diagnosis: Its nature and function. *Journal of Nervous and Mental Disease*, 1955, *121*, 367–373.

Cohen, J. A coefficient of agreement for nominal scales. *Educational and Psychological Measurement*, 1960, *20*, 37–46.

Cronbach, L. J., & Gleser, G. C. *Psychological tests and personnel decisions* (2nd ed.). Urbana: University of Illinois Press, 1965.

Durant, W. *The story of civilization: The life of Greece* (Vol. 2). New York: Simon and Schuster, 1939.

Edwards, G. Diagnosis of schizophrenia: An Anglo-American comparison. *British Journal of Psychiatry*, 1972, *120*, 385–390.

Egan, J. R., Jackson, L., & Eanes, R. H. Study of neuropsychiatric rejectees. *Journal of the American Medical Association*, 1951, *145*, 466–469.

Ehrenwald, J. *The history of psychotherapy: From healing magic to encounter.* New York: Jason Aronson, 1976.

Ellenberger, H. E. *The discovery of the unconscious: The history and evolution of dynamic psychiatry.* New York: Basic Books, 1970.

Endicott, J., & Spitzer, R. L. A diagnostic interview: The schedule for affective disorders and schizophrenia. Paper presented at the meeting of the American Psychiatric Association, Toronto, May 1977.

Ennis, B. J., & Litwack, T. R. Psychiatry and the presumption of expertise: Flipping coins in the courtroom. *California Law Review,* 1974, *62,* 693–752.

Eysenck, H. J. *The scientific study of personality.* London: Routledge, 1952.

Eysenck, H. J. Classification and the problem of diagnosis. In H. J. Eysenck (Ed.), *Handbook of abnormal psychology: An experimental approach.* New York: Basic Books, 1961, pp. 1–31.

Feighner, J. P., Robins, E., Guze, S. B., Woodruff, R. A., Winokur, G., & Munoz, R. Diagnostic criteria for use in psychiatric research. *Archives of General Psychiatry,* 1972, *26,* 57–63.

Felson, B., Morgan, W. K. C., Bristol, L. J., Tendergrass, E., Dessen, E., Linton, O., & Regen, R. Observations on the results of multiple readings of chest films in coal miner's pneumoconiosis. *Radiology,* 1973, *109,* 19–23.

Fisher, J., Epstein, L. J., & Harris, M. R. Validity of the psychiatric interview. *Archives of General Psychiatry,* 1967, *17,* 744–750.

Fleiss, J. L. Measuring nominal scale agreement among many raters. *Psychological Bulletin,* 1971, *76,* 378–382.

Fleiss, J. L., Spitzer, R. L., Cohen, J., & Endicott, J. Three computer diagnosis methods compared. *Archives of General Psychiatry,* 1972, *27,* 643–649.

Foulds, G. The reliability of psychiatric and validity of psychological diagnosis. *Journal of Mental Science,* 1955, *101,* 851–862.

Ginzberg, E., Anderson, J. K., Ginsberg, S. W., & Herma, J. L. *The ineffective soldier: Lessons for management and the nation* (Vol. 1). *The lost divisions.* New York: Columbia University Press, 1959.

Helzer, J. E., Clayton, P. J., Pambakian, R., Reich, T., Woodruff, R. A., Jr., & Reveley, M. A. Reliability of psychiatric diagnosis. II. The test-retest reliability of diagnostic classification. *Archives of General Psychiatry,* 1977, *34,* 136–141.

Helzer, J. E., Robins, L. N., Taibleson, M., Woodruff, R. A., Jr., Reich, T., & Wish, E. D. Reliability of psychiatric diagnosis. I. A methodological review. *Archives of General Psychiatry,* 1977, *34,* 129–133.

Hoiberg, A., Hysham, C. J., & Berry, N. H. The neuropsychiatric implications of illiteracy: Twenty years later. *Journal of Clinical Psychology,* 1974, *30,* 533–535.

Holt, R. R., & Luborsky, L. *Personality patterns of psychiatrists: Vols. I and II.* New York: Basic Books, 1958.

Holtzman, W. H., & Sells, S. B. Prediction of flying success by clinical analysis of test protocols. *Journal of Abnormal and Social Psychology,* 1954, *49,* 485–490.

Hunt, H. F. Clinical methods: Psychodiagnostics. In C. P. Stone & D. W. Taylor (Eds.), *Annual Review of Psychology,* 1950, *1,* 207–220.

Hunt, W. A. An investigation of naval neuropsychiatric screening procedures. In H. Guetzkow (Ed.), *Groups, leadership, and men.* Pittsburgh: Carnegie Press, 1951, pp. 245–256.

Hunt, W. A. A rationale for psychiatric selection. *American Psychologist,* 1955, *10,* 199–204.

Hunt, W. A., Herrmann, R. S., & Noble, H. The specificity of the psychiatric interview. *Journal of Clinical Psychology,* 1957, *13,* 49–53.

Hunt, W. A., Schwartz, M. L., & Walker, R. E. The correctness of diagnostic judgment as a function of diagnostic bias and population rate. *Journal of Clinical Psychology,* 1964, *20,* 143–145.

Hunt, W. A., & Wittson, C. L. The neuropsychiatric implications of illiteracy. *U.S. Armed Forces Medical Journal,* 1951, *2,* 365–369.

Hunt, W. A., Wittson, C. L., & Hunt, E. B. The relationship between definiteness of psychiatric diagnosis and severity of disability. *Journal of Clinical Psychology,* 1952, *8,* 314–315.

Hunt, W. A., Wittson, C. L., & Hunt, E. B. A theoretical and practical analysis of the diagnostic process. In P. H. Hoch & J. Zubin (Eds.), *Current problems in psychiatric diagnosis.* New York: Grune & Stratton, 1953, pp. 53–65.

Kahn, R. L., & Cannell, C. F. *The dynamics of interviewing: Theory, technique, and cases.* New York: Wiley, 1957.

Kandler, H., Plutchik, R., Conte, H., & Siegel, B. Prediction of performance of psychiatric residents: A three-year follow-up study. *American Journal of Psychiatry,* 1975, *12,* 1286–1290.

Kant, I. [*The classification of mental disorders*] (C. T. Sullivan, translator). Doylestown, Pa.: The Doylestown Foundation, 1964. (Originally published 1790.)

Kelly, E. L., & Fiske, D. W. *The prediction of performance in clinical psychology.* Ann Arbor: University of Michigan Press, 1951.

Kelly, E. L., & Goldberg, L. R. Correlates of later performance and specialization in psychology: A follow-up study of the trainees assessed in the VA Selection Research Project. *Psychological Monographs,* 1959, *73,* No. 12 (Whole No. 482).

Kempf, E. J. *Psychopathology.* St. Louis: Mosby, 1920.

Kephart, N. G. *The employment interview in industry.* New York: McGraw-Hill, 1952.

Koran, L. M. The reliability of clinical methods, data and judgments: Part I. *New England Journal of Medicine,* 1975, *293,* 642–646. (a)

Koran, L. M. The reliability of clinical methods, data and judgments: Part II. *New England Journal of Medicine,* 1975, *293,* 695–701. (b)

Kreitman, N., Sainsbury, P., Morrissey, J., Towers, J., & Scrivener, J. The reliability of psychiatric diagnosis. *Journal of Mental Science,* 1961, *107,* 887–908.

London, H. Power and acceptance theory. In B. B. Wolman (Ed.), *International encyclopedia of psychiatry, psychology, psychoanalysis, & neurology.* New York: Van Nostrand/Aesculapius, 1977, Vol. 9, pp. 11–13.

Martorano, R. D., & Nathan, P. E. Syndromes of psychosis and nonpsychosis: Factor analysis of a systems analysis. *Journal of Abnormal Psychology,* 1972, *80,* 1–10.

Martorano, R. D., & Nathan, P. E. *Cluster analysis and multidimensional scaling of psychopathological cues.* Unpublished manuscript, 1978.

Masserman, J. H., & Carmichael, H. T. Diagnosis and prognosis in psychiatry: With a follow-up study of the results of short-term general hospital therapy in psychiatric cases. *Journal of Mental Science,* 1938, *84,* 893–946.

Matarazzo, J. D. The interview. In B. B. Wolman (Ed.), *Handbook of clinical psychology.* New York: McGraw-Hill, 1965, pp. 403–450.

Matarazzo, J. D. The history of psychotherapy. In G. A. Kimble & K. Schlesinger (Eds.), *The history of psychology.* New York: Wiley, 1979, in press.

Mehlman, B. The reliability of psychiatric diagnosis. *Journal of Abnormal and Social Psychology,* 1952, *47,* 577–578.

Melrose, J. P., Stroebel, C. F., & Glueck, B. C. Diagnosis of psychopathology using stepwise multiple discriminant analysis: I. *Comprehensive Psychiatry,* 1970, *11,* 43–50.

Menninger, K., Mayman, M., & Pruyser, P. *The vital balance: The life process in mental health and illness.* New York: Viking, 1963.

Murphy, G. E., Woodruff, R. A., Jr., Herjanic, M., & Fischer, J. R. Validity of the diagnosis of primary affective disorder: A prospective study with a five-year follow-up. *Archives of General Psychiatry,* 1974, *30,* 751–756.

Norden, C., Philipps, E., Levy, P., & Kass, E. Variation in interpretation of intravenous pyelograms. *American Journal of Epidemiology,* 1970, *91,* 155–160.

OSS Assessment Staff. *Assessment of men.* New York: Holt, 1948.

Pasamanick, B., Diniz, S., & Lefton, M. Psychiatric orientation and its relation to diagnosis and treatment in a mental hospital. *American Journal of Psychiatry,* 1959, *116,* 127–132.

Plag, J. A., & Arthur, R. J. Psychiatric re-examination of unsuitable naval recruits: A two-year follow-up. *American Journal of Psychiatry,* 1965, *122,* 534–541.

Plag, J. A., & Goffman, J. M. The prediction of four-year military effectiveness from characteristics of naval recruits. *Military Medicine,* 1966, *131,* 729–735.

Raines, G. N., & Rohrer, J. H. The operational matrix of psychiatric practice. I. Consistency and variability in interview impressions of different psychiatrists. *American Journal of Psychiatry,* 1955, *111,* 721–733.

Raines, G. N., & Rohrer, J. H. The operational matrix of psychiatric practice. II. Variability in psychiatric impressions and the projection hypothesis. *American Journal of Psychiatry,* 1960, *117,* 133–139.

Raines, G. N., Wittson, C. L., Hunt, W. A., & Herrmann, R. S. Psychiatric selection for military service. *Journal of the American Medical Association,* 1954, *156,* 817–821.

Riesman, D., & Benney, M. The sociology of the interview. *Midwest Sociologist,* 1956, *18,* 3–15.

Robins, E., & Guze, S. B. Establishment of diagnostic validity in psychiatric illness: Its application to schizophrenia. *American Journal of Psychiatry,* 1970, *126,* 983–987.

Roe, A. Integration of personality theory and clinical practice. *Journal of Abnormal and Social Psychology,* 1949, *44,* 36–41.

Rotter, J. *Social learning and clinical psychology.* Englewood Cliffs, N.J.: Prentice-Hall, 1954.

Sandifer, M. G., Pettus, C., & Quade, D. A study of psychiatric diagnosis. *Journal of Nervous and Mental Disease*, 1964, *139*, 350–356.

Schacht T., & Nathan, P. E. But is it good for the psychologists? Appraisal and status of DSM-III. *American Psychologist*, 1977, *32*, 1017–1025.

Schmidt, H., & Fonda, C. The reliability of psychiatric diagnosis: A new look. *Journal of Abnormal and Social Psychology*, 1956, *52*, 262–267.

Scott, J. Research definitions of mental health and mental illness. *Psychological Bulletin*, 1958, *55*, 29–45.

Seeman, W. P. Psychiatric diagnosis: An investigation of interperson-reliability after didactic instruction. *Journal of Nervous and Mental Disease*, 1953, *118*, 541–544.

Sharp, W. L. Fate of 395 mild neuropsychiatric cases salvaged from training period and taken into combat. *American Journal of Psychiatry*, 1950, *106*, 801–807.

Spitzer, R. L., Cohen, J., Fleiss, J. L., & Endicott, J. Quantification of agreement in psychiatric diagnosis. *Archives of General Psychiatry*, 1967, *17*, 83–87.

Spitzer, R. L., & Endicott, J. Can the computer assist clinicians in psychiatric diagnosis? *American Journal of Psychiatry*, 1974, *131*, 523–530.

Spitzer, R. L., Endicott, J., Cohen, J., & Fleiss, J. L. Constraints on the validity of computer diagnosis. *Archives of General Psychiatry*, 1974, *31*, 197–203.

Spitzer, R. L., Endicott, J., & Robins, E. Clinical criteria for psychiatric diagnosis and DSM-III. *American Journal of Psychiatry*, 1975, *132*, 1187–1192.

Spitzer, R. L., Endicott, J., & Robins, E. Research diagnostic criteria: Rationale and reliability. Paper presented at the meeting of the American Psychiatric Association, Toronto, May 1977.

Spitzer, R. L., & Fleiss, J. L. A re-analysis of the reliability of psychiatric diagnosis. *British Journal of Psychiatry*, 1974, *125*, 341–347.

Spitzer, R. L., Sheehy, M., & Endicott, J. DSM-III: Guiding principles. In V. M. Rakoff, H. C. Stancer, & H. B. Kedward (Eds.), *Psychiatric diagnosis*. New York: Brunner-Mazel, 1977, pp. 1–24.

Stoller, R. J. Psychoanalytic diagnosis. In V. M. Rakoff, H. C. Stancer, & H. B. Kedward (Eds.), *Psychiatric diagnosis*. New York: Brunner-Mazel, 1977, pp. 25–41.

Van Praag, H. M. The vulnerable brain: Biological factors in the diagnosis and treatment of depression. In V. M. Rakoff, H. C. Stancer, & H. B. Kedward (Eds.), *Psychiatric diagnosis*. New York: Brunner-Mazel, 1977, pp. 153–188.

Wender, P. H. The scope and validity of the schizophrenic spectrum concept. In V. M. Rakoff, H. C. Stancer, & H. B. Kedward (Eds.), *Psychiatric diagnosis*. New York: Brunner-Mazel, 1977, pp. 109–127.

Wilkins, W. L., Anderhalter, O. F., Rigby, M. K., & Stimson, P. *Statistical description of criterion measures for USMC junior officers* (Tech. Rep. No. 5). St. Louis: St. Louis University, Department of Psychology, 1955.

Wilson, M. S., & Meyer, E. Diagnostic consistency in a psychiatric liaison service. *American Journal of Psychiatry*, 1962, *119*, 207–209.

Winokur, G. Genetic patterns as they affect psychiatric diagnosis. In V. M. Rakoff, H. C. Stancer, & H. B. Kedward (Eds.), *Psychiatric diagnosis*. New York: Brunner-Mazel, 1977, pp. 128–152.

Wittson, C. L., & Hunt, W. A. The predictive value of the brief psychiatric interview. *American Journal of Psychiatry*, 1951, *107*, 582–585.

Wolberg, L. R. *The technique of psychotherapy*. New York: Grune & Stratton, 1954.

Wolman, B. B. Schizophrenia and related disorders. In B. B. Wolman (Ed.), *Handbook of clinical psychology*. New York: McGraw-Hill, 1965, pp. 976–1029.

Wolman, B. B. *Call no man normal*. New York: International Universities Press, 1973.

Woodruff, R. A., Jr., Goodwin, D. W., & Guze, S. B. *Psychiatric diagnosis*. New York: Oxford University Press, 1974.

Zigler, E., & Phillips, L. Psychiatric diagnosis: A critique. *Journal of Abnormal and Social Psychology*, 1961, *63*, 607–618.

Zilboorg, G. *A history of medical psychology*. New York: Norton, 1941.

Ziskin, J. *Coping with psychiatric and psychological testimony*. Beverly Hills: Law and Psychology Press, 1975 (Pocket Supplement 1977).

Zubin, J. Classification of the behavior disorders. In P. R. Farnsworth, O. McNemar, & Q. McNemar (Eds.). *Annual review of psychology* (Vol. 18). Palo Alto, Calif.: Annual Reviews, Inc., 1967, pp. 373–406.

4

An Overview of Psychological Measurement

JUM C. NUNNALLY

1. Introduction

Because this book is being written for clinical psychologists, psychiatrists, and kindred professionals, in this chapter it will be assumed that the reader is already familiar with fundamental issues relating to behavioral measurement and, consequently, that there will be no need to discuss low-level principles. Rather, the discussion will center on controversial issues that are of immediate importance to the professional clinician or researcher in the behavioral sciences. Whereas the examples chosen for this chapter to illustrate principles of measurement are particularly applicable to clinical diagnosis, the principles are quite general to empirical science. Because some methods of statistical and mathematical analysis are intimately related to the development and use of measurement methods, critical comments will be made about some prominent approaches to statistical analysis, but details regarding their applications will be left to referenced sources rather than be discussed in detail here. (Any reader who is not already familiar with fundamental principles of psychometric theory and analysis, or would like a refresher course in that regard, might want to consult my book *Psychometric Theory*, 1978.)

I started writing about the generality of measurement problems in science and the usefulness of related methods of mathematical analysis long before I had the actual experience to substantiate the case, e.g., in my first book on psychological measurement (1959). I sensed this generality of principles, and, more importantly, I was told this was so by older and wiser hands who specialized in various aspects of psychological measurement, e.g., in the lectures of the great L. L. Thurstone. As I gradually became involved as a consultant or participant in some manner or another in a wide variety of projects, I came to realize how genuinely true such state-

JUM C. NUNNALLY • Department of Psychology, Vanderbilt University, Nashville, Tennessee 37203.

ments are regarding the generality of measurement methods and attendant methods of analysis. I have found similar principles to apply in an extremely wide variety of scientific issues in psychology, psychiatry, numerous fields of medicine, and law, and in special issues in the physical sciences and engineering, particularly biomedical engineering. Indeed, I have been surprised at the commonality of issues regarding psychological measurement that runs through these various disciplines. I have been even more surprised to find that some research issues regarding what I had thought of as "psychometrics" were more easily testable on physiological variables such as brain waves and pupillary response than on more conventional psychological measures such as achievement tests in arithmetic and personality inventories relating to adjustment.

1.1. Science and Clinical Art

A great deal of ink has been spilled and unkind words have been said regarding the requirements for psychometric methods in research as opposed to clinical practice. Amid unseemly snickers, basic researchers (primarily those who specialize in psychometrics) claim that many of the clinicians' would-be measures lack the refinements of standardization, with all the name implies, and that many of them are at the level of crystal-ball gazing and soothsaying psychologizing. With indignant response, the clinicians have claimed that many of the supposedly well-honed tools of the basic researchers concern only surface-layer trivia and fail to touch the deep richness of human psychological processes. When the partisan rudeness is wrung out of them, both points of view contain a germ of truth; and the outlooks on psychometric theory and analysis for basic science and clinical practice should be compatible.

The squabbles about measurement methods and indeed the inherent problems of measurement themselves relate to the fact that it simply is difficult to study people. The basic scientist is frequently frustrated by the inability to conduct experiments that produce interesting results, and the clinician is frequently frustrated by the intractability of patients to be understood or to lend themselves to successful treatment. Although psychological phenomena are the most intriguing with which any basic researchers or clinical practitioners deal (indeed, one finds this sentiment expressed by people in disciplines far removed from the behavioral sciences), working in the people-oriented disciplines requires tolerance of ambiguity and the ability to operate on low-percentage-of-reward schedules. The difficulties of finding adequate measurement methods for prominent theoretical constructs have had some adverse effects on at least some individuals in both basic science and applied work, or at least so it would seem from my own personal contacts and what is said in print. Some of the more hard-nosed, brass-instrument, basic researchers in psychology (some of the very best ones, so I would judge) have retreated into the study of extremely simple processes relating to memory, reaction time, and perception—as much or more because the phenomena are easily subjected to measurement and experimental control as because they are intrinsically interesting to the investigators or anyone else. In contrast, some of our clinical brethren, in despair of finding standardized measures of truly meaningful human attributes, have retreated into a holistic, existential jargon. In this heady atmosphere, one is not sure whether the goal is to develop clinical practice, a new religion that considers Zen Buddhism as dealing only in low-level abstractions, or a new political movement whose major thrust is to update the Bill of Rights to include the right to be a narcissistic "weirdo." Clinicians who are disposed to these "states of consciousness" are not very accepting of even tried-and-true psychometric hardware such as old-fashioned IQ tests and personality inventories, much less receptive of efforts to measure a broader spectrum of human attributes. In contrast to the fringe extreme of humanistic thinkers with respect to clinical problems, the psychometrician encounters as much "guff" but in a different form from the opposing extreme of behavior-mod zealots. Some of these zealots (usually young professionals who are long on training in techniques and short on seasoned wisdom) see very little need for measures of a broad spectrum of psychological characteristics, for the following reasons: (1) the problems which are attacked are rather easily observed and frequently directly counted or simply measured in some other way (smoking, drinking, eating too much, phobic reactions, etc.); (2) since the "training program" works for everyone, all that is necessary is to manipulate the "parameters" of the Skinnerian-like training program, and it really does not matter much what the individual is like other than for the specific symptom for which he is being treated; (3) since the intention in the training program is to establish a relatively ideal state with respect to the initial problem (bring everyone to "asymptote"), measurement is not a problem with respect to either the specific symptom or the characteristics of the individual more generally.

With the above considerations in mind, one would think that the outlook is dismal indeed for the individual who wants to promote better measurement of a broad spectrum of important human attributes, but such is not really the case. As clinicians we should diagnose and cure ourselves in this regard by realizing that much of the negativistic rhetoric concerning psychological measurement has sprung from rationalization and a variety of other defense mechanisms related to the frustration of not having easily obtained, adequate measurement methods. Actually, I think that better methods of measurement will be readily accepted once they are on the scene.

To make an absolute guess about the matter, I suspect that at least half of the people who end up in a particular profession entered training initially because of some rather unpredictable event. Examples are the clinical psychologist who never would have gone into it at all if a girlfriend had not talked him into auditing a lecture by a spellbinding teacher in introductory psychology or the medical student who had a rewarding set of experiences in his internship training under the tutelage of a wise and kindly old psychiatrist. However, as they evolve in their training, my theory is that "mental professionals" become dominated by one of two semiparanoid fantasies to develop either (1) a mind-reading machine or (2) a mind-controlling machine. To poke fun at my brethren in clinical practice, the former would be represented by analytically oriented clinicians and the latter would be represented by behavior-mod advocates. The mindreader type certainly needs adequate psychological measures, because they constitute the method par excellence for dragging out the very soul of each individual. This is the spirit in which the Rorschach test was developed, and that same spirit was extended into the development of the MMPI and more modern measuring instruments. Although the mind-controlling type tends to be less receptive of the need for standardized psychological measures, both professional experience and the weight of sound argument are convincing that even if excellent controlling techniques are developed (e.g., types of token economies in mental hospitals), there are many needs for psychological measurement in understanding the initial status of the individual, properly assigning the individual to an individualized treatment strategy, progressively adjusting the treatment program in terms of changing status, and assessing overall competence and personality characteristics after treatment. For the above reasons, the present author is inclined to view much of the indifference or hostility toward concepts of standardized measurement as being a defensive reaction to personal frustrations and senses of insecurity on the part of professional people, much as occurred in hostile responses to the innovations of Jenner, Pasteur, Freud, Rogers, and, more recently, advocates of behavior modification techniques.

1.2. The Scientific Study of Personality

The major problem in the study of human personality is not so much that the topic is outside the ken of science but rather that the data-gathering process frequently is so illusive as to make it extremely difficult to put typical scientific methods to work. A primary example that I witness numerous times each day is in the highly metaphorical way in which we communicate to one another in gestures, choices of words, intonations, knowing looks, and many other subtleties which frequently are idiosyncratic to the typical communication pattern of the particular pair of individuals. Frequently, the communicators do not know what they are "saying," what messages they are trying to impart, or the "signaling" devices that are at work, but a brief exchange of such intricately subtle and diverse communication signals will leave the individuals with definite feelings and conceptions of the other person's thoughts.

To me, some of the most interesting things in psychology are matters that I find all but impossible to do anything about scientifically—a primary example being the relevance of dream content for the "scripts" of the daily living circumstances for particular people. I am sure that the reader shares with me hundreds of experiences in which either our own dreams or the dreams of other people were extremely "telling" with respect to important matters in our lives. But after all of these years that men have found dreams interesting (and since Freud we have realized the rich symbolic character of much of the content), it simply has proved very difficult to do anything scientifically in the study of dreams (the exception being the interesting research during the last decade on dreaming in relation to the study of sleep, but that does not get at what is most intriguing to me, namely the processes whereby important daytime ideas and concerns are woven into the fabric of nighttime, self-generated video programs).

I have often found it intriguing that topics are generated by associations (in accordance with principles as old as Aristotle's discussion of the matter). A close friend and I frequently play a game of checking on the association that got us from one topic to a very different one in a matter of a split second, and it is intriguing to find the chance word or thought that propels the conversation in a different direction. However, other than for collecting norms, describing the content of free association, investigating the effects of different measures relating to association in verbal learning, and other matters of that kind, what else is there to study scientifically about association?

So it goes with many of the matters that I find most intriguing in psychology—

either I, and apparently others, find nothing in particular to investigate, or the matters that we think of investigating do not have the types of "data handles" that allow science to move apace. However, the extreme difficulty of investigating some of the more intriguing aspects of human behavior should not lead to the grand non sequitur of assuming that the scientific approach in general is wrong with respect to psychological phenomena. There is ample room for the poet, the biographer, the novelist, and the philosopher in the study of mankind, but there also is a respectable place for the scientist and the tools with which he works. Consequently, those who want to make a scientific study of human behavior should be encouraged to develop as many standardized measures of important human processes as possible, which as I see it is a necessary first step in the data-gathering process. Some psychological processes that prove very difficult to measure now may become susceptible to measurement in the future (there have been breakthroughs in other areas of science, as we all know); other intricate aspects of human behavior may for the great long time be left to the hands of the artist, the poet, the philosopher, and others.

2. Measurement in Science

Although tomes have been written on the nature of measurement and the kernel idea has been smothered in tons of abstruse formal logic, in the end it boils down to something rather straightforward: measurement consists of rules for assigning numbers to objects in such a way as to represent quantities of attributes. No matter how one "cuts it," eventually measurement results in attaching a number to people (or material objects) in such a way as to describe the extent to which a particular characteristic is present. Because of the central importance of this simple definition of measurement, it will be useful to take some of the key terms apart. The object of measurement is to describe a person or material object—to depict, portray, characterize, or by some other word that means the same thing to index particular features. The definition speaks of such description being stated in quantitative terms, which is a matter that we will need to discuss in more detail later. Thus quantitative descriptive indices are IQs, percentile scores on a measure of anxiety, EEG frequency levels in a resting state, average heart rate response to an alerting stimulus, or a rating on a 9-step scale of improvement in psychotherapy ranging from "much improved" to "much worse." In these and many other ways, attributes of persons and material objects are stated in quantitative terms.

In the definition, the word "attribute" implies that quantitative description is with respect to a particular feature of persons or objects, which on first thought sounds like an easy standard to meet but which proves to be one of the major stumbling blocks in the proper measurement of many types of psychological attributes. Thus in measuring the separable attributes of people it is necessary to make a distinction between the individual attributes and the total person. Although the sophisticated reader of this book is well aware of the distinction, he is likely to fall into the semantic trap that we all frequently do of having difficulty in singling out particular measured attributes from more general characteristics of persons, such as in accepting the fact that an individual is highly intelligent, as intelligence is measured by current tests, but also is serving a life sentence for a sickening collection of crimes. Similarly, we frequently employ global terms such as "overall intelligence," "anxiety," and "adjustment," which themselves can be meaningfully broken down into separately measurable attributes that supply differential information about the individual. In this connection, there is always something of a give-and-take between the practical and conceptual advantages of lumping kindred traits together into more general measures, and, on the other hand, taking these more general attributes apart in order to wring the last ounce of explanatory power from a system of trait measures.

Another way of thinking about the definition above is in terms of *descriptors* and *descriptands* (to coin a word). The descriptors constitute the quantitative "yard-sticks" which are used to characterize (depict or portray) the descriptands. An example would be a collection of wildflowers used as descriptands and specified combinations of primary colors used as descriptors. In the usual situation, in a sense, the problem of description is reciprocal in that the descriptors can be used to characterize the descriptands, or the descriptands equally well can be used to characterize the descriptors. Thus the combination of colors that depicts the rose is itself described by the visage of the rose; likewise, whereas a measure of anxiety may serve to describe the panicky state of a particular individual, the visage of the individual serves to characterize the measure itself. This distinction is more than mere hair-splitting because it arises in the generation of "types" as is frequently done in considering various forms of mental illness and in the use of various forms of profile analysis to mathematically induce personality types. However, the distinction between descriptors and descriptands is usually clear in most research, although no one ever stops to make the distinction. In most scientific investigations, the descriptands are complex in terms of the compounds of descriptors. The descriptors are meant to be simple, parsimoniously few in numbers, and broadly useful in accurately depicting and distinguishing among descriptands. Thus, although the color combinations among all flowers may be nearly infinite, this infinitude potentially could be measured by mathematical combinations of a few primary hues and indices of saturation. The same is true of descriptors and descriptands where the latter are people and the former are intended to constitute a parsimonious measurement basis for describing behavior in a particular domain of inquiry, e.g., various measures concerning responses of humans to stressful situations.

The distinction between descriptors and descriptands comes up in issues regarding the study of people in terms of types, as with bodily types, mental illness syndrome types, and personality types derived from cluster analysis. Whereas analysis performed among such descriptands rather than the descriptors frequently has been advocated as having a gestaltlike richness to it, generally it has proved to be less scientifically tractable than the derivation of conceptually and mathematically simpler descriptors. (In essence, this is the argument between the advocates of R technique and Q technique, about which so much fuss was created circa 1950.)

2.1. Measurement and Mathematics

Because measurement and mathematics usually involve quantification (i.e., numbers), it is easy to fall into the trap of confusing the underlying logical bases for the two. Of course, pure mathematics is based on inductive logic and requires no resort whatsoever to the empirical world. Thus a hypothesized approach to solving a particular type of equation rests entirely on manipulations of symbols in the system. At least in principle, all hypotheses are entirely correct or incorrect, and the proof of the pudding is in the symbolic manipulations. Of course, one of the conclusions that one might reach in such manipulations is that the system of rules is faulty, e.g., leads to contradictions. However, in pure mathematics, there is no need to prove deductions by measuring lengths of lumber or heights of clouds, or to make any other appeal to what the real world is like. In contrast, measurements spring from the intuitive processes of empirical investigators. A system of quantification is literally "conjured up" in the hope that it eventually will prove to be useful in explaining a wide variety of phenomena in the real world. Where the twain meet, of course, is in the frequently encountered isomorphism between mathematical systems and characteristics of the real world. Thus the Euclidean theorem relating the sum of squares on the sides of a right triangle to the sum of squares on the hypotenuse holds not only in the context of the axioms in geometry but also in the boards that the carpenter lays in constructing a house (and more importantly for issues in relation to psychological measurement, the same isomorphisms hold with respect to the various forms of multivariate analysis that are so useful for constructing psychological measures and employing them in research). However, it is healthy to keep this distinction in mind, because one frequently sees confusions of the two. Thus one frequently hears people say that scores on a test represent a scale of equal intervals if they are normally distributed (which is nonsense) because they are confusing mathematical distributions with the nature of real human traits. On the other side of the coin, one frequently sees a very amateurish psychometrician attempting to prove the mathematical character of a proposed method of operation with a flurry of data analyses, when instead he should devote his time to a clean mathematical proof relating to the matter.

Where the distinction between mathematics and measurement becomes somewhat blurred is with respect to statistics. The term "statistics" is used far too broadly in referring to almost any process concerning the gathering and analysis of data; as the term will be used here, statistics concerns that branch of applied mathematics relating to useful isomorphisms between mathematics and empirical science, particularly those isomorphisms that help in describing the results of experiments in which various kinds of randomlike processes are "perturbers." Of course, particularly useful in this regard are mathematical systems relating to probability, which in essence are pure forms of mathematics but are readily coupled with the empirical scientist's work of gathering and analyzing data. Even here, however, it is important to distinguish between the rules and procedures whereby measurement methods are generated and the processes whereby various statistical methods are adopted as aids to scientific endeavor. In spite of what should be the obviousness of these hortatory remarks concerning the distinction between measurement and mathematics, it is surprising how frequently one discerns a misunderstanding in this regard in the writings of otherwise highly sophisticated individuals. This is exemplified in the shopworn saying that statisticians thought that the normal distribution of intelligence was an empirical fact and psychologists thought that it was a mathematical fact.

2.2. Precision of Measurement

It was said in the definition above that measurement always involves quantification, but here we will both give a slight demurrer and considerably amplify that point. The demurrer is that it is useful to think of "present-absent" as representing a primitive form of measurement, or at least a prelude to measurement. One could argue that such categorical data really concern "identification" rather than measurement per se. I have found it useful to include categorization as a form of quantification simply to complete the scheme. With that one demurrer, then, it will be claimed that all measurement concerns quantification, that is, "how much" of an attribute is present with respect to a particular descriptor and descriptand. However, as the readers of this book have had beaten over their heads since their early training in research methods, not all measures of human attributes have the same quantitative status, in the sense that the numbers employed with them enjoy the same "rights" with respect to permissible mathematical operations. The litany of reciting nominal, ordinal, etc., "scales" of measurement has occurred ad nauseum in many textbooks and other places since the authoritative admonitions on the topic were given by Stevens (e.g., 1951, 1958). Here we will quickly go back through the common meanings for these "scale types" but only as a reminder to the reader, which will permit me to make some extensions, clarifications, and take some strong stands on controversial issues in this regard. Before quickly reminding the reader of these simple distinctions, it must be strongly pointed out that (1) there is no mathematical or empirical necessity for the classification scheme at all—we might have lived without it, (2) there is nothing sacred about the usually employed scheme— another one might have been better, and (3) it is quite arguable about how one determines which "type" fits any particular measure, e.g., a measure of schizoid tendency or perceptual scanning accuracy.

In building up from the bottom in terms of measurement scales, I typically like to make a distinction between *labels* and *categories*, whereas some authors lump these together under "nominal measurement." By labels I refer to the use of numbers as purely arbitrary symbols for keeping up with things, when there is no quantitative implication intended. An example would be a botanist gathering plants on a newly explored island, in which he would arbitrarily number his specimens, 1, 2, 3, etc., purely to keep up with them. Of course, when numbers are used in this way only as a labeling device, they signify nothing other than individuality or separateness, and there are no legitimate mathematical systems of analysis that usually make any sense. However, in using numbers primarily as labels, it frequently turns out that, for some incidental reason, numbers of different sizes happen to correlate with characteristics of people. I forget the references involved, but 20 or more years ago someone used the example of the numbers on the backs of football players to illustrate numbers employed as labels. Some person who had nothing better to do started adding up these numbers and found that, in the professional leagues, the average numbers on the backs of linemen were larger than those on backfield players (or maybe it was vice versa), and thus a lively but unnecessary controversy was started about the logic of analyzing numbers representing labels. The important consideration is the purpose that the scientist has in mind for employing numbers. If the scientist is using numbers as labels, it really does not matter if there are incidental correlates of these labels. For example, the botanist may have collected his plants in moving from the shore up to the highlands, in which case plants with higher numbers may have been systematically different in some way from those with lower numbers, but that is entirely beside the point. Other than for parlor games, numbers used as labels should not be subjected to any form of mathematical analysis, because obviously nonnumerical symbols would have served the purpose as well. One must inquire about the intent of the scientist in designating a particular use of numbers and question the sensibleness of that designated use.

I mentioned previously that I include present-absent or all-or-none characteristics as representing a form of measurement, even if the term "quantification" must be used in a rather liberal manner. Of course, *categorization* is extremely important to all areas of science, and it certainly is important to the study of abnormal human behavior. Although one can devise more complex rules for categorization, in its simplest form all objects of a specified kind are designated as belonging to one and only one mutually exclusive category. A simple example is one of occupations, in which people are designated as being farmers, plumbers, physicians, and so on. Without further elaboration, categorization itself implies no relations among categories, either qualitatively or quantitatively. Of course, there usually are quantitative and qualitative correlates of categories, but these are matters to determine from empirical investigation rather than built into the categorization scheme itself. Thus, after stipulating a categorization scheme for occupations, one could find many quantitative correlates, e.g., average yearly income, amount of time spent watching television, voting preferences, and many others. Also, categories frequently are dynamically related, in that movement from one to another has a much higher probability than movement between other categories; for example, there is a higher probability that dyslexia will be manifested by individuals in one category of brain damage rather than in another category of brain damage.

Of course, categorization is highly important to the whole "medical model" as employed throughout clinical medicine and as it has been carried over into discussions of various abnormal mental states. In our introductory courses in abnormal psychology, we all learned the elements of the Kraepelinean classification system, the rudiments of which are still with us. All readers have heard the "evils" of employing such systems, including the protests that they (1) dehumanize the person, (2) are simply subject to a great deal of disagreement as regards particular assignments of individuals, (3) lump together people who are very different, (4) say very little about either the origin of the problem or helpful treatment for it, and (5) mainly serve as a gobbledygook language barrier to prevent the average person from finding out what charlatans we mental healers really are. (Just the same, I still think Uncle Louie is a paranoid schizophrenic with strong regressive and phobic characteristics.) In spite of all of these supposed evils, classification schemes simply will not go away, and consequently later in this chapter we will present a more extensive discussion of the art and logic of classification.

Before leaving this discussion of the use of categories for classification, a number of points need to be made clear as regards the place of categories in the traditional scheme of measurement scales. First, in their purest form, category designations have no mathematical implications whatsoever. Thus classification schemes relating to professions or to various types of mental illness do not in and of themselves imply any mathematical relations among the categories in the classification scheme. There are three places in which numbers become involved with respect to categories. First is the trivial instance in which the categories are identified by number. Thus, purely for the sake of convenience, one might identify a number of types of brain damage as evidenced in behavioral symptoms as constituting type 1, type 2, and so on. The numbers might be used instead of employing names in order not to prematurely make assumptions about the etiology and other characteristics of the categories, or the numbers might be used in conjunction with category names. In either case, the numbers are being used purely as labels and have no mathematical implications or uses.

The second place in which numbers become involved with categories is in *enumerating* (or determining the frequency of) subjects from a particular sample of individuals who fall into each category in a classification scheme. Thus, in surveying the patient designations in a mental hospital, one frequently sees enumerations (or "counts") of the numbers of patients of different types, or these are stated in the form of percentages. Such quantification with respect to percentages in categories certainly is very important and leads to various forms of mathematical analysis both in applied work and in research, but it is important to make a careful distinction between quantification regarding relations among the categories and enumerations or frequency counts within the categories. The major point to reiterate is that differences among categories are inherently qualitative rather than quantitative (although a hybrid version will be mentioned subsequently that does involve quantitative relations among the categories).

Going up the scale of mathematical precision allowed in the conventional scheme of discussing measurement scales, the next level is *rank order* or simply the use of ranks. A very simple example would be to ask three therapists who have participated in four different group therapy sets of training sessions to rank-order individuals in each set from most improved to least improved. Thus, if there were four different therapy groups, there would be a total of 12 sets of ranks. Another simple example would be in having a crisis prevention center rank-order the days of the week over a period of 6 months in terms of the number of calls requesting help. Thus, by averaging the ranks or combining them in some other way, one might come to the conclusion that Monday is indeed a "blue day" and that for some peculiar reason Friday appears to be the best day of the week.

Of course, when dealing with measurement that obviously is in the form of ranks, the quantitative implications concern only "greater than" and "less than." This can be very important information (particularly when the data are in forms that lend themselves to models for unidimensional and multidimensional scaling), but obviously in dealing with only ranks one obtains no information regarding how far apart the objects or persons are with respect to the attribute under consideration, and no information is gained regarding the absolute level. Thus, with the therapy example given previously, if patients A and D are ranked 1 and 2 in terms of improvement by one of the three therapists, there is no indication of how far apart patients are with respect to improvement or really whether they have improved at all in an absolute sense. Similarly, if Sunday and Monday are ranked 1 and 2 with respect to numbers of calls to a crisis prevention center, again one has no indication of how far apart they are with respect to any underlying attributes or whether the volume of calls really is relatively large or small as regards expectations of the staff, amount of "traffic" in this regard found in other localities, and other such meaningful comparisons. Numerous authors have referred to rank order as constituting the most primitive form of measurement, primitive in the sense that it underlies all higher form of measurement, but also primitive in the demeaning sense that it provides only very limited information.

Because ranks are defined quantitatively purely in terms of the algebra of inequalities (greater than and less than), some authors have laid down the dictum that only nonparametric statistics can be applied. To a large extent this is true, but there are many exceptions to this overly general rule. For example, it is perfectly meaningful to apply some methods of correlational analysis to ranks that are based on more information than really can be obtained from ranks. Thus, as I have argued elsewhere (Nunnally, 1978), there is nothing wrong with applying the regular product-moment correlation coefficient to sets of ranks (which is identical to the special-appearing version of the formula called "rho"). When this is done, the coefficient ranges from 1.00 through zero to -1.00. This provides an easily understood interpretation of degree of relationship, and auxiliary methods of inferential statistics can be applied. Another consideration with respect to permissible mathematical operations with ranks is that whereas in many cases it makes sense only to apply nonparametric statistics with respect to ranked data themselves, it is entirely permissible to apply powerful parametric methods of analysis to *average* ranks from different categories. An example would be in having patients in an alcohol abuse treatment program rank statements regarding things in daily life from those that bothered them most to those that bothered them least (say in this case there were 40 statements regarding social situations). An average rank could be obtained for each statement, and there would be a distribution of ranks about each such mean. According to well-known theorems in statistics, these average ranks would tend to be normally distributed, and one would anticipate that distributions of ranks about average ranks also would tend to be at least roughly normally distributed. These are all the conditions required for employing analysis of variance, complex correlational methods, and all methods of multivariate analysis. Thus, whereas one may start off with gathering data in the form of ranks, as these are combined by averaging or by some method of psychological scaling, the resulting transformations may lend themselves to much more powerful methods of mathematical and statistical analysis than would have been logical with respect to the original ranks themselves.

A special case of the use of ranks needs to be carefully pointed out because there frequently is confusion about them. Whereas it was said previously that in the simplest form categories have no quantitative relations among them, it is possible to deal with a hybrid metric concerning *ordered categories*. In this case, no quantitative or qualitative distinctions are made among the objects or persons within categories, but the categories themselves are ordered with respect to a particular attribute. An example would be an ordered categorization of new psychiatric patients in terms of severity of illness as linked to recommended modes of treatment ranging, say, from a category 1 relating to short-term supportive treatment and medication down to an extreme of category 5 of immediate, possibly long-term institutional care. When dealing with ordered categories (and the situation arises frequently in the study and treatment of psychopathology), all of the statistics appropriate to rank order can be applied to relations among the categories, but only such analyses as are appropriate to categories can be employed with respect to the "counts" within categories.

Frequently, information that could be obtained on a complete rank-order scale or even a high-order scale is "degenerated" into a set of ordered categories simply by lumping together people at a number of levels—as was done in the old days, lumping together psychiatric patients in terms of intelligence as "normal," "borderline," "morons," etc. Obviously, when some more precise form of measurement is available, one throws away considerable mathematical precision by purposely degenerating information from complete rank order or higher scales into ordered categories. On the other hand, the use of ordered categories may in many situations represent the most precise type of information that is feasible to obtain, e.g., as evidenced previously in the ordered categorization of patients regarding recommended courses of treatment.

The next level of measurement conventionally discussed with respect to scales is the *interval scale*, in which not only rank-order information is available but also information on how far apart persons or objects are with respect to the stipulated attribute. It is now generally recognized that most psychological tests are most sensibly interpreted as constituting interval scales (although this used to be a very controversial point). Thus, in one of the frequently employed tests of general intelligence, one takes seriously not only the rank ordering of people but how far apart they are on the continuum. For example, if three persons have IQs of 100, 110, and 130, respectively, it is generally regarded as sensible to interpret the second interval as at least approximately twice as large as the first. It should be emphasized that such direct calculations of relative sizes of intervals are seldom done in either applied work or research, but rather such comparisons are made as part of overall statistical analyses of results. In performing such statistical analyses, however, any assumptions regarding the exact proportionality of intervals can be taken with a very large grain of salt and have little if any effect on the resulting statistics.

The major information that is lacking on an interval scale is any indication of "how much" in an absolute sense any or all of the objects possess the attribute. However, this proves to be no great loss in most interpretations of test scores in applied situations or basic research in nearly all problems in the behavioral sciences. One can claim that there is no "absolute zero" on an interval scale (e.g., zero intelligence), which is quite true but really not a damning disadvantage in nearly all studies of people. In applied situations, the average score in a normative group usually supplies the necessary benchmark for interpreting scores. Thus the average IQ (conventionally placed at 100) serves as a handy reference point for normatively interpreting scores of people. Similarly, in nearly all of the powerful methods of mathematical and statistical analysis that are useful in research (e.g., factor analysis and analysis of variance), there is no need whatsoever of an absolute zero, and indeed scores are usually equated with respect to the overall mean as part of the statistical analysis. For example, before performing a complex analysis of variance on the results of a multifaceted design, one could subtract the overall mean score from every score in every cell, and, of course, this would in no wise change any of the results of the analysis. So for nearly all problems one could say, "Who needs anything other than interval scales?"

The *ratio scale* is the "queen" of measurement scales in that the resulting "numbers" meet all of the requirements for simple arithmetic as well as the most complex forms of mathematical analysis. Simply put, a ratio scale is an interval scale that has an absolute zero point. Examples of ratio scales in everyday life are the yardstick for the measurement of length and balances for the measurement of weight. Although as was said previously there are not many practical problems or basic research issues where knowledge of the absolute zero is required, there are many measurements in psychology that are sensibly construed as ratio scales. This is the case for any measure based on time of response, such as in a simple reaction time experiment. If one wanted to go out of the way to be troublesome, he could argue that even though one has a ratio scale in the measurement of any type of timed response this does not necessarily constitute a ratio scale for the "underlying attribute" (which frequently is referred to in a tone of reverence). Of course, there would be no difficulty in making the same argument in any of the physical sciences, either—how does one know that the distance of a particular star from us in terms of light-years is a measure of the "real" distance? Workaday science does not have time for such quibbles, and consequently let it be said flatly that any measure in psychology based on response latency can sensibly be analyzed in terms of all of the mathematics employed with ratio scales. It might prove desirable to make various types of transformations of such scales either because they are more sensibly construed in some different manner or because they have a more acceptable distribution, e.g., taking logarithmic values of response latency as is frequently done. In that case, it is equally sensible to perform all of the algebraic manipulations on the transformed scale of latency as were performed on the original scale expressed in seconds.

Any measures in psychology that are based on physical magnitudes of accuracy also are sensibly interpreted as ratio scales. This would be the case in a "tracking" test where an individual attempts to keep an electronic stylus on a randomly wavering line as it passes across the video screen of an automated testing apparatus. It certainly makes sense to refer to zero error when the individual is on the line and to measure amount of error in terms of how far the individual is from the line at any point in time.

There also are many more subtle forms of behavior that quite sensibly can be construed as representing ratio scales. A simple example is given in Table 1, which will serve to illustrate all of the measurement scales discussed so far. This consisted of a "highly elaborate" little demonstration done for a graduate course in psychometric theory. Shortly before classtime, I made up the list of adverbs appearing in the list, e.g., "often," "frequently," "sometimes." These were listed from top to bottom with the aid of a table of random numbers. In that case, the consecutive numbers served as labels and were not meant to represent quantities of attributes. Students were first asked to rank-order the stimuli from most to least in terms of the frequency implied, e.g., the percent of time that it rains on the 4th of July. A very

Table 1. Scaling of 10 Adverbs in Terms of Implied Percentage by 11 Students

Adverb	Rank	Mean percentage	S.D.
Always	1	99.5	1.4
Most of the time	2	85.5	8.1
Usually	3	76.8	10.7
Frequently	4	72.7	6.2
Generally	5	70.5	11.4
Often	6	57.3	12.5
Sometimes	7	39.5	9.2
Seldom	8	15.9	9.2
Rarely	9	7.7	4.5
Never	10	0.0	0.0

high degree of agreement was found among the 11 students, with only three reversals being found with respect to the modal ranking. To illustrate the possibilities of having hybrid forms of measurement scales, students were asked to rank the intervals between the adverbs in the extent to which they implied a high frequency. These data are not shown in the table. After other exercises in "playing around" with the adverbs in terms of possibilities of scaling, students were asked to give an absolute scaling of the adverbs on a ratio ranging from 0% to 100%. The mean and standard deviations are shown in Table 1. (I enjoyed finding that one young lady marked "always" as representing 95% rather than 100% of the time.) A correlational analysis showed a very high degree of disagreement in terms of the ordering of the adjectives, but as can be seen from the standard deviations, the absolute ratings varied somewhat. However, this variation proved to be essentially random error, and the overall amount of agreement was high. The ratio scale shown in Table 1 is as good as that produced anywhere in science, in some ways even better than many. What could be a more meaningful zero point for perceived frequency than "never"? And unlike many of the scales found in the physical sciences, there was an absolute upper limit—"always." Similarly, the perceived ratios in between these end points constitute a very sensible ratio scale relating to the semantics of perceived frequency.

There are many other instances in which human impressions can be converted into sensible ratio scales. Another example comes from a research project currently being undertaken by the present writer on the dimensions of rated emotions. Rating scales are being developed that will employ various emotion-related words such as "pleasant," "frightened," and "angry." Words were collected in such a way as to represent the various factors that have been found in previous factor analytic investigations of emotion ratings, and some additional adjectives were added to cover emotions that seemed not to be represented in the published reports. Using the method of paired comparisons, the subject is required to rate the percentage to which each pair of terms means the same thing. The scale ranges from 100% similarity through 0% to 100% dissimilarity. The percentage scales are marked off in sets of five percentage points each. The matrices of percentage judgments obtained from each subject are then subjected to procedures of multidimensional scaling of a kind that result in underlying factors of rated emotions which are expressed as ratio scales ranging from −100% through 0% to +100%.

Possibilities for developing ratio scales abound in many of the physiological correlates of psychological states, such as in the amount of "power" manifested in the EEG alpha rhythm, pupillary response to activating stimuli, and changes in heart rate as a function of attention-getting stimulation. Whereas 20 years ago there were many individuals who were stating that psychology could not rightly claim the mathematical advantages attendant upon interval scales for much of its research, it is now easy to see in retrospect that the discipline was selling itself short in that regard. Not only is it sensible to employ mathematical operations that befit interval scales with most of our measuring instruments (particularly those that we refer to as constituting psychological tests), but also some of the measurement procedures that relate to psychological attributes stand on as solid a footing with respect to the requirements of ratio scales as do those in any other discipline.

Let me make a number of summarizing comments before leaving the topic of measurement scales in the behavioral sciences. First, to reiterate what was said initially, there is nothing necessary about the particular classification scheme that

has been given here for measurement scales, nor is the behavioral scientist necessarily encumbered to work with this or any substitute scheme of classification. We
might have worked along just as well in applied activities and in basic research if we
had never heard of rank order or interval scales or worried much about the matter.
Second, to the extent to which one chooses to argue about the legitimacy of assuming one type of scale rather than another, in most instances it is sensible to assume
at least interval scales. As was said previously, this permits one to employ nearly
all of the powerful methods of analysis that are needed to keep our science on the
move. Third, and finally, there has been a grand misconception about the logical
status of classification schemes relating to measurement scales. It is true that one
should be self-conscious about the forms of mathematical analysis that are permitted
with respect to the numbers generated by particular measurement methods, but it
is a grand non sequitur to assume that there is an agreed-on method for divining the
particular scale properties of a newly invented measurement method. As I have
argued strongly elsewhere (Nunnally, 1978), the adoption of an approach to scaling
a particular attribute (e.g., reaction time, intelligence, or short-term memory) is a
matter of convention that can be arrived at only after a great deal of circumstantial
evidence is gathered about the most parsimonious "mapping" of a scale into the
system of scientific laws with which it is being investigated.

3. The Characteristics of Good Psychological Tests

Although there are some principles that apply to psychological measurement
in general, there are many forms of measurement in psychology that not only appear
very different in terms of apparatus and procedures but also are constructed and
used for very different purposes (see Nunnally, 1978, for some of the most important
distinctions that can be made among different types of psychological measures).
One important distinction concerns whether objects are used to assign scores to
people or whether people are used to assign scores to objects. The former is the case
where the "objects" consist of problems on an adjustment problem checklist, and
scores for individuals are obtained in terms of how many and what kinds of problems they mark. The latter is exemplified by subjects' rating each problem on the
list in terms of the severity as regards an issue in daily life. In one case the result would
be a distribution of scores relating to individuals, and in the other case the result
would be a distribution of scores relating to the objects (statements in this case).
More typically, when people are used to scale objects rather than vice versa, the
objects are different in appearance from those on most tests of ability, adjustment,
or anything else. Thus all of psychophysics is concerned with employing people as
yardsticks for measuring the perceived characteristics of stimuli of many different
kinds, ranging from the loudness of tones to perceived similarities of adjectives relating to emotions. Conversely, the "objects" employed for scaling people most
frequently are typical test items, and these most frequently consist of printed questions relating to tests of ability or personality. However, it is important to keep
firmly in mind the distinction between using the responses of people to quantify
some characteristic of themselves (e.g., their typical levels of anxiety) and using
people to quantify the perceived attributes inherent in objects or persons other than
themselves (this latter would be the case if people were asked to rate some well-
known United States Senators on a scale ranging from "very liberal" to "very con-

servative"). The importance of the distinction lies in the differences in purposes, data-gathering techniques, typical methods of scaling analysis that are employed, and the arenas of research in which the two basically different types of measurement problems are encountered. In the study of abnormal human behavior, most frequently the interest is in the scaling of people, rather than in psychophysics, which is mainly concerned with scaling of stimuli.

The word "test" is used very broadly to refer to any procedure whereby people are scaled or scored with respect to an attribute—as befits the definition of measurement given earlier. In most uses of tests, the effort is to create large, reliable, individual differences among people on an attribute. Thus in employing a problem checklist to be used with elementary-grade children the effort is to obtain a list of problems and a scoring procedure that will separate children as widely as possible in terms of the supposed trait of adjustment involved. Similarly, in basic research on human abilities (such as in the landmark investigations by the Thurstones of primary mental abilities, 1941), the effort is to obtain as much reliable variance as possible within the limits of the numbers of items or other devices used to generate scores. There are, however, situations in applied work with tests and in research where the effort is not necessarily to create large, reliable, individual differences in scores. Such applied situations occur in the context of "mastery learning," which is similar to Skinnerian behavior modification approaches in general. In essence, the purpose of the training program is to bring all, or nearly all, individuals to a relatively high or satisfactory level of performance (a so-called asymptote). Consequently, the major problem of measurement is to assess how far an individual is below the mastery level initially and to accurately determine when the individual crosses the all-important threshold of satisfactory performance. The special logic and method of constructing tests for mastery learning and for behavior modification programs in general are discussed in Nunnally (1976, 1978). However, it is concluded in most sources that the instruments developed for such special purposes do not tend to be grossly different from those that are constructed specifically to produce a wide range of individual differences among people. Consequently, only tests of the latter type will be discussed here in detail, and the reader will be left to the aforementioned sources for principles relating to the construction of special-purpose tests.

3.1. The Factorial Model

Whether or not one actually employs factor analysis in the development, validation, and use of measures in research, some of the related concepts are fundamental to discussing important issues in psychometrics. Any complex type of performance (which we will symbolize as Y) is potentially explainable by some combination of simple measured variables or tests, which we will symbolize as x_1, x_2, etc. One example would be to think of Y as constituting successful performance on some type of job as numerically indexed in terms of ratings, amounts of sales, or some other index. The x-variables could be thought of as various special tests, including measures relating to general intelligence, particular aptitudes, biographical inventories, and others. In the area of psychopathology, Y could be thought of as response of alcoholics to a training program, and the x's could be thought of as various predictor variables regarding treatment outcome. In this case, the person is the descriptand, the x's are the descriptors, and Y constitutes a combination of the x variables which proves to be particularly useful for some type of applied decision or in analyzing the results of research. In any particular domain of inquiry, such as in the study of anxiety or physiological response to stress, it is useful in continuing research to develop a parsimonious set of descriptors which, when employed generally in practice or research, can be referred to as *factors*. Either such factors are developed on the basis of theory (including just plain hunch), or they are derived mathematically through some type of factor analytic procedure. Whichever the case, the object is to combine the factors mathematically in such a way as to represent hypotheses about complex variables (the *Y*'s in our system) or to actually analyze the results of research. In that case, one frequently performs a simple linear or additive combination as follows:

$$Y = b_1x_1 + b_2x_2 + b_3x_3 + \cdots + b_px_p$$

Thus, in this system of p underlying factors, one would seek differential weights (b_1, b_2, etc.) in such a way as to maximally estimate scores on Y. The model is linear in the sense that the x variables are simply added (after being weighted) rather than being combined multiplicatively. Thus, if the equation embodies a term such as $b_{12}x_1x_2$, then this no longer would be a linear model. By postulating a linear model in this way, it is not assumed that a linear combination provides exactly the best fit for the data, but this has proved frequently to be the case. Also, because the linear model is so simple and so easily extended to complex mathematical developments, it certainly represents a sensible starting point both in conceptualizing a research problem and in performing analyses of actual data. It is important to realize how very general the factorial model is. In addition to including psychological tests and other traditional measuring instruments, the x's could stand for chronological age, sex, measures relating to various physical disease states, and others. Also, some of the x's can stand for various sources of error in Y itself, such as the unreliability inherent in subjective ratings made by clinicians and error from other sources. These forms of error can be included conceptually in the overall factorial model and can be investigated with respect to studies of reliability in the process of instrument development and standardization.

Before making some blanket statements about the fundamental ingredients of psychological measures, it will be important to keep in mind here that the discussion is about measures of *traits*, both the relatively simple descriptors embodied in the *x* factors and the more complex behavior embodied in the dependent variable *Y*. If the effort is to measure individual differences over a wide range of ability or personality characteristics, then it can be said that the total psychometric information in any score distribution is contained entirely in (1) the mean, (2) the standard deviation, (3) the curve shape of the frequency distribution, (4) the reliability, in its various components, and (5) the factorial composition regarding systematic, nonerror components. Thus the efforts in test construction are to employ procedures that optimize various aspects of these characteristics, e.g., to develop a measure that has a near-normal distribution of scores, that is highly reliable, and whose factorial composition relates to anxiety or some other construct of interest.

3.2. The Factorial Bases for Measurement

It is useful to think that in any area of inquiry (e.g., drug treatment programs or research on responses of people to stressful situations) there is a potent group of explainer variables or factors, as illustrated above. It should be made clear that the implication is not that one necessarily "discovers" this group of explainers; rather, it is best if these follow from hypotheses relating to a meaningful theory. At a less sophisticated level of functioning, one frequently derives these empirically and mathematically as a part of continuing research endeavors in an area of investigation. To a large extent, science consists of formulating hypotheses regarding the existence of a sufficient basis of explainers or of mathematically inducing them with factor analysis, although, as was said previously, one can entertain a factorial model without necessarily going through some of the excursions into statistics that frequently are undertaken. An important point about any potential basis of potent explainers is that, at least mathematically, there are an infinite number of transformations of a basis that would serve as well in any program of prediction or in explaining the results of any research project. Thus, rather than employ as a basis the simple variables, or factors, $x_1, x_2, \ldots, x_p$, one equally well could make mathematical transformations of the scores on these factors to achieve another basis, as follows:

$$u_1 = a_1x_1 + a_2x_2 + a_3x_3 + \cdots + a_px_p$$

$$u_2 = b_1x_1 + b_2x_2 + b_3x_3 + \cdots + b_px_p$$

$$u_3 = \cdots$$

$$\vdots$$

$$u_p = p_1x_1 + p_2x_2 + p_3x_3 + \cdots + p_px_p$$

If the original x variables were uncorrelated (orthogonal), then this orthogonality can be maintained in the transformation to the u variables by employing weights that themselves are uncorrelated (e.g., $a_1b_1 + a_2b_2 + \cdots + a_pb_p = 0$). Whether or not the original set of potent explainers or factors were uncorrelated (orthogonal) or whether or not the transformation of them is to an orthogonal basis, the correlations among the resulting u variables can be determined from mathematical procedures inherent in the transformation (see discussions of such matters in books on factor analysis by Comrey, 1973; Gorsuch, 1974; Harman, 1976).

The author is very much in favor of a factorial approach to thinking about the variables in a particular domain of inquiry (e.g., tests concerning reactions to various types of physical stress or attitudinal and cognitive factors relating to programs of compensatory education). Even if one does not go through the statistical intricacies of performing some of the more elaborate methods of factor analysis (and admittedly it frequently is easy to get lost in the sheer statistical maze involved), the factorial model does present a very "clean" way of looking at the necessary descriptors that are thought to be potent explainers with respect to a collection of descriptands. In addition to the other criteria for "good science," one of them is to follow the principle of parsimony as far as the actualities of the domain of inquiry permit, and a factorial model for conceptualizing relevant "yardsticks" for a domain of research or clinical practice fits the criterion of parsimony much better than any other approach of which the author is aware.

3.3. Test Construction

Here as elsewhere in this chapter, the word "test" is being used very widely to refer to any "descriptor." Also, it is usually the case that the purpose of constructing tests is to obtain large, reliable, individual differences among subjects. In applied settings, this is important for differentiating subjects reliably from one another at various points on the continuum of cognitive or affectual traits; in basic research in studying correlations among various traits, it is essential to employ tests that produce large, reliable, individual differences among subjects or else it will not be possible to find substantial correlations. Consequently, in this section on test construction, only those instruments will be discussed which are intended to produce such broad individual differences among people. There are some special types of instruments that are constructed for different purposes (e.g., to measure whether or not a person has reached a certain level of mastery in a training program), but such instruments are by far the exception rather than the rule. Because either whole books or hundreds of pages in other books have been written on particular principles relating to test construction, there will be room here only to make a few summarizing comments, mainly opinions about some of the more controversial issues in test construction.

Previously, it was said that, in this author's point of view, one of the arts of developing and employing measurement methods in science is to obtain a relatively simple set of descriptors in order to make sense out of a relatively much more complex set of descriptands. The examples are having a simple set of color hues that can be combined mathematically to describe an extremely wide variety of colors manifested in samples of flowers and having a relatively small number of tests that could be used to explain the major variance manifested in experiments concerning a variety of forms of physiological and psychological stress.

If a test (using the term very broadly) is constructed in such a way as to measure some unitary function (e.g., a particular type of anxiety or particular types of reasoning), then one can make a very good case that the items (whatever they are like) should be internally consistent. This argument is discussed in detail and illustrated in Nunnally (1978). (As was mentioned previously, however, this runs into a logical stumbling block with the principle which was stated of the innumerable possible transformations or rotations of any factorial basis to an equally acceptable one mathematically. This matter will be discussed subsequently.) The effort to measure a single, unitary attribute leads to an entire logic of test construction based on developing the most homogeneous instrument possible from an item sample relating logically to the domain of the attribute in question. Essentially, what one does is to test out the homogeneity of subsamples of the item pool by looking at the intercorrelations among items, and if these are satisfactorily high (relative to what one can get in this regard in typical collections of items) then one iteratively builds up a test in such a way as to have a very high internal consistency reliability. The entire logic is based on the maxim that a good item for a test is one that correlates highly with total scores on the collection of items being assembled for the test. Essentially, this involves a bootstrap operation in which one starts off with a core of "good" items (say 20 or more) and adds items which correlate relatively highly with the core group.

This approach to test construction would seem to be somewhat at variance with the author's heavy reliance on the factorial model discussed previously for considering measurement variables in a domain of inquiry. However, the author does not consider this really to be the case. As argued considerably elsewhere (Nunnally, 1978), not only is it very tedious to try to construct tests on the basis of a factor analysis of items but also there are many pitfalls involved in this approach. Rather, it is argued that a test should grow from a well-founded hypothesis about the existence of an attribute, which in turn should result in a well-constructed sample of items relating to the hypothesized attribute. Test construction should then be applied to this item pool in such a way as to obtain a homogeneous test. Other authors would argue for applying factor analysis to the item pool, and, whereas some merit can be seen in this argument, the author is strongly of the opinion that in most cases it is better to move directly to procedures for the construction of homogeneous tests. Where factor analysis enters the picture is after a test is constructed by procedures for building homogeneous tests and an instrument is developed that meets the standards for those procedures. After this is done, however, one cannot be sure that the goal of measuring a unitary attribute has been met until the test subsequently is investigated both in a wide variety of experimental settings and in factor-analytic investigations along with other instruments related to the domain of inquiry (e.g., instruments that are thought to be useful for the study of the effects of a program on rehabilitating juvenile delinquents). This approach to constructing summative measures (summing item scores) can lead to an instrument that produces large, reliable, individual difference in scores. Also, the procedure usually produces a reasonable approximation of the normal distribution (the Holy Grail of some psychometricians).

3.4. Explication of Factors

This section is purposefully not entitled "Factor Analysis," because the author definitely feels that it is unwise to emphasize the mathematical procedures of analysis; rather, the strategy of research from which procedures of analysis are selected should be emphasized. It is strongly felt that the better part of wisdom is in conceptualizing the underlying measures required for investigating a domain of inquiry as constituting a set of factors, as illustrated previously. Consequently, after measures are constructed by procedures discussed in the previous section and a number of such measures accrue in continuing research, it is important to investigate the extent to which they serve as a factorial basis of measurement. At the risk of sounding overly apologetic for introducing multivariate statistics in this way, let it be said that factor analysis is very useful at this juncture (discussed in broad outline in Nunnally, 1978, and in detail in Comrey, 1973; Gorsuch, 1974; Harman, 1976). However, factor analysis is a name for a very broad class of "descriptive statistics" including many particular approaches. Some of the approaches are outlandishly complex for most applied purposes and are mainly useful for specialists in mathematical models relating to studies of individual differences. Most of the methods of factor analysis that are required in programs of empirical research, e.g., on drug abuse or compensatory education, are rather easily understood and applied by persons who are not specialists in psychometrics and statistics. Almost all university computer services have readymade factor analysis "packages" available that supply the researcher with the full gamut of statistical results that are needed. Typically, the individual who is not highly acquainted with factor analysis will need the help of a more technically sophisticated friend in making sense out of the results. The obtained factors constitute the measurement basis described previously, the collection of unitary descriptors that can be employed for applied purposes or for research.

The major problem in factor analysis is not mathematical, certainly not a problem in the sheer arithmetic of computation now that computers are available, but rather it is a lingering conceptual problem. The problem lies in the point illustrated previously—that any particular basis, such as the basis of x's used as an example, can be transformed (or rotated) into a perfectly acceptable new system, such as the u variables mentioned previously which are in every way as good statistically. The question then becomes one of the most acceptable transformation of the raw results of a factor analysis. Methods of factor analysis are available for testing hypotheses about the presence and strength of hypothesized factors if a good theory is available regarding the underlying yardsticks in the domain of inquiry; but frequently the investigator is not so sure in this regard, and thus to some extent the factor analysis is exploratory. Almost everyone recognizes that it is inherently poor practice to rely exclusively on methods of statistical analysis to "induce truth," and, indeed, that is correct; however, some methods of exploratory factor analysis do help to indicate possible underlying bases of measurement in terms of groupings of test variables. Frequently, the investigator is surprised, either pleasantly or unpleasantly, by the statistical results, and the basis suggested by the factor analysis is rather different from what had been guessed initially.

Although statistical methods neither generate empirical truth nor even produce theories about empirical truth, some principles regarding parsimonious bases of measurement can be stated partially in statistical terms. Previously it was said that it is both conceptually and statistically fortunate if the basis of measurement consists of relatively unitary or "pure" measures which can be easily interpreted, named, and discussed in the context of relevant theory in the particular area of research or clinical work. Then, from the standpoint of the statistical structure of the descriptor variables, the ideal would be for each descriptor to measure one and only one factor as evidenced in the actual factor analytic results. One of the truly ingenious conceptions of Leon Thurstone (e.g., 1947) was that the desired conceptual simplicity for a measurement basis related to a possible pattern of results obtainable from factor analysis—his well-known concept of *simple structure*. An idealized example of a simple structure is shown in Table 2. There are shown the loadings or correlations of nine tests with three factors. The factor analysis could relate to

TABLE 2. Ideal Set of Rotated Factor Loadings Demonstrating "Simple Structure"

Variable	Factor		
	A	B	C
1	X	O	O
2	X	O	O
3	X	O	O
4	O	X	O
5	O	X	O
6	O	X	O
7	O	O	X
8	O	O	X
9	O	O	X

tests used to study anxiety. Initially, it was hypothesized that tests 1 through 3 concerned anxiety relating to physical violence and bodily harm, tests 4 through 6 related to anxiety concerning embarrassment in social situations, and tests 7 through 9 concerned anxiety relating to feelings of inferiority in situations where success or failure is important. In this idealized factor analytic result, exactly three factors were found, and the three tests in each group had substantial loadings only on one factor. This would have perfectly confirmed the hypotheses of the investigator, if he had held such hypotheses initially. Similarly, if the investigator had held only rather rough ideas about the possible outcomes, he would have been quite pleased by the neatness of the results shown in Table 2. This is simple structure at its best, in that it would have been very simple to measure the three factors either by averaging scores over the three tests relating to each factor or simply by using a representative test from each of the three groups. Also, such neat statistical findings would have lent considerable confidence to the interpretation given of the underlying factors and would have encouraged the investigator to proceed apace in his substantive studies of anxiety. The problem, of course, is that results are almost never this neat. In order to achieve anything approaching a simple structure, one frequently has to perform some outlandish statistical manipulations, some of which are ready made for helping the investigator to confuse himself (see discussion of this matter in Nunnally, 1978). Also, even if one almost burns the computer out in performing statistical gyrations, inevitably the final rotated factors will not display the simple picture shown in Table 2. Rather, many of the tests will have substantial loadings on several of the factors, and some of the factors will be almost uninterpretable because they have almost no "pure" tests with which to define them. Aside from the thousands of pages of technical arguments that have been made about simple structure as a scientific concept and statistical principle, the concept is quite appealing in terms of judging the adequacy of the final measurement basis employed for investigations in an area. It really does not matter whether the tests used for the basis came out of a factor analysis that produced neat results even analogous to those shown in Table 2 or whether they represented only the few relatively pure measures obtained from an exploratory investigation. Also, one frequently can achieve a simple set of descriptors by successively analyzing evolving collections of tests and throwing away the "garbage" at each stage. In other words, one may not find a simple structure in Thurstone's sense of the term on first attempt, but may gradually develop one in the course of successive studies. By these approaches, one can build up a potent set of simple descriptors, potent in the sense that they explain much of the variance in the many tests proposed for use in a domain of inquiry and simple in the sense that each tends to measure one factor only.

A second and somewhat more complex logical problem in seeking a simple basis is that there may be more than one simple basis that could be achieved, such as illustrated previously with our transformation of a simple set of x's into a simple set of u's. This is both good and bad—good from a statistical standpoint but bad from the standpoint of deciding which is the better basis. To the extent to which one can rightly argue that one basis is better or worse than some transformation of it (in factor analytic terminology, a rotation of it), this cannot be answered by purely statistical arguments but rests mainly with the intuitive appeal of the different bases regarding their relevance for theory. If there is no formal theory, then the test of meaningfulness relates to the commonsense language in which the issues are being discussed. Also, there is nothing "wrong" with different investigators' accepting different transformations of the descriptor factors, either because one formulation fits more comfortably into their theoretical language or simply because on intuitive grounds they like one better than the other. Which solution is more workable can only be decided by employing the bases in research or in clinical work, where one basis simply wins out over the others as generally being more acceptable to the majority of investigators.

4. Reliability and Validity of Instruments

Surely no two terms are employed as frequently in discussing psychological measurements as *reliability* and *validity*. In essence, they cover the domain of some crucially important issues regarding measurement methods, but the terms themselves come out of the early days of developing psychological measurement methods going back to the turn of the century. Modern concepts of psychological measurement have far outgrown the original meanings given to these terms, and, consequently, one runs into something of a semantic snarl in trying to discuss modern ideas in the context of old-fashioned terminology. It is tempting to try to do away with both terms altogether and talk about "generalizability theory," "structural models for measurement methods," "scaling paradigms," and other somewhat esoteric terms that give the psychologist who is concerned with logic of science more latitude in pursuing the types of formal discourse required by the issues. However, unless these old-fashioned terms are mentioned, and related modern developments are discussed in their context, the reader would not be sure that he was in the right "ballpark." As we will see, however, this old-fashioned terminology does present some drawbacks to a more freewheeling analysis of the underlying issues in psychological measurement. Ideas change faster than terminology; consequently, we will discuss the major issues under the old rubrics of reliability and validity, respectively.

4.1. Reliability

Traditionally, reliability has been defined in terms of the purely chance element involved in the score made by any particular individual, on any particular instrument, under any particular set of circumstances, at any particular point in time. This is illustrated in Figure 1, which shows the true scores for two individuals, A and B, and hypothetical errors about the true scores. The analogy is frequently used of taking many measurements for the same individual (or material object) on a variety of occasions. Assuming that there is some error (admittedly not well defined at this point), one would expect the measurements to vary somewhat from occasion to

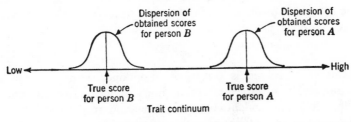

Figure 1. True scores and distributions of obtained scores for two persons.

occasion. An example from physical science would be in repeatedly heating the same metal rod to an observed temperature on a thermometerlike gauge and then measuring the length with a yardstick which was graded in a mechanical way to present a relatively exact "reading." In spite of efforts at precision in controlling all circumstances in the experiment and in accurately measuring and reading the lengths at the specified temperatures, there would be some error in that the results obtained from repeating the experiment many times would not be precisely the same. The results obtained from a relatively long rod can be thought of as analogous to person A in Figure 1; if the rod were relatively short, the results would be analogous to those shown for person B.

Although there is no way to directly measure a "true score," it is useful to think of this as being estimated by the average score in a distribution of obtained scores, such as those shown for persons A and B in Figure 1. The arithmetic means correspond to the two vertical lines. Because errors of many different kinds tend to be normally distributed, the conventional theory of reliability assumes that such errors are normally distributed for all persons (objects) regardless of the type of measurement instrument and regardless of whether scores are relatively high, low, or medium.

The original theory of reliability as it was handed down to us from Spearman (e.g., 1904) and his followers concerns the estimation of true scores and amount of error. This is done by performing experiments in which efforts are made to repeat measurements either under the same conditions or under conditions in which experimental variations are undertaken to purposely introduce a potential source of measurement error. (For a relatively complete description of conventional concepts of reliability, see Stanley, 1971.) The amount of error related to any one true score usually is thought of in terms of the standard deviation of such errors, which is given the special name *standard error of measurement*, σ_e. The standard deviation not only is a very useful descriptive statistic for specifying the variability in any distribution of scores but also is particularly apposite to the normal distribution because of the many related statistics (e.g., the standard deviation is itself part of the equation for the normal curve). Then, the larger σ_e, the more error there is in an *absolute sense*. The words "absolute sense" were italicized because, in most measurement problems in psychology, equally or more important is the *relative* amount of error—that is, the size of σ_e compared to the standard deviation of scores of some group from which the individual is selected (σ_x). The squared ratio of these two is spoken of as the percent of error variance, as follows:

$$\text{Percent error variance} = \sigma_e^2 / \sigma_x^2$$

In the conventional theory, it is assumed that errors of measurement are statistically independent of true scores (which modern theories would challenge in some cases), and thus the σ_e^2 added to the variance of true scores σ_t^2 equals the variance of observed scores as follows:

$$\sigma_x^2 = \sigma_t^2 + \sigma_e^2$$

Then, for example, when one is looking at an obtained set of scores on a measure of memory, anxiety, or sustained attention, one can think of the observed distribution as "hiding" two independent components relating, respectively, to the variance of errors and the variance attributable to true scores. The converse of the percent of error variance is the percent of variance explained by true scores, which is usually spoken of as the reliability coefficient r_{11} as follows:

$$r_{11} = \sigma_t^2 / \sigma_x^2$$

The above extremely simple model for discussing test reliability and the underlying components relating to true and error scores seems quite simple (yet, as we will see, the issues really are more complex), and all that is required is a set of data-gathering procedures for estimating components relating to true and error scores, respectively. This is necessary because, if an instrument tends to be dominated by σ_e^2 rather than σ_t^2, generally the results are untrustworthy. To the extent to which σ_e^2 is large relative to σ_t^2 (and thus r_{11} is low), this will serve to attenuate any type of scientific results that might be obtained; i.e., it will add to the error in analysis-of-variance designs for experiments, and it will lower the size of correlations between scores on different tests. It is important to measure the relative amount of error or, conversely, the reliability r_{11}, as part of the process of test development. Previously, it was said that the major standard for most test construction projects is that of a high level of internal consistency, which will result in a high level of r_{11} as measured by coefficient alpha and KR-20 (see discussion in Nunnally, 1978). Thus the cardinal standard for determining the worth of items that are added consecutively is that of gradually increasing the size of r_{11} as determined by coefficients of internal consistency.

Looking at Figure 1 and thinking about the concepts concerning reliability expressed above, one would think that the ideal approach to estimating true scores and σ_e would be by applying the same measurement instrument over and over to individuals. For example, in a study of simple reaction time, it would be sensible to obtain several hundred measurements and in this way construct a distribution of scores like that shown in Figure 1. However, in nearly all measurement problems, it simply is not possible to repeatedly measure the individual. Either the measurement procedure does not lend itself to repeated application or it would be unfeasible to ask a subject to take the time and effort to undergo repeated measurements. An example would be in determining the ability of brain-damaged individuals to remember the appearances of faces. The test consists of showing the individual pictures on a screen with a timing mechanism attached to a slide projector. The subject is shown 100 faces for 2 sec each and told to remember them as best he can. In the subsequent test session, the 100 pictures that were seen previously are randomly mixed in with another 100 pictures which the subject has not seen. On each trial, the subject says "yes" if he thinks he has seen the picture before and "no" if he thinks he has not seen them before. In this situation, it is logical to think of measurement error as being present as it would be in any other type of psychological measure. However, in order to obtain a distribution of errors and estimated true scores like those shown in Figure 1, one would have to have many such sets of pictures and have the individual come back on many occasions for testing (which, except for special experiments on measurement error, would be totally out of the question). Thus, rather than apply the identical or supposedly comparable measures of the same attribute on many occasions to a relatively small number of people, the measurement procedure repeated once (either in the same form or in a supposedly comparable form) with a relatively large number of individuals (say 300 or more), the product moment correlation coefficient is applied to the two sets of scores, and the reliability coefficient is declared as r_{11}. It is easy to prove that assumptions embodied in this simple theory regarding the nature of reliability would lead to the conclusion that r_{11} indeed represents an estimate of the ratio of true-score variance to obtained-score variance as shown previously. This then can be subtracted from 1.00 to obtain an estimate of the percent of error variance, the square root of which would be σ_e. Thus, traditionally, by correlating the same or supposedly comparable forms of a test on two or more occasions, an estimate of the reliability coefficient is obtained. The reliability coefficient so obtained not only serves as one index of the general worth of an instrument but also leads to many types of statistical corrections (e.g., correcting correlations for attenuation) and serves as a useful part of numerous statistical procedures.

4.1.1. Generalizability Theory

The theory stated above for discussing reliability is fine as long as one skates rapidly over the thin ice of many questions that can be asked. One question that should be asked is "Does one assume that the σ_e is the same for all persons?" The distributions shown in Figure 1 are symmetrical and depict the same size standard deviation or σ_e, and it is conventionally assumed that σ_e is at least approximately the same at all levels of a continuum. This assumption is inherent in estimating the reliability by correlating scores on the same or alternative versions of a test. In that case, what one does is to find a distribution of difference scores (one difference for each person) rather than a distribution of score differences that an individual would have on many occasions. Obviously, what one is doing then is accumulating errors for individuals, one from each individual, to obtain an overall estimate of σ_e, which supposedly holds at least approximately for all persons. However, it is easy to challenge this simple assumption (see discussion in Nunnally, 1978). The size of the σ_e at any point on the score continuum would relate to the way items were chosen for the test. By the procedure recommended previously for constructing tests for most purposes, one would tend to make scores in the middle of the continuum more reliable than those toward either extreme. Also, it is not safe to assume that distributions of scores are "normal." Rather, a more sensible assumption is that only scores that are near average (on conventionally constructed tests) tend to have symmetrical, quasi-normal distributions of errors. Near the extremes, it would be more sensible to assume that errors were skewed—persons with high true scores tending to have distributions of error scores skewed toward the mean and vice versa with individuals who have low true scores. In addition, it can be argued that one loses a great deal of information by lumping together experimental tests of the amount of error all along the continuum and employing overall estimates of reliability. Rather, one should talk about the *precision* of measurement all along the continuum, which may require a statistical rationale that is different from that employed for discussing overall reliability. Whereas in conventional reliability theory r_{11} varies with the size of the distribution of obtained scores σ_x^2, one could argue that a more scientifically respectable index of precision should be independent of the distribution of scores in any particular reference group, because such dependence certainly limits the generality of statements that can be made about measurement error. Thus, if one investigates a group of individuals that is very narrow in terms of individual differences with respect to the trait (e.g., all of the subjects are extremely anxious), one would come to the conclusion that the overall reliability was lower than if one investigated a population that was much broader in that regard (e.g., several hundred students selected more or less randomly from a college population).

Although conventional reliability theory has served rather well as an adjunct to the development and use of psychological measures, it has run into a number of major problems in addition to those cited above. When one looks carefully at the major constructs, it is meaningful to ask questions regarding the true scores and errors being investigated. True scores on what? Errors in what sense? Until psychometricians and other interested persons became restive about the matters, it was commonplace in talking about reliability simply to employ terms like "true scores" and "error scores" without taking the trouble to define them precisely, and indeed the "experts" tended to be annoyed by persons who even raised the issues. Although it was not formally stated as such by most individuals involved, the experimental procedures for measuring reliability implied that true scores could be defined in a circular sense in terms of what was measured in the context of applying an instrument on two or more occasions. Thus, if one had forms A and B of an intelligence test, the correlation between the two was given the name "reliability coefficient" and symbolized as r_{11}. However, when examined closely, employing this procedure infers that these two alternative forms constitute a world unto themselves with respect to the trait in question. Suppose rather than having forms A and B only, one also had forms C and D. Then it would be possible to obtain a total of six correlations among the four alternative forms. Unfortunately, or fortunately as the case may be, these coefficients would not be the same, but rather would vary in any particular sample of all four tests, and the coefficients obtained from one sample would be different from other samples. With these varying estimates of the reliability, what is the r_{11}? Obviously, such Zenoparadoxes were unsettling to those who thought that reliability theory had been all nicely cleaned up by circa 1925, and a continuing debate evolved regarding more explicit and seaworthy conceptual schemes for discussing reliability. Based as they were on the correlation between two testings to obtain an estimate of the reliability, these early theories were collectively referred to in retrospect as the *theory of parallel tests*, or, as it frequently is called, the *theory of platonic true scores*.

Because of the varying coefficients that one could obtain from correlating different forms and from different samples of individuals, it was realized that a broader theory was required. This led to the *domain-sampling* theory of reliability, which has its historical roots in the writings of many persons, even going back to some of Spearman's writings near the turn of the century. The theory was brought out fullblown by Tryon (1957) and later extensively exploited by Cronback (1951). It was made into a fuller theory of reliability by Nunnally (1967) and later supplanted by an even broader theory to be discussed subsequently. In essence, the domain-sampling theory considers any one instrument as constituting a random set of observations from a hypothetical domain (some refer to it as "universe" or even "population") of possible observations. Thus a particular spelling test can be thought of as a random sample of spelling words that could have been selected for a measuring instrument. As described by Nunnally (1978), it is also reasonable to think of items as having been randomly associated with circumstantial factors that influence the extent to which scores obtained from the sample are predictive of scores that would be obtained from the whole domain. Reliability theory, then, became the matter of gauging the extent to which scores obtained from an item sample would lead to efficient estimates of the scores obtainable from the domain as a whole (with the attendant concepts of sampling circumstantial factors to take account of sources of error other than that from content alone). This led to a new generation of thinking about reliability theory, divorced reliability theory from some of the nagging definitional questions that have been present in the more simplistic "platonic" conceptions of true and error scores, and generated a variety of new statistical studies and empirical investigations of reliability (much of this work is summarized in Stanley, 1971).

The importance of the domain-sampling concept of reliability is that it not only provided a more sensible logical basis for doing what had been done previously with respect to the study of reliability but also opened up new vistas and mathematical developments, and suggested interesting experiments with respect to the effects of measurement error on test scores. By dealing with a sampling concept, it permitted one to bring inferential statistics into reliability theory that had not been logically useful before, e.g., applying the ordinary sampling statistics to the precision with which reliability is estimated knowing the average correlation among items and the number of items in a test (see discussion in Lord and Novick, 1968; Nunnally, 1978). Also, when issues relating to test reliability were posed as problems in sampling, this suggested many new statistical estimates of various components of reliability, e.g., the maximum-likelihood estimates, which did not turn out to be very different from the older statistics, but at least shed light on possible statistical ramifications of the domain-sampling concept of measurement error. Actually, as concepts related to domain sampling grew, it came to be realized that the old-fashioned term "reliability" had some restrictive if not misleading connotations and should be replaced by the concept of *generalizability*.

4.1.2. Generalizability Theory

The wide implications of the concept of "observation sampling" from a specified domain led Tryon (1957) to adopt the term *domain validity*, thus dropping the term "reliability" altogether. However, as will be seen subsequently, if anything, the term "validity" has more "surplus meaning" than does "reliability"; consequently, this author does not consider Tryon's shift in terminology to have resulted in any significant clarification of the issues. However, in this and many other ways, Tryon did champion a much broader outlook on the study of measurement error in context with overall issues in psychometric theory and practice. He and others began to evolve a theory of generalizability, which in essence included the study of measurement error but permitted a less restrictive set of terms to be employed and opened up the possibility of more refined and powerful methods of mathematical analysis to be used. Cronbach and his associates (1971) are best known for concentrated work on extending the domain-sampling model into an even broader conception called generalizability theory. Essentially, what reliability theory is about is the extent to which one can generalize from a particular measurement to a broader class of measurements. What was lacking in the original conceptions of reliability grounded in the work of Spearman around the turn of the century and holding on for nearly half a century was a specification of the facets along which generalizability was to be investigated. Thus, although in comparing the measurement of the same individual on two forms of a test, one is in essence studying generalizabilty from one form to the other (and supposedly to some unspecified additional alternative forms), it was never made clear the range of circumstances over which such generalizability was being discussed or to what extent particular experiments were intended to measure the circumstances under which errors of measurement were thought to occur. Although it had been realized for a long time (e.g., see the discussion in Guilford, 1954) that overall measurement error σ_e can be meaningfully broken down into a number of components, most discussions of measurement error in textbooks on psychometrics did not explicitly take account of this matter, nor were multifaceted studies of reliability undertaken either in projects on test construction or in applied projects where tests are used for psychodiagnosis or other purposes.

The need to think about measurement error in terms of a multifaceted theory of reliability and to make appropriate investigations occurs very frequently in clinical practice with abnormal people. An example would be any type of treatment program (say for rehabilitation of parolees) in which adjustment is rated by a number of observers, on a number of traits relating to adjustment, on a number of occasions. This can be thought of as a three-faceted problem concerning measurement error and reliability. In the language in which it is being used here, a facet is simply a "dimension" along which circumstances vary with respect to the ways in which measurements are taken. Thus measurements can vary with respect to the rater making the observations, the traits on which the observations are made, and the occasions on which observations are made. Thus, for each individual, one can think of a cube with the sides designated "raters," "traits," and "occasions." (In this circumstance, it is assumed that the various items are to be summed to obtain a general measure of adjustment, and thus they are intended essentially to be replicates of one another.) Also, to extend the concept of larger numbers of individuals, one can think of the "cells" of this design as being filled with scores obtained from a sample of individuals, where each individual would have a score in each of the cells of the cube.

If one wants to, he can think of even more complex multifaceted designs for specifying the dimensions along which generalizability could be investigated. Indeed, the concept itself can be extended to consider "neighboring" traits that are not intended to be exactly the same as one another but that are thought to share some common core, which shows the "generalizability" of generalizability theory. In other words, this way of looking at it provides a wide-open experimental model for studying variability of scores from circumstance to circumstance and relations among scores on somewhat different trait measures. It also opens a gamut of related statistical procedures in relation to analysis of variance and multivariate analysis in general.

In most of his previous writings, the present author has not pressed heavily the applications of generalizability theory to actual problems of measuring reliability in either basic research or applied problems. However, the full-blown theory and statistical armamentarium of generalizability theory are needed with respect to many problems that are encountered in both research and practice in relation to clinical psychology and psychiatry. The reason it usually is not necessary to go into great detail in taking apart the various facets of measurement error in much psychometric work is that most of the error is due to the sampling of content rather than to variation due to judges, circumstances in which measurements are taken, and other possible sources of measurement error. Thus, in studying the reliability of vocabulary tests, the major limitation on the reliability of the tests is the sampling of words for the instruments, which in turn tends to be rather directly related to the number of words in the test. Thus, with this and many other types of psychological tests, the old maxim holds that a long test is a good test, and one can give primary emphasis to test length in considering sources of reliability. Standard formulas are available showing the expected increase in reliability from lengthening an instrument (these being presented in numerous books on psychological measurement, including Nunnally, 1978). However, as was said above, in the various types of clinical problems one encounters in psychology, psychiatry, and in clinical medicine, one does frequently find that a number of prominent facets must be considered with respect to the "unwanted variability" in measurement.

In actually undertaking generalizability analysis, in essence what one does is to estimate the variance related to the various facets in the generalizability design. Thus, whereas previously with respect to reliability theory it proved sensible to break a particular descriptor x_1 down into a hypothetical true score component t_1 and a general error term for that descriptor e_1, in generalizability theory it is necessary to take a particular measure apart in terms of the various facets of error that can be ferreted out in the design as applied to actual data. Thus, rather than having only one σ_e to stand for the overall error, one would have a series of error terms relating to the various sources of unreliability, e.g., σ_a^2 relating to the error variance attributed to facet a, and σ_b^2 relating to the variance attributable to facet b, and so on. If the general linear model held for explaining these components of error, then the total error could be broken down in terms of additive components as follows:

$$\sigma_e^2 = \sigma_a^2 + \sigma_b^2 + \sigma_c^2$$

Earlier it was said that the simple linear model made good sense in conceptualizing the factor descriptor for studying a domain of variables, but unfortunately it is necessary to consider complex interactions of errors in relation to facet designs in generalizability theory. An example of such an interaction would be that two raters would tend to give a particular patient the same rating on one item relating to anxiety but a very different rating on another item concerning anxiety. Another example of an interaction would be that two patients would receive very much the same rating by a group of judges on one testing occasion but receive very different average ratings by the same group of judges on another occasion. (Although in this instance one could simply say that the patients had changed and thus that measurement error was not at work from the standpoint of generalizing over testing times, such changes would have the effect of introducing error into any mathematical generalization.) Consequently, a total breakdown of the overall error in a facet design must take account of the various possible levels of interaction as follows:

$$\sigma_e^2 = \sigma_a^2 + \sigma_b^2 + \sigma_c^2 + \sigma_{ab}^2 + \sigma_{ac}^2 + \sigma_{bc}^2 + \sigma_{abc}^2$$

The highest order of interaction shown above (σ_{abc}^2) would be the case where one found errors interacting among judges, occasions, and items relating to a trait. Of course, one not only hopes that all of the error as manifested in the size of σ_e^2 will be relatively small, but to the extent to which error is present, one also would rather see this invested in the main effects (e.g., σ_a^2) rather than in the interaction terms. The latter are more difficult to interpret, and they are much more difficult to handle in any applied setting. Thus, if it is found that the facet concerning judges shows a considerable amount of error, one can either select judges who produce less error, train individuals for the rating task, or otherwise reduce this source of error. Similarly, if the error variance is due to the facet concerning items over which ratings are summed to obtain a total trait measure, one can either exchange some better items for ones that are present or seek a more extensive list of items. It becomes much more messy when a considerable part of the error variance is in the interaction terms. For example, if on one occasion judges agree well about the traits of some patients but not about the traits of other patients, and the patients on which agreement is found vary from occasion to occasion, it becomes very difficult to improve the overall measurement operation.

The actual mechanics of taking apart sources of error in a multifaceted design are discussed in detail in Cronbach, Gleser, Nanda, and Rajaratnam (1971) and in a variety of publications since that time scattered throughout the research literature in psychology, education, statistics, and other journals. In situations where there are a number of potentially important facets relating to reliability, it might be necessary to actually conduct the necessary experiments and take apart the error variance statistically in accordance with those procedures. However, in most measurement problems the major admonition is to keep in mind the possible multifaceted character of the measurement error that may be involved. Even though reliance may be placed on simple, more conventional approaches to studying reliability (e.g., only correlating two forms of a test or correlating ratings given by several psychiatrists), the potential complexities of the issues should be kept in mind.

It is easy to see that what started off as an extension of a simple theory of reliability really turned into the rudiments of a molar conceptual and mathematically structural approach to considering scientific generalizability in relation to the theory of measurement error. It is compelling to extend the types of concepts discussed with respect to generalizability theory to include measures of a variety of related constructs, e.g., measures concerning anxiety, stress, and response to specific forms of chemotherapy. The same general ideas and methods of statistical analysis can be applied. There it becomes apparent that the interest is far wider than that of just investigating components of reliability; rather, the interest is in studying generality in terms of the pervasiveness of theoretical principles interrelating variables in a field of inquiry. Looked at in this way, generalizability theory gradually moves over into the topic of *validity*, which is considered in the following section.

4.2. Concepts Concerning Validity

As is true of reliability, the concept of validity initially was discussed in a much oversimplified manner, namely in terms of specific statistical relationships between a measure and other important "dependent" measures. Thus as late as 1955 some of the more well-known experts in psychometric methods still spoke of test validity simply as "the correlation of a test with its criterion." I doubt that anyone with a respectable pedigree in behavioral measurement these days would support such a ridiculously oversimplified point of view. To say that the validity of a test is determined by correlating it with a criterion is an Alice-in-Wonderland statement that says everything while saying nothing.

If anything, the term "validity" has been invested with even more surplus and misleading meanings than has the concept of reliability. As with reliability, one would like to do away with the concept of validity altogether and replace it with terms that are more denotatively apposite for the semantically logical structure that is required for discussing the relevant phenomena; but this author learned long ago that one can change almost anything but terminology. Consequently, here we will use the word "validity" but try to offer numerous demurrers regarding the blind alleys into which the word itself can lead one; also, pains will be taken to delineate different meanings for the term and the different implications that these have for actual research.

Perhaps somewhat better (but not a greal deal) than simply saying that the validity of a test is its correlation with a criterion is to echo the popular phrase that validity consists of the extent to which an instrument measures what it claims to measure. Thus validity implies a degree of "goodness" of the instrument for some stated purpose, e.g., measuring intelligence, anxiety, improvement in therapy, or whatever. However, there is no simple way to do this, and although the present author has struggled with this matter himself and appreciates the efforts of other authors to cleanly delineate the problem and possible solutions, admittedly one does not simply "determine" validity in any straightforward manner. Rather, the so-called evidence for validity usually is a mixture of forms of evidence ranging from complex statistical products of massive experimentation on one extreme to simple impressions of people about the quality of an instrument at the other extreme. However, there are some subprocesses that can be delineated with respect to the topic of validity, and, as most "experts" will agree, some of the standards are more important for some types of instruments than others.

As it stands in the last quarter of this century, major reliance is being placed on three concepts—*content validity*, *predictive validity*, and *construct validity*. Content validity consists of essentially a rational appeal to the appropriateness of the test content for what it is supposed to measure. Content validity is most appropriate and most easily epitomized with respect to achievement testing in elementary school. An example would be a comprehensive battery of achievement tests for the sixth grade, which might include tests relating to reading, measures of other language skills such as punctuation and spelling, one or more tests for mathematics, including computations and arithmetic concepts, and various tests relating to "subject matter" areas frequently lumped into global tests of science and social studies, respectively. Arguing from the negative side, there are no purely empirical procedures that will "validate" instruments of this kind. Although research findings with the instruments are interesting and do add circumstantial evidence to content validity, achievement tests and many other instruments simply cannot be validated by a flight into statistics.

Before it was given a more refined status, content validity was frequently spoken of as face validity, which requires much more than literally "taking a look" at the test content and intuitively judging validity for the stated purpose. Content validity implies something more detailed and elaborate, namely that the domain of variables to be measured should be carefully "blueprinted" in the form of an explicit plan for measurement procedures and the construction of items. Examples of such plans are discussed in detail in many books on educational measurement (e.g., Nunnally, 1972). The plans go into considerable detail regarding the kinds of item content that will be included and the form in which it will be presented. For example, in the computational sections of the mathematical aspects of achievement tests, it would be stated that certain items would relate to long division of particular types (e.g., involving "carrying") and that other items would relate to geometrical concepts concerning the computation of area in figures of different kinds.

Whereas the construction of achievement tests in accordance with principles of content validity exemplifies that type of validity with all other instruments, content validity also is at work quite widely. However, anyone who is interested in the concept of content validity should see the detailed accounts of how the necessary blueprinting and manufacturing process is carried out with standardized measures of achievement. There are many additional details involved, such as having a panel of experts and test users decide on numbers of items of different types that will be included, item formats that are most acceptable, types of scoring units that are most meaningful, and many other details. It is hoped that the final result is an instrument that has been constructed from the ground up in terms of the best judgment possible about the relevant content and the form in which it should be cast. Because it usually is necessary to gather large numbers of responses, which frequently requires testing thousands of children, with most achievement tests many incidental results become available as part of the norming process. These and other statistics obtained from subsequent use of the instrument provide a wealth of incidental information about test validity which complements the primary form of validity, mainly content validity. Thus, as mentioned previously, validity involves a "mix" of concepts and procedures, even though one concept may be of dominant concern with a particular type of instrument. With achievement tests, for example, although they rest primarily on content validity, it is comforting to know that those tests employed in the last 2 years of high school are highly predictive of grades made by students who enter college.

The need for content validity extends far beyond school achievement tests, and, indeed, the more I work with psychological and behavioral measurement generally, the more I realize that many types of instruments are based on content validity either because they logically should be so or because there is really nothing else by which to judge their worth. This is the case for most measures of attitudes, such as attitudes toward the United Nations, abortion, college training, and other issues. This is the case with many important measures of what I call *personal conceptions*, meaning the way in which the individual views the human and material world about him. Thus, in a measure like the Locus of Control Scale, the individual is asked questions pertaining to whether he views success mainly being determined by luck, whom you know, or other forces external to oneself, or by "brains," hard work, or other forces internal to oneself. Although many forms of empirical evidence bear on the validity of the instrument for measuring the construct of Locus of Control, equally or more important is the direct appeal of the content for that purpose. The items simply look as though they relate to the trait name. If everyone agrees that the item content obviously relates to the particular domain of inquiry, this is equally as important as or more important than any type of evidence that can be obtained from experimentation regarding the validity of the instrument. Consequently, many of the instruments that are employed in research and practice in clinical psychology and psychiatry necessarily either rest to a large extent on an informal appeal to content validity or are actually constructed by the more detailed procedures mentioned earlier for ensuring content validity. An example would be in having an individual rate himself on a "happiness scale" in which he is instructed that 50% means about as happy as the average person, 100% means the happiest person in the world, and 0% means the most miserable person in the world. Whereas one might "validate" such a scale empirically from here to kingdom come, nothing could be more important than the obvious content of the item. Although we might not trust the individual or be sure of what implications his rating would have for other forms of behavior, we certainly would know what he was trying to communicate.

4.2.1. Predictive Validity

In some instances, validity does consist quite simply of the extent to which a test variable or other type of measure correlates with some type of criterion in daily life, such as the extent to which a college aptitude test actually is predictive of school grades or how measures of personality characteristics are predictive of successful response to alcoholism treatment. Rather than speak of such simple forms of validation as constituting the validity of the test, it would be more proper to speak of the validity with which the test serves the particular function. This is because an instrument that might be valid in this direct empirical sense for predicting one criterion might be nearly worthless for predicting any other criteria that are not highly related to the one in question. The term "predictive validity" is being used here to refer to empirical relationships between tests and their criteria—past, present, and future. The logic is the same in each case; the difference lies only in the time element. One could, for example, study the extent to which a test was "predictive" of an adult's behavior during childhood, which more grammatically would be referred to as "postdiction." Also, tests frequently are useful for "predicting" a present state, such as "predicting" which individuals do and which individuals do not have brain damage at a particular point in time. Of course, in this instance the tests are not used to predict who will incur brain damage later, but rather they are intended to have a type of "concurrent validity."

Regardless of whether the relationship is formed with some criterion variable in the past, present, or future, predictive validity is simple in concept and rather straightforward in terms of the logic of investigation, even though gathering the necessary data may be very difficult, time-consuming, and expensive. In the end, validity rests entirely on the correlations and other statistical characteristics of the situation that lead to efficient predictions. (Actually, there are other factors in addition to the predictor-criterion correlations themselves that determine the efficiency with which a test can be employed in a particular prediction problem; see discussion in Nunnally, 1978, and Wiggins, 1973.) Prediction problems frequently are at issue in many applied problems and research activities in clinical psychology and psychiatry. For example, if a battery of tests is employed to select people for different programs of treatment, in essence the prediction is that the individual will perform relatively well under the treatment conditions to which he is assigned. Intelligence tests and multifactor test batteries of ability frequently are used in a "negative" predictive sense to indicate the rather low probability of an individual performing very effectively in life, as traditionally has been done in employing IQ tests as adjuncts to diagnosing mentally retarded persons.

The major problem in studying predictive validity is not logical at all but rather lies in the disheartening fact that so many of the efforts to employ predictor tests meet with failure. That is, the tests frequently have near-zero correlations with their criteria. An utter cynic in this regard could with some justification say that predictor tests do an excellent job of predicting success in schools of all kinds but are not very predictive of anything else. This is an exaggeration because predictor tests have been found useful for many purposes; but although no one has kept an accurate count, it probably is so that more people have had disillusioning experiences in trying to employ predictor tests for one purpose or another than have been happily surprised by the degree of predictiveness that was found. This certainly has proven to be the case in a great deal of clinical research and practice. Also, tests are employed in a semipredictive sense with respect to *criterion variables* that are not well conceived, which no one plans really to measure, and, if one did, would have to stretch one's imagination mightily to think of a proper approach. An example would be an inventory in which individuals rated outlooks on their own personal status in life as regards marriage, relations with family members, employment activities, and other sectors of life. Typically, persons who voluntarily call on clinical psychologists and psychiatrists for help are low in some or many of these areas of functioning; it is to be hoped that after the completion of psychotherapy they would be much more optimistic about their performance in these types of personal life goals. One could argue that the validity of the "after" ratings should be validated by some type of predictive validity regarding how well individuals actually perform subsequently in life, but almost no research of that type is undertaken. Usually, the results of such ratings are judged mainly in terms of content validity, as it was described previously. As was said, it is seldom the case that predictive validity is the sole standard for judging an instrument; when such is the case, it certainly is a statistician's delight because the logic is very simple and the possible statistical tools that can be applied are delightfully plentiful.

4.2.2. Construct Validity

The notion of construct validity was adopted and given logical support because there are many uses for measuring instruments that cannot stand on predictive validity alone, content validity alone, or in combination. This is particularly the case for many of the measures that are employed in experiments. An example would be one mentioned previously, that of measures of three types of anxiety to be used in conjunction with research on stress. Such tests could be used as the dependent measures in laboratory-like investigations in which various types of physical stress (e.g., a very loud noise) are manipulated, or more naturalistic investigations could be undertaken of stress created by death in the family, anticipation of serious surgery, and other such potentially traumatic events. Whichever the case, the measures of anxiety are used to index the results of the treatment. Interpretations are then made based on such treatment effects, and such interpretations are wise or foolish only to the extent to which the measures validly tap what they are intended to measure. Now if one will look carefully at this and many other dependent measures employed in experiments, he will find that neither predictive validity nor content validity is completely appropriate for judging the worth of the instruments. Both are important in this regard. Thus, if a test has shown itself to be predictive of numerous behaviors that logically are related to anxiety, this would provide supporting evidence. Similarly, if the content of the tests can be judged to have content validity by the standards mentioned previously, that also is supporting evidence. To further buttress the types of evidence obtained from predictive validity and content validity, however, it is very useful to gather a wealth of circumstantial evidence regarding the extent to which a particular measure acts like it measures what it is purported to measure. Basically, this is nothing more than circumstantial evidence regarding the usefulness of the measuring instruments in relation to their purported underlying traits, but this is given the fancy name of "construct validity."

The present author (e.g., 1978), Cronbach and Meehl (1955), and others have deduced a rather complex logic for investigating construct validity. In the great long run, however, this boils down to something rather homespun, namely accruing evidence from numerous experiments regarding the extent to which measures dependably mirror the trait in question. Actually, there are very few major investigations on record concerning the construct validity of particular measures, and it is quite unlikely that such large-scale programs will be undertaken with respect to most of the measures that are used in research. As was said quite early in this chapter, any consistent set of rules for assigning numbers to objects in such a way as to represent quantities of attributes constitutes a legitimate system of measurement. What is measured may be utterly foolish or worthless, but it is measurement nonetheless. The worth of any measurement method seldom hinges on any tight logic or direct experimentation, as with prediction problems, and consequently construct validity in practice consists mainly of the "reputation" that a measuring instrument develops over much use in the laboratory and in applied settings.

4.3. The Importance of Factors

A topic that is closely akin to that of validity is the importance of factors, either those that are hypothesized and prove to be measures of unitary traits or those that are found in exploratory factor analyses. The virtues of considering measurement problems in any particular area of inquiry as relating to the need for a measurement basis of descriptors were previously discussed. The grinding mills of factor analysis have produced literally hundreds of factors both in the mainstream of human ability and personality and in scattered esoteric domains, e.g., factors relating to the opinions of women about rape. Factor analysis has become a way of life for a small percentage of the total profession, and some of these seem to be bent on factor-analyzing just any collection of variables that is available. In this way an overabundance of factors has been produced, some of these clear-cut and strong in terms of their statistical support, and others rather diffuse and vague in this regard. Typically, one gives names to the factors and provides paragraph descriptions of the apparent content, but how does one know if a test purported to measure a particular factor really is a valid measure of what is named and described? Looking at the issue in another way, validation of measurements can to a large extent be thought of as determining the usefulness of factors of ability, personality, and many special aptitudes and sentiments.

Methods for determining the worth of factors are discussed in Nunnally (1978); only a few summarizing comments will be made here. There are many examples of factors that rear their heads statistically but prove to be utterly trivial in terms of their impact on theory or any form of applied work. An example is a factor of line length estimation, which concerns various tests relating to estimating the length of straight lines, curved lines, lines enmeshed in other lines, etc. However, there is no indication that this factor (which might be better called an "artifactor") relates to anything else, not even other simple problems of estimation such as estimation of area or angular separation. Consequently, it is seriously doubtful that the factor is anything more than a statistical happenstance because of the inclusion in a battery of tests of several relatively trivial measures of essentially the same thing.

In order for a factor to be of any importance, it must meet a number of standards. First, a factor is interesting partly to the extent that it has some surprise value, when some of the tests that belong to it are unsuspected and thus stir investigators to think about the domain of inquiry. Second, a factor is important to the extent that it is predictive of *something*. Although factors cannot be judged entirely in terms of predictive validity, it is comforting to find at least some handsome correlations between measures of a factor and something else that is relatively important. Both content validity and construct validity come into the picture, also. Regarding the former, a factor is important to the extent to which the content looks as though it represents important things to be measured. For example, a factor has been found on numerous occasions which involves various tests concerning the ability to detect hidden figures of many different kinds, actual faces hidden in trees and landscapes, and simple geometrical figures embodied in more complex ones. Because of the interesting-appearing content of the factor (which Thurstone and Thurstone referred to as "flexibility of closure," 1941), many investigations have been undertaken with measures of it. Similarly, construct validity is important in judging the worth of a factor. The previously mentioned factor of flexibility of closure has been found to fit in well in a network of variables concerning the ability to resist distraction, to "see through" irrelevant details, and even to resist misleading cues given in some types of perceptual illusions. To the extent to which a factor weaves itself into a rich fabric of lawful relations of this kind, the attendant construct validity certainly serves to indicate the importance of the factor.

Related to other ways in which a factor helps to prove its worth, a factor is of interest in terms of the breadth of its content. Previously an extremely narrowly defined factor was mentioned, that concerning judging length of lines. On the other hand, some factors are so broad in terms of their "ecological" representation in daily life that it is hard to find an instrument that is not related. This is the case for the verbal comprehension factor, which is a major component in most tests of general ability and scholastic aptitude. A good vocabulary test, frequently posed in the form of verbal analogies, serves well to index this factor, but the factor of verbal comprehension goes well beyond sheer knowledge of words and ability to employ words meaningfully; it seems to be involved very widely not only in any types of items that contain verbal materials but also in some items that are based mainly on pictorial or other symbolic material.

As a final consideration, factors are important to the extent to which they fit in well in particular mathematical models for explaining a domain of ability or personality. Although there is not room in this particular chapter to discuss them in detail, there are numerous mathematical models which have been proposed for structuring collections of variables in particular domains, e.g., for describing various types of reasoning abilities. The simplest and most straightforward of these was illustrated and extensively discussed previously, that of a factor structure based on unitary descriptors. More complex models have been employed, such as hierarchical models which propose general characteristics that successively branch to more and more specific characteristics as one goes down the hierarchy. Various other mathematical models have been proposed for structuring the underlying components of abilities, personality characteristics, and special domains of attributes (see discussion in Nunnally, 1978, and Wiggins, 1973). Then, in the context of a particular mathematical model, a factor might be relatively useful or a downright nuisance in terms of how well it fit into the overall structure. This is a rather subtle matter because the worth of an instrument (measure of a factor) would depend on the nature of the particular mathematical model. Thus a test, such as a vocabulary test measuring verbal comprehension, that correlated with an extremely wide variety of other variables would be quite welcome in some models but would prove awkward in the context of other models. Regardless of this state of affairs, one potential way in which a factor can be important is that it is commensurate with and helps fill out a mathematical model relating to human traits.

After all of the fine things have been said above about the numerous matters concerning validity and the numerous special approaches, let this discussion end on a simple, realistic note. Both reliability theory and all of the possible inroads to the study of validity provide only promissory notes for the general worth of any new measuring instrument. All that a measuring instrument has to do is fit the definition given earlier regarding quantification of an attribute and then it is "in business." Even if it may give the appearance of being the most slapdash of misinventions, this can only be told in the great long run of research. The measure may look utterly silly but prove to be a complete gold mine of information regarding human characteristics; no one knows for sure until a great deal of circumstantial evidence is obtained from employing the measure in many different types of research endeavors.

5. Some Persistent Issues in Psychological Measurement

Looking back over the last century, in which psychological measurement has grown from nearly nothing to the present very large efforts in this regard, one sees a number of persistent "big issues" that arise time and time again. These are the issues that inevitably come up for discussion in a course on psychometric theory, and these are the issues that theoreticians usually face. The major ones are discussed as follows:

5.1. Do Psychological Traits Exist?

Various people have argued that, before starting out to measure psychological traits, it is first necessary to make a conclusive argument that such traits exist. Thus, whereas anyone can invent names for traits such as "intelligence," "abstract reasoning ability," "anxiety," "introversion-extraversion," "dogmatism," and many others, there is no reason to believe that trait names are matched by actual traits that exist among people. This is the old argument between the people who hold *nomothetic* and *idiographic* points of view. Of course, the nomothetic point of view is one in which the scientist "believes in," or at least entertains the possibility of, finding general laws that hold for *all* phenomena in a particular domain of inquiry, such as a set of laws that holds in the field of electricity or with respect to the formation of stellar galaxies. The dream of all science is to find a simple set of principles that could, at least in principle, be used to explain any natural phenomena in a particular domain, even though admittedly specific events may be "caused" by such a complex set of factors that it might prove difficult indeed to pinpoint all of the causal agents involved. Thus, whereas the various principles relating to earthquakes might be known reasonably well, it proves difficult to predict the exact occurrence and form of particular earthquakes. In developing a test (e.g., one of deductive reasoning or anxiety in social situations), there are those who claim that such general traits either do not exist, or, if they do, are unimportant in describing "the totally functioning, dynamic organization of personality" (whatever that is). The proponents of idiography claim essentially that each individual is a law unto himself and that only by ferreting out the particular ways in which an individual is psychically "organized," and only by unraveling the threads of life history of the individual, can the person be understood. Essentially this is the approach of the novelist and the biographer, but it also is an approach that frequently is given credence by personality theorists and workaday practitioners of the clinical arts. Thus many clinicians shun any forms of "objective" test scores as being either unimportant in understanding the individual or unimportant with respect to devising the most effective therapeutic processes.

There is no question but that the whole scientific movement concerned with the use of standardized batteries of tests for various forms of ability, personality characteristics, and others is based on the assumption that some general yardsticks concerning human traits do exist and are, at least in principle, open to measurement. Thus, whether or not it is generally stated as such, when an individual is developing a measure of a particular trait (e.g., anxiety in social situations) he succinctly assumes that it is meaningful to postulate a general yardstick along which all individuals can be ordered from high to low, and perhaps more precise forms of measurement are possible. Again, although the issue frequently is not addressed directly, it is assumed that if two people make the same total score (however individual item scores are combined to obtain a total score) they are alike with respect to the attribute relating to the name of the test. Now admittedly there are some pitfalls in assuming that all of the trait names that can be devised are matched by actual dimensions along which people can be meaningfully ordered, and of course in practice it frequently is difficult to perform measurements properly even where it is sensible to make the attempt.

The danger in postulating a general trait and undertaking the construction of a test to measure it is that in daily life so many instances are encountered in which individuals appear to combine specific modes of behavior in a very idiosyncratic way with respect to the trait names that are employed in psychological measurement. Thus, whereas the psychometrician may employ a general trait name such as "dominance," there are many instances in which an individual is dominant at work but not at home, dominant with women but not with men, dominant in relation to certain areas of living but not with respect to others. And so it goes with many other traits— it frequently proves difficult to describe the individual overall with respect to traits like introversion-extraversion, dominance, and reasoning ability.

For the above reasons, one must grant the idiographists some concessions in relation to their point of view. However, to adopt the idiographists' point of view initially is an antiscience attitude. To enter a domain of inquiry with the assumption that every event is a law unto itself is to postulate chaos in any effort to formulate general laws of nature.

With some types of human abilities, there is ample evidence that general laws prevail in terms of yardsticks for measuring individual differences. An example mentioned previously was that of the verbal comprehension factor, which has been found in many different factor analytic investigations with an extremely wide variety of materials. Also, the factor has shown itself to be extremely important in many applied problems, e.g., as a cardinal aspect of general intelligence, in the diagnosis of mental deficiency, and as an indicator of certain types of brain damage. There are numerous other factors of ability (summarized in Anastasi, 1976, and Guilford and Hoepfner, 1971).

Among noncognitive traits, there also are some factors that have met all of the requirements for broadly indexed, generally useful measurement. This is the case, for example, for the various "problem checklists" that are used widely with school-children for subfactors relating to adjustment in the classroom, with friends, and at home. The same factors hold up in test materials constructed by persons working in very different circumstances, the measures developed by different investigators tend to correlate well with one another, and there is a great deal of circumstantial evidence to indicate that the scales have a substantial degree of validity, in the various senses in which the term was discussed previously.

Where the idiographists can make their strongest case is with respect to measurement in one major sector of personality measurement, namely with respect to the measurement of *social traits*. Social traits are modes of overt behavior in daily life. It is such social traits that are featured widely on many of the personality inventories. For example, on the Guilford-Zimmerman personality test battery (discussed in Guilford, 1959), there are factors relating to friendliness, sociability, aggressiveness, reflectiveness, and other social characteristics. It is in such social characteristics that one so frequently sees examples of individuals who "mix" particular behaviors in an idiosyncratic manner. Consequently, one must admit that the idiographists have a good argument with respect to the difficulty of developing meaningful, general yardsticks with respect to such social traits. However, an important counterargument is that there are individuals on the extremes of all such measures, e.g., individuals who tend to be aggressive in nearly all situations and individuals who tend to be submissive in nearly all situations. It is these extremes that are most important from the standpoint of understanding the trait as well as for much applied clinical work. Consequently, even though the average person tends to be a mixture of habitual modes of behavior with respect to the trait in question (e.g., introverted in some ways but extraverted in other ways), one could argue that such a mixture is, by definition, what one would expect of individuals who are "middling" with respect to the trait; and thus this finding, rather than being an indictment of the nomothetic effort to measure general traits, produces exactly what one would expect. Whatever the eventual outcome of the argument between the nomotheticists and the idiographists in the long run, one should do everything possible to develop measurement instruments on behalf of the effort to find general laws of human behavior.

5.2. Subjective Aspects of Clinical Evaluations

All of us are somewhat battle-weary from the generations of exhortations from hard-nosed psychometricians (or narrow-minded numerologists, depending on your point of view) regarding the lack of *standardization* in some forms of clinical evaluation, such as in some interviewing and projective testing. The recognized father of mental testing, Sir Francis Galton, laid upon us the dictum that the essence of a test is that it be standardized in the sense that the same items be administered to all subjects in the same way, and that there be some uniform method of scoring leading to a quantification of the attribute in question. In this chapter, we have discussed in detail some of the major aspects of the catchall term for scientific measurement, that of standardization; but as the reader knows, there are numerous nitty-gritty details required to arrive at acceptable measurement methods. The reader would quickly become bored with any detailed recitation here of the many examples that could be provided on the breaches of standardization that have occurred in much clinical diagnostic work. Since in my graduate training I cut my teeth on studies of the Rorschach, TAT, SZONDI test, and other projective instruments, I can speak with some time perspective if not with any great wisdom otherwise about this matter. It occurred to me then, as it has occurred to many other individuals, that the so-called measurement involved in much clinical work really was full of holes as regards the requirements for standardization. As brief reminders to the reader, with many of the old-fashioned routines for projective testing, different testers typically obtain different numbers and different kinds of responses, have their own biases in making interpretation, go way out on a limb on the basis of extremely meager item-response material, and usually disagree with one another except for the most obvious of findings.

In a sense, all psychological measurement is "subjective" because, by its nature, it concerns human mental processes. However, some measurement also is highly subjective in that the personality and particular approach of the test examiner influence the subject's responses, and the interpretation frequently is not a profile of scores at all but rather is a "diagnostic picture." Similar efforts are made to provide personality descriptions based on across-the-desk interviews, observations in contrived situations, case history material, and other data bases.

With some of the quasi-objective approaches to measurement from projective tests and interviews, some types of item responses have been scored, such as the various scoring schemes for the Rorschach test, the TAT, and rating scales with respect to interviews and other bases for forming impressions. Frequently, however, the end result is a global description of the individual which is only loosely tied by any set of formal rules to the item responses.

In working closely with some projective testers, I rapidly came to the conclusion that any types of summary statistics obtained from individual responses in various categories (e.g., color responses on the Rorschach) were almost incidental to the overall interpretation that was made. Indeed, I firmly felt that the testers were not entirely sure why they reached certain conclusions about particular patients. In the days when I was working as a graduate assistant for Sam Beck helping perform research on the Rorschach, I was always impressed in watching Sam work his way through a Rorschach record. For example, in thumbing through the responses his eyes lit up when he saw the response "baby deer" to a particular detail on one of the cards. He immediately wanted to look at how the subject responded to a particular part of another card. He raced back and forth through the responses on various cards, and one could almost hear his mind grinding out hypotheses about what type person would give this particular pattern of responses. Although he was careful to enumerate all the statistics that he himself had championed for the Rorschach, I felt quite sure that the overall impression that he gained from any one protocol went far beyond anything that could have come from the summary of responses. In the same way that a gifted composer has a "feel" for what should come next in a composition, so the projective tester's "feel" for the significance of different responses is perhaps beyond his control and comprehension. He literally might not in fact understand his own intuitive processes. Even the most elegant (and some of it is pretty awful) highly subjective personality interpretations that are made in many clinical settings simply do not fit the requirements of true measurement. One can rightly claim that such intuitive judgments frequently are objectively *recorded* with rating scales and other devices, but it must be admitted that the interpretations themselves are highly idio-syncratically intuitive. One might rightly claim that this is all a semantic battle and that an easy way out is to refer to many of the diagnostic techniques as being "aids to diagnosis" and not give further claim for them as standardized procedures. This indeed may be a way out of the problem, but if so it must be laced with a number of "howevers." First, persons who deal with highly informal approaches to arriving at psychodiagnostic descriptions often report their findings as though they were backed up by thoroughly scientific measurement, when indeed that is not the case at all. Second, if one followed the measurement practices inherent in some of the interpretations made on these informal bases, he would break almost every rule of good measurement in the book. For example, there is no way under the sun that 30 responses to the Rorschach will give scientifically valid information about homosexual tendency, free anxiety, ego strength, suicidal tendency, intellectual thinking characteristics, criminal tendency, and many other attributes that frequently enter into interpretations. Indeed, one frequently does the impossible by entering the situation where one could measure more whole traits than there are individual responses given to the instrument, all of which is nonsense of course.

Logically, the major problem in dealing with highly subjective analyses, as with respect to some types of projective tests and some approaches to interviewing, is not that human judgment is required by the test examiner, because to some extent that occurs in many measures that are satisfactorily standardized. For example, an element of human judgment enters into the scoring of items on some of the individually administered tests of intelligence, but the rules for scoring are sufficiently explicit and agreement among scorers is sufficiently high that standardization is achieved. The major problem with many of the subjective analyses of some projective devices and some interviewing procedures is that the *test examiners* are very unstandardized. Not only do they do different things and work in different ways to achieve an overall diagnostic picture, but also they certainly vary widely in terms of their accuracy overall in reaching diagnostic formulations, and their accuracy interacts with the type of patient being considered. (See Nunnally, 1978, and Wiggins, 1973, for evidence on this point.) Then how does one know whether in a particular circumstance he has a good or a bad "measuring instrument"? Obviously it is not possible to perform a validity study for each projective tester or each interviewer, nor is it possible to make any general statement about the validity with which test examiners perform their functions.

The above critical comments about the ways in which some projective testers presently operate definitely are not intended to demean the *concept* of projective testing. To the contrary, on numerous occasions the present author (e.g., 1978) has spoken hopefully about the possibility of developing well-standardized projective tests in terms of the best logic currently available in psychometric theory and practice. What is being criticized is the failure of some projective testers to move on from the initially insightful, but admittedly highly exploratory, approaches to ones that are more fully in comport with the methodological requirements for scientifically acceptable measurement.

In any form of craftsmanship, including clinical psychology and psychiatry, one never simply "talks away" the employment of "bad art," no matter how heavily the evidence weighs against it. Rather, one only supplants bad art with better art. Consequently, until more satisfactory aids to diagnosis are developed, clinicians will continue to use the best that they have and the ones with which they feel most comfortable. Any overly cloistered psychometrician who looks down his nose at this practice is failing to face the realities of the situation; any fuzzy-minded clinician who thinks that some of the presently farcical, unnecessarily intuitive substitutes for scientific measurement are here to stay is a walking anachronism.

5.3. Can Self-Report Be Trusted?

Whereas, as stated above, one can rightly question the intuition of the clinician in arriving at a complex formulation of people's personality (frequently based on absurdly scanty data), one can also rightly question the extent to which the individual can faithfully provide "yardsticks" in gauging his own personality characteristics. Although personologists and psychometricians dream of entirely objective approaches to the measurement of personality (e.g., through brain waves or voice spectra), traditionally most measures of personality have rested either on the intuition of the tester, as in much of projective testing, or on the intuition of the individual in rating himself, as is the case in the multitude of self-inventories that have grown steadily since the end of World War I. All readers are familiar with instruments based on self-report, such as the MMPI for measuring various abnormal states like paranoid tendency and hysteria, and such measures of normal social traits as the Guilford-Zimmerman Inventory, which contains measures of ten traits such as ascendence, objectivity, and friendliness. In addition to the widely used standard batteries of self-inventories both for normal traits and for clinical symptom patterns, there have been literally hundreds of instruments developed with respect to particular aspects of personality.

Many laymen as well as professionals have made fun of self-report inventories as being transparent in purpose, easily fakable, and productive of highly misleading information in most instances in which they are employed. (Evidence regarding this matter is summarized in Guilford, 1959, Nunnally, 1978, and Wiggins, 1973.) Whereas I agree that most people can "see through" most inventories in terms of what is being measured, it is a grand non sequitur to assume that people usually do "fake good" in making self-reports. Even some of the experts in psychometrics have fallen into the trap of assuming that, since both intuition and some research evidence show that self-report inventories frequently can be faked, they actually are faked in research settings and clinical settings. Not only is there almost no evidence to indicate that subjects actually do distort answers markedly to self-report inventories, but also there is a wealth of circumstantial evidence to indicate that self-inventories are at least semivalid in many cases for what they are purported to measure. An example would be any one of the numerous self-inventory measures of overall adjustment (which lump together a variety of aspects of adjustment and maladjustment much as intelligence tests lump together content from a variety of factors of intellect). If one will take 20 persons who have scores far above average on one of these inventories and compare them with 20 people who are far below average, it will be rather obvious that as a group the low-scoring persons are less well adjusted than the high-scoring group. Similarly for many others self-report measures of social traits, forms of mental illness, attitudes, values, and other noncognitive traits, there are many instances in which self-report measures prove to be satisfactorily valid. The grand non sequitur mentioned previously is the assumption that, because people are capable of doing something (faking an inventory), they actually do so. An analogy that I have used on a number of occasions is when someone asks me the time of day: I could easily look at my watch and report an erroneous time, but I never do so.

Another great logical error made by critics of self-report inventories relates to the difference between the effect of faking on the average response and the effect of faking in the factorial composition of variance obtained from the measure. It is so that a considerable amount of circumstantial evidence indicates that people in general tend to paint themselves in a somewhat brighter light than is realistic. I discovered this years ago when employing some self-rating semantic differential scales (e.g., wise-foolish and clean-dirty) with a sample of individuals which was intended to be a miniature of the U.S. population with respect to demographic variables such as age and years of education. Well, of course, if people had been completely knowledgable about their own characteristics and completely frank in responding, then average scores on such traits should have come out in the middle of the rating scales, which in this case would have been 4.00 on a 7-step scale. Somewhat to my surprise, I found that the average person tended to rate himself somewhat above average, because most of the means were closer to 5 than to 4. However, I also found that the *variance* of individual differences in ratings was highly reliable and that the scales evolved statistically into a number of rather obvious factors which made good sense in terms of the research project. I suspect that the same is the case in many uses of self-reporting inventories; whereas the average person may hedge a bit in terms of "faking good," the considerable variance in ratings that typically is found is both reliable and largely valid with respect to the trait in question, e.g., self-report measures of anxiety and dominance.

Another issue with respect to self-report inventories concerns the "social desirability factor," which was forcefully brought to the attention of psychologists by the extensive work of Allen Edwards (e.g., 1957) on the tendency of people to say good rather than bad things about themselves on self-inventories. Although Edwards and others have undertaken some massive, careful research on social desirability, there have been some distinct misunderstandings about the meaning of the findings. As I see it, all of this research adds up to two major conclusions. First, with the types of items employed on most self-report inventories, people tend to agree with one another as to whether particular items are "good" rather than "bad," which means that people in general tend to hold the same conception of social desirability as evidenced in such items. (The illogical, unproven misassumption at this point is that since people can see the good and the bad in such inventories they use this information to purposefully distort their reponses when instruments of this type are employed either in research or clinical practice.) The second major conclusion that follows from this work is that if one will assemble a conglomerate inventory, gathering items from measures of supposedly different traits, with the only stipulation being that they either definitely say good or bad things, and then obtain a total score by adding up numbers of "good" responses and reversing the scoring for "bad" responses, the obtained measure of social desirability tends to correlate highly with many self-inventory measures, such as those found on the MMPI and on the Guilford-

Zimmerman battery of social trait measures. Now this is a much more telling potential fault than the first one. If rating oneself in terms of sheer social desirability is an extremely potent explainer of all self-inventory scales, then it would be rather non-parsimonious to deal with the multifactor inventory and more sensible to just look at the social desirability scores instead. There is a continuing argument about this matter, and psychometricians should be concerned about the dangers inherent in this argument.

However, there are some positive things to be said about the continuing effort to measure a variety of factors of personality other than (or in addition to) social desirability only. First, although a factor of social desirability does go a long way toward explaining the variance in multifactor inventories, the polyglot nature of the item content in social desirability scales is ideal for measuring a general factor, in the same way that the polyglot nature of intelligence tests is ideal for measuring a general factor relating to intellectual abilities. However, with both types of instruments, there is enough separable variance in individual differences to indicate that a variety of different factors can be measured in addition to the conglomerate general factor. As proved to be the case in breaking general intelligence down into a number of more nearly independent traits (e.g., various reasoning factors and spatial abilities), there is enough evidence regarding separately measurable dimensions of personality to indicate that more careful test construction efforts could build up batteries of tests based on self-report that were more nearly independent with respect to their underlying traits. Thus the apparent omnipresence of the social desirability factor may reflect more on previous methods of test construction than on "human nature" in terms of any reification of factorial findings from self-report inventories.

Another point worth making in this regard is that the social desirability factor is important only in inventories where goodness and badness are markedly at work in the item content. There are many domains in which self-report inventories are employed where social desirability logically should not play a very important part (or at least there is no firm evidence so far that it does). This is the case, for example, with a self-inventory concerning the extent to which an individual thinks that "truth" is determined more by fact-finding and logical analysis or by personal sensitivity and intuitive judgment. This represents a very interesting dimension along which people can be ordered, and on the face of it there is no reason to see why an individual should be "ashamed" to rate himself at any point on this continuum. There are many other traits of this kind that can be measured with self-inventories. There simply is no reason to believe that faking would play an important part.

In this section, the author is making a counterattack against those who have strongly criticized self-inventories. Partly this is a rejoinder to what is considered to be a bundle of misassumptions on the part of the critics. A second reason for this counterattack is that the empirical evidence does not support the contention that all self-inventories are fakable, or, worse, that they actually are faked when employed in research or clinical work. Third, and most important, even though self-inventories definitely have their problems as approaches to the measurement of personality characteristics, attitudes, values, and a variety of other noncognitive traits, they represent by far the best approach available. Those who laugh at self-inventories have failed to come up with measures that are one-fourth as good. Although 30 years ago I was prone to poke fun at self-inventories, in the intervening years I have learned that there simply is nothing better, and also I have seen a great deal of research reports which indicate that, although they are far from perfect, we would be in terrible shape without them for the measurement of many types of noncognitive attributes.

5.4. The Mind-Reading Machine

Earlier was mentioned the secret desire of so many persons in psychology to develop a mind-reading machine—something entirely objective, uncontrollable by the subject, revealing all of his secrets, not open to distortion by faking or dependent on the illusive artistry of the projective tester's work. One could establish a whole museum of rusting efforts to develop such mind-reading machines, and in my callow youth as a new Ph.D. I contributed to some of these misinventions. Only a few examples will be given to refresh the reader's memory. Back in the late 1950s and early 1960s, there was a flurry of activity with respect to "cognitive styles," in which personality would be "objectively" determined from the ways in which people's eyes roamed about pictures, the extent to which visual illusions were distorted by distracting stimuli, the amount of negative transfer in color-word naming tests, the numbers and kinds of piles into which objects were placed in an object-sorting test, and many other supposedly objective measures of cognitive style. Except for findings with respect to field dependence (e.g., with the embedded figures test and with the rod-and-frame test), nearly all of these supposed cognitive styles came to naught. Either they did not exist at all in terms of measurable factors, or, if several tests "hung together" to form a factor, they proved to be trivial in terms of any implications for personality. At about the same time, there was a great deal of activity with respect to "response styles," which were by-products of paper-and-pencil tests. Some of these supposed traits were acquiescence, the extremeness tendency, and the tendency to guess when in doubt (supposedly willingness to gamble). Such studies of response styles kept many psychometricians busy for a period of about 10 years in what proved to be a great waste of effort. (See Nunnally, 1978, and Rorer, 1965, for rather scathing reviews of the literature on this topic.)

In spite of the beating that the proponents of mind-reading machines have taken in the empirical arena, the advocates are addicted to the search (and the present author falls victim to this mania on occasion). A more recent effort was to develop a "hedonic thermometer" from pupillary response (work summarized in Nunnally, 1978). Some of the early work of Hess suggested that the pupils of the subject's eyes dilated when he viewed something pleasant and constricted when he viewed something unpleasant. These early reports by Hess not only were incorrect but also led many investigators (including Nunnally and his colleagues, 1967) into hundreds of experiments to determine whether or not the pupil could serve as an adequate mind-reading machine for hedonic values. Foiled again! It turns out that pupillary dilation occurs when the subject views *both* pleasant and unpleasant pictures. Any form of arousal (e.g., from threat of a gunshot or lifting weights) will bring on pupillary dilation. No one found reliable pupillary *constriction* from anything other than turning up the lights. Thus another mind-reading machine was placed in the museum.

I still am hopeful of finding personality correlates in physiological processes such as glandular outputs, vascular activity, various electrical products in the nervous system, and other variables in the province of physiological psychology and physiology. I also am hopeful that some of the by-products of cognitive tests (e.g., certain aspects of memory, reaction time, and perceptual judgment) will prove to be related to personality characteristics. However, admittedly we people who have sought the mind-reading machine have taken quite a beating.

Because of the failures in developing a mind-reading machine for the measurement of personality characteristics, we have had to fall back on some much more homely approaches. When people who are not familiar with the topic ask me how in general one should measure various aspects of personality, my knee-jerk response is "Ask the person or ask someone who knows him well." Previously we have talked about the self-report inventories, which in essence ask the individual about his own personality characteristics. The second half of my admonition—to ask someone who knows him well—is a matter that we need to discuss in more detail. I chastised the seat-of-the-pants school of projective testers specifically because I rather doubt that in general they "know" the subject well. However, it is possible to obtain meaningful ratings from acquaintances of an individual, which is the subject that will be discussed next.

5.5. Observational Methods

As has been true in so many other efforts to measure personality, we have come the long way around to discover that some of the simpler approaches not only are much easier to employ but also are more valid in general than their highly involved counterparts. As an example of the latter, much effort was wasted on so-called situational tests, starting with military experience during World War II. (Wiggins, 1973, discusses this history in detail.) Essentially the situational test consists of placing an individual in a play-acting circumstance that will elicit criterion-relevant behaviors. An example is that four men are given a pile of boards, bricks, and some rope and told that they have exactly one-half hour to build a bridge across a stream. Of course, three of the four individuals are actors who do everything possible to mess up the act, and the "measure of the man" under study is how well he demonstrates his leadership capacity in these trying circumstances. Some of the "sets" for these situational tests would have done Cecil B. DeMille proud, and only military budgets could have afforded putting on such shows. But after 15 years or so of trying out such situational tests in military settings, in selecting clinical psychologists, in studying the characteristics of business leaders, in investigating the behavior of highly creative scientists, and in other such activities, it became obvious that the situational tests largely are a bunch of junk. To make a flat statement, I can compose a simple self-rating questionnaire in a half hour that would be more valid than a monstrous production relating to such situational tests.

To a lesser extent, effort has been wasted (so hindsight shows us) in numerous other efforts to develop observational situations that would elicit relevant behaviors from the individuals to be rated. What gradually dawned on almost everyone working on the problem is that the most reliable and valid rating about people comes from experience with them in real-life situations rather than in contrived situations. Also, far more important than any type of formal training that the rater has is the amount of experience he has had with the ratee in situations that are relevant to the traits under consideration. For example, it has been known now for a quarter of a century that in military ratings men in a barracks who know one another well are far better at rating one another with respect to traits that are important for efficient military functioning than are the men's officers, psychologists who get in on the act, or any other individuals who are not primary members of the group. This finding has led to the wide use of "peer ratings," in which members of some close-knit group (e.g., in a fraternity or members of the same therapy group relating to alcohol abuse) rate each other. When they are feasible to obtain, such peer ratings have been found to be highly reliable and valid for research purposes and for clinical work.

6. Retrospect and Prospect

It is easy to concentrate on the difficulties encountered in certain areas of psychological measurement to the point where one loses sight of the overall achievements that have been witnessed during the last 100 years. We now have available large, well-standardized batteries of tests for various types of human abilities, special abilities, personality characteristics, and psychological disorders, and literally hundreds of special-purpose tests. Indeed, in acting as psychometric consultant on a wide variety of projects, I am usually pleasantly surprised at the amount of "hardware" available to meet the needs for psychological measurement. Only yesterday (while this chapter was being written), I was asked about self-rating and teacher-rating measures of adjustment in elementary schoolchildren. I had recently been acting as a consultant on a large project to develop norms for an excellent pair of instruments for that purpose, and I could tell the questioner of several other excellent instruments that were available. Two weeks ago, I discussed with some educators their needs for the development of scales for the measurement of attitudes and opinions of college students about physical fitness programs. I found that simple approaches to attitude-scale construction and questionnaire development were suitable for their purposes. For the last 8 months I have been consultant to a large-scale project at Vanderbilt on the psychological effects of severe uremia, which results in a general loss of "mental alertness." I found available a wide variety of tests that would be useful for studying the phenomena, ones with a long pedigree in military research, clinical psychology, and other areas. These were tests of various aspects of short-term memory, reaction time, perceptual vigilance, psychomotor skills, and others. Thus, rather than finding the overall picture as regards psychological measurement to be a gloomy one at this point in the twentieth century, my own personal experience leads me to be gratified by the "know-how" that currently is available and optimistic about future developments.

When one will remember that before the turn of the century the major standardized tests (e.g., those employed by Galton in his pioneering work) consisted of such tasks as judging lengths of lines and discriminating strips of colored yarn from one another, one will realize that we have come a long way to the modern multifactor batteries of ability. And the same comparison holds with respect to measurement of personality and many other attributes. For what they are worth, following are some brief suggestions regarding fruitful directions for future research.

With respect to the measurement of human abilities, if anything the major problem is the overabundance of factors that have reared their heads statistically but have never been actually tested out for importance—in terms of the various methods for determining validity discussed previously. Many of these factors should be tried out on a wide variety of problems concerning human competence, and gradually we will be able to separate the wheat from the chaff. So many factors of human ability already have been found that it seems almost superfluous to perform further extensive digging in that regard until the worth of some of the more frequently encountered factors is determined. The same situation exists in the area of self-report measures of personality, both for normal ranges of traits and for diagnostic inventories, but generally the typical evidence there is not as firm as it is in studies of human abilities. It is to be hoped that the factor structures existing in these areas will be further clarified and that the factors that survive the necessary statistical hurdles will be employed more broadly both in research and in clinical practice.

My major hope for the future regarding the refinement of known factors of human ability and personality and the development of interesting new measures lies in the apparent increasing awareness by both psychometric theorists and substantive researchers and clinicians that a strong alliance is beneficial to all. I have seen many examples of how such alliances have grown during the last 20 years. One is in relation to developmental psychology, where psychometricians have "gotten into the act" regarding the developmental sequences and processes proposed by Piaget and other theorists. A second example is in relation to both research and practice in the field of special education, where psychometricians have attempted to develop more flexible measurement methods to fit the goal-referenced approach to individualized instruction and assessment of progress. I have seen this healthy alliance grow in relation to the near explosion of interest in evaluation research throughout the federal government, such as in evaluating the effectiveness of health care programs, mental health clinics, and alcohol abuse programs. There is considerable pressure from the general public exerted through Congress to have all programs of human services "prove their merit," and this requires hitherto unheard of amounts of evaluation research. The psychometrician is offered many challenges, and a close alliance is forced of psychometricians with legislators, program administrators, and clients for the various services. In clinical medicine I have found many examples of partnerships being formed between specialists in psychological measurement and researchers in psychiatry, pharmacology, neurology, physical rehabilitation, and a wide variety of specialties relating to internal medicine. It is coming to be realized that an intrinsic part of the illness, as much as anything that can be found under a microscope or in a chemical analysis, is the fact that people *feel* and *act* sick, and different disorders manifest themselves in different profiles of losses in abilities and social competence.

For over half a century, psychometric specialists could, in many cases, hide behind the rationalization that better methods of measurement were not being developed and employed because of a lack of awareness on the part of the clinical practitioners and administrative officials and a lack of funding for basic psychometric research. There was much merit in that argument 20 years ago, but it is no longer the case. Now the psychometric specialist should either "put up or shut up."

7. References

Anastasi, A. *Psychological testing* (4th ed.). New York: Macmillan, 1976.

Comrey, A. L. *A first course in factor analysis.* New York: Academic Press, 1973.

Cronbach, L. J. Coefficient alpha and the internal structure of tests. *Psychometrika*, 1951, *16*, 297–334.

Cronbach, L. J., & Meehl, P. E. Construct validity in psychological tests. *Psychological Bulletin*, 1955, *52*, 281–302.

Cronbach, L. J., Gleser, G. C., Nanda, H., & Rajaratnam, N. *The dependability of behavioral measurements.* New York: Wiley, 1971.

Edwards, A. L. *Techniques of attitude scale construction.* New York: Appleton-Century-Crofts, 1957.

Gorsuch, R. L. *Factor analysis.* Philadelphia: Saunders, 1974.

Guilford, J. P. *Psychometric methods.* New York: McGraw-Hill, 1954.

Guilford, J. P. *Personality.* New York: McGraw-Hill, 1959.

Guilford, J. P., & Hoepfner, R. *The analysis of intelligence.* New York: McGraw-Hill, 1971.

Harman, H. H. *Modern factor analysis* (3rd. ed.). Chicago: University of Chicago Press, 1976.

Lord, F. M., & Novick, M. R. *Statistical theories of mental tests.* Reading, Mass.: Addison-Wesley, 1968.

Nunnally, J. C. *Tests and measurements—Assessment and prediction.* New York: McGraw-Hill, 1959.

Nunnally, J. C. *Psychometric theory.* New York: McGraw-Hill, 1967.

Nunnally, J. C. *Educational measurement and evaluation* (2nd ed.). New York: McGraw-Hill, 1972.

Nunnally, J. C. Vanishing individual differences—just stick your head in the sand and they will go away. *Journal of Instructional Psychology,* 1976, *3,* 28–40.

Nunnally, J. C. *Psychometric theory* (2nd ed.). New York: McGraw-Hill, 1978.

Rorer, L. G. The great response-style myth. *Psychological Bulletin,* 1965, *63,* 129–156.

Spearman, C. "General intelligence" objectivity determined and measured. *American Journal of Psychology,* 1904, *15,* 201–293.

Stanley, J. C. Reliability. In R. L. Thorndike (Ed.), *Educational measurement* (2nd ed.). Washington, D.C.: American Council on Education, 1971.

Stevens, S. S. (Ed.). *Handbook of experimental psychology.* New York: Wiley, 1951.

Stevens, S. S. Problems and methods of psychophysics. *Psychological Bulletin,* 1958, *55,* 177–196.

Thurstone, L. L. *Multiple-factor analysis.* Chicago: University of Chicago Press, 1947.

Thurstone, L. L., & Thurstone, T. G. Factorial studies of intelligence. *Psychometric Monographs,* 1941, No. 2.

Tryon, R. C. Reliability and behavior domain validity: Reformulation and historical critique. *Psychological Bulletin,* 1957, *54,* 229–249.

Wiggins, J. S. *Personality and prediction: Principles of personality assessment.* Reading, Mass.: Addison-Wesley, 1973.

5

The Rorschach

JOHN E. EXNER, JR., AND BETH CLARK

1. Introduction

Of the large number of diagnostic tools available to clinicians today, perhaps none has been so widely used yet remained so controversial as the Rorschach test. Since the publication of Hermann Rorschach's *Psychodiagnostik* in 1921, dozens of books and more than 5000 articles have been written on the test. Over the almost 60 years of its existence, five major systems of Rorschach administration, scoring, and interpretation have arisen. Each approach offers its own unique postulates, yet each unavoidably adds to the confusion about the uses and the philosophy of the test.

The Rorschach flourished especially during the period of the 1930s to the 1960s, when assessment was seen as the primary role of the clinical psychologist, but the test has so far also stood the challenge of the increasing shift in emphasis toward intervention as the psychologist's main responsibility. Although Biederman and Cerbus (1971) reported a drop in the number of courses offered on the Rorschach in clinical graduate programs, there has been no corresponding reduction in its use in the clinical setting. In 1961, Sundberg surveyed 185 clinical facilities and found that the Rorschach was being used in 93% of them. The proportion of patients given the test was then 80%. Lubin, Wallis, and Paine (1971) replicated Sundberg's study 10 years later. Surveying 251 facilities, they found that the test was being used in 90% of them, even though the proportion of patients given the Rorschach had decreased, perhaps because of more selectivity, to 60%.

For a test that is an integral part of the "standard operating procedure" of most clinical settings, the hue and cry about the Rorschach has never ceased. Echoing the controversies of the early systematizers, empiricists debate phenomenologists as to whether the test is science or art. Demands for evidence of validity are increasing, as is the confusion about just what "the Rorschach" is. Indeed, the assumption that there is a single Rorschach is a naive one. There are perhaps as many Rorschachs as there are examiners. Exner and Exner (1972) surveyed clinicians who use the test and found surprising irregularities. A fifth of the examiners did not score the test at all. Of those who did, 75% personalized their scoring in some way, usually by combining elements

JOHN E. EXNER, JR., and BETH CLARK • Department of Psychology, Long Island University, Brooklyn, New York 11201.

of the various systems, yet maintained that they adhered to one particular system. Of testers, for instance, who claimed allegiance to the Klopfer system, more than half were found to depart significantly from its tenets. Of 166 Klopferians surveyed, 71 administered the test in a face-to-face position and 63 told the subject to report everything he saw. Both of these procedures are strongly cautioned against by Klopfer. Eighty-one used Beck's Form Quality tables instead of Klopfer's Form Level Rating, while another 32 did not score the test at all.

With confusions such as these running rampant, finding any clear-cut approach to the Rorschach has been an extremely difficult task. A first step toward this goal may be the development of a comprehensive, integrative approach to the test, one which uses the best of all systems on the basis of empirical findings. What follows is a discussion of this new approach. Yet, to fully understand the Rorschach, one must understand its foundations and development.

2. History of the Rorschach

The use of inkblots for psychological diagnostic and descriptive purposes was initiated by the young Swiss psychiatrist Hermann Rorschach in 1911; his work on it extended until his death in 1922. It is difficult to tell exactly how Rorschach became interested in the use of the blots. Apparently, inkblots were used in a familiar parlor game called "blotto" in the late nineteenth and early twentieth centuries. They are also known to have been included in numerous research projects in that same era. (Exner, 1969a).

Although Rorschach began experimenting with inkblots in 1911, most of his major work was accomplished between 1917 and 1922. His main interest was in the use of the technique to study perception, and he hoped that it would lead to a more sophisticated tool for psychiatric diagnosis than any that was currently available. With this in mind, he administered the test to both patients and nonpatients, mostly in Switzerland. Rorschach originally used 35 inkblots, but he was forced to reduce this number to the ten currently in use because his publisher was unwilling to invest in the printing of any more. The original blots were not shaded, but a printing error caused the shading effect. Rorschach thought this to be of great interest, and he proceeded to use the shaded blots in the rest of his work.

Rorschach's major monograph, *Psychodiagnostik*, appeared in 1921; unfortunately, he was to die the following year of peritonitis at the age of 38, having made an extremely significant contribution to the fields of psychiatry and psychology, but at the same time leaving the technique of the Rorschach in its infancy. Perhaps most noteworthy is the fact that he never developed a specific theory of the test. He did, of course, make the assumption that the way an individual taking the test interprets the blots is in some way connected to his behavior (Exner, 1969a). He also was committed to an empirical method for studying the test and was cautious about the uses to which it could legitimately be put (Rorschach, 1921). There is some controversy over whether Rorschach would have approved of how the test is used today. Zubin, Eron, and Schumer (1965) maintain that he would not be comfortable with a psychoanalytic theory of interpretation of the test. Rorschach, however, did encourage interpretation of content, and as a member of the Swiss Psychoanalytic Association he was well versed in Freudian theory. It is highly likely that, had he lived longer, he would have developed some sort of integration approach, and that it would have been based on psychoanalytic theory.

Rorschach's work possibly would have been lost to us today if it had not been for the labors of three of his closest colleagues: George Roemer, Walter Morgan-thaler, and Emil Oberholzer. All three continued to teach the technique and to encourage others to carry on research. Of those trained by Oberholzer, a psychoanalyst, one was David Levy, who introduced the Rorschach to the United States. He was responsible for organizing the first Rorschach seminar in Chicago in 1925. Levy, in turn, was a primary influence on Samuel Beck, who became one of the five major systematizers of the technique.

Beginning in the 1930s, the United States became the major source of research on the Rorschach. All of the five systems or approaches to the test that evolved in America incorporate some of the basic ideas that Rorschach first espoused, but each has it own unique position on administration, scoring, and interpretation. The five systematizers are Samuel Beck (1937, 1944, 1945, 1952, 1960, 1967), Marguerite Hertz (1938, 1942, 1951, 1970), Bruno Klopfer (1942, 1954, 1956, 1970), Zygmunt Piotrowski (1947, 1957, 1964), and David Rapaport (1946), together with his pro-tégé, Roy Schafer (1954).

Exner (1969a) suggests two reasons for the emergence of the different systems. One is that none of the systematizers ever had direct exposure to Rorschach himself. Only Beck had had contact with Oberholzer, when he went abroad to study with him in 1933. Rapaport did not complete his doctorate until 1938—16 years after Rorschach's death. Related to this time lapse involved in the development of the systems, a second reason for their divergence is the differences in training and background of the five individuals; these differences led them to emphasize various aspects of the technique.

Samuel Beck was author of the first dissertation of the Rorschach in the United States, completed at Columbia University in the early 1930s. Columbia at that time was a mecca of the traditional form of American behaviorism and positivism. Not unexpectedly, Beck's approach to the technique reflects this cautious and empirically oriented stance. In addition, Beck's later work with Oberholzer brought him closest to Rorschach's original concern for the careful testing of hypotheses concerning the test and to Rorschach's conservatism regarding applicability.

In contrast to Beck, Bruno Klopfer came out of a phenomenological and Jungian psychoanalytic background. He was educated at the University of Munich, where he received his Ph.D. in 1922, but he was forced to flee Nazi Germany in 1933. He then spent a year in Switzerland studying with Jung. It was at this time that he was introduced to the Rorschach. When he came to America a year later, he emphasized an approach to the Rorschach that encouraged more subjectivity of interpretation, in keeping with the German psychological tradition at that time.

Beck and Klopfer may be seen to occupy opposite ends of a continuum representing interpretive positions ranging from empirical objectivity to subjectivity. The other systematizers fall at points between these two extremes.

Zygmunt Piotrowski was, like Klopfer, well versed in the European phenomenological school, having received his Ph.D. in 1927 at the University of Poznan in Poland. Unlike Klopfer, however, his main field of interest was experimental psychology, specifically the areas of perception and mathematical analysis. When he was exposed to the Rorschach in one of Klopfer's seminars, after he had come to the United States as an instructor at the College of Physicians and Surgeons at Columbia University, he came to approach the test from his own position.

Marguerite Hertz's training emphasized basic psychometrics and she was awarded her doctorate in 1932 at Western Reserve University, completing the second Rorschach dissertation. She spent her early career working with children in conjunction with the Brush Foundation. She rather skeptically began a series of studies to determine its value, and this work has continued throughout her career. Although her early psychometric approach would appear to favor Beck's position, her approach to the Rorschach has been marked by a number of shifts over the years, and ultimately she has taken a position that is closer to Klopfer's more subjective approach.

Possibly closest to Klopfer on the continuum is the Rapaport-Schafer position. This approach was never intended to be a formal system by its authors; rather, it evolved gradually from a more general emphasis on the psychoanalytic potential of the test and on the relationship of the examiner to the subject. Much of it is contained in Rapaport's major work, *Diagnostic Psychological Testing* (1946), written while he was affiliated with the Menninger Foundation. Roy Schafer, who worked with Rapaport at the Menninger Foundation, expanded on his work in several landmark works, among them *Psychoanalytic Interpretation in Rorschach Testing* (1954). The Rapaport-Schafer system is, then, almost exclusively psychoanalytically oriented and may be placed nearest the subjective pole on the interpretive continuum.

With so many different backgrounds and orientations, it is not difficult to see why the separate systems developed as they did. Yet they did not do so independently, but in an atmosphere of great controversy and communication. The period of 1933–1940 was the one of greatest activity among the various proponents of the Rorschach, with each trying to make his or her opinions known.

Beck (1935) and Klopfer (1937) were the first of the systematizers to document their respective approaches, and from there the stage was set for often bitter controversy. In two articles, Beck (1935, 1936) expressed dismay that the Rorschach was being treated, he believed, as a device for the artist rather than the scientist. He called for extensive experimental justification before any scoring additions, beyond those that Rorschach had originally used, could be considered. Beck also was concerned that the development of standardization for the test was proceeding too slowly, and that much more work needed to be done in gathering normative data across different clinical populations. In 1937, he published his first book, *Introduction to the Rorschach Method*, in which he proposed a scoring system based on his experimental work.

Beck's appeals for psychometric rigor were not sympathetically received by practitioners of the more phenomenological approach of Bruno Klopfer. Over the years, Klopfer had conducted seminars on the Rorschach, and, as a master teacher and figure of some charisma, he had a considerable following in the United States. At the time Beck was publishing his articles, Klopfer decided that a forum was necessary for the various opinions of those working with the Rorschach. Thus, in 1936, he began publishing the *Rorschach Research Exchange*, which came to evolve into the contemporary *Journal of Personality Assessment*. In the first issue, Klopfer published a refined scoring system based on his past experience and on the discussions that had taken place in his seminars in the 2 years previously (Klopfer & Sender, 1936). In this and in other publications (Klopfer, 1937), he stressed that the examiner's experience should guide him and was thus more sympathetic to a rather subjective approach to the technique, and less concerned with empirical validation. In addition, Klopfer was highly critical of Beck's omission of what Klopfer considered important scoring categories. This prompted a reply from Beck, and a lively traffic of letters and comment began in the *Rorschach Research Exchange*. The battle in print, together with the fact that the two approaches were so differently based, widened a schism that has persisted to the present day.

Marguerite Hertz was in the midst of the controversy. She had published a set of Rorschach norms for various age groups (1935), and had expressed her concern that a method of standard administration for the test be adopted (1936). In 1937, she published an article which placed her in the position of being not only the mediator but also the conscience of the Rorschach community. In that paper, she criticized Beck for failing to provide adequate information about his own standardization and validation procedures. At the same time, however, she was critical of Klopfer for his willingness to accept new scoring criteria without any supporting data base. Hertz also made a plea for compromise and for the development of a uniform Rorschach language. Thus, by taking a firm stand in the middle, Hertz began to develop her own approach, based on her measurement orientation; however, she was later to shift to a position more aligned with Klopfer after Cronbach (1949) criticized her approach to standardization of the Rorschach.

By 1940, there were three separate Rorschach systems. By this time, Piotrowski had become more and more uncomfortable with the subjectivity of the Klopfer approach, but also differed with Beck on scoring, so he worked on his own system. Piotrowski held to no particular theory of personality, but viewed the Rorschach as a visual stimulus that is responded to in various ways by various populations. Piotrowski's thoughts culminated in his 1957 book, *Perceptanalysis*; subsequently, he became involved in the construction of an elaborate computerized system for Rorschach interpretation (1964).

Finally, as mentioned above, the Rapaport-Schafer approach was developed as a system in its own right by 1946. It is the least similar to the other four in that it treats the technique more as a part of a standardized interview procedure, where more importance is attached to the individual's unique response patterns rather than to the stimulus. For Rapaport and Schafer, the Rorschach is a handy tool with which to study psychological process.

Thus, over the years 1936–1957, the five most widely used Rorschach systems developed. For the most part, they are quite different, yet there are similarities among them. They all use some of the basic tenets of Hermann Rorschach in terms of interpretation; all of them tend to incorporate some aspects of psychoanalytic theory into their respective approaches to interpretation of the subject's verbalizations. Differences that do exist among the systems are not merely concerned with fine points, however. Indeed, they extend to such major aspects of the technique as administration, instructions, scoring categories, how far to pursue the inquiry, and how to interpret the resulting data. It is no wonder that this has resulted in a great deal of confusion about what *the* Rorschach test is.

In addition to the chaos created by the lack of congruity among the systems, the Rorschach has been criticized by many on its merits as a diagnostic tool. In a way, many of these criticisms echo the early controversies between Beck and Klopfer, where the merits of the test as an art or a science, or as a nomothetic or idiographic technique, were debated. There were three primary arguments leveled against the Rorschach. The first maintains that the test is unable to accurately predict behavior. The second is that when research findings are attended to, the use of the Rorschach is not supported. The final argument is that the changing role of the clinician obviates the need for such time-consuming tasks as assessment. This issue was discussed above.

Paul Meehl (1954) is a major but by no means the only proponent of the first argument. In comparing actuarial and clinical methods for predicting behavior, he found that the actuarial method was as good as or superior to the clinical method. Holt (1970) objected to conclusions drawn by Meehl and others and pointed out that many of the actuarial vs. clinical prediction studies involve predictions that are not appropriate to clinical assessment, such as interpersonal compatibility and school grades. Holt argues that, in any event, one cannot view prediction, as such, as the goal of assessment; rather, an understanding of the person is a different and equally important goal. A responsible interpretation of the Rorschach considers both nomothetic and idiographic data, and, from the joining of the two, whatever predictions are made will be made in the context of a firm understanding of the subject—his response and cognitive styles, his affective life, and myriad other unique features that constitute him as an individual.

While the issue of predictive validity has appeared extensively in criticisms of the Rorschach technique, a more telling objection has been made by those who cite negative research findings; when the body of the work done on the psychometric value of the Rorschach is taken together, the net result has been seen by reviewers to justify abandoning the test on empirical grounds. However, the methods of the reviewers themselves may be criticized. Literally thousands of articles have been published regarding the Rorschach, especially in the decade from 1950 to 1960. Reviewers citing articles showing the technique to be ineffective have often been selective in their choices, and have neglected other articles that provide evidence favorable to it. For example, in an article concluding that "the clinical status of the Rorschach technique, based on an evaluation of research evidence, is not wholly satisfactory, despite claims to the contrary," Zubin et al. (1965) used only 250 citations, mostly published before 1955.

While most of the research on the Rorschach has been rigorous and well designed, much of it has not been, and data have often been misinterpreted or have been drawn from questionable research designs. One difficulty of general importance may be that standard statistical and psychometric methodologies are inappropriate for studying such a complex technique. Harris (1960) points out that, although the test was never developed or designed to be interpreted by psychometric methodology, it is often approached erroneously in this way. Finally, Wyatt (1968) makes the important observation that the Rorschach is too complex to be taken piece by piece. Each response is given in context and in relation to each other's response. Thus one must view the test as a global configuration. The recent development of multivariate statistical methods may prove to be a boon to a holistic analysis of the Rorschach.

This discussion can only bring us back to one of the most basic difficulties of investigating the Rorschach. With five distinct systems plus any number of idiosyncratic combinations of system in existence, how can research conducted using various approaches ever be compared? The Rorschach has had no common language that would enable researchers to understand one another. There have been no common definitions for scoring symbols. For example, a response influenced by a perception of texture could be scored as T by Beck, c by Klopfer and Hertz, c' by Piotrowski, and Ch by Rapaport-Schafer.

All of these difficulties have created a "chronic Rorschach problem" that has never been resolved. In fact, some of the most basic aspects of the technique have received little or no attention from researchers. Questions such as the effect of where the examiner sits in relation to the subject have rarely been addressed. Types of encouragement given to the subject during free association and the degree to which responses should be inquired have also seldom been studied.

Despite the criticism leveled against it, the techique still flourishes in practice. This, however, can never obviate the need for some sort of resolution of the truly serious problems that exist. Questions as to what, if any, parts of the five major systems work best and provide the most accurate information need to be answered. A system has been needed that will stand up to the requirements of reliability and validity, one based on solid empirical data, one that is relatively easily taught to all levels of practitioners, and one that has a high interclinician reliability. Finally, it should seek to create the common "language community" that Koch (1964) wrote of, to facilitate meaningful research. It is for these reasons that the Comprehensive System has been developed.

In the book *The Rorschach Systems* (1969a), Exner has offered a comparative analysis of the five main systems. This has provided a basis for understanding the similarities and differences among the approaches and has given clues as to which aspects of each are of merit. During the analysis of the systems, the systematizers themselves were extensively interviewed as to their recollections about the early days of the Rorschach and their current opinions in regard to their own and other systems. Also involved in the development of the Comprehensive System were three surveys. The first of these surveys, Exner and Exner (1972), already mentioned, was a questionnaire sent to clinicians and designed to acquire information on specific methods of administering, scoring, and interpreting the test in regard to the various systems. The immense differences in practice that were reported underlined one important problem and served to spur on the development of an integrative approach. The second survey (Exner, 1974) was a 90-item questionnaire sent to a random selection of 200 diplomates of the American Board of Examiners in Professional Psychology (ABPP). A total of 111 questionnaires were returned, and data about the opinions and practices of these eminent psychologists were gathered. The third survey (Exner, 1974) was concerned with research methodology and various difficulties encountered by workers in the field. This was sent to 100 psychologists who had published on the Rorschach since 1960.

An important task has been to create a substantial pool of test protocols administered in a standard manner to use in research. More than 150 psychologists and graduate students initially provided 835 such protocols which were computer-coded along with other normative data to give information on normative baselines. The protocol pool, which has now been expanded to include more than 4000 records, has provided a data base for the study of areas of the test that have been underresearched. Additionally, the accumulated literature on the Rorschach has been carefully reviewed and evaluated, and new research has been conducted where none was found to exist.

What has developed from this work is an attempt to integrate the best aspects of the Rorschach into one system. It has no specific theoretical viewpoint and is designed to be used by clinicians of all persuasions. It does, however, retain much of the same format that the various systems have all used over the years. The Comprehensive System approaches the Rorschach with the belief that, although the technique deserves much of the criticism directed at it, it is still, when used properly, one of the best assessment tools in the clinician's armamentarium. The remainder of this chapter will be devoted to a full description of the system at this stage in its development.

3. The Comprehensive System

3.1. Applicability

It has often been assumed that when testing is called for the Rorschach is automatically included. This assumption is an erroneous one. The technique was never designed to answer all types of diagnostic or descriptive questions, just as it was never designed to predict all or most types of behavior. Those who attempt to describe such things as grades in school or religious or cultural background using the Rorschach could better use any number of other methods, including a straightforward interview with the subject, to more accurately obtain their information. Rather than attempting to perform magical feats of prediction and description, it is extremely important for the clinician to understand what the test can do and what types of information it is best at providing.

First, the test gives a representative view of the person as he is behaving at the present. This may seem to be a limited perspective, but when examined and integrated it can provide a great deal of information. Specifically, a description of a person based on the Rorschach data can include statements about a subject's affective world, his cognitive and response styles, how he related to his interpersonal sphere and to the rest of the environment as a whole, what motivates him and what are his response styles. It can also provide clues as to what type of intervention might prove to be most helpful. Speculation on the etiology of the person's condition and on the likelihood of his making an adequate adjustment is usually included in a Rorschach report. However, it must be remembered that this is speculation only, as it tends to be inferred rather then derived directly from the data provided in the protocol, and, as such, relies on the tester's deductive powers and accumulated knowledge.

It is certainly not uncommon for a psychodiagnostician to receive referral questions that are impossible to answer. Perhaps the most frequent is whether the patient will "act out"; others are requests for estimates of length of hospitalization or the likelihood of commission of a criminal act. Such questions tend to be nebulous, and, because the subject's future environment cannot be accurately predicted by the Rorschach, answers to these questions should not be attempted unless one has a great deal more information.

Questions about intelligence and organicity present another area where, although the Rorschach has proven to be a viable alternative in some respects, it is by no means the best alternative. In terms of intelligence, there are numerous other procedures that specifically address this area and provide more accurate and precise information. Using the Rorschach for detecting the existence of organicity was discouraged by 89 out of the 111 ABPP diplomates surveyed during the development of the Comprehensive System. However, all surveyed used the test for differential diagnosis, in order to provide the psychological data that a simple test for organicity does not include. It becomes clear, then, that the decision to use or not use the Rorschach should be a function of the type of referral question asked.

The same principle also applies to the issue of whether or not to use the technique as a part of a test battery. Rapaport, Gill, and Schafer (1946) make a strong case for the use of a battery in every instance. They cite the need to get a picture of the total individual and stress the importance of having enough data on hand to cross-validate any hypotheses made. Holt (1970) also maintains that the more data that are available, the more likely it is for the examiner to make accurate predictions. While this is true, it has in some instances led to the administration of a standard battery, given in all cases with little regard to the referral questions or the needs of the subject. There are many situations where a full test battery need not be used. The Rorschach is extremely useful on its own when a description of an individual is needed. Such a use for the Rorschach is supported by case material documented by each of the systematizers (Beck, 1937, 1945, 1952, 1960, 1967; Hertz, 1969; Klopfer, 1954, 1956, 1962; Piotrowski, 1957, 1969; Schafer, 1954).

If a test battery is decided on, an important issue becomes the point in the sequence of tests at which to give the Rorschach. Some evidence has indicated that sequencing matters, expecially in relation to the Wechsler Adult Intelligence (WAIS). Grisso and Meadow (1967) found differences in WAIS performance when the Rorschach was given before as opposed to after it. This study suggests that the Rorschach should never be administered before the WAIS. It has been most common for clinicians to give the Rorschach last in the battery. Indeed, 94 out of the 111 ABPP diplomates indicated that they did this and modified the procedure only under special circumstances. Explanations for this practice center around the notion that the Rorschach is usually the most ambiguous test given in a battery and for this reason may prove to be the most threatening and disruptive to the subject.

Thus, the clinician has a number of options to consider and a number of decisions to make on being presented with a subject in need of assessment. When and how to use the Rorschach depend primarily on the type of information requested on referral; however, when a description of the individual is required, it may be that there is no better assessment tool available.

3.2. Administration

After selection of the Rorschach as an instrument of choice in the assessment procedure, the decision process does not stop. There are numerous methods of administration, and each variation can seriously affect the quality and quantity of the responses given, and therefore the conclusions that will be drawn in the report. Many factors that are of importance are neglected by examiners, frequently because they mistakenly become taken for granted or are assumed to be of little consequence. Among these factors are the position of the examiner in relation to the subject, the instructions given to the subject, how the responses are to be recorded, whether the latency and duration of the response should be timed, and how the responses should be inquired so that they yield the most information without inadvertently coaching the subject. Each of these factors deserves to be discussed in some detail.

3.2.1. Seating

Opinions of the five systematizers on the positioning of the examiner in relation to the subject have varied a great deal. Rorschach and Beck recommend that the examiner sit behind the subject, Hertz and Klopfer prefer side-by-side seating, while

Rapaport and Schafer endorse a face-to-face approach; Piotrowski suggests that the subject should be seated in whatever position is most natural, but he believes that this is generally side-by-side with the tester. All of the systematizers explain that the purpose of their particular seating arrangement is to maximize the chance to obtain as much verbal and nonverbal information as possible from the subject while minimizing the possibility that the examiner might influence him in some way.

This issue of examiner influence is quite important and has received considerable attention in the literature. Both Schachtel (1945) and Schafer (1954) discuss the subject's reaction both to the tester and to the test situation as a whole in great detail, indicating that the relationship can influence the content and quantity of responses. Gibby, Miller, and Walker (1953) found that different examiners produced variations not only in the length of the protocols but also in some of the determinants such as pure form, color, and shading. Lord (1950) had her subjects interviewed by three different examiners. One created an environment of general acceptance and feelings of success. The second tester created an environment which made the subject feel like a failure. The third environment was neutral and an attempt was made to give no cues regarding success one way or the other. These three environments did produce significant differences in Rorschach performance. In a later study, Masling (1965) trained two sets of graduate students in a standard administration of the Rorschach. He then told one group that more experienced testers always obtain more human responses than animal responses in their protocols. The other group was told the opposite. Each student then tested two subjects. It was found that each group performed according to the "set" given to it. However, an examination of the sessions showed that the examiners did not verbally reinforce their subjects as such. Instead, Masling maintained that they were being influenced by the tester's gestures, changes in posture, and facial expression.

Although seating arrangement in particular has long been an area that receives little attention from researchers, the findings of the above studies clearly reflect a need to keep the subject from perceiving cues that the examiner may or may not be aware of. It appears that the side-by-side arrangement best serves this purpose. While some types of examiner influence can never be totally eliminated, this seating pattern allows for a comfortable position for both parties, and enables the examiner to have a clear view of the test materials. In addition, it allows the subject to focus his attention exclusively on the test and prevents direct visual access to the examiner's reactions, which at any rate should be kept at a minimum. The side-by-side seating arrangement is also a comfortable one for administering other tests if a battery is given and thereby obviates the need for shifting of positions during a testing session.

3.2.2. Instructions to the Subject

When proper seating and a rapport with the subject have been established, he must be given some sort of basic instructions by which to approach the test. It is agreed by everyone that the subject should not be given the cards without some sort of introduction, even though many subjects have a certain degree of knowledge about testing and indeed may be somewhat familiar with the inkblots. In any event, introductory comments should be kept to a minimum and should be so arranged that they avoid creating any sort of instructional set that might unduly influence the individual taking the test. For example, Schafer (1954) has suggested a brief statement that the test is one developed to study personality. This is usually enough to put the subject at ease and to set the stage for the introduction of the cards. What is recommended by the different approaches to say varies considerably.

Both Rorschach and Klopfer recommend simply handing the subject the first card and asking "What might this be?" Beck adds that the subject should be told that he can keep the card for as long as necessary but should tell everything he sees. Piotrowski uses Rorschach's instructions but also tells the subject that he can turn the card. Hertz follows Beck but uses a trial blot first. Finally, Rapaport and Schaefer encourage the subject to tell everything that "might be." With these differences in degree of information, it is remarkable that there has been only one study (Goetcheus, 1967) which examined the differences in records produced using Klopfer and Beck instructions. Beck instructions occasioned longer protocols; the two sets of instructions also created other significant differences in the type and quality of the responses. Using the inital protocol pool of 835 records, Exner (1974) compared the instructions of all five systematizers. Of the protocols, 329 used the Klopfer system, 310 used Beck, 78 used Rapaport, 66 used Piotrowski, and 52 used Hertz. The Klopfer method was seen to produce the lowest mean number of responses, and the Rapaport system produced the highest. Various other important differences involving location and determinants were also found.

The likelihood that instructional set influences Rorschach responding is buttressed by a number of studies in which the subjects were specifically given clues as to how to respond (Hutt, Gibby, Milton, & Pottharst, 1950; Carp & Shavzin, 1950; Coffin, 1941; Abramson, 1951; Henry & Rotter, 1956). For example, Hutt et al. told their subjects that one of their tasks would be to see as much human movement as possible. In a test-retest design, they found that these instructions increased the incidence of Human Movement (M) by 100%.

With evidence of the power of instructional set in mind, the Comprehensive System has chosen the approach which has the least likelihood of influencing the client. This is the simple "What might this be?" used originally by Rorschach himself and then adopted by Klopfer. There are several other reasons for selecting this approach. First, as shown in the Exner (1974) report, it tends to produce a shorter yet no less rich record. Most importantly, these instructions are brief and to the point, allow little leeway for the examiner, and thus contribute to a standard method of administration.

Even with adequate pretest instructions, subjects often ask questions while the test is in progress. An effort by the examiner to answer these questions should be made, but answers should not be of a directive nature. Generally, it suffices to have the subject understand that various people respond to the inkblots in various ways. There are several answers that will convey this impression. For example, a subject may ask if he can turn the cards or if he is to use all parts of the blot. A simple reply "It's up to you" or "Whatever you like" is usually sufficient. Occasionally a subject will give only one answer to Card I. It is then that the issue of encouragment of responding becomes pertinent. The systematizers have differed greatly on this point, with Klopfer allowing encouragement only on the first card, while Beck recommends doing so through the fifth card. Current practice, as shown by the ABPP and the Exner and Exner surveys, also involves a great deal of diversity. Since there is a dearth of research on this subject to date, the problem must be resolved at this point through logic. In this respect, the Klopfer method has been adopted because it produces the least amount of instructional set. Thus, if only one response is given of the first card, the examiner may say "Most people see more than one thing." This is said only on the first card, and if the subject gives a single response to any of the other nine cards he is not encouraged to give additional responses to that card.

Although it rarely occurs when the subject is properly introduced to the testing situation, he may totally reject a card. This most often occurs with Card IX, a difficult card for many subjects. If this does happen, an indication that there is plenty of time and that everyone is able to see something in the card will usually be enough to encourage a response.

It must be reiterated that the primary task of the examiner is to remain silent as much as possible so as not to contaminate the testing session with unnecessary remarks that might influence the subject. What is said should be limited to the few statements described above unless a truly unusual incident or question occurs. With experience, it can be seen that most subjects are satisfied with a simple statement and the testing session will proceed smoothly.

3.3. Other Procedural Notes

3.3.1. Card Presentation

Cards should be kept out of reach of the subject and should be handed to him right side up. This will ensure that he will hold the card while responding rather than lay it down on the table. Although most of the systematizers advise that the subject should be told to return the card to the examiner or to lay it on the table when he has finished responding, a rule of parsimony in instructions would suggest that this need not be done unless a specific question in this regard is asked.

3.3.2. Timing of Response

How long it takes the subject to produce a response and the total time the subject keeps the card may provide valuable data for the examiner. Therefore, it is recommended that both of these measures be taken. However, of greater importance is that a subject not be overly concerned or influenced by the fact that he is being timed. The common use of a stopwatch is discouraged. Rather, an unobtrusive measurement may be taken by using the sweep-second hand of a wristwatch or even of a wall clock.

3.3.3. Recording of Responses

It is critical that everything that either the subject or the examiner says be recorded verbatim. This will allow the protocol to be more easily read at a later time when the material may not be as fresh in the examiner's mind and will also provide an exact record of what was said. While this procedure may appear to be costly in time and difficult to do, it becomes quite routine as the examiner becomes more experienced. A set of standard abbreviations that can be derived phonetically (such as "r" for "are") or logically (such as "cb" for "could be") facilitates this process.

3.3.4. Inquiry

Except in the Rapaport system, where the Inquiry is conducted immediately after the responses are given to each card, the subject is presented with the cards two times. The first is the Free Association period, discussed above, and the second is the Inquiry, where the subject is questioned about his responses so that the examiner may know exactly what was seen, where on the card it was seen, and what made it look like that to the subject. Thus the examiner's instructions to the subject are brief and to the point, such as

> Now I want to go back through the cards again. I won't take very long. I'll read what you told me you saw and then I want you to help me to see it as you did. In other words, I want to know where you saw it, and what there is there that makes it look like that, so that I can see it just like you did. Understand? (Exner, Weiner, & Schuyler, 1976)

Just as previously cited studies indicate the influence of instructional set on the Free Association section of the test, the same is true for Inquiry. A number of studies (Gibby & Stotsky, 1953; Baughman, 1959; Zax & Stricker, 1960) have shown that the type of questions asked by the examiner influence both the complexity of the scoring of relatively simple responses and the type of responses elicited. Only one study, conducted by Reisman (1970), indicated that direct inquiry has no significant effect on the determinants. It is easy to see how such ill-advised Inquiry questions such as "Which side of the skin is up?" or "Was it the color of the blot or the way it was shaded that made you think it was that?" not only cue the subject as to what is specifically being sought but also will skew the data so that they give more of a picture of the examiner's probing than of what the subject actually saw.

In light of the research, then, the Inquiry used with the Comprehensive System follows four basic rules. First, although there is no directly prescribed set of questions to use, the ones that are decided on by the examiner must be appropriate to the type of information required. Occasionally a response given during Free Association may include enough information so that the examiner can score it confidently with no further Inquiry. For example, a response to Card II might be "I see two people, one here and the other here and they look like they're fighting." This certainly answers the requirements of the examiner, who now knows where the subject saw the percept and how he saw it—as Human Movement, or M. On the other hand, the response "This looks like a bat" to Card I leaves the examiner with several questions he needs to have answered, and so he must inquire.

The second principle is that the Inquiry does not have to include a question concerning each and every determinant. This avoids unnecessary questioning which may influence the subject. Even when the examiner is almost sure that a certain determinant is being used, he sometimes must forego an extensive Inquiry aimed at confirming his hypothesis, and must take the subject at his word. Often, if this occurs, the Rorschacher may want to be sure that this was the case. This can be done by presenting the card a third time and directly inquiring as to whether the subject saw that specific determinant. Although this may prove useful, it must be emphasized that this falls outside the rubric of the Comprehensive System and thus cannot be scored.

A third rule of Inquiry is that the briefer the Inquiry the better. If an unsatisfactory answer to an Inquiry question is given, it is best not to push too much. A final and most important rule is that any questions asked must be nondirective. A maximum of two questions are usually all that is needed to obtain adequate scoring information. The first statement to be made is actually not a question at all, but is a restatement of the Free Association exactly as he gave it. If, at this point, location is not clear, the subject can be asked "Could you show me where you saw that?" Location should be marked on the examiner's own location sheet so that a permanent record of where the subject saw the percept can be made. Then, if more information concerning the determinants is needed, questions should be formulated keeping the four basic rules of Inquiry in mind. Probably one of the most effective and least directive statements that can be made is "I'm not sure I see it as you do." Other viable techniques include repeating a key word such as "hairy?" or other statements such as "I'm not sure what there is there that makes it look like that." While these restrictions may seem frustrating to the Rorschach examiner, how the Inquiry is conducted is perhaps the most important aspect of Rorschach administration, directly influencing the scoring and therefore the interpretation of the test. Overzealous Inquiry may seriously change the entire complexion of the subject's responses, and so, to avoid a disservice to the client, Inquiry must be restrained.

When administered correctly, the test should take 45–55 min. Subjects who are resistant or who compulsively give large numbers of responses per card may take substantially longer, but the Rorschach is generally one of the least time-consuming tests in the usual battery. Using the Comprehensive System, most subjects will give an average of 17–27 responses in total, regardless of whether they are patients or nonpatients.

In order to more easily complete the next step in the Rorschach procedure, that of scoring, a form for the Comprehensive System has been developed. It consists of four pages, three of which are shown in Figures 1, 2, and 3, and the fourth of which is the location sheet spoken of above. As may be seen, the first page provides space on which to list demographic data about the subject, the referral questions asked, and the circumstances of the session. This furnishes a handy data source that is helpful when interpreting the test results. The second page is constructed so that it allows for orderly representation of the scoring of each response to each card in sequence. The third sheet contains the synthesis of the scores and the ratios and percentages derived from them. This page will be discussed briefly in a later section.

4. Scoring

It must be initially pointed out that the term "score" is not really an appropriate one for the Rorschach. To the psychometrician, scoring means that a subject's responses are compared nomothetically against normative data for other individuals matching his general characteristics. This is often done in terms of standard scores and results in an overall value such as an IQ or a percentile rank. Rather than being a psychometric process, Rorschach scoring more resembles data coding, as it involves translating the words used into symbols, each of which contains a certain amount of information but which must be considered in context in order to make sense.

There are several other reasons why the technique is not amenable to traditional scoring techniques. The Rorschach is basically an open-ended test; while one protocol might consist of 35 responses, another subject may give only 14. There is no answer that is right or wrong; rather, answers range on a continuum from good to poor, depending on several scoring variables. It appears that Cronbach (1949) was correct in his critique when he maintained that there are too many interconnecting variables in the test to be able to perform the usual statistical measurements. Holtzman (1961) also made known his dissatisfaction with any attempts to apply nomothetic criteria to the traditional Rorschach. Indeed, he created his own technique, the Holtzman Inkblot Test (HIT), which increases the number of cards to 45 and allows the subject only one response per card. In addition, it comes in two forms, A and B, and thus can be used very easily in tightly designed research. While the Holtz-man is certainly a useful technique, it is a young one and has yet to be widely used, perhaps because it is rather time-consuming to administer and score.

What the critics of Rorschach often neglect is that the complexity of the test is also potentially one of its most attractive points, especially when it is used in idio-

STRUCTURAL SUMMARY BLANK

Developed by John E. Exner, Jr. for use with

THE RORSCHACH: A COMPREHENSIVE SYSTEM

Date: ....

I. SUBJECT DATA

1. Name: .... 2. Age: .... 3. Sex: .... 4. Race: ....

5. Date of Birth: .... 6. Place of Birth: ....

7. Marital Status: 7a. **If** married, divorced or widowed:

Single   ....   Age of Spouse   ....

Engaged   ....   Sex & ages of Children   ....

Married   .... Yrs ....

Divorced   .... Yrs ....

Widowed   .... Yrs ....

8. Father: Mother: Siblings:

Living   .... Living   .... Sex .... Age ....

Deceased   .... Deceased   .... Sex .... Age ....

Age   .... Age   .... Sex .... Age ....

Occupation   .... Occupation   .... Sex .... Age ....

9. Current Employment: .... 11. Education Completed:

           How Long? .... 0 - 8 Yrs .... 13 - 15 Yrs ....

10. Prior Employments: .... 9 - 12 Yrs .... B.A. Degree ....

                             .... H.S. Grad .... Grad Degree ....

II. REFERRAL DATA

1. Purpose: 1a. **If** Psychiatric: 1b. **If** Psychiatric:

Psychiatric   .... Admission   .... In patient   ....

Forensic   .... Progress   .... Out patient   ....

Educational   .... Discharge   .... Day Care   ....

Other   .... After Care   ....

2. What is the referral question? ....

3. What is the presenting problem? ....

....

III. TESTING SITUATION

1. Seating: 2. Cooperation: 3. Other Tests Administered:

Side by side   .... Excellent   ....

Face to face   .... Adequate   ....

Other   .... Reluctant   ....

                          Resistant   ....

© John E. Exner, Jr., 1976

Figure 1

graphic description. No one part of the test, whether it be a verbalization, a score, or a score derivation, can meaningfully stand alone. It must be considered in light of a global interrelation with every other aspect of the protocol. However this does not mean that the scoring is not amenable to some quantitative measure or objectivity. The coded scoring system originally set forth by Rorschach (1921) allows for the construction of frequency distributions for score variables. From these distributions,

SEQUENCE OF SCORES

CARD	RT	NO.	LOCATION	DETERMINANTS (S)	CONTENT (S)	POP	Z SCORE	SPECIAL

Figure 2

ratios and percentages can be derived which denote many of the complex relationships among the various aspects of the single protocol. In addition, these ratios and percentages can be compared to normative data collected via the same method from both psychiatric and nonpsychiatric populations. The Rorschacher, then, actually has four sets of data by which to evaluate his subject. First, there are the quantitative data which can be compared across other records. This is especially helpful when the task is one of diagnosis, because normative data comparing various types of subjects

STRUCTURAL SUMMARY

R =   Zf =   ZSum =   P =   (2) =

Location Features	Determinants (Blends First)	Contents	Contents (Idiographic)
W =	DQ	H =	=
D =	+ =	(H) =	.... =
Dd =	o =	Hd =	
		(Hd) =	.... =
S =	v =	A =	
		(A) =	.... =
DW =	— =	Ad =	
	M =	(Ad) =	.... =
	FM =	Ab =	
	m =	AI =	.... =
	C =	An =	
		Art =	.... =
Form Quality	CF =	Ay =	
	FC =	BI =	.... =
FQx FQf	C' =	Bt =	
	C'F =	Cg =	....
+ = + =	FC' =	CI =	
		Ex =	Special Scorings
o = o =	T =	Fi =	
	TF =	Fd =	
w = w =	FT =	Ge =	PSV =
	V =	Hh =	
— = — =	VF =	Ls =	DV =
	FV =	Na =	
M Quality	Y =	Sx =	INCOM =
	YF =	Xy =	
+ =	FY =		FABCOM =
	rF =		
o =	Fr =		CONTAM =
	FD =		
w =	F =		ALOG =
— =			=

RATIOS, PERCENTAGES, AND DERIVATIONS

ZSum-Zest =		FC:CF+C =	Afr =
Zd =		W:M =	3r+(2)/R =
EB =	EA =	W:D =	Cont:R =
eb =	ep =	L =	H+Hd:A+Ad =
			(H)+(Hd):(A)+(Ad) =
Blends:R =		F+% =	H+A:Hd+Ad =
a:p =		X+% =	XRT Achrom =
Ma:Mp =		A% =	XRT Chrom =

Figure 3

JOHN E. EXNER, JR.,
AND BETH CLARK

do exist (Exner et al., 1976). In addition, the quantitative data allow an interpretation that is free from the bias of the subject's words, which may create a particular set during interpretation. It is interesting to note that all of the original systematizers suggested that protocols be scored "blind," that is, by someone who did not himself administer the test and who knows nothing of the subject, often for this very reason (Exner, 1969a).

The second set of data is made up of the internal comparisons among the subject's own productions. It is here where the most valuable idiographic information is obtained. Such comparisons can shed light on the subject's own unique style of responding, his needs and motivations, and his weaknesses and strengths. In a similar manner, the sequence of the scores can be examined. This helps to illustrate how the subject approaches the testing situation, how a response may be related to a previous response, and how the performance varies as the test progresses. The final set of data is the subject's own words, which are subjected to a qualitative analysis. One of the basic agreements between the systematizers is on the inclusion of an analysis of verbalizations—what words are said and how they are used—all of the richness and subtlety of spoken language. When used with caution, this yields valuable information and allows the examiner to "flesh out" his interpretation and confirm his hypotheses with some of the unique features of the subject.

There are two basic rules that must be followed when scoring the Rorschach according to the Comprehensive System. The first and most important is that only what was perceived during Free Association can be scored. The rationale for this is simple. When the Inquiry is presented after Free Association to all ten cards, it would seem evident that the two sections of the test represent two different thought processes. Levin (1953) describes the difference between the sections as actually two separate processes of test taking. The Free Association is accomplished in a setting of open-endedness and ambiguity, while the Inquiry is much more structured and many more cues are given to the subject by the examiner's questioning. Yet it is a common error in scoring and interpretation to read the protocol horizontally, from Free Association to Inquiry for each response. Instead, the Free Association should be read in its entirety first, and then the Inquiry.

The process of deciding what to score is not simple. For instance, a subject may give a response that seems complete during Free Association, but then add another feature during the Inquiry. An example of this appears below.

Free Association	Inquiry
V. That could be a rabbit in the center, from the way it's shaped.	E: Repeats S's response. S: Well, it's got big ears and skinny little legs like it was standing up sniffing.

The subject initially appears to be using pure Form in this response, but during the Inquiry gives another determinant, that of Animal Movement. The rule for scoring a response such as this is to be conservative. In this case, all the examiner did was to repeat the subject's response. The subject spontaneously introduced the Animal Movement without any further questioning, and thus it can be safely included in the scoring. An example where this would not be the case follows.

| I. That's a bat. | E: Repeats S's response.
S: Yeah, it's shaped like a bat, and now that I look at it, it's dirty.
E: Dirty?
S: The way the edges look dusty, like dust and bat fur. |

It can be seen in this case that the subject introduces a new determinant in the Inquiry, and the examiner is forced to go far afield from the original Free Association, and the rule of conservatism does not allow us to score the additional determinant.

The second rule of Rorschach scoring is to make sure that all determinants given in the Free Association are scored and are given equal weight. This is different from the Klopfer system, which gives a main score and then additional scores. The choice of what symbols and criteria to use has not been taken lightly by the Comprehensive System. As in all aspects of development, several areas have been taken into consideration: The original postulates of Rorschach have been carefully examined, as have the positions of each of the systematizers. The results of the ABPP and the Exner and Exner surveys have been examined for common contemporary practices. Finally, and most importantly, where empirical evidence is available, the criteria most strongly supported by research are the ones that have been selected.

There are five categories of scoring in the Comprehensive System. Four of them, Location, Determinants, Content, and Popularity, were originally postulated by Rorschach and have been used, for the most part, by the other systems. The fifth category, Organizational Activity, was first suggested by Beck (1933) and has been found useful. The first three categories are always scored, while the last two depend for scoring on the specific content of the response. What follows is a more detailed description of each of the five categories. Experienced Rorschachers will see many similarities between the symbols used in the Comprehensive System and those of their own particular system. However, they have been selected with an eye toward integration, standardization, and facility of use, and ideally represent the "best of the Rorschach."

4.1. Location

Location is the first category which is scored for every response given in the protocol. It is probably the easiest score to ascertain. The score simply indicates the area of the blot that the subject used when formulating his response. When the subject looks at the blot, he has basically two choices: to use the whole configuration or to isolate a part of it. If a part is used, it can be either one commonly seen or one that is not so often used by others who have taken the test. In addition, various other combinations which are more unusual can be scored. This creates seven different symbols to select from. The four most commonly used are W or whole, where the entire blot is used, D or common detail, a frequently used area, Dd or unusual detail, an infrequently used area, and S or space response, where a white space is used in the response. An example of how S is used follows:

Free Association	Inquiry
IX. This white part in the middle could be a goblet.	E: Repeats S's response.
	S: It has that goblet shape about it, you see, right here.

Location in this case would be scored DS, for use of a common detail plus white space.

The remaining three scores are seen very infrequently, usually less than once per 1000 records, and are usually considered highly pathological. These are DW, DdW, and DdD. DW and DdW, confabulated whole responses, are scored when the subject attends to a detailed area but then makes a generalization from this area to the entire blot. DdD is a confabulated detail, which is basically the same process, except that an infrequently seen detail is generalized to a more frequently seen one.

W and D are scored in the same way that Rorschach recommended. The cutoff $W(W̶)$ of the Klopfer & Kelly (1942) and Hertz (1942) systems has been discarded because the criteria for its application are somewhat nebulous and there is little research data supporting it. Whether a response is Dd or D is determined from frequency tables largely derived from Beck (1937, 1944), Beck, Beck, Levitt & Molish (1961) indicating how often the areas are seen by large samples of test takers from various clinical and nonclinical populations.

In addition to being concerned with where on the blot the subject has seen something, how he has used the area is of major importance. A selection of location can be highly sophisticated and organized showing considerable cognitive integrative capacity or maturity, or it may be relatively simple and unorganized. For example, a response to Card II that used the whole blot could be "Looks like two beaks." This is relatively unsophisticated when compared with a response such as "This seems like two people at a costume party, like they are dancing, no maybe toasting each other, clinking glasses together." Because of the differences that do occur in the level of sophistication embodied in a response, a "Developmental Quality" score representing this difference has been included in this category of scoring, but several other researchers have shown it to be of great merit in determining developmental levels of cognitive functioning. Friedman (1952) did the pioneering work in this area, and it has been elaborated on by several others (Hemmendinger, 1953, 1960; Goldfried, Stricker, & Weiner, 1971, Chapter 2). In addition, Rapaport et al. (1946) proposed a differentiation of W scoring in order to indicate how the different parts of the blot were integrated. Neither Friedman's nor Rapaport's approach has been popular with contemporary Rorschach practitioners, but the data indicate that it is a valuable addition to the interpretation of the protocol. Thus the two approaches have been combined and distilled in the Comprehensive System to create four categories of Developmental Quality that are scored for each location: a synthesis response (+) that integrates separate areas of the blot into a meaningful, related whole, an ordinary response (o) where a single area is selected and adequately articulated without any gross distortions, a vague response (v) in which no specific form has been articulated and the impression is of a diffuse response, and an arbitrary response (−) where the response given is extremely inconsistent with the structural requirements of the area of the blot that is selected.

4.2. Determinants

The second major group of scoring criteria is intended to shed light on how the subject has used the particular features of the blot to construct his response. These are the Determinants, the most complex and most important scoring category, involving the perceptual-cognitive process that the individual employs in order to select and to organize the various elements in his stimulus world. We all go through this process in every waking moment, and the response given to the inkblot provides a valuable sample of it that can be examined. This perceptual-cognitive process is usually a two-step procedure. First, when the subject is shown a blot, he is presented with a specific sensory stimulus which he must then classify. Stimulus classification is influenced by several factors. Each subject has his own general style of approaching stimulus events. Thus someone who tends to be impulsive would be likely to give a very speedy response that would, perhaps, neglect many of the finer points on the blot. On the other hand, a more cautious or compulsive subject might spend a great deal of time perusing the card from every angle before giving a response. In addition to this general cognitive style, each subject goes through a process of reality testing when classifying the stimulus. That is, the subject makes sure to some degree that what he thinks he sees is really there in the blot. Finally, every subject comes into the testing situation with his own set of needs and expectancies which, of course, influence the way in which the blot stimuli are classified.

The second step in the cognitive-perceptual process is the subject's own evaluation of his possible responses. All that the subject sees is not always what the examiner gets. Subjects give an average of two responses per card in the actual testing situation. However, Exner and Armbruster (1974) had 20 subjects (ten patients and ten nonpatients) give as many responses as they could to each card presented for 60 sec. The nonpatients averaged 104 responses total, while the patients gave an average of 113. Neither group gave fewer than six responses per card. Thus, although we cannot directly measure the actual process, it is likely that some sort of filtering of responses by the subject occurs.

It is this complex process that makes the scoring of Determinants so important. It is not surprising that they are also the point of least agreement among the systematizers. Rorschach (1921) originally suggested three categories: Form, Human Movement, and Color. Each of the other systematizers added other categories with various criteria to the point where there is no single score class that is agreed on by all five of them. Thus a monumental task was in store for the Comprehensive System. Using the criteria discussed previously, 24 symbols have been established, falling into seven broad categories. The first five have been used by most of the systematizers. They include Form, Movement, Chromatic Color, Achromatic Color, and Shading. The other two categories contain elements that have been newly incorporated into the Comprehensive System as a result of the research conducted during its development. These are Form-Dimensionality and Reflections and Pairs.

It has been firmly established that the form features of the inkblot, that is, how the blot is shaped, are included in more than 95% of responses (Baughman, 1959; Exner, 1959, 1961). Form is often used with other determinant categories, especially chromatic and achromatic color. In some cases, form is the primary contributor to the response, as in the case of a percept such as "a red flower." A scoring configuration of FC would indicate this where the subject has indicated that it is primarily the shape of the blot which makes it look like a flower. In other cases, form may be of secondary importance. An example of this would be "That's blood because it's all red and it sort of looks like it's in a drop." This would be scored CF.

Many responses also include some type of movement. There are three symbols used to score it. The first is Human Movement (M), used where the subject indicates that there is some sort of human activity occurring. Responses that include animals involved in human activity are also scored M, as are responses involving perception of human emotion. Second, responses that include Animal Movement are scored FM. Finally, movement occurring in inanimate, inorganic, or insensate objects is scored m. This is most often seen in such responses as rockets blasting off, fireworks exploding, or water falling. Movement responses may be either active (a) or passive (p). For example, "a man jumping" would be scored Human Movement-Active (M^a), while a dog lying down would be scored Animal Movement-Passive (FM^p).

While there are two types of responses involving the use of the color features of the blot, those using chromatic color are much more common. The Comprehensive System includes four scoring categories for color (C, Cn, CF, and FC). It has been previously explained that the *CF* and *FC* scores represent the use of color as either primary or secondary determinant, along with an articulation of form. The Pure Color response (*C*) is much more rare. In this case, there is no attempt to integrate the color with the structure of the blot; thus a formless response is produced. "It all just looks like paint to me" in response to Card X would be an example of a Pure Color answer. *Color Naming* (*Cn*) is seen even more infrequently and indicates a difficulty in integrating the blot as a stimulus. It is scored when the subject simply lists the colors he sees on the blot, e.g., "Blue, red, orange," intending this to be a response.

Subjects also use the blacks, whites, and grays of the blots, the achromatic colors, to formulate their responses. These are scored *C'*, *C'F*, and *FC'*, depending on what degree form plays a part in the construction of the answer. This scoring category does not include instances where achromatic color is used merely to point out a location, e.g., "This black area here looks like a rabbit," but is used only in cases where the response is seen to contain a color, e.g., "A white cloud."

The fifth scoring category is Shading, in which the light-dark features of the blot are used. Several types of shading are scored. Texture (*T*, *TF*, *FT*) is scored when the subject articulates that he conceptualizes the shading features as implying tactile elements. Objects perceived as furry, smooth, grainy, muddy, hot, or cold usually imply and are inquired for the use of texture. When the shading features are used to indicate depth or dimensionality, the Vista response is scored (*V*, *VF*, *FV*). This is the least common response in the shading category. An example of a Vista response follows:

Free Association	Inquiry
VI. The center could be a ditch.	*E:* Repeats *S*'s response.
	S: Well, like an irrigation ditch, it's dug down in, you can tell because it's darker than this other part.

Those responses that use the light-dark features of the blot but do not include reference to either Texture or Vista are simply scored as Diffuse Shading (*Y*, *YF*, *FY*). Silhouettes and X-rays are commonly given answers that are scored as Diffuse Shading.

The sixth scoring category, Form Dimension (*FD*), is a new one, developed during the formulation of the Comprehensive System. It is scored when a response includes reference to a dimensionality or perspective based only on form rather than on shading. It is given most often to Card IV, where the response often involves a figure lying down or where the subject perceives himself as looking up at the figure.

Finally, Pairs and Reflections are scored as a separate category when the symmetry of the blot is a deciding factor in the production of the response. A pair (2) occurs when two of the same object, such as "two mountain lions" on Card VIII, are noted. The Reflection scores (*rF* and *Fr*) developed out of research by Exner (1969b, 1970) on indicators of narcissism but are currently defined more closely as a measure of egocentricity. Reflection is scored when form is used to articulate the response and when it is seen as reflected or as a mirror image because of the symmetry of the blot.

The subject rarely uses the 24 determinants in a simple fashion. For example, he may use more than one in formulating a single response. In the perceptual-cognitive process that finally results in a response, he may synthesize his answer in a successful or an unsuccessful way. Finally, what he sees may be judged as a good fit to the area he is describing, or a poor one. These three aspects of the Rorschach are always scored. They are called, respectively, Blends, Organizational Activity, and Form Quality. All of them give more important information about how the subject uses the determinants.

When more than one determinant is used in a single response, a blend (.) is scored, much in the manner that Beck (1937, 1944; Beck et al., 1961) used it. For example, the response "Two people dancing around a big red fire" on Card II would be scored $M^a.FC$, since both Human Movement and Form Color have been used in the articulation of the answer. Blends are not at all uncommon. During formulation of the Comprehensive System, it was found that they occur in more than 15% of responses, and, depending on the record, may make up as much as 50% of the protocol (Exner, 1974). They can be extremely complex, sometimes using up to five determinants, or relatively simple such as the example given above. It has been found that the blend is related to intelligence and that it gives an index of the complexity of the subject's thinking (Exner, 1974). Thus each response should be carefully examined for use of more than one determinant.

When the subject "selects" a response to a particular area of the blot and articulates it to the examiner, we know that the area looks like that to him. The question the examiner must answer is whether it also looks like that to other people. In other words, he must know how accurate the subject's perception of the reality of the blot is. This question is one of the goodness of fit of the response to the blot, and this fit is scored as Form Quality. While no one can be accurate at all times in his perception of the world, the degree to which accuracy is maintained becomes extremely important as a measure of the reality testing of a subject.

The Comprehensive System uses a variation of Mayman's (1966, 1970) method of evaluating form quality. It involves a 4-point scale by which each response is evaluated. An answer is first judged as either "good" or "poor." This is established by referring to a frequency table derived from Beck (1961) but specifically developed for use in the Comprehensive System. Twelve hundred protocols containing more than 26,000 responses are included in this table. Two thousand more records have been obtained since the first frequency distribution was developed and are currently being incorporated into a revised table to appear shortly. Answers given with high frequency are "good," while those given with very low frequency are judged "poor." However, this dichotomy is not sufficient for making the fine distinctions often required. In addition, it can be easily seen that a simple frequency distribution does not leave much room for responses that are highly idiosyncratic or creative. Therefore, the two broad categories are expanded into two more sections. Responses termed "good" may be scored as superior (+) or as ordinary (o). An ordinary response is one where the content and blot areas are congruent and where the answer is judged superior when the form is articulated very precisely in a way that enriches the quality of the percept. The difference between the two is most easily seen by example. First, an ordinary response:

Free Association	Inquiry
V. A dancer with a costume.	E: Repeats S's response.
	S: It just looks like it. Here's the dancer in the middle, and here's her costume.

Now a response using the same blot and area, but articulated in a superior fashion:

V. It might be a ballet dancer with a cape on.

E: Repeats S's response.

S: You can see the thin legs and this full part would be the arms but covered with a cape, like spread out, and she has a funny hat on too, like a dunce cap or something, it's a costume and she's dancing there.

Answers in the "poor" category are scored as weak (*w*) or minus (−). A weak response is noted when the blot area and the content specified are not congruent but the distortions are few in number. While they are not given frequently, they can usually be seen by most people. On the other hand, the minus response grossly distorts the blot. Often, contours and lines that do not exist are imposed on the blot in an arbitrary manner and the examiner must struggle to get an idea of where and what the subject is seeing. Frequently, the examiner cannot see it at all. Used in relation to other aspects of the Rorschach, then, Form Quality can give a valuable perspective on the subject's willingness to bend reality, or indeed, his inability to perceive his world as others do.

The scoring for Organizational Activity (*Z* score) has been rarely used. Only Beck (1933) and later Hertz (1942) attend to it, while Klopfer (1942) pays it only lip service. In addition, the Exner and Exner (1972) survey found that only 12% of those clinicians responding use it. Yet research indicates that it gives important information about how efficient the subject is at organizing his world (Exner, 1974), and also has some relationship to intelligence (Wishner, 1948; Sisson & Taulbee, 1955; Hertz, 1960). Organizational Activity occurs when the subject integrates two or more areas of the blot into a meaningful relationship. Thus, while one subject may simply see the popular "two people" in Card III, another may see "two people bending over a pot talking to each other." It may be seen that the second subject does more with the blot, imposing a relationship between two separate areas and making the response more complex. This can be done using two detail areas or white space and a detail area. Organizational Activity is also scored when the subject uses the entire blot (*W*). *Z* scores are weighted according to the complexity of the relationship. The table in use for the Comprehensive System is the same as used in the Beck system (Beck, Beck, Levitt, & Molish, 1961).

The 24 scoring categories and the three additional scorings of Blends, Form Quality, and Organizational Activity comprise the backbone of the Rorschach. Although the scoring as described here may seem quite complex and difficult to learn, this is not the case. It can actually be taught quickly, and scoring can be accurate after a relatively brief period of practice. In addition to the Location and Determinant categories, there are three other fairly simple aspects of a Rorschach response that require scoring. These are Content, Populars, and Special Scoring.

4.3. Content

Each response must be coded for its Content. The Comprehensive System uses a list of 22 content categories that have been derived from studying the frequency of use of the various categories employed by the other systematizers in a sample of 300 protocols and including only those used in a great many responses (Exner, 1974). Among the various scoring categories are the familiar *H* (human) and *Hd* (human detail) contents, and *Bl* (blood). What would seem to be rather unique responses, such as "X-ray," have been afforded their own categories because it was found that they were given with a high frequency. Finally, subjects often give answers that are unique and difficult to assign to a particular content category. These responses are instead written out in complete form.

4.4. Popular Responses

All of the systematizers have included a score of Popular (*P*) for objects that are most frequently seen. The Comprehensive System uses a criterion that the response must occur in one in every three protocols in order to be scored *P*. Accordingly, 13 Popular responses are listed and may be found either in Exner (1974) or in Exner et al. (1976).

4.5. Special Scorings

During the original development of the Comprehensive System, Special Scorings were not included, primarily because the research to that date did not show evidence that sufficient interscorer reliability could be obtained. However, since the publication of *The Rorschach: A Comprehensive System* in 1974, research on Special Scoring was resumed. Work to this date has established that two categories can be scored with adequate reliability. These are Perseveration and Unusual Verbalizations, a category including several subcategories. This scoring is useful in indicating disordered thought patterns and faulty cognitive integration. While Special Scores are often seen in subjects manifesting a high degree of psychopathology, it must be kept in mind that a Special Scoring in a record never constitutes enough evidence in itself to make a statement about any particular diagnostic category or type of disorder. Again, it must be emphasized that the protocol must be interpreted in a global, configurational manner and conclusions are to be drawn only through employing this procedure.

4.5.1. Perseveration

Perseveration occurs when the subject persists in the same response inappropriately. This inflexible form of responding may be indicative of a preoccupation or may result from concrete cognitive functioning. The Comprehensive System includes two types of Perseveration. The first occurs within a card; it is noted when a response uses the same scoring categories as its preceding response. This correspondence is exact and thus the two responses are scored exactly the same. The second form of Perseveration, intercard, may occur consecutively, or may be separated by several responses or even cards. It is scored when the subject identifies an object as the same one he had seen at an earlier time and is also called Content Perseveration. An example of this type of response is given by a subject seeing a bat on Card I and on Card V, saying, "Oh, here's that same bat I saw before, but he must have taken off because now he's flying through the air."

4.5.2. Unusual Verbalizations

The category of Unusual Verbalizations is subdivided into three types of responses. All of them indicate that there is something strange about the answer. The first are Deviant Verbalizations (DV). They include responses that have often been termed "queer" or "peculiar" by other systems and are characterized by some type of faulty or disorganized use of language that interferes with clear communication with the examiner. Neologisms or incorrect use of words would be scored DV. "This just looks like an inkblock," "It's a Siamese penis," or "It's a flower, all stilted" are examples of DV responses.

The second category of Unusual Verbalizations includes the Inappropriate Combinations (INCOM, FABCOM, CONTAM). They involve unrealistic relationships or condensations between blot areas and contents. Incongruous Combinations (INCOM) occur when images are inappropriately condensed into a single object. This is frequently seen in such answers as "a person with the head of a rabbit." Responses where color and form are combined inappropriately (e.g., "a pink rat") are also scored INCOM. Fabulized Combinations (FABCOM) involve those responses in which two separate areas of the blot are seen in an absurd or implausible relationship with each other. An example of this would be "a butterfly carrying two rabbits on its wings." The Contamination (CONTAM) response is the most bizarre and the least frequently seen of the Unusual Verbalizations. It occurs when the subject "spoils" his response by fusing two or more impressions of a single blot area so that none of the impressions is adequate, as they would be if reported separately. All CONTAM responses are given a Form Quality of ($-$). An example is "It's like a man jumping up and down and his heart is out here. He must be sick or else why would his heart be sticking out like that?"

The third type of special scoring is Autistic Logic (ALOG), used when the subject uses concrete or circumstantial thinking when justifying his answer. In order to be scored, the subject must volunteer this reasoning spontaneously and without prompting from the examiner. Usually, ALOG answers involve references to the size or spatial features of the blot. Examples of ALOG are "That's a sperm, it's small, so it must be a sperm," and "It must be a man and a woman because they're together and men and women belong together."

The Special Scorings all indicate some form of "slippage" in ideational functioning. However, as mentioned above, not all are of similar quality. CONTAM and ALOG are usually most indicative of serious impairment, but how the subject approaches his answers should always be considered. Subjects who give the impression of being absolutely satisfied with their answers are likely to be more disorganized than those conveying doubt or a knowledge that they are being unrealistic. It is up to the examiner to carefully note the context in which the response is given before jumping to unnecessary conclusions.

4.6. The Structural Summary

Once each response has been scored, it is entered on page 2 of the Structural Summary Blank under Sequence of Scores (see Figure 2). The Structural Summary allows for a handy and orderly listing of the data and, more important, enables the examiner to view the subject's responses in sequence. This can yield valuable information about the subject's general approach to the test and present a picture of where in the record various noteworthy responses or scoring categories occurred.

The next task is to tally the frequency of each particular type of score. The upper part of page 3 of the Structural Summary Blank has been developed for this purpose (see Figure 3). As may be seen, space is provided for entering the total number of scoring Determinants, Locations, Contents, Special Scorings, Form Quality, and Organizational Activity. At the bottom of page 3 is a section of 23 ratios, percentages, and derivations that are produced by using some simple mathematical calculations involving the data already entered in the rest of the Structural Summary. This section is the core of the scoring of the Comprehensive System and provides the bulk of the information used in interpretation and report writing. Some of these derivations were originally used by Rorschach, e.g., Erlebnistypus or EB, or by one or more of the systematizers, e.g., Experience Actual, or EA, introduced by Beck, while others have been developed especially for the Comprehensive System. Because of the large number of these various calculations, an explanation for each one cannot be provided in a chapter of this scope. Those familiar with the Rorschach will no doubt recognize some of the symbols. Those readers wishing for a more extensive discussion may consult Exner (1974) or Exner et al. (1976). However, several are briefly discussed below. For example, the EB and eb are two of the most critical derivations. The EB, or Erlebnistypus, is the sum of all human movement determinants over a weighted sum of all those responses using chromatic color. The eb, or Experience Base, represents the sum of all animal and inanimate movement responses over the sum of all shading and achromatic color determinants. Both of these derivations give the examiner information regarding the subject's ideational and affective world. The $X + \%$ is the proportion of all "good" form responses over the total number of responses and is an indicator of the adequacy of the subject's reality testing. Finally, $3r + (2):R$ is the Egocentricity Index and represents the proportion of reflection and pair answers appearing in the protocol, with Reflections being weighted 3 times that of Pairs.

While this scoring process might appear to require a great deal of time and effort on the part of the examiner, this is not at all the case. With experience, the responses can be scored in about 15 min, and the Structural Summary sheet can be completed in less time. One can administer, score, and summarize the test in about 70–90 min using the Comprehensive System. This should leave the examiner with a sufficient amount of time to complete the most important task, that of interpreting the results and constructing an informative report.

5. Interpretation

While the administration and scoring of the Rorschach are relatively simple, interpretation of the protocol requires much more experience. Simple cookbook approaches fail to glean the subtle nuances of the behavioral and cognitive styles of the individual. The complexity of the process is best illustrated by Piotrowski's masterful computer interpretation which includes hundreds of principles and rules. Interpretation requires a rich knowledge of personality plus the logic necessary to integrate information from the protocol with other data about the subject.

It must be emphasized that a single piece of information is not sufficient to tell us anything about a person. For example, we might note that a particular subject is very meticulous in his approach to the test, making sure that he has viewed the card from every possible angle and taking a great deal of time before completing each card. We might say that he is "compulsive," but what would this mean? Is his meticulous style interfering with his functioning or might it actually be adaptive? Does it help him to produce outstanding responses, or are they grossly distorted? The only way we can know this is to pay close attention to how each bit of information interrelates with the other aspects of the test. This search for configurations is the aim of Rorschach interpretation and gives the only meaningful description of the subject as a unique person.

The interpretive process begins, then, with a review of all of the test data. Free Association, Inquiry, and the entire Structural Summary are included and are analyzed both separately and in configuration. The examiner is here seeking to form hypotheses about the subject, not only from unusual aspects of the test, but also from the general way in which he responds. This is known as the Propositional Stage, because the various hypotheses about the subject are listed in the form of propositions about what might be "going on." This process is not without some normative base, however. During the development of the Comprehensive System, data were gathered on the frequency of each determinant for a number of psychiatric and nonpsychiatric populations. In addition, each ratio, percentage, and derivation were carefully studied, and tables consisting of the mean and standard deviation of each of these components for various adult populations were computed (Exner, 1974). More recently, these tables have also been developed for children (Exner et al., 1976). The examiner may and should refer to these tables when formulating hypotheses, as they give critical information as to whether the subject's responses present a configuration that is within normal limits. This becomes a multifaceted process; for example, on examination of the Structural Summary, the interpreter might note that the subject has an $X + \%$ of .50. On referring to the table, he finds that nonpsychiatric populations usually show good form quality for at least .75 of their responses. This prompts the interpreter to refer to the Sequence of Scores in order to see where the subject responded with poor form. He notes that this most often occurs on responses in which chromatic color is the main determinant. Color has been shown to be connected with the affective world of the subject (Exner, 1974), and so the interpreter might hypothesize that affective stimuli may interfere with the subject's ability to accurately test reality.

The examiner also uses the subject's words as an important piece of interpretive data. Lindner (1943, 1944, 1946, 1947) was one of the first to argue for this approach, and all of the systematizers have included content analysis as a major aspect of their systems. Schafer (1954) has written the most definitive work on content analysis. He recommends examining the verbalizations for logically grouped categories and names 14 themes that are commonly found. In addition, a subject might make a particularly dramatic response to a card, and, while this must be interpreted with caution, it may indicate a particular preoccupation or conflict area. Integrated with the other aspects of the record, analysis of the verbalizations can be a valuable aid in understanding the particular nuances of the subject and helps to "personalize" the data.

The second step in interpretation is called the integration stage. In this stage, all of the propositions are integrated into a description of the person. This is accomplished through a process of both inductive and deductive reasoning. While all of the various pieces of data represent a gestalt that is far too complex in practice to be dealt with here, an example of the kinds of hypotheses generated during integration stage is in order: J. C. is a 28-year-old female with a recurring duodenal ulcer of somatic origin. Surgical intervention is under consideration, and the medical staff asks whether surgical interference with the symptom might endanger her psychological makeup and whether there are other kinds of treatment that they might use that would provide greater success on a short-term basis (Exner, 1974, pp. 386–398). Below are the hypotheses derived from her Rorschach:

1. She has been "overly instilled" with notions of correct and proper behavior.
2. She is currently in a severe and painful conflict concerning her sex role, may have overly identified with her father's role in the family, and may have some homosexual conflicts.
3. She deals with this conflict in a rigidly perfectionistic and obsessive manner. However, this form of defense is not working successfully, as evidenced by her continuing somatic difficulties.
4. Her psychological life is constrained, and she prefers to rely on her high intelligence rather than deal with her inner and outer affective world.
5. She reacts in an irritated and hostile manner when confronted with affect, but prefers to internalize most feelings.
6. This internalizing style is pervasive and constitutes her major form of defense.

While these six hypotheses do not directly respond to the referral questions, they do make important inroads into describing this woman as a unique individual. It will be on the basis of these and other hypotheses that the referral questions will be addressed. The resulting report can confidently describe the subject nomothetically and idiographically, and will make an informed prediction of her likely response to intervention. Work has recently been completed to compile "normative data" to identify those who have a high likelihood of attempting suicide (Exner & Wylie, 1977) or those who are schizophrenic (Exner, 1978).

Implicit in most referral questions, such as those concerning J. C., are requests for treatment plans. The Rorschach was originally developed as a test with great usefulness in differential diagnosis. However, as the role of the psychologist has changed, so too has the function of the Rorschach. It is now used quite frequently to aid in giving an overall picture of the subject so that appropriate treatment objectives can be specified. This area has long been neglected by Rorschachers, and therefore the application of the Rorschach to explicit treatment planning is only in its infancy, but offers a seemingly important potential.

6. Conclusion

The Rorschach is a multifaceted process. The confusion created by five discrete systems and by numerous individual variations, as well as by the lack of empirical justification, has created general skepticism about its continuing utility as a viable method of assessment. Yet the Comprehensive System may be seen as a workable alternative to the "chronic Rorschach problem." By taking the best of the five systems and adding extensive empirical data to that composite, a Rorschach methodology has been created which is both reliable and researchable. This chapter has provided but an overview of the procedure. Information, especially in terms of the interpretive postulates gleaned from the data, can be found in much greater detail elsewhere (Exner, 1978). In addition, work continues in an effort to further examine the validity and the reliability of the test and to extend its clinical utility, with the ultimate objective of placing the Rorschach in its proper perspective in the clinical setting as an empirically sound method of assessment.

7. References

JOHN E. EXNER, JR.,
AND BETH CLARK

Abramson, L. S. The influence of set for area on the Rorschach test results. *Journal of Consulting Psychology*, 1951, *15*, 337–342.

Baughman, E. E. The effect of inquiry method on Rorschach color and shading scores. *Journal of Projective Techniques*, 1959, *23*, 3–7.

Beck, S. J. Configurational tendencies in Rorschach responses. *American Journal of Psychology*, 1933, *45*, 433–443.

Beck, S. J. Problems of future research in the Rorschach test. *American Journal of Orthopsychiatry*, 1935, *5*, 83–85.

Beck, S. J. Autism in Rorschach scoring: A feeling comment. *Character and Personality*, 1936, *5*, 83–85.

Beck, S. J. *Introduction to the Rorschach method: A manual of personality study.* American Orthopsychiatric Association Monographs, 1937, No. 1.

Beck, S. J. *Rorschach's test. I: Basic Processes.* New York: Grune & Stratton, 1944.

Beck, S. J. *Rorschach's test. II: A variety of personality pictures.* New York: Grune & Stratton, 1945.

Beck, S. J. *Rorschach's test. III: Advances in interpretation.* New York: Grune & Stratton, 1952.

Beck, S. J. *The Rorschach experiment: Adventures in blind diagnosis.* New York: Grune & Stratton, 1960.

Beck, S. J., & Molish, H. B. *Rorschach's test. II: A variety of personality pictures* (2nd ed.). New York: Grune & Stratton, 1967.

Beck, S. J., Beck, A., Levitt, E., & Molish, H. *Rorschach's test. I: Basic processes* (3rd ed.). New York: Grune & Stratton, 1961.

Biederman, L., & Cerbus, G. Changes in Rorschach testing. *Journal of Personality Assessment*, 1971, *35*, 524–526.

Carp, A. L., & Shavzin, A. R. The susceptibility to falsification of the Rorschach diagnostic technique. *Journal of Consulting Psychology*, 1950, *3*, 230–233.

Coffin, T. E. Some conditions of suggestion and suggestibility: A study of certain attitudinal and situational factors influencing the process of suggestion. *Psychological Monographs*, 1941, *53*, Whole No. 241.

Cronbach, L. J. Statistical methods applied to Rorschach scores: A review. *Psychological Bulletin*, 1949, *46*, 393–429.

Exner, J. E. The influence of chromatic and achromatic color in the Rorschach. *Journal of Projective Techniques*, 1959, *23*, 418–425.

Exner, J. E. The influence of achromatic color on Cards IV and VI of the Rorschach. *Journal of Projective Techniques*, 1961, *25*, 38–41.

Exner, J. E. *The Rorschach systems.* New York: Grune & Stratton, 1969. (a)

Exner, J. E. Rorschach responses as an index of narcissism. *Journal of Projective Techniques and Personality Assessment*, 1969, *33*, 324–330. (b)

Exner, J. E. Rorschach manifestations of narcissism. *Rorschachiano*, 1970, *9*, 449–457.

Exner, J. E. *The Rorschach: A comprehensive system.* New York: Wiley, 1974.

Exner, J. E. Projective techniques. In I. B. Weiner (Ed.), *Clinical methods in psychology.* New York: Wiley, 1976.

Exner, J. E. *The Rorschach: A comprehensive system. Volume II. Current Research and Advanced Interpretation.* New York: Wiley, 1978.

Exner, J. E., & Armbruster, G. L. Increasing R by altering instructions and creating a time set. Workshops Study No. 209 (Unpublished). Bayville, N.Y.: Rorschach Workshops, 1974.

Exner, J. E., & Exner, D. E. How clinicians use the Rorschach. *Journal of Personality Assessment*, 1972, *36*, 403–408.

Exner, J. E., Weiner, I. B., & Schuyler, W. *A Rorschach workbook for the Comprehensive System*, Bayville, N.Y.: Rorschach Workshops, 1976.

Exner, J. E., and Wylie, J. R. Some Rorschach data concerning suicide. *Journal of Personality Assessment*, 1977, *41*, 339–348.

Friedman, H. Perceptual regression in schizophrenia: An hypothesis suggested by use of the Rorschach test. *Journal of Genetic Psychology*, 1952, *81*, 63–98.

Gibby, R. G., Miller, D. R., & Walker, E. L. The examiner's influence on the Rorschach protocol. *Journal of Consulting Psychology*, 1953, *17*, 425–428.

Gibby, R. G., & Stotsky, B. A. The relation of Rorschach free association to inquiry. *Journal of Consulting Psychology*, 1953, *17*, 359–363.

Goetcheus, G. The effects of instructions and examiners on the Rorschach. Unpublished master's thesis, Bowling Green State University, 1967.

Goldfried, M. R., Stricker, G., & Weiner, I. B. *Rorschach handbook of clinical and research applications.* Englewood Cliffs, N.J.: Prentice-Hall, 1971.

Grisso, J. T., & Meadow, A. Test interference in a Rorschach WAIS administration sequence. *Journal of Consulting Psychology*, 1967, *31*, 382–386.

Harris, J. G. Validity: The search for a constant in a universe of variables. In M. Rickers-Ovsiankina (Ed.), *Rorschach psychology.* New York: Wiley, 1960.

Hemmendinger, L. Perceptual organization and development as reflected in the structure of the Rorschach test responses. *Journal of Projective Techniques*, 1953, *17*, 162–170.

Hemmendinger, L. Development scores. In M. Rickers-Ovsiankina (Ed.), *Rorschach psychology.* New York: Wiley, 1960.

Henry, E., & Rotter, J. B. Situational influences on Rorschach responses. *Journal of Consulting Psychology*, 1956, *20*, 457–462.

Hertz, M. R. Rorschach norms for an adolescent age group. *Child Development*, 1935, *6*, 69–76.

Hertz, M. R. The method of administration of the Rorschach inkblot test. *Child Development*, 1936, *7*, 237–254.

Hertz, M. R. Discussion on "Some recent Rorschach problems." *Rorschach Research Exchange*, 1937–1938, *2*, 53–65.

Hertz, M. R. Scoring the Rorschach inkblot test. *Journal of Genetic Psychology*, 1938, *52*, 16–64.

Hertz, M. R. The scoring of the Rorschach inkblot method as developed by the Brush Foundation. *Rorschach Research Exchange*, 1942, *6*, 16–27.

Hertz, M. R. *Frequency tables for scoring Rorschach responses* (3rd ed.). Cleveland: Case Western Reserve University Press, 1951.

Hertz, M. R. Organization activity. In M. Rickers-Ovsiankina (Ed.), *Rorschach psychology.* New York: Wiley, 1960.

Hertz, M. R. A Hertz interpretation. In J. E. Exner (Ed.), *The Rorschach systems.* New York: Grune & Stratton, 1969.

Holt, R. R. Measuring libidinal and aggressive motives and their controls by means of the Rorschach test. In D. Levine (Ed.), *Nebraska symposium on motivation.* Lincoln, Neb.: University of Nebraska Press, 1966.

Holt, R. R. Yet another look at clinical and statistical prediction: Or, is clinical psychology worthwhile? *American Psychologist*, 1970, *25*, 337–349.

Holtzman, W. H., Thorpe, J. S., Swartz, J. D., & Herron, E. W. *Inkblot perception and personality.* Austin: University of Texas Press, 1961.

Hutt, M., Gibby, R. G., Milton, E. O., & Pottharst, K. The effect of varied experimental "sets" upon Rorschach test performance. *Journal of Projective Techniques*, 1950, *14*, 181–187.

Klopfer, B. The present status of the theoretical development of the Rorschach method. *Rorschach Research Exchange*, 1937, *1*, 142–147.

Klopfer, B., Ainsworth, M. D., Klopfer, W. G., & Holt, R. R. *Developments in the Rorschach Technique. Vol. I. Technique and theory.* Yonkers-on-Hudson, N.Y.: World Book Company, 1954.

Klopfer, B., & Davidson, H. H. *The Rorschach technique: An introductory manual.* New York: Harcourt, Brace & World, 1962.

Klopfer, B., et al. *Developments in the Rorschach technique. Vol. II. Fields of application.* Yonkers-on-Hudson, N.Y.: World Book Company, 1956.

Klopfer, B., & Kelly, D. *The Rorschach technique.* Yonkers-on-Hudson, N.Y.: World Book Company, 1942.

Klopfer, B., Meyer, M. M., & Brawer, F. *Developments in the Rorschach technique. Vol. III. Aspects of personality structure.* New York: Harcourt, Brace, Jovanovich, 1970.

Klopfer, B., & Sender, S. A system of refined scoring systems. *Rorschach Research Exchange*, 1936, *2*, 19–22.

Koch, S. Psychology and emerging conceptions of knowledge as unitary. In T. W. Wann (Ed.), *Behaviorism and phenomenology.* Chicago: University of Chicago Press, 1964.

Levin, M. M. The two tests in the Rorschach. *Journal of Projective Techniques*, 1953, *17*, 471–473.

Lindner, R. M. The Rorschach test and the diagnosis of psychopathic personality. *Journal of Criminal Psychopathology*, 1943, *1*, 69.

Lindner, R. M. Some significant Rorschach responses. *Journal of Criminal Psychopathology*, 1944, *4*, 775.

Lindner, R. M. Content analysis in Rorschach work. *Rorschach Research Exchange*, 1946, *10*, 121–129.

Lindner, R. M. Analysis of Rorschach's test by content. *Journal of Clinical Psychopathology*, 1947, *8*, 707–719.

Lord, E. Experimentally induced variations in Rorschach performance. *Psychological Monographs*, 1950, *60*, Whole No. 316.

Lubin, B., Wallis, R. R., & Paine, C. Patterns of psychological test usage in the United States: 1935–1969. *Professional Psychology*, 1971, *2*, 70–74.

Masling, J. Differential indoctrination of examiners and Rorschach responses. *Journal of Consulting Psychology*, 1965, *29*, 198–201.

Mayman, M. Measuring reality-adherence in the Rorschach test. American Psychological Association Meeting, 1966.

Mayman, M. Reality contact, defense effectiveness, and psychopathology in Rorschach form-level scores. In B. Klopfer, M. Meyer, & F. Brawer (Eds.), *Developments in Rorschach technique. Vol. III. Aspects of personality structure*. New York: Harcourt Brace Jovanovich, 1970, pp. 11–46.

Meehl, P. E. *Clinical versus statistical prediction*. Minneapolis: University of Minnesota Press, 1954.

Meehl, P. E. Wanted—a good cookbook. *American Psychologist*, 1956, *11*, 263–272.

Piotrowski, Z. A Rorschach compendium. *Psychiatric Quarterly*, 1947, *21*, 79–101.

Piotrowski, Z. *Perceptanalysis*. New York: Macmillan, 1957.

Piotrowski, Z. Digital computer interpretation of ink-blot test data. *Psychiatric Quarterly*, 1964, *38*, 1–26.

Piotrowski, Z. A Piotrowski interpretation. In J. E. Exner (Ed.), *The Rorschach systems*. New York: Grune & Stratton, 1969.

Rapaport, D., Gill, M., & Schafer, R. *Diagnostic psychological testing*. Chicago: Yearbook Publishers, 1945, 1946.

Reisman, J. M. The effect of direct inquiry on the Rorschach. *Journal of Personality Assessment*, 1970, *34*, 388–390.

Rorschach, H. *Psychodiagnostics*. Bern: Bircher, 1921 (translation, Hans Huber Verlag, 1942).

Schachtel, E. G. Subject definitions of the Rorschach test situation and their effect on test performance. *Psychiatry*, 1945, *8*, 419–448.

Schafer, R. *Psychoanalytic interpretation in Rorschach testing*. New York: Grune & Stratton, 1954.

Sisson, B., & Taulbee, E. Organizational activity of the Rorschach test. *Journal of Consulting Psychology*, 1955, *19*, 29–31.

Sundberg, N. D. The practice of psychological testing in clinical services in the United States. *American Psychologist*, 1961, *16*, 79–83.

Weiner, I. B. Does psychodiagnosis have a future? *Journal of Personality Assessment*, 1972, *36*, 534–546.

Wishner, J. Rorschach intellectual indicators in neurotics. *American Journal of Orthopsychiatry*, 1948, *18*, 265–279.

Wyatt, F. How objective is objectivity? *Journal of Projective Techniques*, 1968, *31*, 3–19.

Zax, M., & Stricker, G. The effect of structured inquiry on Rorschach scores. *Journal of Consulting Psychology*, 1960, *24*, 328–332.

Zubin, J., Eron, L., & Schumer, F. *An experimental approach to projective techniques*. New York: Wiley, 1965.

6

Thematic Apperception Test and Related Methods

MORRIS I. STEIN

1. Introduction

The Thematic Apperception Test (TAT) was introduced to the psychological world in 1935 by Morgan and Murray. Its conception and birth, as with those of mytho-logical heroes, were cloaked in mystery (Holt, 1949). Conditions surrounding its infancy are clearer, because it was reared at the Harvard Psychological Clinic, in the little yellow house on Plympton Street, with press congenial environment and press nurturance. Doting parents and dedicated disciples clearly saw the newborn infant's power to cast light on the darkest recesses of personality dynamics.

The autonomous infant underwent three revisions to its identity. But changes in structure did not accompany changes in function. It started in life and continued throughout its existence to be both a method and a test for the study of personality. Later, partisan-type psychologists fought for and defended one or the other of these functions. Each side claimed that only it knew what was best.

At one extreme, the method-ists insisted that fundamental truths hidden in the form and content of the stories could be revealed only with the aid of theoretical frameworks assisted occasionally by clinical judgment and experience and not so infrequently by idiosyncratic "intuitive feels." At the other extreme were the test-ists, who turned stories into scores. They were always psychometrizing the TAT down to test size. And when they were accused of making the TAT like any other test, they would say, "Yes, only better."

Partisans strongly defended their cathected positions or strongly cathected their defended positions, but, for our hero, complexity was complexity whether it came from a patient or a psychologist. And, as on so many other occasions, it heroically

MORRIS I. STEIN • Department of Psychology, New York University, New York, New York 10003. This study was supported by a Research Career Award (MH-18679) from the National Institute of Mental Health to the author.

integrated the best of the partisan viewpoints, making available to all who wanted it a rich ambrosia, a self-actualized fulfillment in which one could be both methodist and test-ist, understanding the TAT stories as only an integrated psychologist should.

Early revisions were not traumatic, and our hero was left with few if any emotional scars. The short span of its infant years was rather auspicious, and within 3 years of its introduction to the American scene its budding vita was gloriously crowned by integrated method-test-ist contributions to *Explorations in Personality* (Murray et al., 1938), fulfilling the wildest expectations of its creators and disciples. From then on, its fame spread far and wide—but alas never (or perhaps, hardly ever) again achieving such peaks of glory.

Within the claustral confines of "the Clinic," our hero was king. Outside, it was frequently and unwillingly made to compete with an older peer made of ink. After some minor flurries, the test-of-pictures and the test-of-ink formed an entente cordiale. Under the banner called "projective techniques," they went forth and valiantly set up separate rights of eminent domain in the person and spheres of influence in the environment.

Within the person, 'twas said that the test-of-ink gathered data on the structure or skeleton of the personality and that the test-of-pictures gathered data on the meat and skin. Frequently, it was forgotten which got the meat and which got the skeleton. No one really knew what all this really meant, but everyone understood. Everyone went on using the test-made-of-pictures and the test-made-of-ink without any qualms and in orgies of intuitive delight.

Then it came to geographic spheres of influence. One test took the East Coast and the other the West Coast. Each was nurtured by ocean waters whose broad vistas encouraged fertile creative insights. Between the two, there lay a dustbowl ravaged atheoretically by frenetic hypothetical variables and intervening constructs served up by magnificent chefs who distilled their wisdom by writing cookbooks in which they presented recipes for the perplexed. These recipes, it was claimed, were tested and true ways for the understanding of—people.

To continue with our hero's psychohistory: During early adolescence, for some unexplained reason, our hero began to undergo mitosis. And, while initially it was only white and middle class (religion indeterminate), it was soon not only white but also black, Indian, African, disadvantaged, regressed to childhood, or advanced to old age. It was an identical twin produced by painting its white self black, etc. It was also a fraternal twin sharing its picture quality with another who had scenes different from those in the originals.

At about this same time, a new adversary appeared on the scene. Unlike its earlier adversary, the psychometrician, who tried to annihilate it by cutting it down to test size and who accused it of not possessing characteristics necessary for becoming a member of a test society it didn't even want to join, its new adversary arose from within the tribe called clinical psychologists. Most members of this tribe had initially clutched the truths of projective techniques to their breasts but, later, Judas-like, they accused our hero of a crime it never committed or intended to commit— the evaluation of personality. This denigrating criticism hurt. For the self-concept of our hero was that, no matter what, method or test, it was always on the side of humanistic-empathic nonevaluational understanding.

It was during World War II or shortly thereafter that a significant group of clinical psychologists became disenchanted with diagnosis and sought greener pastures in therapy. Because our hero was establishing its roots as a diagnostic technique, it became one of the straw men marked as a target by this group of clinicians. While many thought the TAT (and even its ink-test ally) were really methods (or even tests) to facilitate understanding of others, the battle cry that resounded throughout the land was that, method or test, the TAT had committed the sin of direct evaluation.

Stalwart disciples of our hero stood by loyally refusing to be confused by verbal barrages nondirectively fired in all directions. But they could not withstand the weight of the sheer numbers who came out against them, and there was a weakening of support and diminution of the ranks. Gradually, the battle cries diminished and peace was established by some verbal magic which erased the onus of "diagnosis" by substituting "assessment" for it. Things were just not the same any longer.

Then, with international peace, our hero had a period of renaissance—one that stemmed from the appearance of a mitotic fraternal twin. TAT-like cards appeared on the scene together with a rigorous scoring system firmly based in theory and psychometrically approved. Furthermore, statistically significant results were produced with actual, real, down-to-earth behavior. And for achievers, affiliators, and power-oriented persons there was a windfall of dissertations and books.

We reckon that our hero is now in its late adolescence. Its auspicious beginnings, we believe, augur well for a maturity in which it will cast new light on and reveal heretofore hidden dynamics of personality and behavior at whatever level they may be found.

2. History

One of the earliest precursors of the TAT, according to Tomkins (1947),* did not involve stories but associations. In 1879, Galton learned from an evaluation of the data in the first free-association experiment that they had much personal relevance. He suggested the possibility that frequently recurring associations could be related to an individual's early life and single associations to an individual's more recent life experiences. Further, he felt that these associations "lay bare the foundations of man's thoughts with more vividness and truth than he would probably care to publish to the world" (Tomkins, 1947, p. 1).

Brittain in 1907 reported sex differences in the stories boys and girls 13–20 years of age told to nine pictures. "Girls' stories revealed more religious, moral, social elements, more interest in clothes and the preparation of food; boys were more interested in the consumption of food. The stories told by the girls were full of pity, sadness, and fear of being left alone" (Tomkins, 1947, p. 2).

Age differences were found by Libby in 1908, who studied adolescents' imagination and found significant differences between the thirteenth and the fourteenth year, with the former more "objective" and the latter more "subjective."

In 1926, Clark became one of the first to study stories as an aid to the psychoanalytic process. Rather than using stories to evoke fantasies, he asked his patients to imagine they were infants and to describe the feelings they might have in the story. Clark, according to Tomkins, found this method useful with narcissistic patients who were unable to develop transference neuroses.

*A more detailed presentation of the historical antecedents of the TAT may be found in Tomkins (1947).

The Social Situation Picture Test was then developed by Schwartz (1931, 1935) as an aid to interviewing juveniles in a court clinic. The test consisted of eight pictures representing situations most frequently found in the histories of adolescents. The subjects were requested to tell stories to the pictures as well as to respond to examiners' questions designed to follow up leads.

It was then in 1935 that Morgan and Murray published their paper introducing the TAT. In 1938, *Explorations in Personality* (Murray et al., 1938) was published, which contained data collected with the TAT and other tests and procedures for understanding personality. All of this was presented in *Explorations* together with an explication of Murray's personology—his theoretical formulations and need-press system.

Many have tried to learn about Morgan's and Murray's creative processes as they developed the TAT, but with little success. Holt, while he was editor of the *TAT Newsletter*, once had a modicum of success. On the basis of correspondence with Christiana Morgan and Harry Murray, Holt (1949) reported that

> Chris had hoped to find time to write up some reminiscences about the TAT's early days, but she got herself completely tied up with work on the study of creative writers . . . as well as another project. Besides, she confesses that she can't remember much that is noteworthy. Harry Murray was good enough to submit the following note as a kind of substitute.
>
> "A conversation I had with a student [Cecelia Roberts—now Mrs. Crane Brinton] was the spark that started us collecting pictures in 1933. At the beginning [Chris Morgan's] part was to help in the selection of pictures [looking through magazines, etc.]*; to redraw a few of the selected pictures; and to administer the test to half our subjects (or half the test to all our subjects, I don't remember which). We wrote the article together rather quickly—in about two weeks, as I remember."

And then, Holt adds: "Perhaps someday one of us will get a chance to draw the original authors out on this topic in an interview; meanwhile this much must satisfy those of us who wonder where brain-children come from."

Since the TAT was first announced and since its related data were published in *Explorations*, it has been used to gather diagnostic data, as an aid to therapy, and in a variety of research studies. It has been used as a complete set of pictures with ten cards, each administered in two test sessions. Parts of it, however, have also been used with effectiveness. It has been used to study normal and psychopathological conditions, child development, attitudes and sentiments, and the interrelations of culture and personality, and it has been used for purposes of assessment in civilian and military life.

The TAT has spawned TAT-like pictures for use with blacks (Thompson, 1949a,b), with American Indian groups (Henry, 1947), interracial groups (Cann,

---

*This is quite an experience. Anyone involved with the TAT, especially in determining the characteristics of a card and the factors related to its "pull," should seek it out.

At the Harvard Psychological Clinic there was a small closet full of picture magazines—*Life, Look, Time, Newsweek*, etc. I spent many an hour in this closet selecting pictures for a Mind Reading Test, a test that would consist of pictures only of faces about the size of those in *Time* or the Szondi Test. The subject was requested to tell in "one liners" about what people were thinking and feeling.

To get some idea of what goes into the selection of pictures, one should try to construct one's own TAT. It wouldn't be long before one would learn that it is not simply a matter of taking pictures out of a magazine. Yet, on an a priori basis, what makes a "good" picture is still unclear. Magazine pictures are frequently only initial stimuli that need to be altered artistically for proper degree of ambiguity, etc., and the final rendition has to be submitted to empirical test to ascertain that the picture actually "pulls" as desired.

1977), etc. Especially noteworthy is a series to gather data on need achievement (McClelland et al., 1953). There is a TAT to study groups (Henry & Guetzkow, 1951; Horwitz and Cartwright, 1953), and there are both slides (Osborne, 1951), and a procedure (Stein, 1955), for group administration. There is a form of administering the test in which the stories are answers (Murray, 1943), and another in which the answers are in the form of multiple choices (Clark, 1944). There are various ways of scoring the TAT and numerous ways of interpreting it. And, last but not least, there are some who work with it as if it were a test and subject it to all sorts of psycho-metric criteria, and there are others who regard it as a method or procedure in which theory and intuition hold sway.

All of this is history—past and current—and only parts of it can be reviewed here. For the reader who wants to know more, I highly recommend work by Tomkins (1947), Murstein (1963), Megargee (1966), and a forthcoming book by Holt (1978). The reader who is interested in TAT history as well as the ambience and flavor of the early days of the TAT should find and read the no-longer-published *TAT News-letter*. It was first published as separately and then as part of the *Journal of Projective Techniques*. Holt was its first editor and its last editor was Shneidman. The warm, informal, chatty style of the *Newsletter* that Holt started reflects the atmo-sphere that permeated the Harvard Psychological Clinic when there were no courses in the TAT, yet everyone learned how to use it through an apprenticeship system of "osmosis." Every so often, usually during an afternoon, everyone at the little yellow house on Plympton Street gathered to discuss a TAT protocol. Hypotheses and in-terpretations were numerous. Depths of personal and collective unconscious were plumbed and levels of personality were explored that even Freud and Jung hadn't heard of. In all instances, data in support of one's idea had to be offered. Many of those around the table in the clinic library at the time I was there would later pub-lish manuals or important works on the TAT (Tomkins, 1947; Wyatt 1947, 1958; Holt, 1971, 1978; Stein, 1955)*, but at this point in history they were still seminar-ians, and at the head of the table sat Harry Murray—listening, urging, challenging, and writing down what everyone said. And when they had pretty much exhausted themselves, Harry pulled together what had been said, frequently rewarding each of his students by selecting a bit of this one's ideas and something more of that one's ideas. Then he contributed his own creative integration in which new insights were revealed, and an understanding of the case would emerge that was more complete than anyone thought possible. This is the unwritten part of the TAT's history in which Harry Murray's charisma and creativity nurtured so many of us who followed in his footsteps.

3. Description

The TAT consists of 31 cards—30 of them pictures in black and white and one blank. There are cards for men and women and cards for boys and girls (under 14 down to 4 years of age). In all, each subject is given 20 cards—ten at each of two sit-tings separated a day apart. The cards in the second set of ten are regarded as more bizarre and more unusual than those in the first set of ten.

The cards currently in use (Murray, 1943) are the third revision of the test. They

---

*Nevitt Sanford, who had done so much of the early work, preceded us. Robert White was with us, and Bellak visited periodically.

were selected by a study of their "stimulating power" or "pull"—operationally defined as the rated contribution of each picture to a final case diagnosis arrived at by a combination of TAT and other psychological tests.

When the TAT is administered, the subject or patient is requested to make up a story in which he will tell what happened before the scene he sees in the picture, what is going on at the present time, what the people are thinking and feeling, and what the outcome will be. The pictures may be administered individually or in groups, and when administered to groups one may ask them to write their stories or to make selections from multiple choices with which they are presented.

Then either the stories are interpreted or their meaning and significance are arrived at by studying the structure and content of the story in the light of theory and clinical experience. The stories may be scored for one or more variables and the results related to some behavioral criterion (e.g., success in school) or applied to some general research problem (e.g., assessment of psychiatrists, the differences between professions, marital choices, etc.) or to the diagnostic category to which the patient belongs, etc.

It should come as no surprise to anyone at all acquainted with this area that practically every statement in the foregoing introductory paragraphs has been the basis for research and study. For example, what are the characteristics of the cards? In what order should they be presented? Would chromatic color have a different effect on the stories produced? How reliable is the test? How valid is it? What scoring systems are there? And so on and so on.

Answers to these questions is what this chapter is all about. However, before we turn in that direction, let us consider a broader issue that must be discussed so that our communication can be clearer.

4. Method or Test

When the TAT is regarded as a test, the emphasis is on its psychometric characteristics. How reliable is the test? Can two or more persons score the test reliably? What variables should be used? Are the pictures more structured than one expected, or is it more important to attend to their ambiguity? How valid is the test? Is it better at concurrent validity than predictive validity?

When the TAT is regarded as a method, it is not that these questions don't matter, but rather that quantifiable answers based on numerous persons are simply not necessary. Can anyone doubt, for example, that data obtained from a person are valid? Of course they are, because they are obtained from a person, and it is not the method that is or is not valid but the expertise of the interpreter. For some interpreters no amount of story data has any meaning, whereas for others the same or even minimal data are full of meaning and information. And when it comes to reliability, is that a method characteristic? Or is it a characteristic of a subject? Are there not some subjects who do exactly the same thing on repeated occasions? And are there not some persons who, just because they told one story once, will tell a different one if they are given another try? Does it make sense to put both groups of individuals together to get an answer? As answers are sought, those who regard the TAT as a method tend to be more personality-theory oriented, and when a preferred theory fails them they become flexibly eclectic and find another theory that will yield some meaning.

In sum, what the method people regard as intuitive inferences about the person they study, the test-oriented people regard as unreliable subjectivity, and what the test-oriented people regard as objective methodology, the method-oriented people regard as misplaced quantification.

This conflict, which has absorbed the energies of many persons, is also to be found among Rorschachers. One might say that the conflict is indigenous to projective technikers. In the Rorschach, testers are represented by those who base their interpretations completely or almost completely on a subject's scores; the method people focus almost completely on the content of the subject's responses and the sequence in which they appear.

The conflict is pervasive, and it finds its way to theory. In this regard, we are tempted to say "A plague on both your houses," and draw upon Kaplan's (1964) statements in another area and say that the method people indulge themselves in a "seductive fallacy" while the test people indulge themselves in a "reductive fallacy." Thus the method people may be constantly chasing rainbows, deluding themselves and disappointing others as they tempt themselves and others that there is always "something more" in the data they have before them. By the same token, the test people restrict themselves and inhibit others by admonishing all who might embark on an exploration in meaning that the data are "nothing but" the manifestation of some basic element—or possibly a series of elements.

Obviously both sides can profit from each other's point of view and from each other's findings. The test-oriented people, without necessarily being short on the development of their own variables, might be stimulated by the variables used by the methods people and the clinicians and theorists among them. The methods people, not unaware of how each of the cards is perceived or misperceived, could nevertheless profit from a set of norms and a systematic study of the pictures' characteristics. These are among the most superficial of the mutual benefits. One can think of many others. It is to be hoped that with the passage of time there will be a greater melding of both approaches—if not necessarily in the same individual, then a greater mutual regard that both groups are contributing to each other and most certainly to the benefit of the field and the subject.

By the very nature of the requirements of this chapter, it is necessary to concentrate on the testlike characteristics of the TAT, although I shall obviously not limit myself to these. As a result, the method point of view as I have conceived of it is not well represented. I hope that what I have just said indicates my awareness of this deficiency and that the reader will compensate for any of the inadequacies by supplementing what is presented with a reading of the manuals written about the TAT and a number of case studies in which the TAT has played a central role. Among the former, the following manuals would be especially helpful: Tomkins (1947), Henry (1956), Wyatt (1958), and Stein (1955). Among the case studies, the following are worthwhile: *Explorations in Personality* (Murray et al., 1938), *Lives in Progress* (White, 1966), and Stein (1955).

With this for background and introduction, let us turn to each of the major problems or areas that have been studied.

5. Instructions

5.1. Individual Administration

In individual administration of the TAT, the subject may sit in a chair, stretch out on a couch, face the examiner, or sit with his back to him. There is no research evidence as to the effect of any position on TAT responses. The position selected has to suit the individual subject, the examiner, and the conditions of the examination.

The TAT may also be group-administered, which will be discussed later.

5.1.1. Individual Instructions

In Murray's (1943) manual accompanying the test, there are instructions for adolescents and adults of average intelligence and instructions for those of low intelligence and psychotics. Essentially, the instructions differ in that those for the first category say "This is a test of imagination, one form of intelligence" and then there is a request for a dramatic story. For less sophisticated and psychotic groups, the test is described as a "story-telling test and the subject is asked to make up a story."

When the second set of ten TAT cards, which is regarded as more unusual and bizarre, is administered to the more sophisticated subject, the subject is asked to "give freer rein to his imagination," to "let your imagination have its way, as in a myth, fairy story, or allegory." The less sophisticated group, when presented with the second set of ten cards, is asked to make up more "exciting" stories than they did the previous time and that they should be "like a dream or fairytale."*

Instructions recommended by others may be found in their respective manuals. In all instances, the instructions are designed so as not to interfere with the subject's own style of responding to the pictures. Nevertheless, research (Summerwell, Campbell, & Sarason, 1958) suggests that Murray's instructions result in stories of sadder emotional tone and outcome than is true of instructions designed specifically to be mental or intellectual.

It is important to bear this finding in mind, especially since, as Murstein (1963, p. 53), who reviewed the Summerwell et al. (1958) as well as other studies presented in this section, says, "these negatively toned stories, usually scored without reference to the eliciting stimulus, are taken to indicate maladjustment." We agree with Murstein that to counteract this effect it is important for TAT workers to keep in mind tendencies of the normal person to shift back and forth in the tone of his stories or in the use of factors which in other records may be pathognomonic but in the normal record are well integrated with other characteristics.

Even without specific instructions to do so, subjects seem to be generally predisposed to appear at their best when telling TAT stories (Weisskopf & Dieppa, 1951; Murstein, 1962). Furthermore, subjects can follow instructions to inhibit stories of negative psychological characteristics (Lubin, 1960, 1961; Murstein, 1961a). Presumably, they can also do so voluntarily, in which case it can be a serious matter for diagnostic purposes, because, as the investigators suggest, clinicians frequently regard the absence of negative signs as an index of adjustment.

Tomkins (1947) and Solkoff (1959, 1960) found that subjects were put off when asked to tell stories in the first person. They did somewhat better with third-person instructions.

---

*Although one is very much aware of the Freudian influence on Murray, it is important to note that he was also influenced by Jung. Such influence is reflected in the emphasis on myths and fairytales in the second set of instructions, which is quite similar to the use of creative imagination by Jungian therapists during the course of therapy.

5.1.2. Length of Stories

Frequently, inexperienced test administrators wonder how long the stories they obtain should be. They are in constant wonderment whether the stories they obtain are long enough. As a rule of thumb, subjects might be told that they should tell stories that are about one page in length (with the examiner writing the story on a sheet of lined typing paper).

Other guidelines reported in the literature are as follows: the average adult gives stories of 300 words in length and the average 10-year-old gives stories of 150 words in length (Tomkins, 1947); in clinical situations, the average story is 100 words in length (Rapaport, Gill, & Schafer, 1968). Murray (1943) says that stories obtained from adults which are less than 140 words "indicate lack of rapport and cooperation, and lack of self-involvement." Probably the briefest protocols which yielded very significant data were those obtained from Navaho and Hopi Indians by Henry (1947).

5.1.3. Inquiry

An inquiry involves one or more questions that the examiner asks of the subject to learn more about what the subject has said or has omitted to say. Stein (1955) suggests the use of two kinds of inquiry. The first type is to be used only with the first two pictures to make certain that the subject understood the instructions. For example, if a subject omits to say what the hero or other characters in the story might have been thinking or feeling, it is suggested that the examiner ask the subject about this and note in the recording of the protocol that this was in response to a direct question. This kind of inquiry makes certain that the subject has not misheard or misinterpreted the instructions.

Stein also suggests a final inquiry. In this instance, the examiner is interested in obtaining additional material about the nature of the feelings, thoughts, and interactions in any one story. It might also be used to inquire into the subject's perceptions or misperceptions of any of the scenes, including objects and people in any of the pictures and stories. This kind of inquiry is reserved for the end so as not to cue the subject as to what might be a desirable story.

Lasaga (1946) used an inquiry to learn about ideas which a subject rejected and had not used to make up a story. He learned that some of the rejected ideas found their way into the stories or were some aspect of the made-up story, but in other instances the rejected ideas did not help in the further understanding of the subject.

5.1.4. Testing the Limits

In testing the limits, a procedure which occurs at the end of the testing, the examiner probes to learn what the subject can do under stressful or extreme conditions. Jones (1956), for example, asked his subjects first to tell stories under standard instructions and then to give their most unlikely stories to each of the pictures. The latter was regarded as reflecting repressed material. Lazarus (1961) investigated whether subjects with sexual problems or problems with aggression would be able to tell erotic stories after they told dramatic stories. After the subjects told erotic stories, they were instructed to tell hostile stories. Case studies indicated that there was little sexual imagery in the latter stories and that they were stilted.

Murstein (1963) summarizes the research on the effects of instructions. He reports the following: (1) When there is stress on imagination, the stories are more negative in tone than stories in which the subjects are encouraged to be on their guard. (2) Negatively toned stories, without due consideration to the characteristics of the picture to which they are told, are often regarded as indicating emotional maladjustment. (3) The preceding is a rather serious problem for studies of normal subjects who indulge in regressive behavior but who also show characteristics and qualities that are more often associated with psychological strength. (4) Testing limits by asking subjects to follow extreme instructions like the sexiest story possible is often a good technique for jarring overly controlled persons.

5.1.5. Recording Stories

One way of recording a subject's stories is for the examiner to write as the subject speaks. To do this effectively means that there has to be rather good rapport between subject and examiner; otherwise, the subject becomes frustrated and irritated. He has to be asked to slow up, speak louder, or otherwise adjust himself to the examiner's writing ability.

While recording a story, the examiner has an opportunity to observe his subject's reactions to his presumed "inferior" or "subordinate" role as "secretary." Some subjects in this relationship behave literally as if they were dictating to the examiner.

Other examiners tape-record stories, or they combine notetaking with tape recording. Students starting to learn the TAT generally prefer tape recordings, but this may result in lost data when the equipment fails to work somewhere in the middle of a test session.

Some persons work with hidden microphones so as not to intimidate subjects. If so, the examiner should write something of the stories because subjects can become quite skeptical if the examiner does nothing. Much embarrassment and anger can be avoided if the recording equipment is kept in full view of the subject and he is told that the stories are being recorded.

Finally, there are examiners who ask their subjects as common practice to write their own stories. Others use this procedure when they are under a great deal of work pressure. Obviously, it is the only procedure used when the TAT is administered to groups of persons.

There are no research studies of the similarities and differences between stories collected by the verbal method with the examiner writing them down and stories written out by the subject. Experience, however, indicates that written protocols are likely to be more formal and have more of the character of schoolroom compositions or English themes. They are more formal, more controlled, and less spontaneous than verbalized stories. Furthermore, verbal stories provide more material in the nature of pauses, changes in tone of voice, side comments, body movement, and interaction with examiner, all of which are lost in the written method.

5.2. Group Administration

For group administration, TAT slides are available. Research comparing group with individual TATs indicates the following:

1. Individually administered TATs yield longer stories with more ideas, but

length of story is not necessarily correlated with its meaning and the content of stories differs little despite number of words involved (Murstein, 1963; p. 46).

2. No differences are found in needs achievement, affiliation, sex, dominance, transcendence, number of themes, involvement, quality, number of figures, and compliance with instruction (Lindzey & Silverman, 1959).

3. It is rather equivocal whether more or less sad stories are obtained with individual or group administration. Eron and Ritter (1951) found somewhat sadder stories with individual administration. Sarason and Sarason (1958) found the opposite result, and Lindzey and Heinemann (1955) and Lindzey and Silverman (1959) found no difference in the emotional tone in the stories.

4. Murstein (1963, p. 46), who reviewed the literature on differences between individual and group administration, reports that group administration results in more rejections while in individual administration there are more alternative themes and comments and there is more opportunity for revealing chinks in the subjects' armor.

5. Considering group administration alone, there is no difference between a 5-min and a 20-sec showing of the pictures (Lindzey and Heinemann, 1955). However, 5 min for writing to each picture is better than 8 min for writing, possibly because the longer time allows for more control to take place and more opportunity for social approval needs to operate. Stories obtained with a 5-min time limit for writing are more similar to those obtained under conditions of individual administration than are those obtained under the longer (8-min) time limit. This holds for such socially approved motives as achievement and happiness, but not for sex and dominance. Murstein (1963, pp. 46–47) believes that there is an optimal amount of time for differentiating any motive. Need achievement, for example, would show a difference between group and individual administration if the length of time for group stories were increased from 5 to 8 min.

6. There are sex differences between individual and group administration; group administration may well be recommended for use in research studies where there is concern with a relatively small number of variables: "It should also be possible to employ it in diagnostic work as a screening device when the consequences of the false positives or false negatives are outweighed by the savings in time and effort" (Murstein, 1963, p. 47). While individual administration allows for important subject observation, it should be borne in mind that there are some subjects who use the anonymity of group administration to be more self-revealing than they might have been if they had to tell TAT stories under conditions of individual administration.

5.3. Group Process

There is another form of group administration which is designed to gather data on group process or the characteristics of a group rather than on the individual members who write out their protocols in a group setting (which was considered above).

In this procedure, a group tells a story to pictures of groups (Horwitz & Cartwright, 1953; Henry & Guetzkow, 1951). The formal and content characteristics of the story are analyzed. Valuable data may also be obtained by analyzing the processes the group went through in developing its story.

6. Number of Cards to Be Administered

As indicated above, the TAT consists of 31 pictures (including the one that is a blank card). In studying any one person, it is recommended that a group of 20 pictures be administered, ten in each session. Those that are to be administered to adult males and adult females are indicated by the letters M and F on the back of the cards, and the order in which the cards are to be shown to the subject is indicated by numbers.

For a long time (Holt, 1947, 1948; Watson, 1951; Dana, 1956b), there has been discussion of a possible shortened version of the test. Generally, the pressures of time and expense have been strong motivators in this regard. Obviously, cards should be selected in terms of how well they provide the user with information that he can use for specific needs or purposes. This would be an almost impossible criterion to meet, and consequently more gross criteria have been favored: a general rating of value and number of different themes.

Hartman (1970) polled a large group of psychologists and asked them to indicate which cards they found most valuable in their practice. Since the pool contained psychologists who worked with children as well as adults, a basic set could be obtained for both age groups. On the basis of his work, Hartman recommended a set of eight cards for clinical, research, and teaching purposes. They were 1, 2, 3BM, 4, 6BM, 7BM, 13MF, and 8BM.

Irvin and Woude (1971) and Newmark and Flouranzano (1973), using a very different criterion and very different populations, corroborated Hartman's work, with some minor exceptions. The criterion they used was Eron's (1950) list of TAT themes, and they studied the number of different themes given to each of the cards. Those that had the largest number of different themes were regarded as most valuable for a basic set. Irvin and Woude studied male college students, and Newmark and Flouranzano studied an adult white hospitalized psychoneurotic population.

7. Order of Administration

The TAT pictures have numbers on the back which indicate the order in which they are to be administered. It is conceivable that the order of cards could affect the kind of material obtained from a person. It is, however, impossible to study this problem with the recommended set of TAT cards. Data do exist on a smaller number of cards and cards that are not of the TAT set.

Atkinson (1950) used four achievement-related and four-affiliation-related cards with college students and varied the order of both sets of cards in the experiment. He found that order affected data on the achievement motive. Cards in the even position had higher achievement scores than those in the odd position. He also found a positive correlation between achievement scores on the first four cards and the amount of decrease in achievement scores in the stories to the last four positions. Lowe (1951) found that the four cards he studied differed in amount of hostility but did not find order effects. Mason (1952), on the other hand, found that order had a significant effect on elation, anxiety and content categories. A study by the Indian Ministry of Defence (1954) did not find order effects, but a study of Dollin (1960) did. The data on order, then, are equivocal.

Reitman and Atkinson (1958) also experimented with four achievement-related and four affiliation-related cards. Their results are important for the relationships between order of cards and the prediction of overt behavior which we shall consider below. They found that when four achievement-related cards came first, a significant relationship with achievement behavior was obtained. Furthermore, if affiliation-related cards came first and were then scored not for affiliation but for achievement, then an even greater relationship with observed achievement was obtained. This relationship based on the achievement score of the four affiliation-related cards was not only stronger than the score obtained for the four achievement-related cards but also stronger for an achievement score based on all eight (achievement- plus affiliation-related) cards. Murstein (1963) finds these results surprising because, from a purely psychometric point of view, when the number of test items is increased the reliability and validity of the test should be improved. In the study just reported, increasing the number of pictures (test items) did not increase the relationship with observed achievement behavior.

The possibility must therefore be considered that the order of the cards is not so important as the cards' characteristics and the variables for which they are scored—factors to which we shall turn later.

8. Administration as Part of Test Battery

Just as one might hypothesize order effects for the sequence of cards, so there may well be order effects when the TAT is administered as part of a test battery. A TAT may be administered at the beginning, middle, or end of a test battery. The question then is whether it will be affected by the tests (e.g., Wechsler-Bellevue, Rorschach, Sentence Completion Test) that precede or follow it. In all instances, the situation is further complicated by the fact that there are two halves of the TAT.

While there is no research evidence to serve as a guide, my personal preference in a case study for diagnostic assessment or teaching purposes is to devote one test to the Stein Sentence Completion Test (1948) and the first ten pictures of the TAT. Since the Stein SCT comes in two parts consisting of 50 sentences each, the first part is administered before the first ten pictures of the TAT, on the (untested) assumption that it helps ease the subject into the process of verbalizing his associations.

The second part of the Stein SCT is administered after the first ten pictures, on the (untested) assumption that the sentences may pick up any data and associations that still remain with the one subject and which have not been verbalized.

Time permitting, the second half of the TAT pictures is administered during a test session reserved all for itself or in conjunction with a partial interview and Rorschach. All of this is contingent on the on-the-spot assessment of the subject's behavior and his readiness for a structured test, a test involving fantasy, or the more unusual cards of the second half of the TAT.

The kind of procedure just recommended is consistent with the belief of clinicians who regard tests in a battery as complementary to each other. Metaphorically speaking, there are those who regard the Rorschach as yielding data for the skeletal structure of the personality and the TAT as yielding data regarding the meat of the personality.

Rosenzweig (1950) provides a conceptual framework for dealing with levels of response from different psychodiagnostic methods. Shneidman (1956) regards the Rorschach as yielding unconscious material, while the TAT, he believes, taps unconscious, preconscious, and conscious material.

On a more concrete level, there are studies in which the relative contribution of the TAT as a test to understanding a case is compared to the contribution of other tests administered to the same person. There have also been studies in which comparisons were made between the same variable scored by the TAT and other tests. The results are hardly consistent; hence it is still to be learned when the results obtained from different tests are complementary or contradictory.

Little and Shneidman (1955) report that clinicians working with a TAT and a MAPS (Make a Picture Story) protocol describe a person as well from this material as they do from the more elaborate material of a clinical folder. The authors are quick to point out, however, that the subject chosen for their study was one for whom there was rather complete clinical material. This statement is reminiscent of Allport's (1953) suggestion that normal individuals are likely to give similar material to combinations of tests, projective and otherwise, while neurotic individuals are likely to give one kind of data to one or more projective tests and different material to the more objective tests. In this regard, it would also be interesting whether highly verbal, highly visual, etc., subjects respond differently to the TAT, the Rorschach, and other tests. Specifically, do individuals who are differentially capable in their different sense modalities respond differentially to different types of personality tests?

Little and Shneidman (1959) also presented a study in which the TAT, MAPS, Rorschach, and MMPI were involved. One of the general conclusions of this study was that projective techniques were not very valid, which was in agreement with a survey of the validity of projective techniques published previously by Little (1957, 1959). With this general finding as background material, there were some specific findings related to the TAT, all of which indicated that results based on the TAT were less reliable than results based on other projective techniques (Megargee, 1966, p. 601).

In the above study by Little and Schneidman (1959), judges interpreted each psychological test individually, but Golden (1964) undertook a study in which he could investigate the reliability and validity of clinical inference based on increasing amounts of information as provided by the Rorschach, TAT, and MMPI. This study also allowed for more comparisons among test data than was possible in Kostlan's (1954) study in which Rorschach, MMPI, Sentence Completion Test, and case history data were studied. The results of the Kostlan study indicated that no combination yielded better results than identifying data (age, sex, etc.) alone. Golden (1964), for his study, had 30 clinical psychologists complete personality questionnaires (the same as those used in the Little and Schneidman study) on the basis of identifying data alone, each test individually (TAT, Rorschach, and MMPI), pairs of tests, and all tests combined. The conclusion was that "reliability and validity did not increase as a function of number of tests nor were there any differences between tests or pairs of tests."

Stone and Dellis (1960) found that data on primitive impulse control systems increased as one went through the following series of tests—Wechsler-Bellevue, Forer Sentence Completion Test, TAT, Rorschach, and Draw-a-Person Test. And Theiner (1962) found more socially acceptable needs on the Rotter Incomplete Sentence Test and less socially acceptable needs on the TAT.

Eron (1972), in his review of the TAT literature for the *Seventh Mental Measurements Yearbook*, reports that the data on needs were not the same when obtained by the Adjective Check List, Edwards' Personal Preference Test, and the

TAT. Aggression scores on the TAT and the Holtzman (1958a, 1958b) Inkblot Technique did not agree. In another study, dreams and TAT responses were scored for needs and press. For some needs, e.g., dominance, there was a negative correlation between TAT scores and dream scores. For other needs, the correlation was positive. As Eron points out, in some instances here we may be concerned with the validity of the TAT but at the same time we should not overlook the possibility that the problem may be with the validity of the technique with which the TAT is being validated or correlated.

Murstein (1963) also points out that data obtained from several projective techniques from the same subject may be contradictory. For example, Shotin (1953, 1955) found that adjustment as measured by the Rorschach correlated with the following variables scored for in the TAT: unpleasant feeling tone, degree of inner conflict, and verbal and emotional aggression.

As in so many other areas, impressions from clinical practice do not always agree with research data. The aforementioned research data notwithstanding, many clinicians would claim that they actually make use of all or most of the data provided by a battery of tests. It is conceivable that this is so and also that clinicians actually differ in their expertise in various techniques. Some may get all they need from a Rorschach, MMPI, or TAT, and others would rely on a whole test battery.

If this is a tenable set of hypotheses, would it not be of interest to preselect clinical judges (who would serve as subjects) in terms of their acknowledged experience rather than persons who simply have some requisite number of years of clinical experience but some unknown set of preferences if they have any at all?

The issue here is not simply one of research or academic interest. It is also one of finances. The more tests administered, the greater the cost. Unless one could justify the number of tests in terms of some direct or indirect benefit to the patient, it would be unethical to administer a battery of tests when less than a battery is what is called for.

Meanwhile, we have to agree with Murstein (1963, p. 67), who, after reviewing various studies on the matter of "levels," said, "The studies considered indicate that, although the 'levels' approach appears intuitively tenable, no conclusive demonstration of the existence of discriminable levels has been made through experimental research." It is to be hoped that more systematic data will be available in the future.

9. Card Characteristics

Among the important contributions to a subject's story are the characteristics of the picture.* As a result, investigators have concerned themselves with varying the figures that appear in the picture, with the presence or absence of color in a picture, with doing without the picture, and with the development of techniques for the study of the structure and ambiguity of a picture.

---

*In his review of the literature on this point, Murstein (1963, p. 195) says, "The stimulus is by far the most important determinant of a TAT response, as is indicated by the work of Eron (1950), Lowe (1951), Mason (1952), Starr (1960), and Murstein (1962c). The last named study will illustrate this point. Though the study investigated the effect of socially evaluated behavior, self concept, different instructions, and sex differences, as well as the various interactions, the stimulus properties of the nine TAT cards accounted for over half of the total variance." This is one point of view and is not necessarily held by all investigators. Campus (1976) finds more variance due to needs.

The structure and ambiguity of a picture relate to a picture's "pull." Some pictures pull only for a certain kind of story, while other pictures pull for a variety of stories. It is important to know this both for the selection of cards congruent with the purposes of the study and for the interpretation of a subject's stories. Stories that are like all other stories are frequently of less interpretive value than stories that are unique to the individual. Furthermore, if one knew the relationships between card characteristics and stories obtained, then one could develop pictures for a variety of purposes.

We shall start this section with a discussion of measures of ambiguity and structure and then turn to the use of color and no pictures at all. Variations in the use of different figures will be presented in Section 18.

9.1. Structure and Ambiguity

To help understand a picture's characteristics, Murstein (1963) differentiates between a card's *structure* and its *ambiguity*. Structure refers to the physical properties of a picture—how many people are in the picture, what is the sex of the people, what makes up the setting or background of the picture, etc. Ambiguity, on the other hand, refers to a card's uncertainty of meaning, or, stated differently, the variety of meanings that may be attributed to a picture.

For example, as Murstein points out, Card 13MF is a highly structured card, because it is clear that it contains a partially nude woman and a man who is standing and has his arm across his face. The background material is also reasonably clear. On the other hand, Card 16, the blank card, is without structure. It contains no figures or background material. (Some might disagree with Murstein on this point because its very lack of material could also be regarded as structure.) It turns out, however, not to be very ambiguous, because it does not pull a wide range of stories.

More investigators seem to be involved in ambiguity than structure. Number of themes, the semantic differential, and needs have been used to gather data on ambiguity, and a Transcendence Index has been developed and used to gather data on structure.

9.1.1. Themes

Both Kenny (1961) and Murstein (1963) provide the basic theoretical discussions and formulas for measuring ambiguity and both stress the use of the themes told to the pictures. They differ, however, as to how to obtain the themes, and the relationship between ambiguity and the kind of data obtained.* Bijou and Kenny (1951) and Kenny and Bijou (1953) focus on judges' ratings of ambiguity in which their experience with the range of themes obtained plays an important role. Murstein (1963, 1972), on the other hand, uses normative thematic data such as that system actually collected by Eron (1950). For purposes of gathering data, Bijou and Kenny (1951) favor cards of medium ambiguity while Murstein (1963) and Kaplan

---

*Kaplan (1969a, 1969b) has been critical of how Murstein measures ambiguity and his criticism has been replied to by Murstein (1969).

(1967) do not believe that increasing ambiguity will increase the amount of information obtained on the subject's personality.

9.1.2. Semantic Differential

Goldfried and Zax (1965) used the semantic differential technique in exploring the stimulus value of the cards. They used ten pairs of polar adjectives which were selected because they were considered proper and relevant for use with TAT cards. Subjects rated the cards using the adjective pairs with a 7-point scale, and in many instances significant differences between cards were obtained. The authors then differentiated between "weak-pull" cards, which did not all pull the same thing from respondents so that subjects were more likely to talk about themselves, and "strong-pull" cards, which were more likely to stimulate stories related to the stimulus cards rather than to the subject's personality.

9.1.3. Needs

A third approach to the study of card "pull" and ambiguity is through the study of needs. This approach was used by Campus (1974, 1976), who studied the pull of cards with 17 different needs. She started with definitions of Murray's manifest needs as used by Stein (1963) to develop her TAT-Adjective Rating Scale. This adjective checklist consists of two adjectives to measure each of 17 needs. To be included in this list, 70% of the 27 judges used had to say that an adjective and a need were in agreement. The second criterion was that the adjectives met the criteria of convergent and discriminant validity (Campbell and Fiske, 1959).

To obtain her data, Campus used 16 TAT cards for males and 15 cards for females. She asked her subjects to make up a story to the pictures, imagining that they themselves were in the picture. For pictures in which there was only one figure, it was obvious who that person was. If there was more than one person, then Campus pointed out who they were to identify with.

After subjects wrote the main points of their story, they then described themselves by assigning ratings from 1 to 7 on each of the 17 needs. Thus, as Campus points out (1976, p. 250), "It should be kept in mind that in this study the TAT cards were used as a self-descriptive rather than as a projective device."

Ambiguity was defined by Campus differently than by other investigators. For her, it was defined as the sum of variances across needs. Using this criterion, her results are consistent with those obtained by Bijou and Kenny (1951) and Kaplan (1967). They are also consistent with Murstein's (1964) data for some cards but not for others; however, they are not in very good agreement with the data obtained by Goldfried and Zax (1965).

To determine the stimulus pull of the cards, Campus used both her definition of ambiguity and the "richness of meaning" found in a card. "Richness of meaning" refers to the number of different needs pulled by a card. (In this regard Campus presents a table, p. 252, that many investigators may find useful.) It is apparent that Campus's definition of card pull is different from that used by others, and, in gathering data on need pull, Campus obtains measures on 17 needs while other investigators generally obtain data on only one. It is therefore of interest to compare her results with those of others. She finds varying degrees of good agreement between her results for aggressive-pull cards and those presented for the same variable by

Murstein, David, Fisher, and Furth (1961), Kaplan (1967), and Goldfried and Zax (1965) for need achievement. Turning to need dominance, there is a fair amount of disagreement between Campus's data and those obtained by Wolowitz and Shorkey (1966).

Finally, in Campus's study, needs (as compared to subjects and cards) accounted for the largest proportion of the variance and "the TAT cards as a set elicit the different needs to varying degrees. The needs evoked most strongly were achievement, autonomy and counteraction for males and achievement and counteraction for females. The needs evoked most weakly for both sexes were exhibition, infavoidance and play . . . there were large individual differences in the needs evoked by the different cards. Perhaps the stimulus is not as important as had been previously claimed since in this study the Cards and Cards × Needs components were not that large" (p. 257).

9.1.4. Transcendence Index

The Transcendence Index was introduced by Weisskopf (1950a) as a measure of the structure of the card. This index is based on what the subject says about TAT stimuli that are not in the picture. Thus the subject is asked to describe the picture, and everything that he says which is not in the picture makes up the Transcendence Index. It is assumed that what the subject says that is not in the picture, and therefore is not directly determined by the picture, is determined by the subject's own characteristics and therefore is likely to be revelatory about the subject.

The Transcendence Index differs from the measure of ambiguity suggested by Murstein (1963) in that it is more directly related to the characteristics of the stimulus while Murstein's measure of ambiguity is based on the variety of themes told to a picture. The two are not equivalent (Murstein, 1963).

In the course of her early work, Weisskopf (1950a) applied the Transcendence Index to both parts of the TAT series. It will be recalled that the first ten pictures are described by Murray (1943) as reflecting everyday situations and the last ten as reflecting fairytale or mythological situations. The result of the study was that the everyday set yielded more fantasy material than did the fairytale series. But when she compared the regular series under normal conditions of exposure with reduced exposure conditions, she did not find any differences in Transcendence Index.

Other studies indicated that the Transcendence Index was higher for completely rather than incompletely traced line drawings (Weisskopf, 1950b; Weisskopf-Joelson & Lynn, 1953). Laskowitz (1959) found that transcendence increased as pictures increased from fuzzy to clear and from incomplete line drawings to complete ones. Weisskopf and Dunlevy (1952) administered three sets of ten cards in which the central figure was obese, crippled, or unmodified to three groups of subjects who were obese, crippled, or normal. The same trend was found for all three groups—the Transcendence Index was lower for the obese figures than for the normal and crippled ones. In still another modification of the stimulus structure, Weisskopf-Joelson and Money (1958) had one series of pictures in which a head was sketched in place of the head in the original series and it was more or less a neutral face. In a second series, there was a head of the subject in place of the one in the regular picture. No differences were found in the data obtained to both series for the Transcendence Index and word content.

Singer and Herman (1954) developed a measure called "voluntary transcendence," which is the difference between the transcendence score obtained from a subject when asked solely to describe the picture and the transcendence score obtained from the same subject when asked to tell a story to the picture using the standard instructions. This new measure was suggested for use as a measure to engage in fantasy in response to experimental instructions.

Prola (1970) provides a scoring scheme for 15 different kinds of transcendence and finds that it can be used reliably. Hartman (1970) found a relationship between the Transcendence Index and the cards recommended as a basic set. The Transcendence Index has also been found to correlate with the M response on the Rorschach, and with a variable called "introspective or ideational dimension of personality" (Prola, 1970).

Slemon, Holzwarth, Lewis, and Sitko (1976) have recently reported an Associative Elaboration Scale which is very similar to the Transcendence Index, in which the subject receives varying credits for descriptive as well as for varying amounts of interpretive comments. They report that with patient groups there was an increase in scale scores up to the age of 11 and then little if any increase. Their scale scores did not relate to IQ.

It may be that an important ingredient in the Transcendence Index is a subject's verbal ability or verbal productivity. Lindzey and Silverman (1959) found a correlation of .84 between word count and the Transcendence Index. Prola (1972) found that the number of transcendent statements in the second half of a description significantly exceeded those in the first half. He believes that subjects low in verbal ability exhaust themselves early in describing the cards, while subjects high in verbal ability are motivated to continue even after they have described the cards.

The Transcendence Index has proven to be an important tool in understanding the TAT, but more work is required if we are to understand the factors that affect it.

9.2. Color

The TAT pictures are in black and white. The original for card 19, the Burchfield painting, is in color and looks quite different structurally with color than without it. While color does not figure in the TAT, it does play a significant and critical role in the Rorschach (1942), where responses to it have been related to control both of impulses and of affect. In a test more similar to the TAT, Van Lennep's (1948, 1951) Four Picture Test color does play an important role and Van Lennep has long been an advocate of its use.

A number of investigators using verbal productivity as the criterion found that it was increased when the cards used were colored rather than black and white (Brackbill, 1951; Thompson & Bachrach, 1951; Lubin, 1955; Lubin & Wilson, 1956). When color was used, an increase in reaction time to the cards was found (Brackbill, 1951) in the responses of psychoneurotics but not in those of normals. In general, Brackbill found that responses to color reflected the subject's current mood and that unpleasant reactions were obtained to it. Thus, while normal subjects did not show any differences in their responses to colored and achromatic cards, the psychoneurotic sample told more depressed stories to the former than to the latter, and showed a decrease in stories classified as Intellectual Destructive or classified in a group characterized as happy, neutral, or shifting in mood.

Other investigators studied the effect of color on children. Atkins (1962), working with a normal sample of kindergarten children, found a group among them that she characterized as disturbed emotionally. These children used more positive and negative emotional words to the colored cards than did the normal children. Color and style interactions were also found in this study—children who told richer stories used more positive emotional words and more intraceptive comments to the colored cards; those who told poorer stories did not have this effect.

Lubin and Wilson (1956) used still another two-children sample—handicapped and normal—and found that the former responded better to the colored cards and the latter responded better to the achromatic cards. If the child was involved in the task, color facilitated identification.

Johnson and Dana (1965) did not find any significant effects attributable to color. However, they, as well as other investigators, did not take into account the characteristics of the cards used. This became the focus of attention for Yudin and Reznikoff (1966); they selected five TAT cards (1, 2, 3BM, 4, and 13MF) on the basis of the work of Goldfried and Zax (1965), who, using a semantic differential technique, found cards 1 and 2 to have "weak pull" and cards 3BM, 4, and 13MF to have "strong pull." The difference in "pull" indicates that a weak-pull card does not impose itself on the subject, and therefore he can tell more about himself, while the stories produced to a strong-pull card are more likely to reflect the picture's characteristics than the characteristics of the subject. These pictures were then administered to student nurses in group settings, and stories were analyzed for emotional tone, outcome, and number of words. "The results indicated a predominant negative tone and outcome for all cards and conditions, but with longer and somewhat more positive stories told to the chromatic pictures. . . . The greatest source of variance, however, was contributed by card differences, per se." And the authors conclude that "color did have at least a subtle effect on fantasy production" (Yudin and Reznikoff, 1966, p. 479).

As in other research aspects of the TAT, there are also problems and inadequacies in scoring which may overshadow the potential usefulness of color as with other modifications. Thus Yudin and Reznikoff (1966, p. 487) say, "What is lacking, of course, is some measure, not of the more formal changes that occur with modification of the stimulus characteristics but of the qualitative and often nonquantifiable aspects that clinicians refer to as having 'interpretive significance.'"

9.3. No Pictures at All

It is probably only fitting in this sequence of studies that have modified the TAT in various ways in an effort to learn about the effects of its structural characteristics to raise the question as to what the effect would be if there were no pictures and if one administered only the descriptions that Murray presents in the manual (Murray, 1943). Lebo and Harrigan (1957) undertook such a study with college women, and Murstein (1963) reports that "Overall analysis of word count, idea count, story mood, outcome mood, level of response, and dynamic content indicated little difference between the presentations. Comparison was made between the normative data of . . . [others] and the response to the pictures, as well as to the spoken description. The correlations on the aforementioned variables were only negligibly lower for spoken descriptions vs. the norm than for the TAT pictures vs. the norm." In another study, rather than the Murray descriptions' being spoken to the subjects (college women), they were written out (Lebo and Sherry, 1959). Once again, with few exceptions, the results were not very different from those previously obtained.

Murstein makes some rather interesting comments on these results:

> The results are a bit trying for the TAT. Apparently, many of the TAT pictures are so unambiguous that it matters little whether a visual or verbal description of the card is presented. It should be interesting to see whether these results would hold if a series of the more highly ambiguous TAT cards were utilized. The Lebo studies, rather than necessarily stressing the utility of nonpicture forms of the TAT, may well have indicated why the highly unambiguous TAT had repeatedly failed to differentiate varying psychiatric groups. Perhaps what it needs for accurate personality diagnosis is a new set of highly structured yet highly ambiguous cards. Another factor is that the results may have been specific to a college population, with the efficacy of the verbal descriptions varying inversely with age and maturity of subjects. (Murstein, 1963, p. 200)

9.4. Norms

It is no mean task to develop proper norms for the stories told to the TAT. Walcott's (1950) personal account is some indication of what one might experience with such an undertaking. He tells us that he started off with 25 stories told by normal male adult subjects to cards 3BM and 4. Then he began breaking the stories down into their component parts. He also used various structural or formal parts of the stories that he considered valuable. After beginning, he realized that "The task was so overwhelming for one person, so it seems to me, that I put the preliminary work aside and conveniently forgot it."

Nevertheless, others have provided helpful normative data. Subjective impressions of the range of themes produced to the various cards may be found in the different manuals written for work with the TAT (e.g., Bellak, 1975; Stein, 1955). A more systematic approach available in the work of Eron (1950) and Dana (1972) provides a series of references to normative data for sex, minority groups, and different IQ groups. Holt (1978) has compiled the published norms, plus a good deal of previously unpublished data covering all of the cards.

A knowledge of the norms is particularly important as an aid to the interpretation of TAT data. Studies of norms are also particularly important for the elucidation of factors that play critical roles in subjects' and patients' responses. This is well reflected in one of the early normative studies by Eron (1948) of the stories told by schizophrenic and nonhospitalized college students. He found that the thematic material is "very much a function of the stimulus properties of the cards themselves and that the specific personality disturbance of the subject is not nearly so important in determining the type of theme that individuals will produce." In this same study, Eron found that the first ten cards of the TAT produce significantly more interpersonal themes than the second ten, which produce significantly more intrapersonal or impersonal themes. The second half of the TAT also elicits more "symbolic, imaginary, fairytale and descriptive stories than the first half."

"In the light of these results," says Eron, "it is felt that the individual examiner might be cautious in using the TAT as a diagnostic instrument and applying cues reported in the literature by various investigators. In making a valid interpretation of any given protocol, due consideration must be given to the stimulus provided by the cards themselves which seem to be a more potent factor in determining the type of theme related than the psychiatric classification of the individual."

While I agree that themes are important in the development of norms for the TAT, it is necessary to keep in mind that the manner in which a theme is dealt with is sometimes of more diagnostic significance than the theme itself.

10. Scoring System

There is no single scoring system for the TAT. The complexity of the stories with their formal and informal content makes for a variety of possibilities. Murray (1952), in his foreword to the manual for Vorhaus's scoring form, said, "For example, there are as many different plots as story tellers are capable of inventing. Consequently, the task of building a comprehensive conceptual system with a place for every possible quality of product of the imagination is so monumental and would result in an instrument so unwieldy and impractical that no one has attempted it."

In addition, the seeming ease of interpretation and opportunity for gathering meaning without scoring (the stories are "after all, only content") lead people to avoid scoring. And finally, of course, there is the fact that Murray himself did not present a scoring system. Many may have thought that he was implicitly suggesting the use of need-press schema for others as he himself and his students had used it (Murray, 1938), but actually few persons have scored all the needs in large-scale studies. At best, one finds that only single needs are scored. It is conceivable that such efforts may eventually lead to separate tests for individual needs. In passing, it should be mentioned that it has been pointed out that needs relate to instrumental activities or secondary process content and should have a more direct relationship to behavior than would be true of clinical assessment procedures which emphasize primary process content (Lazarus, cited in Eron, 1972).

There are a number of quantifiable scoring systems that are available. I shall present some of them in this section, reserving for later the more informal procedures, or procedures that involve theory directly for interpretive purposes of scores. Our discussion of these systems is rather brief. For those who want to know more, it is best that they consult the original sources indicated or other excellent secondary sources, especially Murstein (1963).

McClelland's system (McClelland, Atkinson, Clark, & Lowell, 1953; Atkinson, 1958) for scoring need achievement contains a precise scoring system as well as many good examples to help in learning the scoring procedure. In this system, a story is first judged to determine whether it contains achievement imagery. The story gets 1 point for this; and then can earn up to 10 additional points if it fulfills the requirements of the following variables: need for achievement; successful or unsuccessful anticipatory goal state; instrumental activity with various outcomes, obstacles, or blocks; nurturant press; affective states; and achievement thema.

Pine (1959, 1960) and Eagle (1964) also have systems for scoring thematic drive content which are based on psychoanalytic theory. Both are related to and adapted from Holt's (1970; Eagle and Holt, 1970) technique for scoring primary and secondary process variables in Rorschach responses.

Stephenson developed the Q-sort technique that has so much use in the study of nondirective therapy. It was also applied for use with the TAT (Stephenson, 1953; Friedman, 1957; Silverman, 1959; Little & Schneidman, 1955). When used with the TAT, the Q-sort population of statements is selected from TAT interpretation.

The examiner can distribute these along the preselected normal distribution curve to describe the individual in terms of most and least descriptive characteristics. These can then be correlated with the distribution of the same statements by the subject's therapist, anyone else who knows the subject, someone who knows the subject on the basis of other projective tests, etc. In addition, the data may be factor-analyzed in terms of R- or Q-factor analytic procedures.

While the above scoring procedures have been in the literature for some time, more recent developments include the following: a score for need novelty and variety (Maddi, Propst, & Feldinger, 1965); locus of control, a scoring system for communication patterns that differentiates between parents of schizophrenic patients and parents of neurotic patients (Eron, 1972); a simplified system for scoring needs achievement, affiliation, and power that involves simply counting the stories involving these needs (Terhune, 1969); and even a computer system for scoring purposes (Eron, 1972).

In all likelihood, we have not seen the end of items to be scored. Every variable that is generated for understanding personality is likely to be used in scoring the TAT. Once scores are obtained, they may be used for correlation purposes with other tests, with a criterion for distinguishing between groups, and all other things that one does with scores. Finally, when it comes to interpreting scores, the manner in which this is done depends on the examiner's or investigator's theoretical frame of reference and experience.

11. Examiner-Examinee-Test Interaction

It is apparent from what was said about individual and group administration and it is probably most apparent in individual administration that there is an interaction of examiner, examinee, and test. It is crucial that an examiner "know himself" and be aware of the social interaction occurring between himself and his various subjects or examinees, for all this could affect the nature of the material collected and the understanding of the subject.

Sex differences in examiner effects—the manner in which male examiners respond to female subjects and the manner in which female examiners respond to the testing situation—have been reported (Masling and Harris, 1969). Other examiner effects (Masling, 1957, 1960) and effects attributable to variations in administration technique have also been reported (Eron, 1972). Many good ideas about examiner effects may be extrapolated from Masling (1959), and from Rosenthal's (1966) work on experimenter effects.

Just as there are effects attributed to examiners, so effects may be attributed to certain characteristics of the subjects that relate to the testing situation. Among those reviewed (Eron, 1972), we find sophistication of the subject's attitude to revealing oneself, his conscious control (Holmes and Tyler, 1968), and his socioeconomic status. A review of the factors involved in working with lower-class persons may be found in Levy (1970).

With regard to the matter of class differences, Dana, who has reviewed the studies on examiner-examinee interaction, says:

> Any study making cross-cultural or subcultural comparisons must first demonstrate an equivalence between groups in the functional stimulus meaning, i.e., the existence of similar decoding systems to identify and categorize thematic content. Finally, the survival qualities for the lower class environment are often judged by middle class standards; e.g., lower class persons

have transitory interpersonal relations, and inadequate self concept, a predominantly physical mode of self-expression with primitive defenses, little delay, and much hostility and aggression.

It is mandatory to articulate our own class-typed and sex-typed examiner bias and to look at TAT content as a joint expression of goodness of fit between the examinee and his environmental status and between the examiner and examinee expectancies for interaction. A next logical step is the delineation of personality characteristics that are relevant for participation in our increasingly separate, different, and dissident subcultures. (Dana, 1972, p. 459)

12. Interpretation

The interpretation of TAT material starts from either of two basic sets of data. One set consists of quantified test scores on a specific set of variables, and the other is the TAT protocol itself. In either case, the interpretation of TAT data is dependent on the user's frame of reference. Some workers in the field are quite specific as to what their theoretical orientation is, and others are less so. It is impossible to cover all of the worthy approaches to interpretation. I can cover only a relatively small number here, hoping, at the same time, that the reader will consult various reviews for information on the wide variety of approaches available and from which one might select what is most helpful for one's own purposes.

Murstein (1963) contains a very good critical review of different theoretical orientations, but to see the application of a variety of theoretical orientations in action one should turn to an earlier work by Shneidman, Joel, and Little (1951) in which TAT (11 cards) and MAPS (Make a Picture Story) test (Shneidman, 1949, 1951) protocols, both obtained from the same patient, were interpreted by 15 experts. The book contains a great deal of important detail on how the experts work, the basis for their interpretations, and the interpretations themselves. One wishes that it were possible to see such complete analyses of data on a large number of cases. In this manner, it would be possible to answer numerous questions that have been raised about the TAT in this and other reviews of the test.

In addition to the TAT and MAPS material, the book by Shneidman et al. (1951) contains interpretations of the patient's Rorschach, the Wechsler-Bellevue, the MMPI, the Draw-a-Person Test, and the Bender-Gestalt drawings, each by an expert in the field. And, finally, to complete the richness of this investigation, behavioral data on the patient are also presented.

There are also a number of excellent articles like those of White (1944, 1951) on value analysis, Schafer (1958) on psychoanalytic interpretation of TAT material, and Wyatt (1958) on the synthetic functions of the ego manifest in TAT protocols.

Among the manuals available in book form, there is Tomkins's (1947) manual in which he provides a scoring procedure for vectors, levels, conditions, and qualifiers, and especially good material on inference, level analysis, and the process of diagnosis of personality. Stein (1955) provides definitions of Murray's (1938) needs and press, a guide to the interpretation of the stories, formal characteristics, and an eclectic approach to the interpretation of TAT protocols which is exemplified in a very detailed analysis of a number of cases including protocols of a male before and after psychoanalytic therapy, a woman in nondirective therapy, a young man who came for vocational counseling, etc. Henry (1956) contains a detailed set of variables for the study of the formal characteristics of stories as well as a systematic guide for the study of content characteristics, all of which are intertwined with fine psychodynamic insights. Bellak (1975) presents a method of analysis for the TAT,

CAT, and SAT, as well as a thorough discussion of the relationships of ego psychology, apperceptive distortion, and the basic assumptions for diagnostic inferences to thematic material. The book also contains very helpful illustrations for the use of a form for recording and analyzing thematic material as well as Haworth's (1965) form for the analysis of adaptive mechanisms in stories told to the CAT.

There is hardly a theory or theoretical variable that has not or cannot be applied to the interpretation of TAT protocols. If one wants to keep up with them, one should be current with such reviews as Dana (1972) and others.

13. Self-interpretation

We have focused our attention thus far on interpretations made by others of a subject's or patient's TAT productions. However, a number of investigators have used self-interpretation as a procedure, with varying experiences and varying degrees of success. Bellak, Pasquarelli, and Braverman (1949) have used it in the psychoanalysis of a patient; Deabler (1947) used it in conjunction with nondirective therapy; Bettelheim (1947) used it with students, and Holt and Luborsky (1958a, 1958b) with physicians who were in training to become psychiatrists. Luborsky (1953) has expanded self-interpretation into a general clinical method, which has recently been successfully adapted to research on ego development (Rock, 1975).

14. Reliability*

Interrater reliability, internal consistency, and test-retest reliability have all been studied with the TAT. As we shall see, if one uses the same criteria for the TAT as for objective tests, it is difficult to obtain reliabilities recommended for psychometric tests. There are ways to achieve improvement; however, in general, we should keep in mind, as Murstein pointed out, that "there are many more sources of error variance in dealing with projective media than with true-false type tests. Whereas the latter type of test usually involves only random error, reliability estimates of projective techniques must take into consideration the varying stimulus properties within a test, scoring differences, examiner effects, and the motivation of the subject, to mention but four additional sources of error" (Murstein, 1963, pp. 162–163).

14.1. Interrater Reliability

Sanford, Adkins, Miller, et al. (1943) had four judges score needs and press in ten children's protocols and obtained an average correlation of .57 for the needs and .54 for the press.

Combs (1946) had three judges rate ten protocols which he himself also rated. The average percentage of agreement he obtained was 60%. Combs also studied his own reliability over time, comparing his ratings 6 months apart, and found a 68.8% agreement.

Samuels (1952), studying several variables in the protocols of graduate students, found that his four raters' agreements varied from .16 to .49.

*Murstein (1963) presents a very comprehensive review and evaluation of various reliability measures and their applicability to projective techniques in general and the TAT in particular.

These reliabilities are not very high, but they could be improved. Higher reliabilities are obtained if one uses smaller rather than larger rating scales, if raters work and train together over a period of time, and if the focus is on a smaller rather than longer set of variables.

Insofar as size or the number of rating scale points is concerned, we find a study by Harrison and Rotter (1945) in which 3- and 5-point scales were compared. With the shorter scale, two raters, who scored 70 stories told to five pictures, had complete agreement in 64% of their ratings, partial agreement in 30%, and complete disagreement in 6%.

For the longer 5-point scale, investigators agreed completely in 43% of the cases and disagreed completely in none of them. Later, they defined agreement as a difference of 1 point or less and disagreement as 1 point or more, and they found they agreed in 74% of the cases and disagreed in 26% of them.

Clark (1944) collected two sets of ratings on one story from 50 subjects and found tetrachoric correlations of .90 and above for ratings of effects of the environment, reactions to the environment, the main character's adequacy, and the character of the endings.

Briefer rating scales may not always be the answer, however. While Clark had positive results, he also had some negative ones. For some needs, the correlations were as low as +.30.

In terms of experience together as a factor affecting reliabilities, we find that at the Harvard Psychological Clinic, where raters have lots of experience in working together, interrater reliabilities are as high as +.95 (Tomkins, 1947).

And, finally, intensive experience in scoring needs as well as focused concentration on a small number of needs may also increase interrater reliability. In 1958, Feld and Smith surveyed 14 studies of McClelland's scoring for need achievement, need affiliation, and need power. Reliabilities ranged from .66 to .96, with a median of .89. Persons with only 12 hr of training had a median reliability of .87.

14.2. Internal Consistency

Sanford et al. (1943), working with Murray's need-press analysis of schoolchildren's protocol, reported split-half reliabilities of .46 for needs, .42 for press, and .67 for outcomes. Atkinson (1950) used two sets of four cards and obtained split-half correlations of .48 (raised to .65 by the Spearman-Brown formula). With cards that pulled for need achievement, he obtained higher scores of .64 (and .78 corrected by the Spearman-Brown formula).

Data on ten of Murray's needs were collected by Child, Frank, and Storm (1956). The range of reliabilities was from −.07 to +.34, with an average reliability of .13. The scoring of achievement by the McClelland method yielded values from .32 to .43.

The reliability of .43 was found for a 6-point scale (Auld, Eron & Laffol, 1955) using one statistical technique and .54 using another. Six other variables—Murray's needs—were studied with eight TAT cards by Lindzey and Herman (1955): need achievement .19; need aggression .29; need sex .45; need abasement .28; need nurturance .12; and narcissism .20. The respective reliabilities obtained with the Spearman-Brown formula, which Murstein (1963, p. 142) regards as dubious, are .54, .67, .80, .66, .41, .56.

Hurley, working with the Iowa Picture Interpretation Test involving multiple responses, obtained (with the Spearman-Brown formula) .34 for achievement, .15 for insecurity, .46 for blandness, and .35 for hostility. Johnston (1957), using the 24-card version of the IPIT, reported values of .73, .77, .81, and .73. Murstein (1963) regards the levels of these correlations as due to halo effects. Using the rank method for ordering the choices, Johnston reported correlations ranging from .65 to .82.

Several studies used the coefficient of reproducibility for purposes of reliability. Auld et al. (1955), studying Navy men, obtained a correlation of .93 for their four-card sex scale. Lesser (1958), with a set that pulled for aggression, obtained a coefficient of reproducibility of .91. Murstein et al. (1961) used the Goodenough (1944) method of scaling with the 31 TAT cards for judgments of hostility and obtained a value of .88; using the H technique, the same authors obtained a value of .97.

Murstein's evaluative summary of this material states:

> The internal consistency values for the studies reported are, generally speaking, quite low. They indicate that the portions of the tests compared rarely manifest equal representation of the need they studied. This means that much of the response can be attributed to the stimulus-pull of the cards, and unless the cards are selected on the basis of scaled values, it is unrealistic to expect high internal consistencies. The method described by Jensen (1959) of employing the subject's rank position as the unit, rather than the amount of imagery in the cards, would avoid the dilemma of unequal stimulus-pull.
>
> The use of the coefficient of reproducibility appears promising. The crucial test of its value, however, is whether such scales used with projective techniques have any validity. The dearth of research precludes judgment as yet. (Murstein, 1963, p. 143)

14.3. Test-Retest

Various test-retest reliability studies have been undertaken over varying periods of time. Tomkins (1947, p. 6) collected group-administered TAT protocols from 45 women ranging in age from 18 to 20. He then established three groups of subjects each of 15 selected at random. For one group the test-retest interval was 2 months, for the second group it was 6 months, and for the third group it was 10 months. Correlations of need-press ratings decreased in correlation levels from .80 for the 2-month interval to .60 for the 6-month interval to .50 for the 10-month interval.

One of the problems in studying the test-retest reliability of stories is that subjects on retest may well recall the stories they told to the pictures on the first test administration. To try to remove the effects of memory Lindzey and Herman (1955) asked their subjects (ten highly prejudiced and ten nonprejudiced) not to repeat their stories on the second test administration, which occurred 2 months after the first protocols were collected. The mean of the reliabilities,* which ranged from .00 (for need affiliation) to .94 (for need recognition), was .51.

Auld, Eron, and Laffal (1955) studied Navy men who were confined to a submarine. Elapsed time was 1 month. They obtained a correlation of .13.

Hurley (1955) used a multiple-response technique with a ten-card modification of the TAT and an elapsed time of 6 weeks. Reliability coefficients for the scored variables were insecurity, .46; blandness .57; and hostility .54. Johnston (1957) used

---

*Murstein (1963) believes that these correlations are inflated because the Spearman-Brown formula was used, and it is questionable in this instance, he says.

variations of a similar 24-card set and scored for the same variables a month apart. Correlations ranged from .55 to .78.

For longer periods, we find Sanford et al. (1943) reporting an average repeat reliability for a year between administrations for a 3-year period to be .46. They used Murray's need-press schema.

Using data collected at the Fels Institute, Kagan (1959) studied protocols of subjects when they were 8 years 9 months, 11 years 6 months, and 14 years 6 months. The correlations of data for eight needs and press for all combinations of time period were studied. Four of the 24 tests were significant at the .01 level. These were need achievement .32 between the first and second tests; need physical aggression .34 between first and second tests; need physical aggression again .34 between the second and third tests; and indirect aggression .27 between the second and third tests. No significant correlations were obtained between the first and last test periods. The reliability coefficients for achievement and aggression that were significant were obtained to pictures that quite clearly contained achievement and aggression stimuli.

For need achievement in various studies involving high school and college students, there is a fair degree of variability in reliability coefficients obtained. Morgan (1952) reports a coefficient based on an average of groups that equaled .59. The interval elapsed in the Morgan study was 5 weeks. Shorter intervals did not yield higher correlations—Lindzey and Harman (1955) reported a correlation of .19 over 3-week periods and Lowell (1952) reported a correlation of .22 for an elapsed time of 1 week between test periods. Haber and Alpert (1958) did, however, report a reliability coefficient of .54 for a 3-weeek period.

The second highest coefficient, .56, was reported by Birney (1959) for data collected over a 6-month period. The lowest correlation, .03, was also reported by Birney (1959) for an elapsed time of 1 year 8 months.

Using the multiple-response Iowa Picture Interpretation Test, Hurley (1955) obtained a reliability coefficient of .52 for need achievement over a 6-week period, and Johnston (1957), using the longer version of the test, reported a coefficient of .60 for an elapsed 1-month period and a coefficient of .47 for an elapsed 2-month period.

In evaluating these data, Murstein (1963, p. 140) says there is a "very low but significant correlation between test and retest . . . [there is a] maximum decrease during the first two months, followed by only a slight further decrease over a period of years."

It is likely, at least insofar as need achievement is concerned, that if a stimulus card is structured toward achievement its reliability is increased (Kagan, 1959; Haber and Alpert, 1958). They reported a test-retest reliability of .36 for low need achievement cards and a correlation of .59 for high need achievement cards over a 1-week period, which may or may not be accounted for by the effects of memory.

Skolmick (cited in Eron, 1972) studied the reliability of TAT stories obtained from 92 subjects over a period of 20 years (first when they were 17 and then again when they were 37). Four variables were scored in all stories: achievement, affiliation, power, and aggression. Correlations obtained between judges ranged from .76 to .95. There were also sex differences in reliability scores. For males, raters showed more stability in rating power and aggression ($r = .34$ and .27, respectively); for females, only need achievement showed a significant correlation (.24), but the other three needs showed only trends. These results are consistent with other test results reflecting differences in reliability scores for the sexes (Kogan and Moss, 1962, cited in Eron, 1972).

Murstein, in evaluating these test-retest reliability data says:

> In my opinion, these results indicate that the content of the TAT is strongly influenced by situational factors. yet another factor is the "measurement error." By this I mean that the act of giving a particular theme will to some degree lessen the likelihood of giving a very similar theme again. In short, the situation is analogous to the difficulties in ascertaining the reliability of a response to a joke, as Tomkins (1961) has cleverly pointed out. These studies, therefore, indicate a weakness in the content approach to scoring. (Murstein, 1963, p. 141)

14.4. Stability of the Personality

In the psychometric framework, the focus in a reliability study is on the test, as in test-retest reliability, or on the scorer or rater, as in interrater reliability. In the personological framework, one needs also to consider the individual being studied, the subject, client, or patient.

Consequently, within the personological framework, one would say that, all other things being equal, including the psychometric reliability of the test, the reliability of a subject's response is a function of the subject's personality. Some individuals are more reliable (as a personality characteristic) than others; some people are more consistent (statistically reliable) than others.

Tomkins (1947, p.7), in his manual for the TAT, considered this latter point. Unfortunately, he did not present data from large-scale studies, but he did give examples of the kinds of things that could be probed further in a large-scale study. Thus Tomkins considers reliability scores obtained from individuals of varying degrees of rigidity—low, moderate, and marked.

As an example of a group of persons of low rigidity, Tomkins selected children and adolescents, who, in terms of age alone may be considered to be at an age in their lives when they would be of low rigidity and "maximal plasticity." Such subjects were studied by Sanford (1943). Since Tomkins hypothesized positive correlation between personal rigidity and reliability scores, he then predicted that Sanford's population would have the lowest reliability correlation compared to the other groups of increased rigidity. The evidence supported Tomkins. To start with, the average repeat reliability of TAT test scores given yearly over a 3-year period was .46.

For his example of moderate rigidity, Tomkins selected a single case study, Joseph Kidd by White (1943). This young man was first tested at the age of 19 and later at 22. According to Tomkins (1947, p. 7), this 3-year period "was witness to a spontaneous process of reconstruction of his disorganized personality. Although psychoneurotic, his personality was not particularly rigid. Consequently we might have anticipated marked changes when the TAT was repeated three years later."

White does not present any reliability data, but Tomkins notes that

> In the earlier test there were three main themes: the longing for lost love, the transformation of cruelty and greed by the sympathetic interest of an older man, and a theme of sadism and masochism. In the second set of stories the first two themes had virtually disappeared. The probably reflected Kidd's working through the grief occasioned by an unhappy love affair and the improvement in his relations with his father, with less need for regeneration and a greater tolerance of himself. There was also open expression of the aggressive and acquisitive wishes from which he had previously been rescued by the older man. This represents a modification of the remaining theme. (Tomkins, 1947, p. 7)

On the basis of this kind of information, Tomkins concludes that "although there are continuities between these two sets of stories, it is evident that the repeat reliability is not high, though perhaps higher than the correlation of +0.46 reported for adolescents."

Turning to the third point on the continuum for "marked rigidity," Tomkins presents a case of his own—an 18-year-old psychoneurotic called "Z" who was presented with a different picture for 5 days a week for a period of 10 months and asked to write a story to it. During this same time period, the complete set of TAT cards was administered three times spaced 3 months apart; there was a fourth administration of the TAT with the subject under the influence of alcohol. Dreams were collected from the subject, as well as some 75 hr of additional testing and experimentation. Tomkins reports:

> In general the main themes that appeared in the first 30 stories given at the beginning of the investigation were reported in the second, third, and fourth administrations of the TAT, as well as in the stories written daily. During a two week period of euphoria the subject was presented with very pleasantly toned pictures in an attempt to modify his typically unhappy stories, but despite this change of both pictures and mood the stories remained the same. The writer submitted half of all the stories to one rater and the other half to another rater. This procedure yielded a correlation of +0.91 between approximately 200 stories rated by one interpreter and 200 stories rated by another interpreter. It was clear that the constancy of these stories, despite difference in pictures, time of administration, mode of administration (spoken and written), conditions of the subject (normal, euphoric, intoxicated, fatigued, etc.) was a function of the unusual rigidity of this particular person. (Tomkins, 1947, p. 8)

Tomkins concludes:

> Thus we have seen that for rapidly developing adolescents the repeat reliability of the TAT is approximately +0.46. In the case of a psychoneurotic who underwent a spontaneous process of reconstruction during a three year period there was a relatively low repeat reliability, but when the personality is extremely stable the TAT will reflect such stability in a repeat reliability as high as a coefficient correlation of +0.91, in the case of stories told over a period of ten months. (Tomkins, 1947, p. 8)

14.5. Changes Due to Life Experiences

The reliability of a subject's response may also be affected by life experiences which are more or less novel for the subject and which may intervene between test administrations. For example, in our own experience in the development of the Self Description Questionnaire (Stein, 1963, 1971; Stein & Neulinger, 1968) based on Murray's needs, we studied the reliability of the various needs over varying time periods. On one occasion in a 2-day reliability study, we found in a record of a female college freshman that need exhibition showed a marked increase. Being rather astonished at both the need that changed and the degree of change, we interviewed the young woman to see if we could learn why the change.

She told us that between the first and second administrations of the test there was a student strike. One day she was watching and talking with her friends on the picket line. They coaxed her to join them. At first, she refused, partly because she had never been on a picket line. Finally, her friends and she began to picket. Then she reported that she enjoyed the experience more than she had ever expected. Consequently, when she came to describe herself at the second administration of the test, she had begun to realize that she was more exhibitionistic than she thought the first time. Hence the "unreliability" of her ratings.

Experience with another subject, this time a male freshman, in the same study revealed how experiences which are not so novel as in the case just described may also effect reliability of a test score. In this instance the need involved was need sex. On the first administration of the SDO, the subject said that need sex was less characteristic of him than it was on the second administration. When he was interviewed and asked whether he could account for why he thought need sex was so much more characteristic of him on the second occasion he told the interviewer that the night before the second administration he had gone out on a date and, as he said, "Man, did I have a time."

Similar experience can no doubt occur with subjects taking the TAT who between test administrations have life experiences which affect the content, style, and length of TAT protocols.

14.6. Experimentally Induced Change

Just as important life experiences intervening between test administrations may affect test reliability, so may variables induced experimentally affect test reliability.

Bellak (1944) criticized his subjects before and after TAT administrations and found that there was an increase in aggression in the second TAT which followed criticism. Rodnick and Klebanoff (1942) obtained stories to modified TAT pictures from best-adjusted and more poorly adjusted campers at an institutional camp. The first administrations of the modified TAT preceded and the second followed experimentally induced frustration.

The results indicated that there were differences between the two groups differentiated in terms of adjustment on three variables: themes of superiority, aggression, and "emotional states." The data indicated that, as a result of experimentally induced frustration, more poorly adjusted groups showed a decrease in superiority themes, an increase in aggression, and a decrease in "emotional states" themes. On the other hand, the better-adjusted group showed an increase in "emotional states" themes and no decrease in superiority themes.

15. Diagnostic Classification

The TAT has been applied to the study of various nosological groups both to determine the extent to which they may differ from each other and to determine how they may differ from normal persons. In the main, the results have not been very promising. The TAT, at least insofar as the manner in which it has been used in such situations, and considering the flaws in nosological categories, has not proven a very useful technique.

Here and there one may find some helpful study. Thus Bell, Trosman, & Ross (1953) found that their subjects with diarrhea gave more themes of reconciliation, forgiveness, and punishment than did their subjects with duodenal ulcer. And, in the area of homosexuality, there are studies which "present evidence that homosexual men who acknowledge their homosexuality may be readily differentiated from non-homosexual men" but "whether the same results would occur with homosexual women is unknown, as is the question of whether homosexuality could be predicted from the protocols of persons unwilling to disclose their patterns of sexual behavior" (Murstein, 1963, p. 289).

Turning to studies of other psychopathological cases, there is not much to be sanguine about. Eron (1950), in his content analysis of stories obtained from college students, nonhospitalized neurotics, hospitalized neurotics, hospitalized general neuropsychiatric patients, and hospitalized schizophrenics, did not find any difference that could be attributed to psychiatric classification, but rather that differences were related to hospitalization and nonhospitalization.

In his review for the *Fifth Mental Measurements Yearbook*, Eron (1972, p. 460) reported that he said that "the TAT is probably not a very efficient clinical tool but it has many worthwhile functions and applications in personality research." When he again reviewed the test for the *Seventh Mental Measurements Yearbook* (Eron, 1972), his review was essentially the same:

> It is apparent that many research psychologists interested in personality consider the TAT and its many adaptations as an acceptable procedure for assessing motivation, attitude, and habit, especially when consideration is given to the stimulus value of the pictures and when the analyst takes into account both positive and negative indicates of the variable in question. There is less agreement about the utility and efficiency of the TAT as a clinical diagnostic tool. (Eron, 1972, p. 462)

Murstein is in general agreement with Eron but suggests that the problem may lie with inadequate conceptualization of the behavior studied on the TAT and also on the lack of a refined classification system:

> The attempts at psychiatric differentiation via the TAT have in general led to unsatisfactory results. Most of the studies have managed to yield a sufficient number of significant variables above chance, but to attempt to interpret these findings is more difficult than balancing oneself on a mound of Jell-O. . . . The reason for this predicament resides in the dearth of conceptual thought surrounding the behavior of the various psychiatric classifications on the TAT. . . . In like manner, the rubric "neurosis" may include shy likeable persons, aggressive unlikeable ones, aggressive likeable individuals, etc. Until we evolve a more refined classification system it is unlikely that a fair test of the differentiating power of the TAT can be undertaken. At the same time, the use of more refined scoring procedures, as well as greater cognizance of the stimulus, background, and motivational factors impinging upon the subject, will accelerate the possibility of a fair test of the TAT. For the present at least, the application of the TAT as a medium for psychiatric diagnosis would seem to be an injudicious use of time. (Murstein, 1963, pp. 286–287)

16. TAT in Conjunction with Psychotherapy

Both Tomkins's (1947) and Bellak's (1975) manuals contain material on the use of the TAT in conjunction with psychotherapy. Tomkins points out that it may be used (1) as an adjunct to eliciting repressed memories, (2) to assess attitudes to psychotherapy, (3) to stimulate catharsis of repressed feelings, (4) as a "guide to directive therapy" (Tomkins, 1947, p. 286), and (5) as a kind of play therapy technique with children.

Bellak (1975) points out the following: (1) A patient's stories brought out material that the patient did not bring up in psychoanalytic therapy for about a year. (2) The TAT helps the patient gain "distance" from himself to develop a "psychotherapeutic attitude" (Bellak, 1975, p. 143). (3) The TAT material can help with the development of insight and the working-through process. (4) It can be used with any kind of therapy, especially brief psychotherapy in which the patient is asked to tell stories to pictures directly related to his problems and then these stories are discussed. (5) It is especially useful when the patient has difficulty communicating or free associating "because of lack of familiarity with the psychotherapeutic process, inhibitions, specific resistances, . . . etc." (Bellak, 1975, p. 149).

There are limitations to the use of the TAT in psychotherapy. Tomkins points out the following: (1) It may intensify or precipitate acute attacks of anxiety. (2) For an acutely disturbed individual, it may reflect only his anxiety state, while content, psychodynamics, and origins may be lacking. (3) There are individuals who cannot respond well to interpretations of their TAT stories. Meyer (1951) also indicates that the following are contraindications: if the patient is in an acute anxiety state or psychotic state, if the patient is given to misinterpreting the testing situation, if the patient fears testing, if it is likely that the testing may stir material in the patient that he is unable to cope with, etc.

Research studies have revealed that the TAT does reveal autobiographical material (Combs, 1946) as a possible means for selecting patients for group psychotherapy (Ullmann, 1957) and for evaluating progress in psychotherapy (Fairweather, Simon, Gebhard, Weingarten, Holland, Sanders, Stone, & Reahl, 1960).

17. Prediction of Behavior

One of the major purposes in administering and interpreting a TAT protocol is to provide understanding of the subject or patient. Another crucial purpose is to predict a subject's behavior. Studies in various other parts of this chapter also belong in this section (especially Section 19.3), but for our purposes here we shall limit ourselves to two areas: the prediction of aggression or hostility and the prediction of achievement. The material covered will cast light on the prediction of the related behaviors but will also illustrate some of the factors and difficulties involved in prediction.

17.1. Aggression and Hostility

Sanford et al. (1943), working with children, found that for some needs there were positive correlations between how they were manifest in the TAT and staff ratings of their expression in overt behavior. For other needs, the correlations were negative. They ranged from +.41 to −.41, with an average correlation of +.11.

Murray (1951), studying college men, found a negative correlation between need sex on the TAT and need sex in overt behavior but positive correlations between TAT and overt behavior ratings for abasement, creation, dominance, exposition, nurturance, passivity, rejection, and dejection.

Sanford (1943) suggested that antisocial needs such as aggression may appear in the TAT but not in overt expression because of social prohibitions or inner conflict with regard to their expression. Because such needs receive little or no satisfaction in real life, they would be more intense in the stories. Sanford also suggested that those which occurred both in fantasy and in behavior were those which were encouraged by the culture.

Mussen and Naylor (1954) derived three hypotheses from Sanford's suggestion and found that (1) children from lower socioeconomic groups for whom it is assumed that expression of aggression is permitted had a positive relationship between amount of fantasy aggression and overt aggression; (2) there was mild support for the hypothesis that subjects whose stories contained a great deal of punishment relative to their need for aggression showed less aggression than subjects "whose ratio of punishment press to aggressive needs was low"; (3) there was strong support for the hypothesis that individuals with much fantasy aggression but a low (relatively speaking) ratio of fear punishment to aggression would be more aggressive in their behavior than individuals who have a small amount of aggression in their TAT stories associated with a high degree of fear of punishment.

Lesser (1957) also designed a study in line with the reasoning about environmental support for aggression and found that boys whose mothers encouraged the expression of aggression yielded a higher correlation between aggression in stories and behavior than was true of boys whose mothers did not encourage such expression.

Pittluck (1950) did not find a relationship between aggression in the TAT and aggression as expressed in overt behavior but did find that the predictions improved significantly when she took into account statements in which the subject expressed anxiety about aggression.

Kagan (1956) suggested two hypotheses. The first relates to the kind of material that is scored and the second to the ambiguity of the picture that is used. With respect to the former, Kagan argued that one of the factors involved in the low correlations between fantasy measures and overt behavior is that the TAT measure is usually some undifferentiated measure of aggression. That is, all kinds of acts and goal objects are included in the test measure, but the criterion measure of manifest aggression needs to be more limited in the nature of the aggression expressed or in the goal object toward which it is expressed.

Kagan also developed a second hypothesis. He argued that the prediction of overtly aggressive behavior involves not only a measure of the intensity of aggressive drive but also a measure of the anxiety inhibition associated with its expression. Therefore, subjects' responses to pictures that involve aggression may yield a measure of the subjects' anxiety about their aggression. Thus, if an individual does not give a story with an aggressive theme to a stimulus which regularly elicits aggressive content, he might be assumed to have anxiety about the expression of aggression. Such an individual would be expected to inhibit overt aggressive acts in real interpersonal situations as well. However, Kagan also thought that failure to produce aggressive themes to stimuli that do not regularly elicit aggressive content is not a very sensitive measure of the inhibition of aggressive responses. From this, Kagan suggested the hypothesis that "pictures suggesting aggressive content are more predictive of overt aggression than more ambiguous ones."

The results of the study indicated, first, that children rated as most likely to initiate fighting did in fact produce more fighting themes than children rated extremely nonaggressive. Other categories of aggression were not significantly related to the behavior ratings.

Second, more aggressive subjects than nonaggressive ones produced stories of fighting to the picture most suggestive of a fighting theme. "Occurrence of fighting themes to the picture least suggestive of such content did not result in differences between the aggressive and non-aggressive boys."

Skolnick in his longitudinal study also studied the relationship between fantasy imagery in the TAT and overt behavior. According to Eron (1972), Skolnick says: "The results suggest that it is not possible to make a statement about the relation between TAT fantasy and behavior that will hold for all motives, ages, and both sexes, although the predominant effect seems to be direct rather than inverse." And then Eron adds, "Essentially the same conclusion had been stated by the present reviewer in *The Fifth Mental Measurements Yearbook*."

17.2. Need Achievement

The most important work on the relationship between need achievement in TAT-like cards and behavior is that of McClelland and his associates (1953), which has stimulated the efforts of a large number of individuals. Murstein (1963) has done a rather thorough review of the theory underlying this work, and has covered a wide range of related studies. Those discussed here were selected to be representative of the relationship between need achievement and behavior in the real world as distinct from behavior in laboratory situations.

Moss and Kagan (1961), using the Fels longitudinal data, found that adolescent TAT data predicted adult achievement. Adult TAT data predicted it better. Meyer, Walker, and Litwin (1961) found higher need achievement scores among managers in an industrial setting than among specialists of comparable status. Positive correlations were also reported between need achievement and college grades (McClelland et al., 1953; Atkinson, 1950; Weiss, Wertheimer, & Groesbeck, 1959), and need achievement differentiated between overachievers and underachievers (Morgan, 1952).

On the negative side, Lowell (1952) found a low correlation between need achievement and previous grades, as did Atkinson (1950). Bendig (1959) found that need achievement did not correlate significantly with grades in an introductory psychology course at the end of the semester. As a matter of fact, verbal ability seemed to be much more important. And, indeed, Lindzey and Silverman (1959) also indicated that verbal fluency was related to need achievement.

In reviewing the above material, it is apparent that before the final word is in on the prediction of behavior from TAT material, we will need more work on the contributions of the subjects, the cards, and the situation to which the predictions will be made. Eron says:

> One of the factors which has been shown to affect the relation between TAT and fantasy and overt behavior of the story teller is the stimulus relevance of the picture to the trait in question. The general finding has been that the ambiguity of the picture is inversely related to the degree of relationship between story content and overt behavior. This has been demonstrated particularly for aggression and/or hostility with no difference between men and women, although for achievement motivation, pictures of medium ambiguity seem to be most valuable.... There is some evidence that young children, in contrast to adults, respond more productively to ambiguous pictures . . . however, than to appropriately structured ones. (Eron, 1972)

Considering the work on need achievement, Murstein (1963) does not feel very confident, for example, that it can predict grades with any degree of confidence. He does not feel that the problem is with variations in cards, because studies in this area use the cards recommended by McClelland. He believes that the problems in this area may be related to the populations studied and their interactions with the examiner.

18. TAT-like Tests

The TAT has been altered and modified in a variety of ways for specific purposes. The major efforts have occurred in gathering data on different age groups, on blacks, and on specific needs. Not all these efforts have met with equal success, and it is still not absolutely clear what the ingredients should be in a picture designed to gather data for specific purposes. There are, however, some good ideas. We shall present and discuss a sampling of efforts in this area.

18.1. Children's Apperception Test

MORRIS I. STEIN

While Thompson (1949a, 1949b) assumed that people would identify better with persons the same as or similar to themselves, Bellak and Bellak (1949) and Bellak (1975) worked on another assumption in the test they developed for children, the Children's Apperception Test or CAT. They used animals rather than human beings in situations related to the kinds of problems about which they were interested in gathering data. The idea for using animals was suggested to Bellak (1975, p. 176) by the psychoanalyst Kris on the basis of such information in the psychoanalytic literature as the case of Little Hans. The test is recommended for children from 3 to 10 years of age.

The original CAT was published in 1949, a CAT-S (Children's Apperception Supplement) was published in 1952, and a CAT-H (Children's Apperception-Human) was published in 1965. All of these are described by Bellak (1975).

The CAT and its subsequent revisions were developed with specific problem areas in mind, including "feeding problems specifically" and "oral problems generally," attitude toward parents (including data on the oedipal complex), and children's fantasies about aggression, "about acceptance by the adult world, and about fear of being lonely at night with a possible relation to masturbation, toilet behavior, and the parents' handling of and response to it. We wish to learn about the child's structure, defenses, and his dynamic way of reacting to, and handling, his problems of growth" (Bellak, 1975).

In a number of studies (Biersdorf and Marcuse, 1953; Furyua, 1957; Light, 1954) in which the animal form of the CAT was compared with the TAT or human figures, the data indicated that for such variables as story length the evidence was in favor of the human set. For such variables as the Transcendence Index, there was no difference (Weisskopf-Joelson & Foster, 1962) or a trend favoring the human set (Budoff, 1960). Myler, Rosenkrantz, and Holmes (1972) compared the TAT, CAT, and CAT-H obtained from second-grade girls on five variables: Transcendence Index, initial word count, criterion word count, creativity, and organization. They found no difference between the CAT and CAT-H and also found that the CAT and CAT-H are more productive than the TAT for this age group (of second-grade girls). In contrast, Light (1954) studied older boys and girls and found that they identified better with the human figures in the TAT than with the animal figures in the CAT. Myler et al. (1972) suggest that age may be a factor in this difference in results. Also, Myler et al. (1972, p. 443) suggest that "Tentatively, then, the CAT and CAT-H appear to be more suitable for the younger second and third grade child while the TAT appears to be more useful with the fourth and fifth grade child." Hoar and Faust (1973) found they got more apperceptive responses from preschoolers to a jigsaw puzzle form of the CAT than to the regular form.

While this evidence piles up in favor of the TAT or humanlike tests, one needs to bear in mind the kind of evidence used in favoring one test over another. The CAT may be superior for use with disturbed children with respect to the problems specifically tested for in the CAT and with which children are more likely to be involved than those in the TAT (Murstein, 1963). Also, conceivably, some children may do better with the animal form while others do better with the human form, with preferences being determined by personality differences (Bellak, 1975). Myler et al. suggest that the animal vs. human content may not be so crucial as differences in stimulus content: "Possibly, rather than animal as opposed to human content, the major issues appear to be other stimulus dimensions which make these projective devices more suitable to certain age groups" (Myler et al., 1972, p. 443).

Once again, as in other aspects of this chapter, there is the difference between expected usefulness of a test as presumably indicated by research and as indicated by evidence (research or anecdotal) of a clinical nature. Thus Bellak says: "the usefulness of the C.A.T. does not depend upon whether or not animal pictures produce better or only equally good stories. The C.A.T. and C.A.T.-S pictures were carefully selected to elicit themes relevant to children's growth and emotional problems. There is considerable evidence thus far that the C.A.T. is clinically useful, and the question of animal versus human stimulus will probably remain a more or less theoretical issue" (Bellak, 1975, p. 184).

The CAT has been used, as have the TAT and other TAT-like tests, in a variety of ways. It has been used to gather data of developmental interest: Rosenblatt (1958) studied children in the phallic phase (ages 3–6) and in the latency period (ages 6–10); Nolan (1959) studied needs achievement, affiliation, and power. The CAT has been used in the study of foreign cultures: (Rabin, 1972) with kibbutz and nonkibbutz children in Israel; Chowdhury (1960) used it with children in India; and Earle (1958) used it with Rakau children in a Maori community in New Zealand.

Turning to diagnostic studies and studies more directly related to the clinical area, we find Kagan and Kaufman's (1954) study of speech disorders, Butler's (1961) study of institutionalized mental retardates, De Sousa's (1952) study of emotionally disturbed children, and Gurvitz and Kapper's (1951) study of schizophrenic children.

For material on interpretation, Bellak (1975) is an excellent source, as is Haworth (1963, 1965) on adaptive mechanisms and the review by Haworth (1966) of the literature on the CAT. Moriarty (1972) provides interesting data on normal preschoolers' reactions to the CAT and their implications for later development. Byrd and Witherspoon (1954) present normative data based on stories collected from 38 boys and 42 girls ranging in age from 2 years 8 months to 6 years 5 months. In a later paper, Witherspoon (1968) presents interesting material on an objective scoring system for dealing with longitudinal data generally and specifically the data collected from subjects reported in 1954.

Finally, if one does not have a CAT or CAT-H available but only a TAT, then he might follow a procedure recommended by Kolter (1970). He asks reluctant children to pick out the pictures from the regular TAT series to which they want to tell stories. He also selects some pictures. And, with a modicum of luck, he gets a protocol.

18.2. TAT Pictures for Adolescents

Symonds (1948, 1949) developed 20 cards for use with adolescent boys and girls. The pictures are divided into two sets (A and B) to be administered on successive days. If necessary, only one set (B) can be administered. As with other such sets, the pictures were selected to touch on the problems of adolescents in the hope that they will elicit significant material from the subjects. Some of the scenes in the pictures are leaving home, coming home late at night, social-sexual rivalry about dating, and pictures concerned with delinquency and jail.

MORRIS I. STEIN

18.3. TAT Pictures for Senior Citizens

Two sets of pictures, the Senior Apperception Technique and the Gerontological Apperception Test, have been developed to gather data from persons 65 years of age and older.

18.3.1. Senior Apperception Technique

The Senior Apperception Technique (SAT) consists of 16 pictures which Bellak and Bellak found to be clinically relevant to the problems of persons 65 years and older. The pictures are stimuli that evoke the following kinds of themes: loneliness, illness, and joyous moments such as being with grandchildren, social dance, and playing games. There are several pictures that are sufficiently ambiguous so that they can yield either happy themes or themes reflecting difficulties. Among the latter are pictures of a family setting and a center for the aged.

Bellak (1975) regards the stories told by elderly people, which are concrete and full of self-reference, as an indication of the concerns they have about getting along with their peers, about health problems, and about entering an old folks home.

Bellak prefers using the word "technique" rather than "test" with the SAT because "To the extent that we study each person as an individual, idiosyncratic ideographic ways of dealing with a particular stimulus situation affect the process we are studying. For this reason, Hermann Rorschach's term for his inkblot inquiry was a 'Versuch,' an experiment, and it is still by far the best term and much to be preferred to 'test,' with its normative connotations in American psychology. For this reason, the title Senior Apperception *Technique* is preferable to Senior Apperception Test" [italics in original] (Bellak, 1975, p. 285).

In discussing the technique, Bellak (1975, p. 285) states very directly that no claims are made about the validity or reliability of the technique but that the technique does reveal feelings and thoughts about situations important to the elderly.

No large-scale research studies have been undertaken of the SAT, but Bellak (1975) does present what he calls four pilot studies done by students in fulfillment of degrees. The four include one on hope, despair, and disengagement (Altobello, 1973), one about elderly persons' concerns about psychosexual matters (Ackerly, 1973), one about the world view of elderly people (Toone, 1974), and one about dependency and old age (Garland, 1974).

18.3.2. Gerontological Apperception Test

The Gerontological Apperception Test (GAT) consists of 14 pictures, each of which contains a situation or relationship in which an elderly person might find him- or herself (Wolk, Rustin, & Seiden, 1966; Wolk & Wolk, 1971; Mercer, 1973).

Wolk, Rustin, and Seiden (1966) administered the TAT and GAT to subjects over 65 and presented anecdotal evidence for the superiority of the GAT. Fitzgerald, Pasewark, and Fleisher (1974) also administered GAT and TAT cards to men and women ranging in age from 56 to 94 and studied the frequency with which certain themes expected to be related to the problems of the elderly would show up. For only one theme, physical limitation, was the GAT found to be superior. Pasewark, Fitzgerald, Dexter, and Cangemi (1976) studied the themes obtained from adolescent, middle-aged, and noninstitutionalized elderly females. They did not find that the content of the themes varied significantly with age, nor did they find that the GAT was superior to the TAT in evoking themes related to the problems of the aged. These authors do suggest, however, that "For clinicians specifically interested in provoking age-related themes, there would, of course, be some advantage in including some GAT cards, or cards from another test instrument such as the Senior Apperception Test in their test battery" (Pasewark et al., 1976, p. 590).

18.4. TAT Pictures for Racial and Ethnic Groups: Negro TAT

On the assumption that people find it easier to identify with people in the pictures who are more similar to themselves, Thompson (1949) substituted black figures for the white figures in the regular TAT series. This became known as the Negro TAT or more commonly as the Thompson TAT. The test was group-administered to black students by a black examiner. In a balanced design, Thompson also had his subjects write stories to the regular series. He found that there was a significant increase in story length at .01 level to the black pictures.

These results, however, were not supported by Riess, Schwartz, and Cottingham (1950), who studied both white and black female students with white and black examiners, using the two sets of cards with length of story as the variable. In 1951, Schwartz, Riess, and Cottingham presented another analysis of their data where they dealt with number of ideas appearing in the stories rather than with story length. In this study, they found that, regardless of cards, blacks gave more ideas when their examiner was white, that, regardless of color of examiner, white subjects gave more ideas to Thompson TAT, and that the number of ideas was low when the stimulus, examiner, and test were all of the same color.

Korchin, Mitchell, and Meltzoff (1950) did not find any differences due to color but did find differences due to socioeconomic status, with the middle-class subjects giving stories of longer length than subjects lower in socioeconomic status. Neither was there support for Thompson's data in a study by Light (1955), who found that with white subjects there were themes of low social status and sociopathy. Cook (1953) did not find any differences in how white and black subjects responded to the Thompson and Murray TAT, but rather in how they perceived the people in the two sets. Both black and white subjects saw the regular TAT as dealing with "people in general," but whites saw the Thompson TAT as dealing with blacks and Cook found differences between his black and white subjects on the Thompson-TAT. He therefore suggested the more dissimilar the subject and the figure in the card the greater the opportunity for a diminution in ego defensiveness.

Murstein (1963), who reviewed the studies just cited, comes to a number of conclusions, one of which strikes us as particularly relevant:

> The influence of the stimulus is not a simple function of its similarity to the subject. The culture plays a crucial role in the interpretation of perception. Negroes tended to perceive the Murray TAT characters not as whites but as people in general. Whites, however, perceived the Thompson cards as dealing with Negroes. Thus, majority populations are far more prone to perceive minorities as "different" than vice versa. They also are less likely to have had contact with them. Minority groups such as Negroes, however, must constantly live in a "white" world . . . they must adapt perceptually to the majority white culture if they are to be maximally adjusted to their environment. . . . When, however, Negroes are confronted with the Thompson figures, particularly in the presence of a white examiner, it is apparent to them that something unusual and different is involved, and they tend to be cautious and vague. (Murstein, 1963, p. 206)

Some persons have used the Thompson TAT alone or in conjunction with the Murray TAT to study the behavior of prejudiced persons. Recently, Cann (1977) devised another alteration of the regular cards which seems to have possibilitie in this regard. Rather than limiting himself to an all-black or an all-white series, Cann developed an interracial series.

18.5. Make a Picture Story Test

In the Make a Picture Story Test developed by Shneidman (1949, 1951; Shneidman et al., 1951) the subject has the opportunity to create the scenes to which he then tells stories. The subject makes his choices of backgrounds and figures from materials supplied. Among the variety of backgrounds, some are unstructured (e.g., stage dreams, blank card), some are semi-structured (e.g., forest, grottolike cave), and some are structured (e.g., living room, bathroom, attic). These were selected because they were expected to relate to problems encountered in clinical practice.

The subject may select characters for his scenes from 67 figures that are available. The figures represent those of adults, children, and various ethnic groups, those of indeterminate sex, and legendary and fictitious figures. The figures have different facial expressions and poses; some are clothed and some are partially clothed.

The subject selects 11 backgrounds and as many figures as he wishes and tells a story to each background and its accompanying figures. The instructions for telling the story are very much the same for those used for the TAT. The subject tells who the figures are, what they are doing, thinking, feeling, and how things will turn out.

The examiner has a figure identification card and a figure location sheet on which to indicate the positions of the figures and so have an aid for interpretive purposes.

18.6. Four Picture Test

The Four Picture Test was developed before and independently of the TAT by a Dutch psychologist, D. J. van Lennep (1948, 1951). The first picture shows two people together; the second, one person alone; the third, a person leaning against a lamppost in a dark street; the fourth, two people playing tennis and others watching. The subject arranges the stories in any order he wishes and makes up one story to the sequences he has developed for the four. A unique feature of this test is that it contains color in the pictures.

19. Samples of Research Studies

Among the various ways in which the TAT has been used, one of the most important has been in studies of a variety of psychological issues. Thus, while research on its own characteristics continues, it is used to help cast light on other problems. It is obviously impossible to cover all such problems, and those cited in this section are intended, aside from their content, to reflect the range of problems studied—marital relationships, time, creativity, professional identity, and the prediction of professional effectiveness.

19.1. Marital Relationships

Winget, Gleser, and Clements (1969) adjusted the Gottschalk-Gleser scoring system (Gottschalk & Gleser, 1969; Gottschalk, Winget, & Gleser, 1969) for three variables—anxiety, hostility directed outward, and human relations—for differentiating between well-adjusted and poorly adjusted couples. In both groups, couples told stories to four TAT pictures. The well-adjusted group scored higher than the poorly adjusted group on human relations, the poorly adjusted group scored higher on hostility, and there was no difference between the groups on anxiety.

Murstein (1972a, 1972b) has developed a special TAT-like set of cards for the study of marital choice, and Araoz (1972) uses several of the regular TAT cards for work in marital therapy.

19.2. Time

The matter of time—the subject's attitude toward it, etc.—has also been researched. Lipgar (1969) reports a relationship between the individual's subjective probability notions and how he treats time in the TAT. Wohlford (1968) has studied the extension of personal time in the TAT and found support for the bidirectional (past-future) and cognitive-empirical distinctions. Empirical protension emerged as a quite stable variable, and "structured TAT administration tended to lengthen retrotension and protension scores." Wohlford and Herrera (1970) have also reported on cross-cultural factors (American and Cuban) in relation to personal time.

19.3. Prediction of Professional Effectiveness

One big area of research has been the study of the usefulness of the TAT as well as other projective and nonprojective measures of personality for the prediction of behavior in various kinds of professional situations. With some exceptions, the efforts have not paid off.

Murray and Stein (1943) used a picture different from most that are available. Centered was a military man with an uplifted hand, his mouth open as if shouting, and spread around him on the card were small scenes of war experiences. These smaller pictures might be integrated into a story about the military man's experiences. Stories were obtained from ROTC officers, and scores were correlated against ratings of leadership made by their superior officers. Scores were obtained for various of Murray's needs as well as other of Murray's variables. Some were added and others were subtracted as in the following formula: need achievement + need counteraction + need exposition − need intragression − need change − need deference − need rejection and − inner conflict. The subject's score was the total sum, and this was correlated with the subject's rating on leadership from his superior officer. The resulting correlation was .65.

Murstein (1963) has criticized this study: "The significance of this finding is difficult to judge because of the sparseness of information regarding the study and the failure of the authors to report the number of men tested."

Murstein may be correct. For purposes of the record, I would like to state that the study was undertaken as one of the precursors of some procedures that might be used in the OSS assessment program (OSS, 1948) but was not used. Nevertheless, it should be indicated that the variables were all scored according to the definitions used at that time at the Harvard Psychological Clinic and the scorers were two Radcliffe students who had the most reliable need ratings with Murray. I don't recall the number of subjects and I am sorry that the number of subjects was not reported. If my memory serves me correctly, it was approximately ten or we would have used Pearson r's and not rank-order correlations.

My personal criticism of this study is that it is unfortunate that no cross-validation data were available. It was not possible to carry out any cross-validation since we had exhausted the number of student ROTC officers and did not know how long it would take to get another group. Also, there was the practical matter of a war and matters associated with it that affected certain desirable research goals.

The first really large-scale assessment program in which the TAT was used was the Veterans Administration assessment program of clinical psychologists. (Compared to the VA program, the TAT was only occasionally used in the OSS and therefore it is not reported here.) One hundred and forty students were assessed in groups at Ann Arbor with a variety of techniques, including 10 cards of the group-administered TAT, for a full week. Three years later, criteria data were collected, including evaluations from university and supervisory VA personnel at the end of the second-year status and whether the student was still in training or obtained his Ph.D.

The results of this study were that the TAT was hardly of any use in the prediction of the behavior of the future clinical psychologists. As a matter of fact, neither were any other projective techniques (Kelly & Fiske, 1951).

The second assessment program in which the TAT was used was in the selection of physicians for psychiatric training at the Menninger School for Psychiatry, which was reported by Luborsky and Holt (1957) and Holt and Luborsky (1958a, 1958b). Subjects were studied with a variety of procedures, including the TAT, and the obtained data were correlated with such criteria of success as completing the residency program, establishing a psychiatric practice, judging the success of one's peers, etc. As far as the TAT goes, the results of this study were similar to those in the VA program. Once again, the TAT was of little predictive value, but it may have contributed to the validity of the final, all-data predictions, in interaction with nonprojection data.

While one cannot quarrel with the results of the foregoing research projects, one cannot help but wonder about the nature of the experiences and results of so many consulting firms that use the TAT for selection purposes. These firms make almost daily decisions on the basis of responses to TAT or TAT-like pictures. While it may be that their results, when examined closely, will be no better than the results just presented, it is a little difficult to believe that this will be the case.

One major series of assessment studies in which the TAT contributed to better results was conducted by Stern, Stein, and Bloom (1956). In this series, the TAT was not scored, but was analyzed "clinically." Also, no attempt was made to separate its distinct effects from those of other tests and techniques used in a test battery. Nevertheless, "impressionistically," it was regarded as an important part of the test battery. The critical difference between this series of assessment studies and those reported previously was that the investigators made a direct attack on the criterion problem, differentiating between a standard of performance and a psychological criterion. With this distinction in mind, the investigators made a serious attempt to analyze the psychological environments in which their subjects would be studying or working. Having a picture of the psychological requirements, they then analyzed the TAT and other tests and made their predictions. These predictions in a series of assessment procedures and studies called *Methods in Personality Assessment* (Stern et al., 1955) turned out much more positively than those reported above. One might ask whether without adequate knowledge of the psychological requirements of the situation, the true psychological criterion, but with an emphasis on the standards effected by others (the traditional criterion), proper predictions can be made or should even be tried.

19.4. Professional Identity

Hoffberg and Fast (1966) used two of the TAT cards (11 and 19) to study some psychodynamic aspects of the behavior of "preprofessional" student mathematicians, psychologists, and poets. In describing their goals, they say:

> We have aimed to describe, for three professional groups—mathematicians, poets and psychologists—based on their fantasy productions, their characteristic styles of impulse regulation that may permeate both fantasy life and action: how and where impulse may emerge; its control, management, and integration in behavior, and how these patterns of ego-id integration may dovetail with the activities and satisfactions afforded by a profession. . . .
> We hypothesized, following a preliminary study of fantasy productions, that mathematicians develop a strong ego boundary, focus their interests on activities in the external world and, when confronted by ego alien impulse, experience threat and temporary disorganization. Psychologists also form clear ego boundaries but they retain more awareness of impulse. Their struggles between acceptable and unacceptable, between rational and irrational modes of thought, are carried on more openly and impulse is integrated into behavior or painfully avoided. For the poet, there is no distinct ego boundary; he identified with his own impulse life in fantasy. Rather than defending against the inner-determined and the poorly rationalized, he allows these elements to figure prominently in awareness while he focuses away from external reality upon his inner life. (Hoffberg and Fast, 1966, pp. 488–489)

In summarizing their findings, the authors state:

> The modal mathematician is oriented towards the objective physical world, maintains a clear self boundary, expresses concern and disorganization at emerging hostile impulse. Psychologists deal with inter-individual conflict; the contrast between ego and alien impulse is more neutral and impulse is integrated into behavior. The poet explores and structures identity and self contents, shows greater access to primary process, minimal concern with self boundaries, and his products express the inter-penetration of realistic and unrealistic acceptable and gruesome elements. (Hoffberg and Fast, 1966, p. 488)

Levine (1969) used expression and affect and Pine's (1960) system for rating amount, integration, and directness of drive expression in a study of student mathematicians, creative writers, and physicians. Four of the TAT cards were used. In summarizing his findings, Levine says:

> Writers were most expressive, followed by mathematicians and then physicians. Mathematicians relied heavily upon use of direct, socialized forms of drive content, while physicians emphasized indirect or distinguished forms more than other S's. These emphases appeared to have defensive and integrative functions, as did the physicians' generally suppressive style. The writers showed no comparable emphasis on direct or indirect expression. There were no intergroup differences in overall adjustment. (Levine, 1969, p. 357)

MORRIS I. STEIN

19.5. Creativity

Creativity is also a topic that has come under investigation by researchers using the TAT. There are numerous ways in which it has been used, and the literature is so voluminous that it is, in reality, difficult for one such as I, who is so close to this research area, to make a proper selection of material to be cited. The material that is cited is meant to illustrate the range of uses, rather than to serve as best examples.

To cast light on creativity, the TAT has been used in case studies of persons regarded as creative (Barron, 1968; Stein, Mackenzie, Rodgers and Meer, 1955). It has, of course, been used in large-scale studies where the stories fabricated from the TAT pictures have been scored for originality and have served as part of the criterion (Barron, 1968). Among these studies is the work of Stein and McClelland. In other large-scale studies, the TAT has been used to differentiate between criterion groups in terms of needs or other very interesting variables. Among these studies is the work of Pine and Holt (1960) and Pine (1962) in which primary process scores were used.

Stein found that more creative industrial research chemists rated themselves significantly higher on a self-descriptive personality measure involving need achievement (1963, 1971; Stein and Neulinger, 1968) than did their lesser creative colleagues. The two groups did not differ significantly on McClelland's need achievement score for the TAT. However, when McClelland (1962) scored the TATs for these two groups for need power, he found that the more creative group scored significantly higher on this variable than did the lesser creative group.

While there are scoring problems with the TAT in this area (especially with the reliability of raters), the test is, nevertheless, one of the most versatile of techniques for casting light on the creative process.

20. Conclusion

To summarize the material in this chapter, we shall turn to two papers written some time ago, one by Lindzey (1952) and one by Murstein (1961). Both of these are as good today as they were when first published. Both collated evidence on several assumptions basic to the TAT. Lindzey (1952) considered both the psychological literature and the literature on projective techniques to see what he could learn that was relevant to several basic assumptions, and he came away reasonably satisfied that, in the main, support was found for them. Murstein (1961) stayed a bit closer to the projective test literature and is a bit less sanguine. Because both papers overlap, they will be presented together as they apply.

While reading this material, it is necessary to keep in mind cautions stated by Lindzey with regard to the studies he cites. He says that they cannot be used to validate projective tests but rather to indicate the relationships between assumptions underlying projective tests and empirical findings in the literature. While this, as Lindzey says, may increase the "plausibility" of the tests, "the task of demonstrating the utility of specific rules of interpretation remains" (Lindzey, 1952).

The assumptions that follow were obtained from Lindzey and Murstein, with each author cited in his proper place.

1. *By completing unstructured situations, individuals reveal their personalities.* This assumption, says Lindzey, is a warranted assumption as evidenced by the studies of Sanford (1943), Levine, Chein, and Murphy (1942), and McClelland and

Atkinson (1948) in which relationships were obtained between food deprivation and food responses to ambiguous stimuli; Murray's (1933) work in which a relationship between perceived maliciousness and fear was found; and Katz's work (1950) in which the manner in which a person completes an incompletely drawn face is related to his experience prior to working out the completions. Bruner and Postman (1948) showed that a subject's responses to tachistoscopically presented stimuli are related to his personality or motivational characteristics.

2. *The subject identifies with some figure in the story.* Lindzey says that this assumption cannot be supported at the time of his survey, although evidence points in the direction of support of the assumption.

Murstein, looking at the assumption from the point of view of the stimulus, restates the assumption to say that "the more similar the stimulus is to the subject the greater the degree of projection." To check out this assumption, he reviewed the literature in which pictures of various sorts were designed to resemble the subject— student, adult male, black, crippled, obese, etc. He says that, in general, the data are negative, and do not support the idea that the more central the character is to the subject the more that projection increases. Also, there is no support for the idea that children project more readily to pictures of animals than they do to those of humans.

Murstein (1961), in summarizing his survey on this point, says, "In sum, projection is enhanced by the use of the same species as *S* but within species increased physical similarity to *S* in terms of physical affliction, occupation or appearance does not produce more meaningful objective responses."

3. *The subject's impulses are sometimes represented symbolically in the stories.* The trend is in support of this assumption, although the rules for interpreting symbolic references are not yet clear.

4. *Stories are unequal in their contribution to the diagnosis of a subject's impulses and conflicts.* The evidence is indirect and suggests that the assumption is supported. Stories vary in significance, and the pictures obviously do not always evoke the same responses.

5. *Stimulus-bound stories are less important diagnostically than those that are not directly determined by the stimulus.* According to Lindzey, this assumption seems to be supported—stimulus-bound responses are not as diagnostic as those that deviate from the stimulus.

Murstein (1961) looks at this issue in terms of the stimulus characteristics rather than in terms of the stories' characteristics. He restates the assumption to say that the more ambiguous the stimulus, the more the response reflects the subject's personality. Stating the assumption this way, Murstein (1961) says that extremely ambiguous TAT cards do not produce very evocative stories. Rather, they evoke a "response set" that yields a pleasant response.

Another assumption related to the issue under discussion is presented by Murstein as follows: "Since the stimulus is more or less ambiguous, it is of little importance as compared to the value of the response elicited."

Murstein reports that there is less variation in response to TAT cards than one would believe (Eron, 1950, 1953) and that the cards are not as ambiguous as one might think.

6. *Themes that recur in several stories reflect the subject's personality.* While rational considerations may support this assumption, Lindzey finds little support for it in the literature.

7. *A subject's stories contain evidence for his enduring dispositions as well as momentary impulses, and both are reflected in the same way*. This is a supportable assumption, but there is no evidence that both enduring and momentary factors express themselves in the same way.

8. *Stories may contain events from the subject's past, and these are of diagnostic value*. This, according to Lindzey, is supported by the evidence.

A variant of this hypothesis stated by Murstein is that no response is accidental. Every response that a subject gives is related to an analysis of his personality.

Murstein points out that achievement may be expressed in early but not in later stories because of satiation. "The conclusion is derived that there is considerable variation in the meaningfulness of a response to a projective technique—depending on the effects of S's experience, intelligence, verbal ability and response set."

9. *Stories reflect both individual factors and material related to the subject's group membership or other related cultural and social factors*. There is little material in this area, according to Lindzey, but what there is is in support of this assumption.

10. *There is a relationship between impulses and conflicts found in the stories and overt behavior*. The relationship is an imperfect one, and we still need to know when the correlation is and is not a good one. We shall return to this point later.

11. *One is warranted in making judgments about an individual's personality from a TAT protocol*. Murstein (1961) believes that protocols will vary in the amount of information they contain. As a basis for this, he cites the work of Webb and Hilden (1955), who found a high correlation between a subject's intelligence and the amount of words used in stories. Thus the lack of story or an inadequate story may be a function of personality disturbance, but it may also be a function of intellectual level. Consequently, absence of response may not be as meaningful as presence of adequate number of responses.

12. *The subject is not aware of what he reveals about himself*. This assumption, according to Murstein's (1961) review, cannot be supported. Allport (1953) believes that there is no discrepancy in projective and nonprojective material provided by normals but that there may be a discrepancy in the records of disturbed individuals. According to Murstein, the lack of discrepancy may be equally well applied to normal persons and to persons not so well adjusted.

Subjects can control their responses to ambiguous situations, and, to maintain good relationships with the examiner, they are likely to offer banal responses rather than to reveal themselves. This may be especially true of sophisticated individuals, who, according to Murstein, protect themselves against revealing themselves. They present a picture of themselves consistent with their public images of themselves—a picture in which the clinician is not necessarily interested.

13. *A need's strength is manifest directly or symbolically in a protocol*. This assumption is part of the overall problem of the relationship between fantasy material or projective test material and behavior. It is a matter to which we shall return later.

As stated, the assumption refers only to the strength of a need, omitting the interaction between the need and other aspects of personality. Considered only by itself, the strength of a need (operationally defined in terms of how it manifests behaviorally) is therefore not manifest directly or symbolically in a TAT protocol. The manifestation of its strength is dependent on its relationship with other personality factors.

Pittluck (1950), for example, found that persons whose aggressive needs evoked anxiety and who defended themselves against it by various psychological mechanisms were not likely to manifest their hostility behaviorally.

Murstein (1956) found that two groups who were similar to each other in hostility but who differed in self-concept differed in the projection of their hostility on the Rorschach. One might well assume that similar factors—stimulus properties of the cards, the characteristics of the subject, the environment, and their interaction— all affect the prediction from the protocol to behavior. Intensity of the need alone is therefore insufficient for the prediction of behavior.

And, says Murstein, "Unless the total interaction between person, test and background is quite similar in stimulus value in both projective and overt situations, we have little reason to expect correspondence in behaviors."

14. *There is a relationship between TAT production and overt behavior.* This assumption does have support, but the evidence indicates that the relationships are bound to be rather "complex and idiographic" (Dana, 1972). Furthermore, what evidence is available refers to relatively few of the needs described by Murray (1938).

21. A View to the Future

It is some 40+ years since the TAT was first introduced. Those of us who were involved with it during its early years were quite hopeful and optimistic about its future contributions to the understanding of personality and prediction of behavior. However, after a review such as this and with knowledge of previous reviews, it is apparent that all manner of high hopes have not been fulfilled. Indeed, no major strides have been made since the early days. It is depressing to report no significant breakthroughs even since Murstein's review in 1963. As a matter of fact, the problems he raised then are still problems.

What is the matter? Of course, one can always say it is the fault of the test. This might be so, but it would be too hasty to place all the blame on the test before considering other related matters.

One of the crucial factors affecting the TAT and its usefulness is the change that has occurred in clinical psychology. Clinicians are no longer so involved in diagnosis and the factors affecting diagnostic techniques. They have turned their energies to therapy, utilizing early therapeutic sessions for diagnostic purposes. Without such motivation, it is unlikely that there is going to be much good work.

Clinicians might be convinced to use the TAT for diagnostic purposes if they could be convinced that the data were good enough for differential diagnosis, but, as was indicated, the evidence is not very good on this score. Is the problem with the test? Probably not. The diagnostic categories are a mess, and until the variables that make up the categories are cleared up and until we know more about how these variables manifest themselves in the TAT it is unlikely that any significant contributions will occur. As we turn from practice to research, the situation is quite dismal. There seems to be a lot of "horizontal" research. An investigator thinks up a variable or has an idea, and it is not too long before his students, and related friends begin to apply it in various forms and variations of TAT procedures. And we don't learn very much. As one reviews the research literature, one does not have a sense that studies and research efforts build on top of each other. Even when investigators set out to replicate each other's work, they cannot refrain from adding a new wrinkle to the investigation, which makes comparison of research efforts impossible.

There seems to be a premium on the easy variable, whether it has much signifi-cance or not. After all, students have to get their degrees and they have to get them within a predictable specified period of time. Therefore, why not have them do a word count—it is, after all, a reliable measure, too—and relate it to variations in the picture? Some day someone may make some sense out of it.

Then, too, even when one or more investigators demonstrate that the TAT does predict some sort of behavior related to a criterion (e.g., need achievement and grades), later investigators seem to lose sight of the crucial issues and they get all worked up about the TAT procedure itself. Yes, it is good to know that the TAT pre-dicts grades, but after we know it can be done (even in one experiment and before the contradictory results come in) should we persist in this behavior? It is not crucial to know that crystal-ball gazing through a TAT story yields good predictions. What is crucial is whether the TAT will provide some information that is either qualita-tively or quantitatively different from that provided by other techniques. What is crucial is not whether the TAT predicts a criterion but whether it is the best (consid-ering efficiency, economy, etc.) for predicting the criterion. The investigator with responsibility to the field has also to tell us under what conditions and with what kinds of persons the TAT is the best method to use and when it is the poorest.

These goals are attainable provided that certain things happen in the future. First, we need an agreed-on set of personality variables. Second, we need some cen-tral agency for organizing the research endeavor. Essentially, we need a Bureau of Standards for theory and research. One of the things such an agency would be charged with is getting psychologists together to arrive at a reasonably acceptable set of terms. This can be done with a fair degree of flexibility and without any restric-tions that would limit any changes in existing terms, dropping some and adding others. But the core would be there, and over time it would grow. Without such an agreed-on terminology and set of definitional terms, it is unlikely that we shall ever make much progress.

While the Bureau is calling conferences on terminology and variables, it might also have conferences devoted to the selection and design of research problems. Peri-odic conferences would review the work done during the previous 3 or 5 years and then come up with statements as to what kinds of problems should be considered in the future. Psychologists around the country might engage in cooperative efforts, each testing relatively small numbers of subjects but so selected that when their data are added to those collected by others also involved in the cooperative effort one might see that one is gradually approaching an answer to a problem rather than merely dissipating one's research efforts.

It is easy to say that all this is fantasy and unlikely to occur. If so, then one can predict that future reviews of the TAT and other diagnostic procedures will be the same as this one, as this one is the same as previous ones. If we are to make any prog-ress, we must start by devoting ourselves to a cooperative effort in which variables will be communally defined and selected and research efforts will be so intertwined that future data and results will add significantly to that which already exists.

22. References

Ackerly, L. Sexual fantasies of elderly people. Thesis for the B.S. degree, State University of New York College at Purchase, 1973. Cited in Bellak (1975).

Allport, G. W. The trend in motivational theory. *American Journal of Orthopsychiatry*, 1953, *23*, 107–119.

Altobello, N. Hope and despair in old age. Thesis for the B.A. degree, State University of New York College at Purchase, 1973. Cited in Bellak (1975).

Araoz, D. L. The Thematic Apperception Test in marital therapy. *Journal of Contemporary Psychotherapy*, 1972, *5*, 41–48.

Atkins, M. Color as a variable in a picture-story test for younger children. Senior Honors Thesis, University of Massachusetts, 1962. Cited in Yudin and Resnikoff (1966).

Atkinson, J. W. Studies in projective measurement of achievement motivation. Unpublished doctoral dissertation, University of Michigan, 1950.

Atkinson, J. W. Towards experimental analysis of human motivation in terms of motives, expectancies and incentives. In J. W. Atkinson (Ed.), *Motives in fantasy, action and society*. Princeton, N.J.: Van Nostrand, 1958, pp. 288–305.

Auld, F., Eron, L. D. & Laffal, J. Application of Guttman's scaling method to the TAT. *Educational and Psychological Measurement*, 1955, *15*, 422–435.

Barron, F. *Creativity and personal freedom*. Princeton. Van Nostrand, 1968.

Bell, A., Trosman, H., & Ross, D. The use of projective techniques in the investigation of emotional aspects of medical disorders. II. Other projective techniques and suggestions for experimental design. *Journal of Projective Techniques*, 1953, *17*, 51–60.

Bellak, L. The concept of projection. *Psychiatry*, 1944, *7*, 353–370.

Bellak, L. *A guide to the interpretation of the Thematic Apperception Test*. New York: Psychological Corporation, 1947.(a)

Bellak, L. *TAT blank: For recording and analyzing Thematic Apperception Test stories*. New York: Psychological Corporation, 1947.(b)

Bellak, L. *The Thematic Apperception Test, The Children's Apperception Test and the Senior Apperception Technique in clinical use* (3rd ed.). New York: Grune & Stratton, 1975.

Bellak, L., & Bellak, S. S. *Manual of instruction for the Children's Apperception Test*. New York: C.P.S. Co., 1949.

Bellak, L., Ekstein, R., & Braverman, S. A preliminary study of norms for the Thematic Apperception Test. *American Psychologist*, 1947, *2*, 271 (Abstr.).

Bellak, L., Pasquarelli, B., & Braverman, S. The use of the Thematic Apperception Test in psychotherapy. *Journal of Nervous and Mental Diseases*, 1949, *110*, 51–65.

Bendig, A. W. Comparative validity of objective and projective measures of need achievement in predicting students' achievement in introductory psychology. *Journal of General Psychology*, 1959, *60*, 237–243.

Bettelheim, B. Self-interpretation of fantasy: The Thematic Apperception Test as an educational and therapeutic device. *American Journal of Orthopsychiatry*. 1947, *17*, 80–100.

Biersdorf, K. R., & Marcuse, F. L. Responses of children to human and animal pictures. *Journal of Projective Techniques*, 1953, *17*, 455–459.

Bijou, S. W., & Kenny, D. T. The ambiguity values of TAT cards. *Journal of Consulting Psychology*, 1951, *15*, 203–209.

Birney, R. C. The reliability of the achievement motive. *Journal of Abnormal and Social Psychology*, 1959, *58*, 266–267.

Brackbill, G. A. Some effects of color on thematic fantasy. *Journal of Consulting Psychology*, 1951, *15*, 412–418.

Bruner, J. S., & Postman, L. An approach to social perception. In W. Dennis (Ed.), *Current trends in social psychology*. Pittsburgh, Pa.: University of Pittsburgh Press, 1948, pp. 71–118.

Budoff, M. The relative utility of animal and human figures in a picture-story test for young children. *Journal of Projective Techniques*, 1960, *24*, 347–352.

Butler, R. Responses of institutionalized mentally retarded children to human and to animal pictures. *American Journal of Mental Deficiency*, 1961, *65*, 620–622.

Byrd, E., & Witherspoon, R. L. Responses of preschool children to the Children's Apperception Test. *Child Development*, 1954, *25*, 35–44.

Campbell, D. T., & Fiske, D. W. Convergent and discriminant validation by the multitrait-multimethod matrix. *Psychological Bulletin*, 1959, *56*, 81–105.

Campus, N. Transsituational consistency as a dimension of personality. *Journal of Personality and Social Psychology*, 1974, *29*, 593–600.

Campus, N. A measure of needs to assess the stimulus characteristics of TAT cards. *Journal of Personality Assessment*, 1976, *40*, 248–258.

Cann, A. The effects of the attitudes of whites toward blacks on thematic apperception of racial stimuli. Unpublished doctoral dissertation, New York University, 1977.

Child, I. L., Frank, K. F., & Storm, T. Self-ratings and TAT: Their relations to each other and to childhood background. *Journal of Personality*, 1956, *25*, 96–114.

Chowdhury, U. *An Indian adaptation of the Children's Apperception Test*. Delhi, India: Manasayan, 1960.

Clark, R. M. A method of administering and evaluating the Thematic Apperception Test. *Genetic Psychology Monographs*, 1944, *30*, 3–55.

Combs, A. The use of personal experience in Thematic Apperception Test story plots. *Journal of Clinical Psychology*, 1946, *2*, 357–363.

Cook, R. A. Identification and ego defensiveness in thematic apperception. *Journal of Projective Techniques*. 1953, *17*, 312–319.

Dana, R. H. An application of objective TAT scoring. *Journal of Projective Techniques*, 1956, *20*, 159–163.(a)

Dana, R. H. Selection of abbreviated TAT sets. *Journal of Clinical Psychology*, 1956, *12*, 36–40.(b)

Dana, R. H. Review of Thematic Apperception Test. In D. K. Buros (Ed.), *The seventh mental measurements yearbook* (Vol. 1). Highland Park, N.J.: Gryphon Press, 1972, pp. 457–460.

Deabler, H. L. The psychotherapeutic use of the Thematic Apperception Test. *Journal of Clinical Psychology*, 1947, *3*, 246–252.

De Sousa, T. A comparison of the responses of adjusted and maladjusted children on a Thematic Apperception Test. Unpublished master's thesis, Loyola University, Chicago, 1952.

Dollin, A. P. The effect of order of presentation on perception of TAT pictures. Unpublished doctoral dissertation, University of Connecticut, 1960.

Eagle, C. An investigation of individual consistencies in the manifestations of primary process. Unpublished doctoral dissertation, New York University, 1964.

Eagle, C., & Holt, R. R. Manual for scoring primary process manifestations in thematic material. Appendix C in R. R. Holt, *Manual for the scoring of primary process manifestations in Rorschach responses*. Research Center for Mental Health, New York University, 1970, Mimeo.

Earle, M. Rakau children: From six to thirteen years. Wellington, New Zealand. *Victoria University Publications in Psychology*, No. 11, 1958 (Monographs on Maori Social Life and Personality, No. 4). Cited in Bellak (1975).

Eron, L. D. Frequencies of themes and identification in stories of patients and nonhospitalized college students. *Journal of Consulting Psychology*, 1948, *12*, 387–395.

Eron, L. D. A normative study of the Thematic Apperception Test. *Psychological Monographs*, 1950, *64*, No. 9. (a)

Eron, L. D. Responses of women to the Thematic Apperception Test. *Psychological Monographs*, 1950, *64*, No. 9. (b)

Eron, L. D. & Ritter, A. M. A comparison of two methods of administration of the Thematic Apperception Test. *Journal of Consulting Psychology*, 1951, *15*, 55–61.

Eron, L. D. Review of Thematic Apperception Test. In D. K. Buros, *The seventh mental measurement yearbook* (Vol. 1). New Jersey: Gryphon Press, 1972, pp. 181–182.

Fairweather, G., Simon, R. Gebhard, M., Weingarten, E., Holland, J., Sanders, R., Stone, G., & Reahl, J. Relative effectiveness of psychotherapeutic programs: A multicriteria comparison of four programs for three different patient groups. *Psychological Monographs*, 1960, *74*, No. 5.

Feld, S., & Smith, C. P. An evaluation of the method of content analysis. In J. W. Atkinson (Ed.), *Motives in fantasy, action, and society*. Princeton, N.J.: Van Nostrand, 1958, pp. 234–241.

Fitzgerald, B. J., Pasewark, R. A., & Fleisher, S. Responses of an aged population on the Gerontological and Thematic Apperception Tests. *Journal of Personality Assessment*, 1974, *38*, 234–235.

Fleming, E. A descriptive analysis of responses in the Thematic Apperception Test. Unpublished master's thesis, University of Pittsburgh, 1946.

Friedman, I. Objectifying the subjective—A methodological approach to the TAT. *Journal of Projective Techniques*, 1957, *21*, 243–247.

Furyua, K. Responses of school children to human and animal pictures. *Journal of Projective Techniques*. 1957, *21*, 248–252.

Garland, C. The experience of dependency in the elderly. Thesis for the B.A. degree, State University of New York College at Purchase, 1974.

Golden, M. Some effects of combining psychological tests on clinical inferences. *Journal of Consulting Psychology*, 1964, *28*, 440–446.

Goldfried, M. R., & Zax, M. The stimulus value of the TAT. *Journal of Projective Techniques*, 1965, *29*, 46–58.

Goodenough, W. H. A technique for scale analysis. *Educational and Psychological Measurement*, 1944, *4*, 179–190.

Goodstein, L. D. Interrelationships among several measures of anxiety and hostility. *Journal of Consulting Psychology*, 1954, *18*, 35–39.

Gottschalk, L. A., & Gleser, G. C. *The measurement of psychological states through the content analysis of verbal behavior.* Berkeley-Los Angeles: University of California Press, 1969.

Gottschalk, L. A., Winget, C. N., & Gleser, G. C. *A manual for using the Gottschalk-Gleser content analysis scales.* Berkeley-Los Angeles: University of California Press, 1969.

Gurvitz, S., & Kapper, Z. Techniques for evaluation of the responses of schizophrenic and cerebral palsied children to the Children's Apperception Test (C.A.T.). *Quarterly Journal of Child Behavior*, 1951, *3*, 38–65.

Haber, R. N., & Alpert, R. The role of situation and picture cues in projective measurement of the achievement motive. In J. W. Atkinson, (Ed.), *Motives in fantasy, action, and society.* Princeton, N.J.: Van Nostrand, 1958, pp. 644–663.

Harrison, R., & Rotter, J. B. A note on the reliability of the Thematic Apperception Test. *Journal of Abnormal and Social Psychology*, 1945, *40*, 97–99.

Hartman, A. A. A basic TAT set. *Journal of Projective Techniques and Personality Assessment*, 1970, *34*, 391–396.

Haworth, M. A schedule for the analysis of C.A.T. responses. *Journal of Projective Techniques*, 1963, *27*, 181–184.

Haworth, M. *A schedule of adaptative mechanisms in C.A.T. responses.* Larchmont, N.Y.: C.P.S. Inc., 1965.

Haworth, M. *The C.A.T: Facts about Fantasy.* New York, Grune & Stratton, 1966.

Henry, W. E. The Thematic Apperception Technique in the study of culture–personality relations. *Genetic Psychology Monographs*, *35*, 1947.

Henry, W. E. *The analysis of fantasy, the Thematic Apperception Technique in the study of personality.* New York: Wiley, 1956.

Henry, W. E. & Guetzkow, H. Group projection sketches for the study of small groups. Publication No. 4 of the Conference Research Project at the University of Michigan. *Journal of Social Psychology*, 1951, *33*, 77–102.

Hoar, M. W., & Faust, W. L. The Children's Apperception Test: Puzzle and regular form. *Journal of Personality Assessment*, 1973, *37*, 244–247.

Hoffberg, C., & Fast, I. Professional identity and impulse expression in phantasy. *Journal of Projective Techniques and Personality Assessment*, 1966, *30*, 488–498.

Holmes, D. S., & Tyler, J. D. Direct versus projective measurement of achievement motivation. *Journal of Consulting and Clinical Psychology*, 1968, *32*, 712–717.

Holt, R. R. (Ed.) *The TAT Newsletter*, 1947, *1*, No. 2, Mimeo.

Holt, R. R. (Ed.) *The TAT Newsletter*, 1948, *2*, No. 2, Mimeo.

Holt, R. R. (Ed.) *The TAT Newsletter*, 1949, *3*, No. 3, p. 8.

Holt, R. R. *Assessing personality.* New York: Harcourt Brace Jovanovich, 1971.

Holt, R. R. *Methods in clinical psychology: Vol 1. Projective Assessments.* New York: Plenum, 1978.

Holt, R. R. & Luborsky, L. *Personality patterns of psychiatrists: A study of methods for selecting residents* (Vol. I). New York: Basic Books, 1958. (a)

Holt, R. R. & Luborsky, L. *Personality patterns of psychiatrists: Supplementary and supporting data* (Vol. II). Topeka, Kans.: Menninger Foundation, 1958. (b)

Holtzman, W. H. *Holtzman inkblot technique* (Form A). New York: Psychological Corp., 1958. (a)

Holtzman, W. H. *Holtzman inkblot technique* (Form B). New York: Psychological Corp., 1958. (b)

Horwitz, M., & Cartwright, D. A. A projective method for the diagnosis of groups. *Human Relations*, 1953, *6*, 397–410.

Hurley, J. R. The Iowa Picture Interpretation Test: A multiple-choice variation of the TAT. *Journal of Consulting Psychology*, 1955, *19*, 372–376.

Hurley, J. R. Achievement imagery and motivational instructions as determinants of verbal learning. *Journal of Personality*, 1957, *25*, 274–282.

India, Ministry of Defence, Defence Science Organization, Research Wing. Mood in TAT pictures and its effects. *Indian Journal of Psychology*, 1954, *29*, 125–140.

Irvin, F. S., & Wouds, K. V. Empirical support for a basic TAT set. *Journal of Clinical Psychology*, 1971, *27*, 514–516.

Jensen, A. R. The reliability of projective techniques: Review of the literature. *Acta Psychologica*, 1959, *16*, 108–136.

Johnson, A. W., & Dana, R. A. Color on the TAT. *Journal of Projective Techniques*, 1965, *29*, 179–183.

Johnston, R. A. The effect of achievement imagery on maze-learning performance. *Journal of Personality*, 1955, *24*, 145–152.

Johnston, R. A. A methodological analysis of several revised forms of the Iowa Picture Interpretation Test. *Journal of Personality*, 1957, *25*, 283–293.

Jones, R. M. The negation of TAT; a projective method for eliciting repressed thought content. *Journal of Projective Techniques*, 1956, *20*, 297–303.

Kagan, J. The measurement of overt aggression from fantasy. *Journal of Abnormal and Social Psychology*, 1956, *52*, 390–393.

Kagan, J. Thematic apperceptive techniques with children. In A. Rabin & M. Haworth (Eds.), *Projective techniques with children*. New York: Grune & Stratton, 1960, pp. 105–129.

Kagan, J. The stability of TAT fantasy and stimulus ambiguity. *Journal of Consulting Psychology*, 1959, *23*, 266–271.

Kagan, J., and Kaufman, M. A preliminary investigation of some relationships between functional articulation disorders and response to the Children's Apperception Test. Unpublished master's thesis, Boston University, 1954.

Kagan, J., & Moss, H. A. *Birth of maturity: A study in psychological development*. New York: Wiley, 1962.

Kaplan, A. *The conduct of inquiry*. San Francisco, Calif.: Chandler Publishing Co., 1964.

Kaplan, M. F. The effect of cue relevance, ambiguity, and self-reported hostility on TAT responses. *Journal of Projective Techniques and Personality Assessment*, 1967, *31*, 45–50.

Kaplan, M. F. The ambiguity of TAT ambiguity. *Journal of Projective Techniques and Personality Assessment*, 1969, *33*, 25–29. (a)

Kaplan, M. F. Reply to Murstein's comments on "The ambiguity of TAT ambiguity." *Journal of Projective Techniques and Personality Assessment*, 1969, *33*, 486–487. (b)

Katz, I. Emotional expression in failure: A new hypothesis. *Journal of Abnormal and Social Psychology*, 1950, *45*, 329–349.

Kelly, E. L., & Fiske, D. W. *The prediction of performance in clinical psychology*. Ann Arbor: University of Michigan Press, 1951.

Kenny, D. T. A theoretical and research reappraisal of stimulus factors in the TAT. In J. Kagan & G. Lesser (Eds.), *Contemporary issues in thematic apperceptive methods*. Springfield, Ill.: Thomas, 1961, pp. 288–308.

Kenny, D. T., & Bijou, S. W. Ambiguity of pictures and extent of personality factors in fantasy responses. *Journal of Consulting Psychology*, 1953, *17*, 283–288.

Kolter, N. Self-selection of TAT cards: A technique for assessing test-resistant children. *Journal of Projective Techniques and Personality Assessment*, 1970, *34*, 324–327.

Korchin, S. J., Mitchell, H. B., & Meltzoff, J. A critical evaluation of the Thompson Thematic Apperception Test. *Journal of Projective Techniques*, 1950, *14*, 445–452.

Kostlan, A. A method for the empirical study of psychodiagnosis. *Journal of Consulting Psychology*, 1954, *18*, 83–88.

Lasaga, J. I., & Martinez-Arango, C. Four detailed examples of how mental conflicts of psychoneurotics and psychotic patients may be discovered by means of the Thematic Apperception Test. *Journal of Psychology*, 1948, *26*, 299–345.

Laskowitz, D. The effect of varied degrees of pictorial ambiguity on fantasy evocation. Doctoral dissertation, New York University, 1959.

Lazarus, R. S. A substitutive-defensive conception of apperceptive fantasy. In J. Kagan & G. Lesser (Eds.), *Contemporary issues of thematic apperceptive methods*. Springfield, Ill.: Thomas, 1961, pp. 51–69.

Lebo, D., & Harrigan, M. Visual and verbal presentation of TAT stimuli. *Journal of Consulting Psychology*, 1957, *21*, 339–342.

Lebo, D., & Sherry, P. J. Visual and vocal presentation of TAT descriptions. *Journal of Projective Techniques*, 1959, *23*, 59–63.

Lesser, G. S. The relationship between overt and fantasy aggression as a function of maternal response to aggression. *Journal of Abnormal and Social Psychology*, 1957, *55*, 218–221.

Lesser, G. S. Application of Guttman's scaling method to aggressive fantasy in children. *Educational and Psychological Measurement*, 1958, *18*, 543–550.

Levine, F. J. Thematic drive expression in three occupational groups. *Journal of Personality Assessment*, 1969, *33*, 357–363.

Levine, R., Chein, I., & Murphy, G. The relations of the intensity of a need to the amount of perceptual distortion. *Journal of Psychology*, 1942, *13*, 283–293.

Levy, M. R. Issues in the personality assessment of lower-class patients. *Journal of Projective Techniques and Personality Assessment*, 1970, *34*, 6–9.

Light, B. H. Comparative study of a series of TAT and CAT cards. *Journal of Clinical Psychology*, 1954, *10*, 179–181.

Light, B. H. A further test of the Thompson TAT rationale. *Journal of Abnormal and Social Psychology*, 1955, *51*, 148–150.

Lindzey, G. Thematic Apperception Test: Interpretive assumptions and related empirical evidence. *Psychology Bulletin*, 1952, *49*, 1–25.

Lindzey, G., & Heinemann, S. H. TAT: Individual and group administration. *Journal of Personality*, 1955, *24*, 34–55.

Lindzey, G. and Herman, P. S. TAT: A note on reliability and situational validity. *Journal of Projective Techniques*, 1955, *19*, 36–42.

Lindzey, G., & Silverman, M. Thematic Apperception Test: Techniques of group administration, sex differences, and the role of verbal productivity. *Journal of Personality*, 1959, *27*, 311–323.

Lipgar, R. M. Treatment of time in the TAT. *Journal of Personality Assessment*, 1969, *33*, 219–229.

Little, K. B. Whither projective techniques? Paper read at California State Psychological Association, Los Angeles, March, 1957.

Little, K. B. Problems in the validation of projective techniques. *Journal of Projective Techniques*, 1959, *23*, 287–290.

Little, K. B., & Shneidman, E. S. The validity of thematic projective technique interpretations. *Journal of Personality*, 1955, *23*, 285–294.

Little, K. B., & Shneidman, E. S. Congruencies among interpretations of psychological test and anamnestic data. *Psychological Monographs*, 1959, *75*, No. 6.

Lowe, W. F. Effect of controlling the immediate environment or responses to the Thematic Apperception Test. Unpublished Master's Thesis, University of Louisville, 1951.

Lowell, E. L. The effect of need for achievement on learning and speed of performance. *Journal of Psychology*, 1952, *33*, 41–40.

Lubin, B. Some effects of set and stimulus properties on TAT stories. *Journal of Projective Techniques*, 1960, *24*, 11–16.

Lubin, N. M., & Wilson, M. D. Picture test identification as a function of "reality" (color) and similarity of picture to subject. *Journal of General Psychology*, 1956, *54*, 331–338.

Luborsky, L. Self-interpretation of the TAT as a clinical technique. *Journal of Projective Techniques*, 1953, *17*, 217–223.

Luborsky, L., & Holt, R. R. The selection of candidates for psychoanalytic training. *Journal of Clinical and Experimental Psychopathology*, 1957, *18*, 166–176.

Maddi, S. R., Propst, B. S., & Feldinger, I. Three expressions of the need for variety. *Journal of Personality*, 1965, *33*, 82–98.

Masling, J. M. The effects of warm and cold interaction in the interpretation of a projective protocol. *Journal of Projective Techniques*, 1957, *21*, 377–383.

Masling, J. M. The effects of warm and cold interaction on the administration and scoring of an intelligence test. *Journal of Consulting Psychology*, 1959, *23*, 336–341.

Masling, J. M. The influence of situational and inter-personal variables in projective testing. *Psychological Bulletin*, 1960, *57*, 65–85.

Masling, J., & Harris, S. Sexual aspects of TAT administration. *Journal of Consulting and Clinical Psychology*, 1969, *33*, 166–169.

Mason, B. D. An experimental investigation of the effect of repetition and variation in administration upon the Thematic Apperception Test. Unpublished Master's thesis, University of Louisville, 1952.

McClelland, D. S. On the psychodynamics of creative physical scientists. In H. E. Gruber, G. Terrell, & M. Wertheimer (Eds.), *Contemporary approaches to creative thinking*. New York: Atherton Press, 1962.

McClelland, D. S., & Atkinson, J. W. The projective expression of needs. I. The effect of different intensities of the hunger drive on perception. *Journal of Psychology*, 1948, *25*, 205–222.

McClelland, D. S., Atkinson, J. W., Clark, R. A., & Lowell, E. L. *The achievement motive.* New York: Appleton-Century-Crofts, 1953.

Megargee, E. I. (Ed.) *Research in clinical assessment.* New York: Harper & Row, 1966.

Mercer, M. Review of *Gerontological apperception test*, by R. L. Wolk and Rochell B. Wolk. *Journal of Personality Assessment*, 1973, *37*, 396–397.

Meyer, H. H., Walker, W. B., & Litwin, G. H. Motive patterns and risk preferences associated with entrepreneurship. *Journal of Abnormal and Social Psychology*, 1961, *63*, 570–574.

Meyer, M. M. The direct use of projective techniques in psychotherapy. *Journal of Projective Techniques*, 1951, *15*, 263.

Morgan, C. D., & Murray, H. A. A method for investigating fantasies: The Thematic Apperception Test. *Archives of Neurology and Psychiatry*, 1935, *34*, 289–306.

Morgan, H. H. A psychometric comparison of achieving and nonachieving college students of high ability. *Journal of Consulting Psychology*, 1952, *16*, 292–298.

Moriarty, A. Normal preschoolers' reactions to the CAT: Some implications for later development. *Journal of Personality Assessment*, 1972, *36*, 413–419.

Moss, H. A., & Kagan, J. Stability of achievement- and recognition-seeking behavior from early childhood through adulthood. *Journal of Abnormal and Social Psychology*, 1961, *62*, 504–513.

Murray, H. A. The effect of fear upon estimates of the maliciousness of other personalities. *Journal of Social Psychology*, 1933, *4*, 310–339.

Murray, H. A. et al. *Explorations in Personality*. New York: Oxford University Press, 1938.

Murray, H. A. *Thematic Apperception Test manual*. Cambridge, Mass.: Harvard University Press, 1943.

Murray, H. A. Uses of the Thematic Apperception Test. *American Journal of Psychiatry*, 1951, *107*, 577–581.

Murray, H. A. In E. S. Shneidman (Ed.), *The TAT Newsletter*, 6, 1952, p. 2.

Murray, H. A., & Stein, M. I. Note on the selection of combat officers. *Psychosomatic Medicine*, 1943, *5*, 386–391.

Murstein, B. I. Assumptions, adaptation level, and projective techniques. *Perceptual and Motor Skills*, 1961, *12*, 107–125.

Murstein, B. I. *Theory and research in projective techniques (emphasizing the TAT)*. New York: Wiley, 1963.

Murstein, B. I. A normative study of TAT ambiguity. *Journal of Projective Techniques and Personality Assessment*, 1964, *28*, 210–218.

Murstein, B. I. The stimulus. In B. Murstein (Ed.), *Handbook of Projective Techniques*. New York: Basic Books, 1965. (a)

Murstein, B. I. The scaling of the TAT for n Achievement. *Journal of Consulting Psychology*, 1965, *29*, 286. (b)

Murstein, B. I. Comments on "The ambiguity of TAT ambiguity." *Journal of Projective Techniques and Personality Assessment*, 1969, *33*, 483–485.

Murstein, B. I. A thematic test and the Rorschach in predicting marital choice. *Journal of Personality Assessment*, 1972, *36*, 212–217. (a)

Murstein, B. I. Interview behavior, projective techniques, and questionnaires in the clinical assessment of marital choice. *Journal of Personality Assessment*, 1972, *36*, 462–467. (b)

Murstein, B. I., David, C., Fisher, D., & Furth, H. The scaling of the TAT for hostility by a variety of scaling methods. *Journal of Consulting Psychology*, 1961, *25*, 497–504.

Mussen, P. and Naylor, H. K. Relationships between overt and fantasy aggression. *Journal of Abnormal and Social Psychology*, 1954, *49*, 235–240.

Myler, B., Rosenkrantz, A., & Holmes, G. A comparison of the TAT, CAT and CAT-H among second grade girls. *Journal of Personality Assessment*, 1972, *36*, 440–444.

Newmark, C. S., & Flouranzano, R. Replication of an empirically derived TAT set with hospitalized psychiatric patients. *Journal of Personality Assessment*, 1973, *37*, 340–341.

Nolan, R. A longitudinal comparison of motives in children's fantasy stories as revealed by the Children's Apperception Test. Unpublished doctoral dissertation, Florida State University, Tallahassee, 1959.

OSS Assessment Staff. *Assessment of men*. New York: Rinehart, 1948.

Osborne, R. T. TAT lantern slides. In R. R. Holt (Ed.), *The TAT Newsletter*, 1951, *5*, p. 6.

Pasewark, R. A., Fitzgerald, B. J., Dexter, V., & Cangemi, A. Responses of adolescent, middle-aged, and aged females on the Gerontological and Thematic Apperception Tests. *Journal of Personality Assessment*, 1976, *40*, 588–591.

Pine, F. Thematic drive content and creativity. *Journal of Personality*, 1959, *27*, 136–151.

Pine, F. A manual rating drive content in the Thematic Apperception Test. *Journal of Projective Techniques*, 1960, *24*, 32–45.

Pine, F. Creativity and primary process: Sample variations. *Journal of Nervous and Mental Diseases*, 1962, *134*, 506–511.

Pine, F., & Holt, R. R. Creativity and primary process: A study of adaptive regression. *Journal of Abnormal and Social Psychology*, 1960, *61*, 370–379.

Pittluck, P. The relationship between aggressive fantasy and overt behavior. Unpublished doctoral dissertation, Yale University, 1950.

Prola, M. A re-evaluation of the motor-inhibition fantasy hypothesis. *Journal of Personality Assessment*, 1970, *34*, 477–483.

Prola, M. A review of the transcendence index. *Journal of Personality Assessment*, 1972, *36*, 8–12. (a)

Prola, M. Verbal productivity and transcendence. *Journal of Personality Assessment*, 1972, *36*, 445–446. (b)

Rabin, A. Children's Apperception Test findings with kibbutz and non-kibbutz preschoolers. *Journal of Personality Assessment*, 1972, *36*, 420–424.

Rapaport, D., Gill, M., & Schafer, R. In R. R. Holt (Ed.), *Diagnostic Psychological Testing* (Revised ed.). New York: International Universities Press, 1968.

Reitman, W. R. and Atkinson, J. W. Some methodological problems in the use of thematic apperceptive measures of human motives. In J. W. Atkinson (Ed.), *Motives in fantasy, action, and society.* Princeton, N.J.: Van Nostrand, 1958, pp. 664–684.

Riess, B. F., Schwartz, E. K., & Cottingham, A. An experimental critique of assumptions underlying the Negro version of the TAT. *Journal of Abnormal and Social Psychology*, 1950, *45*, 700–709.

Rock, M. H. Self-reflection and ego development. Unpublished doctoral dissertation, New York University, 1975.

Rodnick, E. H., & Klebanoff, S. G. Projective reactions to induced frustration as a measure of social adjustment. *Psychological Bulletin*, 1942, *39*, 489. (Abstr.)

Rorschach, H. *Psychodiagnostics* (4th ed.) (trans. by P. Lemkau & B. Kronenberg; W. Morgenthaler, Ed.). Bern: Huber, 1942.

Rosenblatt, M. The development of norms for the Children's Apperception Test. Unpublished doctoral dissertation, Florida State University, Tallahassee, 1958.

Rosenthal, R. *Experimenter effects in behavioral research.* New York: Appleton-Century-Crofts, 1966.

Rosenzweig, S. Levels of behavior in psychodiagnosis with special reference to the Picture-Frustration study. *American Journal of Orthopsychiatry*, 1950, *20*, 63–72.

Samuels, H. The validity of personality-trait ratings based on projective techniques. *Psychological Monographs*, 1952, *66*, No. 5.

Sanford, R. N. The effects of abstinence from food upon imaginal processes; a preliminary experiment. *Journal of Psychology*, 1936, *2*, 129–136.

Sanford, R. N. The effects of abstinence from food upon imaginal processes: A further experiment. *Journal of Psychology*, 1937, *3*, 145–149.

Sanford, R. N., Adkins, Margaret M., Miller, R. B., Cobb, E. A., et al. Physique, personality, and scholarship: A cooperative study of school children. *Monograph Social Research Child Development*, 1943, *8*, No. 1.

Sarason, B. R., & Sarason, I. C. The effect of type of administration and sex of subject on emotional tone and outcome ratings of TAT stories. *Journal of Projective Techniques*, 1958, *22*, 333–337.

Schafer, R. How was this story told? *Journal of Projective Techniques*, 1958, *22*, 181–210.

Schwartz, E. K., Riess, B. F., & Cottingham, A. Further critical evaluation of the Negro version of the TAT. *Journal of Projective Techniques*, 1951, *15*, 394–400.

Shatin, L. Rorschach adjustment and the Thematic Apperception Test, *Journal of Projective Techniques*, 1953, *17*, 92–101.

Shatin, L. Relationships between the Rorschach test and the Thematic Apperception Test, *Journal of Projective Techniques*, 1955, *19*, 317–331.

Shepley, T. E., & Veroff, J. A projective measure of need for affiliation. *Journal of Experimental Psychology*, 1952, *43*, 349–356.

Shneidman, E. S. *The Make a Picture Story Test.* New York: The Psychological Corporation, 1949.

Shneidman, E. S. A MAPS test manual. *Projective Techniques Monographs*, 1951, *1*, No. 2.

Shneidman, E. S. Some relationships between the Rorschach technique and other psychodiagnostic tests. In B. Klopper et al., *Developments in the Rorschach Technique.* New York: World Book Co., 1956, pp. 595–642.

Shneidman, E. S., Joel, W., & Little, K. B. *Thematic test analysis.* New York: Grune & Stratton, 1951.

Silverman, L. H. A Q-sort study of the validity of evaluations made from projective techniques. *Psychological Monographs*, 1959, *73*, No. 7.

Singer, J. L., & Herman, J. L. Motor and fantasy correlates of the Rorschach human movement response. *Journal of Consulting Psychology*, 1954, *18*, 325–331.

Slemon, A. G., Holzwarth, E. J., Lewis, J., & Sitko, M. Associative elaboration and integration scales for evaluating TAT protocols. *Journal of Personality Assessment.* 1976, *40*, 365–369.

Solkoff, N. Effects of a variation in instructions and pictorial stimuli on responses to TAT-like cards. *Journal of Projective Techniques*, 1959, *23*, 76–82.

Solkoff, N. Effects of a variation in instructions on responses to TAT cards. *Journal of Projective Techniques*, 1960, *24*, 67–70.

Stein, M. I. The use of a sentence completion test for the diagnosis of personality. *Journal of Clinical Psychology*, *3*, 1948, 47–56.

Stein, M. I., Mackenzie, J. N., Rodgers, R. R. and Meer, B. A case study of a scientist. In A. Burton and R. E. Harris (Eds.), *Clinical studies in personality*, New York: Harper & Row, 1955.

Stein, M. I. *The Thematic Apperception Test*. Cambridge, Mass.: Addison-Wesley, 1955.

Stein, M. I. Explorations in typology. In R. W. White (Ed.), *The study of lives*. New York: Atherton Press, 1963.

Stein, M. I. Ecology of typology, In *Proceedings of the conference on personality measurement in medical education*. Sponsored by the Association of American Medical Colleges, Des Plaines, Ill., June 17–18, 1971.

Stein, M. I., & Neulinger, J. In M. J. Katz, J. O. Cole, & W. E. Barton (Eds.), *The role and methodology of classification in psychiatry and psychopathology*. Washington, D.C.: Government Printing Office, Public Health Service Publication, no. 1584, 1968.

Stephenson, W. *The study of behavior: Q technique and its methodology*. Chicago: University of Chicago Press, 1953.

Stern, G. G., Stein, M. I., & Bloom, B. S. *Methods in personality assessment*. Glencoe, Ill.: Free Press, 1956.

Stone, H., & Dellis, N. An exploratory investigation into the levels hypothesis, *Journal of Projective Techniques*, 1960, *24*, 333–340.

Summerwell, H. C., Campbell, M. M., & Sarason, I. C. The effect of differential motivating instructions on emotional tone and outcome of TAT stories. *Journal of Consulting Psychology*, 1958, *22*, 385–388.

Symonds, P. M. *Symonds Picture-Story Test*. New York: Bureau of Publications, Teachers College, Columbia University, 1948, 20 plates, manual (20 pp.).

Symonds, P. M. *Adolescent fantasy*. New York: Columbia University Press, 1949.

Terhune, K. W. A note on thematic apperception scoring of needs for achievement, affiliation and power. *Journal of Projective Techniques and Personality Assessment*, 1969, *33*, 364–370.

Theiner, E. Experimental needs as expressed by projective techniques. *Journal of Projective Techniques*, 1962, *26*, 354–363.

Thompson, C. E. The Thompson modification of the Thematic Apperception Test. *Rorschach Research Exchange*, 1949, *13*, 469–478. (a)

Thompson, C. E. *The Thompson modification of the thematic apperception test*. Cambridge, Mass.: Harvard University Press, 1949. (b)

Thompson, C. E., & Bachrach, H. J. The use of color in the TAT. *Journal of Projective Techniques*, 1951, *15*, 173–184.

Tomkins, S. S. *The thematic apperception test*, New York: Grune & Stratton, 1947.

Tomkins, S. Discussion of Dr. Murstein's paper. In J. Kagan & G. S. Lesser (Eds.), *Contemporary issues in thematic apperceptive methods*. Springfield, Ill.: Thomas, 1961, p. 279.

Toone, D. Is old age accompanied by a constricted view of the world? Thesis for the B.A. degree, State University of New York College, Purchase, 1974.

Ullmann, L. Selection of neuropsychiatric patients for group psychotherapy. *Journal of Consulting Psychology*, 1957, *21*, 277–280.

van Lennep, D. J. *Four-picture test*. The Hague: Martinus Nijhoff, 1948.

van Lennep, D. J. The four picture test. In H. A. Anderson & G. L. Anderson (Eds.), *An introduction to projective techniques and other devices for understanding the dynamics of human behavior*. New York: Prentice-Hall, 1951.

Watson, R. I. The Thematic Apperception Test. In R. I. Watson, *The clinical method in psychology*. New York: Harper & Row, 1951.

Webb, W. B., & Hilden, A. H. Verbal and intellectual ability as factors in projective test results. *Journal of Projective Techniques*, 1953, *17*, 102–103.

Weiss, P., Wertheimer, M., & Groesbeck, B. Achievement motivation, academic aptitude, and college grades. *Educational Psychology Measurement*, 1959, *19*, 663–665.

Weisskopf, E. A. A transcendence index as a proposed measure in the TAT. *Journal of Psychology*, 1950, *29*, 379–390. (a)

Weisskopf, E. A. An experimental study of the effect of brightness and ambiguity on projection in the TAT. *Journal of Psychology*, 1950, *29*, 407–416. (b)

Weisskopf, E. A., & Dieppa, J. J. Experimentally induced faking of TAT responses. *Journal of Consulting Psychology*, 1951, *15*, 469–474.

Weisskopf, E. A., & Dunlevy, G. P. Bodily similarity between subject and central figure in the TAT as an influence on projection. *Journal of Abnormal and Social Psychology*, 1952, *47*, 441–445.

Weisskopf-Joelson, E. A., & Foster, H. C. An experimental study of stimulus variation upon projection. *Journal of Projective Techniques*, 1962, *26*, 366–370.

Weisskopf-Joelson, E. A., & Lynn, D. B. The effect of variations in ambiguity on projection in the Children's Apperception Test. *Journal of Consulting Psychology*, 1953, *17*, 67–70.

Weisskopf-Joelson, E. A., & Money, L. Facial similarity between subject and central figure in the TAT as an influence on projection. *Journal of Abnormal Psychology*, 1958, *48*, 341–344.

White, R. K. Value-analysis: A quantitative method for describing qualitative data, *Journal of Social Psychology*, 1944, *19*, 351–358.

White, R. K. *Value analysis: The nature and use of the method.* New York: Society for the Psychological Study of Social Issues, 1951.

White, R. W. *Lives in progress: A study of the natural growth of personality* (2nd. ed). New York: Holt Rinehart & Winston, 1966.

Williams, J. E. Mode of failure, interference tendencies, and achievement imagery. *Journal of Abnormal and Social Psychology*, 1955, *51*, 573–580.

Winget, C. N., Gleser, G. C., & Clements, W. H. A method for quantifying human relations, hostility, and anxiety applied to TAT productions. *Journal of Personality Assessment*, 1969, *33*, 433–437.

Witherspoon, R. Development of objective scoring methods for longitudinal C.A.T. data. *Journal of Projective Techniques*, 1968, *32*, 407.

Wohlford, P. Extension of personal time in TAT and story completion stories. *Journal of Projective Techniques and Personality Assessment*, 1968, *32*, 267–280.

Wohlford, P., & Herrera, J. A. TAT stimulus-cues of extension of personal time. *Journal of Projective Techniques and Personality Assessment*, *34*, 1970, 31–37.

Wolk, R. L. Refined projective techniques with the aged. In D. P. Kent, R. Kastenbaum & S. Sherwood (Eds.), *Research, planning, and action for the elderly; The power and potential of social science.* New York: Behavioral Publications, 1972.

Wolk, R. L., Rustin, S. L., & Seiden, R. A custom-made projective technique for the aged: The Gerontological Apperception Test. *Journal of the Long Island Consultation Center*, 1966, *4*, 8–21.

Wolk, R. L., & Wolk, R. B. *The Gerontological Apperception Test.* New York: Behavioral Publications, 1971.

Wolowitz, H. M., & Shorkey, C. Power themes in the TAT stories of paranoid schizophrenic males. *Journal of Projective Techniques and Personality Assessment*, 1966, *30*, 591–596.

Wyatt, F. The scoring and analysis of the Thematic Apperception Test. *Journal of Psychology*, 1947, *24*, 319–330.

Wyatt, F. A principle for the interpretation of fantasy. *Journal of Projective Techniques*, 1958, *22*, 173–180.

Yudin, L. W., & Reznikoff, M. Color and its relation to personality: The TAT. *Journal of Personality Assessment*, 1966, *30*, 479–487.

7

Holtzman Inkblot Technique

WAYNE H. HOLTZMAN

1. Introduction

For several generations the most used psychodiagnostic technique in clinical assessment has been the Rorschach. Working with mental patients in Switzerland, Rorschach developed a system of analysis for inkblots which, in its broad outlines, still stands today. The ten inkblots constituting the Rorschach test are the same today as they were over 50 years ago when first published following Rorschach's death in 1922. Until the early 1940s, the mainstream of academic psychology looked askance at the Rorschach movement, criticizing its cultist character and lack of scientific discipline. Primarily working outside of academic circles, the Rorschach practitioners developed their own ideas and interpretive systems, relying mainly on intuitive insights and clinical confirmation rather than on hard scientific evidence. World War II changed this situation rather dramatically when the sudden urgent need for new devices for personality assessment and clinical diagnosis arose in the armed services. By 1945, the Rorschach was firmly established as the leading clinical instrument for psychodiagnosis.

In spite of its popularity as a diagnostic instrument, the Rorschach technique was heavily criticized by a growing number of clinical psychologists and academicians who had experimented with the technique in the immediate postwar years. Typical of these criticisms were the critical attacks leveled by Zubin (1954), in which he charged seven major failures as follows: (1) failure to provide an objective scoring system free of arbitrary conventions and showing high interscorer agreement, (2) lack of satisfactory internal consistency or test-retest reliability, (3) failure to provide cogent evidence for clinical validity, (4) failure of the individual Rorschach scoring categories to relate to diagnosis, (5) lack of prognostic or predictive validity with respect to outcome of treatment or later behavior, (6) inability to differentiate between groups of normal subjects, and (7) failure to find any significant relationships

WAYNE H. HOLTZMAN • Hogg Foundation for Mental Health, The University of Texas at Austin, Austin, Texas 78712.

between Rorschach scores and intelligence or creative ability. While few Rorschach specialists would agree with Zubin, even the most enthusiastic advocates of the Rorschach were increasingly aware of the limitations of the method, especially when scored by conventional systems.

The Holtzman Inkblot Technique (HIT) was developed in the late 1950s as a major research program aimed at overcoming the weaknesses noted in the Rorschach.* Much of the controversy over the Rorschach at this time arose from failure to distinguish between the Rorschach as a projective technique in the hands of a skilled clinician and the same set of inkblots when viewed as a psychometric device that could yield scores for personality assessment. Various systems for the analysis of responses to inkblots have ranged widely from considering the technique as a structured depth interview to be analyzed in a purely qualitative manner to focusing primarily on objective scores that deal with the content or the characteristics of the inkblots that determine the response. Associations to inkblots, when analyzed qualitatively from a strictly phenomenological point of view, represent a purely projective approach. The use of a highly structured multiple-choice inkblot test such as Harrower-Erickson's multiple-choice version (1945) or Stone's Structured-Objective Rorschach (1958) yields an objective personality test that has only the stimulus materials in common with the standard Rorschach.

The Holtzman Inkblot Technique attempts to capture the best qualities of both the projective and psychometric approaches to the Rorschach. The method consists of two parallel forms, each containing 45 inkblots as well as two practice blots, cards X and Y. The subject gives only one response to each card rather than as many or as few responses as he wishes, the standard approach with the Rorschach. Instead of a separate performance and inquiry phase of the examination, the subject is asked simple questions at the time of his initial response to each blot. The examiner's questions are designed to find out where the percept reported by the subject is located in the inkblot, what there is about the inkblot that suggests this percept, and anything else that the subject may wish to report. Each response can be scored for up to 22 standardized variables with a high degree of reliabilty.

The 92 inkblots composing the two parallel forms are the best of thousands of inkblots constructed over a period of 4 years. Systematic variation in form, color, shading, and symmetry resulted in a much richer set of inkblots than the original ten Rorschach plates. The first 30 inkblots in both Forms A and B were carefully paired on both stimulus and response characteristics to assure the equivalence of the two parallel forms. The last 15 blots were also balanced across the two forms, although they are not precisely matched in pairs. In a large number of studies, no differences in the two forms have been discovered for the standardized set of scoring variables.

The final order of presentation for the inkblots in each form is arranged so that many of the best inkblots appear early in the series. The two trial inkblots, X and Y, are identical in both Forms A and B. Card X is commonly seen as a winged creature (butterfly, bat, or moth) and is black and white in color with considerable inner detail shading. This card tends to establish a response set for giving whole responses which use the entire inkblot. It is very easy for most individuals. Card Y is black and symmetrical with a blotch of bright red in the center. A common response is "Two people" (ignoring the color) or "Spots of blood" (focusing only on the color). This

---

*Plates for Forms A and B, *HIT Administration and Scoring Guide*, individual and group Record Forms and Summary Sheets, and slide sets for group administration can be obtained from The Psychological Corporation, 757 Third Avenue, New York, New York 10017.

card tends to break up the whole response set and also introduces the subject to color in a "shocking" form for the first time. The regular test cards start with a black and white inkblot which is highly symmetrical and rather stylized and generally yields a popular response in one of the detailed areas, breaking up still further the tendency to give only a whole response. The remaining series have both achromatic and chromatic inkblots as well as symmetrical and asymmetrical blots arranged in a sufficiently random order to minimize any undesirable sequential effects. The details of the early developmental work on the HIT are described by Holtzman, Thorpe, Swartz, and Herron (1961). A summary of the development and standardization follows.

2. Development and Standardization of the Holtzman Inkblot Technique (HIT)

From the thousands of inkblots constructed over a period of several years, 135 were selected as the most likely to elicit diverse rich associations useful in personality assessment. Preliminary work had indicated that 45 inkblots with one response per card was about the limit for a standardized procedure. Preliminary testing of the blots was undertaken by administering random sets of 45 inkblots to a large number of patients in a local state mental hospital, as well as to a large number of college students. These two groups were selected because they represent opposite extremes on several broad personality variables of interest. Any inkblots which failed to differentiate these two extreme groups would probably be too insensitive for inclusion in any final version of the test.

Item statistics for the 135 blots were developed, paying closest attention to location of the response, appropriateness of the form, use of color and shading, specificity of the form in the response, and amount of movement projected into the response. The 135 inkblots were rated on a 5-point scale as to the extent to which they differentiated the college from hospital groups and as to the variability of response on the initial set of scored variables. All of these stimulus and response characteristics were taken into account for each of the 135 inkblots. The blots were paired according to the similarity of their characteristics, and one blot from each pair was assigned randomly to Form A while the other was placed in Form B. Only the best 90 blots were used in this manner to construct two parallel sets.

Standardized copies of the test required an expensive, slow process of photoengraving to ensure that the subtle shading nuances, blending of colors, and richness of the original blots were fully preserved. Standardization involved the specification of detailed procedures for administering and scoring the test, the collection of test protocols from large numbers of individuals representing a wide variety of well-defined populations, both normal and abnormal, and the development of extensive statistical information on the reliability and validity of measurement.

Using standard administration and scoring procedures developed for the purpose, nearly 2000 individual protocols were collected from a variety of institutions. Fifteen different populations were sampled to provide the basis for standardizing the HIT. One set of samples was chosen to represent a developmental continuum ranging from preschool children to mature adults. A second set of samples dealt with important nosological groups such as chronic schizophrenics, severe depressives, mental defectives, and organics. The initial standardization samples are outlined in Table 1.

Table 1. Summary of Initial Standardization Samples for the HIT[a]

Sample	Number of individuals	Number of protocols		
		Form A	Form B	Total
5-year-olds	122	62	60	122
Austin elementary	60	45	60	105
4th graders	72	—	72	72
7th graders	197	—	197	197
11th graders	72	72	72	144
Austin firemen	80	39	41	80
Housewives	100	50	50	100
UT college	143	143	143	286
UT superior	92	92	—	92
Austin college	66	66	48	114
Waco schizophrenic	99	—	99	99
Montrose schizophrenic	41	19	22	41
Woodward retarded	50	—	50	50
Austin retarded	50	—	50	50
VA depressed	90	48	42	90
Total	1334	636	1006	1642

[a]Adapted from Table 5-1 in Holtzman, Thorpe, Swartz, & Herron (1961).

3. Administration and Scoring

Standard procedures have been developed for administering the HIT so that reported normative data can be used as an aid in interpretation. Instructions to the subject have been designed to make the task as simple as possible while eliciting sufficient information to score major variables reliably. The basic problem is one of encouraging the subject to respond fully without at the same time revealing to him the specific nature of the variables to be scored.

A Record Form and a Summary Sheet are available for the examiner to use in recording responses and scoring. Schematic diagrams for the inkblots are reproduced in miniature on the Record Form so that the specific area used for a given response can be outlined by the examiner at the time of the response. Scores for the 22 standardized variables are recorded in the appropriate boxes on the Summary Sheet after completion of the administration. Reaction time is entered on the Record Form at the time of administration and transferred later to the Summary Sheet.

After establishing initial rapport with the subject, the examiner picks up the cards, one at a time, handing each one in upright position to the subject. Instructions should be informal, somewhat along the following lines:

> I have here a set of inkblots which were made by dropping ink on paper and folding it. I'd like you to look at each inkblot and tell me what it might look like, what it might represent, or what it could be. Since these are only inkblots, there are no right or wrong answers and each blot looks like different things to different people. It's possible for a person to see several things in each inkblot, but I want you to give me only *one* response for each card. After you see something and tell me about it, I'll ask you some questions, because I want to see it in the same way you do. I'll be writing down what you say and making note of the time, but you may take as long as you wish on each card. Do you have any questions?

Immediately following each response, the brief inquiry by the examiner informally stresses some variation of the following three questions: "Where in the blot do you see a _____?" "What is there about the blot that makes it look like a _____?" and "Is there anything else you care to tell me about it?" The actual inquiry can be kept to a minimum for most subjects, who comprehend the nature of the task very quickly. A skilled examiner, sensitive to subtle nuances in the examiner-subject interaction, can control the flow of conversation by stimulating a reticent individual and slowing down a verbose person.

Most of the 22 standardized variables for the HIT can be readily traced to earlier systems of analysis employed in coding and scoring the Rorschach. Four criteria were especially important in formulating variables for the scoring system. First, a variable had to be one which could be scored for any legitimate response, making it at least theoretically possible for a score to range from 0 to 45 when given unitary weight. Second, the variable had to be sufficiently objective to permit high scoring agreement among trained individuals. Third, the variable had to show some a priori promise of being relevant to the study of personality through perception. And, fourth, each variable had to be logically independent of the others wherever possible so that the maximum amount of information could be coded in the most flexible, efficient manner. The name, abbreviation, brief definition, and scoring weights for each of the 22 variables when applied to a single response are given below:

Reaction Time (*RT*). The time in seconds from the presentation of the inkblot to the beginning of the primary response.

Rejection (*R*). Score 1 when subject returns inkblot to examiner without giving a scorable response; otherwise, score 0.

Location (*L*). Tendency to break down blot into smaller fragments. Score 0 for use of whole blot, 1 for large area, and 2 for smaller area.

Space (*S*). Score 1 for true figure-ground reversals; otherwise, score 0.

Form Definiteness (*FD*). The definiteness of the form of the concept reported, regardless of the goodness of fit to the inkblot. A 5-point scale with 0 for very vague and 4 for highly specific.

Form Appropriateness (*FA*). The goodness of fit of the form of the percept to the form of the inkblot. Score 0 for poor, 1 for fair, and 2 for good.

Color (*C*). The apparent primacy of color (including black, gray, or white) as a response determinant. Score 0 for no use of color, 1 for use secondary to form (like Rorschach *FC*), 2 when used as primary determinant but some form present (like *CF*), and 3 when used as a primary determinant with no form present (like *C*).

Shading (*Sh*). The apparent primacy of shading as response-determinant (texture, depth, or vista). Score 0 for no use of shading, 1 when used in secondary manner, and 2 when used as primary determinant with little or no form present.

Movement (*M*). The energy level of movement or potential movement ascribed to the percept, regardless of content. Score 0 for none, 1 for static potential, 2 for casual, 3 for dynamic, and 4 for violent movement.

Pathognomic Verbalization (*V*).   Degree of autistic, bizarre thinking evident in the response as rated on a 5-point scale. Score 0 where no pathology is present. The nine categories of *V* and the range of scoring weights for each is as follows: Fabulation, 1; Fabulized Combination, 2, 3, 4; Queer Response, 1, 2, 3; Incoherence, 4; Autistic Logic, 1, 2, 3, 4; Contamination, 2, 3, 4; Self Reference, 2, 3, 4; Deterioration Color, 2, 3, 4; Absurd Response, 3.

Integration (*I*).   Score 1 for the organization of two or more adequately perceived blot elements into a larger whole; otherwise, score 0.

Human (*H*).   Degree of human quality in the content of response. Score 0 for none, 1 for parts of humans, distortions, or cartoons, and 2 for whole human beings or elaborated human faces.

Animal (*A*).   Degree of animal quality in the content. Score 0 for none (including animal objects and microscopic life), 1 for animal parts, bugs, or insects, and 2 for whole animals.

Anatomy (*At*).   Degree of "gutlike" quality in the content. Score 0 for none, 1 for bones, X-rays, or medical drawings, and 2 for visceral and crude anatomy.

Sex (*Sx*).   Degree of sexual quality in the content. Score 0 for no sexual reference, 1 for socially accepted sexual activity or expressions (buttocks, bust, kissing), and 2 for blatant sexual content (penis, vagina).

Abstract (*Ab*).   Degree of abstract quality in the content. Score 0 for none, 1 for abstract elements along with other elements having form, and 2 for purely abstract content ("Bright colors remind me of gaiety").

Anxiety (*Ax*).   Signs of anxiety in the fantasy content as indicated by emotions and attitudes, expressive behavior, symbolism, or cultural stereotypes of fear. Score 0 for none, 1 for questionable or indirect signs, and 2 for overt or clear-cut evidence.

Hostility (*Hs*).   Signs of hostility in the fantasy content. Scored on a 4-point scale ranging from 0 for none to 3 for direct, violent, interpersonal destruction.

Barrier (*Br*).   Score 1 for reference to any protective covering, membrane, shell, or skin that might be symbolically related to the perception of body-image boundaries; otherwise, score 0.

Penetration (*Pn*).   Score 1 for concept which might be symbolic of an individual's feeling that his body exterior is of little protective value and can be easily penetrated; otherwise, score 0.

Balance (*B*).   Score 1 where there is overt concern for the symmetry-asymmetry feature of the inkblot; otherwise, score 0.

Popular (*P*).   Each form contains 25 inkblots in which one or more popular percepts occur. "Popular" in the standardization studies means that a percept had to occur at least 14% of the time among normal subjects. Score 1 for popular core concepts (or their precision alternatives) as listed in the scoring manual; otherwise, score 0.

Summary scores for the 22 variables are obtained by adding the weights for a given variable across the 45 inkblots. Three variables, Form Definiteness, Form Appropriateness, and Pathognomic Verbalization, are corrected for the number of rejections in order to provide an estimate of what the score would have been if the subject had given a response to each of the 45 cards. This correction can be done either by formula or by a printed table. Earlier studies indicated that such a correction was not necessary for the remaining variables in the system.

Studies conducted as part of the initial standardization for the HIT reveal a high degree of interscorer agreement for all 22 variables. Only Penetration and Integration fall below reliabilities of .95, and in many cases the reliability approaches 1.00. Because the system is different from the Rorschach, some experienced clinicians have difficulty shifting to the HIT. In most cases, however, the published scoring manuals provide all the information needed for either a neophyte or an experienced clinician to learn the scoring system in a matter of a few hours.

Extensions of the original scoring system have also been reported by various investigators. In most cases, these consist of minor differentiations of additional content such as "explosions" or "eyes" which are of special interest in certain cases. In her extensive clinical work with the HIT, Hill (1972) has differentiated color and shading to a higher degree than in the original standardization. Clinical application of the vista, texture, and film subscores for the shading response and of color responses relative to high and low stimulus strength of the inkblot has been described in some detail by Hill in her handbook on the HIT.

4. Reliability of Scores

Both internal consistency and test-retest reliability for the standardized scores in the HIT have been reported extensively by Holtzman et al. (1961). Split-half reliabilities determined by computing the correlations between scores based on odd-numbered and even-numbered blocks are generally high. Median values for 50 different samples in the initial standardization work were generally in the .70s and .80s. Only Anxiety, Penetration, and Popular fell below this level, while Reaction Time, Rejection, and Location had average reliability coefficients of .90. These initial results have been repeatedly confirmed in more recent studies in the United States, Mexico, and elsewhere (Holtzman, Diaz-Guerrero, & Swartz, 1975).

The initial standardization studies included four samples in which both Form A and B were given to the same subjects, with intervals ranging from 1 week to 1 year between the two testing sessions. Test-retest correlations generally ranged from .36 for Popular to .81 for Location for normal adults. Similar results were obtained in a cross-cultural longitudinal study of large numbers of schoolchildren in the United States and Mexico, as reported by Holtzman et al. (1975).

Location, Reaction Time, Form Definiteness, Movement, and Human are the most stable of the inkblot scores across repeated testing with a year's interval between sessions. Rejection, Form Appropriateness, Shading, Pathognomic Verbalization, Barrier, and Penetration tend to have lower stability coefficients, values ranging from the .30's to the .50's, with occasional coefficients as high as the .60's and .70's. Test-retest stability increases with an increase in the age of a child and is highest for adults.

The longitudinal study also reveals that after an interval of 5 years between testing, stability coefficients for Shading, Pathognomic Verbalization, Animal, and Penetration dropped to an insignificant level. Location, however, showed a higher degree of stability over a 5-year period (.51) than was true of any of the subtests of the Wechsler Intelligence Scale for Children, which had also been given to the Mexican and American children in this extensive study. With an interval of 3 or 4 years between testing sessions, all variables showed significant stability over time.

The 6-year longitudinal study of schoolchildren also yielded some interesting information concerning practice and adaptation effects for HIT scores when the test is used repeatedly on the same individuals, alternating Forms A and B. Children of all ages in both cultures tended to use smaller detailed areas more frequently as the test was repeated. Most of this adaptation took place between the first and second years of testing. On the average, about 5 points on the Location Scale could be attributed to adaptation even though the interval between testing was an entire year. In spite of such adaptation, however, the stability of individual differences through time was very high. Most of the other scores revealed no adaptation effects with repeated testing.

In summary, it can be concluded that the reliability of the HIT scores is generally as high as the reliability of mental test scores, whether considered in terms of internal consistency measures or in terms of test-retest stability over time.

5. Dimensions Revealed by Factor Analysis

Intercorrelations were routinely computed among the 22 inkblot variables, and factor analyses were carried out independently for each of the 15 basic standardization samples to determine the common dimensions underlying inkblot perception and how they may differ in patterning from one population to the next. Almost invariably, five or six factors are necessary to explain the obtained intercorrelations. The first three factors are the most important and have emerged repeatedly, regardless of the population studied. It is useful to keep in mind the six most common factor groupings of HIT variables when considering clinical applications of the HIT in personality assessment of individuals. Highlights of these six factors follow, with particular reference to recent replications on children in the United States and Mexico.

5.1. Factor I

Movement, Integration, and Human invariably have high loading on Factor I. Form Definiteness and Popular tend to vary somewhat from one population to the next. Location, Anxiety, Hostility, and Barrier often show high loadings on this factor, although in no consistent fashion. For younger children, Anxiety and Hostility are more likely to be high on Factor I than for teenagers or adults. A high amount of Factor I is generally interpreted as indicative of well-organized ideational activity, good imaginative capacity, well-differentiated ego boundaries, and awareness of conventional concepts.

5.2. Factor II

Color, Shading, and Form Definiteness (reversed) generally have high loadings on Factor II in every population. Occasional negative loadings for Location are consistent with findings that high use of color and shading is associated with use of the whole inkblot rather than small areas. Among younger children, significant negative loadings on Factor II appear for Animal, suggesting that children tend to use color and shading as stimulus determinants only when they cannot find a familiar animal form. The positive pole of Factor II indicates overreactivity to color or shading, while the negative pole shows primary concern for form alone as a determinant.

5.3. Factor III

Pathognomic Verbalization, Movement, Anxiety, and Hostility are the primary variables defining Factor III. Very high scores on these variables can be considered strong evidence of psychopathology and uncontrolled bizarreness (Holtzman et al., 1961; Connors, 1965; Hill, 1972). Among children, Factor III tends to be correlated with Factor I, making separation of the two factors in an orthogonal solution difficult. Among normal children, moderately high scores on Factor III are indicative of affective expressivity and loose imagination in fantasy productions. Two other variables, Penetration and Anatomy, are also often associated with the primary variables in Factor III.

5.4. Factor IV

Location and Form Appropriateness generally appear as defining variables for Factor IV. The more an individual delves into small detail while responding to inkblots, the more likely that he will find a percept for which the form of the blot is highly appropriate. Anatomy, Barrier, and Penetration tend to have negative loadings on this factor. Factor IV is bipolar in nature, the positive pole tending to indicate perceptual differentiation coupled with a critical sense of good form, while the negative pole appears indicative of immaturity, diffuse bodily preoccupation, and possibly psychopathology.

5.5. Factor V

Minor Factor V is defined primarily by Reaction Time and Rejection, which tend to be closely associated for obvious reasons. The longer a person takes to look at an inkblot before he gives a response, the more likely he is to reject the card without seeing anything in it. It is interesting to note that Factor V is a significant dimension orthogonal to the first four factors, indicating that an individual's performance on other inkblot scores is generally independent of his reaction time or the number of cards he rejects.

5.6. Factor VI

Factor VI appears most strongly among schizophrenic populations and is usually defined by Anatomy, Sex, and Abstract. The factor rarely appears among children, and only occasionally is present for other adult samples.

5.7. Variance of Clusters

These factors demonstrate empirically what many earlier clinicians intuitively interpreted as logical clusters of inkblot variables for purposes of personality assessment. Although the amount of variance common among the defining variables for such factors is sizable, in nearly every case each of the 22 variables still has sufficient, reliable, unique variance to justify consideration of the variable in its own right. For this reason, it is still useful in clinical analysis to examine performance on the individual variables rather than considering only the factors themselves.

6. Variations in Standard Form

Two standardized, group-administered variations of the HIT have been developed and published. One involved the use of colored slides and a special booklet for group administration (Swartz & Holtzman, 1963). A short form of this particular method using only 30 cards rather than all 45 has been developed and shows promise for training purposes (Herron, 1963). The other major group method that has been standardized uses the same colored slides but substitutes a streamlined record form on which the subject writes a brief response and checks the amount of the blot used for the percept (Gorham, 1967).

Gorham, Moseley, and Hill have developed a system for scoring 17 of the HIT variables by high-speed computer (Moseley, Gorham, & Hill, 1963; Gorham, 1967; Gorham, 1970).* An empirically derived dictionary containing about 4000 words has been compiled in English, Spanish, and Portuguese to facilitate cross-cultural studies. Each word in the dictionary has been assigned multiple scoring weights by an individual experienced in scoring HIT variables. The weights have been double-checked and refined by independent expert review. Stored in the computer, the dictionary provides an automatic scoring system in any language for which words and weights have been compiled. Agreement between hand and computer scoring of the same protocols is very high in spite of the fact that syntax is taken into account by the computer program only in a rudimentary way.

The group method of administration is particularly effective because the HIT has a simple format involving only one response per card. Some of the most important clinical variables, however, cannot be dealt with except in the individual method of administration. Form Appropriateness, Pathognomic Verbalization, Reaction Time, Space, and Balance are not scorable in the group method. The method is also limited to individuals who are sufficiently literate and cooperative that they can follow the simple directions and write out their responses properly on the record form.

Split-half reliability and test-retest stability using parallel forms with a 1-week interval are as high for the group method as for the individual. In one study comparing the two methods given to the same subjects 1 week apart, only five of the 18 ink-blot scores that were analyzed showed any significant mean differences attributable to method of administration (Holtzman, Moseley, Reinehr, & Abbott, 1963). Location, Space, and Color scores were higher for the group method, while Barrier and Popular scores were higher for the individual method. Standard deviations of scores were the same for all variables except Anxiety, which had a higher variance in the group method. Comparing the cross-method correlations in a multitrait-multimethod matrix revealed a striking degree of similarity across the two methods.

A more recent extension of the computer-scored HIT involves a computer-based system for personality interpretation that uses extensive normative data and studies of group differences among psychiatric patients as a basis for the system. Evidence from studies with both the Rorschach and the HIT supports some person-

---

*Information on computer scoring services can be obtained from HIT Scoring Service, ARBEC, Inc., 3909G North I.H. 35, Austin, Texas 78722.

ality interpretations while refuting others. The availability of objective norms for HIT scores based on large samples provides a basis for codifying complex patterns of scores to derive new configural scores that are close to those often used in the clinical assessment of personality (Holtzman & Gorham, 1972).

Several hundred rules dealing with various aspects of personality that are purported to be revealed by patterns of inkblot scores were constructed on the basis of Hill's handbook for interpretation of the HIT (Hill, 1972). These patterns were then refined by panels of experienced clinical psychologists and reduced to 60 carefully defined patterns which were then coded and stored in a specially constructed computer program. An exploratory study of their validity was undertaken using 58 normal men (naval enlistees), 78 neurotics, and 100 depressed patients as criterion samples. A large reference group of normals provided percentile norms for decision points on each score in a given pattern. Whenever the specific conditions for a given rule were met, the computer printed out the accompanying interpretive statement. A set of such statements constituted a "personality description" for a given individual.

Analysis of the frequency of occurrence of each rule among individuals in the three samples revealed highly significant differentiation for 28 of the rules. Diagnosing normality in a positive sense was the most difficult to achieve; only two statements proved to be highly significant. Good Form Definiteness coupled with high Integration and whole responses cleanly differentiated 10% of the normals while yielding no false positives among the neurotics and depressed patients. High achievement motivation was revealed by above-average Integration coupled with high Barrier, a predominance of whole responses, and low Rejection; this pattern correctly diagnosed 10% of the normals while picking up 2% of the neurotics and 1% of the depressed patients.

A slightly easier task was the differential diagnosis of depressed patients from normals and neurotics. Five configurations of scores produced no false positives among the normals and neurotics, but unfortunately the frequency of occurrence among depressed patients was less than 10%. A high number of rejections, revealing minor blocking of ideational activity, occurred among 26% of the depressed as contrasted to only 12% or 13% of the normals and neurotics, respectively.

Diagnosing the neurotics was the easiest task. Very high Shading plus very high Anxiety (greater than the 98th percentile for normals) was characteristic of 25% of the neurotics and only 1% of the other subjects. High Human, Color, and Shading, high Penetration coupled with low Human, and several other patterns were also diagnostically significant for neurotics.

This completely objective scoring of the HIT and the generation by the computer of personality patterns that are significant for differential diagnosis constitute a promising approach for large-scale screening purposes. It also sheds considerable light on the meaning of inkblot variables and the clinical validity of interpretations as summarized in Hill's handbook for clinical applications of the HIT. A much more detailed description of this approach has been presented elsewhere (Holtzman, 1975).

Specialized sets of inkblots and deliberately altered methods of administration can be readily developed from the extensive item-analysis information available on each inkblot (Holtzman et al., 1961, for individual form; Swartz, Witzke, & Megargee, 1970, for group form). It is a fairly simple matter to establish experimental subsets for the study of unusual variables such as Space, Abstract, or Balance. For example, Sanders (1976) developed a special set of inkblots by choosing only those blots from the set of 92 for which Space responses were given with a reasonable frequency in the item-analysis tables. He found a significant positive correlation between Space and aggression as measured by the Jackson Personality Research Form. A negative correlation was obtained between Space and autonomy.

The item-analysis information can also be employed to establish smaller subsets of parallel forms. For example, Palmer (1963) constructed six sets of 15 cards for each repeated measurement in the study of sleep deprivation over many days in a small number of subjects.

Still another variation in the standard form involves the development of a multiple-choice method. Fisher and Cleveland (1968) were among the first to develop a series of multiple-choice items using 40 of the HIT blots for measuring Barrier and Penetration. The particular inkblots were selected on the basis of preliminary item-analysis data prior to completing and printing the final versions of Forms A and B. Each of the 40 items has three fairly acceptable choices—one representing a Barrier response (such as "Knight-in armor"), one representing a Penetration response (such as "X-ray"), and one which is neutral (such as "Flower"). A more recent example of a multiple-choice inkblot test is the Atypical Response Scale for measuring form-inappropriate whole responses, developed by Mendelsohn and Linden (972). Such multiple-choice forms are of interest only where there is a specific variable for which an objective measure is needed.

7. Studies of Validity

What can be said about the psychological meaning of inkblot variables? How do such variables relate to each other and to independent measures of personality? Are they of value in a differential diagnosis of mental or emotional disorders? The question "What is the validity of the HIT?" has no meaning unless the purpose for which the method is to be used can be specified in some detail. Since conceivably a technique may be used for many purposes, it may prove highly valid in one situation and totally invalid in another.

Initial studies of validity were conducted as part of the original standardization of the HIT. Three general methods were employed. First, intercorrelations and factor analyses were carried out for all of the standardization samples to determine the common dimensions underlying inkblot perception and how they may differ in patterning from one population to the next. The general results of this set of factor analyses have already been summarized. Second, external correlates of inkblot variables were determined and used as a basis for testing earlier hypotheses taken from the Rorschach, as well as for providing new empirical data bearing on the interpretation of personality. And, third, numerous significant differences among well-defined samples were discovered which shed further light on the meaning of inkblot variables while also providing a basis for psychodiagnosis of the individual.

As indicated earlier, the six dimensions typically found in factor analyses of the HIT are very similar to earlier work with the Rorschach, although the dimensions themselves are more clearly defined in the HIT. These factor analyses form the primary basis for most interpretive systems that have been developed for the HIT (see Hill, 1972).

Several hundred studies have been reported in the past 15 years dealing with external correlates of HIT variables. Only the highlights of these studies can be presented here. One obvious comparison is that involving the standard Rorschach and the standard HIT. In one study by Bock, Haggard, Holtzman, Anne Beck, and Samuel Beck (1963), a systematic comparison was made between Rorschach and HIT protocols obtained from 72 eleventh graders on two different occasions 3 months apart—a total of four inkblot protocols per subject. The Rorschachs were scored by Beck, using Beck's system of analysis. Eight scores within the two systems were sufficiently comparable in a priori definitions to justify direct correlations between them. While no really satisfactory method is available for partialing out R in the Rorschach because of its complex, curvilinear correlation with most other scores, each score was converted into an average value per response by dividing the score by R, thereby overcoming a major component of confounding. In every case, the obtained correlation between the HIT and the Rorschach was significant beyond the .01 level in the expected direction. When corrected for attenuation due to unreliability, correlations ranged from .51 to 1.00 for Shading, Human Movement, Color, Human, and Animal (Holtzman et al., 1961).

Correlations between inkblot scores and scores in self-report personality inventories generally are low. The largest number of studies have compared Anxiety and Hostility from the HIT with various questionnaire measures of anxiety and hostility. Typical of these studies is one by Fehr (1976) in which the IPAT Anxiety Scale Questionnaire (ASQ) and the Manifest Hostility Scale (MHS) were correlated with Anxiety and Hostility scores from the HIT for 72 college students. The ASQ correlated .35 with Anxiety, but only .17 with Hostility, while the MHS correlated .43 with Hostility and only .19 with Anxiety. Cook, Iacino, Murray, and Auerbach (1973) found that Anxiety correlated significantly with a measure of state anxiety but not one trait anxiety from the State-Trait Anxiety Inventory. In a later study, Iacino and Cook (1974) found a significant correlation between Anxiety on the HIT and a measure of trait anxiety from the State-Trait Anxiety Inventory. Experimental studies of adults under stress by Kamen (1971) demonstrate the ability of the HIT to detect state anxiety. High scores on HIT Anxiety are also significantly correlated with poor tolerance for pain (Nichols & Tursky, 1967).

One would not expect much correlation between fantasy measure of anxiety and hostility in the HIT and self-report measures of similar traits using paper-and-pencil questionnaires. Nor is it likely that peer ratings of socially observable traits would have much in common with inkblot scores except in unusual circumstances. Scales from self-inventory personality questionnaires usually have high reliability and often correlate with socially observable behavior. Such correlations, however, can generally be traced to the fact that the individual has a conscious self-concept that dominates his test responses and is not unrelated to his social behavior as judged by others. It should be kept in mind that Anxiety and Hostility from the HIT are strictly ratings at a fantasy level which are not necessarily related in any simple, direct way to overt behavior that is judged to be anxious and hostile. More to the point is the fact that HIT Anxiety and Hostility are useful in the psychodiagnosis of neurosis, as evidenced by the study mentioned earlier differentiating neurotics from normals and depressed patients. Of interest also is the study by Rosenstiel (1966) indicating that Anxiety and Hostility increased substantially for individuals who were exposed experimentally to gruesome passages from a Poe story.

The most extensive study involving external correlates of inkblot variables is the cross-cultural longitudinal investigation involving over 800 children in Mexico and the United States reported by Holtzman et al. (1975). Several inkblot scores proved to be significantly associated with certain scales from the Jackson Personality Research Form. High color scores were correlated with high scores on Exhibitionism, Impulsiveness, and Nurturance, all in the expected direction based on Rorschach's theory concerning the meaning of color. Integration was positively correlated with the Understanding scale, a finding also in the expected direction since Understanding relates to intellectual capacity.

Many studies indicate that Movement has a significant cognitive component. Repeatedly significant correlations ranging as high as .42 were obtained between Movement and WISC Vocabulary in all the age groups in both Mexico and the United States in the cross-cultural study. This bivariate relationship is about as high as the internal correlation among certain of the WISC subtests. Factor analytic studies of the same populations reveal that Movement deals particularly with the expressive, imaginative aspects of verbal ability rather than with factual information, word meanings, and analytical problem solving. Consistent with this interpretation is the earlier finding by Mueller and Abeles (1964) that Movement possibly is related to the degree of empathy in counselors. Clark, Veldman, and Thorpe (1965) found that Movement is correlated with divergent thinking ability in talented adolescents, a finding corroborated by Insua (1972) in a study of problem-solving processes in college students. Movement rises markedly with increasing age until early adolescence (Thorpe & Swartz, 1965).

The underlying meaning of Movement has been clarified in part by a series of experimental studies. Lerner (1966) found that dream deprivation in sleep produced an increase in quantity of projected movement, offering support for Rorschach's views on the fundamental similarity between movement and dreams due to the centrality of kinesthetic experience in both. A series of studies by Greenberg and Fisher (1973) demonstrated that, in women, Movement increased markedly in a variety of conditions involving heightened muscle awareness.

Barrier and Penetration have also been studied extensively because of their direct relevance to body image and personality. Increased Barrier scores were found to result from body awareness training in schizophrenics (Darby, 1970). Low Barrier scores together with high Color were found to be predictive of poor performance in the Peace Corps (Holtzman, Santos, Bouquet, & Barth, 1966). Decreased Penetration scores were discovered after body awareness training in mental retardation (Chasey, Swartz, & Chasey, 1974). Fisher (1970) has reviewed additional literature concerning Barrier and Penetration as measures of body image and personality.

The third method of assessing the validity of HIT variables is the most relevant to clinical application and involves studies of intergroup differences and differential diagnosis. The initial standardization studies included mental retardates, chronic schizophrenics, and depressives, as well as normal individuals ranging in age from 5-year-old children to middle-aged adults. Additional normative data have been published by Hill (1972) for emotionally disturbed children, emotionally disturbed adolescents, juvenile delinquents, neurotic adults, and alcoholics. Differences in means and standard deviations across these groups are often striking and are in a direction to be expected from earlier Rorschach theory. Similar results have been obtained by Shukla (1976), who worked primarily with Pathognomic Verbalization in the differential diagnosis of organics, schizophrenics, neurotics, and normals in India.

Using data from the initial HIT standardization studies, Moseley (1963) developed an objective approach to differential diagnosis by finding the best linear combinations of HIT variables and then cross-validating them on independent samples. He was able to classify accurately 82% of the normals from schizophrenics, 71% of the normals from depressed patients, and 78% of the depressives from schizophrenics. When Pathognomic Verbalization was added to his model for use with doubtful middle-range cases, the efficiency of differential diagnosis was improved even more.

Differentiating patients with chronic brain syndrome from normal aging adults is possible with the HIT, using the procedures developed by Overall and Gorham (1972) based on over 300 Veterans Administration domiciliary members. A different patterning of test scores was identified with the separation of the chronic brain syndrome group from the normal aging groups. While results based on the Wechsler Adult Intelligence Scale subtests and on the 17 HIT variables for the group method were substantially similar, a discriminant function analysis using both sets of data provided maximum separation of aging and chronic brain syndrome groups. Differentiating brain-damaged patients from schizophrenic patients is more difficult, as evidenced by the failure of HIT variables to differ significantly between small samples of heterogeneous brain-damaged patients and heterogeneous schizophrenics (Velez-Diaz, 1976). Large samples of well-defined, organically impaired patients are needed in order to develop more effective psychodiagnostic procedures based on HIT scores.

Developmental norms for preschool children, elementary and secondary children, as well as normal adults provide a useful basis for interpretation of an individual protocol. Norms for the computer-scored HIT (Gorham, Moseley, & Holtzman, 1968) based on over 5000 cases have been presented for schizophrenics, depressives, psychoneurotics, alcoholics, and chronic brain syndrome patients, as well as normal adults from the United States and 16 different countries around the world. These reference groups provide a strong basis for the development of systems of differential diagnosis.

The best single variable for revealing pathology in thought processes is Pathognomic Verbalization, the one variable in the HIT that requires some clinical experience and can be scored only for the individual method of the HIT, not the group. In a study of normals vs. schizophrenics, Swartz (1970) found that normals tend to produce more fabulation and fabulized combinations, while schizophrenics tend to give more contaminations, autistic logic, and self-reference responses. Among normal children, fabulized responses increase with increasing age, while autistic logic, contamination, and absurd reponses drop significantly. Qualitative differences in Pathognomic Verbalization are quite striking among the various populations for which norms have been compiled. As one would expect, schizophrenics give far more Pathognomic Verbalization than other groups. Among gifted normals, artists yield significantly higher scores on Pathognomic Verbalization, Anatomy, and Sex than do engineers or architects (Holtzman, Swartz, & Thorpe, 1971). It is also interesting to note that engineers obtained significantly lower scores on Human while architects obtained higher scores on Integration and Balance in this comparison of HIT scores for artists, architects, and engineers, highly significant differences in the predicted direction.

Still another kind of validation involves the longitudinal study of individuals who have been given the HIT initially and for whom criterion data are obtained at a later date. Such predictive validity is difficult to establish, usually requiring years of study and careful research planning. A 9-year follow-up investigation of 46 first-grade children was reported by Currie, Holtzman, and Swartz (1974). School counselors and teachers who knew the children well were interviewed and were asked to rate each child on a 4-point scale of personal adjustment ranging from "well-adjusted" to "serious problems," focusing mainly on the child's self-concept and relationship with others. Children with high scores at age 6 on the Factor III variables Pathognomic Verbalization, Anxiety, and Hostility were those who developed severe problems of emotional adjustment or behavior disorders 9 years later.

Four of the variables in the HIT—Space, Sex, Abstract, and Balance—generally have been overlooked in most of the research to date. These variables are relatively uncommon, although they do occur with sufficient frequency in some populations to justify more systematic efforts aimed at improving the measures. One approach is to select subsets of inkblots chosen specifically to elicit these particular variables, as was done by Sanders (1976) in his study of Space. Additional variables can also be derived from the HIT, particularly where there is a special interest in selected aspects of inkblot perception, such as Color (Hill, 1966). The content of inkblot responses is especially well suited to such treatment, as evidenced by Endicott's Suspiciousness score (1972) and "eye" responses (Coleman, 1966; Fernald & Stolurow, 1971). A great deal of work has been done with the body image scores, Barrier and Penetration, and there is no reason why other specialized content scores would not prove equally useful.

8. Conclusion

Many investigations using the HIT have been omitted in this brief review of the technique. An annotated bibliography of over 400 articles, monographs, and books on the HIT has been stored on magnetic tape in computerized form where frequent updating and printout on demand can be done easily (Swartz, Witzke, Holtzman, & Bishop, 1978). A handbook for clinical application (Hill, 1972), a workbook for the HIT (Hill & Peixotto, 1973), and clinical interpretation forms (Megargee & Velez-Diaz, 1971; Hill, 1972) have greatly augmented the original materials published in 1961. Extensive reviews of studies dealing with the HIT have also been published by Holtzman (1968, 1975) and Gamble (1972). Translation of the original materials and supplementary manuals into a number of other languages has extended the possibilities for cross-cultural studies and clinical applications in other societies.

The steadily growing acceptance of the HIT as an important assessment technique to be used in a wide variety of practical situations as well as for research speaks well for its future. The basic stimuli are unusually rich. The standardized HIT has clear psychometric advantages over the Rorschach, and yet the subtle qualitative nuances essential for a deeper clinical interpretation are fully present.

9. References

Bock, D. R., Haggard, E. A., Holtzman, W. H., Beck, A. G., & Beck, S. J. *A comprehensive psychometric study of the Rorschach and Holtzman Inkblot techniques.* Chapel Hill: Psychometric Laboratory, University of North Carolina, 1963.

Chasey, W. C., Swartz, J. D., & Chasey, C. G. Effect of motor development on body image scores in institutionalized mentally retarded children. *American Journal of Mental Deficiency*, 1974, *78*, 440–445.

Clark, C. M., Veldman, D. J., & Thorpe, J. S. Convergent and divergent thinking abilities of talented adolescents. *Journal of Educational Psychology*, 1965, *56*, 157–163.

Coleman, K. A. The significance of eye responses on the Holtzman Inkblot Technique as measured by the Minnesota Counseling Inventory. *Springfield College Studies*, 1966, *1*, 41

Conners, C. K. Effects of brief psychotherapy, drugs, and type of disturbance on Holtzman Inkblot scores in children. *Proceedings of the 73rd annual convention of the American Psychological Association*, 1965, pp. 201–202.

Cook, P. E., Iacino, L. W., Murray, J., & Auerbach, S. M. Holtzman Inkblot anxiety and shading scores related to state and trait anxiety. *Journal of Personality Assessment*, 1973, *37*, 337–339.

Currie, S. F., Holtzman, W. H., & Swartz, J. D. Early indicators of personality traits viewed retrospectively. *Journal of School Psychology*, 1974, *12*, 51–59.

Darby, J. A. Alteration of some body image indexes in schizophrenics. *Journal of Consulting and Clinical Psychology*, 1970, *35*, 116–121.

Endicott, N. A. The Holtzman Inkblot Technique content measures of depression and suspiciousness. *Journal of Personality Assessment*, 1972, *36*, 424–426.

Fehr, L. A. Construct validity of the Holtzman Inkblot anxiety and hostility scores. *Journal of Personality Assessment*, 1976, *40*, 483–486.

Fernald, P. S., & Stolurow, K. A. Projected eye responses and sensitivity to the opinion of others. *Journal of Clinical Psychology*, 1971, *27*, 258–259.

Fisher, S. *Body experience in fantasy and behavior*. New York: Appleton-Century-Crofts, 1970.

Fisher, S., & Cleveland, S. E. *Body image and personality* (2nd rev. ed.). New York: Dover, 1968.

Gamble, K. R. The Holtzman Inkblot Technique: A review. *Psychological Bulletin*, 1972, *77*, 172–194.

Gorham, D. R. Validity and reliability studies of computer-based scoring system for inkblot responses. *Journal of Consulting Psychology*, 1967, *31*, 65–70.

Gorham, D. R. Cross-cultural research based on the Holtzman Inkblot Technique. *International Congress of the Rorschach and Other Projective Techniques*, 1970, *7*, 158–164.

Gorham, D. R., Moseley, E. C., & Holtzman, W. H. Norms for the computer scored Holtzman Inkblot Technique. *Perceptual and Motor Skills Monograph Supplement*, 1968, *26*, 1279–1305.

Greenberg, R. P., & Fisher, S. A muscle awareness model for changes in Rorschach human movement responses. *Journal of Personality Assessment*, 1973, *37*, 512–518.

Harrower-Erickson, M. R., & Steiner, M. E. *Large scale Rorschach techniques*. Springfield, Ill.: Thomas, 1945.

Herron, E. W. Psychometric characteristics of a thirty-item version of the group method of the Holtzman Inkblot Technique. *Journal of Clinical Psychology*, 1963, *19*, 450–453.

Hill, E. F. Affect aroused by color, a function of stimulus strength. *Journal of Projective Techniques and Personality Assessment*, 1966, *10*, 23–30.

Hill, E. F. *The Holtzman Inkblot Technique: A handbook for clinical application*. San Francisco: Jossey-Bass, 1972.

Hill, E. F., & Peixotto, H. E. *Workbook for the Holtzman Inkblot Technique*. New York: The Psychological Corporation, 1973.

Holtzman, W. H. The Holtzman Inkblot Technique. In A. I. Rabin (Ed.), *Introduction to modern projective techniques*. New York: Springer, 1968, pp. 136–170.

Holtzman, W. H. New developments in Holtzman Inkblot Technique. In P. McReynolds (Ed.), *Advances in psychological assessment* (Vol. 3). San Francisco: Jossey-Bass, 1975.

Holtzman, W. H., Diaz-Guerrero, R., & Swartz, J. D. *Personality development in two cultures*. Austin: The University of Texas Press, 1975.

Holtzman, W. H., & Gorham, D. R. Automated scoring and interpretation of the group-administered Holtzman Inkblot Technique by computer. *Proceedings of the 80th annual convention of the American Psychological Association*, 1972.

Holtzman, W. H., Moseley, E. D., Reinehr, R. C., & Abbott, E. Comparison of the group method and the standard individual version of the Holtzman Technique. *Journal of Clinical Psychology*, 1963, *19*, 441–449.

Holtzman, W. H., Santos, J. F., Bouquet, S., & Barth, P. *The Peace Corps in Brazil: An evaluation of the Sao Francisco Valley project*. Austin: International Office, University of Texas, 1966.

Holtzman, W. H., Swartz, J. D., & Thorpe, J. S. Artists, architects, and engineers: Three contrasting modes of visual experience and their psychological correlates. *Journal of Personality*, 1971, *39*, 432–449.

Holtzman, W. H., Thorpe, J. S., Swartz, J. D., & Herron, E. W. *Inkblot perception and personality*. Austin: The University of Texas Press, 1961.

Iacino, L. W., & Cook, P. E. Threat of shock, state anxiety, and the Holtzman Inkblot Technique. *Journal of Personality Assessment*, 1974, *38*, 450–458.

Insua, A. M. The Holtzman movement variable in relation to problem-solving processes of college students. *Journal of Clinical Psychology*, 1972, *28*, 199–202.

Kamen, G. B. A second look at the effects of a stress-producing film on adult test performance. *Journal of Clinical Psychology*, 1971, *27*, 465–467.

Lerner, B. Rorschach movement and dreams: A validation study using drug-induced dream deprivation. *Journal of Abnormal Psychology*, 1966, *71*, 75–86.

Megargee, E. I., & Velez-Diaz, A. A profile sheet for the clinical interpretation of the Holtzman Inkblot Technique. *Journal of Personality Assessment*, 1971, *35*, 545–560.

Mendelsohn, M. B., & Linden, J. D. The atypical response scale: An objective assessment of form inappropriateness. *Journal of Clinical Psychology*, 1972, *28*, 204.

Moseley, E. C. Psychodiagnosis on the basis of the Holtzman Inkblot Technique. *Journal of Projective Techniques and Personality Assessment*, 1963, *27*, 86–91.

Moseley, E. C., Gorham, D. R., & Hill, E. Computer scoring of inkblot perceptions. *Perceptual and Motor Skills*, 1963, *17*, 498.

Mueller, W. J., & Abeles, N. The components of empathy and their relationship to the projection of human movement responses. *Journal of Projective Techniques and Personality Assessment*, 1964, *28*, 322–330.

Nichols, D. C., & Tursky, B. Body image, anxiety, and tolerance for experimental pain. *Psychosomatic Medicine*, 1967, *29*, 103–110.

Overall, J. E., & Gorham, D. R. Organicity versus old age in objective and projective test performance. *Journal of Consulting and Clinical Psychology*, 1972, *39*, 98–105.

Palmer, J. O. Alterations in Rorschach's experience balance under conditions of food and sleep deprivation: A construct validity study. *Journal of Projective Techniques and Personality Assessment*, 1963, *27*, 208–213.

Rosenstiel, L. v. Zur Frage der Angst- und Feindseligkeitsinhalte in Formdeutverfahren. *Zeitschrift für experimentelle und angewandte Psychologie*, 1966, *8*, 611–631.

Sanders, J. L. Aggression and autonomy as correlates of the space response on Holtzman Inkblot Technique. *Perceptual and Motor Skills*, 1976, *42*, 1049–1050.

Shukla, T. R. Pathological verbalization on inkblots and psychodiagnosis. *Indian Journal of Clinical Psychology*, 1976, *3*, 17–21.

Stone, J. B. *Structured-objective Rorschach test*. Los Angeles: Test Bureau, 1958.

Swartz, J. D. Pathognomic verbalization in normals, psychotics, and mental retardates. *Dissertation Abstracts International*, 1970, *30*, 5703–5704.

Swartz, J. D., & Holtzman, W. H. Group method of administration of the Holtzman Inkblot Technique. *Journal of Clinical Psychology*, 1963, *19*, 433–441.

Swartz, J. D., Witzke, D. B., Holtzman, W. H., & Bishop, C. *Holtzman Inkblot Technique annotated bibliography* (revised). Austin, Tex.: Hogg Foundation for Mental Health, 1978.

Swartz, J. D., Witzke, D. B., & Megargee, E. I. Normative item statistics for the group form of the Holtzman Inkblot Technique. *Perceptual and Motor Skills*, 1970, *31*, 319–329.

Thorpe, J. S., & Swartz, J. D. Level of perceptual development as reflected in responses to the Holtzman Inkblot Technique. *Journal of Projective Techniques and Personality Assessment*, 1965, *29*, 380–386.

Velez-Diaz, A. Schizophrenic vs. brain-damaged performance on the Holtzman Inkblot Technique. *Journal of Clinical Psychology*, 1976, *32*, 177–178.

Zubin, J. Failures of the Rorschach technique. *Journal of Projective Techniques*, 1954, *18*, 303–315.

8

The Sentence Completion Method

ROBERT I. WATSON, JR.

1. Introduction

The sentence completion method of projective testing encompasses a wide variety of tests, all of which share a common format. In each instance, individuals being studied by this method are required to complete a number of sentence stems which are presented to them. Since the origination of this testing technique, a great many stems have been used, various methods of administration have been attempted, and a good deal of diversity has developed in the interpretation of the resulting material. The ease with which a sentence completion test can be constructed has proven to be both one of the strengths and one of the weaknesses of this method. Since the generation of the stems is not complicated, a great many sentence completion tests have been authored. While this often leads to the valid use of a test for the particular question it has been designed to answer, the number of such instruments has precluded the development of an extensive body of literature on a single sentence completion test. Without one dominant test on which to focus, it has been deemed expedient to deal with the method in general for the first part of this chapter. This is then followed by the specifics of a number of the most popular sentence completion tests in clinical use.

As a method of testing, the sentence completion has been classified as projective, objective, and "semiprojective" in nature. Relatively few psychologists view the test today as an objective measure, but there is still an open question as to how much the instrument allows the subject to project and how much conscious control there is of the responses. Campbell (1957) in his more exact typology of testing procedures classifies the method as voluntary, free response, and direct, indicating that he views the method as one in which the subject understands that any answer is acceptable (voluntary) and that the range of response is not limited (free response). According to Campbell, however, the method is not one that offers a façade. Rather, it is direct

---

ROBERT I. WATSON, JR. • Institute of Advanced Psychological Studies, Adelphi University, Garden City, New York 11530.

in that subjects are aware that they are revealing aspects of themselves in a fairly straightforward fashion. Many others (cf. Rohde, 1957) would disagree with the last aspect of this typology. They see the method as voluntary and free response but also as indirect, as allowing subjects to remain unaware that they are presenting aspects of their own personalities and attitudes to the examiner. This question will be dealt with at some length when the issues of validity and the levels hypothesis are presented.

2. History

The use of the sentence completion technique as a psychological test is considered to have its origin with the work of Ebbinghaus (1897) in his studies of mental abilities. Binet and Simon (1905) found the method to be useful for measuring intellectual abilities and included sentence stems as one of the tests in their first battery. While others (Kelly, 1917; Trabue, 1916) also used the testing technique as a measure of intellectual capacity and some investigators (Copple, 1956; Piltz, 1957; West, 1958) have recently used it as such, the sentence completion method is primarily thought of as a technique for assessing personality and attitudes. In terms of the use for personality assessment, the heritage of the test can be traced to the word association technique, which originated with the work of Jung in 1904 and 1906 and also in the United States with the usage of Kent and Rosanoff (1910) and Wells (1911). While valuable material can be gathered through the word association technique, it was soon realized that there are limitations to this method and that longer and possibly more structured stimuli and responses would be useful for the investigation of personality.

The first use of a sentence completion test for personality assessment was by Payne (1928), who used it as one of a number of tests to aid in questions of guidance. Tendler (1930) used the method to study emotional reactions and found that a wide variety of emotions could be investigated using even a rather limited number of sentence completion stems. Again, as part of a battery of tests, Cameron (1938) found the sentence completion technique useful for exploring more formal aspects of language and thought. He compared the thought processes of senile and disorganized schizophrenic subjects in terms of their responses to causal statements such as "I get warm when I run because _____." There began to be more and varied applications of the method to personality assessment, although not all studies reported its usefulness positively (Lorge & Thorndike, 1941a, 1941b).

With the beginning of World War II, there came a demand for relatively quickly administered psychological tests which could be presented to large groups and which would deal with general and specific issues of assessment. The sentence completion method soon became a part of psychological batteries in military settings. It was used in the Air Corps as a screening device (Flanagan, 1947), but was probably best know for its use in the Office of Strategic Service (OSS). Selection of personnel was one prime concern of this branch of the service, and the sentence completion test was one of a number used by the staff (Murray & MacKinnon, 1946). The OSS test consisted of 100 items, referring to both the first person and the third person, 50 of which were given at each of two sessions (U.S. Office of Strategic Services, OSS Assessment Staff, 1948). The design of the test allowed for responses in 12 different aspects of personality: Family, Past, Drives, Innerstates, Goals, Cathexes, Energy Reactions to Frustration and Failure, Time-Perspective, Optimism, Pessimism, Reactions to

Others, Reactions of Others. The interpretation of the data involved the application of two rather elementary but seemingly effective criteria:

> Two fundamental assumptions were constantly kept in mind even though they were held only as tentative hypotheses: (1) the rarer the response of the subject, in comparison with the responses given by other subjects to the same item, the more significant; and (2) the more frequently a response is given by any one subject to different items, the more significant it is, presuming that the repetition is not the result of perseveration. (U.S. OSS, 1948, p. 383)

The information gathered from the sentence completion test was treated tentatively by the staff and was used primarily as an aid in subsequent interviews. It gave a preview of the individual and allowed certain personality aspects to be emphasized in the interview. Esteem for the test was very high. According to the assessment staff, although it was "one of a number of projective techniques tried out in the program, it was the only one in use at the end." The test was translated into Chinese and Korean, and following the war Stein (1947) developed a civilian version.

The sentence completion method also came to be used with clinical populations in various military hospitals as a basic assessment tool. Holzberg (1945) reported that it was used extensively and was especially helpful in deciding who should be given more thorough psychological testing with other devices such as the Rorschach. Rotter and Willerman (1947), out of the earlier work of Hutt (1945), Shor (1946), and Holzberg, Teicher, and Taylor (1947), developed a rather unstructured 40-item test to be used in Air Force hospitals. As well as being brief, the test lent itself to a relatively objective method of interpretation, including the assigning of each response to one of three categories—conflict, neutral, or positive—as defined by a scoring manual. This test was also adopted for civilian use after the war (Rotter, Rafferty, & Schachtitz, 1949), and the Incomplete Sentence Blank (ISB) has proven to be one of the most widely used sentence completion tests.

Following World War II there was an increased interest in the development of sentence completion tests, the work of Rohde (1946, 1947), Holsopple and Miale (1954), and Forer (1950) being the most noteworthy for the development of standard tests that could be used in clinical settings or for the general study of personality. Rohde's (1946) test was actually a refinement of a testing procedure first used to study high school students in 1939. Rohde (1957) developed the test further using a system of interpretation based on Murray's need-press system. Holsopple and Miale were primarily interested in demonstrating the usefulness of the technique in discovering underlying dynamics of the individual's personality. They attempted to select those items with the "minimum of threat or obvious exposure" (1954, p. 10) so that the responses could be used to study "unconscious and semi-conscious desires, motives, conflicts, and systems of personality organization" (1954, p. 11). Forer (1950), as well, was interested in personality dynamics but took a different direction in developing the sentence stems. He chose his sentence stems so that they would be quite highly structured in order to avoid preoccupations and to some extent defensive reactions of the subject. The structure also directed the subject toward revealing certain attitudes and dynamics that Forer considered important.

These were but the major sentence completion tests developed to study personality. The method was also employed in a number of different areas of psychological investigation, and tests began to be designed for use in specific research projects. The method has especially been productive in the study of attitudes in a great number of areas and groups—school life (Costin & Eiserer, 1949), mental hospitals (Souelem,

1955), career choice (Getzels & Jackson, 1960), peers and parents (Harris & Tseng, 1957), and the elderly (Golde & Kogan, 1959). Sentence completion tests have also been used to make comparisons of differences between a wide variety of groups. MacBrayer (1960) reviewed the difference between males and females in the perception of the opposite sex. Farber (1951) studied the national character of English and Americans using a sentence completion test. The method has been used to predict success in such varied fields as clinical psychology (Kelly & Fiske, 1950, 1951), the Air Force (Holtzman & Sells, 1954), and more recently civilian airline piloting (Lunneborg & Olch, 1970). Other studies have attempted to relate specific personality variables (i.e., self-concept, need for achievement) ascertained from sentence completion tests to overall academic achievement (Irvin, 1967b; LaPlante & Irvin, 1970). Specialized sentence completion forms have been used in academic settings to discover such divergent aspects of students' personality and behavior as their potential for self-actualization (McKinney, 1967) and for disruptive behavior in the classroom (Feldhusen, Thurston, & Benning, 1966). Certain tests have also been designed to explore such personality issues as egocentricity (Exner, 1973) and the motives of safety and esteem (Aronoff, 1972; Wilson & Aronoff, 1973).

3. Present Status of the Sentence Completion Method

As the range of psychological investigations undertaken with the sentence completion method has broadened, its reputation as a useful, valid testing technique has also grown. Goldberg (1965), reviewing the method as a whole, was laudatory in his comments on the usefulness of the technique for a variety of purposes. Murstein (1965), commenting on this review, states: "The Sentence Completion Method is a valid test, generally speaking, and probably the most valid of all the projective techniques reported in the literature" (p. 777). Murstein feels that the reasons for this are that the test is designed to produce specific evaluations of personality aspects, that it is not a "broad-band" instrument, and that on the whole it is validated with criteria that emphasize verbality and behavior which is under conscious control. One other reason for its validity may be the large number of custom tests that are designed to study one specific personality aspect. Yet more general tests have been found to be extremely useful as well. Following his extensive review of the testing method, Goldberg (1968) studied its status as a test—the regard in which psychologists held the sentence completion method. He obtained ratings, rankings, and comments from 69 members of the Society for Projective Techniques and Personality Assessment on ten commonly used psychological tests and found that the sentence completion method was ranked "slightly below average" in its actual clinical use but still among the most popular clinical tools and "decidedly below average" in its use as a research instrument (p. 216). Its ranking in clinical use was comparable to its ranking by both earlier and later studies that found it second only to the MMPI as a group personality test (Sundberg, 1961; Lubin, Wallis, & Paine, 1971). It is unclear why it was not accepted more as a research instrument, especially since it has good psychometric properties when compared to other projective techniques such as good reliability based on its greater number of items. There was, however, a great deal of agreement among Goldberg's respondents that the test is especially useful in the evaluation of interpersonal attitudes, personality evaluation, and assessment of adjustment for both adults and children, and in assessing anxiety and aggression, all of which have generally been borne out in the literature. The respondents thought that the method was not useful for assessing such factors as organicity and intellectual capacity and were evenly divided on its use for psychiatric diagnosis. Those surveyed may feel its use to be limited in diagnosis because of consideration of the conscious control of the material elicited and the alleged undynamic nature of responses. Although there has been no definitive study on its use for differential diagnosis, there have been extremely encouraging reports in the literature on its use in diagnosis (Rotter and Willerman, 1947; Sacks, 1949; Wolkon & Haefner, 1961) as well as its obvious use in many other clinical questions.

One indirect and recent measure of the method's perceived popularity in psychology is the fact that in the most recent *Psychological Abstracts*, that of 1976, the method does not receive a separate section in the index, but is placed within the broad category of "projective techniques." This is somewhat discouraging for the reputation of the method as a separate testing procedure, since most popular tests do receive a separate heading, (e.g., the Holtzman Inkblot Test), but there is one additional note—the Rotter Incomplete Sentence Blank does receive a separate heading. Perhaps the method as a whole is once again suffering from the great variety of tests using it as a basic method.

Overall, the method appears to be held in relatively high regard by psychologists and has been shown to be useful in the assessment of a wide variety of aspects for personality and clinical study.

4. Clinical Use of the Sentence Completion Method

Having established that the sentence completion method does have a good reputation as a testing instrument, it is now important to examine its actual usefulness in a clinical setting. As will be discussed, the sentence completion test, used in conjunction with other instruments in a battery, can provide the clinican with additional information about the dynamics of a patient. Yet, as with all projective techniques, the amount of awareness or conscious control that the patient exerts in the production of responses is a major consideration in determining how much reliance the clinician can place on the data obtained. Because of its structure, the sentence completion test has been more subject to such considerations, and some reservation has been attached to its use in diagnosis.

Such concerns are reflected in the concept of the levels hypothesis as it pertains to projective testing. Two studies which bear directly on the relationship of the levels hypothesis to the sentence completion method have been undertaken by Stone and Dellis (1960) and Murstein and Wolf (1970). Stone and Dellis tested the levels hypothesis in terms of the stimulus structure of different testing procedures. They reasoned that the less a test was structured the more chance the test would have of revealing primitive impulse controls. Conversely, more structure would result in less of the patient's pathology being revealed. They proceeded to evaluate the records of 20 pseudoneurotic and pseudocharacterological schizophrenics, reviewing the protocols of these patients, which included the WAIS, Forer Structured Sentence Completion Test, TAT, Rorschach, and Draw-a-Person Test. Stone and Dellis thought these ranged in order from most to least structured. The protocols were then submitted to judges who rated them on the Menninger Health-Sickness Rating Scale. The results were that the impulse control rating followed the same order as Stone and

Dellis's judgment of the tests' structure, but with only two adjacent tests, the TAT and Rorschach, differing significantly.

Murstein and Wolf (1970) followed much the same hypothesis but used a widely varying psychiatric population and a normal population. The levels hypothesis in terms of less stimulus structure leading to increased judgment of pathology was again substantiated but only for the normal population. In this study the patient population showed no significant differences in their rating on pathology as the structure of the tests was lessened. Therefore, although the levels hypothesis in terms of structure was supported for the normal subjects in the study, it was not for the psychotic patients, which differs from the Stone and Dellis results. Murstein and Wolf offer the possible explanation that their results are based on differing sensitivity to the test stimuli by these two groups. The normal subjects respond primarily to external stimuli and therefore closely follow the stimuli. They project less pathology on the more structured test, but begin to respond to the ambiguity in the less structured tests, with more pathology. Psychiatric patients, conversely, are responding to a greater extent to internal stimuli and ignore external cues unless they are quite strong, as they would be in the more structured tests.

> The ego controls of these Ss have broken down, and their sensitivity and/or desire to respond to the cue properties of the outside world is minimal. They project their problems to all tests, manifesting a supreme indifference to the varying stimulus properties found from test to test unless they are extremely clearly structured. (Murstein & Wolf, 1970, p. 43)

The implication of Murstein and Wolf's interpretation of the results is quite interesting in terms of the use of moderately structured projective tests such as the sentence completion. It may be that just those tests that offer a middle range of structure are the best aids to differential diagnosis, in that they allow normal individuals to follow the structure of the stimuli and thereby give less pathological responses while at the same time giving less forceful cues to disturbed subjects, who then project more of their dynamic issues onto the moderately structured stimuli of the test. In any battery of tests, test structure should be varied, and the structure of the stimuli within a test should also be taken into account when judging the projected material of any patient or subject.

There is, however, an additional aspect to the levels hypothesis which perhaps confuses the issue as it relates to the sentence completion method and to the work of Stone and Dellis and Murstein. As Coleman (1969) has pointed out, the levels hypothesis implies a theory of personality involving varying levels of personality structure and differing levels of fantasy productions. Projective testing is often thought of as being intimately related to a psychoanalytic understanding of the individual and yet, as Holt (1961) has stated, projective testing is considered to be qualitatively different from fantasy in psychoanalysis, especially in terms of secondary process thinking. It would seem best, as Coleman has suggested, not to speak of different levels of fantasy resulting from different projective tests but rather to think in terms of the varying structure of these tests and the resulting awareness or unawareness on the part of the subject in regard to his or her own response to test stimuli. Sentence completion tests are usually considered to have more structure than a Rorschach or TAT and therefore to involve more awareness on the subject's or patient's part. This issue also relates to Campbell's (1957) point, put forth earlier, that the test should be considered a direct test, although once again there is disagreement on this point with a great number of clinicians, considering the test to be indirect and therefore implying that the subject is not fully aware of the purpose and possible meaning of his or her responses. It must also be remembered that directions do vary for different sentence completion tests, some calling on more conscious controls than others. The structure of items also varies from such items as "I_____" to "As a child my greatest fear was _____." Overall, some awareness must be involved in the performance on any sentence completion test. How much awareness there is and whether this is significantly greater on a sentence completion test than on many other projective techniques are still open questions. What appears to be the case is that the patient does project some meaningful dynamic material in a sentence completion test, and the patient's response to the relative structure and awareness engendered on the test may be a diagnostic tool in itself. Some dynamic issues can be discerned from the material, and the process which the ego of the patient brings to bear on the stimuli can give the diagnostician some indication of the ego controls available to the patient. How this material is then used and integrated with the material gathered from other testing procedures is still a question to be answered by the individual clinician.

Related to these questions is the extent to which the sentence completion test agrees with and adds to other diagnostic tools. Nystedt, Magnusson, and Aronowitsch (1975) reviewed the contribution of the Rorschach, TAT, and Sentence Completion Test using a multitrait-multimethod matrix. They found that the three tests demonstrated low levels of convergent validity and concluded that each test added different information to clinician's understanding of the patient. They put forth the idea that each test tapped a subvariable of a global variable and that each test was then important to a thorough understanding of the individual. Gardner and Harrison (1967) carried out an experiment comparing the qualitative interpretation of a sentence completion test with the in-depth interview of a single patient. Twenty-four questions were posed to 16 judges, six clinicians, and ten psychology graduate students, who had only the patient's responses on the Sack Sentence Completion Test with which to work. The questions covered the areas of childhood and family relations, psychosexual development, attitude toward people and worth, personality traits, and general adjustment. These same questions were then answered by two experienced interviewers (one a clinical psychologist and one a psychiatrist) who had worked extensively with the patient and had access to all the previous testing. The mean Pearson r of the clinicians with the psychologist ratings was .82 ($p < .01$) and with the psychiatrist .73 ($p < .01$). The students' correlations were not so high, .65 with the psychologist and .41 with the psychiatrist, but were still significant. Five of the six clinical psychologists were also able to correctly diagnose the patient. Certainly for this study of a single case it is evident that a sentence completion test can be used qualitatively to reach a high degree of agreement with the experienced clinicians' views of a patient.

5. Research and Clinical Scoring Systems

As stated in Section 2, the sentence completion method was first most highly valued as a tool to aid in structuring patient interviews and as a device which could be quickly administered and which would indicate the need for further psychological testing. It has subsequently been used as a primary screening device to determine if an individual is in need of counseling or psychotherapy. The best known of these screening scoring systems is the one developed by Rotter and Rafferty (1950) which is applied to the Incomplete Sentences Blank (ISB). The scoring of the 40 items in this version of a sentence completion test gives the clinician a simple overall adjustment score. A specific cutting score is reported in the test manual, suggesting that those above it be thought of as "maladapted" and should be referred for psychological help. In the original sample the cutting score correctly identified nearly two-thirds of the already classified "maladjusted" subjects and screened out almost 80% of the adjusted subjects. These results have also been cross-validated by Churchill and Crandall (1955) and have been used as well in a great number of studies as indicators of adjustment. Although it is realized by the authors that their adjustment score is only a general indicator, they believe that it is useful for basic screening and as a research tool.

Other objective scoring systems have been developed to study much more specific issues of interest to clinicians. Bartz (1968) has studied identification using a sentence completion test, while Rothaus, Johnson, Hanson, Brown, and Lyle (1967) have used the method to investigate issues of patient attitudes to group orientation. Two scoring systems, developed separately, have dealt with the areas of dependency, anxiety, and hostility (Renner, Maher, & Campbell, 1962; Lanyon, 1972). The Renner et al. (1962) measures are based on the use of the ISB and have been shown to have construct validity by use of a multitrait-multimethod matrix. The basic comparisons were carried out with peer- and self-ratings of these personality aspects. Lanyon (1972) has constructed a sentence completion test and scales to study these same issues of hostility, anxiety, and dependency, but in junior high school students. Working with the rating criteria of teachers, she constructed sentence stems reflecting ten specific behaviors indicated as being important by the teachers. The responses of the students on these stems were then judged by the use of a 3-point scale indicating the degree of the personality variable. The final selection of sentence stems was shown to differentiate children judged by their teachers to be high or low on the relevant criterion rating. Both of these scoring systems therefore are able to determine and differentiate high and low subjects on important behaviors pertaining to hostility, dependency, and anxiety.

Exner (1973) has formulated a new test, the Self Focus Sentence Completion test, and has devised a scoring system of egocentricity for it. Normative data have been developed from the protocols of nearly 3000 normal subjects and psychiatric patients. The scoring system involves four categories—Self Focus, External World Focus, Ambivalence, and Neutral—with which scorers have been able to obtain high levels of interscorer reliability. Exner implies that there should be a balance between Self Focus and External World focus in normal individuals. In his sample all psychiatric patient groups had greater difference scores between these two categories than did any of the adult nonpsychiatric groups. Six validity studies are reported involving such criteria as change in SFSC score after and during interventions, or its relationship to specific behaviors such as use of personal pronouns in an interview setting.

Harvey (1964, 1965), working with the concepts developed by Harvey, Hunt, and Schroder (1961), has also designed a custom sentence completion test. The This I Believe test (TIB) was developed to study the level of conceptual systems functioning ranging over four levels from concrete to abstract conceptualization. It is somewhat different in format than other sentence completion tests in that the statement "This I believe about _____" is the beginning of each stem and is followed by a stimulus word such as "sex," "religion," or "people." Subjects are asked to respond with at least two sentences to nine or ten of the statements and are given 2 min for each of the stimulus words. Scoring judgments are then made dealing with the response absolutism, evaluativeness, normativeness, and simplicity-complexity. Each response is assigned to one of the four major categories or to a mix of two systems. Relatively good interrater reliability and test-retest reliability have been reported (Greaves, 1971). The test and scoring system have been used to explore such varied issues as dissonance resolution (Harvey & Ware, 1967) and teacher effects on classroom atmosphere (Harvey, Pratter, White, & Hoffmeister, 1968). The most interesting clinical use of conceptual complexity was carried out by Reilly and Sugerman (1967). Using a test similar in format to the TIB, developed by Schroder and Streufert (1962), they studied the conceptual level of hospitalized male alcoholics. Although most of these patients were concrete, there was a differentiation made between System I patients, the most concrete, and System II patients, the more differentiated in functioning, who also avoid dependency and question control. Reilly and Sugerman suggest that the System I patients can benefit most from directive therapy and affiliation with Alcoholics Anonymous, while System II individuals would rebel at such treatment and be dropouts from such a program. It would appear that this testing procedure could prove quite useful in the differentiation of other patient groups and should have implications for the choice of treatment.

The most elaborate and extensive research using a sentence completion test that should be of interest to clinicians has been undertaken by Loevinger and her colleagues at Washington University. Using her concepts (Loevinger, 1966) and those of Sullivan, Grant, and Grant (1957), she and her colleagues have developed a detailed evaluation system for the levels of ego development. Seven basic levels of ego development are delineated, six of which along with transitions from one level to another are scored in their ego developmental system (Loevinger & Wessler, 1970). The levels are Presocial-Symbiotic (which cannot be scored), Impulsive, Self-Protective, Conformist, Conscientious, Autonomous, and Integrated. Each individual is assumed to have one of these as the core level of his or her functioning. Using the Washington University Sentence Completion test, they then rationally devised and empirically verified scoring of the different responses demonstrating the level of ego functioning. An extensive and detailed scoring manual for female subjects is the result of these endeavors, with a number of examples of each level being presented (Loevinger, Wessler, & Redmore, 1970). Scorers trained in the use of this manual can then apply the system to each of the 36 responses to the sentence stems. Since the hoped-for result is an overall estimate of the core functioning of an individual, ogive scoring rules have been formulated to best estimate the primary level of the subject's ego functioning. Validity studies of the scoring system reported by Loevinger and Wessler (1970) involve structured interviews of adults and comparison of children at different age levels. Ego development ratings, from the interview and the sentence completion levels scored, correlated quite highly (.58 and .61 for the two raters), indicating an agreement between the two techniques. Age differences for children between 9 and 18 also reflect differences in ego development, with correlations between age and ego level of .74 for boys and .69 for girls. The investigation also found no overlap between the ogive curves of the various age groups, indicating rather distinctive ego functioning for the different age levels. While high levels of interrater reliability have been reported, Redmore and Waldman

(1975) have discovered some difficulty with the test-retest reliability of the measure, with correlations being significant but of a low order. They offer the explanation that there was a restricted range in their sample and that the responses to the second testing were banal, lowering the scores. This is understandable since the tests were given only 1 week apart. Redmore (1976) has also investigated the test's susceptibility to faking and found generally that, when directed to, subjects can lower their ego levels on the test but have great difficulty in increasing them. Only when subjects had studied ego development intensively could they significantly fake an increase in their scores. Raters could also identify most faked protocols. This problem of faking does raise a question for use of the test with uncooperative subjects or patients who wish to appear as if they have a lower level of functioning. Overall, this test and scoring system would appear to have great potential for use with patients in various diagnostic categories and for further investigation of psychopathology. Loevinger apparently has data on psychiatric patients but has not published any of this material. She has pointed out a number of cautions for using the scale with psychiatric patients. Primarily, in itself it does not deal with pathology and might both underestimate certain patients who have learned to verbalize impulsive thoughts more and overestimate patients who give unique responses to the stems. The only safeguard against this is to have experienced and insightful raters carry out the scoring of the protocols. Even with these difficulties, the system for evaluating ego development may prove to be of great use for the study of the developmental ego levels of patients in different diagnostic categories.

All of these studies imply that the sentence completion method can be useful for better understanding of general diagnostic issues and of specific personality factors. While all of the existing sentence completion tests are considered to be more structured than the other projective tests, and material from them is therefore closer to the patient's awareness, this does not preclude the patient's indicating many important diagnostic issues on the test. Also, the very nature of the test's being more highly structured can be used as a diagnostic indicator with patients. The test can be a useful addition to a test battery and can add meaningful information on a variety of clinical questions.

6. Methodological Considerations

As with any projective testing device, there are certain changes that can be made in the test material and its administration that should aid in its general usefulness. The clinician should be aware of these methodological considerations and how they may affect the data gathered from an individual patient before choosing a particular form of sentence completion test and deciding how to interpret the resulting data. Opinions have been stated and some empirical studies carried out that deal with issues of both sentence stem content and test administration. Unfortunately, few definitive answers have been reached.

Concerns over variation in stem content have focused primarily on two areas: (1) person reference in the stem and (2) stimulus pull and structure of the stem. Person reference involves the use of either a first person pronoun in the stem or a third person pronoun. The use of the third person referent is logically consistent with the projective hypothesis that a subject should give more revealing information when responding as if talking about another and be more defensive when giving important information about him- or herself. Following this concept, some investigators use few, if any, first person stems (e.g., Holsopple & Miale, 1954) while others ignore or do not believe in the value of this projective assumption and use primarily first person stems (e.g., Rotter & Rafferty, 1950). Others, such as Stein (1947), use both forms, possibly thinking as Stein does that the first person stems are "personal" ones while the third person stems are "projective" and will allow the subject to reveal more threatening information. Each form then complements the other.

A number of studies have been carried out to determine the difference between first and third person referents in sentence completion tests, but no consensus has been reached. One of the first projects to deal with the question was done by Sacks (1949). He constructed two forms of a 60-item sentence completion test, with one form using only first person referents and the other using only third person stems. Both forms were then given to 100 psychiatric patients. Ratings of psychological disturbance were obtained from psychiatrists treating these patients and were compared to similar ratings by three psychologists who had only the sentence completion material with which to work. The results clearly demonstrated a greater degree of agreement between the ratings based on first person stems and the psychiatrists' rating than with those obtained from the third person form. A majority of psychologists in the study stated that they preferred the first person form of the test for clinical use. Preference for first person stems was evident in a study carried out by Cromwell and Lundy (1954). In this study, 39 clinical psychologists formulated hypotheses and personality inferences for 60 protocols. The psychologists also indicated which of the sentence stems had made the most contribution to their evaluation. Since the psychologists had been given both first and third person stems, Cromwell and Lundy were able to tell which form was most clinically useful in the judgment of the psychologists in the study. They found that the first person stems were judged to be more productive in formulation of clinical hypotheses. Since this study involved only the perceived clinical usefulness of the two types of stems, no validity criterion was included in it. A difficulty with this study has been pointed out by Murstein (1965). Reviewing the actual stems in the study, he found that the most productive were all negatively toned stems and that all the negation stems that had a person reference used the first person pronoun. Therefore, it is difficult to attribute the productiveness of the first person stems to the use of the first person pronoun alone.

More recent research has also dealt with this issue of the use of first or third person referents. Irvin (1967a) used a custom-designed sentence completion test of 35 items, ten of which were neutral or third person references such as "Boys are _____," "School is _____," "Most mothers _____," while the other 25 were first person references. This test was presented to 40 male subjects and was evaluated in terms of acceptance or rejection demonstrated in the responses to the stems. He found that the first person stems elicited a significantly greater degree of negative expression with more rejection aspects, suggesting that the use of first person referents elicits more meaningful emotional material. Murstein (1965) had certain reservations about the methodology of earlier studies of person reference. He therefore designed an experiment to determine what effect the person reference has on projection on the sentence stems and adjustment as judged in terms of them (Murstein, Colon, Destrexhe-deLeval, & VanHoof-VanParys, 1972). A custom 36-item sentence completion test was designed which varied both respondent and stimuli pull (more about stimuli pull will follow) and was presented to 120 subjects in Brussels. Projection was rated on a 4-point scale from revealing responses to those devoid of projection and are simply elaborations of the stem. Adjustment was also rated on a simple 4-point scale judging conscious manifestation of adjustment or maladjustment. What was discovered in the study was that the first person stems were more projective than the contrasting impersonal stems and that they also yielded high adjustment scores. Seemingly, more meaningful material came from the first person stems, but it was also material that led the raters to see the subject as more adjusted. It may be that subjects are more willing to say meaningful things about themselves when given first person stems but what they say is under more conscious control and is said to make themselves appear better to the examiner.

Not all studies have demonstrated superiority of first person stems. Stricker and Dawson (1966) used the Incomplete Sentence Blank (Rotter & Rafferty, 1950) as the basis of their study. Two alternate forms were constructed, one using the 22 items of the ISB which contained a first person referent and the other a modified form in which all the first person referents were changed to corresponding third person pronouns. The first person form or the third person form was presented to each of 144 psychiatric patients. All indications as to the form from which the response was obtained were removed. The investigators applied an objective scoring system for the areas of dependency, anxiety, and hostility (Renner et al., 1962) to the protocols. Separate analyses of variance were carried out for each of the scores for dependency, hostility, and anxiety. No significant effects were found in comparing the forms. Both first and third person forms were equally effective in eliciting the responses which were subsequently scored for these three important areas. In this study it did not make any significant difference which referent was used. Wood (1969) has also based his investigation of referents on the ISB using the 20 first person referents and 20 neutral nonpersonal items and then constructing 20 stems replacing the personal pronouns with proper female names (a substitute for third person pronouns). A total of 144 female subjects took one of these forms of the ISB, which was scored using the adjustment criterion of Rotter and Rafferty (1950). An analysis of variance was applied to the resulting data, and it was found that each form differed significantly on the adjustment criteria. The form using proper names elicited the responses which were seen as most maladjusted while the form containing the nonpersonal-neutral material produced the least amount of maladjustment, with the first person form being between these two. Indications of pathology may be more easily projected onto other referents, as the projective hypothesis would predict. When these last two studies are taken into account, there cannot be a clear-cut preference for first person referents, especially in dealing with issues of pathology.

The other important consideration in constructing a sentence completion test is the amount of structure and the stimulus pull found in the stems. The method is considered generally to have more inherent structure than other projective tests, but structure can be varied in different forms of stems. Some investigators (e.g., Forer, 1950) believe that a good deal of structure is necessary to produce responses that are unambiguous and that are related to important clinical issues. Others (e.g., Rotter & Rafferty, 1950) believe that the test should be unstructured to allow the patient or subject to bring his or her own projected material to the test more easily. Preference for one format or the other generally depends on the opinion of the test author.

Relatively little research has been carried out on the question of structure. Some studies, such as that of Peck and McGuire (1959), have reported that more highly structured stems result in less ambiguous material from subjects. However, the issue becomes one of having unambiguous material but also material that may be less significant in its meaning. Closely related to this issue of content is the area of stimulus pull. What effect does the tone of the content of the stimulus itself have on the resulting response to it? Meltzoff (1951) carried out the first investigation of the stimulus-pull properties of a sentence completion test. He regarded the pull as negative if the stem involved unhappy or unpleasant connotations and as positive if it had happy or satisfying connotations. These stimulus-pull properties were then compared to adjustment and affect ratings of the resulting responses. He found, not surprisingly, that positive-pull stimuli resulted in more positive responses and gave less indication of maladjustment, while negative-pull stimuli resulted in negative responses with more indication of poor adjustment. The stimulus of the stem was then determining to some extent the subject's response. While stimulus pull must be considered when constructing the stem for a test, it is not a truly damaging property of the test so long as it is recognized as a factor in the subject's response. All classifications of subjects should react equally to the stimulus pull, so differences in responses can be attributed to individual differences.

Stephens (1970), however, has found that stimulus pull apparently influences some subjects more than others. Using the ISB he factor-analyzed the responses of 345 male and 245 female subjects and found that stimulus-pull factors were present for males but were not clearly present for females. Male subjects were reacting to the negative-, neutral-, and positive-pull factors, while female responses involved a mix of stimulus-pull and content factors. Implications of the study are that data from male and female subjects may not be comparable since their reaction to stimulus pull differs and that any broad test should involve stems with all three stimulus-pull characteristics.

Murstein et al. (1972) studied the effects of positive, neutral, and negative pull on the projection and adjustment of the resulting responses. (This was part of a study cited earlier that also included the person reference of the stem.) Again, using a 4-point projection scale, they found that neutral stems elicited more projection than either positive or negative items. It is just these neutral items that should allow for more meaningful projections since they do not have strong affect cues and should allow the subject to project more of his or her own meaning into the stem. The investigation also found, using a 4-point adjustment scale, that subjects obtained higher adjustment scores with the positively toned stems. Again, the stimulus pull of the item can affect the judgments made about the responses, primarily with positive items giving them a positive "set" and not allowing for so much projection. Both Stephens (1970) and Murstein et al. (1972) imply that the stimulus pull of the sentence stems might be a consideration when judging the context of the sentence completion. Murstein et al. hypothesized that the different pull may be a diagnostic tool in itself. For example, negative responses to positive-pulling stems may have more diagnostic import than similar negative responses to negative stimuli. Apparently, the best format for a test would include some positive and negative stimuli in the stems while consisting primarily of neutral stimuli to allow for a greater projection on the test.

Another important methodological issue is how the sentence completion test is actually administered to the subject or patient. Instructions have been formulated so that the subject's response will be as revealing and meaningful as possible. Test authors favor different types of instructions. Some emphasize "real feelings" in the instructions (e.g., Rotter & Rafferty, 1950) while others attempt to make the material as revealing as possible by emphasizing the speed of response (e.g., Stein, 1947). Still others do not ask for either speed or truth, instead telling subjects to "complete each sentence in whatever way you wish" (Holsopple & Miale, 1954). These differences in directions are primarily based on the author's opinion on how best to aid the projection process. The use of the different instructions has, however, been explored in a number of empirical studies. Cromwell and Lundy (1954) were among the first to deal with this issue in a study. They presented an extended version of the Incomplete Sentence Blank (Rotter & Rafferty, 1950) with either a set of instructions saying it was a test of "speed of thinking" or instructions emphasizing the expression of "real feelings." No difference was found in the productivity resulting from either form of instructions. The authors feel that significant differences may have been masked by uncontrollable judge variability.

Other empirical studies have been carried out more recently using essentially the same variation in instructions and have found that they resulted in no significant differences. Wood (1969) used two sets of instructions for the ISB, calling it a timed "verbal speed test" or an untimed "personality test," and got no difference on Rotter and Rafferty's (1950) adjustment scores. Similarly, Flynn (1974) presented the ISB twice to 40 psychiatric patients, once as an oral test with the instructions to respond immediately and once in the usual written manner, emphasizing "real feelings." Again no significant differences were obtained when the two versions were scored for maladjustment. Stricker and Dawson (1966) used the standard "real feelings" instructions of the ISB but also asked half of their 144 patients to respond with the "real feelings of the average person of your sex and age" (p. 170). The protocols were then scored for dependency, anxiety, and hostility (Renner et al., 1962), and again the instructions did not affect any significant difference in the scores. Another study used four forms of instruction (Irvin & Johnson, 1970). One form asked for "real feelings," another for responses "as fast as you can," a third for a combination of real feelings and immediate responses. The fourth allowed subjects to complete the stems in whatever way they wished. Responses were then judged on an acceptance-rejection dimension, and again no significant differences were found for any of the instructions.

Only one study has demonstrated significant differences due to variations in instructions. Siipola (1968) presented an 80-item custom-designed sentence completion test to normal female subjects with either the instructions to write "the very first thing that comes into your mind," emphasizing speed, or the instructions to work at one's "own pace," emphasizing that it was not a speed test. The investigator was interested in the ego-alien quality of the responses. She had subjects judge their own responses by asking if each response reflected the way the subject personally felt or acted and whether it applied to herself. A significantly greater number of responses were judged ego-alien by the subjects when they had taken the test with the time-pressure instructions. Conflict or maladjustment in the material was also rated by judges using only the most extreme degree of conflict from the Rotter and Rafferty (1950) scale. Only 20 of the items were judged, and a low percentage of the items proved to be conflicted, but the difference between the two variations in instructions was again significant. Time pressure apparently leads to more ego-alien material that also contains more indications of conflict. Given these last findings, it cannot be definitely stated that instructions make no difference in responses to sentence completion tests.

One of the most interesting variations in the administration of a sentence completion test has been carried out by Wood (1967). Half of the items of the ISB were presented in the conventional manner to 80 subjects. The other half of the stems were then presented using a tachistoscope. Subjects believed that they were reading a full sentence and would attempt to repeat it, while what they saw was a sentence stem followed by letters selected and grouped at random. The speed of the exposure was set so that the stem could be perceived correctly but the random letter combinations were not. This technique was carried out to disarm the subjects and to see if they would then give responses to the tachistoscopic "sentence" that would reflect higher levels of maladjustment. Once again, no significant difference was found between the two techniques of administration. Overall, it would appear that the sentence completion method is rather impervious to changes in administration procedures. What is necessary is to see if this robust aspect of the method is true for all diagnostic categories since the format may make a difference for more defensive patients.

7. Clinical Sentence Completion Tests

The following section contains descriptive and interpretive guidelines for several representative sentence completion tests in clinical use. These are but brief descriptions, and the reader is encouraged to turn to the original sources for detailed accounts of the interpretive systems and the tests themselves. It is also only a representative sample, and some useful tests have had to be excluded because of limitations in space.

7.1. The Rotter Incomplete Sentence Blank (ISB)

7.1.1. The Test

The ISB consists of 40 items which are presented to the patient or subject with the following instructions: "Complete these sentences to express *your real feelings.* Try to do every one. Be sure to make a complete sentence" (Rotter & Rafferty, 1950, p. 5). A few representative items are

> I like _____.
> Back home _____.
> What annoys me _____.
> I can't _____.
> Marriage _____.
> I secretly _____.

Most items are short and relatively unstructured, and many use first person pronouns. The test has been published with three parallel forms: for college students, high school students, and adults. Each is essentially the same form with certain items modified so that they are more appropriate for the particular age group (e.g., "Men _____" is used in the adult form instead of "Boys _____").

ROBERT I.
WATSON, JR.

7.1.2. Evaluation and Interpretation

Rotter and Rafferty (1950) make it quite clear in their manual that the test was developed for two purposes—as a basic screening device and as a diagnostic tool that will aid the clinician in structuring further interviews and, possibly, treatment. It was not thought of as a tool that would expose fundamental personality functioning. As a screening device, the ISB is used primarily with the scoring criteria set forth in the manual, giving each patient a simple overall adjustment score. This adjustment score is based on a summation of the scored levels of conflict in the patients' responses to the stem. Conflict or maladjustment is portrayed in the responses in many different ways. As Rotter and Rafferty have stated,

> These include hostility reactions, pessimism, symptom elicitation, hopelessness and suicidal wishes, statements of unhappy experiences, and indications of past maladjustment. Examples of these types of reactions follow. "I hate . . . almost everyone." "People . . . destroy what they build." "I suffer . . . from dizzy spells." "Sometimes . . . I wonder what's the use." "I wish . . . I were dead." (Rotter & Rafferty, p. 15)

Three levels of conflict are then rated and given weighted scores corresponding to their severity. Not all responses, of course, are conflicted; descriptive responses are scored neutral and responses that are hopeful and healthy responses are scored as positive, again with three levels and corresponding weights for the scores given to them. The manual contains a number of examples for the varying levels of conflict, neutral, and positive responses for each stem. For example: "I regret _____": the highest level of conflict, $C3$, is given for a response like "being born," a lesser level of conflict, $C1$, for "wasted time," while a positive response, $P1$, is "not being a millionaire." All responses are to be scored independently of other responses. The final adjustment score is obtained by totaling all of the weighted scores. A cutting score is also suggested as a basic demarcation between adjustment and maladjustment. This cutting score was used to identify a majority of already identified maladjusted subjects while also identifying over three-fourths of the adjusted subjects, and, therefore, can be used as a rough screening device for pathology.

Rotter and Rafferty (1950) do not propose an actual system for qualitative interpretation of the protocols, but do suggest some general guidelines and give a number of case examples in their manual as an illustration of the potential use of the ISB. They indicate that the interpretation depends to a great degree on the preference and experience of the clinician, and the data can lend themselves to interpretation "from a common sense point of view or at a symbolic psychoanalytic level" (p. 30). The case example analyses they present are organized around the lines of Familial Attitudes, Social and Sexual Attitudes, General Attitudes, and Character Traits. Material for these aspects of the patient's functioning can come from any stem, and the manual does not organize them in any way, but obviously certain stems are more likely to pull for information in one of these areas (e.g., "My father _____" will usually give some indication of a family attitude). The material in the manual also demonstrates how the information can be interpreted to formulate a diagnostic understanding of the individual and make recommendations for psychotherapy. For example, one protocol has a great number of conformity responses such as "Reading . . . is good for broadening the mind," or "The happiest time . . . in my life was when I got married," combined with a number of dependency responses such as "When I was a child . . . I had everything I needed" and "A mother . . .'s love is the greatest in the world." The manual states that in therapy,

271

THE SENTENCE
COMPLETION
METHOD

> One would expect to receive from this patient a great many conformity responses and find
> quick acceptance of superficial insights; but the patient would not be likely to take any real re-
> sponsibility for changing his patterns of behavior. (Rotter & Rafferty, 1950, p. 40)

Overall, the ISB has proven to be an excellent tool for research and can add to the diagnostic understanding of a patient.

7.2. The Rohde Sentence Completion Method (SCM)

7.2.1. The Test

The SCM consists of 65 items plus an open-ended question at the end of the testing procedure. Rohde (1957) has taken great pains to delineate why the stems she uses were chosen and to make comparisons of her stems with those in already existing tests. Her thoughts on test construction were essentially that the stems should represent a broad range of stimuli and that conflict should be stimulated but the stem should not be so highly structured that the pull dominates the responses. She also arranged the order of the stems "to lead the subject away from everyday life to more inaccessible areas of personality, in order to avoid engendering resistance" (p. 46).

Instructions are as follows: "Kindly complete the following sentences as rapidly as possible. Try to express your real feelings and opinions"—combining the speed criteria with the expression of "real feelings." A few representative items are:

> The future _____.
> I feel _____.
> I remember _____.
> My mother _____.
> God _____.
> Most people _____.
> My worst _____.
> Suicide _____.
> I try to get _____.

The open-ended question is simply "Write below anything that seems important to you." This test, like all sentence completion tests, can easily be administered in a group setting as well as in an individual session.

7.2.2. Evaluation and Interpretation

Rohde (1957), in her book on the test, delineates three approaches to interpretation of the material and suggests that all three be applied to each protocol. The approaches are as follows: "(1) overt content, (2) formal aspects of the protocol, and (3) personality dynamics inferred from overt and latent content" (p. 70). Reviewing the overt content such as attitudes and values does have some clinical use since it portrays the main conscious elements of the patient's functioning but is usually not a primary concern for a diagnostician. The formal aspects, such as sentence structure or grammar, can be very useful diagnostic indications, especially of brain dysfunction syndromes and schizophrenia. Rohde points to perseveration as an especially important formal aspect of the responses, being the result of preoccupation with an issue or some forms of organic deterioration. The main interest of the diagnostician is, of course, the personality dynamics of the patient. Rohde believes that the most valuable method for understanding diagnosis is by an analysis of the motivational forces of the individual. To aid in organizing the basic motivational components, she has suggested the use of Murray's (1938) conceptual scheme. She has produced a great many illustrative case examples in her book (Rohde, 1957) but has purposely not attempted a formal scoring manual, feeling that such a device might lead to only mechanical scoring without any genuine understanding of the individual. She does, however, offer advice and organization for the evaluation of protocols. Each response of an individual should be evaluated and assigned to a need category or combination of categories (e.g., need autonomy or need affiliation). Inner states, general traits, inner integrates, and environment presses should also be judged from the responses and used in final determination of the individual's dynamic functioning. Rohde demonstrates how, with a great number of examples, the material can be integrated to better understand the dynamics of neurotic personality disorder and schizophrenic patients. She also presents norms of the various need categories obtained from different psychiatric populations. Her system for interpretation is well integrated and consistent with her view of understanding the personality functioning of a patient through the need-press system of motivational variables.

7.3. The Sacks Sentence Completion Test (SSCT)

7.3.1. The Test

The SSCT consists of 60 items that are somewhat more structured than those of many of the other sentence completion tests. The instructions are as follows: "Below are sixty partly completed sentences. Read each one and finish it by writing the first thing that comes to your mind. Work as quickly as you can. If you cannot complete an item, circle the number and return to it later" (p. 377). Representative items are:

> I feel my father seldom _____.
> To me the future _____.
> At work, I get along least well _____.
> I wish I could lose the fear of _____.
> If I had sex relations _____.
> The worst thing I ever did _____.

Sacks and Levy (1950) also suggest than an inquiry should be conducted. Both especially significant and cryptic responses can then be elaborated and should aid in the understanding of the patient.

7.3.2. Evaluation and Interpretation

Unlike Rohde (1957) or Rotter and Rafferty (1950), Sacks and Levy (1950) believe that it is important to organize the sentence completion material in terms of the stems representing specific attitudes. Fifteen different attitudes were used in the construction of the test, with four stems being designed for each attitude. A rating sheet has been devised which groups each set of attitude responses together. For example:

> Attitude toward Women:
>
> My idea of a perfect woman _____.
> I think most girls _____.

I believe most women _____.
What I like least about women _____.

The 15 attitudes involve Mother, Father, Family Unit, Women, Heterosexual Relationships, Friends and Acquaintances, Superiors at Work and School, People Supervised, Colleagues at Work and School, Fears, Guilt Feelings, Abilities, Past, Future, and Goals. The degree of disturbance for each specific attitude is rated on a 3-point scale from none to severely disturbed. Through this organization, the most prominent areas of disturbance can be delineated and the interrelationships between the various attitudes can be reviewed to aid in understanding the dynamic factors in the case.

Sacks and Levy believe that the material obtained from the "SSCT may reflect conscious, preconscious or unconscious thinking and feeling" (1950, p. 375). They also urge that it be used in conjunction with other projective techniques such as the Rorschach and TAT.

7.4. The Forer Structured Sentence Completion Test (Forer)

7.4.1. The Test

The Forer Structured Sentence Completion Test consists of 100 items, making it one of the longest tests in general use. Instructions emphasize speed: "Complete the following sentence as rapidly as you can. Write down the first thing you think of" (Forer, 1950, p. 18). Forer has purposely structured his stems to force the patient to deal with specific material that can be useful in diagnosis. Representative items are:

When he was completely on his own, he _____.
I was most depressed when _____.
When he met his boss, he _____.
While he was speaking to me, I _____.
Most women act as though _____.
When I think of marriage _____.

A male and a female form are used, with the gender reference being appropriate for the patient taking the test. A wide variety of issues are covered in the 100 items, and the highly structured quality of the stems is thought to make clear the use of evasiveness and defense mechanisms of the patient as they relate to specific issues.

7.4.2. Evaluation and Interpretation

Forer (1950) suggests the use of a specially designed checksheet to help organize the material gathered from the test. It is not a formal scoring system but is a way of organizing the descriptive material to aid in formalization of the patient's dynamics and diagnosis. Seven major areas are delineated in the checksheet:

1. Attitudes toward important interpersonal figures.
2. Dominant needs or drives.
3. Types of environmental conditions that lead to emotional responses.
4. Reactions in interpersonal situations.
5. Summary of all predominant attitudes and moods.
6. Aggressive tendencies, amount and direction.
7. Affective level.

The structure of the test has allowed Forer to assign specific items to specific attitudes, reactions, or motivational areas. The structure of the items also makes the impact of any deviation from the formal aspects of the completion more pronounced, usually indicating "the presence of highly personalized elements in the associative processes" (p. 25). It is suggested that careful comparison be carried out, reviewing the different aspects of attitudes and reactions to the interpersonal figures portrayed on the items, with special attention to issues of transference, displacement, and differential attitudes to males and females. Forer's hope is that the checksheet will encourage the systematic interpretation of the material and lead to better diagnostic inferences.

7.5. The Miale-Holsopple Sentence Completion Test

7.5.1. The Test

The Miale-Holsopple Sentence Completion Test consists of 73 items, most of which are quite unstructured. Holsopple and Miale (1954) summarize the criteria they used to select the stems, choosing those which

> threaten least and expose least obviously; permit variety of expression and flexibility of interpretation; lie within the experience and understanding of the subject; are relatively unstructured; invite completions which can be interpreted similarly by different clinicians; and invite completions from which the inference drawn can be checked against external fact. (Holsopple & Miale, 1954, p. 15)

A few representative items are:

> Children are usually certain that _____.
> A large crowd _____.
> When fire starts _____.
> Few children fear _____.
> People shouldn't _____.
> A woman's body _____.

The quality of these stems is quite different from that of stems in the more structured tests, and the instructions given with them also have a much more unstructured quality:

> Complete each sentence in whatever way you wish. If you have trouble thinking of a completion to any sentence, put a circle around the number, and return to the sentence when you have finished the rest. (Holsopple & Miale, 1954, p. 175)

The authors expressly discount the use of time-pressure instructions, believing that unconscious defense mechanisms may be even more effective in rapid responses.

7.5.2. Evaluation and Interpretation

No formal scoring system is offered, Holsopple and Miale (1954) stating that such an endeavor would be premature at this time. Instead, they believe that the clinician should carry out "a process of interpretation sentence by sentence until an acceptable global description is achieved" (p. 6). They offer a number of suggestions of how to go about this interpretive process. First, one should read through the complete protocol without attempting any interpretation. This will give the clinician a global impression of the individual and also stop him or her from overre-acting to the responses to the first few items. Next, one should read only the re-sponses—ignoring the stems, getting a feel for clusters of responses, and seeing dominant themes which emerge without any specific relationship to the stems to which the patient is responding. Last, one should explore the significance of the individual completions. Especially important are responses which are unusual for the specific stem. So that clinicians can make such comparisons, a great number of characteristic responses are given for each stem (Holsopple & Miale, 1954). Certain aspects of phrasing that they feel have special importance are also outlined:

(1) Is the completion positive or negative?
(2) Is the statement a "should" or "may be" response?
(3) Is the subject in the response passive or active?
(4) Is the response imperative or a simple declarative statement?
(5) What is the time orientation of the response?
(6) What are the differences in identification with the material of the stem?
(7) Is there a wholehearted commitment in the response?
(8) Are there differences in definiteness or vagueness of the different responses?
(9) What is the amount of verbalization in the responses and is it different from other responses?

Holsopple and Miale also describe the basic interpretive process very well:

> As one proceeds through the sentences, vague structures and outstanding properties begin to emerge. These clarify themselves gradually with full use of the examiner's insight, empathy, and experience, until a personality picture in terms of basic conflicts, ways of handling con-flict, limitations and defects, as well as positive resources, has developed. (Holsopple & Miale, 1954, p. 43)

They illustrate their process with a number of case reports taken from many diag-nostic categories which they hope will help with the interpretation of other patients' protocols. Overall, the Miale-Holsopple is the least structured of the sentence com-pletion tests and depends on the subjective interpretive skills of the clinician more than any of the other tests. It is also true, however, that none of these tests can or should be used in a mechanical-unthinking manner. There is no substitute for a well-trained clinician making interpretations based on the data the patient presents. No matter which test the individual clinician chooses to use and no matter what form the interpretation of the material takes, experience with the test is a key element in the effective and valid use of it.

8. Conclusion

The sentence completion method has, on the whole, been shown to be a flexible and useful clinical and research tool. A number of interesting scoring systems for clinically relevant issues have been presented and have proven to be valid and to possess as good reliability as any other projective technique. Although there are still disagreements over what level of personality functioning the tests tap and how much the patient is able to censor responses, the method is still considered by most clinicians to involve projection of at least some dynamic aspects of the indi-vidual. The structure of the test itself can be used as a diagnostic indicator, revealing how closely the patient is able to follow the cue properties of the stems. No definitive answer is possible at this time to the question of how best to encourage projection in terms of both instructions and stem structure. There are a number of popular clinical sentence completion tests, each differing in terms of the items used and the suggested method of interpretation, with no one test clearly superior to the others.

9. References

Aronoff, J. *A manual to score safety, love and belongingness, and esteem motives.* Technical Report, unpublished, 1972.

Bartz, W. R. Identification on the sentence completion test. *Journal of Clinical Psychology*, 1968, *24*, 351–355.

Binet, A., & Simon, T. Méthodes nouvelles pour le diagnostic du niveau intellectuel des anormaux. *Année Psychologique*, 1905, *11*, 191–244.

Cameron, N. A study of thinking in senile deterioration and schizophrenic disorganization. *American Journal of Psychology*, 1938, *51*, 650–664.

Campbell, D. T. A typology of tests, projective and otherwise. *Journal of Consulting Psychology*, 1957, *21*, 207–210.

Churchill, R., & Crandall, V. J. The reliability and validity of the Rotter incomplete sentences test. *Journal of Consulting Psychology*, 1955, *19*, 345–350.

Coleman, J. C. The levels hypothesis: A re-examination and reorientation. *Journal of Projective Techniques and Personality Assessment*, 1969, *33*, 118–122.

Copple, G. E. Effective intelligence as measured by an unstructured sentence-completion technique. *Journal of Consulting Psychology*, 1956, *20*, 357–360.

Costin, F., & Eiserer, P. E. Students' attitudes toward school life as revealed by a sentence completion test. *American Psychologist*, 1949, *4*, 289.

Cromwell, R. L., & Lundy, R. M. Productivity of clinical hypotheses on a sentence completion test. *Journal of Consulting Psychology*, 1954, *18*, 421–424.

Ebbinghaus, H. Über eine neue Methode in Prüfung geistiger Fähigkeiten und ihre Anwendung bei Schulkindern. *Zeitschrift für Psychologie und Physiologie des Sinnsorganen*, 1897, *13*, 401–457.

Exner, J. E. The self focus sentence completion: A study of egocentricity. *Journal of Personality Assessment*, 1973, *37*, 437–455.

Farber, M. L. English and Americans: A study in national character. *Journal of Psychology*, 1951, *13*, 241–249.

Feldhusen, J. F., Thurston, J. R., & Benning, J. J. Sentence completion responses and classroom social behavior. *Personnel and Guidance Journal*, 1966, *45*, 165–170.

Flanagan, J. E. (Ed.) *The aviation psychological program in the AAF* (Aviation Psychology Research Report No. 1). Washington, D.C.: Government Printing Office, 1947.

Flynn, W. Oral vs. written administration of the Incomplete Sentences Blank. *Newsletter for Research in Mental Health and the Behavioral Sciences*, 1974, *16*, 19–20.

Forer, B. R. A structured sentence completion test. *Journal of Projective Techniques*, 1950, *14*, 15–30.

Gardner, J. M., & Harrison, R. Reliability and validity of the qualitative interpretation of sentence completions. A single case statistical study. *Journal of Projective Techniques and Personality Assessment*, 1967, *31*, 69–73.

Getzels, J. W., & Jackson, P. W. Occupational choice and cognitive functioning. *Journal of Abnormal and Social Psychology*, 1960, *61*, 119–123.

Goldberg, P. A. A review of sentence completion methods in personality assessment. *Journal of Projective Techniques and Personality Assessment*, 1965, *29*, 12–45.

Goldberg, P. A. The current status of sentence completion methods. *Journal of Projective Techniques and Personality Assessment*, 1968, *32*, 215–221.

Golde, P., & Kogan, N. A sentence completion procedure for assessing attitudes toward old people. *Journal of Gerontology*, 1959, *14*, 355–360.

Greaves, G. Harvey's "This I Believe" test: Studies of reliability. *Psychological Reports*, 1971, *28*, 387–390.

Harris, D. B., & Tseng, S. C. Children's attitudes toward peers and parents as revealed by sentence completions. *Child Development*, 1957, *28*, 401–411.

Harvey, O. J. Some cognitive determinants of influencibility. *Sociometry*, 1964, *27*, 208–221.

Harvey, O. J. Some situational and cognitive determinants of dissonance resolution. *Journal of Personality and Social Psychology*, 1965, *1*, 349–355.

Harvey, O. J., Hunt, D., & Schroder, H. *Conceptual system and personality organization.* New York: Wiley, 1961.

Harvey, O. J., Prather, M., White, J. B., & Hoffmeister, J. K. Teachers' benefits, classroom atmosphere and student behavior. *American Educational Research Journal*, 1968, *5*, 151–166.

Harvey, O. J., & Ware, R. Personality difference in dissonance resolution. *Journal of Personality and Social Psychology*, 1967, *7*, 227–230.

Holsopple, J. Q., & Miale, F. *Sentence completion*. Springfield, Ill.: Thomas, 1954.

Holt, R. D. The nature of T.A.T. stories as cognitive products. In J. Kagen & G. Lesser (Eds.), *Contemporary issues in thematic apperception methods*. Springfield, Ill.: Thomas, 1961.

Holtzman, W. H., & Sells, S. B. Prediction of flying success by clinical analysis of test protocols. *Journal of Abnormal and Social Psychology*, 1954, *49*, 485–490.

Holzberg, J. Self-idea completions test. *Bulletin of the Menninger Clinic*, 1945, *9*, 89–93.

Holzberg, J., Teicher, A., & Taylor, J. L. Contributions of clinical psychology to military neuropsychiatry in an army psychiatric hospital. *Journal of Clinical Psychology*, 1947, *3*, 84–95.

Hutt, M. L. The use of projective methods of personality measures in army medical installations. *Journal of Clinical Psychology*, 1945, *1*, 134–140.

Irvin, F. S. Effects of stem reference on sentence completion responses. *Psychological Reports*, 1967, *21*, 679–680. (a)

Irvin, F. S. Sentence completion responses and scholastic success or failure. *Journal of Counseling Psychology*, 1967, *14*, 269–271. (b)

Irvin, F. S., & Johnson, M. L. Effect of differential instructional set on sentence completion responses. *Journal of Consulting and Clinical Psychology*, 1970, *34*, 319–322.

Jung, C. G. *Diagnostische Assoziationsstudien*. Leipzig: Barth, 1904.

Jung, C. G. Diagnostische Assoziationsstudien. *Jahrbuch für Psychologie und Neurologie*, 1906, *8*, 25–60.

Jung, C. G. Diagnostische Assoziationsstudien. *Jahrbuch für Psychologie und Neurologie*, 1907, *9*, 188–197.

Kelly, E. L., & Fiske, D. W. The prediction of success in the VA training program in clinical psychology. *American Psychologist*, 1950, *5*, 395–406.

Kelly, E. L., & Fiske, D. W. *The prediction of performance in clinical psychology*. Ann Arbor: University of Michigan Press, 1951.

Kelly, T. J. Individual testing with completion test exercises. *Teacher's College Records*, 1917, *18*, 371–382.

Kent, G. H., & Rosanoff, A. A study of association in insanity. *American Journal of Insanity*, 1910, *67*, 37–96, 317–390.

Lanyon, B. J. Empirical construction and validation of a sentence completion test for hostility, anxiety, and dependency. *Journal of Consulting and Clinical Psychology*, 1972, *39*, 420–428.

LaPlante, M. J., & Irvin, F. S. Sentence-completion responses and academic performance re-examined. *Journal of Projective Techniques and Personality Assessment*, 1970, *34*, 219–222.

Loevinger, J. The meaning and measurement of ego development. *American Psychologist*, 1966, *21*, 195–206.

Loevinger, J., & Wessler, R. *Measuring ego development 1. Construction and use of a sentence completion test*. San Francisco: Jossey-Bass, 1970.

Loevinger, J., Wessler, R., & Redmore, C. *Measuring ego development 2. Scoring manual for women and girls*. San Francisco: Jossey-Bass, 1970.

Lorge, I., & Thorndike, E. L. The value of the responses in a completion test as indications of personal traits. *Journal of Applied Psychology*, 1941, *25*, 191–199. (a)

Lorge, I., & Thorndike, E. L. The value of the responses in a free association test as indications of personal traits. *Journal of Applied Psychology*, 1941, *25*, 200–201. (b)

Lubin, B., Wallis, R. R., & Paine, C. Patterns of psychological test usage in the United States: 1935–1964. *Professional Psychology*, 1971, *2*, 70–74.

Lunneborg, P. W., & Olch, D. Sentence completion correlates of airline pilot attitude and proficiency. *Journal of Projective Techniques and Personality Assessment*, 1970, *34*, 497–502.

MacBrayer, C. T. Differences in perception of the opposite sex by males and females. *Journal of Social Psychology*, 1960, *52*, 309–314.

McKinney, F. The sentence completion blank in assessing student self-actualization. *Personnel and Guidance Journal*, 1967, *45*, 709–713.

Meltzoff, J. The effect of mental set and item structure upon response to a projective test. *Journal of Abnormal and Social Psychology*, 1951, *46*, 177–189.

Murray, H. A. *Explorations in personality*. New York: Oxford, 1938.

Murray, H. A., & MacKinnon, D. W. Assessment of OSS personnel. *Journal of Consulting Psychology*, 1946, *10*, 76–80.

Murstein, B. I. (Ed.). *Handbook of projective techniques*. New York: Basic Books, 1965.

Murstein, B. I., Colon, R. M., Destrexhe-deLeval, N., & VanHoof-VanParys, M. Influence of stimulus properties of the sentence-completion-method on projection and adjustment. *Journal of Personality Assessment*, 1972, *36*, 241–247.

Murstein, B. I., & Wolf, S. R. Empirical test of the "levels" hypothesis with five projective techniques. *Journal of Abnormal Psychology*, 1970, *75*, 38–44.

Nystedt, L., Magnusson, D., & Aronowitsch, E. Generalization of ratings based on projective tests. *Scandinavian Journal of Psychology*, 1975, *16*, 72–78.

Payne, A. F. *Sentence completions*. New York: Guidance Clinic, 1928.

Peck, R. F., & McGuire, C. Measuring changes in mental health with the sentence completion technique. *Psychological Reports*, 1959, *5*, 151–160.

Piltz, R. J. Problems in validity for the Copple sentence completion test as a measure of "effective intelligence" with Air Force personnel. *Dissertation Abstracts*, 1957, *17*, 1914–1915.

Redmore, C. Susceptibility to faking of a sentence completion test of ego development. *Journal of Personality Assessment*, 1976, *40*, 607–616.

Redmore, C., & Waldman, K. Reliability of a sentence completion measure of ego development. *Journal of Personality Assessment*, 1975, *39*, 236–243.

Reilly, D. H., & Sugerman, A. A. Conceptual complexity and psychological differentiation in alcoholics. *Journal of Nervous and Mental Disease*, 1967, *144*, 14–17.

Renner, K. E., Maher, B. A., & Campbell, D. T. The validity of a method for scoring sentence completion responses for anxiety, dependency, and hostility. *Journal of Applied Psychology*, 1962, *46*, 285–290.

Rohde, A. R. Explorations in personality by the sentence completion method. *Journal of Applied Psychology*, 1946, *30*, 169–181.

Rohde, A. R. *Sentence completions test manual*. Beverly Hills, Calif.: Western Psychological Services, 1947.

Rohde, A. R. *The sentence completion method: Its diagnostic and clinical application to mental disorders*. New York: Ronald Press, 1957.

Rothaus, P., Johnson, D. L., Hanson, P. G., Brown, J. B., & Lyle, F. A. Sentence-completion test prediction of autonomous and therapist-led group behavior. *Journal of Counseling Psychology*, 1967, *14*, 28–34.

Rotter, J. B., & Rafferty, J. E. *Manual: The Rotter Incomplete Sentences Blank*. New York: Psychological Corporation, 1950.

Rotter, J. B., Rafferty, J. E., & Schachtitz, E. Validation of the Rotter incomplete sentences blank for college screening. *Journal of Consulting Psychology*, 1949, *13*, 348–366.

Rotter, J. B., & Willerman, B. The incomplete sentences test as a method of studying personality. *Journal of Consulting Psychology*, 1947, *11*, 43–48.

Sacks, J. M. The relative effect upon projective responses of stimuli referring to the subject and of stimuli referring to other persons. *Journal of Consulting Psychology*, 1949, *13*, 12–20.

Sacks, J. M., & Levy, S. The sentence completion test. In L. E. Abt & L. Bellak (Eds.), *Projective Psychology*. New York: Knopf, 1950.

Schroder, H. M., & Streufert, S. The measurement of four systems varying in levels of abstractiveness (sentence completion method) [Technical Report No. 11 on project R-171-055]. Princeton, N.J.: Princeton University, 1962.

Shor, J. Report of a verbal projective technique. *Journal of Clinical Psychology*, 1946, *2*, 270–282.

Siipola, E. M. Incongruence of sentence completions under time pressure and freedom. *Journal of Projective Techniques and Personality Assessment*, 1968, *32*, 562–571.

Souelem, O. Mental patients' attitudes toward mental hospitals. *Journal of Clinical Psychology*, 1955, *11*, 181–185.

Stein, M. I. The use of a sentence completion test for the diagnosis of personality. *Journal of Clinical Psychology*, 1947, *3*, 46–56.

Stephens, M. W. Stimulus pull as a determinant of individual difference in sentence completion responses. *Journal of Projective Techniques and Personality Assessment*, 1970, *34*, 332–339.

Stone, H. K., & Dellis, N. P. An exploratory investigation into the levels hypothesis. *Journal of Projective Techniques*, 1960, *24*, 333–340.

Stricker, G., & Dawson, D. D. The effects of first person and third person instruction and stems on sentence completion responses. *Journal of Projective Techniques and Personality Assessment*, 1966, *30*, 169–171.

Sullivan, C., Grant, M. Q., & Grant, J. D. The development of interpersonal maturity: Application to delinquency. *Psychiatry*, 1957, *20*, 373–385.

undberg, N. D. The practice of psychological testing in clinical services in the United States. *American Psychologist*, 1961, *16*, 79–83.

endler, A. D. A preliminary report on a test for emotional insight. *Journal of Applied Psychology*, 1930, *14*, 123–126.

rabue, M. R. *Completion test language scales.* New York: Columbia University Press, 1916.

U.S. Office of Strategic Services, OSS Assessment Staff. *Assessment of men.* New York: Rinehart, 1948.

Wells, F. L. Practice effects in free association. *American Journal of Psychology*, 1911, *22*, 1–13.

West, J. T. An investigation of the constructs "effective intelligence" and "social competence" with the Copple sentence completion test utilizing a school of social work population. *Dissertation Abstracts*, 1958, *19*, 1121.

Wilson, J. P., & Aronoff, J. A sentence completion test assessing safety and esteem motives. *Journal of Personality Assessment*, 1973, *37*, 351–354.

Wolkon, G. H., & Haefner, D. P. Change in ego strength of improved and unimproved psychiatric patients. *Journal of Clinical Psychology*, 1961, *17*, 352–355.

Wood, F. A. Tachistoscopic vs. conventional presentation of incomplete sentence stimuli. *Journal of Projective Techniques and Personality Assessment*, 1967, *31*, 30–31.

Wood, F. A. An investigation of methods of presenting incomplete sentence stimuli. *Journal of Abnormal Psychology*, 1969, *74*, 71–74.

9

Projective Drawings: Two Areas of Differential Diagnostic Challenge

EMANUEL F. HAMMER

1. Introduction

My experience in conducting the annual American Projective Drawing Institute summer workshops suggests that clinicians and clinical students, using projective drawings for differential diagnostic assessment, experience the most uncertainty in two areas: (1) in the differentiation of the vague and shimmering spectrum from schizoid to borderline and latent schizophrenia onto schizophrenic conditions, and (2) in the differentiation of organic brain damage from the former group. With respect to this problem, there are several broad points that may be made in observation of the mixed results that research studies yield in validating projective drawings (as they similarly yield on the other projective techniques).

2. Issues Concerning Research Findings

Projective drawings have been attacked and defended vigorously, with a sizable literature resulting. The balance of positive vs. negative research results has not changed much since previous reviews. What has emerged are more promising directions of research and an increasing sophistication concerning the defects of previous research designs. These promising directions may be seen in the following:

1. Levy, Minsky, and Lomax (1977) found that the accuracy or inaccuracy of the proportions within the figure drawings correlated highly—and in the expected direction—with the degree of pathology of the subject executing the drawing. Thus the relationships between the elements of the drawing, more than the individual de-

---

EMANUEL F. HAMMER • 381 West End Avenue, New York, New York 10024.

tails, may prove to be the validating dimensions. This promising lead, of comparative dimensions within the sets of drawings of an individual, is illustrated by the carefully scored and analyzed work of Irgens-Jensen (1971). Comparing the male and female human figure drawings of male problem drinkers, he found that alcoholics to a statistically significant degree, more frequently drew male figures with abnormal (blurred, disturbed, or omitted) heads and caricatured eyes. Thus, using the heads of the female figures drawn by alcoholics as a baseline, Irgens-Jensen could discern the emergence of distortions concerning the self-figure. These male subjects also drew female figures, again to a statistically significant degree, larger than male figures. The females were drawn in an obscene manner and were rated by judges as more typically a sex object, in the style of drawings in men's rooms. Based on this cluster of findings, Irgens-Jensen engaged in a multivariate analysis which accounted for 60% of the variants associated with alcoholism. The direct interpretations from the projective drawings revealed the problem drinker as having hostile and conflicted attitudes toward females, a less differentiated and articulated conception of his own body, a diminished lack of self-confidence, a reduced control of emotional impulses, and a reliance on both punitive and crude defense mechanisms. The study stands as an example of how careful research with projective drawings can be done, with mutual illumination of the subject population and of the validity of the projective instrument.

The central findings of this study concerning validity of several dimensions of projective drawings are consistent with findings of Craddick and Leipold (1968), who also investigated the hypotheses that alcoholics will draw same-sex figures smaller than will a control group and that male alcoholics will draw male human figures smaller than female figures since more anxiety is attached to their own body image (and, according to my own work with alcoholics, because of their feeling threatened by females). The statistical differences were significant at better than the .01 level. The more impressive difference was within the sets of each subject's drawings, between the comparative size of his male and female drawings.

2.   The introduction of dynamic stimuli (rather than the investigation of static relationships), by intensifying the reactions caught by projective drawings, puts the variable in question under a magnifying glass, as it were, to enhance the emergence of data for validity studies. Ludwig (1969) investigated the relationship between one's self-image and one's projective drawing of a person. Negative feedback, in the form of criticism of a male subject's physical abilities, produced a highly significant corresponding decrease in the height of the male figure drawn. That criticism from "experts" resulted in constriction of the height of the person drawn underscores the validity of height of drawing as a reflection of self-esteem.

An interesting collateral effect was the significant increase in the athletic appearance of the male figure drawn as the height decreased. The threat to the ego that a lowered self-image produces seems to give rise to a compensatory increase in the athletic quality drawn onto the person. This suggests, we may read from the data, that the deeper feelings about the self will be expressed in the more basic qualities of the drawing, such as height, whereas the secondary or defensive maneuver—in this case, compensation—will be projected via secondary qualities such as the exaggeration of muscles and the introduction of athletic equipment.

Another core hypothesis involved in projective drawing assessment was also verified: the higher a subject's state of self-esteem the more likely a "happy" mood will be drawn on the projected figure, and the lower the self-esteem the more likely a dysphoric mood will be projected.

In a study investigating the hypothesis that extensive shading in the drawing serves as an index of anxiety, Goldstein and Faterson (1969) showed films to male subjects; these included an anthropological one, from Geza Rohein's study of Australian aborigines, depicting a subincision rite. The film showed an incision being made on the surface of the penis with a sharp stone, the bleeding penis being held over a fire, and the faces of the initiates reflecting their pain. The control situation included nonstress films, one a travelogue of the Far West and one of London. The findings dramatically supported the hypothesis of the relationship between anxiety and shading for the self-sex figure. This study illustrates the principle of dynamic stimuli in research and, at the same time, the earlier principle mentioned involving comparative assessment within the set of drawings. In terms of the latter, the proportionately greater anxiety concerning the self was directly correlated with the greater shading laid onto the self-figure in contrast to the opposite-sex figure.

In experiments such as these, the issues of ethics and immediate alleviation of the induced anxiety or of the negative feedback (as in the experiment before the current one cited) are self-evident. Employing the dynamic stimuli already provided by eugenic sterilization, Hammer (1953), without subjecting individuals to negative stimuli for the purpose of the experiment, found striking support for the hypothesis of sexual symbolism. Elongated objects in the House-Tree-Person drawings, such as chimneys, branches, arms, nose, and feet, were utilized as phallic symbols. Circles, triangles, and objects with a vertical split down the center were employed as vaginal symbols, and served as reflections of felt castration in the drawings of males. Feelings of genital inadequacy were presented via the phallic symbols drawn as damaged, cut through, broken, or otherwise impaired.

3. Studies which avoid the hazards of employing the pigeonholes of psychiatric diagnosis (themselves lacking in established reliability and validity) have better chances at establishing projective technique validity. Griffith and Peyman (1965) found support for the hypothesis that eye and ear emphasis in the drawing of a person is associated with ideas of reference. This study is memorable in drawing to our attention the superiority of actual overt behavior to official psychiatric classification in attempts to validate projective techniques. Had psychiatric diagnosis been the criterion in this study, nonsignificant rather than statistically significant results would have been yielded. Also avoiding psychiatric diagnosis as the criterion, Schmidt and McGowan (1965) demonstrated the relationship between drawn Persons and the traits of the subject offering the drawing; judges operating "blindly" could distinguish figure drawings by physically disabled persons from figure drawings by physically normal persons.

4. Content and global dimensions are proving more valid as projective drawing indicators than are formal or expressive characteristics. In a noteworthy study, Coopersmith, Sokol, Beardslee, and Coopersmith (1976) obtained figure drawings from 97 preadolescents who differed in self and behavioral assessment of self-esteem. The figure drawings were scored for formal characteristics, content, and global-interpretations of the total drawings. Content and global-interpretive categories proved more differentiating between self-esteem groups than did the formal qualities. The advantage of content interpretation over the scoring categories has clearly been emerging in studies of the Rorschach, and as Klopfer (1972) summarized, "It

283

PROJECTIVE
DRAWINGS: TWO
AREAS OF
DIFFERENTIAL
DIAGNOSTIC
CHALLENGE

has become amply evident that content is that aspect of the Rorschach which has shown the greatest success as a predictor of other behavior."

5.   The validity of projective drawing hypotheses is being established in children's drawings in advance of adults' drawings. In addition to the study by Coopersmith et al. on preadolescent subjects, one by Vane and Eisen (1965) may serve as illustration. In this study, kindergarten children served as subjects. Those rated as showing poor adjustment in school produced figure drawings differentiated, to a statistically significant degree, from the other children's on four signs: "grotesque" (the drawing has gross distortions), "no body," "no mouth," and "no arms." A follow-up the next year, with first-grade teachers' ratings, served to validate all four signs. These qualities in children's drawings thus have predictive value as indices of maladjustment (and as clues for consideration of referral for preventive therapy).

In a study of samples of disturbed and of normal children, disturbed youngsters showed considerably greater tendencies toward barrenness in their drawings and toward the inclusion of only minimal details (Davis & Hoopes, 1975).

A series of studies was undertaken by Koppitz (1968) to select a list of valid "Emotional Indicators" for children's drawings "from the hypotheses of Machover (1949) and Hammer (1958)." Comparisons of the Emotional Indicators on the projective drawings of well-adjusted pupils with those of clinic patients validated the Emotional Indicator technique for spotting emotional difficulties. As one example, shy children drew tiny figures more often than did others. Another study showed that anxiety or threat, too, produced constriction in the size of drawings (Craddick, 1963). Generally, we are finding that experiments on validity of projective drawings employing child subjects more easily establish the hypothesis in question. This may be because children's drawings, as with children's behavior in general, are more transparent and less defensively covered. As we find important leads about adults by studying children, and as we find out much about the universal in people by studying neurotic and psychotic behavior, we may initially seek those situations where the issue is more obviously laid bare. More concentrated research efforts with the young subject first may be the wisest sequential program to pursue at this point of development of our understanding of the language of projective drawings.

6.   Apfeldorf, Walter, Kaiman, Smith, and Arnett (1974) focused on the affectively toned associations that occur when an observer first sees a drawing, and from this developed a system for measuring two components: emission of emotional associations and evaluation of affective associations. This method was applied with significant success in studying individuals who had represented in their drawing an image correlated with their actual physical appearance. The research suggested that the affective tones and their evaluation may contribute more to the assessment of the subject who did the drawing than do the usual components focused on. It is for this reason, of course, that the Post Drawing Inquiry, with its many emotionally toned searching questions, is traditionally employed to obtain the subject's emotional and associational elements to enrich the drawing analysis.

7.   We are learning to separate the data within any study for possible sex linkage operating in the study. One such finding occurred, for example, in a study (Roback, 1966) of the relationship between figure drawing size and depression. In this investigation, there was a significant difference (.01) in the height of drawings between depressed and control-group females, although not in their male counterparts. Keeping the male and female data combined in an aggregate had obscured the significant difference for female subjects. We similarly don't know whether keeping the

285

PROJECTIVE
DRAWINGS: TWO
AREAS OF
DIFFERENTIAL
DIAGNOSTIC
CHALLENGE

data in one mass may in many other studies have spuriously masked the significant validity of the investigated dimension for one sex or the other.

8. The use of a battery of drawings is suggested for research purposes, as it is used clinically by those who employ the House-Tree-Person-Person (one of each sex), both achromatic and chromatic, and the Draw-a-Family technique combined as the minimal drawing battery, rather than only the drawing of a male and a female Person. A drawing of just two people is, after all, a very small sample. This might be much like testing the validity of a Rorschach examination by employing only the first two cards. The conflicting results of research studies based merely on the Draw-a-Person technique suggest that for a more valid test we should employ a wider projective drawing net than just the paired drawings of the human figure. Caligor (1952) found that paranoid trends could be detected in only 25% of a group of paranoid schizophrenics when only one drawing was used but could be detected in 85% when a series of eight drawings was employed.

We know—not only as clinicians but as readers of novels, as play watchers, and as viewers of art (think, for example, of Kafka, of Tennessee Williams, and of Van Gogh, particularly his later work)—we know, in our bones, that every creative product draws in part from the psychic innards of the creator. We receive, and resonate to, the person revealed in the work, the tenderness of J. D. Salinger, the sympathy of Rembrandt, the strength of Michelangelo as well as his bisexuality, the gloom of El Greco, the fury of Beethoven, the macho of Hemingway, the agony of Toulouse-Lautrec, or the wit of Picasso. Nor does it have to be art to embody the artist, for even more apparent is the sadism in the non-art novels of Mickey Spillane.

Shy children draw shyly, aggressive children aggressively, impulsive people impulsively, and controlled people tightly. Part of the difficulty revealed in our experiments is expressed in the truth offered by Saul Bellow. The recent Nobel laureate tells us, in *Herzog*, that human life "is far subtler than any of its models."

Many of our experiments do not catch the elusive variables because these clues do not always appear in the same place. A person may reveal trait X in the type of line with which he draws, another may reveal the same trait in the contents he draws, another person in the placement of the drawing on the page, another in its size, another in the color employed, another in the pressure, i.e., the savage digging of the pencil into the paper vs. the hesitant, uncertain, timid line pressure, and so on. In one set of projective drawings a diagnostic hint emerges, in another a personality need, in still another psychodynamics, and in still another something of expressive personality style. It is the rare experiment that can throw out so fine and so comprehensive a net as to catch such complexity for which the clinical approach is, thus far at least, more flexibly geared. It is, perhaps, in part for this reason that studies employing global analysis of projective drawings prove more effective than those resting on item analysis.

As we continue with our research efforts, the above guideposts may point the way toward a more sophisticated and more refined program. With this in mind, let us turn now to the clinical.

3. Schizoid to Schizophrenic Continuum

Figures 1 to 21 illustrate the continuum from schizoid to schizophrenic on which the clinical psychologist is most often asked to make his diagnostic contribution.

Figures 1 and 2 represent the drawing of a male and a female by a schizoid patient. The drawn male (Figure 1) is more mannequin-like than human and actually suggests a store dummy. Figure 2 was described as "She looks like a paper doll." The patient's projections thus are not of flesh-and-blood beings, but of derealized humans who cannot engage in emotional give-and-take. Within the patient, the sap of affect has grown thin. He feels himself to be a synthetic being rather than a full living person. This is an individual who does not seem to be buoyed by any connection he feels with the human. He appears to have lost the sensations of spontaneity, play, warmth, autonomy, and even emotional authenticity. The bloodless man and woman drawn suggest feelings of alienation within the subject. A sense of isolation—of distance, aloneness, and separateness from the human environment—appears central to his portrait of himself. He lives beside life more than in it.

Consistent with his drawings, on the TAT he demonstrated a failure to include much about the relationship between the people shown in the stimuli. On the Rorschach, the number of his Movement responses was diminished, and, when they were given, the Forms were static. The humans or animals did not act, but were only about to act or were acted upon. Color was also absent, vitality low, and zest for living muted. Emphasis was almost exclusively on Form as a determinant, again implying minimal feelings of emotional life within.

The implications for therapy are that his sterility and restriction of personality, and his markedly schizoid structure, will limit and define his behavior in the therapeutic situation. A long period of treatment would be necessary to achieve a gradual

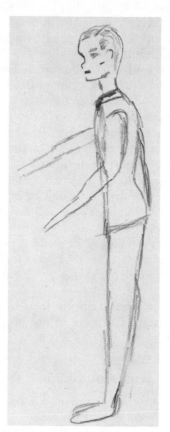

Figure 1

287

PROJECTIVE
DRAWINGS: TWO
AREAS OF
DIFFERENTIAL
DIAGNOSTIC
CHALLENGE

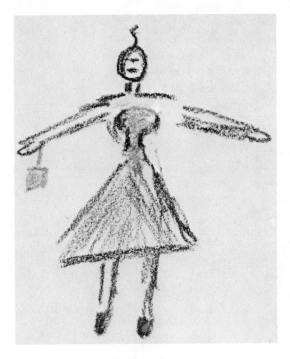

Figure 2

melting through the wall of his detachment by human warmth and interest, and would have to be extended with care to avoid stimulating further protective withdrawal.

Further along the continuum of feelings of depersonalization, we find the subject who drew Figures 3 and 4 as her respective achromatic Persons and Figure 5 as

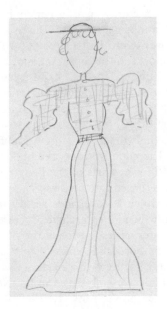

Figure 3

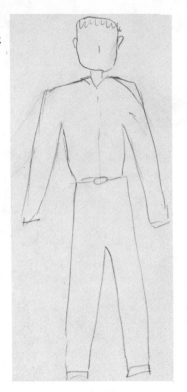

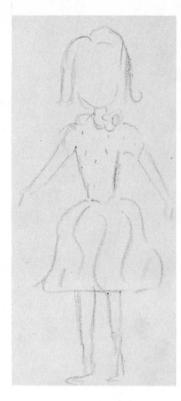

Figure 4   Figure 5

her chromatic Person (executed in blue). These drawn Persons express, and reiterate the expression of, the patient's feeling that she does not exist at all behind her surface façade.

The subject who offered the drawing of a Person in Figure 6 communicates the same existential feeling of nonbeing. Perhaps this is all the more so because his obsessive compulsive defenses cause him to emphasize such rare extremes of detailing as the cufflinks, the clocks in the socks, the shoelaces, and even the shoe soles, against which the expected human details of hand, eyes, nose, mouth, and ears are all the more strikingly absent and meaningfully communicative in their absence. His Rorschach projection of a butterfly "as if pressed in a book in someone's collection" approaches stating the same theme, but nowhere as strikingly.

Along the continuum, the woman who drew Figure 7 is situated further into the schizophrenic process. The ghoulish tone, the hollow-eyed quality of an empty, baglike head, the upper and lower parts of the body regressed to mere nonspecific circles, and the arms and legs turned into arrows as a reflection of the raw, primitive, primary-process-like anger which so overrides reality testing as to replace human limbs all show the degree to which inner, archaic processes are overflooding logically based perceptions. Distortive qualities approach the rampant here.

To backtrack, within the borderline span of the continuum, we may next observe Figure 8. The patient who drew this person was a well-built, immaculately dressed, 37-year-old black man. He had served in the Navy and received an honorable discharge, having attained officer rank. He then attended college and received

289

PROJECTIVE
DRAWINGS: TWO
AREAS OF
DIFFERENTIAL
DIAGNOSTIC
CHALLENGE

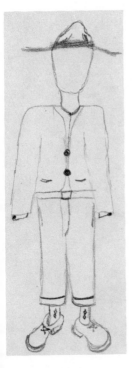

Figure 6

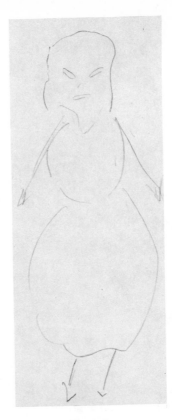

Figure 7

his B.A. After this, he was an assistant preacher in a Southern church for several years, and then came to the North. He was referred for examination because he had been convicted on three counts of assault, involving two men and a woman. The police officer had found a straight razor, a packing knife, and a penknife on the defendant's person. The complainants had never seen the defendant before. One man and the woman had been standing near a candy booth when the defendant pushed his way between them, knocking the woman off balance and causing her to fall. The man—according to his story—shouted "Are you crazy or something?" which enraged the defendant, who then struck the man on the side of the head and struck the woman about the mouth. At that point, the second man appeared and came to their assistance, and the defendant pummeled him with his fists.

The defendant's version was that the man who had exclaimed "Are you crazy or something?" had added "you black nut!" Thus the referring probation officer raised some question concerning a racial issue having inflamed the defendant's reaction. The diagnostic query which accompanied the referral for an examination was "Is this man emotionally sick, is there any presence of significant pathology, and is he capable of peculiar reactivity?"

On the Rorschach, the patient emerged as a borderline schizophrenic individual. Primary thinking processes seeped through to color his perception of the world. His Person drawings were both of nudes, his drawn female a massive, threatening figure and his drawn male (Figure 8) a timid figure with hands behind his back, eyes suspiciously and paranoidally alerted, and chin exaggerated in a demonstration of

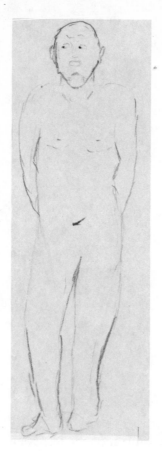

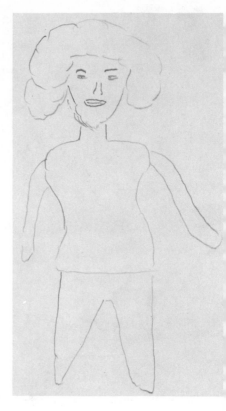

Figure 8

Figure 9

needs to prove himself assertive. What is more important, however, is the reality-testing impairment. He described his drawn male as "standing there and talking . . . talking to a neighbor or someone he sees passing on the street." Here, the strikingly inappropriate description of a nude male standing and talking to a neighbor or passerby on the street conveys the impaired reality testing and dissociative capacities of the subject.

Figure 9, an adult male subject's depiction of a woman with a clear implication of a beard on her face, suggests the borderline process his entire projective technique picture conveyed. Reality testing is impaired but not sweepingly so. It tends, rather, to exist in a circumscribed area. In contrast, Figure 10, also representing a male subject's perception of women, tends to push further into the schizophrenic area. We find not only the beard-depicting (otherwise ununderstandable) line protruding from the woman's chin but also the transparent arm, the empty eye socket, and the suggestion of the beginning of a penis before the lower page edge interrupts the drawing. Here, of course, the reality-distorting confusion of sexual identity goes considerably further than in the preceding illustration.

Contaminated thinking and fabulized combinations may express themselves in drawings as on the Rorschach. Figure 11 shows a contamination of arms and cape,

291

PROJECTIVE
DRAWINGS: TWO
AREAS OF
DIFFERENTIAL
DIAGNOSTIC
CHALLENGE

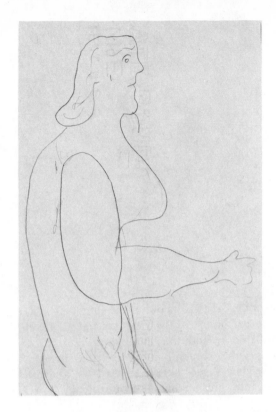

Figure 10

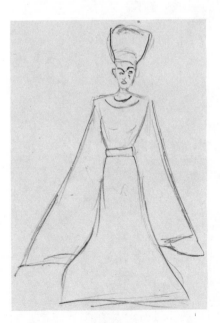

Figure 11

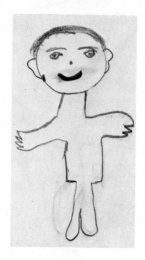

Figure 12

where it appears as if the cape grows out of the shoulders where arms should. This is to be understood in the context of the Egyptian figure offered, a symbol of a long-since-dead person distant in both time and place. Figure 12, drawn by a 14-year-old girl, also presents us with a contamination, this time carried a bit further. Arms become wings, legs become suggestive of tail feathers, and the entire figure appears ready to fly upward into, presumably, autistic realms.

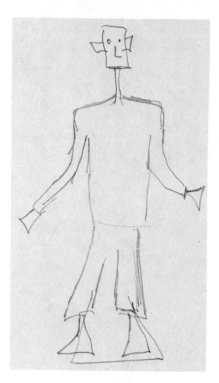

Figure 13

293

PROJECTIVE
DRAWINGS: TWO
AREAS OF
DIFFERENTIAL
DIAGNOSTIC
CHALLENGE

Well into the schizophrenic domain, Figure 13 stands as a reflection of frank pathology. The geometric rendition of hands, feet, and ears suggests an arbitrary perceptual tendency (to overabstract and possibly also to rely on magical signs). The robotlike head and neck add to the depersonalized quality, while the absence of a mouth and the pupilless eyes reflect the communication difficulties schizophrenics so agonizingly experience. The ears alerted so conspicuously out from the head convey a strong tendency to ideas of reference, if not actual auditory hallucinations. The line for the ground suddenly comes up in a rather peculiar way as if to add some stability to the figure's footing, no matter how artificially. This patient is an individual who, at the most, has a pseudointegration of personality, with the frail links barely keeping him together. His illness appears to serve, at best, as a mere expedient for survival amid the contradictions within him. The patient appears to have constructed an unreal world into which he is retiring.

Figure 14, drawn by a frankly paranoid schizophrenic man, carries this process much further and expresses the automatonlike experience of being controlled by hallucinatory voices telling him what to do. The compensatory grandiosity, at the same time, is embellished across his chest in the purple band across the green.

Figure 15 carries the reflection of the depersonalization process still further. This patient's identification is with a fluid and formless being, a truly tragic conception of personal identity. Ego boundaries fade, and the figure melts away. Haunted by a picture of himself as a creature whose outlines blur, he has eventually given in, and now, a back-ward patient in a mental hospital, he has lost sight of who and

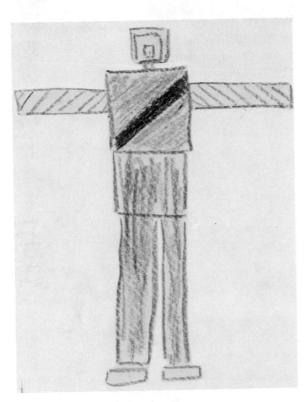

Figure 14

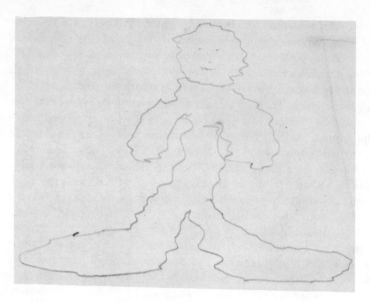

Figure 15

what—and if—he is. A search through the hospital folder revealed a Draw-a-Person projection done, on admission, many years earlier. His Person was standing rigidly at attention, body and head very stiff, legs pressed closely together, arms straight and held to the body. The kinesthetic emphasis was on the rigid stance and on the tension with which the body was held, keeping the self closed off against the world. The overall impression was of a person frozen into a posture, unable to move over the threshold of exchange or action.

Still further along the continuum to massive deterioration, Figure 16 reflects

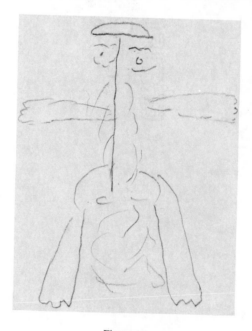

Figure 16

an individual with body image totally shot, with peripheral lines no longer present around the face, and a body wall through which the intestines have spilled.

Figure 17 stands as an extreme example of paranoid schizophrenic reaction. The savage mouth expresses the rage-filled projections loosened from within. The emphasized eyes and ears, with the eyes almost emanating magical rays, reflect the visual and auditory hallucinations the patient actually experiences. The snake in the stomach points up his delusional sensations of a reptile within, eating away and generating venomous evil.

Two other issues of schizophrenic expression in projective drawings deserve mention before closing this section: anthropomorphism and the prediction we extend when we offer the diagnostic impression of preschizophrenia.

An anthropomorphic version of the House may be seen in that drawn by the subject offering us Figure 18. The front of the House conveys a quality of two eye-positioned windows, a circular "nose," and a door which in this context serves as a mouth, all then set off by the "bangs" which hang down like hair from the crown of the house. Anthropomorphism, in drawings, appears to represent the schizophrenic diminishment of reality testing, on the one hand, but all the more the totally projective coloring of the outer world due to insufficient ego boundaries and an inability to sense where the self ends and the outer world begins. (The regression often draws from the infantile stage of the baby in its psychic connection with the mother.) As an illustration of the process, I recall a 6-year-old girl I was treating who in leaving

295

PROJECTIVE
DRAWINGS: TWO
AREAS OF
DIFFERENTIAL
DIAGNOSTIC
CHALLENGE

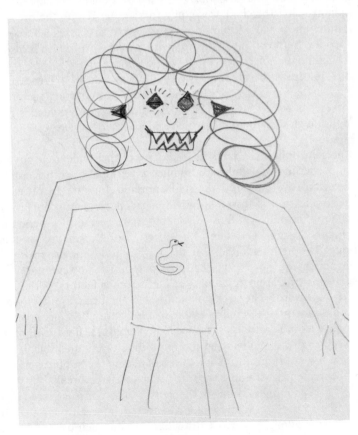

Figure 17

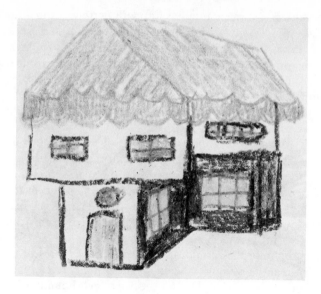

Figure 18

the office after a session one day, kicked the leg of a chair. When I inquired about this, she explained that the chair was going to kick her. Here, the projective mechanism is so much more global than in mere paranoid processes where projection is onto other people. In the anthropomorphic process, the projection is also indiscriminantly onto inanimate objects.

In Figure 19, drawn by an adult, we find a depiction of a Tree which becomes more humanlike than treelike. The branches extend out as exaggerated ears, the foliage becomes bushy hair, and all the more unequivocably a face is put onto the trunk. The full-blown schizophrenia, which is all too evident here, can be more subtly sensed in Figure 18.

As to "preschizophrenia": here, as stated, we chance a clear-cut prediction. The diagnosis of borderline schizophrenia implies a reasonably stable condition positioned with partial overlap onto the schizophrenic domain. In preschizophrenia, however, the implication is that the individual, while presently not overtly schizophrenic, will soon, usually within a reasonably short period of time, manifest open pathology. Figure 20 may be taken as a reflection of "normality" in almost every regard but one. The figure is intact, the detailing is good, the proportions are accurate, and distortions do not exist. The one thing amiss, however, and that a most striking one against the appropriateness of all the other factors, is that the figure is toppling over backward. The eyes go blank, and the arms are kept rigidly at the side without any potential flexibility to break the figure's fall. Because the drawing is so well done, the imbalance is all the more meaningful. That the imbalance is one of falling over *backward* renders the figure all the more vulnerable. The imminent loss of personality equilibrium, of psychic balance, is the subjective experience of an individual threatened with an impending schizophrenic break.

Figure 21 is even more extreme in this regard. The figure is placed up on the top of a mound as if to use it as a launching pad away from reality. Something I advise students to do in "reading" projective drawings is to put their own bodies in the position of the drawn figure and thus experience kinesthetically, as a supplement to the visual taking in of the data, what the drawing communicates. (This is much like the

297

**PROJECTIVE
DRAWINGS: TWO
AREAS OF
DIFFERENTIAL
DIAGNOSTIC
CHALLENGE**

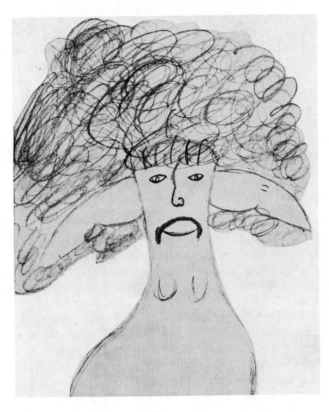

Figure 19

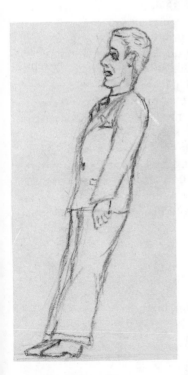

Figure 20

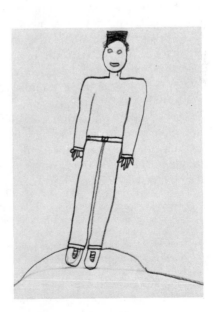

Figure 21

kinesthetic method used in remedial reading, which adds a modality to the visual learning.) If one places oneself in the same position as the drawn Person, one can feel in the upward and sideways tug of the shoulders the pull within the body away from the ground. It is as if the figure, with perhaps a faint suggestion of a nosecone hat and fingers trimmed for trailing behind, is ready to soar up and away. The empty eye sockets add a depersonalized quality to the autism and psychic imbalance. Figure 21 is a more extreme expression than is Figure 20, in that in Figure 20 the loss of emotional balance, while clear, is a statement of losing equilibrium and falling; Figure 21 is a statement of abandoning groundedness altogether and going off into one's own idiosyncratic, delusional orbit, leaving reality behind.

4. Organicity Reflected in Projective Drawings

In practice, much as it may surprise the uninitiated, the responsibility for the assessment of the presence of organic brain damage is often passed along, by both the psychiatrist and the neurologist, to the clinical psychologist. EEG's are generally vague and ambiguous except in the more severe cases, and neurological examination cannot pick up the subtleties which organic damage produces in alterations of the perceptual processes.

The clinical psychologist often finds that his greatest uncertainty in differential diagnosis is in separating the organic from the schizophrenic in their respective expressive-perceptual performances. Goldworth (1950) found that 32% of his sample of schizophrenics and 58% of his sample of people with organic brain damage drew heads which were characterized by the judges as "bizarre" or "grotesque." In contrast, none of his sample of 50 normals and only four of his group of 50 neurotics drew heads so characterized. Thus, where the projective technique interpreter quite easily determines that the case before him is "sicker" than normal or neurotic, he's often left with the dilemma "But is it schizophrenic or organic?"

In meeting this assessment challenge, in the projective battery usually the H-T-P (particularly the drawings of House and Tree) is the most determining. The H-T-P, I find, is superior to the Bender-Gestalt for detecting organicity in that with the Bender the patient has something specific and concrete to lean on, to copy from. These Bender figures are relatively simple, and the patient has to be fairly organically impaired before he, with the organic's concrete orientation, cannot merely reproduce the elemental figure directly before him. The kinds of performance on the Bender-Gestalt that have established their association with brain dysfunction—problems in spatial organization, difficulty in forming angles, omission of parts in the service of simplification—are more readily picked up in their subtler variety of expression when there is nothing from which to copy. With the House-Tree-Person drawings, the patient has a blank page before him and merely a vague conceptual stimulus—"house," "tree," or "person"—to build from. This is directly parallel to what Landisberg finds comparatively with H-T-P and Rorschach:

> Evidence of organicity is discerned in a more clear-cut fashion with the H-T-P than with the Rorschach, and such evidence may be reflected earlier on the former technique. This is a result of the fact that the H-T-P, comparatively speaking, forces the individual to use his mental resources in a more independent and volitional manner. Blots are blots. The patterns and boundaries may be ill defined, but they do serve as props. And the organic, concrete as he is, has at least a little to build from. But with just a blank sheet of paper in front of him and just a word to conceptualize from, his basic weakness and shakey responses are more prone to come to the fore. (Landisberg, 1973)

299

PROJECTIVE
DRAWINGS: TWO
AREAS OF
DIFFERENTIAL
DIAGNOSTIC
CHALLENGE

In a study comparing the Rorschach, the Bender-Gestalt, and projective drawings, it was found that the drawings exceeded both the Bender and the Rorschach in detecting organicity (*Proceedings*, 1960).

Let us turn now to the task of differentiating organic from schizophrenic conditions, a task all the more complicated in subjects of relatively lower intellectual functioning. Since the emphasis of the responsibility within the projective drawing battery is borne by the subtasks of the drawing of House and Tree, we may keep in mind the relatively representative schizophrenic drawings of lower-IQ subjects (Figures 22 and 23), which will stand in contrast to those we will later inspect of the organic. The drawing of a House with its obvious anthropomorphic quality of wide-mouthed door, eyelike-placed windows, and curlicue-of-hair chimney, embellished further with tielike pathway, seems to look more like a schematic face than a house. The "classic" split Tree, which is essentially two one-dimensional trees side by side, reflects the shattering or disintegration of self experienced by the schizophrenic. To add another House drawing illustrating anthropomorphism, Figure 24 embodies leglike walkways, earlike laterally placed chimneys, and hairlike fence on the roof.

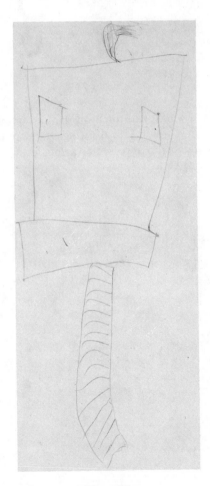

Figure 22

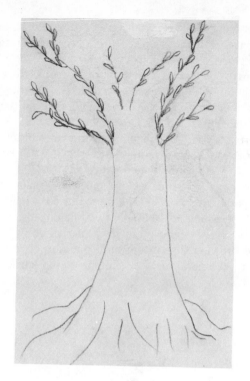

Figure 23

The gestalt is more like a walking automaton than a house. Not all schizophrenics anthropomorphize, or "split" their Tree drawings, but simple organics do not!

General principles which run across the various drawings of the H-T-Ps of organic patients are found to be as follows:

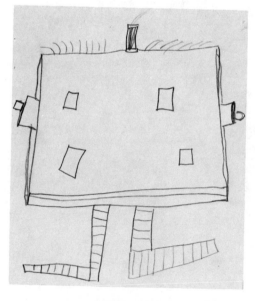

Figure 24

301

PROJECTIVE
DRAWINGS: TWO
AREAS OF
DIFFERENTIAL
DIAGNOSTIC
CHALLENGE

1.   There is a preoccupation with symmetry and balance in the drawing. The marked need for the maintenance of symmetry may be shown in the House drawing, for example, by a window drawn on one side calling for the immediate drawing of a window on the other side to maintain exact balance, by a door to the right matched by one to the left, etc. Sometimes a chimney at the top of a House must be balanced by steps, which look exactly like the chimney, at the bottom of the House and positioned exactly beneath it. If the House is turned upside down, the steps then look just as much like a chimney, and the chimney looks just as much like steps. The drawing of each and every branch on the left side of the Tree calls for the exact mirror image branch on the right side of the Tree, and so on.

2.   Equally striking is the separation of the parts within the drawing. This is often reflected in the Tree branches constituting separate units, rather than fluidly interrelating with the trunk. Thus a space appears between each branch and the trunk. If a ground line is drawn, a space usually separates it from contact with Tree trunk. "Segmentalization" designates such rendition of each major detail drawn in and of itself rather than integrated with the rest of the drawing.

3.   Oversimplified, unidimensional figures are offered in place of more complex ones. Stark, barren, mere skeletal representation of this Tree and just the outline of the House reflect the concreteness of the organic's thinking. This is most graphic in the drawing of the Tree, where a one-dimensional trunk with an elementary one-dimensional, symmetrically placed branch system (and usually with no secondary or tertiary system) gives the impression of an entity reduced to its most simple representation. This is equivalent to a stick figure for the drawing of a human (although few organics suffer such impairment as to have to do this for the Person drawing on the basis of the still more exaggerated concreteness which would require this). Goldstein and Sheerer (1941) earlier demonstrated that the brain-damaged patients, with their concretistic tendencies, reorganize gestalts in the direction of simplification. Bender (1949) also utilized this principle of simplification in her scoring of the Bender-Gestalt.

4.   As an extension of the tendency toward simplification, we find that organically damaged patients tend to omit one or more of the essential details within the drawing.

5.   Perseveration, a well-known sign of organicity, occurs noticeably in the drawings. Thus cross-hatching put into a window, indicating window sashes, is then carried uncritically into the drawing of a chimney, which is left looking like a window protruding off the roof top. On the chromatic drawings, perseveration may be seen in the use of the same single color from one drawing to the next, so the House, Tree, and Person are all drawn in whichever color was chosen for the first one drawn. In the drawing of the Tree, each branch is drawn just like the preceding one, and sometimes the perseveration extends to the roots as well. In Figure 25, an entire border of branches and roots around the trunk makes the Tree look more like a centipede.

6.   Verbal expressions of impotency are frequent. There is much greater perplexity and "catastrophic" anxiety in the expressions of impotency than we ordinarily get from the neurotic, who may be expressing mere feelings of inferiority relative to the task. Whereas the neurotic will erase and improve his or her drawing, the organic, feeling massively impotent, does not even envision the possibilities of improvement. He rarely will erase no matter how poor the drawing, or cannot achieve any improvement by his erasing and redrawing efforts. Thus the finished drawing looks just as it did before the erasing and redoing attempts.

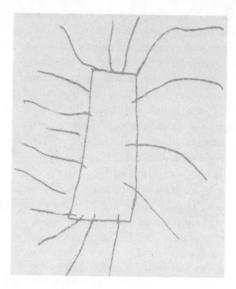

Figure 25

7. Excessive pressure is generally employed, and this excessive pressure tends to be accompanied by poor union of the lines (as is also seen in the Bender-Gestalt).

8. An excessive amount of time is generally employed, not in absolute terms, but in relative terms; the organic has labored, as it were, to produce a molehill. Thus, fully 3 min may be taken for a simplified drawing which a nonorganic subject could readily produce in 15 sec.

9. Ineptness in terms of the form of the drawing will reflect both the organic's reduced ability to synthesize and his rigidity of approach.

10. Difficulties in abstracting may be seen in response to the questions of the Post Drawing Interrogation. When asked how old the Person drawn might be, the organic patient will respond literally and concretely, "He's only a few minutes old," meaning that he was drawn only a few minutes ago, or "It's only on a piece of paper."

11. Buck (1970) points out: "Where organicity is far advanced, the quality of the responses on the Post Drawing Interrogation will, of course, be affected as well as the drawings, but where organicity is in the earlier stages, there is often a striking disparity between the quality of the subject's verbalization (which remains high) and the quality of the drawn concepts (which is far lower).".

When we look at the particular drawings, we find the following leads in that of the House:

1. There is usually a sharp contrast between the quality of House and Person drawings, with the House far inferior. This may be because the House represents a more difficult challenge, a more clearly three-dimensional object, with its aspect of greater depth, to be translated by the patient suffering cerebral pathology onto the two-dimensional page.

2. There is, therefore, a strong propensity to present the House in façade, that is, as merely a front without any indications of side walls.

3. A boxlike rendition of the House is frequently offered, sometimes looking, additionally, like a blueprint of the rooms has been superimposed on the front of the House. See Figures 26 and 28, respectively, for a severe and a somewhat less se-

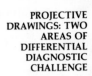

303

PROJECTIVE
DRAWINGS: TWO
AREAS OF
DIFFERENTIAL
DIAGNOSTIC
CHALLENGE

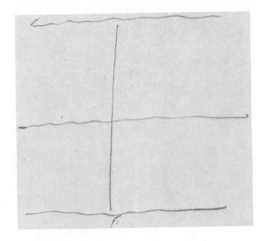

Figure 26

vere instance of such organic damage. (Figure 27, drawn by the same subject who drew the House in Figure 26, represents the "classic" type of organic's Tree with its unidimensional trunk and branches, its segmentalization of at least two of the branches not touching the trunk, its absence of secondary and tertiary branch systems, its total barrenness, and the exact symmetry of each branch on the left balanced by an almost identical branch on the right.)

4. The organic will often write in verbal designations of the various elements within the drawing (see Figure 29). Feeling insufficient to convey the required concept in drawing, he retreats to the use of an inappropriate second medium to buttress the graphic. (Figure 30 by the same subject, a less classic type of organic's Tree, still serves to convey the exact symmetry of such patients' Tree drawings.)

The characteristics of organics' Tree drawings having been cited and illustrated, we now consider drawings of Persons by this group. As mentioned earlier, the drawing of a Person is less differentiating between organics and nonorganics than are the other drawings.

Disproportionately large heads were found by Vernier (1952) to distinguish

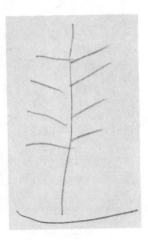

Figure 27

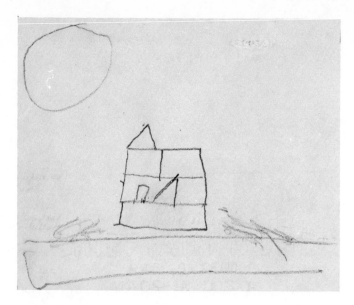

Figure 28

brain-damaged subjects from other subjects, as he also found head and neck distortions to do.

Machover (1947) found that frontal lobe injury produced a decrement in the quality of the drawing of the human figure. In line with this, Bender (1949) found that postencephalitic patients demonstrate a lower Goodenough mental age (scored on the drawing of a Person) than their Stanford-Binet mental age. This was also demonstrated by Neal (1942) and by Shaskan, Yarnell, and Alper (1943). Hence the Goodenough scoring of the drawing of a human figure can serve as a "Don't Hold" test item, with the standard IQ test serving as the "Hold" or baseline from which to judge the discrepancy. Thus, to take the broader span of behavior as the configura-

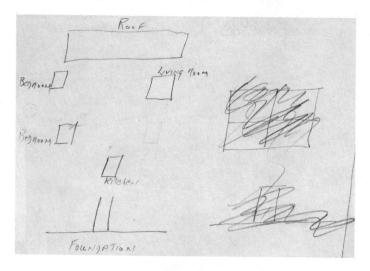

Figure 29

305

PROJECTIVE
DRAWINGS: TWO
AREAS OF
DIFFERENTIAL
DIAGNOSTIC
CHALLENGE

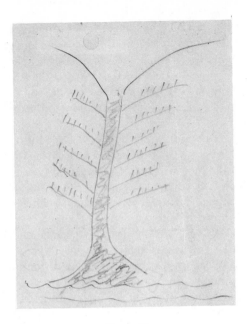

Figure 30

tion, an IQ level which appears to fall increasingly lower as one goes from a standard IQ test to the Goodenough scoring of the figure drawing, and then progressively still lower on the drawing of House and Tree, presents us with a relationship which should always make the examiner suspect the presence of an organic condition.

To conclude the examples, we might examine the consistency of the organic indicators we have been discussing by seeing their emergency in a single case across the various drawings of the battery. The subject, an adult male of 38 years, was examined because of an offense of rape and forced oral sodomy. The psychiatric examination ended with "diagnosis deferred" and a request for psychologicals. Following the suggestion of organic brain damage elicited by the drawings, referral for further and extensive medical examination uncovered a traumatic brain damage resulting from a car injury many years before.

The pencil drawing of a House (Figure 31) shows the barrenness, simplicity, and elementalness characteristic of the Houses we have been discussing. The exact symmetry of the upper window on the left balanced by the upper window on the right, the lower window on the left balanced by the lower one on the right, and their attachment to the side wall itself are typically organic. Sometimes organics will attach the window to the inside of the side wall and sometimes even to its outside.

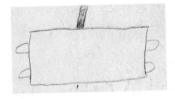

Figure 31

Figure 32, the achromatic Tree, is almost "classic" in its concrete simplicity, its one-dimensional branches, and its elemental, exact balancing of left and right.

The Person drawing (Figure 33) is not necessarily organic (as for the most part the Person drawings of organics are not) except for the characteristically larger head (perhaps reflecting feelings of compensation in the site of experienced impairment) and the specific and rare indicator of a trauma to the head in the damage expressed between the eyes.

What is so typical of organics is that the chromatic House and Tree are so little different from their achromatic counterparts. The chromatic House (Figure 34) here makes the same statement of brain damage expressed in the pencil-drawn House, except for the writing-in to label parts of the drawing and for the fact that now the symmetry is extended even further. To left-right symmetry there is now added a top-bottom symmetry, and the chimney above is exactly balanced by a "door" extending below the House. Even the ground is treated in segmentalized, fractionated, concrete fashion in the chromatic drawings where it is introduced. The ground does not run off to each side in a continuous horizon line, as a minimum capacity for abstraction would ordinarily suggest it does.

The chromatic Tree (Figure 35) is again just about what its pencil counterpart was. The "buglike" appearance of the Trees of organic subjects, earlier mentioned, is perhaps all the more graphically conveyed here. Ground and Tree are segmentalized rather than joined. The chromatic Person was a repeat of the achromatic one, again as organics tend to do.

The drawings here combine to reflect the patient's impairment of ego functions by the initiating cortical damage. Cerebral incapacity, in turn, serves largely to weaken the coordinating and integrating mechanisms of the ego, to reduce inhibitory powers, and thereby to open the floodgates to the impulses which, in this case, led to rape.

A last point: The more consistency we find in the broad sweep of the H-T-P signs of organicity appearing in the other tests too, the more confidence, of course, we place in our diagnostic impression. Thus, excessive time employed in making the drawings relative to the quality of the drawing produced should make us look for long reaction time on the Rorschach, with meager content offered. Insufficiency of the drawn content should make us look for low form percent on the Rorschach, the verbal writing in of the parts of the drawing ("window" or "door," etc., written over

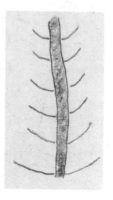

Figure 32

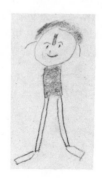

Figure 33

307

PROJECTIVE
DRAWINGS: TWO
AREAS OF
DIFFERENTIAL
DIAGNOSTIC
CHALLENGE

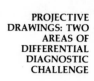

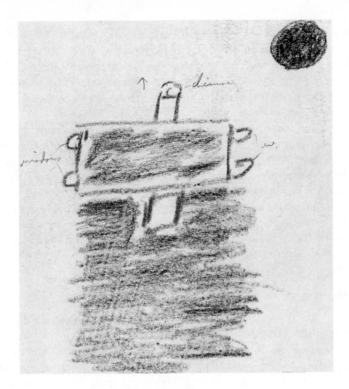

Figure 34

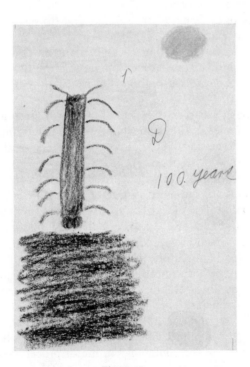

Figure 35

its drawn counterpart) for its related correlate of color naming on the Rorschach, and the expressions of impotence, perplexity, repetitiveness, or perseveration running across the various tests. The "catastrophic" feelings of mental impairment and damage are likely to be countered by a frantic effort, again in all the tests, to cling to the specific, the actual, the static, and the literal—all generically encompassed in the mental set we term "concretistic."

Conversely, the possibility of cerebral damage is contraindicated when the H-T-P and Bender-Gestalt are, respectively, well organized and effectively executed, and their component parts are well integrated with each other; when the drawings show good body-image organization, requiring, in turn, ego controls and adequate eye-hand coordination; when Rorschach, TAT, and H-T-P reflect imagination, reality-testing intactness, and cognizance of the requirements of conventional thinking; and when the projectives and the Wechsler demonstrate the capacity for abstract levels of thought. Cortical intactness is consistent with the ability to perceive and to psychomotorically produce things accurately.

5. Conclusion

Three interrelated areas of relevance to, and within, projective drawings have been addressed in this chapter.

1. Directions of promising validation research were focused: (a) comparative relationship between dimensions or elements within the drawings rather than the individual details, (b) introduction of dynamic stimuli, (c) avoidance of the unsubstantiated criterion of psychiatric diagnostic pigeonholes, (d) content and global evaluation, (e) children's drawings, (f) affective associations to the drawings, (g) use of a larger battery of drawings as the sample, and (h) separation of the data of studies for possible sex relatedness.

2. The complexities of the shifting variables along the continuum where schizoid adaptations shade into the borderline domain and the borderline gives way to schizophrenic processes were discussed and illustrated in their projective drawing expression.

3. Cerebral damage was seen to reflect itself in projective drawings via (a) exaggerated, exacting symmetry, (b) segmentalization, (c) oversimplified, unidimensional presentations, (d) omission of essential details, (e) perseveration, (f) impotency, perplexity, and "catastrophic" feelings, (g) excessive pressure, (h) time employed for the drawing particularly long for the product resulting, (i) ineptness, reduced ability to synthesize, and rigidity, (j) difficulty abstracting on the Post Drawing Interrogation, (k) subject's verbalizations of a strikingly higher quality than that of the drawings, (l) quality of House and Tree drawings noticeably inferior to that of Person drawing, (m) House presented as façade, with no sides evident, (n) boxlike House with blueprint effect superimposed on front, (o) verbal designation of various items of the drawing written in, (p) disproportionately large heads, occasionally with head and neck distortions, (q) lower Goodenough IQ than IQ obtained on a standard intelligence test, and (r) concretistic emphasis.

Some investigators have endorsed the view that impaired perception is the hallmark of the organic (e.g., Niebuhr & Cohen, 1956), while others have minimized the role of perception in favor of the "outgoing" or motor processes (Stoer, Corotto, & Curmutt, 1965). The present writer's experience is that both stand as sensitive radar, catching the subtleties of cerebrally impaired expression on the drawing page.

6. References

309

PROJECTIVE
DRAWINGS: TWO
AREAS OF
DIFFERENTIAL
DIAGNOSTIC
CHALLENGE

Abel, T. M. Figure drawings and facial disfigurement. *American Journal of Orthopsychiatry*, 1953, *23*, 253–261.

Apfeldorf, M., & Smith, W. J. The representation of the body self in human figure drawings. *Journal of Projective Techniques and Personality Assessment*, 1966, *30*, 283–289.

Apfeldorf, M., Walter, C., Kaiman, B., Smith, W., & Arnett, W. A method for the evaluation of affective associations to figure drawings. *Journal of Personality Assessment*, 1974, *38*, 441–449.

Bender, L. Psychological principle of the visual motor gestalt test. *Transactions of the New York Academy of Sciences*, 1949, *70*, 167–170.

Buck, J. N. Personal communication, 1970.

Caligor, L. The detection of paranoid trends by the 8 Card Redrawing Test (8 CRT). *Journal of Clinical Psychology*, 1952, *8*, 397–401.

Cauthen, N., Sandman, C., Kilpatrick, D., & Deabler, H. D-A-P correlates of *Sc* scores on the MMPI. *Journal of Projective Techniques*, 1969, *33*, 262–264.

Coopersmith, S., Sokol, D., Beardslee, B., & Coopersmith, A. Figure drawing as an expression of self-esteem. *Journal of Personality Assessment*, 1976, *40*, 368–374.

Craddick, R. Size of Halloween witch drawings prior to, on, and after Halloween. *Perceptual and Motor Skills*, 1963, *16*, 235–238.

Craddick, R., & Leipold, W. Note on the height of Draw-a-Person figures by male alcoholics. *Journal of Projective Techniques*, 1968, *32*, 486.

Cramer-Azima, F. J. Personality changes and figure drawings: A case treated with ACTH. *Journal of Clinical Psychology*, 1956, *20*, 143–149.

Cutter, F. Sexual differentiation in figure drawings and overt deviation. *Journal of Clinical Psychology*, 1956, *12*, 369–372.

Davis, C., & Hoopes, J. Comparison of H-T-P drawings of young deaf and hearing children. *Journal of Personality Assessment*, 1975, *39*, 28–33.

Goldstein, H., & Faterson, H. Shading as an index of anxiety in figure drawings. *Journal of Projective Techniques and Personality Assessment*, 1969, *33*, 454–456.

Goldstein, K., & Sheerer, N. Abstract and concrete behavior. *Psychological Monograph*, 1941, *43*, 1–151.

Goldworth, S. A. A comparative study of the drawings of a man and a woman done by normal, neurotic, schizophrenic, and brain damaged individuals. Doctoral dissertation, University of Pittsburgh, 1950.

Gray, D. M., & Pepitone, A. Effect of self-esteem on drawings of the human figure. *Journal of Consulting Psychology*, 1964, *28*, 452–455.

Griffith, A., & Peyman, D. Eye-ear emphasis in the DAP Test as indicating ideas of reference. In B I. Murstein (Ed.), *Handbook of projective techniques*. New York: Basic Books, 1965.

Gutman, B. An investigation of the applicability of the human figure drawing in predicting improvement in therapy. Unpublished doctoral thesis, New York University, 1952.

Hammer, E. An investigation of sexual symbolism: A study of H-T-P's of eugenically sterilized subjects. *Journal of Projective Techniques*, 1953, *17*, 401–413.

Hammer, E. F. (Ed.). *The clinical application of projective drawings*. Springfield, Ill.: Thomas, 1958.

Hammer, E. Critique of Swensen's "Empirical evaluation of human figure drawings. *Journal of Projective Techniques*, 1959, *23*, 30–32.

Irgens-Jensen, O. *Problem drinking and personality: A study based on the Draw-a-Person Test*. Oslo: Universitetsforlaget, 1971.

Kamino, D. K. An investigation of the meaning of the human figure drawing. *Journal of Clinical Psychology*, 1960, *16*, 429–430.

Klopfer, W. "Will the real Rorschach please stand up?" *Contemporary Psychology*, 1972, *17*, 25–26.

Koppitz, E. M. *Psychological evaluation of children's human figure drawings*. New York: Grune & Stratton, 1968.

Lakin, M. Formal characteristics of human figure drawings by institutionalized and non-institutionalized aged. *Journal of Gerontology*, 1960, *15*, 76–78.

Landisberg, S. Personal communication, 1973.

Levy, Minsky, and Lomax. In preparation, 1978.

Lord, M. Activity and affect in early memories of adolescent boys. *Journal of Personality Assessment*, 1971, *35*, 418–456.

Ludwig, D. Self-perception and the Draw-a-Person Test. *Journal of Projective Techniques*, 1969, *33*, 257–261.

310

EMANUEL F. HAMMER

Machover, K. A case of frontal lobe injury following attempted suicide. *Rorschach Research Exchange*, 1947, *11*, 9–20.

Machover, K. *Personality projection in the drawing of the human figure*. Springfield, Ill.: Thomas, 1949.

Neal, J. *Encephalitis: A clinical study*. New York: Grune & Stratton, 1942.

Niebuhr, H., Jr., & Cohen, D. The effect of psychopathology on visual discrimination. *Journal of Abnormal and Social Psychology*, 1956, *53*, 173–177.

Phillips, L. *Human adaptation and its failures*. New York: Academic Press, 1968.

Proceedings of the 16th International Congress of Psychology, Psychological testing in diagnosing cerebral pathology. 1960, 811–812.

Roback, R. Depression and size of the drawn human figure. *Journal of Abnormal Psychology*, 1966, *71*, 416.

Schmidt, L. D., & McGowan, J. F. The differentiation of human figure drawings. *Journal of Consulting Psychology*, 1965, *23*, 129–133.

Shaskan, D., Yarnell, H., & Alper, K. Physical, psychiatric and psychometric studies of post-encephalitic Parkinsonism. *Journal of Nervous and Mental Disorder*, 1943, *96*, 653–662.

Stoer, L., Corotto, L., & Cormutt, R. The role of visual perception in the reproduction of Bender-Gestalt designs. *Journal of Projective Techniques and Personality Assessment*, 1965, *29*, 473–478.

Swensen, C. H. Empirical evaluations of human figure drawings. *Psychology Bulletin*, 1957, *54*, 431–466.

Swensen, C. H., & Sipprelle, C. N. Some relationships among sexual characteristics of human figure drawings. *Journal of Projective Techniques*, 1956, *30*, 224–226.

Tolor, A. Teachers' judgments of the popularity of children from their human figure drawings. *Journal of Clinical Psychology*, 1955, *11*, 158–162.

Vane, J., & Eisen, V. The Goodenough D-A-P test and signs of maladjustment in kindergarten children. In B. I. Murstein (Ed.), *Handbook of projective techniques*. New York: Basic Books, 1965.

Vernier, C. M. *Projective test productions: I. Projective drawings*. New York: Grune & Stratton, 1952.

10

The Minnesota Multiphasic Personality Inventory (MMPI)

JOHN R. GRAHAM

1. Introduction

The MMPI deserves inclusion in this volume because it is the most widely used personality inventory in the United States (Lubin, Wallis, & Paine, 1971). In contrast to projective techniques such as the Rorschach and Thematic Apperception Test, which have ambiguous stimuli and unstructured response formats, the nonambiguous stimuli (self-reference statements) and structured response format (true/false) of the MMPI qualify it for classification as an objective technique. While much has been written about the differences between projective and objective techniques, the two categories of tests probably are more alike than different. Both kinds of tests have as a primary goal the prediction of important nontest behavior of examinees. In addition, the interpretation of both objective and projective test data is "a highly subjective art which requires a well-trained and experienced practitioner to give such 'scores' predictive meaning in the life of any given human being" (Matarazzo, 1972, p. 11).

The purpose of this chapter is to introduce mental health professionals and students to the rationale, development, and interpretation of the MMPI. It should be understood clearly that the information included here is not sufficient to qualify the reader as the "well-trained and experienced practitioner" that Matarazzo sees as necessary for MMPI interpretation. The reader who wants to learn more about the MMPI should consult *The MMPI Manual* (Hathaway & McKinley, 1967), critical reviews in the *Seventh Mental Measurements Yearbook*, (Buros, 1972), basic texts on personality assessment (e.g., Weiner, 1976; Sundberg, 1977), or the books devoted exclusively to MMPI use and interpretation (e.g., Dahlstrom, Welsh, & Dahlstrom, 1972, 1975; Graham, 1977a).

JOHN R. GRAHAM • Department of Psychology, Kent State University, Kent, Ohio 44240.

JOHN R. GRAHAM

2. Rationale and Scale Development

The MMPI was developed in the late 1930s and early 1940s and was published in 1943 (Hathaway & McKinley, 1943). Earlier personality inventories, such as the Woodworth Personal Data Sheet (Woodworth, 1920) and the Bernreuter Personality Inventory (Bernreuter, 1931), which had been constructed according to intuitive or logical keying procedures, had fallen into disrepute. Assessments of psychiatric patients typically involved an individual interview or mental status examination and the administration of individual intellectual and projective personality instruments. Hathaway and McKinley were involved in diagnostic assessments at the University of Minnesota Hospitals. They conceptualized the MMPI as a more efficient, and perhaps more reliable, way of arriving at appropriate psychodiagnostic classification of patients.

The empirical keying strategy was utilized in the construction of the original MMPI scales. The test authors collected a large number of self-reference statements from textbooks, psychological reports, and other sources. The pool of items was examined, and 504 of these statements were judged to be relatively nonambiguous and independent of each other.

Next, appropriate criterion groups were identified. The "normal" group consisted of relatives and visitors of patients at the University of Minnesota Hospitals, high school graduates attending precollege conferences at the University of Minnesota, medical patients, and Work Progress Administration workers. The "clinical" group was made up of patients representing the following major psychiatric diagnostic categories: hypochondriasis, depression, hysteria, psychopathic deviate, paranoia, psychasthenia, schizophrenia, and hypomania. The 504 items were administered to the normal and clinical groups, and for each diagnostic group item analyses were conducted to identify items that discriminated between that diagnostic group and normal subjects and between that diagnostic group and other diagnostic groups combined. Such items were selected for the scale and were keyed in the direction (true or false) most often chosen by the diagnostic group in question. Each clinical scale was developed in this manner and was cross-validated by comparing scores of new groups of normals, general psychiatric patients, and patients in the appropriate diagnostic group.

At a somewhat later time, two additional scales were constructed and have come to be considered as standard clinical scales. The Masculinity-femininity (*Mf*) scale originally was intended to identify homosexual males. However, when very few items could be identified that differentiated between homosexual and heterosexual males, items also were included in the *Mf* scale if they differentiated between normal males and females. In addition, 46 items from the Masculinity-femininity scale of a previously published interest inventory were added to the item pool and included in the *Mf* scale.* The Social Introversion (*Si*) scale was developed by Drake (1946) by comparing the item responses of college women who participated in many extracurricular activities with the responses of college women who were not very socially participative.

Hathaway and McKinley were sensitive to the criticism that earlier inventories could easily be faked or distorted to create an impression of greater adjustment or maladjustment than was really the case for individual subjects. Thus the test authors

---

*The addition of these 46 items brought the total number of items to 550.

developed four validity indicators to detect deviant test-taking attitudes. The Cannot Say scale simply is the number of omitted items in a test protocol. Obviously, the omission of large numbers of items tends to lower the scores on the clinical scales and calls into question the interpretability of scores on those scales. The L scale was rationally constructed to detect a naive, global attempt to present oneself in an extremely favorable light by denying minor flaws in character to which most subjects would be willing to admit. The F scale was developed by selecting items very infrequently endorsed by subjects in the normal criterion groups. Thus high F scale scores are suggestive of deviant responding and may indicate that the subject has not read the test items, that he is trying to appear to be very disturbed, or that he has approached the test-taking task with some other deviant attitude. The K scale originally was conceptualized as a measure of clinical defensiveness. Items were selected for the scale by comparing responses of subjects who were quite disturbed clinically but who produced average scores on the clinical scales of the MMPI with responses of subjects who were essentially normal and who also produced average scores on the clinical scales. Higher K scores were thought to be more indicative of clinical defensiveness. Later the K scale was used to develop a correction factor for some of the clinical scales. Scores on the clinical scales are increased to the extent that defensiveness is suggested by a subject's K scale score. The appropriate correction for each clinical scale was determined empirically by comparing the ability of scores on each clinical scale to discriminate between subjects in the appropriate diagnostic group and other subjects when various proportions of subjects' K scale scores were added to their raw scores on the clinical scale. The K-correction has come to be used routinely in MMPI scoring and interpretation.

Through the procedures described above, 14 standard scales were developed from the MMPI item pool. Four scales were designed to assess test-taking attitudes, eight scales were associated with diagnostic categories, and two scales (Mf and Si) were developed to assess other important aspects of behavior and personality. While many additional scales subsequently have been developed using the original MMPI item pool, the scores on these 14 standard scales constitute the data base from which most MMPI interpretive approaches are derived.

3. Administering and Scoring the MMPI

A major positive feature of the MMPI is that it is easy to administer and to score. The basic task confronting the test subject is to indicate whether each of 550 self-reference statements is true as applied to him or false as applied to him. The subject also is given the option of not answering items that do not apply to him or that deal with something that he doesn't know about, but he is encouraged to try to make a true or false response to most of the items.

The MMPI has several different test forms and answer sheets available, ensuring that the test can be administered to a broad spectrum of subjects. While *The MMPI Manual* (Hathaway & McKinley, 1967) suggests that the MMPI is appropriate for subjects who are 16 years old or older and who have at least a sixth-grade reading level, there is evidence that younger subjects and subjects with lower reading levels can complete the test satisfactorily if they are carefully supervised.

Originally, the MMPI items were printed on individual cards and subjects were instructed to sort the cards into three categories—TRUE, FALSE, and CANNOT

SAY. The examiner then recorded the responses on an appropriate answer sheet. While it is not very frequently used currently, this individual or box form of the test is still available.* It is most appropriate for very disturbed subjects or others who might find it difficult to complete other forms of the test. The group or booklet form of the test is by far the most commonly used one. The statements are printed in reusable paper booklets, and the subject marks his responses on one of several different answer sheets. Form R of the test is becoming increasingly popular. It involves a hard-cover booklet with step-down pages. As with the group form, answers are marked on a separate answer sheet. In Form R, all of the items necessary for scoring the standard validity and clinical scales appear as the first 399 items in the booklet.

From the MMPI's inception, there have been efforts to develop abbreviated, less time-consuming forms of the test. Graham (1977a) reviewed many of these abbreviated forms and concluded that most are not adequate for use with individual subjects. However, all of the standard validity and clinical scales can be scored from 399 items. As indicated above, these items are conveniently placed first in Form R of the test so that a subject can be instructed to stop after completing 399 items. In the booklet form of the test, the subject must complete the first 366 items plus 33 additional items scattered throughout the remainder of the booklet. A major problem in using any abbreviated version of the test is that most of the additional or special scales cannot be scored unless all items are completed. Before deciding to use an abbreviated form of the MMPI, the clinician should consider whose time is being saved. In most instances, it is the time of the test subject and of a nonprofessional person who supervises test administration.

There also are some other less frequently used forms of the MMPI. In addition to the standard tape recording of the items, the test has been translated into numerous foreign languages.† For more information about these special test forms, the reader should consult Volume I of *An MMPI Handbook* (Dahlstrom et al., 1972).

Because of the ease with which it can be administered, some MMPI users tend to become careless in administering the test. Subjects are given the test by a secretary, with little or no explanation about why they are taking the test or how the results will be used. Sometimes subjects are encouraged to complete the test at home, on the hospital ward, or elsewhere. As with any assessment procedure, test users should ensure that the MMPI is completed according to standardized procedures. The test should be administered in the clinician's office or in some other professional setting. The subject should be given clear instructions for completing the test and should be told who will see the results and how they will be used. When these procedures are followed, the subject is more likely to take the test seriously and to produce a valid, interpretable protocol.

Once the test has been administered, using test forms and answer sheets most convenient for the examiner and the test subject, several alternatives are available for scoring. Most clinicians find it convenient to score the test by hand, but for high-volume users machine scoring is available. Specially designed templates are available for hand scoring. For more information about hand and machine scoring, the reader is referred to Chapter 2 of *The MMPI: A Practical Guide* (Graham, 1977a).

---

*All MMPI materials are available exclusively from the Psychological Corporation, 757 Third Avenue, New York, New York 10017.

†Butcher and Pancheri (1976) and Butcher and Owen (Chapter 15, this volume) have summarized and evaluated cross-cultural MMPI data.

After raw scores for the scales have been determined, the next step is to construct a profile of these scores. A standard profile sheet is commercially available for this purpose. After the appropriate K-correction, if any, has been added to each raw score, the raw scores are plotted on the sheet, which allows them to be converted readily to T scores. T scores are standard scores with a mean of 50 and a standard deviation of 10. The scores of normal subjects in the original derivational samples serve as the basis for the T score conversions. The standardization sample consisted of males and females with about a tenth-grade education. Recently, special norms have been published for adolescent subjects (Marks, Seeman, & Haller, 1974). It is recommended that these special norms be used routinely with subjects younger than 18 years of age. Hathaway (1947) and Welsh (1948) developed systems for coding most of the relevant information about the profile in a concise manner.

4. Interpreting the MMPI

4.1. Current Approach to Interpretation

Soon after the original scales were developed, it became apparent that the MMPI was of only limited utility for the major purpose for which it was designed, i.e., assignment of patients to appropriate psychodiagnostic categories. Patients with particular diagnoses (e.g., schizophrenia) often obtained high scores on the corresponding clinical scale, but they also were likely to have high scores on other scales as well. In addition, many nonclinical subjects obtained high scores on one or more of the clinical scales. Several factors have been suggested as contributing to the limited success of the MMPI in psychodiagnosis. One important factor is the limited reliability of psychiatric diagnosis. Also, subsequent research has indicated that the MMPI clinical scales are highly intercorrelated, making it highly unlikely that only one scale would be elevated for any given subject. In his Foreword to the first edition of *An MMPI Handbook* (Dahlstrom & Welsh, 1960), Hathaway concluded that "if the validity views of 1941 were the only support for the inventory, it could not survive."

Why, then, has the MMPI survived and become the most popular personality inventory in the United States? When it became apparent that the test is of only limited utility for psychiatric diagnosis, a new approach to MMPI utilization began to emerge. Since reliable differences in scores on the clinical scales have been found among subjects, it can be assumed that the scales are measuring something. In the current approach to MMPI interpretation, no assumptions are made about what the scales are measuring. Only through clinical experience and empirical research are nontest correlates of the scales identified. When a subject obtains a score on a scale, the inference is made that the subject will have characteristics and behaviors similar to other persons who have scored similarly on the scale. Thus there has been a shift away from the predictive validity of the 1940s toward an emphasis on construct validity. To lessen the likelihood that excess meaning will be attributed to scores because of the original clinical labels, current practice encourages the clinician to replace the labels with numbers. The numbers assigned to replace the original labels are listed in Table 1.

To be able to interpret MMPI protocols accurately, the clinician must familiarize himself with the large number of empirical research studies that have been conducted with the MMPI. To facilitate this learning process, several attempts have

Table 1. Sample Interpretive Inferences for Standard MMPI Scales

Scale name	Scale abbreviation	Scale no.	Interpretation of high scores	Interpretation of low scores
—	*L*	—	Trying to create favorable impression by not being honest in responding to items; conventional; rigid; moralistic; lacks insight	Responded frankly to items; confident; perceptive; self-reliant; cynical
—	*F*	—	May indicate invalid profile; severe pathology; moody; restless; dissatisfied	Socially conforming; free of disabling psychopathology; may be "faking good"
—	*K*	—	May indicate invalid profile; defensive; inhibited; intolerant; lacks insight	May indicate invalid profile; exaggerates problems; self-critical; dissatisfied; conforming; lacks insight; cynical
Hypochondriasis	*Hs*	1	Excessive bodily concern; somatic symptoms; narcissistic; pessimistic; demanding; critical; long-standing problems	Free of somatic preoccupation; optimistic; sensitive; insightful
Depression	*D*	2	Depressed; pessimistic; irritable; dissatisfied; lacks self-confidence; introverted; overcontrolled	Free of psychological turmoil; optimistic; energetic; competitive; impulsive; undercontrolled; exhibitionistic
Hysteria	*Hy*	3	Physical symptoms of functional origin; lacks insight; self-centered; socially involved; demands attention and affection	Constricted; conventional; narrow interests; limited social participation; untrusting; hard to get to know; realistic
Psychopathic Deviate	*Pd*	4	Asocial or antisocial; rebellious; impulsive; poor judgment; immature; creates good first impression; superficial relationships; aggressive; free of psychological turmoil	Conventional; conforming; accepts authority; low drive level; concerned about status and security; persistent; moralistic
Masculinity-femininity	*Mf*	5	Male: aesthetic interests; insecure in masculine role; creative; good judgment; sensitive; passive; dependent; good self-control	Male: overemphasizes strength and physical prowess; adventurous; narrow interests; inflexible; contented; lacks insight
			Female: rejects traditional female role; masculine interests; assertive; competitive; self-confident; logical; unemotional	Female: accepts traditional female role; passive; yielding to males; complaining; critical; constricted

Table 1. *(Continued)*

317

THE MINNESOTA
MULTIPHASIC
PERSONALITY
INVENTORY (MMPI)

Scale name	Scale abbreviation	Scale no.	Interpretation of high scores	Interpretation of low scores
Paranoia	*Pa*	6	May exhibit frankly psychotic behavior; suspicious; sensitive; resentful; projects; rationalizes; moralistic; rigid	May have frankly psychotic symptoms; evasive; defensive; guarded; secretive; withdrawn
Psychasthenia	*Pt*	7	Anxious; worried; difficulties in concentrating; ruminative; obsessive; compulsive; insecure; lacks self-confidence; organized; persistent; problems in decision making	Free of disabling fears and anxieties; self-confident; responsible; adaptable; values success and status
Schizophrenia	*Sc*	8	May have thinking disturbance; withdrawn; self-doubts; feels alienated and unaccepted; vague goals	Friendly, sensitive, trustful; avoids deep emotional involvement; conventional; unimaginative
Hypomania	*Ma*	9	Excessive activity; impulsive; lacks direction; unrealistic self-appraisal; low frustration tolerance; friendly; manipulative; episodes of depression	Low energy level; apathetic; responsible; conventional; lacks self-confidence; overcontrolled
Social Introversion	*Si*	0	Socially introverted; shy; sensitive; overcontrolled; conforming; problems in decision making	Socially extroverted; friendly; active; competitive; impulsive; self-indulgent

been made to summarize and to synthesize the appropriate interpretive data in a form most useful to the clinician. The reader who aspires to become proficient in MMPI interpretation should consult one or more of the following sources: *An MMPI Handbook*, Volume I (Dahlstrom et al., 1972), *The MMPI: A Practical Guide* (Graham, 1977a), *MMPI Interpretive Manual for Counselors and Clinicians* (Duckworth & Duckworth, 1975), and *The Physician's Guide to the MMPI* (Good & Brantner, 1961). These sources present interpretive information for high and low scores on the standard MMPI scales singly and for configurations of high scores on these scales.

4.2. Codebooks

In 1956, Paul Meehl presented a plea for a "good cookbook" for psychological test interpretation. Responding to research indicating that, in many situations, actuarial treatment of test data resulted in more accurate inferences than did interpretation of the same data by trained clinicians, Meehl proposed a system that would eliminate, or at least minimize the importance of, the clinician's judgment process.

His proposed system involved the formulation of rules for classifying test data into categories and the empirical determination of behavioral correlates of each category.

In response to Meehl's plea, several codebooks for MMPI interpretation were developed. Marks and Seeman (1963) and Gilberstadt and Duker (1965) used a similar approach in developing their codebooks. First, complex rules were stated for classifying profiles into rather homogeneous categories. Gilberstadt and Duker provided 19 categories, and Marks and Seeman listed 16 categories. For each profile category, interpretive data were provided. These data were derived from empirical study of persons whose profiles met the rules for the various categories.

Initially, practicing clinicians were very excited about the codebook approach to interpretation. The prospect of having extensive, empirically determined, interpretive information on which to base psychological test reports was quite appealing. Unfortunately, the excitement and optimism were short-lived. Clinicians soon became frustrated with the approach as profile after profile encountered in clinical practice did not fit any of the available code types. Research has indicated that if either the Marks and Seeman or Gilberstadt and Duker codebook is used individually, only 20–30% of the profiles obtained in a psychiatric setting can be classified (Fowler & Coyle, 1968; Huff, 1965; Meikle & Gerritse, 1970; Pauker, 1966; Schultz, Gibeau, & Barry, 1968). The classification rate rises to 35–45% if the codebooks are used jointly.

4.3. Behavioral Correlates of Simple Code Types

More recently, there has been a trend toward classifying profiles according to much simpler rules and determining empirical correlates for the code types (Lewandowski & Graham, 1972; Gynther, Altman, & Sletten, 1973; Boerger, Graham, & Lilly, 1974). Typically, code types are defined in terms of scores on individual scales or in terms of the two highest scales in the profile. When individual scales are utilized, a distinction is made between high scores and high point code types. High scores are defined in terms of some absolute cutoff point, such as a T score greater than 70. Other scales in the profile are not considered, and a test subject can have high scores on more than one scale. A high point code is identified according to which scale is the highest one in a test subject's profile, regardless of the absolute score on the highest scale. Obviously, there can be only one high point code for any particular test subject. Using simpler code types has the obvious advantage of being able to account for virtually all profiles encountered in clinical practice. The major disadvantage of the approach is that the resulting categories are rather heterogeneous, and it is less likely that each and every descriptor will apply to every subject with a given code type.

Marks et al. (1974) revised the earlier codebook of Marks and Seeman. For their adult subjects, they replaced the complex code types with codes based primarily on configurations of two high scales and concluded that there was no appreciable loss of accuracy in shifting to this simpler system of classification. Marks et al. also defined code types for their adolescent subjects in terms of configurations of the two highest scales in the profile.

While it is not feasible in this chapter to present exhaustive interpretive data for each MMPI scale and for various configurations of scales, Table 1 summarizes some of the most salient nontest characteristics of high and low scorers on the standard validity and clinical scales, as presented by Graham (1977a). In utilizing data such as those in Table 1, T scores greater than 70 usually are considered to be high scores and T scores less than 40 are considered to be low scores. However, some demographic variables, such as age, sex, education, and race, must be taken into account in determining if T scores should be considered high or low for individual test subjects. For example, scores on the K scale are related to education level. While a T score of 70 on the K scale would be considered a high score for someone with a tenth-grade education, such a score would be about average in a college population.

Gynther and Gynther (1976) and Graham (1977a) summarized the relationships between demographic variables and scores on the MMPI scales. In addition to obtaining higher scores on the K scale, more educated persons tend to score higher on scales 3 and 5 and lower on the L scale. Older subjects tend to score higher on scales 1, 2, and 0, while younger subjects tend to score higher on the F scale and on scales 4, 8, and 9. Black subjects score higher than white subjects on the F scale and on scales 4, 8, and 9. In addition, Gynther, Altman, and Warbin (1973a, 1973b) found that empirical correlates of profile types for white patients did not replicate for black patients. The experienced MMPI interpreter takes demographic variables into account in determining the significance of score levels on the MMPI scales.

In utilizing data such as those in Table 1, it should be understood that each and every correlate will not always be characteristic of every subject with a high or low score on a particular scale. In general, the more extreme the scores are, the more likely it is that descriptors presented for high and low scorers will apply to a particular examinee. In addition, the intensity or salience of the inferred behaviors is likely to increase for more extreme scores.

Careful examination of the data in Table 1 reveals several important factors. First, while some of the interpretive statements are consistent with the original clinical labels of the scales, the scales are not pure measures of the symptom syndromes suggested by the labels. Also, one should not assume that low scorers on a scale will be characterized in ways opposite to high scorers. While this simplistic view seems appropriate for some of the scales (e.g., scale 1), on other scales (e.g., scale 6) low scores can be interpreted similarly to high scores. It should also be noted that different interpretations are made for males and females who obtain high or low scores on scale 5.

4.4. A General Interpretive Strategy

Within the general framework of generating inferences from scores on individual scales and configurations of scales, many different approaches to profile interpretation are possible. Graham (1977a) suggested a general interpretive strategy that should prove useful to beginning MMPI users. His strategy centers around trying to answer the following questions about each MMPI protocol:

1. What was the test-taking attitude of the examinee, and how should this attitude be taken into account in interpreting the protocol?
2. What is the general level of adjustment of the person who produced the protocol?
3. What kinds of behaviors (symptoms, attitudes, defenses, etc.) can be inferred about or expected from the person who produced the protocol?

4. What etiology or set of psychological dynamics underlies the person's behaviors?
5. What are the most appropriate diagnostic labels for the person who produced the protocol?
6. What are the implications for the treatment of the person who produced the protocol?

Graham suggested that the major sources of data for trying to answer these questions are the manuals that summarize interpretive inferences for the validity and clinical scales singly and in configuration. However, he also discussed some special MMPI scales and indices that are relevant to the questions. In some instances, it is necessary to rely on higher-order inferences in trying to answer the questions.

4.5. Computerized Interpretations

Currently, there are more than a half-dozen commercial services in the United States that offer computerized scoring and interpretation of MMPI protocols. Computers are more reliable and more efficient than human clinicians in scoring protocols, classifying profiles into categories, and assigning appropriate interpretive statements to each category. Such utilization of computers can free the clinician's time so it can be spent on other activities such as therapy and consultation.

Several steps typically are involved in the computerized interpretation process. First, rules for scoring and classifying protocols are stored in the computer's memory. Next, appropriate interpretive statements for all possible categories are stored in the computer. After a subject completes the MMPI, the responses are fed into the computer, where they are scored. Classification rules then are applied to determine the appropriate categories for each protocol, and the computer searches its memory and prints out the interpretive statements designated for the categories.

Obviously, this process requires that appropriate classification rules be determined and that interpretive statements be generated for the various categories. Both of these functions are performed by the human clinician. In most existing interpretive services, protocols are classified according to score levels on individual scales and according to configurations of scores on two or more scales. The interpretive statements for each category typically are generated by experienced clinicians based on their clinical experience and knowledge of MMPI research findings. While these statements will not always be accurate for all individual subjects, the computerized services do make expert MMPI interpretation available to all MMPI users.

The computerized interpretation services currently available differ considerably in terms of cost, test materials required, and completeness of the resulting report. Readers who may be interested in using such services should refer to the detailed reviews of the various services that have appeared in the literature (Dahlstrom et al., 1972; Butcher, 1978; Eichman, 1972; Kleinmuntz, 1972; Graham, 1977a; Butcher & Owen, Chapter 15, this volume).

Graham (1977a) and Butcher (1978) have pointed out several potential limitations of the computerized interpretation services. There is a tendency to attribute greater scientific authenticity to the interpretations than is warranted simply because they have been generated by a computer. Also, computerized interpretations tend to "fix" interpretations that have not been adequately validated. While most of the services caution against reaching conclusions solely on the basis of their reports, in many settings the computerized interpretation is used instead of a more complete psychological assessment procedure. In spite of these potential limitations, the computerized interpretation services can serve as a valuable tool to the clinician if they are understood completely and are used appropriately as *part* of the assessment process.

5. Psychometric Considerations

5.1. Temporal Stability

Temporal stability data for the individual MMPI validity and clinical scales have been reported for several different normal and clinical populations and for varying test-retest intervals. These data have been summarized by Dahlstrom et al. (1975), Schwartz (1977), and Graham (1977c). Graham reported that for normal subjects the typical test-retest coefficients for relatively short intervals (1 day to 2 weeks) range from .70 to .85 and that for considerably longer intervals (1 year or more) the typical coefficients are much lower (.35–.45). For psychiatric patient samples, test-retest coefficients are quite similar to those for normal subjects. For criminal and delinquent subjects, coefficients based on short intervals range from .60 to .80. No data have been reported for criminal and delinquent subjects for longer intervals. Schwartz (1977) concluded that there do not seem to be any systematic relationships between temporal stability and sex or MMPI form utilized. Further, no MMPI scale appears to be consistently more stable than other scales. In summary, the temporal stability of individual MMPI scales over short periods of time compares favorably with that of scores from other personality instruments.

Fewer data are available concerning the temporal stability of configurations of scores on the MMPI scales. Graham (1977c) and Schwartz (1977) pointed out that many clinicians emphasize configural aspects of MMPI interpretation and that interpretations based on these configurations often are such that an assumption of configural stability is necessary. Data reviewed by Graham (1977c) suggest that profile configurations are not so stable as many clinicians assume them to be. Typically, about 40–60% of subjects will have the same high point code for two separate administrations of the MMPI. For 2-point codes, only about 20–40% of the subjects repeat the same code on retest, and only 20–30% of subjects repeat the same 3-point code on retest. When absolute level of high and low scores and differences between the extreme scores and scores on other scales are taken into account, the configurations tend to be somewhat more stable (Schwartz, 1977). Although profile configurations tend to be somewhat unstable, the extent to which the instability should be attributed to error variance and the extent to which it reflects actual changes in the behaviors being assessed have not yet been determined.

5.2. Internal Consistency

Data concerning the internal consistency of individual MMPI scales also have been summarized (Dahlstrom et al., 1975). While specific internal consistency estimates vary considerably (from −.05 to .96), typical values range from .60 to .90. Internal consistency seems to be lower for college students than for psychiatric patients. Scales 3, 5, and 9 appear to have the least internal consistency, while scales

1, 7, and 8 appear to be the most internally consistent. Factor analyses of items within each standard scale indicate that most of the scales are not unidimensional (Comrey, 1957a, 1957b, 1957c, 1958a, 1958b, 1958c, 1958d, 1958e; Comrey & Margraff, 1958). The one exception seems to be scale 1, where most of the variance is associated with a single dimension. Since no attention was given to internal consistency when the MMPI scales were constructed, it is not at all surprising that the scales are not so internally consistent as some other personality measures.

5.3. Factor Structure

When scores on the basic validity and clinical scales have been factor-analyzed, two major dimensions have emerged consistently (Welsh, 1956; Eichman, 1961, 1962; Block, 1965). One of these two factors has high positive loadings for scales 7 and 8 and a high negative loading for the K scale. Welsh and Eichman both labeled this factor "Anxiety," while Block scored items in the opposite direction and labeled the factor "Ego Resiliency." While subsequent research has indicated that manifest anxiety is characteristic of high scorers on this scale, the factor probably can more accurately be labeled "General Maladjustment" (Graham, 1977b).

The second major factor that has been identified has high positive loadings for scales 1, 2, and 3 and a high negative loading for scale 9. Welsh and Eichman labeled this factor "Repression," and Block called it "Ego Control." The Repression factor seems to be tapping denial, rationalization, lack of insight, and overcontrol of needs and impulses.

Some investigators have factor- or cluster-analyzed responses to individual MMPI items (Barker, Fowler, & Peterson, 1971; Chu, 1966; Stein, 1968; Tryon, 1966; Tryon & Bailey, 1965). Barker and his colleagues identified nine major factors and constructed scales to assess them. The resulting scales were demonstrated to be as reliable as the standard MMPI scales and to be as good as or better than the standard scales in discriminating among diagnostic categories. Stein and his associates used cluster analytic procedures and identified seven clusters that were judged to be significant and meaningful. Tryon (1966) reported high internal consistency estimates for scales constructed to assess the seven cluster dimensions, but no temporal stability data have been reported for the cluster scales. Stein (1968) reviewed studies indicating that some of the cluster scales seem to be measuring characteristics that also are reflected by scores on the standard MMPI scales, while other cluster scales are tapping characteristics not assessed by the standard scales. Graham (1977a) has offered some tentative interpretive information for the cluster scales.

5.4. Response Sets

Some critics have suggested that the standard MMPI scales are of limited utility because most of the variance in scale scores can be attributed to response sets or styles. Jackson and Messick (1961) argued that high scores on the standard MMPI scales reflect primarily an acquiescence response style, i.e., a tendency for subjects to agree passively with inventory statements. A major factor used in support of their argument is that the standard MMPI scales are not balanced for proportion of items keyed true and false. Further, it was demonstrated that scores on Welsh's Anxiety scale correlated highly with an acquiescence measure.

Edwards (1957, 1964) maintained that scores on the standard MMPI scales are grossly confounded with a social desirability response set. He felt that high scores on the scales simply indicate that a test subject is willing to admit to socially undesirable traits and behaviors. Edwards reasoned that if the social desirability effects were removed from the MMPI then scores on the scales would not be related to important nontest behaviors. Major support for the social desirability response set positions came from data indicating that scores on the standard MMPI scales and on Welsh's Anxiety factor scale were highly correlated with a social desirability scale.

While a number of persons have argued against the acquiescence and social desirability interpretations of MMPI scales, Block (1965) systematically reviewed the arguments offered in support of the positions, pointed out some statistical and methodological problems with data used to support the positions, and developed new evidence that clearly rebutted the positions. Block modified the standard MMPI scales in order to balance the number of items keyed true and false in each scale. Contrary to the prediction of Jackson and Messick, when these modified scales were factor-analyzed, the resulting factor structure was essentially the same as that previously identified for the standard MMPI scales. Block also developed a social desirability free measure of Welsh's Anxiety factor scale. Scores on his revised scale correlated with the same MMPI scales and to a similar degree as was the case when the original Anxiety factor scale was utilized. Finally, Block refuted the arguments that scores on the MMPI factor scales are unrelated to important nontest behaviors. Using ratings of five different samples of subjects, Block was able to identify reliable and meaningful nontest correlates of the two MMPI factor scales.

5.5. Validity

In addition to the cross-validational work completed when the original MMPI scales were constructed, much additional research concerning the validity of the MMPI has been completed. In Volume II of *An MMPI Handbook*, Dahlstrom et al. (1975) cited over 6000 studies involving the MMPI. Most of the MMPI validity studies can be grouped into three general categories.

First, there are studies that compared the MMPI profiles of relevant criterion groups. Most of the studies of this kind have identified significant differences on one or more of the standard validity and clinical scales among groups formed on the basis of diagnosis, severity of disturbance, treatment regimes, and numerous other criteria. Lanyon (1968) has published average or typical MMPI profiles for a large number of criterion groups. Also included in this category is the work on profile discrimination of Meehl and Dahlstrom (1960), Peterson (1954), Taulbee and Sisson (1957), Henrichs (1964), and Goldberg (1965).

A second category of validity studies includes efforts to demonstrate reliable nontest correlates of scores on MMPI scales considered singly and in configuration. Some of the earliest MMPI research studies were of this kind. Hathaway and Meehl's atlas (1951) presented case histories of patients having various profile types. Nontest correlates of high scores and low scores and for high point and low point code types were identified for adolescents (Hathaway & Monachesi, 1953), normal college students (Black, 1953), student nurses (Hovey, 1953), normal adults (Hathaway & Meehl, 1952), normal Air Force officers (Block & Bailey, 1955; Gough, McKee, & Yandell, 1955), medical patients (Guthrie, 1949), and college counselees (Mello &

Guthrie, 1958). Correlates of 2-point codes were reported for normal adults (Hathaway & Meehl, 1952), normal college students (Black, 1953), medical patients (Guthrie, 1949), and psychiatric patients (Meehl, 1951). The nontest correlates identified in these studies have been summarized by Dahlstrom et al. (1972) and Graham (1977a). The reader who wants to become familiar with these data should consult these sources.

The approach of studying profiles classified in simple ways (single scales or two highest scales) very quickly came under fire. Critics argued that such simple classification resulted in very heterogeneous groups of people. The behaviors of persons within a particular group tended to be so variable that it would be difficult to find behaviors shared by persons within one group but absent in other groups. Apparently this criticism was very convincing, because the research utilizing simple criteria for classifying profiles was short-lived, covering a period from 1949 to 1958.

As an alternative to the simple criteria, a number of investigators (e.g., Marks & Seeman, 1963; Gilberstadt & Duker, 1965) developed lengthy and complex rules for classifying profiles. They maintained that the behaviors of persons whose profiles fit one of the complex code types would be more homogeneous than when the simple criteria were utilized. Thus it would be much easier to identify behaviors more likely to be associated with one code type than with others. As stated earlier, the major problem with the complex code types was that most profiles encountered in clinical settings could not be classified using the available code types. In addition, when efforts were made to determine the accuracy of the correlates of complex code types in other settings, the results were quite discouraging (Gynther & Brillant, 1968; Palmer, 1970). Thus the practicing clinician was forced to return to using data based on simple classification of profiles.

More recently, there has been a renewed interest in determining nontest correlates for simple code types. Lewandowski and Graham (1972) and Gynther, Altman, and Sletten (1973) studied nontest correlates of 2-point code types, and Boerger et al. (1974) classified profiles according to high and low scores on individual scales. These studies included replication as an integral part of the designs. While the results of these investigations indicated some difficulties in replicating some correlates in new samples, they also demonstrated that reliable and meaningful correlates could be identified for profiles classified according to simple criteria. Also, as noted earlier, in their revision of the Marks and Seeman codebook, Marks et al. (1974) abandoned the more complex classification schema in favor of a simpler one.

A third approach to studying MMPI validity has been to consider the MMPI protocol and the clinician who interprets it as an integral unit and to study the accuracy of inferences based on the MMPI. Studies of this kind typically employ a design in which a test judge is given an MMPI profile and is asked to generate inferences about the test subject using a Q-sort procedure or some other technique that ensures that a standard set of descriptors is used. Similar descriptors are rated for each test subject on the basis of criterion information. In some studies, therapists provide criterion data for patients with whom they have familiarity. Other studies ask judges to generate criterion descriptions after reviewing clinical records and/or interviewing relatives of the subject. Accuracy of MMPI-based inferences is determined by comparing them with the criterion data.

Goldberg (1968) summarized the clinical judgment research and concluded that, in general, clinical judgments tend to be rather unreliable, only minimally related to the confidence and to the amount of experience of the test judge, relatively unaffected by the amount of information available to the judge, and rather low in validity on an absolute basis. While Goldberg's pessimistic outlook for clinical inferences cannot be overlooked, it should be pointed out that some positive results also can be cited. For example, compared with the Rorschach and other projective techniques, personality descriptions based on the MMPI were relatively more accurate (Little & Schneidman, 1959). Also, descriptors based on MMPI data were more accurate than descriptions based on the judge's stereotype of the "typical patient" (Graham, 1967). When MMPI data were used in conjunction with social history and/or interview data, the resulting descriptions were more valid than when the MMPI data were used alone (Kostlan, 1954; Sines, 1959). Finally, there are data suggesting that when test judges are asked to predict a reliable criterion and when there are valid relationships between test data and the criterion, a high level of descriptive accuracy can be achieved with limited experience (Cohen, 1975).

While it is difficult to reach very definitive conclusions about the validity of the MMPI, this writer believes that the validity data suggest that the MMPI is the most valid personality assessment instrument of those that have been studied empirically and that MMPI data can add significantly to the understanding of individual cases. Especially when the MMPI is used in conjunction with other test data, history, and observational data, it represents a valuable assessment tool for the clinician.

6. Additional MMPI Scales

Subsequent to the development of the standard validity and clinical scales, the basic MMPI item pool has been utilized to construct many additional scales. In their two-volume *MMPI Handbook*, Dahlstrom et al. (1972, 1975) listed 500 such scales. These scales vary considerably in what they were designed to measure, in the care with which they were constructed, in the extent to which they have been cross-validated, and in their popularity among clinicians and researchers. Graham (1977a, 1977b) summarized some of the more potentially useful of these additional scales. Only several of the more comprehensive efforts to construct new scales from the MMPI item pool will be discussed in this chapter.

6.1. Subscales

Recognizing that the standard MMPI scales are not homogeneous in content and that any given score on a scale can be obtained by endorsing different combinations of items within the scale, Harris and Lingoes (1955, 1968) developed subscales for six of the ten standard MMPI clinical scales (2, 3, 4, 6, 8, and 9). Each subscale was constructed rationally by grouping together items within a scale that seemed similar in content or seemed to reflect a single attribute. Thirty-one subscales were constructed in all, but three summary scales typically are not used in clinical interpretation of the MMPI. The remaining 28 subscales are listed in Table 2. Graham (1977a, 1977b) reviewed the reliability and validity data for the Harris and Lingoes subscales and concluded that the subscales represent a potentially useful addition to the standard MMPI scales and that the subscales may be especially useful in understanding what kinds of items a test subject endorsed in obtaining a high score on a standard clinical scale. Graham also offered some tentative interpretive data for the Harris and Lingoes subscales.

Serkownek (1975) utilized factor analytic data reported by Graham, Schroeder,

Table 2. Subscales for the Standard MMPI Clinical Scales

Standard MMPI scale		Subscales
1—Hypochondriasis	None	
2—Depression	D1	Subjective Depression
	D2	Psychomotor Retardation
	D3	Physical Malfunctioning
	D4	Mental Dullness
	D5	Brooding
3—Hysteria	Hy1	Denial of Social Anxiety
	Hy2	Need for Affection
	Hy3	Lassitude-Malaise
	Hy4	Somatic Complaints
	Hy5	Inhibition of Aggression
4—Psychopathic Deviate	Pd1	Familial Discord
	Pd2	Authority Problems
	Pd3	Social Imperturbability
	Pd4A	Social Alienation
	Pd4B	Self Alienation
5—Masculinity-femininity	Mf1	Narcissism-Hypersensitivity
	Mf2	Stereotypic Feminine Interests
	Mf3	Denial of Stereotypic Masculine Interests
	Mf4	Heterosexual Discomfort-Passivity
	Mf5	Introspective-Critical
	Mf6	Socially Retiring
6—Paranoia	Pa1	Persecutory Ideas
	Pa2	Poignancy
	Pa3	Naiveté
7—Psychasthenia	None	
8—Schizophrenia	Sc1A	Social Alienation
	Sc1B	Emotional Alienation
	Sc2A	Lack of Ego Mastery, Cognitive
	Sc2B	Lack of Ego Mastery, Conative
	Sc2C	Lack of Ego Mastery, Defective Inhibition
	Sc3	Bizarre Sensory Experiences
9—Hypomania	Ma1	Amorality
	Ma2	Psychomotor Acceleration
	Ma3	Imperturbability
	Ma4	Ego Inflation
0—Social Introversion	Si1	Inferiority-Personal Discomfort
	Si2	Discomfort with Others
	Si3	Staid-Personal Rigidity
	Si4	Hypersensitivity
	Si5	Distrust
	Si6	Physical-Somatic Concerns

and Lilly (1971) to construct subscales for scales 5 and 0 of the MMPI. The six clusters of items from scale 5 and the six clusters from scale 0 are listed in Table 2. While no reliability and validity data have been reported for Serkownek's subscales, Graham (1977a) has offered some tentative interpretive data for the subscales based on examination of item content.

6.2. Content Scales

While initially little or no importance was attached to the content of items within the standard MMPI scales, more recently some investigators (e.g., Hase & Goldberg, 1967; Jackson 1971; Koss & Butcher, 1973) have suggested that examination of item content can add significantly to MMPI interpretation. The content scales developed by Wiggins (1966) represent the most systematic effort to assess the important content dimensions of the MMPI. The scales were developed rationally by grouping together items that were judged to have similar content and were refined using internal consistency procedures. These procedures yielded a final set of 13 content scales judged by Wiggins to be mutually exclusive, internally consistent, moderately independent, and representative of the major content dimensions of the MMPI item pool. See Table 3 for a list of the content scales. Reliability data, norms, and validity data for the Wiggins content scales have been summarized by Graham (1977a, 1977b). The reader should also refer to Butcher and Owen (chapter 15, this volume). Graham (1977b) concluded that the Wiggins content scales are psychometrically sound measures of the content dimensions of the MMPI and are related to important nontest behaviors different from the ones assessed by the standard MMPI scales. When used in conjunction with the standard scales, the content scales can add significantly to the understanding of test subjects.

7. Conclusion

While the MMPI has not lived up to its original purpose—the diagnosis of psychiatric patients—subsequent construct validity studies have yielded a wide array of nontest correlates for the original MMPI scales. Such information is of great value to clinicians faced with the task of assessing personality. While the MMPI by no means is a perfect test instrument, it is the writer's opinion that no better one currently is available. As Hathaway stated in his Foreword to the second edition of *An MMPI Handbook* (Dahlstrom et al., 1972), we cannot lay down even a Stone-Age axe if we have no better one to hew with.

Table 3. Wiggins Content Scales
for the MMPI

Scale abbreviation	Scale name
SOC	Social Maladjustment
DEP	Depression
FEM	Feminine Interests
MOR	Poor Morale
REL	Religious Fundamentalism
AUT	Authority Conflict
PSY	Psychoticism
ORG	Organic Symptoms
FAM	Family Problems
HOS	Manifest Hostility
PHO	Phobias
HYP	Hypomania
HEA	Poor Health

8. References

Barker, H. R., Fowler, R. D., & Peterson, L. P. Factor analytic structure of the short form MMPI in a Veterans Administration hospital population. *Journal of Clinical Psychology*, 1971, *27*, 228–233.

Bernreuter, R. G. *The Personality Inventory*. Palo Alto, Calif.: Consulting Psychologists Press, 1931.

Black, J. D. The Interpretation of MMPI profiles of college women. Unpublished doctoral dissertation, University of Minnesota, 1953.

Block, J. *The challenge of response sets: Unconfounding meaning, acquiescence, and social desirability in the MMPI*. New York: Appleton-Century-Crofts, 1965.

Block, J., & Bailey, D. Q sort item analyses of a number of MMPI scales. Officer Education Research Laboratory, Technical Memorandum, OERL-TM-55,7, 1955.

Boerger, A. R., Graham, J. R., & Lilly, R. S. Behavioral correlates of single-scale MMPI code types. *Journal of Consulting and Clinical Psychology*, 1974, *42*, 298–402.

Buros, O. K. (Ed.). *The seventh mental measurements yearbook*. Highland Park, N.J.: Gryphon Press, 1972.

Butcher, J. N. Present status of computerized MMPI reporting services. In O. K. Buros (Ed.), *Eighth mental measurements yearbook*. Highland Park, N.J.: Gryphon Press, 1978.

Butcher, J. N., & Pancheri, P. *Handbook of cross-national MMPI research*. Minneapolis: University of Minnesota Press, 1976.

Chu, C. Object cluster analysis of the MMPI. Unpublished doctoral dissertation, University of California, Berkeley, 1966.

Cohen, R. Accuracy level and confidence level in clinical inference as a function of feedback, cues, and specific practice. Unpublished doctoral dissertation, Kent State University, 1975.

Comrey, A. L. A factor analysis of items on the MMPI depression scale. *Educational and Psychological Measurement*, 1957, *17*, 578–585. (a)

Comrey, A. L. A factor analysis of items on the MMPI hypochondriasis scale. *Educational and Psychological Measurement*, 1957, *17*, 566–577. (b)

Comrey, A. L. A factor analysis of items on the MMPI hysteria scale. *Educational and Psychological Measurement*, 1957, *17*, 586–592. (c)

Comrey, A. L. A factor analysis of items on the F scale of the MMPI. *Educational and Psychological Measurement*, 1958, *18*, 621–632. (a)

Comrey, A. L. A factor analysis of items on the MMPI hypomania scale. *Educational and Psychological Measurement*, 1958, *18*, 313–323. (b)

Comrey, A. L. A factor analysis of items on the MMPI paranoia scale. *Educational and Psychological Measurement*, 1958, *18*, 99–107. (c)

Comrey, A. L. A factor analysis of items on the MMPI psychasthenia scale. *Educational and Psychological Measurement*, 1958, *18*, 293–300. (d)

Comrey, A. L. A factor analysis of items on the MMPI psychopathic deviate scale. *Educational and Psychological Measurement*, 1958, *18*, 91–98. (e)

Comrey, A. L., & Margraff, W. A factor analysis of items on the MMPI schizophrenia scale. *Educational and Psychological Measurement*, 1958, *18*, 301–311.

Dahlstrom, W. G., & Welsh, G. S. *An MMPI handbook: A guide to clinical practice and research*. Minneapolis: University of Minnesota Press, 1960.

Dahlstrom, W. G., Welsh, G. S., & Dahlstrom, L. E. *An MMPI handbook. Volume I: Clinical interpretation*. Minneapolis: University of Minnesota Press, 1972.

Dahlstrom, W. G., Welsh, G. S., & Dahlstrom, L. E. *An MMPI handbook. Volume II: Research applications*. Minneapolis: University of Minnesota Press, 1975.

Drake, L. E. A social I.E. scale for the MMPI. *Journal of Applied Psychology*, 1946, *30*, 51–54.

Duckworth, J. C., & Duckworth, E. *MMPI interpretive manual for counselors and clinicians*. Muncie, Ind.: Accelerated Development, Inc., 1975.

Edwards, A. L. *The social desirability variable in personality assessment and research*. New York: Dryden, 1957.

Edwards, A. L. Social desirability and performance on the MMPI. *Psychometrika*, 1964, *29*, 295–308.

Eichman, W. J. Replicated factors on the MMPI with female NP patients. *Journal of Consulting Psychology*, 1961, *25*, 55–60.

Eichman, W. J. Factored scales for the MMPI: A clinical and statistical manual. *Journal of Clinical Psychology*, 1962, *18*, 363–395.

Eichman, W. J. Minnesota Multiphasic Personality Inventory: Computerized scoring and interpreting services. In O. K. Buros (Ed.), *The seventh mental measurements yearbook* (Vol. I). Highland Park, N.J.: Gryphon Press, 1972.

Fowler, R. D., & Coyle, F. A. Overlap as a problem in atlas classification of MMPI profiles. *Journal of Clinical Psychology*, 1968, *24*, 435.

Gilberstadt, H., & Duker, J. *A handbook for clinical and actuarial MMPI interpretation*. Philadelphia: Saunders, 1965.

Goldberg, L. R. Diagnosticians vs. diagnostic signs: The diagnosis of psychosis vs. neurosis from the MMPI. *Psychological Monographs*, 1965, *79*, 9 (whole No. 602).

Goldberg, L. R. Simple models or simple processes? Some research on clinical judgments. *American Psychologist*, 1968, *23*, 483–496.

Good, P. K., & Brantner, J. P. *The physician's guide to the MMPI*. Minneapolis: University of Minnesota Press, 1961.

Gough, H. G., McKee, M. G., & Yandell, R. J. Adjective check list analyses of a number of selected psychometric and assessment variables. Officer Education Research Laboratory, Technical Memorandum, OERL-TM-55-10, 1955.

Graham, J. R. A Q-sort study of the accuracy of clinical descriptions based on the MMPI. *Journal of Psychiatric Research*, 1967, *5*, 297–305.

Graham, J. R. *The MMPI: A practical guide*. New York: Oxford University Press, 1977. (a)

Graham, J. R. The stability of MMPI profile configurations. Paper presented at the Twelfth Annual MMPI Symposium, St. Petersburg Beach, Fla., 1977. (b)

Graham, J. R. A review of some important MMPI special scales. In P. McReynolds (Ed.), *Advances in psychological assessment* (Vol. IV). Palo Alto, Calif.: Jossey-Bass, 1977. (c)

Graham, J. R., Schroeder, H. E., & Lilly, R. S. Factor analysis of items on the social introversion and masculinity-femininity scales of the MMPI. *Journal of Clinical Psychology*, 1971, *27*, 367–370.

Guthrie, G. M. A study of the personality characteristics associated with the disorders encountered by an internist. Unpublished doctoral dissertation, University of Minnesota, 1949.

Gynther, M. D., Altman, H., & Sletten, I. W. Replicated correlates of MMPI two-point code types: The Missouri actuarial system. *Journal of Clinical Psychology*, 1973, *29*, 263–289.

Gynther, M. D., Altman, H., & Warbin, R. W. The interpretation of uninterpretable MMPI profiles. *Journal of Consulting and Clinical Psychology*, 1973, *40*, 78–83. (a)

Gynther, M. D., Altman, H., & Warbin, R. W. Behavioral correlates for the MMPI 49/94 code type: A case of the emperor's new clothes? *Journal of Consulting and Clinical Psychology*, 1973, *40*, 259–263. (b)

Gynther, M. D., & Brillant, P. J. The MMPI *K+* profile: A reexamination. *Journal of Consulting and Clinical Psychology*, 1968, *32*, 616–617.

Gynther, M. D., & Gynther, R. A. Personality inventories. In I. B. Weiner (Ed.), *Clinical methods in psychology*. New York: Wiley, 1976.

Harris, R., & Lingoes, J. Subscales for the Minnesota Multiphasic Personality Inventory. Mimeographed materials, The Langley Porter Clinic, 1955.

Harris, R., & Lingoes, J. Subscales for the Minnesota Multiphasic Personality Inventory. Mimeographed materials, The Langley Porter Clinic, 1968.

Hase, H. D., & Goldberg, L. R. Comparative validity of different strategies of constructing personality inventory scales. *Psychological Bulletin*, 1967, *67*, 231–248.

Hathaway, S. R. A coding system for MMPI profiles. *Journal of Consulting Psychology*, 1947, *11*, 334–337.

Hathaway, S. R., & McKinley, J. C. *Manual for the Minnesota Multiphasic Personality Inventory*. New York: Psychological Corporation, 1943.

Hathaway, S. R., & McKinley, J. C. *The Minnesota Multiphasic Personality Inventory Manual*. New York: Psychological Corporation, 1967.

Hathaway, S. R., & Meehl, P. E. *An atlas for the clinical use of the MMPI*. Minneapolis: University of Minnesota Press, 1951.

Hathaway, S. R., & Meehl, P. E. Adjective check list correlates of MMPI scores. Unpublished materials, 1952.

Hathaway, S. R., & Monachesi, E. D. (Eds.). *Analyzing and predicting juvenile delinquency with the MMPI*. Minneapolis: University of Minnesota Press, 1953.

Henrichs, T. F. Objective configural rules for discriminating MMPI profiles in a psychiatric population. *Journal of Clinical Psychology*, 1964, *20*, 157–159.

Hovey, H. B. MMPI profiles and personality characteristics. *Journal of Consulting Psychology*, 1953, *17*, 142–146.

Huff, F. W. Use of actuarial description of abnormal personality in a mental hospital. *Psychological Reports*, 1965, *17*, 224.

Jackson, D. N. Response styles on the MMPI: Comparison of clinical and normal samples. *Journal of Abnormal and Social Psychology*, 1962, *65*, 285–299.

Jackson, D. N. The dynamics of structured tests: 1971. *Psychological Review*, 1971, *78*, 239–249.

Jackson, D. N., & Messick, S. Acquiescence and desirability as response determinants on the MMPI. *Educational and Psychological Measurement*, 1961, *21*, 771–790.

Kleinmuntz, G. Minnesota Multiphasic Personality Inventory: Roche MMPI computerized interpretation service. In O. K. Buros (Ed.), *The seventh mental measurements yearbook* (Vol. I). Highland Park, N.J.: Gryphon Press, 1972.

Koss, M. P., & Butcher, J. N. A comparison of psychiatric patients' self-report with other sources of clinical information. *Journal of Research in Personality*, 1973, *7*, 225–236.

Kostlan, A. A method for the empirical study of psychodiagnosis. *Journal of Consulting Psychology*, 1954, *18*, 83–88.

Lanyon, R. I. *A handbook of MMPI group profiles.* Minneapolis: University of Minnesota Press, 1968.

Lewandowski, D., & Graham, J. R. Empirical correlates of frequently occurring two-point MMPI code types: A replicated study. *Journal of Consulting and Clinical Psychology*, 1972, *39*, 467–472.

Little, K. B., & Schneidman, E. S. Congruencies among interpretations of psychological test and anamnestic data. *Psychological Monographs*, 1959, *73*, 6 (whole No. 476).

Lubin, B., Wallis, R. R., & Paine, C. Patterns of psychological test usage in the United States: 1935–1969. *Professional Psychology*, 1971, *2*, 70–74.

Marks, P. A., & Seeman, W. *Actuarial description of abnormal personality.* Baltimore: Williams & Wilkins, 1963.

Marks, P. A., Seeman, W., & Haller, D. L. *The actuarial use of the MMPI with adolescents and adults.* Baltimore: Williams & Wilkins, 1974.

Matarazzo, J. D. *Wechsler's measurement and appraisal of adult intelligence.* Baltimore: Williams & Wilkins, 1972.

Meehl, P. E. *Research results for counselors.* Minneapolis: University of Minnesota Press, 1951.

Meehl, P. E., & Dahlstrom, W. G. Objective configural rules for discriminating psychotic from neurotic MMPI profiles. *Journal of Consulting Psychology*, 1960, *24*, 375–387.

Meikle, S., & Gerritse, R. MMPI cookbook pattern frequencies in a psychiatric unit. *Journal of Clinical Psychology*, 1970, *26*, 82–84.

Mello, N. K., & Guthrie, G. M. MMPI profiles and behavior in counseling. *Journal of Counseling Psychology*, 1958, *5*, 125–129.

Palmer, W. H. Actuarial MMPI interpretation: A replication and extension. Unpublished doctoral dissertation, University of Alabama, 1970.

Pauker, J. D. Identification of MMPI profile types in a female, inpatient psychiatric setting using the Marks and Seeman rules. *Journal of Consulting Psychology*, 1966, *30*, 90.

Peterson, D. R. Predicting hospitalization of psychiatric outpatients. *Journal of Abnormal and Social Psychology*, 1954, *49*, 260–265.

Schultz, J. D., Gibeau, P. J., & Barry, S. M. Utility of MMPI "cookbooks." *Journal of Clinical Psychology*, 1968, *24*, 430–433.

Schwartz, G. F. An investigation of the stability of single scale and two-point MMPI code types for psychiatric patients. Unpublished doctoral dissertation, Kent State University, 1977.

Serkownek, K. Subscales for scales 5 and 0 of the Minnesota Multiphasic Personality Inventory. Unpublished materials, 1975.

Sines, L. K. The relative contribution of four kinds of the data to accuracy in personality assessment. *Journal of Consulting Psychology*, 1959, *23*, 483–492.

Stein, K. B. The TSC scales: The outcome of a cluster analysis of the 550 MMPI items. In P. McReynolds (Ed.), *Advances in psychological assessment* (Vol. I). Palo Alto, Calif.: Science and Behavior Books, 1968.

Sundberg, N. D. *Assessment of persons.* New York: Prentice-Hall, 1977.

Taulbee, E. S., & Sisson, B. D. Configural analysis of MMPI profiles of psychiatric groups. *Journal of Consulting Psychology*, 1957, *21*, 413–417.

Tryon, R. C. Unrestricted cluster and factor analysis with application to the MMPI and Holzinger-Harman problems. *Multivariate Behavioral Research*, 1966, *1*, 229–244.

Tryon, R. C., & Bailey, D. (Eds.). *Users' manual of the BC TRY system of cluster and factor analysis* (taped version). Berkeley: University of California Computer Center, 1965.

Weiner, I. B. (Ed.). *Clinical methods in psychology*. New York: Wiley, 1976.

Welsh, G. S. An extension of Hathaway's MMPI profile coding system. *Journal of Consulting Psychology*, 1948, *12*, 343–344.

Welsh, G. S. Factor dimensions A and R. In G. S. Welsh & W. G. Dahlstrom (Eds.), *Basic readings on the MMPI in psychology and medicine*. Minneapolis: University of Minnesota Press, 1956.

Wiggins, J. S. Substantive dimensions of self-report in the MMPI item pool. *Psychological Monographs*, 1966, *80*, 22 (whole No. 630).

Woodworth, R. S. *Personal Data Sheet*. Chicago: Stoelting, 1920.

11

The Hutt Adaptation of the Bender-Gestalt Test: Diagnostic and Therapeutic Implications

MAX L. HUTT

1. Introduction

The unique values of a perceptual-motoric test for personality assessment have been sensed by many but realized by relatively few clinicians. I shall attempt to explicate this statement in later sections of this chapter but wish to introduce some preliminary observations first. The Bender-Gestalt Test, with its many forms and assorted scoring systems, has certainly captured the interest of clinical psychologists and others: it is reported to be one of the three or four most widely used testing devices (Schulberg & Tolor, 1961; Sundberg, 1961; Crenshaw, Bohn, Hoffman, Matheus, & Offenbach, 1968; Lubin, Wallis, & Paine, 1971; Lerner, 1972; Hutt, 1977). These reports have also indicated the widespread use of objective methods of evaluating test findings. Many clinicians use the test either to harvest projective inferences about the personality or to provide information useful for purposes of differential diagnosis. Yet there have been relatively few publications dealing extensively with the unique nature of projections as manifested in perceptual-motoric behavior or of the almost limitless possibilities of employing what I have called the "experimental-clinical method" with such behavior. More often than not the Bender-Gestalt Test has been employed for supplementary or marginal purposes in the total clinical evaluation rather than for examination in depth of underlying dynamics, of areas of conflict, or of specific defense hierarchies.

MAX L. HUTT • 21 Regent Drive, Ann Arbor, Michigan 48104.

These marginal purposes to which I have referred may have value, but the clinician who is content merely to look for grossly abnormal perceptual-motoric phenomena in a test record—perhaps in an effort to detect "signs" of psychosis or "signs" of cerebral dysfunction, or even "signs" of perceptual immaturity—may not only misinterpret such phenomena, turning up false positives, but also miss entirely the richer lode of the test protocol. First, any test sign, no matter how validly it may discriminate known groups of patients from each other, may in any given instance be the product of other factors than it usually and presumably indicates. Second, a test sign can be properly understood only in the light of the total pattern of the behavioral response of which it is an integral part. Thus the clinician who, to coin a phrase, "putters with the test record," hoping thereby to come to some quick insight about the patient, not only is abandoning the relevant evidence which the patient reveals but also is abandoning his role as a "scientist-clinician." As Beck (1968) suggests on improper use of the Rorschach test: "Many use the test simply for thematic content which it evokes . . . what these examiners are doing is no more than free associating to the patient's free associations."

Another horn of the dilemma of using the HABGT (or other versions of the Bender-Gestalt Test) is that of employing solely some objective scale in evaluating the test protocol. Objective scales have their value, and I do not wish to derogate them, but, as we shall see later, such scales, when taken out of the context of the behavioral process which led to the test phenomena, and without proper consideration of intrapersonal and situational factors which may have significantly affected the score on the scale, can be grossly misleading. Whether objective scales are employed as the major method of test analysis or whether they are used as part of the total set of behavioral data, the clinician's task always involves the critical function of evaluating their meaning by scientific rules of evidence. This involves, in part, an analysis of the applicability of the assumptions germane to the derivations of the scales in the particular instance, as well as an examination of alternative explanations of the behavior of the patient which produced the score in that case. One method of conducting such an examination is through the "experimental-clinical method" which is presented later in this chapter.

As we shall see, perceptual-motoric behavior can offer significant evidence of personality disorganization and organization, but this evidence can be neglected unless the nature of perceptual-motoric behavior is thoroughly understood. Hence we shall discuss this aspect of the HABGT at various points in later sections.

2. HABGT Test Materials

The HABGT consists of nine test cards, 3 inches by 5 inches, on each of which is a simple gestalt design (see Figure 1). Each card is presented to the subject in a designated sequence, with the longer axis of the card parallel to the frontal plane of the subject. (Details of administration will be discussed in the next section.)

These cards* are significantly different in several respects from those furnished by other publishers of test materials. They were developed by Hutt, with the cooperation of F. L. Wells, in 1945, and were made available to clinical psychologists and psychiatrists who were members of the armed services. Unlike other sets of cards,

*The HABGT test cards may be purchased from Grune & Stratton, Inc., 111 Fifth Avenue, New York, N.Y. 10003.

they are designed to follow the gestalt principles and the criteria employed by Wertheimer (1923) in his original work on gestalt aspects of visual perception. The nature of the curves, features of size, and angle crossings, for example, are designed to maximize certain features of the integrative process in perception. Moreover,

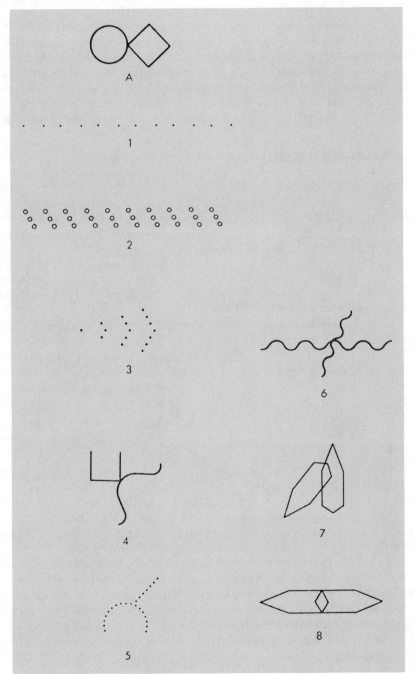

Figure 1. The Hutt Adaptation of the Bender-Gestalt Figures. This illustration has been reduced about 45% from the original size. From Hutt, Max L., *The Hutt Adaptation of the Bender-Gestalt Test*, 3rd edition, 1977. Reprinted with the permission of Grune & Stratton, Inc., New York, N.Y.

and especially important, the criteria for evaluating deviations in size and distortions of the gestalt in the test protocols of subjects are based on these test stimuli in particular. The test scales and the criteria for scoring, discussed later in this chapter, are likewise based on these test cards. Hence the use of other sets of cards with such criteria is inapplicable.

Other test materials include a stack of white, unlined, 8½- by 11-inch paper and medium-soft pencils with erasers for use by the subject. Again, in conjunction with my criteria for analysis of line quality and pressure, deviations from the use of such materials must be considered in any clinical evaluation of a test record. It should also be obvious that a smooth and comfortable surface for copying the designs, adequate light, and appropriate conditions of rapport with the subject are required if the criteria for scoring and analysis suggested by this writer are to be employed.

3. Methods of Administration

Administrative procedures that have been employed with Bender-Gestalt Test stimuli have varied considerably when employed by some psychologists. I shall not attempt to review these different procedures; each has its own value. However, in my use of the test materials, I have attempted to coordinate the methods of administration with the general and specific objectives of the examination. In order to maximize the emergence of projective phenomena, my basic method of administration involves three phases, each of which has its own rationale. In addition, whenever there is a critical question involving differential diagnosis, I frequently employ my experimental-clinical method. Each of these features will be discussed briefly. The reader who wishes to have a more complete discussion of them is advised to consult Hutt (1977), in which they are discussed in detail.

The first phase of the basic method of administration is designed, as already noted, to maximize the emergence of projective phenomena. In the Copy Phase, the subject is presented with a stack of paper, placed near him on the examining table, along with pencils and erasers. He is then told that he will be asked to copy, as well as he can, each of a number of simple designs. One sheet of paper is placed in front of him, with the long axis perpendicular to his frontal plane. The first test card is then presented to him with the long axis parallel to his frontal plane. This sets up a discrepancy between the spatial orientation of the two sets of materials, which tends to increase perceptual rotation, elongation of reproductions in the horizontal plane, and so on. Moreover, the subject is given no guidance with respect to methods of procedure. For example, when he asks "Where shall I draw this?" he is told to do it the way he wishes or feels is best. When the second card is presented after the first card has been copied, he may inquire about where he should place it or how large he should make it. In this, as in all other instances in which the subject inquires about how he should proceed, he is given no structuring but simply told to do it as well as he can and as he wishes. Each card is presented sequentially to the subject in the same manner. Subjects frequently ask whether they should draw all of the designs on a single sheet, especially when they see that they may be running out of space on the first sheet. Here, as in all similar instances, the examiner refers the problem back to the subject with some comment such as "That is up to you."

The essential feature of this method of procedure is to require the subject to adapt in his own unique way. His use of space, his spacing of the figures on the page, his size of reproductions, and his sequence of placement of the figures on the page are thus products of his own need system and his own conflicts. The availability of a stack of paper, instead of the availability of only a single sheet, tends to maximize his degrees of freedom and thereby helps us to understand how he sees himself in relation to space (which may represent his life space in some respects) and how he adapts progressively as the test proceeds.

337

THE HUTT
ADAPTATION OF THE
BENDER-GESTALT
TEST: DIAGNOSTIC
AND THERAPEUTIC
IMPLICATIONS

Of course, the subject's methods of work as well as his product are matters of considerable clinical import. In Hutt (1977), there is discussion of these aspects of the test record.

The second phase of the test is called the Elaboration Phase. After the subject has completed his nine drawings, they are removed from sight. The test cards, or a sampling of them, are then reintroduced and a new stack of paper is provided, with a single sheet again presented in front of the subject. The subject is then told something to this effect: "This time I am going to show you the cards (or some of the cards) again, but this time I should like you to draw them in any way you wish so as to make them more pleasing to you. You can change them as much or as little as you wish." (The wording may be varied in accordance with the maturity of the subject.) As in the Copy Phase, each card is presented individually and in the same sequence.

The intent of this procedure is to obtain derivatives of conflict-loaded material which the stimuli may evoke. Some subjects are severely threatened by the Elaboration Phase; they require guidelines for support; they wish to satisfy the authority figure and do what is expected. Other subjects feel free to exhibit their creativity and their independence. Still others are threatened by anxieties evoked by the stimuli or their drawings, or by the symbolic meaning they attach to these. Some subjects stick very closely to the original directions of the Copy Phase, feeling anxious about revealing themselves. In these and many other ways, the Elaboration Phase provides rich sources of data which help to confirm trends that may have been evident in the Copy Phase, to reveal new nuances of the subject's potential, or to reveal aspects of ego functioning more clearly. Both structural and process aspects of functioning may be clarified by the new material elicited in the Elaboration Phase.

The third phase of the basic method is called the Association Phase. In this phase, the test cards are separately presented alongside of the drawing made for that card in the Elaboration Phase. The subject is asked, in turn, for each pair of stimuli (the card and the elaboration of the card, even when they are similar): "Now tell me what each of these reminds you of, or what each looks like." The examiner makes note of which stimulus is responded to first (card or elaboration) and the content of the associations. If the subject, as frequently happens, gives an association only to the test card or only to the elaboration, the additional question asked is "And what does this other one look like or remind you of?" Some subjects give few associations, while others give many.

The purpose of placing the test card alongside the elaboration is to confront the subject with the differences in the two and thereby to assist in maximizing the evocation of idiosyncratic and derivative data. Frequently, the subject first becomes aware that there is something especially meaningful and perhaps threatening about the stimuli when he sees the contrast between the test design and what he has done with it. Sometimes, repressed and isolated fragments of personal experience are evoked by this method. It is my belief, based on many experiences in clinical work with this test, as well as on clinical and research literature, that some repressed material comes to the surface in apparently aimless and meaningless perceptual-motoric behavior. Or, put another way, many of our traumatic experiences, especially those of early formative periods, have become "bound" in perceptual-motoric phenomena and are subsequently released in nonpurposeful perceptual-motoric behavior, thereby becoming more available to conscious awareness.

These three phases of the test can, in most cases, provide a rich lode of clinical data. Some of these data are not readily available in verbal projective tests, in which intellectualization may obscure the particularly relevant phenomena. Moreover, as will be seen in later sections, tentative hypotheses formulated on the basis of the basic method can be tested in the experimental-clinical method.

Let us now examine the nature of these test data and derived hypotheses.

4. Nature of the Test Data

The test data may be categorized in a number of ways.

4.1. Behavioral Data

As with any test used in clinical evaluation, one broad category of test phenomena has to do with behavior elicited in the course of testing. The experienced clinician, and particularly the clinician experienced with the particular test, will observe and record such data. Moreover, the "locus of the behavior" (i.e., the point and stimulus in the test sequence where such behavior emerges) may be especially significant.

I can specify only some of the more important of such behaviors which can be observed on the HABGT. Of primary importance is the kind of motivation (and involvement with the task) which is displayed. Does the individual exert maximum effort? Is he easily fatigued? Does he respond regressively to difficult items or the buildup of stress? Does he work carefully or impulsively? Does he plan and anticipate adequately? Does he seek a dependent relationship with the examiner? Do some of the test stimuli cause "blocking"? Does he show confusion or display feelings of "impotence"? Most of these behaviors can be observed during any projective test. Some of them may have particular diagnostic significance, and others may lead to reexamination of the usual meanings of test scores and configurations.

The HABGT is a nonverbal, perceptual-motoric test. Consequently, some individuals may display more of themselves on such tests since they are less aware of what it is they are displaying and they tend to be less defensive. More particularly, since performance on the Copy Phase of the test involves both perception and motoric behavior, as well as a delicate synthesis of these functions, certain types of behaviors are especially relevant. I cannot take the space to itemize all of these phenomena, but shall present some illustrative examples. First, the items of the test range in difficulty (or levels at which adequate reproduction is normally expected) from the 6–7 year level to about the 11-year level in terms of perceptual-motoric performance. Hence we note whether the subject performs with less difficulty on the easier items and with greater difficulty on the more difficult items. Any discrepancy in such progression is suspect; discrepancies may be caused by cerebral dysfunction, traumatic reaction to the symbolic meaning of a design, differential difficulty with open vs. closed figures or with curved vs. straight-line figures, difficulty

339

THE HUTT
ADAPTATION OF THE
BENDER-GESTALT
TEST: DIAGNOSTIC
AND THERAPEUTIC
IMPLICATIONS

with overlapping figures, fatigue or loss of motivation, and so on. The reader is referred to the basic text (Hutt, 1977) and an atlas of test protocols (Hutt & Gibby, 1970) for examples of such discrepancies and their probable clinical significance.

The latter two phases of the test offer considerable evidence for further evaluation of inferences derived from observations of the kinds of behavior we have been discussing. Consistency of particular types of difficulties and the associative material offered during the Association Phase often provide confirmation of preliminary inferences.

Two other general features of observational data may be noted. One of these involves the spontaneous verbalizations offered by the subject during the course of the test. Often the subject will explain some aspects of the difficulties or feelings he is experiencing. The other concerns the tendency of some subjects to rotate either the test card or the drawing paper. Perceptual rotation (i.e., perception of the stimulus as having a different axis than the one in which it is presented) can have many meanings. The degree of rotation is also important. Some of the common causes of perceptual rotation are the discrepancy between the long axis of the test card and the long axis of the paper (which mature, integrated individuals compensate for easily), oppositional tendencies, narcissistic needs which impel the subject to rotate the drawing centripetally, and many types of cerebral dysfunction. This latter type of phenomenon is most striking and always needs serious evaluation. Perceptual rotations occur more frequently in young children (say, below 9 years of age), and are rarely present in older persons unless one of the types of factors noted is present. Rotations by young children are often due primarily to immaturity in perceptual development.

Rotation of the test paper is quite different in significance. The most common causes are prior experiences with drawing materials, cultural factors in the use of drawing and writing materials, oppositional tendencies, and anxiety which produces some type of avoidant behavior. The clinician will seek to determine the precise cause of the rotation through inquiry as well as through other indicators on the test of the presumed hypothesis.

I wish to stress the importance of behavioral data, which, too often, are neglected by the clinician. They enable us to interpret the test data much more sensitively and relevantly than when they are overlooked. This consideration is especially important on a nonverbal perceptual-motoric test, but it is highly relevant on all individually administered tests, because test findings do not occur *in vacuo:* they are influenced by set, motivation, examiner-examinee relationship, current anxiety level, and so on.

4.2. Test Factors and Test Signs

On the basis first of clinical experience and then of research data with a great variety of normal and psychiatric populations, I have selected those test factors and test indicators which have been shown to predict certain outcomes or to differentiate various nosological groups or dynamic patterns of behavior. The primary evidence on the test for such phenomena is culled from the test productions on the Copy Phase. It is this phase which yields configuration scores characteristic of various psychiatric conditions, the Psychopathology scale, and the Adience-Abience scale. I shall discuss each of these in a subsequent section.

Each of the 26 test factors is usually related to one or more types of behavior processes and thus contributes to the process of inferential analysis presented in the following section. Seventeen of the test factors are incorporated, with weights assigned in terms of differential capacity, in the Psychopathology scale. Twelve test factors, with somewhat differing weights and definitions, are incorporated into the Adience-Abience scale. A few of the most relevant test factors are included in each Configuration score, each with appropriate weights to provide a rapid means of screening for particular psychiatric conditions. Thus the basic test data are derived from the Copy Phase protocol.

However, in addition to the findings from the Copy Phase, there are important test indicators to be derived from the Elaboration Phase and the Association Phase. As we have already indicated, these phases furnish corroborative data which serve to reinforce findings derived from the Copy Phase, but they also serve to provide additional sources of significant clinical data. Strength of defense, degree of spontaneity, accessibility of marginal and unconscious phenomena, and idiosyncratic meanings of test productions can be more adequately evaluated on the basis of such data and a comparison with findings from the Copy Phase.

Finally, there are highly important, sometimes crucial, data to be obtained from the experimental-clinical method. The objective of this method is to test the precise antecedents of specific aspects of test phenomena and to learn under what conditions, if any, such phenomena are modifiable. Hence we can think of this method as one which enables us to test inferences and probable conclusions about the individual. It enables the astute clinician to check his findings and to clarify their meanings.

The rich harvest of data obtained in the course of administering the HABGT is often sufficient to provide an extensive description of the individual's personality, of the severity of his psychopathology, and of prognostic indicators. However, like any clinical instrument, despite objective scores and projective findings, the findings may still have limited value in some cases. Just as an interview, or a Rorschach evaluation, or a Minnesota Multiphasic profile, or a Thematic Apperception Test protocol can offer a distorted view of the person or a limited sampling of his difficulties and potential, so the HABGT has its limitations. Its unique contribution is that it attempts to provide an assessment via perceptual-motoric behavior—an area of behavior that is rich in its own right, and one that is neglected in most other assessment approaches. It is especially useful in a battery of tests or clinical procedures precisely for this reason.

5. HABGT Test Factors

As I have indicated, there are 26 test factors which have been selected on the basis of clinical and research evidence for use in evaluation of test protocols. Only 17 of these have stood the test of empirical findings in showing differentiation among several psychiatric categories. Twelve factors have been selected, redefined, and given new weights to contribute to the Adience-Abience scale. Nine of the factors which are not included in my present objective scales because they do not provide sufficient statistical contribution to them are, nevertheless, significant in some clinical cases. In some instances, they occur with insufficient frequency in a random sampling of records to warrant their inclusion in a scale; in others, differentiation was not sufficiently great. However, when these factors do occur they usually are

341

THE HUTT
ADAPTATION OF THE
BENDER-GESTALT
TEST: DIAGNOSTIC
AND THERAPEUTIC
IMPLICATIONS

quite important and can be utilized in the individual case to refine hypotheses about the nature of the pathology or to contribute to an enriched understanding of the record.

I shall not attempt, in this brief presentation, to do more than list the factors and offer some comment on them. The basic text dealing with the HABGT (Hutt, 1977) offers precise definitions of each factor and suggests possible interpretation for each.

5.1. Factors Related to Organization

The eight factors related to organization have to do with the individual's use of space and the organizational features of his work. In general, they tend to reflect how the individual sees himself in relation to life space and to capacity for anticipatory planning.

1. Sequence. This factor is scored on the basis of the degree of regularity with which the subject places his successive drawings on the page (or pages). Persons with poor impulse control or with poor anticipatory planning reveal irregular or confused sequences in their placements.

2. Position of the First Drawing. This is scored as either normal or abnormal, according to defined criteria. Abnormal placement of the first drawing indicates something about the subject's anxiety level and his rapport with the world of reality. Paranoid patients, especially, frequently reveal abnormal placement of this figure.

3. Use of Space I. This refers to the spacing between successive or adjacent figures. Such spacing can be normal, constricted, or excessive. Spacing, like Position of the First Drawing, tells us about the individual's mode of adaptation.

4. Use of Space II. The separate figures can be compressed in size or expanded. Based on statistical criteria that are provided, one can score for Use of Space II and use the data in clinical interpretation, but this factor is included only in the Adience-Abience scale and not in the Psychopathology scale.

5. Collision. This factor relates to the actual running together of the drawings, or to a tendency toward such overlap. It is a highly significant factor in evaluating disturbance of ego functions. There are seven scaled steps for this factor. Collision or collision tendency is rare in well-adjusted adults but is more frequent among children below the age of 7 years.

6. Use of Margin. Although this factor is not included in my objective scales, it is an important indicator of anxiety and of how the individual "enters the test situation." Excessive use of the margin as a "crutch" or support suggests the presence of at least covert anxiety. It is sometimes found in the records of brain-damaged patients.

7. Position of the Paper. Some subjects shift the paper on which they make their drawings so that the long axis of the paper is parallel to the long axis of the test card. Others shift their paper for each drawing. Still others shift the paper only for drawings which they find difficult to execute. The factor contributes to the Psychopathology scale and is usually indicative of some form of oppositional behavior, although other explanations are, of course, possible.

8. Shift in Position of Stimulus Card. Although not so frequent as factor 7, shifts in the position of the stimulus card may also be indicative of oppositional tendencies. This factor is not scored in our test scales.

5.2. Factors Related to Size

9. Overall Increase or Decrease in Size. Drawings that are either larger than the stimulus by one-quarter (in either axis) or smaller by one-quarter are considered to show an excessive change in size. When five or more of the drawings meet this criterion, the condition is abnormal. Such abnormal changes in size of the drawings, depending on whether they are expanded or constricted, reveal feelings of anxiety or impotency, and, in extreme cases, even paranoidal suspiciousness.

10. Progressive Increase or Decrease in Size. Such changes in the size of the drawings are correlated with poor impulse control and acting-out tendencies.

11. Isolated Increase or Decrease in Size. Such changes in size of individual figures usually pinpoint some specific anxiety associated with that figure—either for symbolic reasons or because of the complexity of the figure for the subject. Such indications warrant further analysis in terms of data furnished in the Elaboration Phase and Association Phase of the test.

5.3. Factors Related to Changes in the Gestalt

The following factors relate to ways in which the subject distorts or modifies the drawing but still retains essential gestalt features.

12. Closure Difficulty. This factor relates to difficulty in making the "join-ings" of the figures. Criteria are provided for scoring these closure difficulties and obtaining scaled scores. This factor has been found to relate to adequacy in inter-personal relations.

13. Crossing Difficulty. This factor relates to difficulty in executing the cross-ings on figures 6 and 7. Crossing difficulty, when not caused by immature motoric or perceptual development, is usually attributable to psychological blocking of some kind.

14. Curvature Difficulty. This is scored when there is some obvious change in the nature of the curvature—e.g., flattening, spiking, or increased curvature. Changes in curvature, as scored on the basis of my criteria, reflect some form of emotional disturbances. One example of such a disturbance is that of persons who have difficulty in expressing aggression; they usually do better on straight-line figures than on curved figures.

15. Change in Angulation. A change in angulation is counted when the angula-tion in the drawing differs from that in the test designs by 15° or more. Increased angulation generally reflects increased affectivity, whereas decreased angulation reflects the reverse.

5.4. Factors Related to Distortion of the Gestalt

The following factors relate to more severe manifestations of psychopathology. Some of these factors occur only in records of psychotic or brain-damaged individuals.

16. Perceptual Rotation. A shift in the major axis of the drawing even though the stimulus design is in the correct position is indicative of problems in perceptual rotation. In my scales, I score only for the severity of the rotation, although in clinical work one takes note of both frequency and severity of rotational difficulties. Severe perceptual rotation (i.e., 80° or more) suggests that some profound disturbance is present, assuming of course that the subject has adequate cognitive and general

perceptual maturity. It reflects a severe impairment of ego functions. Considerable research evidence is available concerning this factor.

343

THE HUTT
ADAPTATION OF THE
BENDER-GESTALT
TEST: DIAGNOSTIC
AND THERAPEUTIC
IMPLICATIONS

17.   Retrogression. This factor refers to the substitution of more primitive gestalten for those presented on the test cards. Retrogression suggests some severe disturbance in ego-integrative functions.

18.   Simplification. This factor may seem similar to factor 17, but refers only to the substitution of a simpler figure (not necessarily more primitive) in that the drawing is easier to execute. This finding is also indicative of a severe disturbance in ego functions, but more specifically refers to a decrease of cathexes in relation to the external world.

19.   Fragmentation. This factor is scored when there is a destruction of the gestalt caused by separation of that gestalt into separate parts. It represents a very severe disturbance in perceptual-motoric functions. Fragmentation occurs most frequently in the records of chronic psychotics and brain-damaged individuals.

20.   Overlapping Difficulty. This factor refers to specific types of difficulties in executing the drawings of contiguous figures (figure A) and overlapping figures (figure 7). These types of difficulties are defined in my criteria for this factor. Although other conditions may cause overlapping difficulty, the most common explanation is that of diffuse brain damage.

21.   Elaboration or Doodling. Here we are dealing with impulses which are out of control and which are manifest in the "fantasy" work that doodling, as defined, indicates. The subject has lost contact with the reality of the test requirements and has "let himself go."

22.   Perseveration. Perseveration refers to either the inability to shift from one set to another or the inability to inhibit the inappropriate continuation of a response pattern once it has begun. In either case, the individual displays interference in inhibitory and excitatory functions. As scored on my two objective scales, it can be categorized as "none present," "mild," "moderate," or "severe." Both psychotics and organics manifest severe perseverative tendencies more frequently than neurotics or normals do. Heroin users frequently show a high degree of perseverative tendencies.

23.   Redrawing of the Total Figure. As scored, this factor is indicative of either poor anticipatory planning or an overly self-critical attitude.

5.5.   Factors Related to Movement and Drawing

None of the following factors is scored on any of the scales, but their presence in a record (at least when present to a severe degree) is likely to be clinically significant. Movement factors are clearly related to cultural experiences but also reflect, to a degree far more than is usually thought, aspects of personal style in relating to others and to the world. Thus, for example, centripetal movement is usually indicative of an egocentric orientation, while centrifugal movement is indicative of other-orientedness and self-assertion. I shall simply list the several factors in this general category and refer the reader to my text on the HABGT or to other works dealing with expressive movement.

24.   Deviation in Direction of Movement. This factor is scored in terms of deviation from the usual or expected line movement for the particular figure.

25.   Inconsistency in Direction of Movement. Here we are dealing with inconsistencies within the record. Frequently, such shifts in the person's typical direction

of movement are indicative of some temporary "traumatic" reaction which the test figures or the reproduction of them stimulates.

26. Line Quality. This factor refers to the qualitative aspects of the line quality of the drawings: excessively heavy, excessively light, poor coordination, sketching. Each of these qualities may reflect important aspects of the personality: tension, anxiety, overcompensation and defensiveness, and neuromuscular difficulties. I do not provide any scoring scheme for these test characteristics, but suggest possible conditions that might give rise to them.

6. The Process of Inferential Analysis

The most rewarding aspect of HABGT analysis resides in the inferential analysis of test behavior, particularly in the Copy Phase.

I have provided detailed and extensive illustration of this method of analysis, both in "blind" analysis of test records furnished by clinicians who supplied the records for research or comparative clinical studies (Hutt, 1949, 1951, 1963) and in my own work (Hutt & Gibby, 1970; Hutt, 1977). I can do no more, in this short presentation, than to suggest some of the most important features of this approach.

Inferential analysis attempts to follow the process through which the subject proceeds as he takes the Copy Phase of the test, noting the specific features of his test performance, his adaptations to successive tasks and differing stimuli, his methods of coping and defending as the test progresses, and the stylistic and specific perceptual-motoric aspects of his performance on the various test stimuli. It involves the postulation of alternate hypotheses about this performance, based on research evidence concerning the meanings to be attributed to the test factors that are evident as well as on the clinical evidence which has been accumulated by me and by many others.

Usually one first takes note of the general style of the test protocol, so as to gain some orientation of a general nature concerning the subject. Such issues are addressed as the spatial arrangement of the drawings on the page (or pages), the sequence or disturbance in sequence which characterizes the placements of the successive drawings, the size of the drawings and regularity or irregularity in size, and the spacing between drawings. Each of these stylistic features leads to hypotheses (first-order hypotheses) about the performance. Thus compressed use of space suggests anxiety which tends to be internalized. The use of excessive space for the total set of drawings suggests "acting out," or, if each drawing is centered on a separate sheet, narcissism or egocentrism. Sequence suggests hypotheses related to the order or disturbance in organizing tasks over time, i.e., particular ego functions. Irregularities in the size of the several figures connote some degree of irregularity in expending energy or in adapting in an orderly fashion to requirements. These are but a few of the hypotheses which are generated. The placement of the first figure of the test (figure A) provides some special sets of hypotheses: the subject's orientation vis-à-vis the world, the degree of paranoid attitude which may be present, etc.

These and other features of the subject's style lead to many hypotheses, some of which may be contradictory and some of which may be supplementary. The clinician's task is to attempt to reconcile these, to modify them, and to integrate them in the light of all of the evidence from the test, and, later, in actual clinical work, with other sources of evidence. It cannot be overemphasized that the hypotheses

345

THE HUTT
ADAPTATION OF THE
BENDER-GESTALT
TEST: DIAGNOSTIC
AND THERAPEUTIC
IMPLICATIONS

are only hypotheses—not conclusions—and that the clinician must be able to entertain as many hypotheses as possible, discarding none, even if some appear to be based on apparently flimsy evidence, until there is confirming or contradictory evidence. It should also be noted that the hypotheses are not "wild analysis," but are based on clinical and research evidence which I have culled over many years and presented in my volume (Hutt, 1977).

Following the analysis of general stylistic features of the record, one then proceeds, step by step, with the subject as he has progressed through the several test cards. Each drawing is examined in turn as the clinician attempts both objectively and subjectively to empathize with the subject's performance. From the objective perspective, one notes the distortions or modifications which the subject has performed on each figure. These features, which may be subsumed under several major headings, are organizational factors, changes in the gestalt, distortions of the gestalt, direction of movement, and quality of line drawing. Thus when the subject places his successive drawings so that they "hug" the margin of the page, one may infer some type of insecurity; if "hugging" is severe, one may suspect extreme anxiety. As another example, if severe perceptual rotation occurs (as defined in the text) one may infer oppositional qualities, organic brain dysfunction, perceptual immaturity, and the like. As still another example, difficulty with curved-line drawings suggests difficulty in handling affect: reduced curvature connotes flattened affect, and excessive curvature connotes heightened affect.

I noted that one tries to empathize with the subject as he progresses through the test. The progressive adaptation of the subject tells the clinician more than the simple notation of "errors" made on each drawing. Does he, for example, meet difficulty for the first time when he has to deal with a more difficult test design (evidence of perceptual immaturity)? Does he show disturbance on "open figures" (need for structure)? Does he have problems with phallic symbols? Does he have difficulty with overlapping designs (organic insult)? This type of analysis offers important leads to confirming, rejecting, or integrating the separate hypotheses formulated and based on the test factors alluded to above. They reveal how the subject deals, over a time period, with tasks of different kinds.

Thus the Copy Phase data are analyzed inferentially as the clinician works through the test "as if" he were in the subject's place. One utilizes all of the known findings about the significance of one's test factors (and others) as one develops and modifies one's hypotheses. One further "hones" the hypotheses on the basis of test observations of the subject's behavior, including his spontaneous comments. Finally, one has a set of fairly well-defined and revised hypotheses which seem reasonable. But one is not through yet.

Although one's inferential analysis is based primarily on data from the Copy Phase, it is checked and modified further in the light of the data from the Elaboration Phase and the Association Phase. The Elaboration Phase offers confirmatory and additional data. Are stylistic features the same? Do some of the test distortions reappear and, if so, do they occur in the same sequence? Do the subject's associations help to confirm or explain inferences one has derived previously? And are there other assets in the subject's personality which give us a better understanding of his performance?

If one's analysis has been rigorous and complete, it will yield very strong hypotheses and some probable conclusions, based on the rationale which has been employed and on the test factors (with their unique meanings) as the individual has demonstrated them. As with any psychological test, however, a "test is only a test is only a test." It is a sample of behavior only, no matter how adequate. The wise and careful clinician will extend his analysis based on other test findings, the history of the individual, and other pertinent information such as physical and medical findings. One of the special features of the HABGT, however, is that further "within-test" data are available. The HABGT also yields configuration patterns and scores as well as scores on two objective scales. Of special significance, it is relatively simple to test probable hypotheses or to refine them by means of the experimental-clinical method. Let us examine this method next.

7. The Experimental-Clinical Method

There are two questions which the experimental-clinical method is particularly useful for. One is: can the test phenomena be explained by other hypotheses than those which seem most likely in most cases? The second is: what is the precise nature of the problem which is causing the difficulty noted on the test? The first question asks whether some other factor than one the clinician would have assumed to be relevant accounts for the data. For instance, when an individual shows "perseveration" on the test, is this phenomenon attributable to an inability to shift "set"? Although this is likely to be the case in most instances, other factors might account for it. If one suspects that this might be the case, one can conduct an experimental-clinical test to check this out. The perseveration might have been due to the subject's unwillingness to leave that particular task and continue with the next task, i.e., to some form of resistance. It might have been caused by inattentiveness in which the individual, having taken a quick glance at the test card, then projected what he thought he had seen. It might have been due to a misunderstanding of test directions! These or other conditions might have produced the "perseveration." The same is possible for any test factor. (I have not indicated another type of alternate explanation, i.e., malingering. My basic text deals with this special problem at some length.)

The second problem is even more important from the viewpoint of clinical evaluation. Here, one is concerned with the nature of the functions which are interfering with an accurate response. Is the individual's difficulty due to lack of perceptual and/or motoric maturity? Is it due to a lesion in a particular part of the brain? Is it the result of disturbance in some cortical integrative function? Is it a consequence of difficulties with the symbolic meaning of the stimulus for the subject? Is the problem one of dealing with fine coordinations, spatial configurations, open figures, or curved figures? These are the types of problems with which a clinician is especially concerned. The HABGT easily lends itself to exploration and analysis of such issues. Unfortunately, "clinicians" who have been overly impressed with objective scales and with normative data neglect or are unaware of the potential for investigating clinically the precise nature of the problem in the individual case. As I have indicated, scores are based on certain assumptions which are, as often as not, violated in a given clinical case. Hence the clinician must explore experimentally the precise antecedents of the response.

I have suggested elsewhere (Hutt, 1977) some methods that are applicable in pursuing the analysis of the factors which have interfered with or produced a particular test response. In brief, these involve interview analysis, test performance analysis, and card sorting. The first procedure involves interviewing the subject

347

THE HUTT
ADAPTATION OF THE
BENDER-GESTALT
TEST: DIAGNOSTIC
AND THERAPEUTIC
IMPLICATIONS

about the nature of his response: inquiring whether he perceives the error or distortion he has made, what his motivation was for performing in that manner, and what special conditions led him to perform as he did. The second involves varying the stimulus so that the precise factor contributing to the difficulty can be determined: if it is suspected that there is difficulty due to the complexity of the figure, it might involve offering him a simpler figure to copy; if the difficulty is with curved lines or open figures, the subject might be asked to copy similar figures with straight lines or closed figures; if the problem appears to be one of difficulty with spatial configurations (field-ground difficulty such as might be due to parietal lesion), the subject might be offered the separate elements of the figures to be copied; etc. In the third (card-sorting) procedure, the subject might be asked to sort the kinds based on some central issue (i.e., those you like vs. those you dislike; those that are easy vs. those that are difficult; those that disturb you vs. those that are bland; etc.). Such methods as these enable the clinician to help determine, in the individual case, what the nature of the problem is or what cortical dysfunction may be involved.

I cannot emphasize too strongly that, when the clinician employs such an experimental-clinical approach, he is less likely to overlook the idiosyncratic factors that are critical in a given case. The clinician is far more likely to gain a more precise understanding of the nature of the subject's difficulty and begin to learn whether it may be possible to provide some appropriate rehabilitative (therapeutic) correction.

8. Configurational Analysis

Based on, first, clinical findings, and, later, research data, I have developed a number of Configurational Patterns which assist in the process of differential analysis. At the present time, such configurations are available for organic brain damage, schizophrenia, essential psychoneurosis, depression, and mental retardation. Each configuration is based on those test factors, with appropriate weights, which research has demonstrated are applicable to the particular syndrome. The factors are those defined in the Psychopathology scale (see below), but weights are assigned to each factor in terms of its differential strength. For example, in the case of the configuration for organic brain damage (although it is clearly recognized that different types of damage produce different sequelae), the test factors of marked angulation difficulty, severe perceptual rotation, collision, severe fragmentation, perseveration, and overlapping difficulty each receive a weight of 2 points. In the same configuration, the test factors of simplification and line incoordination each receive a weight of 1 point. The Configuration score is simply the total of the weights which apply in a given record.

Critical scores are offered for each syndrome. Research findings indicate that, for adults, the critical scores differentiate neurotics from both organics and schizophrenics at the probability level of $p < .001$, while among organics, schizophrenics, and depressives these scores produce differences significant at the probability level of $p < .01$ (Hutt, 1977). Thus these Configuration scores appear to offer statistically significant differentiation, as indicated, for groups of patients. It is not claimed that such scores are sufficient to yield adequate clinical diagnosis for the individual case. Rather, they are useful for screening purposes and for further clinical investigation. Taken together with other clinical findings, they can be quite useful.

9. The Psychopathology Scale

The Psychopathology scale is based on 17 test factors, each defined in a particular way, and each assigned scores ranging from 1.0 (least degree of psychopathology) to 10.0 (highest degree of psychopathology), with the exception of one test factor on which scores may range from 1.0 to 3.25. The total Psychopathology score is the sum of the separate scores on the 17 test factors.

The psychopathology scale represents an attempt to derive an objective measure, based on nonverbal, perceptual-motoric behavior, of the severity of general psychopathology. It is easily scored (especially with the use of a Scoring Template which is furnished with the Revised Record Form) and has been shown to have a high degree of reliability. Several studies have explored interscorer reliability (Miller & Hutt, 1975; Hutt, 1977; Hutt & Dates, 1977). Interscorer reliabilities have ranged from .90 to .96, indicating considerable objectivity for the method of scoring. Moreover, these same studies have indicated that the three major components of the Psychopathology scale are also highly reliable. Test-retest reliability has also been investigated over both short-term intervals (2 weeks) and longer-term intervals (40 weeks). Typical of these findings have been a test-retest reliability of .87 over a 2-week interval with hospitalized schizophrenic patients (Miller & Hutt, 1975) and a test-retest reliability of .91 for a male adolescent delinquent population over a 40-week interval.

A variety of studies have explored the scale's validity. Deaf retarded individuals were studied (Hutt & Feuerfile, 1963), and the scale was found to be effective in differentiating more severe from less severe pathology in this population. Significant degrees of differentiation were shown in the case of various psychiatric populations and in differentiating organics from nonorganics (Hutt, 1977). The scale was found to be useful in predicting improvement among schizophrenics (Hutt, 1969a). It was shown to have utility in predicting recidivism among delinquents (Hutt, Dates, & Reid, 1978). Some aspects of the scale's construct validity were confirmed in another study (Credidio, 1975).

Since the Psychopathology scale, based entirely on the Copy Phase of the HABGT, is nonverbal, it is particularly useful with subjects from bilingual background and deprived cultural experience. It provides a unique type of measure which other scales of psychopathology do not offer and hence is helpful in many kinds of clinical situations. However, I do not believe that any measure of psychopathology, no matter how sophisticated and valid, is sufficient by itself to provide adequate data for clinical conclusions about an individual. Such conclusions should rest on confirmatory data from several sources, particularly on case history and clinical observational data.

The scale is largely independent of level of intelligence (at least above the 10-year level) and of sex and educational attainment. Normative data are available for children above 10 years of age and for a wide variety of clinical groups at the adult level.

10. The Adience-Abience Scale

The Adience-Abience scale was derived on the bases of clinical hunches and theoretical formulations, and later revised a number of times on the basis of empirical data. It provides a measure of perceptual-motoric approach-avoidance. It is believed that an individual's perceptual style is developed during the formative experiences of infancy and is quickly reinforced during early childhood, although genetic factors cannot be ruled out. Infants who experience a supportive and stimulating early experience tend to develop "adient" perceptual mechanisms, actively seeking out and exploring their immediate environment and learning and adapting more quickly and effectively. They become "open" to new experience. On the other hand, infants whose early experiences are highly inconsistent, or who suffer traumatic or impoverished early experiences, tend to develop "abient" perceptual mechanisms, shunning new experiences and becoming closed off perceptually to them. These early perceptual adaptations become integrated into a general adient or abient perceptual style, and, it is believed, underlie the formation of other primitive mechanisms of defense. Once a perceptual style has been developed, it tends to persist, and is highly resistant to modification. If my theory is correct, those who are perceptually adient should be healthier psychologically, more easily able to adapt and to profit from new experience, and generally more able to learn effectively. As we shall see, there are data which support these theoretical formulations (Hutt, in press).

349

THE HUTT
ADAPTATION OF THE
BENDER-GESTALT
TEST: DIAGNOSTIC
AND THERAPEUTIC
IMPLICATIONS

The revised Adience-Abience scale is based on 12 test factors drawn from the Psychopathology scale but defined differently and scored with different weights. The measure is derived entirely from data obtained in the Copy Phase of the test. Normative findings are available for children and for adults; normative data are available for different psychiatric populations (Hutt, 1977).

A number of reliability studies have been published. In one (Hutt & Miller, 1975), it was found that interscorer reliability on a group of hospitalized schizophrenic patients was $\rho = .912$. In another, with delinquent subjects, Kendall's Coefficient of Concordance for three scorers was about .90. Test-retest reliability has been found to be quite high for both short-term and long-term intervals, ranging from Pearson r's of .84 for schizophrenics to .93 for delinquents (Hutt & Miller, 1975; Hutt & Dates, 1978).

Validity has been investigated in a number of studies. In a population of deaf retardates (Hutt & Feuerfile, 1963), 18 predictions were made, of which 15 reached statistical significance at or above the .01 level. In another study (Hutt, 1969b), it was shown that adults differing in degree of therapeutic change were significantly different in score on Adience-Abience ($p = .01$). It was also found (Hutt, 1969b) that the difference in Adience-Abience scores between schizophrenic patients hospitalized for less than 6 months as compared with patients with comparable diagnoses, ages, and sex distributions who had been hospitalized for 5 years or more was, as predicted, significant at the .01 level. In a much more rigorous study, matched groups of hospitalized schizophrenics ($N = 80$) who differed in our measure of Adience-Abience were significantly different on measures of creativity and memory functions. Adience-Abience scores were shown to be significantly related to measures of recidivism in a delinquent population (Hutt et al., 1978). Credidio (1975) demonstrated that there was evidence for the construct validity of our measure.

Other studies have explored the interrelationship of psychopathology and Adience-Abience (Hutt & Miller, 1976). It has been found that there is relatively little commonality between these measures in less severe cases of psychopathology, but the degree of commonality increases (as predicted) when psychopathology is severe. Adience-Abience has only a moderate to small relationship with field dependence-independence (Kachorek, 1969; McConville, 1970), and with altruism (Meyer, 1973), as predicted. These and other studies have shown that adience-abience is largely independent of other measures of personality, and thus tend to support our theory of the uniqueness of this phenomenon.

Much more research is needed to explore the meaning and predictive power of the measure of adience-abience, and more research is needed to evaluate the process of development of this phenomenon. However, it is believed that the measure is clinically quite useful and that it has considerable potential for research in a variety of clinical and experimental situations.

11. The Clinical Use of the HABGT

My brief presentation of the various aspects of the HABGT as a clinical instrument can only hint at the ways in which a resourceful clinician may utilize this instrument. I have not discussed the many ways in which test administration can be modified to highlight certain kinds of behavior which may be illuminating with respect to various clinical conditions. For instance, if the problem concerns possible cerebral dysfunction, administration can be altered so as to maximize the effects of possible organic insult. Some of these ways include utilization of the recall method (Hutt, 1977; Armstrong, 1965; Rogers & Swenson, 1975), the tachistoscopic method (Snortum, 1965), and the background interference procedure (Pardue, 1975). I have not discussed the many projective hypotheses and findings which may be specifically obtained with the use of the Elaboration and Association procedures (Hutt, 1977), nor have I discussed specific utilization of the test with retarded, depressive, and character types of problems. The interested reader will wish to consult other sources of reference for these and other conditions reported by me and other workers whom I have cited in my book about this method.

There are, however, a number of problems which deserve special comment. One of these concerns the relative merits of utilizing this procedure to evaluate perceptual-motoric maturity vs. evaluation of personality disturbance. Koppitz (1963, 1975) and others prefer to use the test in its former aspect, particularly with young children. I have no quarrel with the use of the test as a measure of perceptual-motoric maturity; it surely deserves a place here. One might note, however, that if this is the objective, there are available a number of more extensive tests which tap a greater variety of aspects of perceptual-motoric maturity. The use of this procedure simply as a test of perceptual-motoric maturity leaves many important questions unanswered. What is causing the perceptual-motoric immaturity: is it organic, developmental, or emotional in character? Can the perceptual-motoric immaturity be modified? If so, under what conditions? Are the perceptual-motoric abnormalities related to traumatic effects of the symbolic meanings of some of the figures? What does perceptual-motoric immaturity mean in terms of specific learning difficulties or in terms of adjustment problems? These are only a few of the questions that remain to plague us once we have determined that there is some disturbance in the perceptual-motoric area. The rich lode of clinical data which the procedure provides is discarded if only a measure of perceptual immaturity is obtained.

I have preferred to utilize this procedure, instead, as a projective device. As such, it can yield data which are not readily available, or even available at all, from other test procedures or from other clinical methods. The counterbalancing of data derived from the Copy Phase, the Elaboration Phase, and the Association Phase not only provides a rich source of significant clinical material but also offers many

351

THE HUTT
ADAPTATION OF THE
BENDER-GESTALT
TEST: DIAGNOSTIC
AND THERAPEUTIC
IMPLICATIONS

opportunities of checking out hypotheses about the patient and of exploring leads for therapeutic and other rehabilitative procedures. If, in addition, one utilizes the three objective measures (Configuration scores, Psychopathology scale scores, and Adience-Abience scores), one can "verify" probable conclusions about degree of psychopathology, sources of conflict, and stratagems of defense. It is unfortunate, in my opinion, that we have become "so addicted to our scores" in this country that we have invested them with validity far beyond their limits. A score is only a beginning in clinical work; it tells us only how the individual compares on this test with others, and assumes that, if we are to take this comparison seriously, conditions for the testee and the normative populations are not significantly different. Even when these assumptions are reasonable, the score is only an indication of present status. It does not tell us how the score was achieved, how it might be modified, and even whether or not to take it seriously. One might say that, at best, a score is an "indicator," but never a clinical finding!

The clinical and projective use of the HABGT, on the other hand, can tell us much we need to know in evaluating the patient's condition and in proposing certain remedies for it. For example, suppose we are dealing with a 12-year-old youngster who is retarded in his school work, and has, as we now phrase it, a "learning disability." On the WISC, he obtains an IQ score of 86, confirming the indication that he is below average in intellectual ability. Now he is given the Bender-Gestalt Test and obtains a perceptual-motoric score of 8 years. We thus have confirmation that, in the perceptual-motoric area, he shows some degree of retardation. But now we examine the test protocol (as administered on the HABGT) to evaluate projective and other objective features. We find that he performs the more difficult figures (say, figures 7 and 8) quite well, suggesting that on these figures he attains a perceptual-motoric level commensurate with his age, but he does poorly on figures A (about 7-year level) and 4 (about 8-year level). This inconsistency in his pattern of performance on the Copy Phase of the test suggests that something is interfering with his performance on the test (and in school as well as in life). We now examine the Elaboration Phase and Association Phase of the test and learn that he is "blocked" on figures with curves and that these figures have strong sexual meanings for him. We learn further that he "sees" women as authoritarian, castrating, and otherwise forbidding. Further study of the record reveals that he likes men, gets along comfortably with them, but still shows a low aspiration level. An examination of his Configuration scores suggests that he falls within the neurotic category, and his Psychopathology scale score confirms this finding. However, his Adience-Abience score is 28 (well above the norms for his age and far beyond that of "disturbed" children).

Although I have only suggested some of the most superficial aspects of HABGT analysis and I have not presented any findings from a possible inferential analysis of the test data, we already have considerable evidence that, although one might still wish to "categorize" this boy as having a "learning disability" (I would not), there is far more than first meets the eye. He is not, in the usual sense, perceptually immature; rather, he is "disturbed" (i.e., he can do well on difficult perceptual tasks when these do not trigger aberrant emotional reactions). One would guess that he is not unintelligent. His Adience-Abience score suggests that he can profit considerably from some form of learning (especially therapeutic learning). His Psychopathology score indicates that he is not, apparently, psychotic or organically brain damaged, but is rather "neurotic." The content of his associations and his elaborations suggests important leads to his school difficulties (and to possible difficulties with women—female teachers?).

Thus an internal and projective analysis of the test performance, with full utilization of the possible meanings of each of the test factors, with evaluation of the objective findings from the several objective scales, and with additional data from the social history and from other tests, can provide a highly meaningful clinical evaluation, and can suggest leads that might be very useful in any program developed to assist this boy. And, after all, if clinical evaluation does not lead to appropriate remedial measures or to appropriate administrative decisions, what function does it really serve?

The many ways in which HABGT records can be evaluated clinically are illustrated in other works (Hutt & Gibby, 1970; Hutt, 1977). Other test procedures can, of course, serve similar functions. However, the HABGT has certain unique characteristics which make it particularly useful in many clinical situations.

12. References

Armstrong, R. G. A re-evaluation of copied and recall Bender-Gestalt reproductions. *Journal of Projective Techniques and Personality Assessment*, 1965, *29*, 134–139.

Beck, S. J. Reality, Rorschach, and perceptual theory. In A. I. Rabin (Ed.), *Projective techniques in personality assessment*. New York: Springer, 1968.

Credidio, S. G. A construct validity study of a measure of perceptual approach-avoidance. Unpublished doctoral dissertation, University of Detroit, 1975.

Crenshaw, D., Bohn, S., Hoffman, M., Matheus, J., & Offenbach, S. The use of projective methods in research. *Journal of Projective Techniques and Personality Assessment*, 1968, *32*, 3–9.

Hutt, M. L. The Bender-Gestalt Test: The case of Gregor. Interpretation of test data. *Rorschach Research Exchange and Journal of Projective Techniques*, 1949, *13*, 443–446.

Hutt, M. L. The Bender-Gestalt drawings. In E. S. Shneidman, W. Joel, & K. B. Little (Eds.), *Thematic test analysis*. New York: Grune & Stratton, 1951.

Hutt, M. L. The Bender-Gestalt Test. In D. Rosenthal (Ed.), *The Genain quadruplets: A study of heredity and environment in schizophrenia*. New York: Basic Books, 1963.

Hutt, M. L. *The Hutt Adaptation of the Bender-Gestalt Test* (2nd ed.). New York: Grune & Stratton, 1969. (a)

Hutt, M. L. The potentiality of a measure of perceptual adience-abience in predicting inner psychological adaptability. Paper presented at American Psychological Association, Annual Meeting, Washington, D.C., September 1969. (b)

Hutt, M. L. *The Hutt Adaptation of the Bender-Gestalt Test* (3rd ed.). New York: Grune & Stratton, 1977.

Hutt, M. L. Adience-Abience. In R. H. Woody (Ed.), *Encyclopedia of Clinical Assessment*. San Francisco: Jossey-Bass, in press.

Hutt, M. L., & Dates, B. Reliabilities and interrelationships of two of the HABGT scales in a male delinquent population. *Journal of Personality Assessment*, 1977, *41*, 353–357.

Hutt, M. L., Dates, B., & Reid, D. M. The predictive ability of HABGT scales for a male delinquent population. *Journal of Personality Assessment*, 1977, *41*, 492–496.

Hutt, M. L., & Feuerfile, D. The clinical meanings and predictions of a measure of perceptual adience-abience. Paper presented at American Psychological Association, Annual Meeting, Philadelphia, September 1963.

Hutt, M. L., & Gibby, R. G. *Patterns of abnormal behavior*. Boston: Allyn & Bacon, 1957.

Hutt, M. L., & Gibby, R. G. An atlas for the Hutt adaptation of the Bender-Gestalt Test. New York: Grune & Stratton, 1970.

Hutt, M. L., & Miller, L. J. Further studies of a measure of adience-abience. *Journal of Personality Assessment*, 1975, *39*, 123–128.

Hutt, M. L., & Miller, L. J. Interrelationships of psychopathology and adience-abience. *Journal of Personality Assessment*, 1976, *40*, 135–139.

Kachorek, J. Relationships between measures of adience-abience and field independence-dependence. Unpublished master's thesis, University of Detroit, 1969.

Koppitz, E. M. *The Bender-Gestalt Test for Young Children*. New York: Grune & Stratton, 1963.

353

THE HUTT
ADAPTATION OF THE
BENDER-GESTALT
TEST: DIAGNOSTIC
AND THERAPEUTIC
IMPLICATIONS

Koppitz, E. M. *The Bender-Gestalt Test for Young Children. Volume II: Research and applications, 1963–1973.* New York: Grune & Stratton, 1975.

Lerner, E. A. *The projective use of the Bender-Gestalt Test.* Springfield, Ill.: Thomas, 1972.

Lubin, A. M. Bender-Gestalt Test and background interference procedure in discernment of brain damage. *Perceptual and Motor Skills,* 1975, *40,* 103–109.

Lubin, B., Wallis, R. R., & Paine, C. Patterns of psychological test usage in the United States: 1935–1969. *Professional Psychology,* 1971, *2,* 70–74.

McConville, M. G. Perceptual adience-abience and social field-dependence: An attempt at construct validation. Unpublished master's thesis, University of Windsor, 1970.

Meyer, R. Altruism among male juvenile delinquents related to offense committed and parents' cultural status. Unpublished doctoral dissertation, University of Detroit, 1973.

Miller, L. J., & Hutt, M. L. Psychopathology scale of the Hutt Adaptation of the Bender-Gestalt Test: Reliability. *Journal of Personality Assessment,* 1975, *2,* 129–131.

Pardue, A. M. Bender-Gestalt test and background interference procedure in discernment of organic brain damage. *Perceptual and Motor Skills,* 1975, *40,* 103–109.

Rogers, D. L., & Swenson, W. M. Bender-Gestalt recall as a measure of memory versus distractibility. *Perceptual and Motor Skills,* 1975, *40,* 919–922.

Schulberg, H. C., & Tolor, A. The use of the Bender-Gestalt Test in clinical practice. *Journal of Projective Techniques,* 1961, *25,* 347–351.

Snortum, J. R. Performance of different diagnostic groups in the tachistoscopic and copy phases of the Bender-Gestalt. *Journal of Consulting Psychology,* 1965, *4,* 345–351.

Sundberg, N. D. The practice of psychological testing in clinical services in the United States. *American Psychologist,* 1961, *16,* 79–83.

Wertheimer, M. Studies in the theory of Gestalt psychology. *Psychologische Forschung,* 1923, *4,* 301–350.

12

Clinical Contributions of the Wechsler Adult Intelligence Scale

JOEL ALLISON

1. Ego Psychology

The emergence of a psychoanalytic ego psychology secured a firm place in clinical diagnosis for the Wechsler Scales and solidified the substantial efforts already begun in exploring the nonintellective aspects of intelligence. The Wechsler Scales were well suited to the ego-psychological program to provide an integrated theory of personality organization that would include normal as well as abnormal activity, that would include not only the expression of wishes and fears associated with varying psychosexual levels but also the individual's various skills, aptitudes, and achievements and his processes of perceiving, conceptualizing, remembering, and judging. If the major task of projective testing until then was to probe into the lower depths of personality, into highly personalized fantasies and imagery, the task now also included the more "surface" aspects of personality, and aimed to provide a "general psychology." Various assets or functions which until then had been exclusively the province of a cognitive psychology of normal persons now became of increased interest and were systematized into a broad theory. And, in particular, it was the development of ego psychology that supplied the basis for this broad theory, beginning with Hartmann's conceptualization of structures of primary or secondary autonomy, structures, that is, which either are relatively free of drives and conflicts from the outset or develop that way over time (Hartmann, 1958).

In large measure, this development meant an extension of the projective hypothesis that all acts of the individual are reflections or expressions of his unique personality. Interest was no longer focused exclusively on the deeper motivations and on the inner world but also on aspects of style that were organized into particular patterns. If the motto of the previous focus was access to the unconscious, the newer orientation had as its motto *"Le style, c'est l'homme."*

JOEL ALLISON • Department of Psychology, Yale University, New Haven, Connecticut 06520

In terms of diagnosis, the newer orientation reflected a shift toward emphasizing thought organization as the most basic and reliable foundation for clinical assessment. While clinical manifestations, symptoms in particular, might or might not be present or might have different meanings in different contexts, style of thinking was held to remain invariant. Hysterical organization, for example, was not solely characterized by a particular content related to the Oedipal phase of development but also involved specific ways of perceiving, remembering, judging, and conceptualizing. Even in the absence of dynamic content, one could observe the imprint of characteristic modes of experience and cognition, and patterns of thinking could be detected prior to the development of overt symptomatology, a fact which led to the formulation of such concepts as borderline, incipient, or latent psychosis. The intelligence test, rather than being viewed as a catalogue of relatively independent, specific traits or abilities, now could be seen as reflecting meaningful clusters or configurations of personality organization. For certain abilities were likely to receive relative emphasis or deemphasis over the course of development, and their patterning would reveal various ways of coping and/or defense. Moreover, it appeared possible that coping and defense developed from a common matrix and that intelligence and personality were intertwined if not inseparable aspects of a unified phenomenon.

From the standpoint of ego psychology, the Wechsler Scales served new and various purposes. The expanded interest in thought processes and the extensions of the projective hypothesis led to an interest in situations which deemphasized elaboration of personal concerns and instead emphasized more detached functioning (the "highly differentiated quasi-stable ego contents and functions") (Mayman, Schafer, & Rapaport, 1951). In terms of a battery of tests, the WAIS yielded greater access to functioning in a type of everyday situation where conventional logic is highlighted, where one is expected to be relatively impersonal and detached, to restrict personalization, fantasy, imagery, and dynamic content, and where routine, habituated, often overlearned responses are appropriate.

Analysis of the scatter or patterning of the various abilities (tapped by the different subtests) was the method which yielded reliable clusters of relationships associated with specific diagnostic categories. Diagnosis was also facilitated by analysis of the person's manner of coping with problems, by study of the sequences of passes and failures, by the degree of disruption of an ability, and by the specific personalized content involved in the disruptions. An additional advantage that accrued from application of a unified theory to testing was the possibility of internal cross-validation. Since certain patterns were expected to be accompanied by specific content or by specific approaches to task solution, one could validate hypotheses by the degree to which divergent test findings converged in a particular direction. For example, a hypothesis of hysterical defense based on a test scatter that reflected overdevelopment of conventionality (high Comprehension) in contrast to a more meager development of a fund of discrete knowledge (low Information) would receive additional support by the appearance of indications of naiveté, avoidance of active ideational efforts, difficulty with items concerning marriage and sexuality, repressive signs of global, impressionistic thinking such as a failure to know the names of recognized missing items (on Picture Completion), the reliance on childlike cute language, and any additional suggestions of content oriented toward Oedipal dynamics. Moreover, one could look for internal consistencies not only within the WAIS but also across the battery of tests. Inasmuch as a freer encouragement of fantasy occurs

357

CLINICAL
CONTRIBUTIONS OF
THE WECHSLER
ADULT
INTELLIGENCE
SCALE

on the other tests (TAT and Rorschach), even minor personalizations on the WAIS could be seen as harbingers of what would appear in bolder relief in other situations. As in clinical work generally, the possibility of cross-validation, the establishment of patterns with common factors, is what makes interpretation possible at all.

Despite the mostly salubrious influence of ego psychology in relation to testing, one negative consequence of its application to the Wechsler Scales has been a tendency to exaggerate the significance of "purely reality-oriented thought processes" (Waite, 1961) and to take as the model of ideal intelligence the "clean" intelligence test (Shapiro, 1954) that is free of so-called interfering regressive trends. It was recognized that while correct responses are fixed the routes to them can be variable; it was also acknowledged that some aspects of the test provide a range of more or less possible responses and vary in their latitude for unique but task-appropriate and successful response. And Schafer advised that "any test response has both a past achievement aspect and a current creative aspect." Nonetheless, the literature on intelligence testing from the viewpoint of ego psychology has tended to emphasize as an ideal the perfect uncontaminated test, free of idiosyncratic preoccupations and defensive orientations. This emphasis can be seen as a direct extension of the ego-psychological emphasis on functions that possess primary or secondary autonomy from the drives and conflict. Cumbersome concepts such as regression in the service of the ego seemed a way of smuggling in and making acceptable experiences that appeared at variance with a purified but essentially sterile ego. The Wechsler Scales were regarded as measures of various ego skills or functions somehow expected to operate in their ideal form in the absence of drives—free of manifestations of a seemingly disruptive id.

One recent attempt (Blatt and Allison, 1968) to challenge the model of the "clean," impersonal intelligence test pointed out the essential banality and constriction of the well-intact intelligence test. On the basis of Rapaport's (1951, 1958) discussion of autonomy, it was argued that the intelligence test does in fact clarify the degree of autonomy from drives as a consequence of its emphasis on habituated, logical thinking. But it was also suggested that the solely perfect intelligence test protocol might at the same time reflect a disturbed sense of autonomy from the environment. Accordingly, manifestations of drives whether in personalization of response or in unique strategies would, in effect, protect the person from a slavish adaptation to the environment. In this manner of discussion, it appeared possible to stick to a basically ego-psychological approach and simultaneously to rescue individuals from an idealized goal that loomed as overly detached and machinelike perfect. Clinicians, of course, in their daily work recognized that high-level efficiency could be primarily defensive while leading to elevated IQ scores. Clinical improvement sometimes meant the lowering of IQ scores. The previously hyperalert person whose concentration was now more relaxed and less anxiously vigilant failed to reach as great heights of success on items which rewarded vigilance. Hence theory and clinical practice seemed out of joint.

Gradually, it has become clear that the theoretical orientation to psychological testing based exclusively on the ego-psychology proposed by Hartmann, Rapaport, and others may have overextended its usefulness and is in need of revision or replacement. Although the recent theoretical criticisms and revisions have not been directed at psychological testing per se but rather apply to the theory in general, they have major implications for our views of clinical testing.

Apfelbaum (1966), for example, has supplied a critique of the very structural theory that provided the framework for conceptualizing the clinical role of the Wechsler Scales. In particular, Apfelbaum has suggested that recent ego-psychological theory has relied on an early notion of drives prior to Freud's later emphasis on the mutual regulation between the ego and id. This early notion of drives implies a basic antagonism between ego and id, between the forces of control and inhibition and the essentially infantile, undeveloped, maladaptive urges. In this view, only the ego develops, and the id is identified with primitive content and modes of ideation and affect. One consequence of this view is the concept of regression in the service of the ego by which a controlling ego allows itself access to alien processes and content as a respite from reality. Such a concept is far removed in its language from the acknowledgment of a fully unified psychological activity (Schachtel, 1966). Invariably, in ego-psychological discussions, id phenomena seem disruptive, undeveloped forces which, on special occasions, are granted a temporary and restricted emergence. An illustrative example occurs in Blanck and Blanck's (1974) discussion of Hartmann's theoretical understanding of reciprocal relationships. They cite the example of an adult woman's relationship with her infant and state that it is not sufficient for the woman to have reached "psychological adulthood" in order to relate to her infant. She must also possess "a capacity for partial and temporary regression in order to become a partner in the mother-infant dyad. *Temporarily abandoning her higher forms of development*, mother and infant fit together, serving both the maternal requirements and the infant's needs" (Blanck and Blanck, p. 31). It is clear from this example that the language used to describe the mother's psychological contributions implies a model that elevates in importance the more detached, "higher forms of development," presumably those levels that are uncontaminated by more dynamic relatedness. Considerations such as these led Apfelbaum to conclude that current ego theory caricatures obsessive-compulsive neurosis with its emphasis on "control over the outer world, its concept of objectivity as detachment from drive, and its interest in issues of autonomy." In this regard, Shapiro's use of the word "clean" to describe Wechslers that are free of personalization may reflect a similar obsessively phrased view of efficient detached functioning as clean in contrast to what is instead messy or dirty. Apfelbaum continues to argue that, if one takes any ego function, one can show how there is structural development of the id as well, that only repressed drives remain infantile, that there is little ego functioning without connections with id processes. Hartmann's discussion of synthesis as a pure ego function is cited, and an alternative view of synthesis as partaking of the id aim of unity is offered by Apfelbaum. In another context, Schafer (1968) has also highlighted the intertwining of ego and id processes in his discussion of defense mechanisms. He reminds us that Freud also took a dynamic approach to defense mechanisms in his discussion of the defenses of isolation and undoing by suggesting that obsessional isolation is a dynamic psychic means of not touching for fear of associated aggressive and sexual meanings.

Apfelbaum's solution is to reemphasize the concept of the ego as "an aim-organization in dynamic equilibrium." More recent criticisms of psychoanalytic metapsychology, however, have advocated a more thoroughgoing revision of psychoanalytic theory in an attempt to narrow the gap between the clinical situation and the metapsychological theory used to describe and explain clinical phenomena. In particular, the aim is to omit from theory its mechanistic aspects, to alter an approach in which "reasons become forces, emphases become energies, activity becomes functions, meaningful thoughts become representations, affects become dis-

359

CLINICAL
CONTRIBUTIONS OF
THE WECHSLER
ADULT
INTELLIGENCE
SCALE

charges or signals, deeds become resultants, and particular ways of struggling with inevitable diversity of intentions, feelings and situations become structures, mechanisms and adaptations" (Schafer, 1973). Schafer has endeavored to place the "sentient, self-determining, choice-making, responsible, active human being" at the center of his theory, to move toward a more phenomenological and intentionalistic outlook, to exclude the view of people "as organisms or apparatus with functions," and yet to retain the basic clinical methods and findings of psychoanalysis (such as the significant role of unconscious infantile sexuality and aggression). The concept of action is forefront in Schafer's view, and he has begun to clarify the application of his model to various clinical phenomena and to rewrite basic psychoanalytic concepts.

Another attempt to rebuild psychoanalytic theory anew without relying on its prior metapsychological foundation was in progress until it was stopped short by George Klein's death in 1971. Klein listed three guidelines in his revision of psychoanalytic theory: "First, an effort to point to the concepts that are constructed from the patient's standpoint; second, an emphasis on phenomenological experience; and third, an emphasis on the dynamic principles that account for this experience in terms of motive and aim" (Klein, 1976, p. 5). Although his ground rules overlapped with Schafer's, Klein's theoretical reconstruction pointed in different directions and showed promise of embracing broader psychological phenomena than Schafer's philosophically derived revision.

The increasing dissatisfaction with the theoretical model that played such a major part in conceptualizing the role of the Wechsler Scales in clinical assessment demands a reconsideration of our view of these scales in assessment. From the point of view of Schafer's and Klein's suggested revisions, it is clear that the various subtests of the Wechsler would have to be described as assessing certain activities in which people engage and that the language used to describe such activity would refer to the person's emphases, intentions, actions, thoughts, and feelings. Description would have to be devoid of mechanistic terms such as "energies," "mechanisms," and " structures." In effect, we would be shifting to a point of view which has probably always characterized good clinical work in the sense of defining what is unique about each person, how he experiences himself, his life, others around him, how he relates to various situations, what is more or less important, pleasurable, or desirable to him, and how he is an active agent in his own life. Moreover, it would still be possible to try to categorize people in various ways in terms of shared, preferred modalities of experience, shared emphases, and the like. What would be crucial would be the consistent emphasis on meanings and on the view of persons as active agents. One could still talk of styles of experience in the way Shapiro (1965) has presented them, i.e., "ways of thinking and perceiving, ways of experiencing emotion, modes of subjective experience in general, and modes of activity that are associated with various pathologies," without subscribing to an ego-psychological understanding of the meaning or origins of these styles. Shapiro (1970) more recently has in fact also emphasized the central role of volition in human activity and has described the role of assessment procedures in clarifying the "characteristic kinds of volitional experience" and "modes of action" of the individual.

2. The Test

The WAIS is presented in the test battery as the test involving the most structure in order to clarify the characteristics of the person's responses in relatively routine, often overlearned, habituated, detached situations. It bears emphasis that structure is both a function of the instructions of a task and a function of the attitude of the person in approaching the task. The WAIS asks for detailed facts, conventionally held judgments, specified manipulations of material. Meanings and definitions are requested, not associations, not what could be, but what is, not an imaginative account, but a faithful reproduction. From Schachtel's (1966) perspective, the development of a geometric-technical, detached outlook of the kind tapped by the Wechsler Scales may be relatively unalive, narrow, and specialized, but may be relevant at certain times and in certain tasks. Similarly, a capacity for a more dynamic outlook, while permitting a "fuller, closer and deeper relatedness between perceiver and percept," may not be sufficient or relevant in all situations. Schachtel concludes that "the insufficient development of either leaves man impoverished in his relatedness to the world." Flexibility of orientation, the capacity to respond (adapt) to diverse situations, to be able to shift one's intentions and alter them according to different situational requirements, may reflect an important value of our society and may also constitute an underlying dimension of mental health in any culture (Boyer, 1964). In large measure, the capacity to shift successfully among different modes of experience is assessed by studying results across a battery of tests, each of which tends to highlight a particular mode. As was indicated earlier, however, even within a specific situation like the WAIS, there are variations in task expectations, in the degree of habituation or novelty, in the degree of latitude of possibilities of response, strategy, or personalization, that are not associated with inefficient performance. The person who reveals little or nothing of himself, moreover, may obtain his superior efficiency at the price of constriction, inhibition of personal expression, and affective inaccessibility.

For clinical purposes, the administration of the WAIS follows the general instructions set down in the manual, with some modifications intended to clarify diagnostic issues. It is recommended that one obtain a verbatim account of the subject's responses and of his various strategies of approach for which an alternate lengthier recording form is often necessary. It is essential, moreover, that all ambiguities of communication be questioned, cryptic comments understood, personalization attended to, particular approaches clarified. Especially in the instance of early or incipient psychosis, what might look unusual and relatively minor may be too easily passed over. For beginning testers in particular and as a principle in careful clinical inquiry generally, the usual tendency to cover over ambiguities, to normalize them and fail to take note of their essential idiosyncracy, must be rigorously resisted. [This tendency may reflect the wish to unite and merge with others in order to counter the anxieties of recognizing and acknowledging one's essential difference and separation from others (Tarachow, 1963).] An added benefit for the clinician of training in psychological testing is that it gives the student a unique opportunity to study the complexities of communication at close hand. In terms of administration of the tests, it is also recommended that the tester give graded help and devise ways of encouraging reluctant people to stick to the task and try to improve their performance. Through such methods one learns ways of working with a person and the conditions under which his efficiency or relatedness is disrupted or can be maximized. Clearly, such information will have a direct carryover to educators, therapists, or others who will be working with the individual.

Only two specific alterations to the test procedure are advocated. One involves

361

CLINICAL
CONTRIBUTIONS OF
THE WECHSLER
ADULT
INTELLIGENCE
SCALE

asking subjects to explain their incorrect Picture Arrangement stories and routinely to explain the basis for their sequences on the last two items even if they are correct. For seemingly efficient performance on this task often veils idiosyncratic understanding. While the bulk of our inquiries tend to concern what is unusual, inquiry into the logic and methodology of every response would convert testing into an unduly arduous procedure. Yet the finding that correctly arranged sequences on Picture Arrangement may sometimes occur on the basis of idiosyncratic or illogical reasoning reminds us of the degree to which everyday conventionality frequently ignores the understanding of underlying process in favor of focusing on final results. A compelling example of this finding appears in Wechsler's account of a schizophrenic person who correctly asserted that it is 3220 miles from New York to Paris and who explained his answer as follows: "Well, it takes about a week to get from Paris to New York. There are seven days in a week and twenty-four hours in a day; so multiply 24 by 7 and you get 161 which equals the hours in seven days or one week. Now there are 20 blocks in a mile; so multiply 161 by 20 and this gives you 3220. The distance from Paris to New York is 3220 miles" (Wechsler, 1944, p. 167).

An additional test alteration involves the inclusion of a test of memory for meaningful content. With this end in mind, it has been customary to use the following short passage from the Babcock Test.

> Dec. 6/ Last week/ a river/ overflowed/ in a small town/ 10 miles/ from Albany./ Water covered the streets/ and entered the houses./ Fourteen persons/ were drowned/ and 600 persons/ caught cold/ because of the dampness/ and cold weather./ In saving/ a boy/ who was caught/ under a bridge/ a man/ cut his hands./

This passage is presented following Similarities with the instructions: "I am going to read you a short passage. Listen carefully. After I am finished I am going to ask you to repeat as much of it as you can from memory." Following the subject's recall, he is told, "I am going to ask you to repeat this passage later so I am going to reread it now to refresh your memory." Subsequent to the rereading, the subject is presented with Digit Span, Digit Symbol, and Picture Completion (an interval of approximately 10 min). He is then asked to repeat the passage. Each element is scored 1 point. Because the delayed recall comes after two presentations of the story, the immediate recall is given a bonus of 4 points to make it equivalent with the delayed or second recall. The total score should fall several points above the Vocabulary scaled score. Scores below Vocabulary must be evaluated in terms of memory disturbance.

In questions of organic brain pathology, where assessment of memory is uniquely important, one would ordinarily want to include supplementary memory measures such as the Wechsler Memory Scale in the test battery. As a rough screening measure, however, where organicity has not been anticipated on the basis of current clinical information, the inclusion of this brief memory test can serve critical assessment purposes. Because of the violent content of the passage, which could in itself be disruptive to some persons on a psychological rather than organic basis, it would seem desirable to include a passage for memory which is more neutral in content. While Talland's (1965) study of Korsakoff syndrome patients shows no differences in memory ability associated with variations in content, his findings may be restricted to the case of organic pathology and its ubiquitous impairment of memory efficiency. The possibility exists that memory efficiency in nonorganic groups like schizophrenics may be more selectively variable in terms of differences in content. Disruptive performance on this task therefore cannot be taken as an unambiguous indication of organic pathology.

3. Diagnostic Usefulness

In order to illustrate the diagnostic usefulness of the Wechsler Scales, examples of WAIS protocols of different diagnostic classifications will be presented. Diagnosis in itself, of course, cannot be the sole aim of extensive individual testing when rough screening methods which are shorter, self-administered, easily scorable, and easily interpretable are available. More extensive testing is in order when interest is in a more careful description of an individual's significant emphases, thoughts, and affects and in the unique ways in which this particular person struggles "with inevitable diversity of intentions, feelings and situations" (Schafer, 1973, p. 161). Diagnostic labels are a summation of various styles and contents which cluster together into a meaningful pattern, and diagnostic testing has as its primary aim the description of the styles and patterns. The further the inferential distance from phenomenological data, the greater is the likelihood of disagreement. Whereas a final diagnostic label may be in dispute, a precise description will be more likely accurately to reflect the person's psychological position. Ideally, therefore, test interpretations should start with careful description of styles and contents and then proceed to diagnosis. In this way, if there are disagreements in diagnosis between clinicians, at least the basis of the evidence will be clear. For example, there is considerable current controversy surrounding the diagnosis of borderline schizophrenia. Some see the borderline condition as a specific entity characterized by particular features and by a relatively stable character organization. Others, however, take some sort of core schizophrenic experience to be the crucial diagnostic criterion and argue that, in the context of such core experience (whether of a sense of unreality, inner emptiness and deadness, and/or boundary instability), the preferred diagnosis is schizophrenia. One must in effect choose whether one prefers a diagnostic clarification in which a person can be viewed as "somewhat" or borderline schizophrenic or whether with schizophrenia, as with pregnancy, you either have it or you don't. Whichever side one takes in this diagnostic controversy, it is possible nonetheless to provide a detailed description of the person's ways of coping with varied experiences, situations, feelings, and thoughts.

Experiences with testing have shown that certain test content, approaches, or scores can be associated with particular diagnostic categories. Inasmuch as the focus of this book is diagnosis, the approach of this chapter will be to review specific test expectations of various diagnostic categories. For this task, it will be necessary to clarify the diagnostic criteria which provide the bases for the specific signs.

No attempt will be made either to be exhaustive in covering all diagnostic categories or to restate the underlying rationales of the individual subtests. The reader is referred to Rapaport, Gill and Schafer (1945, 1946), Schafer (1948, 1954), Mayman et al. (1951), Waite (1961), Allison, Blatt, and Zimet (1967), and Blatt and Allison (1968). Rather, particular WAIS protocols will be presented in detail in order to demonstrate the process of clinical interpretation. Moreover, certain of the WAIS protocols have been chosen in which scores, content, and style of response appear inconsistent in order to demonstrate how such seeming discrepancy can be integrated

363

CLINICAL
CONTRIBUTIONS OF
THE WECHSLER
ADULT
INTELLIGENCE
SCALE

into a unified clinical picture. What appears on the surface as inconsistency will be viewed instead as an instance of clinical complexity.

3.1. Hysterical Personality Organization

The definition of hysterical personality in the *Diagnostic and Statistical Manual of Mental Disorders* (1968) is as follows: "These behavior patterns are characterized by excitability, emotional instability, over-reactivity, and self-dramatization. This self-dramatization is always attention-seeking and often seductive, whether or not the patient is aware of its purpose. These personalities are also immature, self-centered, often vain, and usually dependent on others" (p. 43). By contrast, the more psychoanalytic approach has attempted to supply a theoretical rationale and constructs that account for these various personality characteristics. From the perspective of psychoanalytic ego psychology, the essential feature of hysterical organization is the reliance on the defense of repression as a generalized strategy in dealing with thoughts, feelings, and situations. The defensive emphasis on being unaware carries with it associated personality characteristics which give hysterics "the appearance of grown-ups with the egos of children" (Schafer, 1954). (One hysteric person, for example, referred to the missing tuning key of the violin on Picture Completion as "the tuning goody.") From an alternate view, the various characteristics of hysterical cognition are the consequences of an essentially impressionistic style which is "global, relatively diffuse and lacking in sharpness, especially in sharp detail" (Shapiro, 1965, p. 111). This style sets the stage for but is not equivalent to the defense of repression from which Schafer deduced the various characteristics of hysterical personality. Yet both Shapiro and Schafer are in essential agreement as to the nature of the hysterical characteristics. These include labile, relatively diffuse emotional experience, impulsive action, unreflectiveness, naiveté, and avoidance of intellectual curiosity and active thinking. The basis for organizing these various characteristics as a style (or generalized defense) is their occurrence in neutral as well as in emotionally charged areas. As a consequence of a diffuse impressionistic style, these features of hysterical thinking are highlighted by Shapiro: "The relative absence of active concentration, the susceptibility to transient, impressive influences and the relatively nonfactual subjective world" (p. 116). The subjective world of the hysteric is further described by Shapiro as being "romantic and sentimental," lacking in detail, and instead impressionistically occupied with "nostalgic and idealized recollection of past figures and places and to a sentimental view of the present" (p. 118). Schafer, on the other hand, is likely to view such nostalgic idealization and sentimentalizing of the past as the gratification aspect of repressive defense insofar as it may permit a continuation of infantile, Oedipal gratifications. From the point of view of emotional experience, Shapiro also sees the predominance in hysterics of response to "the vivid, the colorful, the emotionally charged, and the emotionally provocative" (p. 119). One consequence of their impressionistic style of response is to feel "struck" by things rather than to seek out specific facts. The labile affect, the emotional storms that subside quickly without being experienced as being fully participated in, also follows from a style that is "impressionistic, relatively immediate, and global."

In terms of specific test indications, one would look for manifestations of these various characteristics in the scores, in the manner of approach, in the content of response, and in the relationship to the tester. The various test expectations can best be explicated by turning to an actual test protocol.

Patient is a 23-year-old single white woman, a graduate of a 2-year junior college who is in outpatient psychotherapy. The referring therapist is concerned with diagnosis, treatment, and her fragility, especially with whether her current anxiety and depression might mask a psychosis. There is a history of a psychotic episode on the part of her mother.

Verbal Subtest Score		Performance Subtest Score	
Comprehension	12	Picture Arrangement	12
Information	13	Picture Completion	16
Digit Span	12	Block Design	12
Arithmetic	11	Digit Symbol	8
Similarities	10		

Verbal IQ—109   Performance IQ—112   Full Scale IQ—111

Typically, in a hysterical picture one would expect to find an underdevelopment of the range of factual knowledge (low Information), in contrast to other abilities and especially in contrast to an often emphasized proficiency with conventional, stereotyped, here-and-now situations (high Comprehension). Besides the Information-Comprehension relationship, there are few reliable features of test scatter that routinely suggest hysterical personality organization. Performance IQ is at times superior to Verbal IQ as a reflection of the more restricted development of verbal modes. In this example of scatter, the elevation of Performance over Verbal IQ might be suggestive of hysterical organization, but the absence of the usually reliable Information-Comprehension discrepancy makes this scatter inconclusive. Instead, what is noteworthy in the scatter are the high Picture Completion and the low Digit Symbol scores. Low Digit Symbol is most likely to indicate depressive features associated with sluggish energy output and retarded motor efficiency. A high Picture Completion score is most consistent with hyperalertness. The combination of low Digit Symbol and high Picture Completion therefore would suggest some intermingling of both depressive and hyperalert, possibly paranoid features and the likelihood, therefore, of a mixed neurosis.

After the first 12 Information items, her efficiency becomes variable; she seems unsure even on correct answers (e.g., Temperature: "212° F., I can't remember these things") and has difficulty recalling information which in one instance (Faust) she retrieves much later, toward the end of testing. She corrects one temporary inefficiency of memory (referring to President Johnson as Johnston) and voices concern about the adequacy of her performance (Population: "Three billion I guess. Do I get into college?"). Her style here is not depressive in terms of being overly self-disparaging but is more concerned with retrieving information that is not readily accessible. Nor is her style overly paranoid in terms of externalizing blame for her difficulties onto the test situation and/or the tester. Rather, taken by itself, her Information subtest suggests that, beyond an average level (i.e., beyond the 16th question), her style emphasizes memory difficulties, temporary or permanent inability to recall facts, or else a sense of unsureness about what she does remember. Blood Vessels: "I don't know what that means, like arteries and veins? Those aren't vessels. Arteries and veins. [Do you know another?] Capillaries?" Faust: "Several different authors wrote versions of it. I have one by, I can't think of the name. Milan? I don't know. I'm going to go home and find out."

365

CLINICAL
CONTRIBUTIONS OF
THE WECHSLER
ADULT
INTELLIGENCE
SCALE

It would appear that her acquisition of information may not have been disturbed—a fact also suggested by her high Picture Completion score and its attendant hyperalertness and attentiveness to external forms—but that her recollection is interfered with. Thus, although she obtains her highest Verbal subtest score on Information, a qualitative analysis of her responses suggests the type of memory disturbance typically connected with repressive defense (especially given the absence of signs of organicity). In other words, she simultaneously wants to be aware and also unaware of factual information she could have available. Her high score alone, seemingly unrepressive, belies her qualitative repressive style. The discrepancy between score and style of response serves to highlight a critical aspect of test analysis. It is not that one source of information is correct and another inconclusive or misleading. It is not in this instance that her scatter is basically unreliable because it would not place her in a hysterical-repressive category. The task of clinical analysis is to take such seeming discrepancies and inconsistencies and try to make sense out of them, to form a hypothesis which can account for how someone can obtain factual information and can even recall it yet in the process make herself seem unreflective and unaware. This woman has already graduated from junior college, yet she wonders aloud, "Can I get into college?" Although her IQs are not extraordinary, she gives the impression of being less bright than she actually is. Her eagerness to know or to remember is offset by a desire to be unaware, unknowledgeable.

At the outset, her Arithmetic answers are crisp and efficient. Then, when she is incorrect, she has difficulty correcting her response, she comments on her slowness, her concentration wavers ("There are six fifteens in 60"). She ends by saying "I don't know" and on the last item states her need for paper and pencil. As on Information, here, too, when items get beyond the overlearned level, she retreats from active, effortful ideation and internal elaboration to focus finally on an external aid. Thus far, an interesting pattern is emerging of a woman who may initially appear efficient but who, with increased task difficulty, begins to demonstrate the type of repressive style and flight from active ideation associated with hysterical personality organization. Again, these characteristics are evident in the qualitative analysis rather than in the scores or their specific patterning.

Several noteworthy aspects of Comprehension expand other characteristics of this woman's style. Taxes: "So that others less fortunate and who don't have jobs can clothe and house themselves and so we can have better roads and buildings and our cities nicer." Her response to this item reflects an initial emphasis on destitute people and she ends with a global, unspecific comment about making cities "nicer." Taxes, of course, are used for these purposes, but what is unique is the sequence, emphasis, and style of verbalization. Her starting out with destitution as an issue may reflect this theme as of particular concern to her, and it is of interest that she affiliates herself with the more fortunate people. When we consider this representation of herself in the light of the suggestion of depressive features in her scatter, it may be that what we are witnessing is an attempt to counter a view of herself as less than fortunate. Having things "nice" indicates a similar wish for things to be pleasant, reflects the unspecific style of the sort associated with a repressive-hysterical orientation, and further elaborates the hypothesis derived from Information and Arithmetic.

Iron: "I can't put it into context. I would say like if you are going into battle or war is to . . . It could also mean to do something while you are thinking about it, while it is fresh in your head. Not to put it off." She has difficulty getting started on this item; she starts to say something about battle or war, trails off, and shifts to a more abstract level but one that highlights inner urgency as the basis for action rather than an interplay between urge and opportunity. Her fumbling approach may reflect initial repressive efforts; while she ultimately shifts to a more abstract level, her increased efficiency may also reflect a move away from the unpleasant aggressive content which she blocks in midsentence. On the Forest item, when asked what she would do if she did not know in which direction to go, she discounts the likelihood of getting lost ("I used to play in the woods and never got lost"). Might this response be an additional reflection of a wish to try to deny unpleasantness and especially to counter depressive feelings such as loneliness, neediness, or feeling lost? It may bear reemphasis that this formulation follows from an attempt to integrate the content of her responses with features of the test scatter and that each type of data might by itself yield different conclusions.

Similarities is variable in efficiency (2-2-2-2-0-1-1-0-2-2-0-0-0), as was Information, which suggests a higher level of potential than her scores reveal. In terms of the original discussion of Information, therefore, several things are operating. She both knows more than her style of verbalization would suggest and is capable of even higher levels of proficiency. Her response to Dog-Lion, that they are both dependent, is highly unusual and therefore was inquired into. Dog-Lion: "Um . . . both are in the animal family and both are dependent. [What do you mean about their being dependent?] Like a male lion is dependent on the female to provide everything for him. I guess a dog or human could care for itself but is better off if it has others caring for them." [She begins to joke about men she knows.]

Her answer demonstrates a deprecatory view of men as needy and dependent on women—a clear minimization of the male lion's kingly power, authority, and strength. Disparagement of men, while not an exclusive characteristic of hysterical women, is frequently met with. Her reversal of traditional roles and the implicit disclaiming of her own dependency may corroborate further the earlier indications of denial of her own neediness. She may habitually disparagingly put men into a dependent position. The poverty of the quality of her verbalization is evident at other times in her responses, especially in Egg-Seed, where again she shows an approximate, searching quality, never quite zeroing in on target. "Both come from inside something, like a seed inside a peach and an egg inside a chicken before it hatches, not hatches but before it lays it. And both produce another what it came from."

Picture Completion is almost perfect. Yet she refers to car door handles as "knobs," the bridge of the glasses as "the thing," the tuning peg of the violin as the "little tuner," the oarlock as the "little thing to put the oar in, bracket," the base threads of the bulb as "little rivets." The theme is diminution accompanied by imprecision in language. Such imprecision in language is the hallmark of a repressive orientation that has kept out articulated knowledge; diminution, similarly, in such a context is likely to reflect efforts to keep her experience manageable, small, childlike, and unthreatening. Her one error involves misperceiving the horn on the saddle as missing and then claiming never to have seen a saddle with a horn—a likely repressive interference in which she asserts and disclaims her perception because of possible unconscious associations with horns, such as the penis. A repressive theme on this item and its phallic significance would fit with the generally repressive style

367

CLINICAL
CONTRIBUTIONS OF
THE WECHSLER
ADULT
INTELLIGENCE
SCALE

and the suggestion of Dog-Lion of an underlying fear of male assertion and aggression. On Blocks, she gives her first response suggestive of mistrust in accord with the hyperalertness suggested by her high Picture Completion—that is, when she says "tricky," which she explains by diminutive reference to "all these little things."

On Picture Arrangement, her incorrect sequence to Enter (Opesn) was questioned: "He can't get in. He sees someone else go in so he tries and bumps his head or something. [You seem puzzled about it.] There is a man going out who resembled the man who went through the door so I don't know if it is meant to be the same man or not. Oh, Marlowe wrote Faust. Oh, that's awful. Also, Goethe [pronounced "gaytah"]. I knew that would bother me." Her response emphasizes not just inability to figure out a method of entry, but painful bodily response. This may constitute a representation of a disturbance at the periphery of perceptual or motor action and may refer to the difficulty of penetrating across a firm repressive barrier; it may have referents to sexual difficulty around penetration; it may represent men again as especially incompetent. It is of interest that she then seems unclear whether there are two men or one man—the sort of confusion that is found in people having trouble with separation and individuation. At this point, she recalls the authors of Faust for unclear reasons (the association with two men, the possible unconscious connection between entry and Faust's immorality?).

This WAIS reflects an essentially hysterical picture. Although she is a bright woman (Full Scale IQ of 111 with higher potential), her repressive style often gives her the impression of being less bright. Thus she will forget what things are called, claim unfamiliarity with certain information she obviously knows, restrict her active ideational efforts (when pressed), and emphasize what is pleasant, cute, and diminutive. Images of strength or potential aggressivity are minimized and weakened into images of "little" things. One clear aspect of this trend is her wish to minimize male strength and aggressivity by a reversal of dependency relationships coupled with disparagement.

She is brighter than she makes herself appear at times. The fact that she strives to figure things out, is persistent, and is bothered by her repressive orientation are positive indices of a degree of perseverance and critical self-evaluativeness that contrast with her repressive, minimizing style. Underlying depressive issues are suggested, which may be countered by an alternate representation of herself as the one who is strong, who feeds and cares for (especially with men).

I have selected this WAIS largely because of its illustration of discrepancies between scores and style and content of responses. It is suggested that such discrepancy has dynamic meaning. In terms of personality description and diagnosis, the other tests would be viewed from the perspective of all the varied WAIS test indications. In this instance, the other tests confirm, expand, and augment the varied hypotheses offered here.

3.2. Schizophrenia

The term "schizophrenia" shall be restricted in its meaning to apply only to those people who show "an impairment in experiencing, perceiving and representing boundaries" (Blatt, Wild, & Ritzler, 1975). This has variously been referred to as a disruption of ego boundaries, a deficiency in self-other differentiation, a tendency toward merging inner and outer experience. It would take us too far from the present task to explore the controversy among the various deficit and conflict theories of schizophrenia (Gunderson & Mosher, 1975). A specific style of thinking—the tendency to blend or merge together usually distinct characteristics of experience in a troubled and conflicted manner—shall be taken to be a core characteristic of schizophrenia. It shall be assumed that a subtle interaction of endowment, early developmental dilemmas, and later conflict most likely accounts for this state of affairs so that what may be a deficiency in development may also operate in the service of conflict. Schizophrenia, like all other diagnostic categories, is treated here as an active mode of relatedness to self and others by a choice-making, intentional person.

The manifestation of blending or merging may be evident in affects, cognitions, or behavior. Certain test features such as poor judgment (low Comprehension) and widely fluctuating scatter are usually taken to be signs of schizophrenia, but from the present position they will constitute signs of psychosis and not necessarily schizophrenia. Without indications of merging (Contamination), schizophrenia will not be diagnosed. Since merging as such is not revealed directly in the scatter, it will have to be established on the basis of qualitative analysis. From the perspective of scatter, there are three indications relevant here. The first two, low judgment and great fluctuation in abilities, have already been mentioned. The third is a pattern first described by Bleuler and later elaborated by Rapaport et al. as the out-of-pattern relationship in which the Digit Span score is elevated above the Arithmetic score. This pattern reflects a superiority of attentional over concentration activities. With an anxious person, one usually sees interference of passive attention, which is then shored up by more active concentration. In the case of schizophrenia, however, concentration is disrupted; it fluctuates or is effortful, whereas attention is heightened as if the schizophrenic unselectively registers all experience like a camera, takes in everything but disclaims efforts to more actively employ his powers of concentration. In terms of diagnosing schizophrenia from test scatter, the out-of-pattern relationship, given a context of other suggestions of psychosis, is the only dependable sign.

Beyond test scatter, the qualitative features associated with schizophrenia consist of the various deviant verbalizations which were categorized by Rapaport with special reference to the Rorschach test but which are applicable to all clinical situations. According to the diagnostic stance toward schizophrenia taken here, the most telling verbalizations involve the blurring of boundaries of separate thoughts, feelings, or experience. For example, there will appear signs of a basic unsureness as to what is animate or inanimate, real or artificial, singular or plural, up or down, male or female, etc. Or what is presented will be overly infused with elaboration by inner urges and misrecognitions. Sudden shifts will also occur in the level of organization of responses.

Patient is a 21-year-old single white female college junior. Her therapist reports that, for several months prior to testing, things seemed to go downhill, with increased depression, sleep disturbance, nightmares, and hallucinatory-like phenomena of voices (that patient describes as "nightmares in my head, screaming in my head"). The diagnostic question is of borderline to incipient or overt psychosis and with whether the therapist can continue with her without hospitalization since she gives the impression of just making it on an outpatient basis. Reality testing is said to be largely intact.

Scatter is here unrevealing of psychosis. The lower Performance IQ may suggest a depressive lowering of motoric energy. The Digit Span score suggests subjective distress, anxiety, and attentional difficulties which are being countered by active

369

CLINICAL
CONTRIBUTIONS OF
THE WECHSLER
ADULT
INTELLIGENCE
SCALE

efforts at concentration (high Arithmetic). Concentration on external forms (Picture Completion), however, may be less effective than more inwardly directed concentration. Scatter is not particularly variable overall and might on the surface suggest a person who is anxious and depressed only to a neurotic degree because of the absence of any of the three psychotic scatter indicators (low Comprehension, widely variable scatter, out-of-pattern relationship between Arithmetic and Digit Span).

Verbal Subtest Score		Performance Subtest Score	
Comprehension	13	Picture Arrangement	12
Information	14	Picture Completion	11
Digit Span	11	Block Design	11
Arithmetic	15	Digit Symbol	11
Similarities	12		

Verbal IQ—118   Performance IQ—107   Full Scale IQ—114

On Information, her responses are verbalized tersely and efficiently; she guesses when encouraged if she has some approximate idea of the answer but refrains from taking wilder guesses. If anything, her Information responses seem styleless and her lapses in knowledge are not especially revealing. Her response to Movies seems highly unreflective for someone as bright as she is, and it may reflect feelings that she has difficulty containing her reactions, especially in a frightening situation. Movies: "Yell. [Do you think that is the best thing to do?] Probably ring the alarm but I'd yell first." Iron: "Act while something is still happening and alive . . . right and the right moment." Her use of the word "alive" to the Iron item is odd; she tries to explain herself as meaning the "right moment" but "alive" here in view of its oddness has an ominous ring to it. Is she concerned about things remaining in an alive state? Could this represent suicidal thoughts? While its meaning is as yet conjectural, its intrusive, peculiar quality is striking, as is its contrast with the usual terseness of her verbalization. One hypothesis thus far is that she may express old thoughts sporadically and in the context of otherwise effective functioning.

Arithmetic is generally smooth and quick. Most of Similarities is also relatively efficient, clear, and precise except for her response to Wood and Alcohol: "They're both inorganic . . . both organic. I don't know. Are you still waiting? Well, they're both made up of molecules. [You seem unsure whether they are organic or inorganic.] Wood is organic and alcohol comes from a lot of organic things but I don't know if it is organic itself." Her confusion whether the two are inorganic or organic continues the concern on Comprehension about things in an alive state. At her level of intelligence, such unclarity must be viewed as exceptional and can only reflect the introduction of a personalized, conflictful issue. The fact that her personalizations thus far are markedly peculiar by being grossly out of line with expectations from her intellectual level would argue for their having psychotic rather than neurotic import. Moreover, this is not depressive content in the sense of being gloomy, sad, or unhappy; rather, it partakes of an uncertainty about the basic categories of existence, indicates some blurring of these categories, and therefore is suggestive of schizophrenia.

Some of her errors on Picture Completion reinforce the theme of unsureness of reality. At her intellectual level especially, it is odd that she does not seem to recognize with confidence either oarlocks or the American Flag ("Is that supposed to be the American Flag?"). The introduction and emphasis on eyes several times may also suggest a preoccupation with feelings of being looked at, criticized. Nose Piece: "I don't see anything missing unless it's the bottom of the eyes. It may be the drawing." Crab: "The eyes and the third claw. [Which is more important?] I guess it's supposed to have three on each side."

Blocks contains temporary inefficiencies like leaving one block incorrect on No. 7 or else making an incorrect design, recognizing it as an error yet feeling unable initially to correct it. Again, the problem seems to lie with some difficulty in concentration.

Picture Arrangement is of particular interest. She has the Fish sequence correct and with a time bonus but has no idea of the meaning of her arrangement. [What is your story?] "I have no idea. [What do you imagine?] I don't really know. I was arranging by the size of the fish and the number in the basket but I couldn't figure out what the guy in the skindiving suit was doing." Such behavior suggests that she may at times be able to follow logical sequences without appreciation of the meaning of events. Her behavior on this item is paradigmatic of her WAIS protocol in general. That is, she follows the general structure or outline or routine of a situation but feels basically unsure as to what her behavior or experience means. Her designation of the diver as "the guy in the skindiving suit" may be a mild perceptual misrecognition that comes close to her unsureness of the American Flag on Picture Completion. Her last item is incorrect, and her story is uniquely schizophrenic. She arranges Taxi as LESAMU, and, when asked her story says, "I don't know what's going on. [On what basis did you arrange it?] It looked like he was riding with someone real and was embarrassed to sit close to her. Then he wasn't, when he had the mannikin. [Could you review the specific order?] First he was riding with someone and embarrassed. Then there is a gap because I couldn't figure out how he got the mannikin and got rid of the real person. Then he was not embarrassed because it was not real." She envisions the one figure as two, both as mannikin and as real woman. At some point, the woman is gotten rid of and the mannikin is substituted, and the man's embarrassment subsides. The direction of the sequence of the content of this story from vitality and emotional response to lifelessness and affectlessness may have ominous implications in that it may suggest a move away from relatedness and participation to detachment and unreality. In the context of the other responses of this record, it would be hypothesized not only that there are sporadic indications of schizophrenic preoccupations in a record that is often crisply intact but also that this woman may actively be moving in a more detached, lifeless, schizoid direction.

While the overall scatter in this instance suggests psychological disturbance, it is only the qualitative features that permit understanding of the full extent of this disturbance. Again, it is not that the scatter is inaccurate or invalid. Rather, the relatively intact scatter, like her Picture Arrangement sequence of Fish, demonstrates that she is able and willing to adhere to the general organization and sequence of experience by reasoning on the basis of specific—at times even confused or misrecognized—details without showing a full grasp of the meaning of her experience. She adheres to the form rather than the substance of experience.

A WAIS record of this nature with the added suggestion that the direction of psychological movement is toward greater depths of psychosis is likely to be found in incipient or early schizophrenic states.

With regard to the diagnosis of schizophrenia, it is apparent that, to the degree

371

CLINICAL
CONTRIBUTIONS OF
THE WECHSLER
ADULT
INTELLIGENCE
SCALE

indicators of schizophenic thinking become more pervasive throughout the different tests of the test battery and make their presence abundantly known on the WAIS, to that degree one is confronted with a more full-blown schizophrenic orientation. Borderline and incipient or latent schizophrenics manifest the least disruption on the WAIS. Stable borderline states show the least turmoil and anxiety, whereas acute states show the most anxiety. Paranoid schizophrenics would also show minimal intellectual disruption. As with diagnoses generally, the varied test indicators in each category will be a function of the clarity of conceptualization of the specific diagnostic category. Test indicators are translations of theory into practice; for any particular theory, the tester will have to make predictions about test signs that could be associated with that theory. If one understands that, in the early stages of affective withdrawal, schizophrenics "sense the emotional emptiness as rather painful so that they may easily be mistaken for melancholias" (Bleuler, 1950, p. 51), one will be alert to the differentiation between schizophrenic and depressive indicators. Concerns about animate vs. inanimate states such as we saw in our test example, in the context of schizophrenic thinking, will be taken to indicate a reflection of the active move of a schizophrenic person away from full affective interrelatedness and the consequent experience of frozenness and inner deadness.

Careful inquiry is in no instance more crucial than in the diagnosis of schizophrenia when conventional or overlearned forms are adhered to but perceptions and meanings have become idiosyncratically odd. Clinical experience in the case of schizophrenia has also shown the power of inquiry into the Picture Arrangement sequences. The basis for this power lies in the presentation of social interaction to a greater extent than the other test items and in the introduction (on the last Picture Arrangement item) of the theme of what is or is not realistic, animate, or inanimate. Inasmuch as a definitional characteristic of schizophrenia is the experience of unsureness of reality, this test item has an unusually potent pull toward eliciting the expression of a uniquely schizophrenic preoccupation. Frequently, odd aspects suggesting schizophrenia involve initial perceptions of the mannikin as a real woman or transformations where the mannikin becomes alive. Misrecognitions of affective states such as the man's embarrassment can also point to the kind of affective disharmony of schizophrenia. The introduction of a helping relationship on Fish also makes this item informative about therapeutic transference expectations. Witness the young man who described the diver as "someone trying to steal his fish." Or the schizophrenic man who arranged Fish correctly, but offered the following as his story: "The King was fishing. Then the fisherman caught another fish and whistled to him. [Whistled to whom?] The three men in a tub. [I don't follow.] He caught another fish and in the last picture was whistling to the men who had a fish in their boat. [What did you mean about the men in a *tub*?] I thought the thing was a tub with shower curtains." Since inquiry is done without the cards present, the last card was reshown and he was able to see the diver accurately. A young woman with a relatively smooth WAIS made one of her few odd verbalizations when she described the fisherman as holding "a sword to fight the fish with."

3.3. Obsessive-Compulsive Personality

From the psychoanalytic perspective, obsessive-compulsive personality is characterized by its anal-sadistic emphasis and by a clustering of the defenses of intellectualization, isolation, reaction formation, and undoing. In terms of style, the obsessive-compulsive contrasts dramatically with the hysteric. Attention is sharply focused, details are emphasized, cognition tends to be rigid and technical, and experience is characterized by "tense deliberateness" (Shapiro, 1965), with a consequent restriction of relaxed, free, or spontaneous feelings, thoughts, or actions. Self-awareness is heightened, but in the service of moral and work imperatives as to what "should" be done, felt, or thought. Such people "caricature the logical thinker" (Schafer, 1954); show themselves to be "driven, hardworking automatons" (Shapiro, 1965); tend to be ruminative, overly conscientious, orderly, tedious, and hypercritical.

In terms of test expectations, the most reliable feature of scatter is the pattern in which Information is clearly superior to Comprehension. This reflects the obsessive's investment in details of a factual nature, by contrast with a more restricted ability to take a broad overview of a situation. Frequently, it is the obsessive's indecision and qualification which interferes with his judgment or ability to get a general feel for immediate life situations. Often, because of the heightened emphasis on words and symbols, obsessives achieve high IQs and especially high Verbal IQs.

The person to be discussed is a 31-year-old graduate student who was referred for a routine evaluation. He had reported increasing feelings of worthlessness, incompetence, and suicidal ideation, as well as inability to think or concentrate. Some suspiciousness was also noted.

Verbal Subtest Score		Performance Subtest Score	
Comprehension	15	Picture Arrangement	9
Information	14	Picture Completion	12
Digit Span	14	Blocks	17
Arithmetic	15	Object Assembly	13
Similarities	12	Digit Symbol	8
Vocabulary	15		

Verbal IQ—124   Performance IQ—112   Story Recall I—16
Full Scale IQ—119   Story Recall II—15

The scatter is not suggestive of obsessive-compulsive personality. What are striking are the drop in Picture Arrangement and Digit Symbol scores and the heightened Blocks score. Low Digit Symbol suggests depression, while the high Blocks in addition to a relatively high Digit Span score suggests tendencies toward blandness and acceptance of symptomatology (by virtue of lack of anxiety). This scatter raises the question of the sort of person who simultaneously might appear depressed and relatively unanxious. Such a person might experience his depressive concerns as alien intrusions rather than experience them ruminatively and anxiously. The low Picture Arrangement score, when viewed in conjunction with Comprehension, indicates lip-service adherence to social forms and understanding accompanied by reduced effectiveness in putting his understanding into action to serve future plans and interpersonal relationships. Such a pattern could be suggestive of psychosis.

Information (1–4 not administered)

5. Rubber   Tree: sap from; as latex.

6. Presidents   I'm not very good at history. Roosevelt, Truman, Wilson, Bryan I guess—no, Harding. Probably was wrong on last one.

373

CLINICAL
CONTRIBUTIONS OF
THE WECHSLER
ADULT
INTELLIGENCE
SCALE

7.	Longfellow	Writer.
8.	Weeks	52.
9.	Panama	South.
10.	Brazil	On eastern half of bulge in north part of South America. Would comprise about one-third of continent.
11.	Height	5′3″.
12.	Italy	Rome.
13.	Clothes	Because they absorb heat, do not reflect it.
14.	Washington	January 12 or 22. I always get them mixed up. I'd guess the 12th. I don't know which month. I said January. I'm not positive. I'll stick with it.
15.	Hamlet	William Shakespeare.
16.	Vatican	Organization connected with Catholic Church. Identified with Pope. Just how it fits in precisely, I do not know, quite frankly.
17.	Paris	About 5500 miles.
18.	Egypt	In eastern part of Africa, in similar position to . . . as Brazil is to South America, but not as large. Area would be approximately 10% of whole continent. Would be north, northeast part.
19.	Yeast	Yeast is an enzyme which reacts with starch, forming CO_2, forming air holes . . . I'll take that back. Yeast is not an enzyme, but a bacterium.
20.	Population	170 million . . . plus.
21.	Senators	Roughly 100 (smile) plus or minus zero.
22.	Genesis	Evolution of man . . . evolution not right word. The coming of man, creation of man. Creation of world. Creation. I'll rest on simply creation.
23.	Temperature	212 F. at sea level.
24.	Iliad	Homer.
25.	Blood vessels	Arteries, veins, capillaries.
26.	Koran	It's the . . . would be analogous to the Bible in Mohammedan philosophy. It's a text, tract . . . written word.
27.	Faust	Goethe . . . Johann Wolfgang Goethe.
28.	Ethnology	The study of . . . I'm afraid you've got me on this one, people . . . allied to social customs. It's in sociology. I may be all wet on this one.
29.	Apocrypha	It again is a religious tract. Associated with the Near East. Don't think I can get closer than that. I'd guess its origin would be Arabic. I'm in the realm of guesswork now so I won't go much further.

Qualitative features of Information show an obsessive-compulsive preoccupation with details, accuracy, and self-observant monitoring of responses. The response to Brazil, for example, is an illustrative example of obsessional attention to detail. His efforts to attend to how positive he is and whether or not he is guessing also reflect a type of obsessional attention to the response process. Only on the Senators item does he show a temporary capacity for humorous display of his overexactness. In addition, his verbalization "you've got me" suggests suspicious features.

Comprehension (1 and 2 not administered)

3.	Envelope	Put it in a mailbox. [Gives me a condescending look.]
4.	Bad Company	This is not necessarily true. If one felt this strongly it would be because of the danger that bad influence would rub off on oneself. One would be associated with them, would tend to become bad himself. But I do make the point that this is not necessarily desirable.
5.	Movies	Get up calmly, walk out, and inform an usher or someone in an administrative position. But in no case reveal what you have found out, which would lead to catastrophe. As a corollary, I would offer my services in any way that would be helpful.
6.	Taxes	[Smile] People have to be governed as history has proven. Government has to have money. This is a painless way to do it and also one of the most equitable ones. According to our own socialistic beliefs this is the most desirable way to run a country.
7.	Iron	Don't let a situation become cold, or you will lose your grasp of the facts, or even of the situation itself.
8.	Child Labor	To prevent exploitation of children because of their inability, defenselessness, which is due to their not being mature individuals.
9.	Forest	If sun is shining, this is helpful. If not . . . sun rises in the east, sets in west . . . Wind direction is also helpful . . . can count on prevailing wind currents. If land has topography . . . will have mental picture of it. Aside from that, little! Position of moss on trees can be relegated to old wives tales. Also I'll add a corollary. Follow a stream . . . down stream. Civilization always near water. Also, of course, you have to walk in a straight line, etc.
10.	Deaf	Because deafness and dumbness tend to be hereditary and through alleles and genes they go together. Also associated is if you cannot hear, it is difficult to learn to express, however, it can be done through sight training . . . if a person has a palate which is capable of delivering a sound.
11.	City Land	Simply because it's all relative. People tend to be gregarious, living in association with one another. Land in city becomes more valuable. [I have to ask him to slow down here] I'll reduce this. In city, land is used by large number of people per square unit of area . . . the potential for investment of large sums of money in small area

375

CLINICAL
CONTRIBUTIONS OF
THE WECHSLER
ADULT
INTELLIGENCE
SCALE

is relatively large. The counterpart would be in the country where it is spread out, potential for investment is much less.

12. Marriage
As far as the state is concerned, this would be more for reasons of preventing immoral exploitation of normal association between men and women. It's a legalistic thing rather than a religious thing as far as the state is concerned.

13. Brooks
People with superficial character tend to talk too much.

14. Swallow
In other words . . . it would have to do with evidence. Rudimentary evidence is worthless. Thorough evidence is necessary to prove a point.

Comprehension continues the overdetailed, qualified, intellectualized (e.g., "as a corollary") style. It is of interest that he brings up losing one's "grasp of the facts" on the Iron item, a typically obsessive emphasis on retaining factual information in preference for the more general and more appropriate response involving action. Losing one's grasp of a situation may also refer to his present experience of losing hold of things. The emphasis on proving one's point to Swallow has a disputational, legalistic quality and relates back to the suspiciousness observed on Information. In retrospect, the comment "I'll rest . . ." to Genesis (on Information) may have meant "I'll rest my case" as if he felt he was making points or proving things, although it may also reflect some expansive identification with a God who rested after creation. On the Marriage item, the phrase "immoral exploitation" should have been inquired into. It may have a cryptic, odd meaning and could suggest that he may become odd around themes of marriage and sexuality.

On Arithmetic, another instance of suspiciousness occurs on the second item when he says, "I'm wondering why the simplicity of the questions. I hesitate because I assume some catch."

Similarities

1. Orange
Fruit.

2. Coat
Both coverings for the body. Both full length coverings. Not necessarily! Both are coverings for the body, I'll stick to that.

3. Axe
Perform same type of work, though not necessarily the same job. [?] Both used essentially with wood, cutting down, and cutting trees to length. Axe is more suitable to do section of smaller materials than a saw.

4. Dog
Both carnivores. Do you want all similarities that I can think of? [Just essential ones.] Both carnivores.

5. North
Both cardinal directions.

6. Eye
Sensory mechanisms.

7. Air
Both are matter.

8. Table
Furniture.

9. Egg
Both basic to life, embryonic . . . well, preembryonic forms of life . . . *proto*-embryonic, not preembryonic.

10.	Poem	Both require artistic sense in their composition.
11.	Wood	Wood can be used to make alcohol.
12.	Praise	They are most unlike. I can see no similarity. If anything, they're antonyms. I see little relationship between the two.
13.	Fly	Again, both are forms of life: one botanical, the other zoological.

Reference to "full length coverings" on Similarities, even though modified later, may suggest wishes to hide his sensuousness and may link up with usual obsessive inhibition and restriction. The word "mechanisms" in reference to sensory organs elaborates a technical affectless approach to bodily experience. And the general lack of joyful zest and aesthetic emotionality of obsessives is revealed in his picking out as central only the compositional aspect of Poem and Statue rather than their fuller aesthetic appeal.

Several other test responses of relevance include the following. After recalling the first Story Recall, he says, "From that narrative you can deduce that one of my main troubles is comprehension and retention of current facts." Again, he emphasizes highly logical processes and reveals his apprehension lest he not retain factual details. On Picture Completion, to the man with the missing finger, he comments, "Feminine left arm, masculine right arm . . . forearm and hand. Also the third finger on the left hand which I didn't see at first which gave rise to my misinterpretation and my early floundering." This is a classic instance of self-observation. On Picture Arrangement, he gets the comic book sequence 10 sec over time and loses credit. His story to Fish is correct but he reverses the order of H and I. To Taxi, his sequence is correct, as is his story, but he says of the man that "his thought process was embarrassed." This description of the detached reaction of a thought process rather than the emotional reaction of a person is a supreme illustration of the impersonal, affectively detached, mechanistic quality of obsessional personality. He repeats his detached approach in his definition of Tangible as "Ability to be visualized. Quality of being visualized, not the ability." Here he becomes doubting, meticulous, distanced, and observational from something direct and concrete. Freud's discussion of the defense of isolation as the avoidance of touch has particular bearing on the interpretation of this response.

The summary of this man's WAIS already reflects various obsessive-compulsive characteristics. Paranoid features (suspiciousness and legalistic verbalization) are also evident to some degree, and their significance, along with a few odd verbalizations, would have to be determined in the context of the entire test battery. Depressive features, interestingly, are suggested primarily in the test scatter but seem absent from the content of his responses; it was suggested earlier in the test scatter that depression might be present but would be accompanied by efforts at rigorous containment.

3.4. Organicity

If the contribution of the WAIS were to the diagnosis of organic brain disorder or dysfunction alone, its significance as a clinical instrument would be assured. Although these scales were not planned with the intention of neurological evaluation, "the subtests sample the majority of the abilities relevant to cerebral function" and are "neurologically relevant" (McFie, 1975, p. 14). The major exceptions are tests of verbal fluency and memory for visual material, which must be supplemented by other sources.

377

CLINICAL
CONTRIBUTIONS OF
THE WECHSLER
ADULT
INTELLIGENCE
SCALE

Organicity will be dealt with here in terms of its varied psychological deficits rather than in terms of correlating deficits with specific types or locations of organic damage. In the absence of extensive neurological knowledge, the tester is wise to use a more cautious descriptive approach without going out on a limb and trying to predict exact type and location of damage. Efforts to develop systematic correlations of the loci of neurological damage with specific psychological dysfunction are also still in their early stages, and the known correlations may not be readily applicable to the bulk of test referrals which are likely to stem from neurological ambiguity. Moreover, in those instances where neurological evidence is unambiguous, the purpose of testing is usually less with specificity than with charting the current state of the varied psychological capacities or dysfunctions. It is also in this area that the differentiation between intentionality and deficit often becomes difficult to establish with any certainty. But even here, in terms of intentionality, it is apparent that the individual may cope with his deficit in any number of ways and that the task of testing is only in part to assess the extent of deficit. The purpose of testing is also to establish the psychological context in which the deficit has occurred and the style with which the deficit is being dealt.

The broad class of CNS disorders is associated with various types of difficulties in concept formation, memory, and perceptual and visual-motor activity. Concept formation is likely to be more concrete than abstract; the ability to shift from one thought or activity to another is restricted; analytic and synthetic abilities and hypothetical thinking are diminished. Memory and learning ability show impairments in the intake and retention of stimuli, in overall amount recalled, and in qualitative aspects. Organics show difficulty in keeping track of a train of thought or a task, and grope toward concepts and ideas with great effort. Ordinary words become unavailable even with considerable search for them; or responses of poor quality are recognized but there is little ability to alter and improve them. Various perceptual, spatial rearrangements may occur such as figure-ground reversal, rotations of designs, confusion as to directionality (up-down, left-right, east-west). Responses are repeated perseveratively without acknowledgment of their repetition. At times, there is a conspicuous filling in or elaboration of ideas unrelated to the material at hand (confabulation). Procedures may be known but cannot be put into action, and there may be a persistent sense of inability to evaluate one's performance. With organically disturbed persons, generally, there is a sense that the regularity and expectability of everyday life are disrupted, that the organics are struggling to supply order and reestablish a hold on conventional reality. Hence their activity is oriented toward groping toward reality and feeling unable to reach it. Consequently, they may appear odd at times, confused, uncertain, or constricted, but they generally lack the sort of psychological embellishment and thematic richness one finds in psychic disturbances like schizophrenia. There are, of course, instances in which schizophrenic and organic features may interweave and present formidable diagnostic lack of clarity. Typically, the most difficult differential diagnostic issues involve organicity and psychosis because they share some marked cognitive disturbances that are uncommon in neurosis. One rule of thumb to help resolve such diagnostic uncertainty is that, in the presence of extensive cognitive disruption, most psychotic persons will introduce strange, morbid, otherworldly content, whereas the organic person will give the impression that he is struggling to crystallize a rather mundane concept or thought. Furthermore, the cognitive disruptions of the psychotic person will be more likely to have a dynamic significance, whereas the organic person will show equivalent disruption both with dynamic and with more neutral, ordinary experience. Organics will be bothered about where they are in space and with keeping tabs of their train of thinking but usually without rich embellishment and without withdrawal from conventional modes of experience. For example, an organic patient routinely walked behind his therapist, who tentatively viewed this behavior as indicative of suspicious, paranoid trends. Testing revealed marked problems in spatial orientation, and further questioning led this patient to explain that he followed behind his therapist as a way of orienting himself in space.

As a consequence of the particular disturbance with abstract conceptual thinking, the Similarities and Block Design subtests are the most indicative of organicity, and there may also be particular difficulty with the proverbs on Comprehension. Where perceptual and perceptual-motor efficiency is most disrupted, the Performance IQ may fall significantly below the Verbal IQ. Low scores on Story Recall, as a test of memory, are suggestive of organicity. Marked disturbance of attention and concentration may also be indicative, especially in the context of lowered Similarities or Block Design. A lowering of motor tasks such as Object Assembly or Digit Symbol may be relevant, although by themselves they may reflect either the personalization of marked bodily concerns (Object Assembly) or depressive retardation (Digit Symbol). Qualitative features include the variety of organic aspects referred to above.

Verbal Subtest Scores		Performance Subtest Score	
Comprehension	11	Picture Arrangement	6
Information	10	Picture Completion	8
Digit Span	9	Blocks	6
Arithmetic	8	Digit Symbol	3
Similarities	5		
Vocabulary	10		

Verbal IQ—97   Performance IQ—81   Story Recall I—10
Total IQ—94   Story Recall II—7

This is the WAIS record of a 59-year-old, married white male, a laborer who, 1 year prior to testing, suffered a head injury with clear neurological signs. Psychological testing was requested in order to document the pattern of loss of mental abilities.

The scatter shows noteworthy organic signs: Performance is significantly below Verbal IQ (i.e., by more than 8–10 points, Wechsler, 1944, p. 147); Similarities is the lowest Verbal subtest; Digit Symbol is low, which may also suggest depressive features; and Story Recall is poorer on the second recall.

Information (1–4 not administered)

    5. Rubber   A mixture. It comes from the Far East, something like that. [What does rubber come from?] It grows on trees . . . some kind of liquid.

    6. Presidents   1900 . . . Truman, Eisenhower, Kennedy, Johnson, Hoover, Harding. [How many did I ask for?] Four.

379

CLINICAL
CONTRIBUTIONS OF
THE WECHSLER
ADULT
INTELLIGENCE
SCALE

7.	Longfellow	A writer or poet or something.
8.	Weeks	52.
9.	Panama	Roughly south.
10.	Brazil	In South America.
11.	Height	About 5'4".
12.	Italy	Of America? [of Italy.] Rome.
13.	Clothes	[He repeats question.] Maybe with wool it's made with.
14.	Washington	. . . I think January something.
15.	Hamlet	Could you repeat? [I repeat question.] Would that be Shakespeare?
16.	Vatican	Connected with the Church of Rome. [Could you explain?] Pope goes there, Swiss guards are outside.
17.	Paris	From where? Harris? Is that Hearris? [Paris.] Paris, about 3200 miles
18.	Egypt	In the Far East, Mediterranean. [Continent.] In Africa.
19.	Yeast	Could you repeat? [I repeat.] The sun rises in the east and sets in the west. [I repeat again. Do you know what yeast is?] Oh yeast! That's for making bread, yeast in dough. [Repeat.] The heat would make it rise.
20.	Population	Population? I think 300 million.
21.	Senators	Senators . . . 104. [How did you get that?] Two from each state, 52 states.
22.	Genesis	That would be . . . start of the Bible. [What is it about?] Something to do with . . . Moses is in Genesis; it leads up to the present. It leads up to a world crisis, everything going back. [What do you mean about a world crisis?] I was thinking back to when the Jews had to leave and crossed the Red Sea.
23.	Temperature	180 degrees I think.
24.	Iliad	I beg your pardon. [Repeat.] I don't know.
25.	Blood Vessels	I don't know that.

(26–29 not administered)

Information reflects various qualitatively organic features, including numerous mishearings and requests to have questions repeated. He misinterprets questions, states *where* rubber comes from rather than *what*, and offers too many Presidents even though he then correctly states how many were requested. Even when he is correct, his initial orientation is often uncertain or involves mishearing words that sound similar. This indicates a receptive organic impairment that may include responding by virtue of a clang association ("east" or "yeast") and on the basis of a segment of the question (the words "east" and "rise") alone. His giving more Presidents than requested yet recalling the correct number reflects a disharmony between understanding expectations and putting them into action. His response to Genesis may offer insight into more dynamic depressively toned issues in the emphasis on "world crisis" and on exodus and departure rather than beginnings.

On Comprehension, his response to the Forest item is correct, but he concretely equates summertime and sunshine when he states that "in summertime" one can watch where the sun rises. It is as if it is only then that one can rely on the sun for direction. This response combines both organic concreteness and a depressive sense of gloominess. He misses the last two proverbs and wavers between a functional and concrete definition to Iron.

On Arithmetic, he has trouble answering how much $4.00 and $5.00 are. First he says, "5 would be one more than 4." When asked how much they are together, he says, "If adding, $9.00; but if you are writing it down it would be $45.00." This is another example of a type of concreteness in his emphasis on visualizing the two numbers as placed together.

Similarities

1. Orange	I beg your pardon. [Repeated.] An orange is round and a banana is a straight object. [How are they alike?] One could be yellow and the orange skin would be a different color, not much different. [Any way they are alike?] Banana is in branches and oranges are packed in crates.
2. Coat	I beg your pardon. [Repeated.] A dress if you put it on and can go around the house and a coat you put on if you are going out, if it is raining or something like that. [How are they alike?] Color and style, short or long.
3. Axe	I beg your pardon. [Repeated.] A saw is a thing for sawing wood and an axe is good for chopping wood and other stuff that a saw can't do. [Alike?] They could at times do the same job. If there were no saw, an axe maybe could help you out. And if no axe, a saw could help.
4. Dog	Both are animals.
5. North	Cold weather countries. [What do you mean?] If you go north it gets colder and if going south you are going to the South Pole. [What was the question?] North and south [North and west!] West . . . coming from south that would be on your right. [North and west—how alike?] In cold weather so from the west . . . would be warm weather.
6. Eye	One . . . ear for hearing, an eye for seeing. [Alike?] You got me beat there, an ear for hearing, an eye for seeing.
7. Air	Air is the thing that gives you life. Water is to help yourself out . . . if you take water when walking . . . Water and air inside your body keep you alive. [Alike?] I think there is a certain amount of air in the water.
8. Table	Both have four legs, a chair for sitting on and a table for putting things on . . . books or dishes.
9. Egg	I beg your pardon. [Repeated.] An egg before it is hatched matures life and a seed would too if planted.
10. Poem	What? [Repeated.] Poem and . . . [Poem and statue.] A poem is something someone wrote and can look at. A statue is the same; it is made and you can look out the window and see it.
11. Wood	I think you get some kind of alcohol from wood—wood alcohol.

381

CLINICAL
CONTRIBUTIONS OF
THE WECHSLER
ADULT
INTELLIGENCE
SCALE

12. Praise   If you do something wrong you can be punished. Before you are punished you can pray to see if that could help.

13. Fly   A tree . . . there might be a likelihood for a fly to go there and feed off the leaves, something like that.

Although he gets some credit, he is highly variable and is unable to take a consistently abstract orientation. He does not seem to understand how to relate things together even when he appears to be engaging in conceptual thinking. Many of his answers are concrete, specific descriptions of separate objects or aspects of objects. In addition, he frequently needs to have questions repeated, mishears "north and south" instead of "north and west," and interprets "praise" as "prays." This subtest performance is an unambiguous demonstration of an organically based impairment of conceptual thinking. Notice how he gets mixed up on "north and west," tries to orient himself concretely in terms of locating himself spatially in terms of left and right, yet without getting peculiar, cryptic, or overly symbolic. Schizophrenics would not lose their capacity for abstraction in this manner but would instead infuse symbolic, personalized meaning. Organics, as in the case here, lose their capacity for abstraction, although not necessarily without dynamic factors entering in. For his hearing "prays" may reflect feelings of being a supplicant in particular need of help and consolation.

On Picture Completion, five items are answered overtime, which suggests a potential scaled score of 11 and indicates a slowing down of concentration rather than a more basic impairment. He at first says a "place for holding the paddle" is missing on the rowboat before correcting himself. His response that "the superstructure to carry the captain" is missing on the ship probably reflects feelings of needing a strong, guiding, directing force in his life in order to counter feelings of lacking in these qualities, possibly as a result of his organic difficulties.

On Story Recall, the amount of recall is impoverished without any personalization.

On Blocks, as on Picture Completion, he goes on to complete a number of items correctly but beyond the time limit, and he also checks and rechecks each completed design for a long time. If we take into consideration his overtime items (No. 6 through No. 9), he would obtain a scaled score of 11 on Blocks. Thus it is apparent that when he is allowed extra time he can significantly improve his efficiency on a task involving concentration on external forms (Picture Completion) and on a motoric task involving abstraction and synthesis (Blocks). This finding is in accord with a comment he made at the outset of testing, that he does "better if left alone," and that he "needs time." By contrast, he does not show similar improvement with verbal abstract material.

He gets the first Picture Arrangement overtime, and misses Nos. 4, 5, 7, and 8. His stories to Nos. 4, 5, and 7 are correct but not odd. On 4, he describes a man who is reading a book and sees two small boys fighting; he separates them and they shake hands and become friends. On No. 5 (Enter), he describes a man "making for the bathroom and the door is locked or something. The first guy tried to push it; then somebody came out and he went in." On Fish, he sees "a man fishing and after he fished he shouted and a diver came up. I think he said wait a minute, I'll see if I can get you out of the water." This response of a person stranded in the water is a likely personalization of feelings of needing to be rescued from a difficult situation. On Taxi, he sees "a man carrying the statue of a woman. He puts the statue in the back seat. It looks like a man and woman in there. See him looking out the back window, *like* he was kissing the statue." He enjoys telling this story of a man putting on a show of sexual prowess. While the details are incorrect, there is nothing here that is odd in a psychotic way. It is most likely, therefore, that whatever difficulty is suggested by his low Picture Arrangement score involves problems in planning and anticipation on the basis of his cognitive organizing deficit. Furthermore, the discrepancy between his Comprehension and Picture Arrangement scores would suggest someone whose grasp of conventional judgment will mask difficulties in putting things into action. His feelings of needing rescue from a stranded and helpless situation (Picture Arrangement: Fish item) and the need for a guiding, orienting captain (an executive function) can be understood in this light. His depressive feelings may well be a consequence of a recognition of the impairment in his cognitive equipment.

3.5. Psychopathic Character

Under the classification of impulsive styles, Shapiro brings together several different diagnostic categories which appear to share certain stylistic characteristics. Included are "Those persons usually diagnosed as impulsive characters or psychopathic characters, some of those who are called passive-neurotic characters and narcissistic characters, and certain kinds of male homosexuals, alcoholics, and probably addicts" (Shapiro, 1965, p. 154). Although hypomania is not directly included, Shapiro considers it to exhibit some aspects of the impulsive style. The characteristics of the impulsive style are egocentricity and concreteness, a shortsighted restricting of interests, attention, aims, and values to what is immediate and personally relevant, and action that is unself-critical and glib. From the perspective of an interest in intentionality, the impulsive style converts experiences of "whim, urge or impulse, and giving in" (p. 37) into a thoroughgoing, dominant style rather than having them as occasional experiences that fit into a context of ongoing, organized, developed goals, aims, wishes, and intentions. While there is a similarity between impulsive and hysterical people, the affects and interests of the hysteric are less "transient and essentially exploitative," and are more developed and integrated. The emphasis of the impulsive person is entirely on the immediate moment, and even though he may possess social charms, be aware of conventional mores, and be emphasically astute to interpersonal nuances, such skills are most likely to be used in the pursuit predominantly of momentary interests and immediate personal gains.

The psychopathic person shows these specific features which overlap with narcissistic disorders but will be more compliant and ingratiating and lack the narcissist's affective lability, demandingness, blatant self-centeredness, and preoccupation with ornate, sensuous display.

This is the WAIS record of a 17-year-old white young man with a history of antisocial activities involving theft. From the scatter, it is clear that he is very bright. At this level of verbal intellectual efficiency, it is more usual for the Performance IQ to fall below the Verbal IQ so that his higher Performance IQ may suggest tendencies in a more motoric, action-oriented direction (e.g., hysteria, narcissism, psychopathy). This pattern may be indicated even though it is clear that he has achieved significant verbal skills as well. The perfect Picture Completion score indicates hyperalertness

383

CLINICAL
CONTRIBUTIONS OF
THE WECHSLER
ADULT
INTELLIGENCE
SCALE

Verbal Subtest Score		Performance Subtest Score	
Comprehension	15	Picture Arrangement	17
Information	14	Picture Completion	18
Digit Span	9	Blocks	12
Arithmetic	12	Object Assembly	13
Similarities	15	Digit Symbol	10
Vocabulary	12		

Verbal IQ—122   Performance IQ—128   Story Recall I—10
Total IQ—126   Story Recall II—8

to details, which, in the context of high Similarities and its emphasis on relating things together, might also suggest paranoid tendencies. Similarly, the attentiveness to nuances of social interaction and to anticipation evident in the high Picture Arrangement score would point in a paranoid direction. Saving features of the scatter are the low Digit Span and Digit Symbol, which indicate the likelihood of subjective anxiety and depression rather than a bland or chronic settling in. Thus we see a combination of an emphasis on social judgment, social interaction, anticipation, and hypervigilance without indications of psychosis. Although the diagnosis may be in question, there can be little doubt that this young man is likely to be a very watchful, cautious, socially tuned-in person, possibly a schemer. It is also clear that, unlike other action-oriented people, his verbal skills have developed to a high degree, including his fund of information.

His politeness was immediately evident during Information, e.g., to Brazil he answered, "South America, the continent of South America, *excuse me*, to be more specific." He later excuses himself as well after giving an initially incorrect response before correcting it. On Senators, which he misses, he excuses his lack of knowledge on the basis of his not being "too hep on the government" and thereby offers personal liking as the basis for acquiring information. His politeness and precision on Information and his attention to the sureness of his responses might seem obsessional. Obsessives, however, would not be so ready to try to excuse a lack of knowledge purely on the basis of personal inclination, nor would they be this colloquial. In other words, what we see here is a style that combines a polite, measured tone with a more colloquial, self-centered communication. Colloquialism is inconsistent with obsessionality, but the cautious, diligent, measured tone could be an aspect of a psychopathic or narcissistic effort to impress others and engage in intellectual display.

Comprehension (1 and 2 not administered)

3. Envelope   I would take it to the mailbox, probably mail it. I'd figure if it was addressed to the right place it would go to the person it was meant for. Someone probably dropped it. If it was the wrong address, it would at least go back to the sender.

4. Bad Company   I can answer that one from experience. When you're with bad company sometimes you're put in an environment where you can easily get in trouble and join them. Another reason is they can influence your whole life in a way which wouldn't be beneficial.

5. Movies	I'd immediately get up cautiously so I wouldn't excite other people and I'd go to the movie people and tell them there was a fire and then I'd go to the fire doors and open them so people could escape if they had to. I think it would keep people from panicking if they could see an open door. Then I'd try to help put out the fire if I could.
6. Taxes	Why should they? Well, number one, it's required by the government. Number two, It's for their own good. The money really goes back in their own . . . benefits them.
7. Iron	. . . well, if you're in a situation where it becomes a crisis, to take care of it at the moment, at a time that would be most beneficial, using foresight and judgment.
8. Child Labor	To protect children from being abused.
9. Forest	Could you be more explicit? In other words, what would I have with me? If I had nothing I'd pick up all the pebbles around, anything I could use to mark a trail. I'd start walking, marking my path from a point I would use as a home base. And then, if it was a wrong trail, I'd follow my path back to home base and start again till I reached the right direction. If I had a compass or a map it would be easier, but if I didn't this is the best way. Then again it depends on the situation. I'd usually tell my parents or someone when I was coming home. So I'd wait until they came to get me. Or if I had matches I'd clear an area and start a fire. But if I were alone I'd do that first. If there was a tall tree I'd climb it and survey the area. Maybe I'd see signs of civilization.
10. Deaf	They never have heard *human* sounds; therefore, they don't know how to imitate.
11. City land	Supply and demand.
12. Marriage	Well, number one for recording, records. Number two, for society. It's just a part of society and our civilization. A requirement. I mean it's to protect, in the long run, both parties concerned and it also has something to do with if there are any children, you'd have any legal involvement.
13. Brooks	Means people who talk only when they have something to say are usually the smartest. People who are always jabbering are the ones who really don't have that much knowledge.
14. Swallow	In other words, don't jump to a conclusion before you completely analyze the situation and all the facts that can be obtained.

On Envelope, he introduces the theme of whether something is right or wrong—here, whether the envelope is addressed to the right or wrong place. His introduction of this theme is irrelevant to the question, and there is also no reason for hesitancy

385

CLINICAL
CONTRIBUTIONS OF
THE WECHSLER
ADULT
INTELLIGENCE
SCALE

and deliberation. His "probably mail it" and concern with right and wrong may reflect a response to an implicit temptation, but in any case his response is overly specific, and it introduces a theme suggestive of a moral preoccupation. His manner of response suggests he may be covering himself against all possible alternatives. His next response, to Bad Company, is confessional and has the style of a repentent sinner, someone who has been there and seen the light. His next answer (Movies) introduces massive constraint after the immediate response of getting up and then conscientiousness and helpfulness regarding every detail of the evacuation from the theater. Taxes, too, illustrates an emphasis on doing things that are required and the personal benefit that will result. All these responses have a seemingly obsessive-compulsive diligence except that they appear exaggerated and caricatured, especially when viewed in terms of the suggestions in the scatter that we are here confronting a rather hyperalert, watchful person. The sense of caricature is especially evident on Iron in his highlighting doing what is "beneficial" and "using foresight and judgment."

On Arithmetic, he asks to have No. 7 repeated, then apologizes, saying, "I'm sorry; my mind just wandered off." On No. 9, he says "46¢, wait wait . . . 36¢, excuse me. Did you put 36 down?" Here he introduces a conspicuous mistrust of the tester, which conforms to the suggestion from scatter. (He has trouble on No. 13 ($60 less 15%), says, "I'm not too good in multiplication. Funny thing, I'm good in algebra but not in that." Is he covering up for himself by offering a positive achievement, or is he raising a real discrepancy in ability that he is trying to account for? He misses the last question (8 men—6 days) and gives 32 as his answer. ". . . 32? I ain't too sure [How did you get it?] I figured if 6 people can do a job in 6 days, multiply; that is what you said. [I said 8 men.] I multipled 8 × 2, that would cut it down to 3 days and then by 2 again and that would make it 1½ and then, oh, I got it all wrong. Forget it. Mark me wrong. [Try.] Forget it. I can't work without paper. I'm not too bright in math. [Try.] I can't, man. Hell! [You were on the right track.] 8 men 6 days. That's 8, 16, 32 . . . 36? [How'd you get that?] I just took a guess. 32 was 1½ days. I just added on an extra 4. Wait, I did it wrong again; 46. I don't know, I just took a guess. I'm not too good at this." His style of verbalization shifts here from his polite, cautious tone to a more colloquial style. He has to be kept to the task and, unlike the obsessive-compulsive person, is too ready to take flight in the face of a difficult concentration task or call for an external support (paper on which to compute his answer). Also, his avowal of not being too bright seems a way of eluding further concentration rather than a depressive revelation. Thus it appears that when pressure is put on him to concentrate he begins to get more self-critical, negativistic, escapist, and feels put upon. His statement "I can't, man. Hell!" had the sound of "What the hell are you putting me through, ease off!"

On the Story Recall, he attributes his difficulty in remembering the passage to the manner in which the tester read it to him—an externalization of his difficulty. He becomes angry and says, "If you read it faster I could repeat the whole damn thing to you." After it is reread for the delayed recall, he claims to be able to remember it better right then, but his delayed recall is also low. It is not clear why his recall is this low compared to his general intellectual level. It should be at least 4 or 5 points higher. There is little else that is suggestive of organicity in the WAIS. One possible dynamically based difficulty is manifested on Story Recall II where he refers to the man as having "sawed his finger, or hurt his finger." Perhaps it is the specific content of the story and his response to a castration theme that is here interfering with recall. Response to other more neutral passages or passages with different content would help clarify this hypothesis.

Blocks is perfect, with time bonuses on Nos. 7, 8, and 9. When he has trouble with No. 10, he claims to be getting confused, and when urged to try longer, he says, "The hell with it." Thus we see again his anger and intolerance with frustrating situations. His intellectual resources are substantial enough so that most of the test is not overly challenging to him, but when a considerable challenge is introduced there is a distinct change in his style, and his sense of frustration, anger, and avoidance comes to the fore.

Picture Arrangement sequences are all correct, with time bonuses. He quickly catches on to the cues on the back of the cards that show the tester how to put out the cards and what sequence is given. On Janet, he suspiciously asks, "Is that the comment I made that you just wrote down? [Where?] Oh forget it. I was just curious." He arranges Fish with two bonus credits, yet when asked his story he claims not to have been concentrating and as having arranged the order by the number of fish. When pressed, he says, "He was catching fish and apparently somebody was putting fish on the hook. I'm not sure. That was wrong wasn't it?" His approach to quickly and correctly arrange the cards on the basis of appropriate details but without consideration of meaning is of interest. It may be that he assumes he is wrong because of the tester's questioning, or it may be that he is revealing an aspect of his approach to situations, that he quickly may seem to size up a situation and base his behavior on certain cues while lacking full appreciation of the meaning of the situation. What seems like planning and anticipation may reflect his hyperalertness.

He defines Terminate as "start out from . . . starting position. You know, it's a place where you start." Calamity is "excitement, wait, excitement, uh, due to an incident." Compassion is "an emotion of . . . love?" His reversal of Terminate as start is unclear in meaning, but his difficulty with Calamity and Compassion reflects imprecision with emotionality. Also, he may be striving to limit aggressive themes by toning down Calamity and later restricting Ominous to "something overpowering." His definitions otherwise are generally precise and terse.

This young man is clearly possessed of superior intelligence, but it is suggested that with pressure beyond his level of facility he externalizes, becomes angry, is barely tolerant of difficulty, and takes flight. He is cautious and hyperalert and may use his superior intelligence to cover and justify himself. He presents himself as reasonable, helpful, and cooperative, but his compliance seems exaggerated, caricatured, ingratiating, and scheming. More so than some people with this kind of impulsive style, he shows anxious and depressive trends which are evident in his scatter. He shows more acknowledgment of difficulty with tasks and also does not reveal the more reckless guessing one may find with psychopathic people.

This WAIS record also illustrates the importance of attending to the various sources of information supplied by the test—to the scores, the style of verbalization, the content of responses, the relationship to the tester. For we find once again that some hypotheses are suggested more by one source than by another, or else that the convergence of impressions from different sources maximizes the strength of a particular hypothesis. His watchfulness and hyperalertness, for instance, appear at times in the content of his responses, but the extent of his hyperalertness is indicated primarily by the scatter of his subtest scores. His compliance is belied by his annoyance when tasks become difficult, but the juxtaposition of compliance (suggested by his manner) with hyperalertness (suggested by the scores) is a major lead in diagnosis. Furthermore, his high Picture Arrangement score, which by itself would suggest a high capacity for long-range planning and anticipation, is, on inspection, a consequence (at least on occasion) of a hyperalertness to immediately given specific cues rather than a necessary involvement with meanings and goals. His high Picture Arrangement score raises a larger issue discussed by Shapiro. Shapiro (1965), it will be recalled, emphasizes the psychopath's restriction of interest to what is of "immediate practical gain or advantage." According to Shapiro, excellent efficiency on a task which measures the capacity to plan action over time and to be oriented toward the future is inconsistent with the psychopathic style. My impression is that some psychopaths fit Shapiro's description, but others—like the young man under discussion—may have a more developed capacity for planning and the pursuit of long-range goals. What is unique is that the style of pursuit will be manipulation and scheming and will involve the subjugation of all aims to those of particular personal interests. Persistent, long-range wishes and goals may be present, and what looks like momentary whim or urge on surface appearance may mask chronic specific unsatisfied longings.

3.6. Hypomania

The aim of the hypomanic is to disclaim dysphoria. The psychoanalytic approach to hypomania has stressed its major reliance on defense by denial. What is essentially threatening is reversed and made unthreatening. Inasmuch as the major emphasis on denial is associated with very immature psychological development, denial is typically associated with content from the earliest psychological stages of development, especially with oral content. A regular connection with hypomanic states and underlying depression is suggested by the fact that the hypomanic style seems in all its aspects a direct refutation of essentially depressive modes of action, feelings, and ideation. If depression can be described as a preoccupation with feelings of sadness, worthlessness, self-recrimination, depletion, and decay, with limited abilities, energies, and resources, with withdrawal, apathy, or inertness, with retardation and sluggishness of thoughts and actions, then the hypomanic state is a reversal of each of these characteristics. For the hypomanic person feels happy, guiltless, full of energy and enthusiasm, unlimited in his resources, affable and extrovertish, hyperactive, and bursting with ideas and plans. His experience is playful, gay, exciting, colorful, and untroubled. The depressed person feels needy whereas the hypomanic seems overflowing with nurturance. The sense of abundance often applies to all areas including sexuality or more abstract ideation, but, whatever its content, it often turns out to represent an attempt to ward off experiences of depletion and depression. As the psychotic range of experience is approached, the hypomanic person's denials increase in intensity and unrealistically attempt to forcefully alter the perception of even unambiguously dysphoric situations to a more positive vein. With some people, the underlying depressive orientation is countered more by neutralizing it than by converting it into its opposite. Their experience will end more bland, serene, mild, and tame than exciting, boundlessly energetic, and enthusiastic. Nonetheless, even with such people, one can often view the basically unhappy feelings they are trying to deny.

387

CLINICAL
CONTRIBUTIONS OF
THE WECHSLER
ADULT
INTELLIGENCE
SCALE

Verbal Subtest	Score	Performance Subtest	Score
Comprehension	16	Picture Arrangement	9
Information	14	Picture Completion	9
Digit Span	15	Blocks	9
Arithmetic	9	Object Assembly	7
Similarities	13	Digit Symbol	9
Vocabulary	15		

Verbal IQ—121   Performance IQ—91   Story Recall I—15
Total IQ—109   Story Recall II—15

Patient is a 33-year-old married woman, the mother of two children, who is described as showing gradual diminution of outside activity over the past year, increasing feelings of inadequacy, aggression toward husband and children, many crying spells, and compulsive eating.

The discrepancy between Verbal and Performance IQ is outstanding and would most likely reflect organicity or depression. Organicity, however, would not routinely affect all Performance subtests, and, in addition, the high Digit Span and Story Recall are inconsistent with organicity. A massive interference with visual and visual-motor tasks is evident, along with a noteworthy difficulty in concentration (low Arithmetic). With Digit Span higher than Arithmetic, the out-of-pattern psychotic attention and problematic concentration are suggested. The high Comprehension indicates that, if psychosis is present, there is a strong investment in conventional judgment and understanding in contrast to more limited success in putting this understanding into practice (low Picture Arrangement). What we are left with are the possibilities of both psychosis and depression in a woman who shows a surface adherence to and interest in conventional social mores and whose concentration is likely to be disrupted. With Comprehension above Information, the possibility of repressive trends is also suggested, which would indicate that her lowered concentration reflects an avoidance of active modes of ideation.

On Information, she responds to Height with "I think she's about 5′5″, 5′6″. She's getting taller all the time, that's for sure." Her response is correct, but her verbalization implies rapid changeability (almost before one's eyes) and unlimited growth. Her tone is expansive and quite at variance with the suggestion of depression in the scatter. Although positive mood and grandiosity may be suggested, this response may also, in a negative light, reflect feelings of her experience as being unstable and rapidly fluctuating. She answers Paris correctly, but first says, "Pish-posh"—the first of various "cute" comments. Senators is also correct, but before answering she asks, "Now, today?" and again her specificity with regard to time implies a notion that things change from day to day. Of course, some things do fluctuate from day to day but the number of Senators in the United States Senate is not one of these. She is variable after question 17, which suggests an even higher intellectual potential.

On Comprehension, to Bad Company she says, "Well, I personally wouldn't enjoy it and it depends on what you mean by bad. I suppose we're influenced by it and I don't know that I would necessarily keep away." This is another correct response but one that contains the telling initial egocentricity of making her decision on the basis of enjoyment. She then goes on to acknowledge the conventional response but refuses to commit herself. She seems, therefore, to say she will base her decision

389

CLINICAL
CONTRIBUTIONS OF
THE WECHSLER
ADULT
INTELLIGENCE
SCALE

on what is fun for her, but she begrudgingly admits she recognizes the conventional response. It is in such an instance that hypomanic style is similar to impulsive style, because decisions are represented as being made in terms of immediate personal interest. Her answer to Taxes is "in order to maintain what we have and improve what we have and in order to pay for all the things within the bounds of the country we supposedly need. [What things?] Roads, seaways . . ." Foreign affairs are totally excluded in preference for domestic dealings, which express an egocentric desire to limit transactions to those which pertain to home and self. In addition, the emphasis on the bounds of the country may reflect a need to establish a firm, nonpermeable psychological boundary to counter more fluid experiences of instability and fluctuation as was suggested on Information and Comprehension (Bad Company). According to this latter view, her narcissistic concern might also stem from a wish to establish a firmer sense of her own limits and boundaries. Her reference to things that are "supposedly" needed may imply a sense of hypomanic sufficiency.

She starts out Child Labor with reference to "many *of us*" who would cruelly put children to work but quickly attempts to disassociate herself from such people by shifting instead to "many *people*." She both affirms and disclaims her view of herself as a cruel parental figure.

The Forest item is significant. "Well, if the sun sets in the west, and I know I could be helped in the west I would go, I would use the sun as a guide. I hope it is a sunny day. Or a river sometimes can be used, follow it." The sense of instability of experience hinted at previously is here given full voice in her uncertainty about where the sun will be setting. There is apparently no framework of security and reasonable expectability in this woman's life. When on City Land she talks of the "greater demand for land in the city and therefore the principles of supply and demand go up," she further elaborates her feelings of insecurity by suggesting it is the principles themselves that change rather than recognizing the operation of an invariant, stable principle. Little seems dependable and stable. On Brooks, she complains of the coldness of the room and asks if she can wear the tester's jacket. To Swallow, she says, "I've never heard of it before; it doesn't mean anything to me at all. [What might it mean?] It might mean a person swimming during summer might swallow a gulp of water but he has yet to anticipate more swallows because he has lots more swimming." She is here more in the realm of speculation because of her unfamiliarity with the proverb, and personalization therefore is more expectable. Her response involves a disrupted oral state, a succession of unpleasant oral intakes, a sense of relentless oral misery. Intake is not insufficient but is rather a surfeit of discomfort. The oral interpretation of Swallow is a frequent hallmark of depressive and hypomanic preoccupation. Her comment about feeling cold and needing the tester's warmth seems depressive, but she more actively requests help than depressed people usually do. She may be able to request the jacket because she externalizes blame for her experience of coldness onto the tester ("Couldn't you have picked a warmer spot for these tests?"). Thus she may be indicating that she is a person who may actively seek consolation only when she can externalize the source of a need.

She has considerable trouble after the ninth Arithmetic problem, needs repetition of questions, claims she does not know how to figure out the problems, feels lost, and tries to "give up," but with pressure she continues to work and gets two answers overtime with encouragement from the tester to be persistent. Given difficulty, she needs encouragement to persist and is compliant with external demands.

On Similarities, she relates air and water as ". . . free, no that's not the way. Nature's elements. [What did you mean by free?] Boundless quantities of air and water, salt water anyway, yeah fresh water too." Freedom and "boundless quantities" are distinctly hypomanic in quality, with the emphasis on excess as opposed to depressive lack and depletion. Her experience thus far shows primarily hypomanic (including narcissistic) features and also depressive elements such as the gulps of water (on Similarities) that intrude into the pleasant summer of swimming. On Forest, she could also only voice hope for a sunny day. A confirmed depressive would assume gloominess, and a thoroughgoing hypomanic would assume an optimistic position. She shows instead a more depressively toned desire for pleasantness and a basic unsureness as to what each day will bring. She introduces the theme of "durability" when relating Poem and Statue, which takes us back to her earlier concern with the stability, reliability, and trustworthiness of experience. One wonders at this point what sort of person it is whose visual and visual-motor efficiency is generally retarded, who emphasizes her personal enjoyment in situations of morality, who represents much of experience as unstable and undependable, who shows disrupted oral imagery, and who is simultaneously oriented toward boundless, unlimited quantities of things. A purely depressed person would not emphasize enjoyment or expansively highlight limitless amounts of anything (except misery). Nor would a depressed person dwell so much on the undependability of experience, since gloominess would regularly be expected. Rather, a person who emphasizes unpredictability would experience unpredictability both in her sense of herself and in her sense of things external to her. Most probably, she would be unable to anticipate how she would feel at any time. In this regard, might her low Picture Arrangement score also reflect her limited capacity to experience continuity over time and to plan ahead? Inasmuch as a major aspect of unpredictability is likely to be inconsistency in the anticipation of affective experience, the variable indications of mood in this WAIS record, narcissistic at one moment and expansive, depressive, or externalizing at other times, would be concomitant to the general emphasis on instability and unreliability in her experience.

Her next response of interest is to Fly and Tree, which she describes as "something man isn't responsible for, something nature created, not man created." Why does she show a need to excuse man from responsibility unless she is somehow preoccupied with the issue of responsibility? A speculation here—in view of her earlier disapproval of cruelty toward children—is that issues of responsibility regarding what one creates (one's offspring) are distressing to her and that an aspect of depressive, guilty concerns may revolve around her relationship with her children. Her way of dealing with such issues may be less a guilty depressive style than unstable efforts to disclaim responsibility.

Her Story Recall is efficient, but before the passage is read she asks like a little girl if it is a bedtime story. Before Blocks, she asks if there is a manicurist available and is described by the tester as excited and childlike, but this hypomanic quality is offset on the last design by her statement that she is exhausted.

Her last arrangement on Picture Arrangement (Taxi) is of interest. She describes the man as seeing someone watching and therefore moving the bust away, but when he looks back again and sees no one watching he brings it close to him out of a "sense of propriety." The concern here is primarily on an externally derived source of standards of behavior. As long as no one is looking, she will feel free to do as she pleases. Other verbalizations are also consistent with narcissistic and egocentric features.

391

CLINICAL
CONTRIBUTIONS OF
THE WECHSLER
ADULT
INTELLIGENCE
SCALE

For example, she states, on Object Assembly, "Come on fellows, this is silly" and when asked the meaning of Plagiarize she comments in a naive, unrealistic, cute way, "That's not nice" before offering a definition.

Thus we see here a woman who shows many clearly hypomanic features but who does not sustain a hypomanic position. Instead, depressive aspects are evident both in the scatter of her subtest scores and in the content of some of her verbalizations. Trends toward externalization are also present. The degree of her instability around experience that ought to be regular and dependable and her degree of ambiguity in this regard suggest sufficient disarticulation with external events to warrant a diagnosis of at least borderline psychotic trends. Moreover, one can see the various ways in which the hypomanic style overlaps with the impulsive style. For, despite her depressive tone, at times she by contrast appears actively oriented toward action based on personal gain and fun, especially as long as no one is looking. She suggests therefore that her experience of morality is not bound up with strict, internalized standards that operate relatively independently. Her ethics emphasize the narcissistic gratification of more immediate aims and pleasures. In view of her experience of instability, however, her moods are likely to fluctuate widely, and feelings of positive experience may be fleeting and transient.

4. Conclusion

I have attempted here to discuss the Wechsler Scales from the point of view of their role in diagnostic assessment. All diagnostic possibilities have not been covered; rather, the highlights of some of the major diagnostic classifications have been presented. Inasmuch as the tester's theory regarding personality organization and the tester's view of diagnostic categories have a thoroughgoing effect on the sense he will make out of test responses, I have tried to be as clear as possible about my own views, their origin in psychoanalytic ego psychology, and the influence on them of recent trends in psychoanalytic theorizing. I have also stressed the necessary reliance on all aspects of test data—scores, style and content of response, and interpersonal test behavior. With that end in mind, specific cases have been selected, some of which lack consistency in their varied sources of data, in order to demonstrate the process of integrating diverse information into a coherent picture. The primary focus must always be on the characteristics of the person who would give these particular test results. Inconsistencies among scatter of scores, style of response, and content do not invalidate the importance of each of these, but rather present a task for clinical conceptualization and integration.

ACKNOWLEDGMENTS

I am grateful to George H. Davis, Ph.D., and Millicent Allison, M.S., for their comments. The Yale Psychiatric Institute also generously made its test material and resources available for preparation of this chapter.

5. References

Allison, J., Blatt, S. J., & Zimet, C. N. *The interpretation of psychological tests.* New York: Harper & Row, 1967.

Apfelbaum, B. On ego psychology: A critique of the structural approach to psycho-analytic theory. *International Journal of Psychoanalysis*, 1966, *47*, 451–475.

Blanck, G., & Blanck, R. *Ego psychology: Theory and practice*. New York: Columbia University Press, 1974.

Blatt, S. J., & Allison, J. The intelligence test in personality assessment. In A. I. Rabin (Ed.), *Projective techniques in personality assessment*. New York: Springer, 1968.

Blatt, S. J., Wild, C. M., & Ritzler, B. A. Disturbances of object representations in schizophrenia. *Psychoanalysis and Contemporary Science*, 1975, *4*, 235–288.

Bleuler, E. *Dimentia praecox or the group of schizophrenias*. New York: International Universities Press, 1950.

Boyer, L. B. Comparisons of the Shamans and pseudo-Shamans of the Apaches of the Mescalero Indian Reservation: A Rorschach study. *Journal of Projective Techniques*, 1964, *28*, 173–180.

Diagnostic and statistical manual of mental disorders (2nd ed.). Washington, D.C.: American Psychiatric Association, 1968.

Gunderson, J. G., & Mosher, L. R. (Eds.). *Psychotherapy of schizophrenia*. New York: Jason Aronson Press, 1975.

Hartmann, H. *Ego psychology and the problem of adaptation*. New York: International Universities Press, 1958.

Klein, G. S. *Psychoanalytic theory: An exploration of essentials*. New York: International Universities Press, 1976.

Mayman, M., Schafer, R., & Rapaport, D. Interpretation of the Wechsler-Bellevue Intelligence Scale and personality appraisal. In H. H. Anderson & G. L. Anderson (Eds.), *An introduction to projective techniques*. New York: Prentice-Hall, 1951.

McFie, J. *Assessment of organic intellectual impairment*. New York: Academic Press, 1975.

Rapaport, D. The autonomy of the ego. *Bulletin of the Menninger Clinic*, 1951, *15*, 113–124.

Rapaport, D. The theory of ego autonomy: A generalization. *Bulletin of the Menninger Clinic*, 1958, *22*, 13–35.

Rapaport, D., Gill, M., & Schafer, R. *Diagnostic psychological testing* (Vol. 1). Chicago: Year Book Publishers, 1945.

Rapaport, D., Gill, M., & Schafer, R. *Diagnostic psychological testing* (Vol. 2). Chicago: Year Book Publishers, 1946.

Schachtel, E. G. *Experiential foundations of Rorschach's test*. New York: Basic Books, 1966.

Schafer, R. *The clinical application of psychological tests*. New York: International Universities Press, 1948.

Schafer, R. *Psychoanalytic interpretation in Rorschach testing*. New York: Grune & Stratton, 1954.

Schafer, R. The mechanisms of defense. *International Journal of Psychoanalysis*, 1968, *49*, 49–62.

Schafer, R. Action: Its place in psychoanalytic interpretation and theory. *The Annual of Psychoanalysis*, 1973, *1*, 159–196.

Shapiro, D. Special problems of testing borderline psychotics. *Journal of Projective Techniques*, 1954, *18*, 387–394.

Shapiro, D. *Neurotic styles*. New York: Basic Books, 1965.

Shapiro, D. Motivation and action in psychoanalytic psychiatry. *Psychiatry*, 1970, *33*, 329–343.

Talland, N. *Deranged memory*. New York: Academic Press, 1965.

Tarachow, S. *An introduction to psychotherapy*. New York: International Universities Press, 1963.

Waite, R. R. The intelligence test as a psychodiagnostic instrument. *Journal of Projective Techniques*, 1961, *25*, 90–102.

Wechsler, D. *The measurement of adult intelligence*. Baltimore: Williams & Wilkins, 1944.

13

Diagnostic Applications of the Hand Test

EDWIN E. WAGNER

1. Introduction

The Hand Test, a comparatively new projective technique, probably owes its clinical utility to the following practical features: simplicity of stimulus material, brevity of administration and scoring, and amenability to straightforward validation. The test was first introduced in the form of a research monograph as a promising technique for predicting overt aggressive behavior (Bricklin, Piotrowski, & Wagner, 1962), but it soon became apparent that the instrument was suitable for general diagnostic purposes, and a Hand Test "kit" was put together, made up of the stimulus cards, manual, and scoring tablet (Wagner, 1962b).

The stimuli consist of ten cards approximately $3\frac{1}{2}$ by $4\frac{1}{2}$ inches in size. Nine of the cards portray simple line drawings of a hand in various ambiguous poses; the last (tenth) card is blank. Reviewers have commented on the roughness of the renditions, but experience has shown that the artistic crudity actually has clinical merit: normal subjects ignore the imperfections, while critical comments, when they do occur, are apt to be evinced by negative or obsessive individuals.

The testee is handed the cards one at a time, right side up, and is simply requested to "Tell me what it looks like the hand could be doing." When the last (blank) card is turned over, the subject is asked to "Imagine a hand and tell me what it might be doing." If only one response is given to the first card, the subject is prompted with "Anything else?" If a hand is merely acknowledged or described, then the first time this occurs the subject is reminded of the instructions with "What is it doing?" If the subject cannot muster any response at all to a particular card, then, just once, he is asked "Can you take a guess?" It is always permissible to ask for further elaboration or explanation of a response with "Can you explain that?" or "Can you tell me more?" The initial reaction times to each card and the responses themselves are copied verbatim on the special answer sheet or on any convenient piece of paper. Following

EDWIN E. WAGNER • Psychology Department, University of Akron, Akron, Ohio 44325.

the administration, the responses are scored and summarized. Median administration time is approximately 10 min, and scoring takes about another 5 min.

2.1. Basic Rationale and Scoring

The Hand Test was first developed in an attempt to reveal, for all subjects, tendencies associated with the Rorschach human movement or *M* response. Piotrowski had specified that the Rorschach *M* represents prototypal actions which are apt to be expressed in behavior (Piotrowski, 1957, p. 141). However, not everyone produces *M* on the Rorschach, although the great majority of people *do* behave. Therefore, it seemed advantageous to construct a projective technique which would directly epitomize the kind of behavior people habitually display. After the test was tried on a number of nonplussed human guinea pigs (mostly patients, associates, and relatives), it became obvious that the stimuli did evoke tendencies close to the motor system, so much so that actions involving "things" as well as people were easily obtained. It was also noted that, at times, difficulty in effectively relating to people and/or things due to incapacity of the hand and/or inhospitable environmental circumstances was projected; furthermore, some subjects, usually patients, were unable to come up with meaningful action tendency at all, merely describing the hand, visualizing bizarre percepts which were not in fact hands, or failing to respond at all. Therefore, on both logical and empirical grounds, the following four major scoring categories were derived: Interpersonal responses (INT) involving relations with other people, Environmental responses (ENV) representing actions directed toward impersonal objects, Maladjustive responses (MAL) reflecting difficulty in successfully carrying out various action tendencies because of internal weaknesses or external difficulties, and Withdrawal responses (WITH) representing an inability to relate to the personal or impersonal world in a meaningful and effective manner. Therefore, the Hand Test can be precisely defined as a projective technique which elicits responses connoting the presence or absence of various prototypal action tendencies necessary for relating to the world of reality.

The four major scoring categories were further subdivided into 15 basic scores to further refine the action tendencies manifested by a given subject so that personality descriptions could be individualized and differential diagnosis maximized. As is always the case when an attempt is made to reduce the implications and nuances of projective responses to a set of scores, a compromise had to be achieved: too few scores would fail to take advantage of the diagnostic potential of the instrument; too many notations could become cumbersome and prohibitively difficult to learn. The final 15 scores were compromises arrived at on the basis of conceptual clarity, general familiarity (e.g., many of the terms are similar to those associated with the Thematic Apperception Test), and differential implications for understanding personality and predicting behavior. The 15 categories are as follows:

A. Interpersonal
   1. Affection (AFF): Interpersonal responses involving the interchange or bestowment of pleasure, affection, or friendly feeling, e.g., "Shaking hands with an old friend."
   2. Dependence (DEP): Interpersonal responses which express or imply the reception of or need for succor, e.g., "A beggar asking for a handout."
   3. Communication (COM): Interpersonal responses in which information

is expressed or exchanged either verbally or by gesture, e.g., "Telling some-body where a certain classroom is located."

4. Exhibition (EXH): Interpersonal responses which stress some positive attribute of the hand (or the action) and which involve a display or per-formance which elicits attention, e.g., "A rich lady holding her hand out to be kissed."

5. Direction (DIR): Interpersonal responses which dominate or directively influence the activities of others, e.g., "A policeman giving a command."

6. Aggression (AGG): Interpersonal responses where pain, hostility, or ag-gression is dealt to others, e.g., "Punching somebody in the mouth."

B. Environmental

1. Acquisition (ACQ): Environmental responses involving an attempt to acquire an object or goal where the issue is still somewhat in doubt and/or an unusual expenditure of energy is required, e.g., "Jumping up to catch hold of a tree branch."

2. Active (ACT): Environmental responses involving the construction, manipulation, or attainment of a goal or an object. ACT responses are distinguished from ACQ responses in that the object or goal has been (or will be) accomplished with a normal expenditure of effort and the issue is not in doubt, e.g., "Pulling a lever on a machine."

3. Passive (PAS): Environmental responses involving an attitude of rest and/or relaxation and an appropriate temporary withdrawal of energy from the hand, e.g., "Like someone fell asleep in an armchair and their hand is just hanging down."

C. Maladjustive

1. Tension (TEN): Energy is exerted but little or nothing is being accom-plished, accompanied by a feeling of anxiety, strain, or malaise, e.g., "Person is nervous and is clenching her fist."

2. Crippled (CRIP): The hand is unable to deal effectively with the world because it is crippled, sore, dead, disfigured, sick, injured, or incapacitated, e.g., "That hand's got arthritis."

3. Fear (FEAR): The hand is threatened with or is receiving pain, injury, incapacitation, or destruction from another person. A FEAR is also scored if the hand is seen as meting out aggression to an imaginary person with whom the testee clearly identifies, e.g., "Person is about to get hit and she's raising her hand helplessly."

D. Withdrawal

1. Description (DES): There is no action tendency imparted but, instead, the hand is merely acknowledged, with perhaps a few accompanying in-consequential details or feeling tones, e.g., "That's just a hand, palm up."

2. Failure (FAIL): No scorable response is given to a particular card. A FAIL is tabulated in computing summary scoring but is not included in the response total, R.

3. Bizarre (BIZ): The subject "sees" something other than a hand, e.g., "An octopus," or projects a response of unusual and idiosyncratic mor-bidity, e.g., "Smashed to smithereens with blood dripping out."

After the responses have been scored, they are summarized and integrated into the following major scoring categories: ΣINT, the sum of AFF + DEP + COM +

EXH + DIR + AGG; ΣENV, the sum of ACQ + ACT + PAS; ΣMAL, the sum of TEN + CRIP + FEAR; ΣWITH, the sum of DES + FAIL + BIZ; R, the sum of all scoring categories minus the number of FAILS; AIRT, the sum of all initial reaction times to the cards divided by the number of cards responded to; H − L, the lowest initial reaction time subtracted from the highest; PATH (Pathology score), the sum of MAL + 2 times the sum of WITH (MAL + 2 WITH); ER (Experience ratio), the ratios among the sums of Interpersonal, Environmental, Maladjustive, and Withdrawal scores (ΣINT : ΣENV : ΣMAL : ΣWITH); and the AOR (Acting-Out Ratio), which is the ratio of Affection, Dependency, and Communication responses to the Direction and Aggression responses: (AFF + DEP + COM) : (DIR + AGG).

In all, then, there are 15 scoring categories which are converted to 10 additional summary scores. With experience, the process becomes automatic and seldom takes more than 5 min.

Some psychologists have felt the need to provide further scoring annotation in order to call attention to qualitative nuances of diagnostic import. Again, the question arises as to how much to score and how much to leave to the clinician's tacit evaluation. For those who prefer further scoring refinements, a variety of "content" scores were developed. These scores can be placed in parentheses alongside any of the original 15 scoring categories, where applicable, but are not included in the summary scoring. The psychological implications of these parenthesized scores, like the regular Hand Test variables, are obvious to the sophisticated clinician. A list of the more popular parenthesized content scores is presented below:

1. Sexual (SEX), e.g., "Well, looks like a hand reaching for a woman's breast. (Q) To grab a feel."
2. Immature (IM), e.g., "A mother taking her little child by the hand to lead him across the street."
3. Inanimate (INAN), e.g., "Looks like the hand of God giving life to Adam in that painting."
4. Hiding (HID), e.g., "Covering something with his palm so you can't see it."
5. Sensual (SEN), e.g., "Been crushing grapes and the hand is covered with sediment."
6. Cylindrical (CYL), e.g., "Has something long and round in his hand like a pipe."
7. Denial (DEN), e.g., "Would be shaking hands except that it is the wrong hand."
8. Ambivalent (AMB), e.g., "Look's like he's hitting someone but there's not too much force to it."
9. Movement (MOV), e.g., "Just shaking his hand up and down. (Q) For no reason, just doing it."
10. Orality (ORAL), e.g., "Drinking a glass of water."
11. Gross (GROSS), e.g., "Smashing a dude over the head with a rock."
12. Emotion (EMO), e.g., "Thrusting his hand out to shake—he's just busting with joy to see his friend again."
13. Original (O). This auxiliary score is reserved for responses which are appropriate as well as "different" and does not include percepts which are highly idiosyncratic or bizarre. The implication of an "original" is that the respondent is both bright and creative. Diagnosticians should refrain from scoring an O until they have administered many protocols and have a "feel" for what constitutes a truly original response.

This list is partial and somewhat arbitrary, and additional parenthesized scores could easily be added according to taste if they serve to call attention to relevant clinical nuances. It is also permissible to parenthesize any one of the regular scoring categories where significant overlap in meaning occurs. For example, the response "He's shaking his fist at someone to tell 'em he's gonna hit 'em" could be scored AGG (COM) since the intent is primarily aggressive, but communication is also involved. In this case, as with other parenthesized scores, the (COM) would not be included in the summary scoring.

3. Norms, Reliability, Validity, and Clinical Usefulness

When the Hand Test Manual was first published, it contained norms on 1020 cases, including normal adults, Air Force pilots, college students, student nurses, high school students, children, schizophrenics, patients with organic psychoses, neurotics, depressed patients, mental retardates, male parolees, male prisoners, female prisoners, and delinquents. By the time the third edition of the manual was published, thanks to many contributors throughout the world, an additional 1628 cases were reported in the appendix covering imbeciles, morons, three separate groups of normal children, technical high school boys from Australia, dyslexic children, three separate groups of delinquents, engineers and technicians, Guamanians, Japanese junior high school students, inpatients from a receiving hospital, neurologically handicapped children, and an entire police department. Admittedly, this rather heterogeneous assemblage of normative groups falls short of the ideal random or stratified-random sampling advocated by statistical textbooks, and much remains to be done. Still, the Hand Test must be considered among the best-normed projective techniques, particularly when its relatively young age is taken into account.

Surprisingly, there have been few reliability studies on the Hand Test. The manual reports interscorer reliabilities of from .86 to .92, and split-half reliabilities of from .84 to .85 computed against the PATH score (which is reasonably parametric), and percentages of interscorer agreement on all scoring categories varying from 78% to 83%. Ronald K. Andrea, a school psychologist whose study is summarized in the appendix of the manual, reports agreement between two independent scorers of 86%. It has been the author's experience that well-trained graduate students will consistently produce agreements in the 80% range and that disagreements, when they occur, tend to be within rather than between major scoring categories. For example, it is more likely to find a disagreement in scoring a response an ACT or an ACQ, both ENV, than an ACT or an AGG, which would entail cutting across the ENV and INT major scoring categories.

In order to objectively assess the validity of the Hand Test, the author made an attempt to survey the literature, coming up with a total of 56 studies, 42 originating in the United States and 14 of foreign origin. Of the 56 studies, 16 involved either a description of the test or a presentation of its usefulness in a diagnostic setting, while 40 were directly concerned with issues of validity. Of these 40, a total of 35 revealed positive findings while five reported negative results, which means that over 87% of the validity studies have been in the predicted direction. This enviable track record is, however, mitigated by the fact that the author of the test has a hand (no pun intended) in 30 studies reported in the literature. Obviously, more independent verification would be desirable.

Because of its brevity, simplicity, and nonthreatening nature, the Hand Test has proved amenable for administration to subjects belonging to a diversity of ages and nosological groupings. It has been administered, for example, to children (Selg, 1965), juvenile delinquents (Azcarate & Gutierrez, 1969), old persons (Panek, Sterns, & Wagner, 1976), mental retardates (Wagner & Capotosto, 1966), deaf persons (Levine & Wagner, 1974), schizophrenics (Fornari & Gasca, 1971), neurotics (Wagner, 1962a), drug users (Wagner & Romanik, 1976), karate students (Greene, Sawicki, & Wagner, 1974), policemen (Rand & Wagner, 1973), and hypnotized subjects (Hodge & Wagner, 1964).

While no scientific data have been assembled on the extent to which the Hand Test is actually being employed in diagnostic practice, it does appear to be gaining in popularity, and it seems appropriate at this juncture to list some caveats governing its use.

1. The test is intended for use as part of a battery. It can serve as a short screening technique and/or an interview supplement when necessary but is much more effective when integrated into the context of a general assessment battery.
2. Experience has indicated that the Hand Test measures what it purports to measure, i.e., prototypal action tendencies. While there is often "bleed-through" from other aspects of the psyche such as intellect and emotion, the test is limited in scope and does not reflect the "whole personality."
3. While the test is in some ways ideal for children, who often treat it as a game, it should not be used below the age of 6. From 6 to puberty, the interpretive implications of the responses are the same as with adults (although the total number of R's tends, on the average, to be fewer with children), but under 6 the relationships among scoring categories are altered and meaningful interpretation breaks down.
4. The Hand Test is deceptively simple, and neophytes can lose sight of the fact that it is a projective technique and that optimum interpretation requires knowledge of personality dynamics, clinical insight, and a good bit of experience with the instrument.
5. The total number of responses is diagnostically significant, but it is also sensitive to the way the test is administered. Therefore, the examiner should be careful not to deviate from the basic rules of administration presented in the manual.
6. Personality disorders can present an intact picture on the Hand Test, particularly if interpretation is confined to quantitative scoring. Qualitative analysis often reveals the typical superficiality of the personality disorder, along with other telltale nuances which can help in making a differential diagnosis; but experience and expertise are required to make this discrimination.

4. Basic Interpretation: The Characteristic Features of Normals, Neurotics, Schizophrenics, Organics, and Subjects with Personality Disorders

Normal, reasonably intelligent adults produce an average of about 15 responses to the Hand Test. Anywhere from 10 to 25 responses is within the normal range. R's under 10 or over 30 are definitely abnormal. Underproduction of R is indicative of a lack of behavior resources and is found mostly in organics, retardates, and custodial schizophrenics. An overproduction of R is indicative of serious compulsivity, often overlying an organic or schizophrenic condition. The ideally adjusted adult would have no MAL, no WITH, about 60% INT, and about 40% ENV. He should produce at least 5 INT responses distributed throughout no less than three scoring categories and a minimum of 3 ENV responses, mostly ACT. His AIRT should be between 10 and 20 sec, and his H − L should be 20 or less. Our paragon of adjustment would have a 0 PATH score, and his AOR would be approximately balanced. If there is an imbalance in the AOR, it should be in favor of the responses which are positively oriented toward people (AFF, DEP, COM) rather than those which are designed to manipulate (DIR) or hurt (AGG) others. This is not to say that DIR or AGG is necessarily unhealthy, but, other things being equal, it is easier to get along when one relates to others with warmth, deference, or a willingness to communicate. Qualitatively, there should be no "time shocks" (unusually long initial response times to any of the cards) and the responses themselves should be clearly articulated and of reasonable length. Neither short, "skeletal" reactions nor long, idiosyncratic, highly embellished descriptions are desirable. The former are characteristic of organics, retardates, long-term schizophrenics, and subjects with personality disorders; the latter are frequently found in certain neurotic, schizoid, and borderline types.

The protocol of AB, a 29-year-old, single woman, is an example of a reasonably normal Hand Test. AB is a college graduate and a librarian. She had no history of mental problems, she appeared to be well adjusted, and she certainly did not feel that she was suffering from any emotional difficulties when tested. AB had been recruited to take part in research involving driver safety and consented to take the Hand Test as part of an additional normative study.

AB produces 16 responses, none of them with MAL or WITH. She shows 4 INT and her AOR is fairly balanced. Her ENV is greater than her INT, which is a little unusual, and, in light of her 8 ACT responses, indicative of a good energy level and perhaps some compulsivity. Her AIRT is also a little fast, presenting a picture of a woman who reacts quickly, energetically, and maybe compulsively to environmental challenges—not bad attributes for a librarian. Qualitatively, there are a number of interesting features to her protocol (for example, the response to Card IX), but the record is essentially within the range of normality and provides a general idea of what can be expected from adjusted subjects.

The possibilities of individual variations within the quantitative parameters of normality are, of course, astronomical, and they allow for differential personality appraisals of individuals free of psychopathology. Furthermore, even when signs of maladjustment appear, such as a TEN or a CRIP, the personality is not necessarily "abnormal," especially when compensatory "healthy" features are present. As a rule, a protocol with a goodly number of responses would be preferable to one with a paucity of R, because, within limits, the greater the psychological energy available for behavior, the greater the adjustive potential. Other things being equal, a MAL of 3 would have more serious implications if the R were 10 than if it were 20.

To oversimplify, the normal protocol shades into a neurotic record as the amount of energy available for behaving falls off, producing a proportionate rise in MAL and sometimes DES. Neurotics tend to give more MAL and also less ENV than normal subjects. "Shocks" in the form of long initial reaction times to certain cards (and a resultant high H − L score) are common. DES or FAIL could occur, but two or more such responses increase the possibility that the condition is more serious than a neurosis. Since most neuroses are somewhat "mixed," any of the MAL scores

*To aid in recording, the following standard abbreviations can be used, most of them already familiar to the reader who has worked with the Rorschach or T.A.T.:

   ⑤   Subject turns card.

   V   Card held upside down.

   <   Top of card turned to the left.

   >   Top of card turned to the right.

a.t.e. Examiner asks, "Anything else?"

 (Q)   Examiner asks a question.

  E   Subject emulates the card with his own hand.

  D   Subject demonstrates his response with his own hand.

  ✔   A "check" can be placed beside a score to show that it is a repetition of or similar to a previous response. "Repetitions" are often indicative of retardation and/or organic brain syndromes.

_____ Words or phrases of particular import can be underlined for future reference.

could be expected; but, as a general rule, CRIP is associated with feelings of inferiority, TEN with anxiety and/or tension, and FEAR with apprehension over aggression (either external or internal), a condition more typical of conversion hysteria. INT holds up well, as does R: the total amount of psychological energy available to the neurotic does not decrease; it becomes blocked or dissipated, resulting in a rise in MAL. The neurotic's sensitivity to people remains constant or may even increase, hence INT usually does not suffer; but the neurotic's environmental efficiency often falls off, a phenomenon reflected in a reduction in ENV.

Clues to the nature of the neurotic's difficulties can often be adduced from shocks to various cards, which could take the form of long reaction times, hesitancies, obvious discomfort with the image, and the projective implications of the response itself. Each card does have its own "pull"; therefore, symbolic interpretations and differential analyses of shock, pacing, and sequencing should take into account the card characteristics listed in Table 1.

CD exemplifies a serious neurotic condition. CD is a 13-year-old boy who was rejected by his peers and who left a plaintive note on his mother's bureau stating that he was "queer." The Hand Test indicates a severe neurosis and a decided sexual problem, a diagnosis confirmed by the psychiatrist to whom the boy was subsequently referred for psychotherapy. Note that, out of ten responses, there are 5 MAL—a pronounced obstruction of productive psychological processes. The ENV category is seriously depressed, and the H − L score is indicative of neurotic shock. The long reaction time plus the qualitative shock to card IX is clearly indicative of a psycho-

CARD	IRT	HAND TEST RESPONSES	SCORE
I	4	Telling someone to stop. (a.t.e.?)	DIR
		Closing a door.	ACT
II	3	Getting ready to catch a ball.	ACT (ACQ)
III	2	Pointing. (Q) The way to go.	COM
		Or ready to ring a doorbell.	ACT (COM)
IV	4	Getting ready to pat a little boy on the head.	AFF (IM)
		Looks like he's getting ready to pick up something like a telephone.	ACT (COM)
V	12	This hand is at leisure-- resting.	PAS
VI	5	Ready to pound something. (Q) Like making something.	ACT
		Punch someone.	AGG
VII	3	Shaking hands. Or holding his hand out to help someone.	AFF / AFF (DEP) (AMB)
		Karate chop.	AGG
VIII	2	Going to pick something up. (Q) A pencil.	ACT
IX	10	This person is about to receive a secretly passed note. They have their hand behind their back to take it.	ACT (COM,HID)
X	12	Hands making something. (Q) With tools. Making a bird house.	ACT (CYL)

sexual conflict, and the TEN on card X probably reflects the boy's awareness of and consternation over neurotic problems with which he cannot cope.

While the neurotic's action tendencies are restricted, his orientation toward the world is at least reality-oriented as attested to by responses which are appropriate and conform to the contours of the drawn hands. In contradistinction, the reactions of the schizophrenic to the Hand Test connote a lack of reality contact which

The Hand Test

SUMMARY SHEET

by Edwin E. Wagner, Ph.D.

PUBLISHED BY

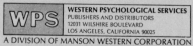

WESTERN PSYCHOLOGICAL SERVICES
PUBLISHERS AND DISTRIBUTORS
12031 WILSHIRE BOULEVARD
LOS ANGELES, CALIFORNIA 90025

A DIVISION OF MANSON WESTERN CORPORATION

DATE 3/5/76

NAME AB   SEX F   AGE 29   RACE W

ADDRESS 111 Merry Lane

OCCUPATION Librarian   DIAGNOSIS Normal

AFF = 3	ACQ = 0	TEN = 0	DES = 0	R = 16
DEP = 0	ACT = 8	CRIP = 0	FAIL = 0	AIRT = 5.7
COM = 1	PAS = 1	FEAR = 0	BIZ = 0	H-L = 10.0
EXH = 0	Σ ENV = 9	Σ MAL = 0	Σ WITH = 0	PATH = 0
DIR = 1				
AGG = 2	ER = Σ INT: Σ ENV: Σ MAL: Σ WITH = 7 : 9 : 0 : 0			
Σ INT = 7	AOR = (AFF + DEP + COM):(DIR + AGG) = 4 : 3			

QUALITATIVE ADMINISTRATIVE OBSERVATIONS Cooperative; business-like

CASE HISTORY AND DIAGNOSTIC DATA

EXAMINER P. Panek

can be manifested in a variety of ways depending on the progress of the psychotic process. Long-term, "burnt-out," chronic schizophrenics tend to produce a paucity of responses composed mainly of the short DES but also sometimes showing BIZ and FAIL. In the extreme, the records of this "type" tend to resemble those of patients with severe organic impairment. In periods of relative remission, the responses,

Table 1. Card Characteristics

Card No.	"Pull"	Symbolic meaning
I	DIR, COM, AFF	Reactions to new situations
II	ACT, ACQ	Possible neurotic shock
III	COM, DIR, ACT	An "easy" card and a FAIL is pernicious
IV	No strong pull	"Father" card; masculinity; aggression
V	ENV	Possible neurotic shock; attitudes toward passivity
VI	AGG, ACT	Attitudes toward aggression
VII	No strong pull	May be a reaction to the aggression elicited on VI
VIII	ACT	An "easy" card (like III) and a FAIL here is therefore serious
IX	ACT	Psychosexual implications; but be careful because it is also a "difficult" card
X	No strong pull	Readiness to bring into play imaginal resources; conception of one's future role in life

while bordering on descriptions, may be nominally scorable, and, in terms of strictly quantitative indices, the protocol could seem "normal." It takes a little experience to get used to this stylistic feature because it is the qualitative weakness, even more marked than the bland responsivity characteristic of the personality disorder, which is the critical factor in making the differential diagnosis. Occasionally, emotionally impoverished schizophrenics can produce records with little or no INT but with a high ACT score, reflecting a compulsive attachment to things instead of people which permits them to retain a circumscribed relationship to the environment.

Another kind of schizophrenic record, much more obvious and a good deal more interesting, is the "blatant" type—so named because aberrated thinking is projected directly onto the stimulus cards. This "type" is associated mainly with ambulatory, paranoid, and fulminating types of schizophrenics who are actively hallucinating and/or thoroughly enmeshed in delusional processes, and is characterized by one or more of the following: genuine BIZ; embellished and idiosyncratic DES; dysphoric and/or morbid subject matter; and a combination of both MAL and WITH, which usually results in a high PATH. EF has produced such a protocol. She is a 20-year-old, single female with a high school education who has been hospitalized three times with a repeated diagnosis of schizophrenia. When tested, she was being seen for psychotherapy on an outpatient basis. She spoke in a barely audible whisper, claiming she had laryngitis; yet, at times, her voice sounded quite normal. She earned a FS WAIS IQ of 113, which could well be potentially higher judging from some of the interesting percepts, including an "original," which she produced on the Hand Test. EF's protocol is unmistakably schizophrenic, with 4 genuine BIZ responses, an odd DES which borders on a BIZ, a generally idiosyncratic tone throughout the entire protocol (there is hardly a percept which is not different in some way from a "normal" or "popular" response), and the high PATH score. In general (if benchmarks are desired), a PATH of 3 can be considered indicative of at least some psychopathology, while a PATH of 10 or over is very serious. There is no doubt that EF is seriously disturbed.

It is obvious that, for the type of schizophrenia represented by EF, the Hand Test cards merely serve as triggers which readily release pathological processes. The subject uses the stimulus as a highly plastic medium which he drastically molds to represent his own autistic view of the world. Little attention is paid to the sub-

CARD	IRT	HAND TEST RESPONSES	SCORE
I	6	Saying stop. (a.t.e) Don't think so.	DIR
II	19	Got cut or something. He's in pain.	CRIP (TEN)
III	2	Giving a direction. (Q) Telling somebody to go someplace.	DIR
IV	12	Reaching out to grab something. (Q) Anything.	ACQ
V	16	Show deadness. No life in it.	CRIP
VI	5	Holding his grip: trying to control his anger (E).	TEN
VII	4	Ready to shake hands with another person.	AFF
VIII	6	Just got done snapping his fingers. (Q) Nervous I guess.	TEN
IX	54	I don't know... Kinda funny... This guy looks like he's saying stop too... But I don't know...	DIR (AMB)
X	10	Scratching. (Q) My head. (Q) Thinking... got a problem.	TEN (PERS)

stance inherent in the drawings themselves. The act of projection is schizophrenically creative inasmuch as the final product is subjective, original, and often symbolically pregnant with meaning, but it is simply too far divorced from reality to have coinage for concourse based on consensual validation.

The patient suffering from an organic brain syndrome usually exhibits a com-

The Hand Test

SUMMARY SHEET

by Edwin E. Wagner, Ph.D.

PUBLISHED BY

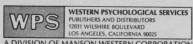

WPS WESTERN PSYCHOLOGICAL SERVICES
PUBLISHERS AND DISTRIBUTORS
12031 WILSHIRE BOULEVARD
LOS ANGELES, CALIFORNIA 90025

A DIVISION OF MANSON WESTERN CORPORATION

DATE **14/2/65**

NAME **CD**   SEX **M**   AGE **13**   RACE **W**

ADDRESS **222 Maple Rd.**

OCCUPATION **student**   DIAGNOSIS **Neurotic**

AFF = 1	ACQ = 1	TEN = 3	DES = 0	R = 10
DEP = 0	ACT = 0	CRIP = 2	FAIL = 0	AIRT = 13.4
COM = 0	PAS = 0	FEAR = 0	BIZ = 0	H-L = 52
EXH = 0	Σ ENV = 1	Σ MAL = 5	Σ WITH = 0	PATH = 5
DIR = 3				
AGG = 0	ER = Σ INT: Σ ENV: Σ MAL: Σ WITH = 4 : 1 : 5 : 0			
Σ INT = 4	AOR = (AFF + DEP + COM):(DIR + AGG) = 1 : 3			

QUALITATIVE ADMINISTRATIVE OBSERVATIONS **Tense and toned down. Seemed bothered by the test stimuli.**

CASE HISTORY AND DIAGNOSTIC DATA

EXAMINER **E.E.W.**

pletely opposite orientation toward the cards than the freewheeling schizophrenic. The brain-damaged individual views the stimulus materials concretely as representations of real problems, the solutions to which require effort, caution, and careful consideration. The schizophrenic uses the card as a launching pad for flights of fancy; the organic is anchored to the card itself, holding fast to the only reality he sees lest

CARD	IRT	HAND TEST RESPONSES	SCORE
I	5	Giving a point-- stressing a point, actually.	DIR
		(a.t.e) Pointing to the person. (Q) The person who owns the hand: like an egotistical person	EXH
		saying "me!". Or it's saying stop.	DIR
II	7	It's reaching or grasping. (Q) It wants to scratch someone (D) but doesn't have finger-nails. And it's like a poor hand-- it's broke.	AGG(ACQ,TEN)
			CRIP
III	3	Pointing out another person or a place or a thing.	COM
		There's a little face in the hand too. It's a sad face.	BIZ
IV	3	It's going to pat a head.	AFF
		There's a happy face on it... There's also a	BIZ
		kidney bean. (pause) And a bridge, and water	BIZ
		and waves, lots of waves.	BIZ
V	3	It's reaching over the edge of something. (Q) Oh, maybe for a cat...	ACQ (IM)
		Getting a kleenex.	ACT
VI	4	He's got a mouse. (Q) He's got a mouse in his hand. It's a big hand and a little white baby mouse. Maybe he's squashing it... maybe he's hurting it.	AGG (BIZ?)
VII	4	It's a boyscout hand shake. It's an aged boy scout cause he's got spots on his hand.	AFF (CRIP)
		It could be a hand holding a crock pot. He's got a potter's wheel and he's molding a pot.	ACT (EXH) (O)
VIII	6	It's either sprinkling spices into a skillet	ACT (ORAL)
		full of spagetti sauce or it's somebody giving a tid bit to a cat or a starving bird.	AFF (IM, ORAL)
IX	4	Making his hand walk...like through the Yellow Pages, making his fingers do the walking. Or	EXH
		making like a ballerina. I see a Chinese hand.	EXH
		(Q) It has the look of a Chinaman's hand.	DES (BIZ)
X	3	Peace sign to a friend: "Peace."	AFF (COM)

it slip away. Consequently, the typical brain-damaged record will show DES, FAIL, low R, and the various qualitative indices of effort and ineptitude which Piotrowski (1936) first observed with the Rorschach as organic indicators such as impotence, perplexity, perseveration, and automatic phrases. If desired, repetitions of responses can be duly noted with a check mark; impotence and perplexity can be designated,

The Hand Test

SUMMARY SHEET

by Edwin E. Wagner, Ph. D.

PUBLISHED BY

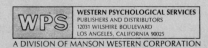

WESTERN PSYCHOLOGICAL SERVICES
PUBLISHERS AND DISTRIBUTORS
12031 WILSHIRE BOULEVARD
LOS ANGELES, CALIFORNIA 90025

A DIVISION OF MANSON WESTERN CORPORATION

DATE __12/27/76__

NAME __EF__   SEX __F__   AGE __20__   RACE __W__

ADDRESS __333 ShadyLane St.__

OCCUPATION __Unemployed__   DIAGNOSIS __Schizophrenia__

AFF = 4	ACQ = 1	TEN = 0	DES = 1	R = 22
DEP = 0	ACT = 3	CRIP = 1	FAIL = 0	AIRT = 4.2
COM = 1	PAS = 0	FEAR = 0	BIZ = 4	H-L = 4.0
EXH = 3	Σ ENV = 4	Σ MAL = 1	Σ WITH = 5	PATH = 11
DIR = 2				
AGG = 2	ER = Σ INT: Σ ENV: Σ MAL: Σ WITH = 12 : 4 : 1 : 5			
Σ INT = 12	AOR = (AFF + DEP + COM):(DIR + AGG) = 5 : 4			

QUALITATIVE ADMINISTRATIVE OBSERVATIONS __Argued over unimportant details.__
__Made comments designed to shock the examiner. Described herself as__
__"schizophrenic" and "a nervous twit".__

CASE HISTORY AND DIAGNOSTIC DATA __High school education. Has worked as a__
__nurses aide, waitress and cashier. Hospitalized at Akron General__
__Psychiatric Unit and twice at Fallsview.__

EXAMINER __T. Walter__

respectively, with the parenthesized scores (IMP) and (PERP), and automatic phrases can be underlined. The reaction times of organic subjects will vary and may cluster at either extreme: quick responsiveness from those who have become labile and impulsive, and very slow reactivity from those who are overwhelmed by uncertainty, circumspection, and hesitancy. The record of GH is fairly typical of subjects with

HAND TEST: GH

CARD	IRT	HAND TEST RESPONSES	SCORE
I	18	I don't know. I don't know any of these things. I never had anything like this. (can you take a guess?) Just up like this (D,E). (Q) I give up.	DES (IM,PERP)
II	7	(E) I don't know how to describe what it's doing. It's doing the same thing my hand is doing. (Q) Just laying here like this. (D)	DES (IMP, PERS
III	4	Pointing. (Q) (E) Well, I point my fingers... to... ah... If I saw somebody I knew, you know, to say "hi" to 'em. (lights cigarette) Another cigarette... calms my nerves.	COM (PERS)
IV	5	It's got the thumb up. Some of these I don't know how to describe.	DES (IMP)
		And could be thumbin' a ride	DEP
V	6	Could be wavin'... I guess... (Q) Uh huh, hello. To me it doesn't look like it'd be doing anything... but...	COM (AMB)
VI	12	I don't know what that'd be doing. You're a fast writer.	FAIL
VII	9	It's just... I don't know what that finger's doing. I have several other tests to take yet? I should have brought lunch.	FAIL
VIII	25	(E) Same thing I'm doing with my finger. (Q) Holdin' my cigarette because I'm tense. (subject laughs) You writin' down what I'm sayin'?	TEN (PERS) (ORAL)
IX	42	I don't know what these fingers do: Do you know what they do? That finger's holdin' on to my pot holder when I'm gettin' something out of the oven.	(PERP) ACT (PERS, ORA
X	8	Ah, windin' my watch. One finger? Yeh, two fingers windin' my watch.	ACT (PERS)

moderate to severe brain impairments. GH is a 30-year-old, married woman with three children. About a year prior to testing, she tried to commit suicide because of marital difficulties and was comatose for 6 weeks due to carbon monoxide poisoning. She has an R.N. degree but is now obviously incapable of pursuing that career, showing a FS WAIS IQ of only 63. During testing, she was distractible, nervous, and labile, obviously a shell of her former self.

The Hand Test

SUMMARY SHEET

by Edwin E. Wagner, Ph.D.

PUBLISHED BY

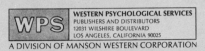

WESTERN PSYCHOLOGICAL SERVICES
PUBLISHERS AND DISTRIBUTORS
12031 WILSHIRE BOULEVARD
LOS ANGELES, CALIFORNIA 90025

A DIVISION OF MANSON WESTERN CORPORATION

DATE _8/21/73_

NAME ___GH___ SEX _F_ AGE _30_ RACE _Chicano_

ADDRESS ___444 Rose Lane___

OCCUPATION _Housewife (R.N.)_ DIAGNOSIS _OBS (carbon monoxide poisoning)_

AFF = 0	ACQ = 0	TEN = 1	DES = 3	R = 9
DEP = 1	ACT = 2	CRIP = 0	FAIL = 2	AIRT = 14.4
COM = 2	PAS = 0	FEAR = 0	BIZ = 0	H-L = 38
EXH = 0	Σ ENV = 2	Σ MAL = 1	Σ WITH = 5	PATH = 11
DIR = 0				
AGG = 0	ER = Σ INT: Σ ENV: Σ MAL: Σ WITH = 3 : 2 : 1 : 5			
Σ INT = 3	AOR = (AFF + DEP + COM):(DIR + AGG) = 3 : 0			

QUALITATIVE ADMINISTRATIVE OBSERVATIONS _Smoked heavily. Related to examiner in a dependent, child-like manner. Distractable, nervous, labile._

CASE HISTORY AND DIAGNOSTIC DATA _Feels memory is coming back after suicide attempt and that she can return to nursing with retraining. Has now been released by psychiatrist and neurologist._

EXAMINER _E.E.W._

GH's protocol shows many of the features commonly associated with brain impairment: DES, FAIL, low R, impotence, and perplexity. She also demonstrates her concrete attitude toward the task by using her own hands to emulate and describe the drawings. Personalizations (PERS) are also common (although not exclusive) to persons with organic brain syndromes. She still seems able to handle a few environmental tasks (ACT = 2), but her INT score is low, suggesting that the organicity has seriously interfered with interpersonal relationships. Note that the dependenc observed during the test administration was confirmed by the DEP on the Hand Test. The high H − L score may reflect a delay occasioned by intellectual difficul ties rather than "neurotic shock," although she did give a TEN response which sug gests that she is experiencing some inner strain due perhaps to her lowered efficiency

Inasmuch as personality disorders are fundamentally shallow, people with self centered attitudes and limited behavioral repertoires tend to produce Hand Tes protocols with the following features: relatively low R, seldom exceeding 15 in num ber; comparatively banal responses lacking in individuality and uniqueness; and action tendencies directly mirroring their personality distortions, so that, for example acting-out sociopaths usually give grossly aggressive responses. WITH is usually absent, although a FAIL may occur among those personality disorders subject to episodic outbursts beyond conscious control, and DES could crop up with inade quate personalities, especially those with a low IQ. Personality disorders are seldom bothered by guilt and neurotic conflicts; hence, unless the individual is being sub jected to current environmental pressures such as the threat of jail or a disruptive marriage, MAL is absent or sparse. Clues to the specific nature of the personality disorder can often be detected in the content as well as the regular scoring. For in stance, dependent characters often produce (ORAL) content, and sociopaths are prone to (CYL) because of their weak masculinity. The Hand Test can be useful for diagnosing the presence and nature of the personality disorder, but the cliniciar must be alert to those cases which superficially resemble normal records. The use of a test battery is very helpful in this respect.

IJ, a 29-year-old divorced female, is a good example of how a passive-aggressive personality might show up on the Hand Test. IJ was receiving psychotherapy osten sibly because of emotional problems following her divorce, and had been diagnosed as passive-aggressive with dependent and inadequate features. She was described as adopting a "poor me" attitude and playing the role of the abandoned wife and loving mother. Efforts to get her back to work had proved unsuccessful despite average intelligence, a high school education, and reasonably good scores on a variety of vocational tests.

That this woman has limited energy for constructive accomplishment can be inferred from the R, which is a little on the low side, and from the complete absence of ACT, a rather unusual feature. As might be expected in a passive-aggressive, IJ shows both AGG and PAS (two of each). Qualitatively, passive-aggressives also tend to produce AGG responses which are underhanded. That is, they seldom give a direct "punch in the nose" AGG, preferring a more surreptitious expression of hostility. IJ's response to card II is of the "sneaky" variety and is fairly typical. She also shows some ambivalence with aggression on card VI. Qualitatively, she demon strates orality, dependency, and immaturity. In view of the difficulty which has been encountered in galvanizing this woman into action, her PAS response to card X is of interest. It is merely a feeble repetition of the response to card VII after what appears to be a time shock, and does not bode well for the future. Data from the Hand Test seem to coincide with the case history material and psychiatric description.

The foregoing material is not intended as an exhaustive explication of the many Hand Test patterns associated with various nosological groupings. Its purpose is to point up the logical relationships among some major diagnostic categories and an ticipated projective responses to the Hand Test as a precursor to differential diagnosis. The rules which have been outlined are empirically verifiable, but they cannot be generalized to every case and should not be used rigidly. Best results will accrue when the above precepts are used as a springboard from which the experienced clinician can develop his own expanded interpretations. And, of course, the efficacy of the Hand Test will be greatly enhanced when it is integrated with case history, interview impression, and data from other psychological tests.

5. Some Theoretical Considerations

The oft-repeated platitude that projective techniques measure the "whole personality" is patently absurd, for, if that were so, there would be no need for more than one such test. Thoughtful writers (e.g., Korner, 1950; Rapaport, 1952) have pointed out that there are probably different kinds of projection and that various projective techniques can be expected to measure divergent aspects of personality. The logic of this position is inescapable, and, obviously, it would be of theoretical and practical value if a system could be devised which could apportion the variance measured by a given test to relevant aspects of the personality. Because the Hand Test is a "narrow-band," one-dimensional instrument which, since its inception, has been narrowly defined as revealing prototypal action tendencies apt to be behaviorally expressed, it has been possible over the years to use it as a vantage point, a "home base" from which to compare and evaluate other projective techniques. It has been found, for example, that there is a significant overlap between the F or form response on the Rorschach and the general integrity of the Hand Test. A low $F\%$ and/or a low $F+\%$ is invariably correlated with some sort of Hand Test weakness. Furthermore, action tendencies associated with the Rorschach M tend to be reflected in the Hand Test INT scores (Wagner & Hoover, 1971). On the other hand, the impact of emotion as measured by the color response on the Rorschach, or the kind of fantasy material evoked by the TAT, has no direct Hand Test analogue. After studying thousands of cases in this manner, and comparing the overlaps as well as the differences among various projective techniques, particularly as they related to the Hand Test, it was possible to formulate a paradigm which seemed capable of accommodating and integrating the divergent contributions of each test to personality assessment (Wagner, 1971, 1976b). The "theory" is referred to as Structural Analysis to indicate that personality, although dynamic, also consists of various components or "structures" which are differentially measured by various projective techniques. The theory is discussed at this point because it has a direct bearing on the circumspect use of the Hand Test, but it is also hoped that Structural Analysis will be of heuristic value for the reader in terms of stimulating a fresh look at the relationship between psychopathology and projective testing.

Structural Analysis posits two major psychological structures, the Façade Self and the Introspective Self. The Façade Self consists of learned and readily available attitudes and action tendencies designed to cope with the external world; it is primarily this structure which the Hand Test measures. The Façade Self interfaces with reality through physiological receptors and effectors termed the Perceptual-Motor Screen. The Introspective Self, conversely, is composed of covert, internal processes which can be expressed only through the mediating function of the Façade Self. The workings of the Introspective Self can be viewed along a dynamic continuum, ranging from clearly conceptualized life roles likely to be actualized, through

EDWIN E. WAGNER

CARD	IRT	HAND TEST RESPONSES	SCORE
I	15	You mean ah... (pause) Holding, ah, telling someone to stop. (a.t.e.) Waving. Or telling someone "Bye".	DIR COM COM
II	4	Sneaking up... getting ready to scratch someone. (Q) (laughs) Should I say whatever comes to my mind? Well getting ready to scratch someone.	AGG
III	2	Pointing. (Q) Ahem... Like showing someone where they could sit down.	COM (DIR)
IV	8	Getting ready to put your hand around something. (Q) A person.... or a baby.	AFF (DEP) (IM)
V	11	Looks like a hand pulling up. A child pulling up to something. (Q) Like a counter top in a candy store.	ACQ (IM, ORAL)
VI	3	A fist. (Q) Looks like it's getting ready to hit. Hit a table or something.	AGG (AMB)
VII	12	I don't know, it's just a hand laying there resting. (laughs) Doesn't look like it's doing anything.	PAS
VIII	9	Ah, looks like it's snapping it's fingers. (Q) (Q) To get someone's attention... tell 'em to get something.	DIR
IX	12	If it was turned the other way it could be someone holding up four fingers. (Q) Well if it was a kid, could be telling you they were four years old.	COM (IM)
X	22	Could be a hand just laying there resting.	PAS ✓

the Façade Self to fantasies and ruminations seldom (if ever) manifested in behavior. To function effectively in the real world, a person must have a viable Façade Self, i.e., the Hand Test has to be reasonably intact. However, the Introspective Self can be overdeveloped, underdeveloped, or even nonexistent, and the personality can still operate. The two structures are viewed as being activated by emotion and intellect, the final product observable in terms of behavior which, terminally, depends

The Hand Test

SUMMARY SHEET

by Edwin E. Wagner, Ph.D.

PUBLISHED BY

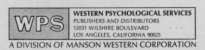

WPS WESTERN PSYCHOLOGICAL SERVICES
PUBLISHERS AND DISTRIBUTORS
12031 WILSHIRE BOULEVARD
LOS ANGELES, CALIFORNIA 90025

A DIVISION OF MANSON WESTERN CORPORATION

DATE _6/4/74_

NAME _IJ_   SEX _F_   AGE _29_   RACE _W_

ADDRESS _555 Orange Blossom Lane_

OCCUPATION _Housewife_   DIAGNOSIS _Personality Disorder, Pas-Agg_

AFF = 1	ACQ = 1	TEN = 0	DES = 0	R = 12
DEP = 0	ACT = 0	CRIP = 0	FAIL = 0	AIRT = 9.8
COM = 4	PAS = 2	FEAR = 0	BIZ = 0	H-L = 20
EXH = 0	Σ ENV = 3	Σ MAL = 0	Σ WITH = 0	PATH = 0
DIR = 2				
AGG = 2	ER = Σ INT: Σ ENV: Σ MAL: Σ WITH = _9_ : _3_ : _0_ : _0_			
Σ INT = 9	AOR = (AFF + DEP + COM):(DIR + AGG) = _5_ : _4_			

QUALITATIVE ADMINISTRATIVE OBSERVATIONS _Sought feedback from examiner._

CASE HISTORY AND DIAGNOSTIC DATA _Receiving Psychotherapy from Dr. Zilch_
following a divorce. BVR reports that efforts toward vocational reha-
bilitation have been unsuccessful despite normal abilities.

EXAMINER _J. Daubney_

W-110A

on the Perceptual-Motor Screen for expression. The entire system can be represented topologically as a triangle consisting of Emotion, Intellect, and Behavior as the three sides enclosing both the Façade Self and the Introspective Self (Figure 1). Only Behavior is directly observable.

Once having established this framework, it becomes possible to partial out the relative contributions of various projective techniques to personality assessment.

EDWIN E. WAGNER

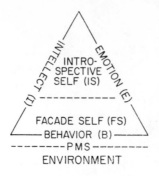

Figure 1. Showing how Façade Self attitudes and action tendencies are close to Behavior and hence apt to be expressed through the Perceptual-Motor Screen. Introspective Self processes are pictured as occupying a "deeper" level of personality since they must pass through the Façade Self in order to become actualized. The modalities of Behavior, Intellect, and Emotion are represented as an interlocking tripartite system, positioned to show that it is only Behavior which is observable in the environment while the remainder to the psyche must be inferred. From Wagner (1976b). Reprinted with permission of the publisher.

As can be seen in Figure 2, projective techniques are pictured as lying somewhere in between the space formed by the Emotional and Intellectual vectors, which is one of the characteristics which differentiates them from the more objective personality tests which are primarily intellectual in orientation. Furthermore, projective techniques vary in terms of the "depth" of measurement, so that the TAT can be portrayed at the apex of the triangle, assessing fantasy material, while the Hand Test lies at the base directly involved with Façade Self activities. The Rorschach occupies a larger middle ground, overlapping both techniques to some extent, and is thus a more versatile or broader-based instrument. Other projective techniques could easily have been substituted for the three portrayed in the illustration. For example, the Bender-Gestalt Test would be assigned mainly to the Perceptual-Motor Screen.

It is also postulated that psychopathology can be described in terms of the strength of and the articulation among the major dimensions of personality as stipulated by Structural Analysis, i.e., Façade Self, Introspective Self, Emotion, Intellect, Behavior, and Perceptual-Motor Screen. Schizophrenics are always characterized by a weak Façade Self, but the strength of the Introspective Self can vary to any extent, which is why there are so many schizophrenic "types." Patients with personality disorders show very little in the way of Introspective Self resources, but their Façade Self, albeit rigid and stilted, is viable. Neurotics usually exhibit conflicts between the Façade Self and the Introspective Self and/or imbalances among Intellect, Emotion, and Behavior. These interrelationships can be pictured topologically by varying their lengths of the sides of the triangle and simultaneously altering the amount of space encompassed by the Façade Self and the Introspective Self. If this schema is even approximately valid, important repercussions for diagnostic testing will ensue, because it follows that the amount of information which

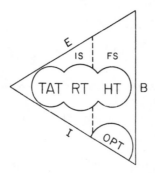

Figure 2. Showing unique areas of personality measurement as well as overlap for some representative projective techniques, the Hand Test (HT), Rorschach Technique (RT), and Thematic Apperception Test (TAT), according to Structural Analysis levels of personality depicted in Figure 1. Objective personality tests (OPT) are portrayed as lying mainly along the intellectual vector. From Wagner (1976b). Reprinted with permission of the publisher.

can be gleaned from a technique depends not only on the projective characteristics of the test itself but also on the psychological status (structure) of the person being tested. Figure 3 illustrates that point using the TAT. As can readily be seen, the TAT would yield a great deal of information on certain schizoid types, with an abundance of Introspective Self processes, but could be expected to elicit very little material from a conversion hysteric, who simply doesn't fantasize very much.

The author has tried to show how it might be possible to enhance clinical prediction by specifying, through the use of Structural Analysis, what tests will elicit what material from what diagnostic category (Wagner, 1973, 1974b, 1976a; Wagner & Heise, 1974). It is contended that intertest patterning is an extremely powerful method for arriving at a differential diagnosis once the mutual interrelationships among the tests and psychopathological conditions are explicated. By the same token, it should be possible to indicate the diagnostic strengths and weaknesses of a specific test vis-à-vis a particular mental disorder.

Applying Structural Analytic principles to the Hand Test permits certain logical inferences to be made, many of which have been confirmed by clinical experience. First of all, if the Hand Test does indeed measure the Façade Self, a readiness to respond in a habitual manner, it should reflect the kind of behavior manifested in diurnal activities—what the person does (or doesn't do) as he interacts daily with his environment. Therefore, the patient's interview behavior should to a certain extent overlap with tendencies noted on the Hand Test; case history data should be understandable in relation to the Hand Test; other people should describe the client in terms which correspond to what appears on the Hand Test. Consequently, discrepancies between what is known about the patient and what he seems to be on the Hand Test might be looked at very closely, because a great deal can be learned from such apparent inconsistencies. For example, consider a man who has functioned as an executive in a big company for 20 years and is referred for testing because of depression following heart surgery. The Hand Test is full of doubt, hesitancy, and descriptions—completely contrary to what might be expected from hard-driving, managerial personalities. The diagnostician should immediately be alerted to the possibility of an organic brain syndrome associated with the depression and perhaps the operation itself.

While the Hand Test's capacity for mirroring overt behavior is a distinct advantage for conducting validity studies and for seeing the subject as others see him—for obtaining a concise description of how he can be expected to behave under cus-

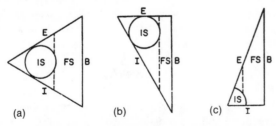

Figure 3. A topological representation according to Structural Analysis of (a) an idealized personality with full and balanced development of the Introspective Self, Façade Self, Intellect, and Emotion; (b) a schizoid type with a predominance of Introspective Self and Intellect and underdevelopment of Emotion and Façade Self; and (c) conversion hysteria with underdevelopment of the Introspective Self and Intellect. The circular areas indicate how the Thematic Apperception Test would differentially measure these three personality structures. From Wagner (1976b). Reprinted with permission of the publisher.

tomary circumstances, it provides relatively little information about deeper personality resources such as fantasies, self-regard, internalized life roles, and motivational level. It furnishes little insight into Introspective Self and depicts the individual as a one-dimensional being. This presents no problem when dealing with subjects having personality disorders, impoverished schizophrenics, and most mental retardates, who are, in fact, Façade Self people bereft of depth. Their behavior is essentially their personality. But when it comes to answering questions such as resources for psychotherapy or motivation for long-term training, the Hand Test is less efficacious. Furthermore, assuming that the personality does have depth, the Hand Test will miss out on the emotional and intellectual resources associated with the Introspective Self and thus elude much of what makes the individual personality unique and complex. The Hand Test will reflect to some extent intellectual and emotional processes feeding into the Façade Self, but only indirectly, because, as can be seen from Figure 1, the two Façade Self segments representing Intellect and Emotion are small in comparison to the Behavior sector which is served by the Façade Self. Feeling tone can be projected into the Hand Test responses (e.g., "That looks like a very warm and friendly hand"), and intelligence can often be inferred from verbiage, diversity of percepts, originality, and other subtle chords which will resonate in the "third ear" of the experienced clinician, but these are qualitative nuances which will not grace every record. Individuals with well-developed, smoothly functioning personalities will express their Introspective Self effortlessly through the Façade Self, but the final product is an integrated percept which is sometimes difficult to distinguish from a response which is primarily Façade Self in nature.

When introspective processes start to break through a weakened façade, the responses take on a primitive, idiosyncratic tone which can vary from "strange" to outright bizarre. Topologically, a weak Façade Self can be depicted by two dotted (instead of straight) lines interfacing with both the Introspective Self and the environment. The boundaries can now be conceptualized as being overly permeable so that forces from the Introspective Self impinge directly on Behavior, and the Façade Self simply becomes a mouthpiece for emotions, thoughts, and desires, untrammeled by reality testing. An outpouring of idiosyncratic material, while pathological, does at least establish the presence of an Introspective Self. Strange, autistic percepts stopping short of being genuinely bizarre responses are often produced by highly ideational schizoids; a true BIZ is indicative of schizophrenia; and borderline cases fall somewhere in between.

The fewer the R and the more stereotyped and skeletal the responses, the greater the probability that the testee is lacking in Introspective Self processes. With such subjects, the Hand Test comes closer to reflecting the "whole" personality: "What you see is what you get." The Hand Test is particularly effective for catching the essence of those "façade" individuals who rely on a thin, circumscribed set of action tendencies to deal with reality such as a repetitive veneer of compulsivity or a patina of learned social skills.

To iterate, the Hand Test does not measure the entire personality, and, for best results, it is incumbent on the diagnostician to become familiar with the relative strengths and weaknesses of the instrument, especially in relation to various psychopathological conditions. Structural Analysis provides a convenient paradigm for envisioning what the Hand Test does; but, for those who are not enamored with new theoretical systems, it may suffice to keep in mind the following generality: the Hand Test measures prototypal action tendencies which are apt to be expressed in behavior; therefore, other things being equal, the more complex the individual, the less the instrument will reveal about the "whole personality."

6. Special Clinical Applications

Because Hand Test scores are easily converted into behavioral predictions, the test lends itself to direct experimental validation. For example, ceteris paribus, lawbreakers who habitually perpetrate crimes against their fellow man such as assault or armed robbery can be expected to produce AGG responses. Nevertheless, the history of projective testing surely indicates that the popularity of a test is not necessarily dependent on positive findings in the research literature. In some cases, the complex patterning within a projective technique militates against simplistic behavioral predictions, naive experimental designs, and fractionization of composite data into component parts. In other cases, the data reflect psychological rather than psychometric principles and are not well suited to standard statistical analyses. In still other cases, research has been instituted by investigators lacking insight into and extensive clinical experience with a technique, who, in all good faith, conduct experiments which are poorly conceived and foredoomed to failure. But, whatever the reason, diagnosticians have grown wary of accepting negative research data at face value, and hence a projective technique will be judged by its clinical usefulness as well as by the weight of the published evidence for validity. In this respect, then, it would be instructive to review what appear to be the major clinical advantages of the Hand Test as perceived by working diagnosticians.

Because of the ease of administration, nonthreatening nature, simplicity, and portability of the Hand Test, many clinicians view it as a convenient screening technique, applicable for a variety of situations where time is limited and where a quick estimate of psychopathology is desired. The present author, committed to the belief in the superiority of a test battery, deprecates such an approach; however, under certain circumstances, the use of the Hand Test to screen subjects can probably be justified, provided that it is undertaken with due caution and some attempt is made to integrate the findings with whatever other data are available. The following comments from a psychiatrist, Dr. James R. Hodge, who has used the Hand Test for quite some time and probably qualifies as an "expert," testify to the versatility of the instrument for screening purposes but properly place it in context as just part of the total picture, "rounding out" a diagnostic impression.

> Psychiatrists rarely administer psychological tests, yet having available a simple, quick, and reliable instrument can be of immense value in rounding out a mental status examination and supplementing case history and interview data.
>
> I can get a quick estimate of intelligence and some mental functioning by using selected questions from the WAIS, and an estimate of organicity from the Bender-Gestalt. I can get both of the above and more by using the Hand Test, a projective test which also gives a personality assessment, indications of current emotional states and conflict areas, and types of psychological defense mechanisms.
>
> The greatest advantage of the Hand Test for me is that it is relatively easy to learn, is quick and easy to interpret, takes only a short time to administer, and I can do it myself. This permits me an immediate assessment of the patient's clinical status without having to wait for a more comprehensive test battery.
>
> I keep two sets of the Hand Test, one in my office desk drawer and one in my hospital consultation kit. (I can even put it in my pocket if I choose.) Administration of the Hand Test, with or without the Bender-Gestalt and WAIS selections, often permits a diagnostic impression and treatment recommendations in one session instead of two or more. Further, because

of its brevity and simplicity, it can be administered at any time during the process of therapy in order to clarify the current clinical picture or to evaluate the progress of therapy. Sometimes its greatest value is to indicate that further tests are necessary.

In using the Hand Test for screening purposes, caution must also be exercised to avoid a strictly psychometric approach, falling back on Summary Scores such as the PATH or the AOR, and establishing some arbitrary cutoff point as an expedient tactic for separating normal from disturbed patients. The Hand Test is a projective technique which can furnish many qualitative clues for interpretation; if it is treated like an objective personality test, much discriminatory power will be lost. There is no substitute for a careful, serious, insightful clinical analysis.

A second major clinical asset which sets the Hand Test somewhat apart from other techniques is that, because it reflects motoric tendencies, it has special application for situations in which a particular kind of behavior per se, regardless of the motivation behind it, is of primary importance. There are at least two such behavioral manifestations to which the Hand Test is particularly sensitive, acting out and compulsivity.

"Acting out," i.e., aggressive, antisocial behavior, has been a concern of the Hand Test since the publication of the original monograph, and much of the research reported in the literature has been oriented toward testing the efficacy of the Acting-Out Ratio, or a "score" derived from that ratio (the Acting-Out Score, which is the algebraic difference between AFF + COM + DEP and DIR + AGG), in predicting various kinds of overt hostility varying from irascible behavior in the classroom to violent criminal acts. In general, the research has yielded moderately positive results (Azcarate & Gutierrez, 1969; Brodsky & Brodsky, 1967; Fornari, 1971; Gutierrez & Sanchez, 1970; Oswald & Loftus, 1967; Selg, 1965; Wagner & Medvedeff, 1963; Wagner & Hawkins, 1964; Wetsel, Shapiro, & Wagner, 1967; Wagner, 1974a). However, negative studies have also been reported (Breidenbaugh, Brozovich, & Matheson, 1974; Drummond, 1966; Higdon & Brodsky, 1973). It is in some ways unfortunate that a disproportionate amount of effort has been devoted to the Acting-Out Ratio because (1) this tends to represent the Hand Test solely as a test of acting-out behavior rather than a general diagnostic instrument, (2) there is a tendency to place too much reliance on a single quantitative score, treating the test as an objective rather than projective technique, and (3) it ignores other indices of possible aggressive behavior which the experienced clinician can glean from a perusal of the entire protocol. In regard to the third point, experience has shown that the following features should also be taken into account when estimating the likelihood of aggressive behavior:

1. Grossly aggressive content, usually scored AGG (GROSS), indicates tendencies toward behavior which is no longer even an appropriate display of hostility but which, instead, inflicts grievous hurt upon another and denotes inveterate antisocial tendencies, e.g., "Smashing somebody in the face with a brick."

2. The content score (MOV) is given by individuals who display random, inappropriate behavior, usually to relieve tension, but which can be antisocial in nature, e.g., "Just waving his hand back and forth because he has a cramp."

3. The FAIL response, especially if the failure appears to be due to "shock" rather than the impotence associated with retardation, connotes a lack of conscious control over action tendencies. In some cases this will result in a

complete absence of behavior, but in other instances dissociative reactions, often aggressive, may supervene.

4. Fast reaction times indicate impulsivity, "acting without thinking," and therefore an AIRT under 5 sec could contribute to antisocial behavior by releasing precipitous actions without due consideration of possible undesirable consequences.

5. Up to a point, MAL tends to depress all action tendencies, including aggression, but the relationship is nonlinear. When the MAL score is high—about 4 or 5—psychological defenses can become paralyzed by intrapsychic conflicts, and temporary breakdowns in habitual constraints can ensue, permitting acting-out behavior to occur.

6. EXH responses, especially when they occur in connection with other acting-out indicators, can increase the probability of aggressive behavior, especially with teenagers where delinquency may, to some extent, be motivated by a desire to show off or attract attention through social misdeeds.

7. Generally speaking, a dearth of responses is taken to indicate a lack of psychological flexibility, an inability to choose appropriately from among a reservoir of diverse action tendencies, and hence a more rigid approach to life's challenges. Therefore, any of the acting-out indicators mentioned above take on added import when R is low.

KL's protocol is an extreme example of how aggressive inclinations can be manifested on the Hand Test—so much so that it is almost a caricature. KL is a convicted murderer who committed a heinous and cold-blooded crime. He claimed that he had been urged by voices to perpetrate the killing and, indeed, there was plentiful evidence that this man was schizophrenic as well as frighteningly hostile. For example, on the WAIS Comprehension subtest, he answered as follows:

Q. Why do we wash clothes?
A. "You have to keep the devils out."
Q. What is the thing to do if you find an envelope in the street that is sealed, and addressed, and has a new stamp?
A. "Find out what's in it."
Q. Why should we keep away from bad company?
A. "Because they throw water on you and call you names."

Notice how the "throw water on you" theme which appears on the Comprehension question (No. 4) reappears on card X of the Hand Test and probably represents a delusional leitmotif. The psychotic origin of KL's aggression is corroborated not only by the BIZ on card V but also by the very fact that he produced 9 AGG responses, a rarity for even highly aggressive individuals. The acting-out indicators are rife: 9 AGG out of a limited total of only 10 R (in fact, there would be 10 AGG were it not for the bizarre aggressive response on card V); (GROSS) aggressive content on at least 4 cards; a completely unbalanced AOR in favor of acting out; and fairly fast IRTs with no prolonged time shocks to mitigate the expression of hostile impulses. The total preoccupation with aggression, a deeply embedded behavioral cachet, is vividly revealed on KL's protocol and illustrates how trenchantly the Hand Test can reflect such tendencies.

Another set of behavioral tendencies to which the Hand Test is particularly

HAND TEST: KL

CARD	IRT	HAND TEST RESPONSES	SCORE
I	8	Well, it looks like it's gonna hit something. (Q) Ah, it looks like it's gonna hit a person. (a.t.e.?) I don't think so.	AGG
II	12	Looks like... oh, it's gonna... choke something or somebody.	AGG (GROSS)
III	4	Ah, it's pointin' at somebody. (Q) Ah, it looks like the way... that the person points at somebody whose smarter than they are, making fun at them.	AGG (COM)?
IV	20	It looks like... it's going to... hit something. (Q) I don't know, it looks it's going to hit a head.	AGG (GROSS)
V	7	That hand just used a knife. It's got blood on it and everything... just killed somebody.	BIZ (AGG) (GROSS)
VI	14	That hand's squeezing somebody's arm I think. (Q) They don't like the person.	AGG
VII	6	Looks like it's gonna use karate. (Q) It looks like it's gonna chop somebody's neck or something. Or their arm.	AGG (GROSS)
VIII	7	That hand's pinching. It's pinching somebody's arms and legs. (Q) They just don't like 'em.	AGG
IX	9	That hand's hitting somebody... digging, digging the thumb in.	AGG
X	12	Ah... it has, ah.. a cup of water in its hand and it's throwing the water on the other person, 'cause the other person's smarter than it is and it doesn't like it.	AGG (BIZ?)

sensitive is the "compulsive façade" (Levine & Wagner, 1974; Wagner, 1976a). The word "façade" seemed apposite because what is being referred to is not the more widely known obsessive-compulsive neurosis where reoccurring thoughts are associated with repetitive acts, but rather perseverative behavior relatively independent of ideation. This behavior can be considered "thin" inasmuch as quantity is substituted for quality. There is always repetition, often on COM or ACT, which attests

The Hand Test

SUMMARY SHEET

by Edwin E. Wagner, Ph.D.

PUBLISHED BY

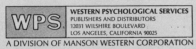

WPS — WESTERN PSYCHOLOGICAL SERVICES
PUBLISHERS AND DISTRIBUTORS
12031 WILSHIRE BOULEVARD
LOS ANGELES, CALIFORNIA 90025

A DIVISION OF MANSON WESTERN CORPORATION

DATE 2/13/75

NAME KL   SEX m   AGE 25   RACE W

ADDRESS County Jail

OCCUPATION Unemployed   DIAGNOSIS Paranoid schizophrenia

AFF = 0	ACQ = 0	TEN = 0	DES = 0	R = 10
DEP = 0	ACT = 0	CRIP = 0	FAIL = 0	AIRT = 9.9
COM = 0	PAS = 0	FEAR = 0	BIZ = 1	H-L = 16
EXH = 0	Σ ENV = 0	Σ MAL = 0	Σ WITH = 1	PATH = 2
DIR = 0				
AGG = 9	ER = Σ INT: Σ ENV: Σ MAL: Σ WITH = 9 : 0 : 0 : 1			
Σ INT = 9	AOR = (AFF + DEP + COM):(DIR + AGG) = 0 : 9			

QUALITATIVE ADMINISTRATIVE OBSERVATIONS   Sat with chin on chest, rarely looking at the examiner. Subdued, toned down, little affect.

CASE HISTORY AND DIAGNOSTIC DATA High school dropout. Committed murder and
claimed voices told him to do it.

EXAMINER   Tom Walter

to the fact that the overproduction of responses is not a manifestation of rich, powerful psychological resources but rather a compulsive attempt to structure the environment and discharge energy through stereotyped rather than creative behavior.
Coupled with this compulsive façade is an absence of internal living which can easily
be detected by noting the relative dearth of material on other projective tests such
as the Rorschach and TAT, which measure deeper psychological resources. The

CARD	IRT	HAND TEST RESPONSES	SCORE
I	3	Getting ready to shake. (a.t.e.?) Getting ready to grip something? (Q) Some type of tool... hammer, saw.	AFF ACT (CYL)
II	3	That one, I'd say... like catching something that was falling off a shelf. Or feeling along a rug trying to get something.	ACT (ACQ) ACQ (SEN)
III	1	Pointing... (Q) I don't know, a lot of things- "Look at him", something of that nature. Dialing a phone; pushing a button; flipping a light switch.	COM ACT ACT ACT
IV	4	That one could be getting ready to shake a hand. Reaching for a doorknob. Reaching down to pick something up.	AFF ✓ ACT (QCQ) ACT (ACQ)
V	2	That one looks like it's climbing up over a wall- reaching to pull himself up. Or like reaching up into your gutter to feel where something is at.	ACQ ACQ (SEN)
VI	3	Getting ready to punch somebody. Ah, hitting a desk. (Q) Why? Mad at somebody and want his attention. Guess he could be holding something like a bill-club if it were in the picture.	AGG DIR (AGG) ACT (CYL) (AGG)
VII	5	Karate chop- breaking a board. Could be getting ready to shake hands. About all for that one.	AGG (IM) AFF ✓
VIII	2	Reaching down to pick up a coin. Holding a pencil... Ah, just gripping something small like a pin or small screwdriver.	ACT (ACQ) ACT ACT (CYL)
IX	11	(E) Reaching down to pick up a bucket. Going to paddle somebody. Reaching down to pick up a table-- something of that nature.	ACT (ACQ) AGG (IM) ACT (ACQ)
X	29	Imagine a hand... Reaching for a book. Reaching for the telephone. Picking something up.	ACT (ACQ) ACT (ACQ) ACT

syndrome can, therefore, be described as a thin layer of compulsive behavior which constitutes the individual's first and only line of defense; once this shell is pierced, there is nothing behind it to cushion reality, and in that respect the personality is rather fragile.

The compulsive façade as a behavioral syndrome is found mainly in individuals with mild to moderate brain damage. It is almost a "flight into behavior" and con-

The Hand Test

SUMMARY SHEET

by Edwin E. Wagner, Ph. D.

PUBLISHED BY

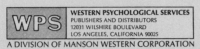

WESTERN PSYCHOLOGICAL SERVICES
PUBLISHERS AND DISTRIBUTORS
12031 WILSHIRE BOULEVARD
LOS ANGELES, CALIFORNIA 90025

A DIVISION OF MANSON WESTERN CORPORATION

DATE___4/3/76___

NAME___MN___ SEX__M__ AGE_22_ RACE__W__

ADDRESS___666 Blueberry Patch___

OCCUPATION___Assistant salesman___ DIAGNOSIS___Aphasia; compulsive overlay___

AFF = 3	ACQ = 3	TEN = 0	DES = 0	R = 27
DEP = 0	ACT = 16	CRIP = 0	FAIL = 0	AIRT = 6.3
COM = 1	PAS = 0	FEAR = 0	BIZ = 0	H-L = 28
EXH = 0	Σ ENV = 19	Σ MAL = 0	Σ WITH = 0	PATH = 0
DIR = 1				
AGG = 3	ER = Σ INT: Σ ENV: Σ MAL: Σ WITH = 8 : 19 : 0 : 0			
Σ INT = 8	AOR = (AFF + DEP + COM):(DIR + AGG) = 4 : 4			

QUALITATIVE ADMINISTRATIVE OBSERVATIONS___Friendly, cooperative. Applies himself
diligently and energetically to task.___

CASE HISTORY AND DIAGNOSTIC DATA___Feels he should be going to college and that
he is good at math. Has high school education. Worked previously as a
panel board wirer.___

EXAMINER___E.E.W.___

stitutes one strategem for coping with reality when only limited psychological resources are available. MN, a 22-year-old male, working as an assistant salesman,
is a good example of a reasonably intact compulsive façade. He was mildly aphasic,
exhibiting the usual substitutions of words like "were" for "where" in his writing
and coming up with spelling errors such as "emmossions" (for "emotions"), but his
IQ was average and his energy level, at least superficially, was high. He had managed

to hold down a number of medium-level jobs but was dissatisfied with his vocational progress, believing he was "good at mathematics" and should become an accountant. On the College Qualification Tests series, he could not complete the Verbal items in the allotted time limit, placing at the tenth percentile and further confirming the aphasia. He also did poorly on the Numerical test despite his putative mathematical ability.

The Hand Test is fairly typical of the compulsive façade, showing 27 responses with a perseveration on ACT. Perseverations are also observable on the "shaking hands" response designated by a checkmark and on the word "reaching" which is interspersed throughout the protocol and has been underlined for emphasis. There is also a decided proclivity toward the ACQ response with the implication of striving for environmental success which, in this case, will probably elude MN since he doesn't have the wherewithal to achieve his goals. There are no MAL responses, suggesting that MN is not neurotically conflicted, but neither does he possess much insight, blithely insisting that he is college material despite evidence to the contrary. He does appear to have psychosexual problems as attested to by the (CYL) content. This seemed to be corroborated by the fact that he felt constrained to emphasize during his interview that he was engaged to be married. He also made statements on the Incomplete Sentences Blank such as "The happiest time . . . is when I am with my fianca [sic]," and "The best . . . time I've had is meeting fianca [sic]." MN's lack of insight and judgment is additionally betrayed by his generally impulsive reaction times, the only "shock" coming, understandably, on the last (future) card.

The Hand Test of MN would stand on its own merits as a compulsive protocol, but all doubt is dissolved when even a cursory comparison is made with his Rorschach. He produced only nine responses, failing card VII, and presenting a picture of a fairly "empty" personality. In general, responsivity on the Rorschach is correlated with the Hand Test except that the latter would have a lower index of central tendency. For example, a person giving about 25 R on the Rorschach would be expected to produce about 15 R on the Hand Test. Therefore, when this relationship is reversed and responses to the Hand Test greatly exceed the number of responses to the Rorschach (in this instance by a ratio of 3:1), the diagnosis of a compulsive façade becomes even more certain.

As can be gathered from the case of MN, the Hand Test can yield important information on its own, but its effectiveness increases when it is juxtaposed against other tests, either reinforcing and developing similar data or providing unique information which can fill in a diagnostic hiatus. Because of its brevity, the Hand Test can readily be integrated into any standard diagnostic battery and therein lies its major appeal to the practicing clinician.

In integrating the Hand Test data into a battery, it may be convenient, if desired, to conceptualize the interrelationships among tests in terms of Structural Analysis, but this approach is by no means necessary provided that it is always recognized that the Hand Test deals with prototypal action tendencies and should be compared with other tests on that basis. Test data from OP exemplify such an approach.

The protocols of OP represent what might be termed a "façade-type" schizophrenic in a Structural Analytic framework: that is, a schizophrenic where both the Introspective Self and the Façade Self are impoverished, as opposed to the "introspective type" where the Façade Self is weak but the Introspective Self is active, producing florid symptomatology. Test data from these two "types" are very different, and, consequently, lumping norms together yields measures of central tendency which would be quite misleading. The schizophrenic who is a façade type on the Hand Test is usually labeled psychiatrically as a simple, chronic, or process schizophrenic. The subject's behavior is generally inefficient and withdrawn but not fulminating or symptomatically spectacular, and, despite pervasive deficiencies in reality contact, during relatively intact periods, the subject can establish a nominal interaction with reality and even appear superficially normal. To people who know him well, he seems strange and unable to cope but not necessarily bizarre.

OP was a 29-year-old, single male who attended college and flunked out. He worked as a school bus driver, custodian, and clerk but had remained unemployed for about 5 years following his first "break." When tested, he expressed interest in becoming a male nurse or driving a tank(!). When first hospitalized, he was classified as a paranoid schizophrenic, but after repeated hospitalizations this diagnosis was changed to schizophrenic, chronic undifferentiated type.

OP is a tall, slender man with short brown hair and glasses; he was dressed in brown slacks, a white shirt, and a maroon cardigan when tested. He presented a neat, clean appearance. He was physically rigid, socially stilted, and restless, finding it necessary to pace about the office. He spoke in a high-pitched monotonous voice. He seemed self-centered, guarded, thinly held together, and without insight.

On the Wechsler Adult Intelligence Scale, OP earned a Verbal IQ of 101, a Performance IQ of 105, and a Full Scale IQ of 103, which places him within the average range of intelligence. His general fund of knowledge was good (Information), but otherwise his performance was just average and, in fact, he showed weaknesses in subtests dealing with social judgment (Comprehension, Picture Arrangement) and immediate recall (Digit Span). His answers were long and rambling, and he sometimes "spoiled" a response by saying too much and contradicting himself. He had trouble staying on the subject, and his thoughts seemed to wander.

Subtest scatter was as follows:

Subtest	Scaled Score
Information	14
Comprehension	8
Arithmetic	12
Similarities	11
Digit Span	7
Vocabulary	10
Digit Symbol	10
Picture Completion	11
Block Design	12
Picture Arrangement	8
Object Assembly	12

The general diagnostic picture of OP presented by three projective techniques (Rorschach, Draw-A-Person Test, and Hand Test) is in agreement with the final psychiatric diagnosis inasmuch as he does appear to be a chronic undifferentiated schizophrenic who, at a comparatively young age, almost seems to be approaching a "burned-out" state. He interacts minimally with his surroundings and is disinterested in activities that require physical or mental exertion. He feels inferior, yet

HAND TEST: OP

CARD	IRT	HAND TEST RESPONSES	SCORE
I	1	Stop. (Q) Uh huh, like a cop. (a.t.e.?) (pause) No, just looks like a hand signal that says stop to me.	DIR
II	2	It looks like a sick hand...hand crippled with arthritis.	CRIP
III	4	A hand pointing the way for someone.	COM
IV	7	Looks like a working hand. ((Q) Grasping for something. (Q) Tool.	ACT (CYL)
V	3	That looks like a sick hand...looks like a crippled hand. Crippled with arthritis.	CRIP ✓
VI	3	Hand clenched in a fist. (Q) I don't know.	DES (AGG)
VII	4	This looks like a hand at rest.	PAS
VIII	3	Hand snapping fingers. (Q) I don't know. Maybe tension.	TEN (IMP)
IX	3	That looks like a sick hand again. (Q) Arthritis.	CRIP ✓
X	12	Oh... making a slow down signal.	DIR (COM) ✓

there is little he can do about it because he is detached from the world and unable to constructively alter his life. He is an empty shell of a man whose hold on reality is marginal at best. Social relationships are very difficult for him, and it is interesting to note that he refused to fill out the Incomplete Sentences Blank except for question 18, where he wrote, "My nerves . . . are good"(!).

The Hand Test.

SUMMARY SHEET

by Edwin E. Wagner, Ph.D.

PUBLISHED BY

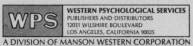

WESTERN PSYCHOLOGICAL SERVICES
PUBLISHERS AND DISTRIBUTORS
12031 WILSHIRE BOULEVARD
LOS ANGELES, CALIFORNIA 90025

A DIVISION OF MANSON WESTERN CORPORATION

DATE _3/6/72_

NAME _OP_   SEX _M_   AGE _29_   RACE _W_

ADDRESS _777 Heaven Path_

OCCUPATION _Unemployed_   DIAGNOSIS _Schizophrenia, chronic Undiff._

AFF = 0	ACQ = 0	TEN = 1	DES = 1	R = 10
DEP = 0	ACT = 1	CRIP = 3	FAIL = 0	AIRT = 4.2
COM = 1	PAS = 1	FEAR = 0	BIZ = 0	H-L = 11
EXH = 0	Σ ENV = 2	Σ MAL = 4	Σ WITH = 1	PATH = 6
DIR = 2				
AGG = 0	ER = Σ INT: Σ ENV: Σ MAL: Σ WITH = _3_ : _2_ : _4_ : _1_			
Σ INT = 3	AOR = (AFF + DEP + COM):(DIR + AGG) = _1_ : _2_			

QUALITATIVE ADMINISTRATIVE OBSERVATIONS _Seems to be trying hard yet to be_
terribly impotent.

CASE HISTORY AND DIAGNOSTIC DATA _Hospitalized at least five times over the_
past few years. Most recent diagnosis by Dr. XYZ: Schizophrenic, chronic
undifferentiated. Doesn't feel he can return to college but wants a job.

EXAMINER _E.E.W._

W-110A

OP's Rorschach is extremely impoverished, with many failures. The form level is weak and characterized by vague W's and a low $F + \%$. Psychological complexity is absent, with form responses predominating at the expense of movement and color. On card IV, the response borders on schizophrenic contamination, shifting from a "sea monster" to "seaweed" to a "seaweed-monster."

<pre>
                        Rorschach : OP

I.   11" Oh, a butterfly. (Anything else?) ⑥   W   F A   P

        Some kinda insect or something. That's   W   F± A

        all I can get out of it. That's a hard

        one. (Q) The outside shape of 'em.

II.   ⑭ I don't know what to say about it...   FAIL

        I can't make heads or tails out of it.

        (Nothing?) No.

III.   ⑮ I can't make heads or tails out of   FAIL

        number three either.

IV.   7" Looks like some kinda deep sea monster   W   F± (A)   , pl

        ...and seaweed. (W?) Uh huh. (Q) The

        way it's shaped. (Q) Seaweed-monster.

        (Q) Uh huh.

V.   11" Looks like a...some kind of...bat,   W   FM A   P

        a flying bat. (Q) Oh, just looks like it

        has wings...just looks like a bat. Or

        some kinda insect. (Q) Moth. (Q) Just   W   F A

        shapes.

VI.   ⑭ I don't know what it would be.   FAIL

VII.   11" Can't make anything out of number seven   WS   F± geog

        either. Looks like an island or a cave...

        or a peninsula. (Q) Well...there's the

        island (W) and there's the cave (Center S).

VIII.   ㉔ I don't know what to say.   FAIL

IX.   ② I don't know what to say about this   FAIL

        one either.

X.   ② Just an ink blot.   FAIL
</pre>

The Hand Test, like the Rorschach, is impoverished. OP shows only 10 responses; his PATH score is high; he gives just 1 ACT; and his INT has dropped to 3, a sure sign of a severe withdrawal from reality. However, the Hand Test supplies some additional information which can provide a little better picture of how OP actually appears to others. OP's lack of internal resources has caused him to fail many Rorschach plates; hence, while it is obvious that he is psychotic, it is difficult

W = 5	FM = 1	A = 4	R = 6
WS = 1	F = 2	(A) = 1	P = 2
FAIL: II, III, VI ⎫	F± = 3	pl = 1	airt = 10.0
VIII, IX, X ⎭		geog = 1	W:D = 6:0
Partial contamina-			W:M = 6:0
tion on IV?			FM:M = 1:0
			ΣC:M = 0:0
			ΣC:Σ_{c^-} 0:0
			FC:CF:C = 0:0:0
			A% = 83
			F% = 83
			F+% = 40

*Scored according to Piotrowski.

to detail his everyday functioning. The Hand Test, however, does reflect his enfeebled attempts to maintain some semblance of reality interaction, and, furthermore, it indicates some awareness of and concern with his precarious mental state by way of the heavy MAL score. The 3 CRIP denote feelings of inferiority, and the TEN shows that OP does experience strain and disharmony in his abortive attempts to cope with a world which is too complex for him. This high MAL should not be construed as "neurotic," however, since OP possesses neither the depth nor the affect (note how he failed all of the Rorschach color plates) to be regarded as neurotically conflicted. He is apparently cognizant of his psychological impotence and suffers keenly because of it, but this is all on the surface and, in this case, does not imply insight or inner resources which might be utilized in psychotherapy. Note that the 3 CRIP responses are repetitions and practically identical. This is an indication of inferiority born of rigidity and impotence rather than neurotic discord.

The two figure drawings of OP are also in accord with the psychiatric diagnosis (Figures 4A and 4B). Both the man and the woman are empty, diagrammatic, and impoverished, with little differentiation between the sexes. The empty eyes and the relative absence of facial features connote withdrawal from social relationships, and the two lines which seemingly separate the neck from the body and the head of the man may indicate the dissociation between thought and bodily impulses. The ground-line on which the male figure stands may reflect the need for a reference point in order to retain a semblance of reality contact. Both figures are oriented toward the bottom of the page, which is often construed to denote insecurity and inadequacy. The hands of the woman and one hand of the man are placed behind the back, which may indicate problems in constructively dealing with the environment. The DAP test seems to come a little closer to the Hand Test than the Rorschach in mirroring the isolation, detachment, and feelings of inferiority which pervade OP's personality. However, without further knowledge of the client's case history, it might be difficult to arrive at a definitive diagnosis of schizophrenia with the DAP alone, inasmuch as an inadequate personality disorder could conceivably produce similar drawings.

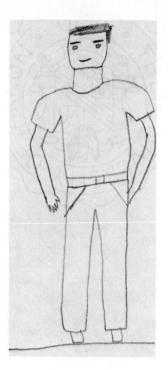

Figure 4A.   Man.

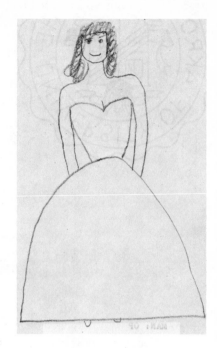

Figure 4B.   Woman.

In this instance, the fact that the INT score on the Hand Test dropped down to 3 provides the clinching argument for the schizophrenic diagnosis.

The case of OP is an illustration of a diagnostic situation in which there is extensive overlap among tests, yet each technique does provide a little extra color in painting the composite personality picture. The case of QR is different in that the psychodiagnostic contribution of the Hand Test is more unique.

QR, a 20-year-old, single male matriculated to college but dropped out after a semester because of what he described as a "conflict of interest." He then worked briefly as a press operator until he injured his thumb. He remained idle for about a year but expressed his intention of returning to college as a journalism or architecture major. He believed he had talent for "writing, art, imagination, persuasion, and positive thinking." His parents, disturbed by what they considered to be QR's idiosyncratic attitudes toward life, referred the client to a psychiatrist. Initial psychiatric impression, based on what appeared to be QR's eccentricity and detachment, was schizoid personality.

QR is a tall, slender man with long brown hair and glasses; he looked younger than his stated age when tested. He was dressed in blue jeans and a plaid flannel shirt. He was quiet and nominally cooperative, but he was bereft of warmth or affability, and he tended to stare wide-eyed at the examiner. He displayed excessive concern for executing graphic tasks and required a good deal of time to complete the battery.

On the Wechsler Adult Intelligence Scale, QR earned a Verbal IQ of 105, a Performance IQ of 115, and a Full Scale IQ of 110, which places him within the bright-normal range of intelligence. Subtest scatter was beyond normal limits, and he showed a sharp declension on Digit Span which may reflect underlying test-taking anxiety. Generally speaking, his Performance IQ was better than his Verbal IQ, and he did well on subtests involving spatial perception (Block Design, Object Assembly), suggesting that he is probably a better risk for training in the graphic arts than in journalism (his Vocabulary score was only slightly above average). Subtest scatter was as follows:

Subtest	Scaled Score
Information	13
Comprehension	10
Arithmetic	10
Similarities	13
Digit Span	7
Vocabulary	12
Digit Symbol	12
Picture Completion	11
Block Design	16
Picture Arrangement	16
Object Assembly	17

On the Hand Test, QR produced a relatively low number of responses (11), with only 4 INT. Furthermore, the EXH on card III is an inanimate response which, qualitatively, suggests ruminatory origins and detracts from the direct behavioral impact of the action tendency. He reacts quickly (AIRT = 4.4), and he is exhibitionistic, but his relationships with people are limited. His ACT score is comparatively high and may account for his turning to a job such as a press operator when he left college. The responses are relatively brief, yet there is an odd flavor to some of them, particularly on cards III, VI, and IX. The (HID) response on card VII suggests that QR is prone to concealing his inner intentions (see also the mask responses to the Rorschach), and the response to card X seems unusually immature and prosaic for a supposedly "arty" individual. There is no MAL, and a neurosis is contraindicated. The overall impression would be consistent with a schizoid personality disorder—withdrawn, rigid, and individualistic.

QR deliberately turned the paper sideways when copying the Bender-Gestalt cards (Figure 5), possibly indicating oppositional tendencies (see also the many space responses on the Rorschach). He was concerned with accuracy, carefully executing each figure. He seemed to have a little trouble getting the sine curves correct, perhaps reflecting a deliberate effort to keep his emotions under wraps. There is no evidence of a perceptual-motor problem, but the renditions do seem to reflect rigidity and in this respect would go along with the Hand Test.

On the DAP, the narcissism, autistic facial expressions, lack of free movement, delineation of joints, tight stance, and sketchy line quality are all characteristic of the schizoid (Figures 6A and 6B). The exhibitionism noted on the Hand Test is corroborated on the DAP: the man is dressed in bathing trunks and the woman in leotards. The lack of legs and feet in the drawing of the man provides further evidence of rigidity and constriction.

EDWIN E. WAGNER

CARD	IRT	HAND TEST RESPONSES	SCORE
I	3	It looks like a policeman's hand stopping traffic. (a.t.e.?) Oh sure, it could be like "hi". Be like a wave (D) but you know be like a half circle kind of thing.	DIR COM^
II	5	He's ah, grasping a rock or something like he's climbing.	ACQ
III	4	That looks posed. (Q) Like if I saw a sculpture, you know, a posed hand.	EXH (INAN) (DES)
IV	5	Kinda scooping something off a table or something. (D)	ACT (ACQ)
V	4	It looks like he has his hand over his chest. (Q) Resting.	PAS
VI	5	He's ah, holding something in his hand. (Q) a pea.	ACT (FOOD)
VII	3	Looks like a magician when they do their hand tricks you know, concealing something.	EXH (HID)
VIII	3	He's picking something up. (Q) Something small.	ACT
IX	3	He's pushing a frog or something, a little animal, prodding them.	ACT (IM, DIR)
X	9	He's ah, holding his finger up, counting 'em.	ACT (IM)

On the Incomplete Sentences Blank, QR's idiosyncrasy seems to come more into the open. He waxes humorous, philosophical, and critical. He is reasonably literate and gives his intelligence more free play. He confesses to a few failings, but on the whole the comments are "upbeat," self-centered, and positive. He presents himself

The Hand Test

SUMMARY SHEET

by Edwin E. Wagner, Ph.D.

PUBLISHED BY

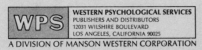

WESTERN PSYCHOLOGICAL SERVICES
PUBLISHERS AND DISTRIBUTORS
12031 WILSHIRE BOULEVARD
LOS ANGELES, CALIFORNIA 90025

A DIVISION OF MANSON WESTERN CORPORATION

DATE __4/19/74__

NAME _____QR_____ SEX __M__ AGE __20__ RACE __W__

ADDRESS_____888 Straightgate_____

OCCUPATION____Unemployed____ DIAGNOSIS __Schizoid__

AFF = 0	ACQ = 1	TEN = 0	DES = 0	R = 11
DEP = 0	ACT = 5	CRIP = 0	FAIL = 0	AIRT = 4.4
COM = 1	PAS = 1	FEAR = 0	BIZ = 0	H-L = 6.0
EXH = 2	Σ ENV = 7	Σ MAL = 0	Σ WITH = 0	PATH = 0
DIR = 1				
AGG = 0	ER = Σ INT: Σ ENV: Σ MAL: Σ WITH = __4__ : __7__ : __0__ : __0__			
Σ INT = 4	AOR = (AFF + DEP + COM):(DIR + AGG) = __1__ : __1__			

QUALITATIVE ADMINISTRATIVE OBSERVATIONS___Seemed self assured, almost supercil-
ious.

CASE HISTORY AND DIAGNOSTIC DATA__College dropout. Psychiatric impression--
schizoid.

EXAMINER____E.E.W.

as wise, cynical, and basically capable. Occasionally, he includes a somewhat cryptic remark which sets him off from the common herd, e.g., "I suffer . . . from pausing before the gun." The general tone is certainly not neurotic, and in this respect the Incomplete Sentences Blank complements the Hand Test; but QR now appears more

Rorschach : QR

I. 10″ I see ah...looks like ah...Halloween mask with four eyes. (Q) Well, 'cause it, ah...top portion here seemed to come out like ears; something like horns. I don't see anything human in the features. And four eyes - how many people have four eyes? (Anything else?) Well...first it looked like a crab with	WS F mask eyes
diamonds on the back or whatever it is, tri-angles on the back. (Q) This part in here reminds me of the antenna and the small mouth that clasps together, it's not a human mouth and these up here they really don't look like claws but if they were open...(Q) The general form.(subject stares at examiner) You want more? I can go on forever. (pause) Well, I don't see anything else in there. Can I turn it upside down or anything? (Yes). **V** Well,	WS F A
that does make a difference. Looks like a space-ship. (rocket?) Spaceship not a rocket! A landing craft more or less, 'cause when I turn it over it has the landing gear and those space probes. I was thinking of those space probes that landed on the moon...I was thinking of Von Daniken. (pause) You want me to say some-thing else? Oh...looks like a phoenix rising out of a fire. (Q) The head I guess. It just brought about the symbol of a bird, eagle you know. Looks like the indian firebird and it seemed like it was rising out of something so I thought of fire or something 'cause it seemed	W F imp
like this was bursting. (Q) I think the im-portant thing was the head, I really didn't see the fire. And it looks like a Japanese	WS (FM) (Ad)

architecture. That's all I'm gonna say. (Q)
It's wide at the base and Japanese architecture
has those eaves that jut out with the point at
the top. (Q) No, no particular one, just a
vague impression.

W	F±	arch

II. 14" Looks like ah...Nineteenth century man
with ah...he's got the large goatee and open
mouth...large mutton chop sideburns. (Q)
Well, just a vague impression. The eyes here
with a goatee at the bottom and the space
framing the mouth maybe. (long pause) And ah...

WS	F±	Hd

V Oh, if I turn it over it looks like a picture
of, what's that short French artist? (Lautrec?)
Yeah, like a Lautrec painting of the dancing
girl, holding up her dress. (Q) Well, I see

W	M	art H O

it in motion. (Q) No, I don't know about the
color. And it looks like a pelvis. (Q) The

D	F±	anat

dark part here, something like it. (Q) No,
just the shape.

III. 10" Looks like two people holding on to
the same object or trying to pull it apart.

W	M	H	P
	F±	obj	

(Q) Don't know what the object could be.
V Turning it over it looks...vaguely...like
a baboon. (Q) Well, turned over you can see
the eyes...should have a nose coming out.

WS	F±	eyes Ad

This thing might be a nostril. Could be.

IV. 3" The skull of ah...an elephant. Skeletal
skull. In these two outlines you can see the
eye sockets coming off of the cranium. These

W	F	eye anat

two parts coming out when they have the
thick, heavy jaw. (Q) Uh huh, the shape. ⑤
And it looks like walking into really dark
woods. (Q) Has depth but it's dark. V

W	cc'F	N

And it could be like some sort of dried up

W	cF	fl

leaf or flower. (Q) Looks dry and crumbly.

V.	25" Well...looks like ah...a butterfly with his wings down. (Q) No, it'd be impossible for a butterfly to get his wings down in that position. (Q) The shape of it. Mostly the tail structure on the bottom and the antenna on top.		W	F	A
VI.	3" Looks like a caricature of a cat meowing. (Q) The top part. It looks like you could see the bottom of his jaw and he's sticking		D	(FM)	(Ad)
	his head straight up and you can see the hair on his jaw. (Q) The top part looks like his head, the bottom part looks like an animal skin on the wall. (Q) It looks like it's been flattened out and dried like a skin you'd hang on a wall.		D	F	obj
VII.	6" They look like two indian maidens facing each other...squaws. (Q) Just looking at each other. **V** (pause) The other way it looks like		W	M	H
	two ladies dancing, facing each other's backs with large hairdos.		W	M	H
VIII.	14" Looks like whales with legs on each side of it crawling up a precipice of some kind. (Q) The long shape, the small eye. (Q) General shape of mountains. (pause) Or it		D	$\left\{\begin{array}{l}\text{(FM)}\\\text{F}^{\pm}\end{array}\right.$	(A) geol
	looks like two animals tearing a piece of blue cloth between 'em. (Q) It does look like it's ripping, definitely.		D	$\left\{\begin{array}{l}\text{FM}\\\text{CmF}\end{array}\right.$	A app
IX.	30" Well, it looks like a clown with, ah, some sort of a...mask...The green things look like some sort of a...thingies...something he's looking through. (Q) Mostly, I can see the hair here, this orange...it reminds me of Bozo. This green part is a mask or something he's looking through. There's the bald				

spot with the hair on the sides.   (Q) The pink   WS $\Big\{$ MC   app Hd

at the bottom could be part of the costume   CF   mask

because it's a wild color. (pause) And it looks

like parts of it could be part of a map or

globe. (Q) Oh, well right here (orange) it

could be part of a northern country, it juts

out with bays (space) and things and this part   DS F$^{\pm}$ geog

here (green) looks like another country.   (Q)

No, not the color. (Q) The bottom part doesn't.

X.   10" Looks like a flea circus. (Q) Well, the

colors look like a circus...and the figures   W $\Big\{$ (M)$^{\pm}$ (H)

couldn't be human but they're like acrobats   CF   decor

building like a pyramid or something. (Q)

Well there's decorations all around. (pause)   W   CF   fl

Or some kind of hanging garden. Tropical.

(Q) Yes, the whole thing, and the colors.

W = 12		M = 5		A = 3		R = 24
WS = 6		(M)$^{\pm}$ = 1		(A)= 1		P = 3
D = 5		mF = ½		Ad = 1		O = 1
DS = 1		FM = 1		(Ad)= 2		airt = 12.5
		(FM)= 3		H = 4		W:D = 18:5
		cF = 2		(H)= 1		W:M = 18:6
		F = 6		Hd = 2		FM:M = 4:6
		F$^{\pm}$ = 7		obj = 2		ΣC:M = 4¼:6
		c'F = ½		eyes = 3		ΣC:Σc= 4¼:3
		FC = ½		mask = 2		FC:CF:C = ½:4:0
		CF = 4		anat = 2		A% = 24
				app = 2		F% = 45
				fl = 2		F+% = 46
				art = 1		
				imp = 1		
				arch = 1		
				N = 1		
				geol = 1		
				geog = 1		
				decor = 1		

freewheeling and there is less evidence of the rigidity and constriction noted previously.

QR becomes even more expansive on the Rorschach, his imagination apparently stimulated by the greater ambiguity of the inkblots. He produces 24 responses, over twice as many as on the Hand Test. Imaginal resources are revealed in the goodly number of movement responses, particularly the 6 M, and he also shows some emotional responsivity in terms of his reactions to color. There is much less rigidity, his color responses are mostly CF, and his $F+\%$ is only 46. His human movement responses are highly exhibitionistic ("... dancing girl, holding up her dress; ... two ladies dancing; ... a clown; ... acrobats building like a pyramid ..."), and it seems likely that these kinds of tendencies will be actualized on the Hand Test through the EXH responses. Some paranoid leanings are evidenced in the masks, eyes, generally feminine use of color, and the full face on card IX. QR's idiosyncratic proclivities are apparent in the original response, use of space, high M, and individualistic percepts.

How can we account for the differences among these tests, and, in particular, how can we reconcile what appears to be the rigidity manifested on the Hand Test with the looseness and expansiveness which comes through to some extent on the Incomplete Sentences Blank and to a greater extent on the Rorschach?

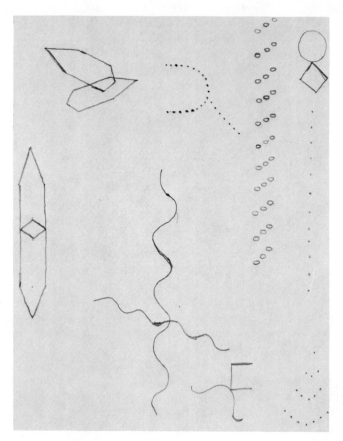

Figure 5

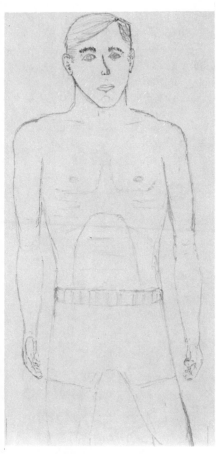

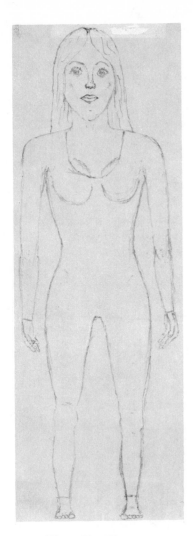

Figure 6A.   Man.   Figure 6B.   Woman.

The answer is quite simple: QR is a schizoid individual whose rigid, brittle exterior conceals a rich, imaginative, autistic inner life replete with paranoid ideation. Outside, he is buttoned down, but inside he is wide open. Were his façade to give way, a borderline or schizophrenic condition would supervene. He produces some rather practical, mundane ACT responses on the Hand Test, which anchor him to reality but are far removed from the imaginative and emotional latitude he permits himself on the Rorschach. The Hand Test betrays little tension, while, on the DAP, the sketchiness and light retracing could reflect anxiety. On the Incomplete Sentences Blank, he admits "My nerves . . . get the better of me when I let them," and, on the Rorschach, anxiety can be detected in the two diffuse light shading responses given to card IV, which, interestingly enough, is often viewed as the "father card." The same situation is encountered in regard to hostility. On the Hand Test, he does not allow himself an AGG response, not even to card VI. But on the Incomplete

INCOMPLETE SENTENCES BLANK — ADULT FORM

Name___QR_____ Sex _M_____ Age___20_____ Marital Status___S___

Place _____Office_____ Date_4/19/74____

Complete these sentences to express <u>your real feelings</u>. Try to do every one.
Be sure to make a complete sentence.

1. I like _tapioca pudding, but there's a limit to everything._

2. The happiest time _is when everyone around me is positive._

3. I want to know _all I can._

4. Back home _things are changing._

5. I regret _I wasn't there during the change._

6. At bedtime _I wish someone I love is with me._

7. Men _have a "y" chromosome, whereas women do not._

8. The best _part of my life is still ahead._

9. What annoys me _most is narrow-mindedness._

10. People _are the greatest books I've ever read._

11. A mother _is the one thing we all have in common._

12. I feel _different everyday, and the change is refreshing._

13. My greatest fear _in life is time._

14. In school _I do not accept everything as truth._

15. I can't _beare children._

(TURN PAGE OVER AND CONTINUE)

Ⓥ

Printed in U.S.A. 71-181AS   JULIAN B. ROTTER, AUTHOR

Sentences Blank he indicates that "I can get pretty pissed off," and on the Rorschach he produces two anatomy responses indicative of repressed hostility. In other words, while some interaction does take place between his behavior and his inner living, QR is much like an iceberg, and the world sees only a small portion of him.

Integration of all the test data reveals a young man who is ideational and has internalized most of his affect. He has the capacity for creativity and originality and may well be brighter than he shows on the WAIS. He fancies himself a clever and independent thinker, and he enjoys being unconventional and controversial, but his eccentric life-style has its limitations inasmuch as he is actually too rigid in

16. Sports <u>are more enjoyable if I participate in them.</u>

17. When I was a child <u>I was not as healthy as I should have been.</u>

18. My nerves <u>get the better of me when I let them.</u>

19. Other people <u>shouldn't be called "other".</u>

20. I suffer <u>from pausing before the gun.</u>

21. I failed <u>few things only to correct them later.</u>

22. Reading <u>causes me to think, while experience causes reaction to thoughts.</u>

23. My mind <u>needs a filing system.</u>

24. The future <u>is for some a strict design, while for me it is a free form.</u>

25. I need <u>new experiences and a change in the old ones.</u>

26. Marriage <u>is not in my near future.</u>

27. I am best when <u>I convince myself to be.</u>

28. Sometimes <u>I'm hot, sometimes I'm cold, because mediocrity is not my bag.</u>

29. What pains me <u>is some people just don't care.</u>

30. I hate <u>no one, but I can get pretty pissed off.</u>

31. This place <u>is not where I want to be.</u>

32. I am very <u>independent.</u>

33. The only trouble <u>with normalcy is that it infers truth.</u>

34. I wish <u>the Bible hadn't been written, money hadn't been printed, and greed meant a lust for life.</u>

35. My father <u>is extremely intelligent about the wrong things.</u>

36. I secretly <u>kept most of myself to myself until recently.</u>

37. I <u>can fit no other mold than the one I was born in.</u>

38. Dancing <u>is good exercise and relieves tension.</u>

39. My greatest worry is <u>trying not to worry when I know I should.</u>

40. Most women <u>think similarly about fashion, but who knows how they determine love.</u>

his behavior to effectively utilize the potential that is locked up in his head. He is more comfortable wallowing around in his own thoughts because his social skills are limited, and this only serves to maintain the distance between himself and other people. When he does interact, it is often in a dull, stereotyped manner and therefore he will be inclined to work beneath his potential at jobs which require little intellectual effort.

Again, the overlap among the Hand Test and the other tests used to evaluate QR is apparent. But this time the disjunction between QR's inner life and his overt behavior has created a diagnostic situation where, perforce, the Hand Test yields some almost unique information which could be crucial in understanding how this young man functions. It faithfully mirrors the rigid life-style which he pursues, together with some interesting schizoid paradoxes: he is interpersonally exhibitionistic, yet socially stilted; ideationally individualistic, yet environmentally common-place; free of overt anxiety, yet full of internal stress. The case of OP revealed a significant overlap among the Hand Test and other diagnostic tests; with QR, there was less diagnostic mutuality among the instruments, and the Hand Test, therefore, had a more unique role to play. Obviously, these delicate interrelationships will vary with the nature of the patient's psychopathology, and, to use the Hand Test effectively, the clinician should keep in mind what the test measures and how it is likely to be refracted through various types of personalities.

7. Conclusion

The Hand Test is a projective technique consisting of ten cards portraying hands in different positions. The subject "projects" prototypal action tendencies by telling what the hands appear to be doing. It is easily scored, and the categories can be reduced to numbers, but the instrument works best when approached clinically rather than psychometrically. The Hand Test is quick and nonthreatening, does not require literacy, is applicable over most of the life span, can be administered to almost any kind of patient regardless of diagnosis or IQ level, reveals overt behavior (and some special behavioral syndromes), and is easily integrated into a test battery. Like any other diagnostic instrument, the Hand Test has limitations: it requires knowledge and experience to be used optimally in a clinical setting, despite its apparent simplicity; it does not measure the entire personality; and it is not yet rooted in a deep data base in terms of currently available reliability and validity studies. On balance, because of its brevity, the Hand Test would seem to recommend itself for inclusion in the diagnostician's armamentarium.

8. References

Azcarate, E., & Gutierrez, M. Differentiation of institutional adjustment of juvenile delinquents with the Hand Test. *Journal of Clinical Psychology*, 1969, *25*, 200–202.

Breidenbaugh, B., Brozovich, R., & Matheson, L. The Hand Test and other aggression indicators in emotionally disturbed children. *Journal of Personality Assessment*, 1974, *38*, 332–334.

Bricklin, B., Piotrowski, Z. A., & Wagner, E. E. *The Hand Test: A new projective test with special reference to the prediction of overt behavior*. Springfield, Ill.: Thomas, 1962.

Brodsky, S. L., & Brodsky, A. M. Hand Test indicators of antisocial behavior. *Journal of Projective Techniques and Personality Assessment*, 1967, *31*, 36–39.

Drummond, F. A failure in the discrimination of aggressive behavior of undifferentiated schizophrenics with the Hand Test. *Journal of Projective Techniques and Personality Assessment*, 1966, *30*, 275–279.

Fornari, U. Studio su alcune correlazioni tra il test di Rorschach e il test della mano, somministrati ad un gruppo di minori dissociali. *Annali di Freniatria e Scienze Affini*, 1971, *84*, 220–226.

Fornari, U., & Gasca, G. Il test della mano studiato in un gruppo di schizofrenici cronici. *Annali di Freniatria e Scienze Affini*, 1971, *84*, 62–73.

Greene, R. S., Sawicki, R., & Wagner, E. E. Hand Test correlates for karate students: A preliminary interpretation based on structural analysis. *Perceptual and Motor Skills*, 1974, *38*, 692–694.

Gutierrez, J. L. A., & Sanchez, E. C. Valoracion de la agresividad con el Hand Test. *Revista de Psicologia General & Aplicada*, 1970, *20*, 535–541.

Higdon, J. F., & Brodsky, S. L. Validity of Hand Test Acting-Out Ratio for overt and experimentally induced aggression. *Journal of Personality Assessment*, 1973, *37*, 363–368.

Hodge, J. R., & Wagner, E. E. The validity of hypnotically induced emotional states. *American Journal of Clinical Hypnosis*, 1964, *1*, 37–41.

Korner, A. F. Theoretical considerations concerning the scope and limitations of projective techniques. *Journal of Abnormal and Social Psychology*, 1950, *45*, 619–627.

Levine, E. S., & Wagner, E. E. Personality patterns of deaf persons: An interpretation based on research with the Hand Test. *Perceptual and Motor Skills*, 1974, *39*, 1167–1236 (monograph supplement).

Oswald, O., & Loftus, P. T. A normative and comparative study of the Hand Test with normal and delinquent children. *Journal of Projective Techniques and Personality Assessment*, 1967, *31*, 62–68.

Panek, P. E., Sterns, H. L., & Wagner, E. E. An exploratory investigation of the personality correlates of aging using the Hand Test. *Perceptual and Motor Skills*, 1976, *43*, 331–336.

Piotrowski, Z. A. On the Rorschach method and its application in organic disturbances of the central nervous system. *Rorschach Research Exchange*, 1936, *1*, 23–29.

Piotrowski, Z. A. *Perceptanalysis*. New York: Macmillan, 1957.

Rand, T. M., & Wagner, E. E. Correlations between Hand Test variables and patrolman performance. *Perceptual and Motor Skills*, 1973, *37*, 477–478.

Rapaport, D. Projective techniques and the theory of thinking. *Journal of Projective Techniques*, 1952, *16*, 269–275.

Selg, H. Der Hand-Test als Indikator für offen aggressives Verhalten bei Kindern. *Diagnostica*, 1965, *4*, 153–158.

Wagner, E. E. The use of drawings of hands as a projective medium for differentiating neurotics and schizophrenics. *Journal of Clinical Psychology*, 1962, *2*, 208–209. (a)

Wagner, E. E. *Hand Test: Manual for administration, scoring and interpretation*. Los Angeles: Western Psychological Services, 1962. (b)

Wagner, E. E. Structural analysis: A theory of personality based on projective techniques. *Journal of Personality Assessment*, 1971, *35*, 422–435.

Wagner, E. E. Diagnosis of conversion hysteria: An interpretation based on structural analysis. *Journal of Personality Assessment*, 1973, *37*, 5–15.

Wagner, E. E. Projective test data from two contrasted groups of exhibitionists. *Perceptual and Motor Skills*, 1974, *39*, 131–140. (a)

Wagner, E. E. The nature of the psychopath: Interpretation of projective findings based on structural analysis. *Perceptual and Motor Skills*, 1974, *39*, 563–574. (b)

Wagner, E. E. The façade compulsive: A diagnostic formulation derived from projective testing. *Journal of Personality Assessment*, 1976, *40*, 352–362. (a)

Wagner, E. E. Personality dimensions measured by projective techniques. *Perceptual and Motor Skills*, 1976, *43*, 247–253. (b)

Wagner, E. E., & Capotosto, M. Discrimination of good and poor retarded workers with the Hand Test. *American Journal Mental Deficiency*, 1966, *1*, 126–128.

Wagner, E. E., & Hawkins, R. Differentiation of assaultive delinquents with the Hand Test. *Journal of Projective Techniques and Personality Assessment*, 1964, *28*, 363–365.

Wagner, E. E., & Heise, M. R. A comparison of Rorschach records of three multiple personalities. *Journal of Personality Assessment*, 1974, *38*, 308–331.

Wagner, E. E., & Hoover, T. O. Exhibitionistic M in drama majors: A validation. *Perceptual and Motor Skills*, 1971, *32*, 125–126.

Wagner, E. E., & Medvedeff, E. Differentiation of aggressive behavior of institutionalized schizophrenics with the Hand Test. *Journal of Projective Techniques*, 1963, *1*, 111–113.

Wagner, E. E., & Romanik, D. G. Hand Test characteristics of marijuana-experienced and multiple-drug using college students. *Perceptual and Motor Skills*, 1976, *43*, 1303–1306.

Wetsel, H., Shapiro, R. J., & Wagner, E. E. Prediction of recidivism among juvenile delinquents with the Hand Test. *Journal of Projective Techniques and Personality Assessment*, 1967, *31*, 69–72.

14

The Measurement of the Self-Concept

LEONARD D. GOODSTEIN AND
DEBORAH LEE DOLLER

1. Introduction

The self is typically defined as the total, essential, or particular being of a single individual or person. That is, the self involves those qualities that differentiate or distinguish that person from other persons. The study of the self has been a continuing preoccupation for both philosophy and psychology.

2. A Historical Overview

Early in the nineteenth century, when American psychology was breaking away from philosophy and establishing itself as an independent discipline, the self was perhaps the most important theoretical concept. Because early psychologists were concerned with the nature of conscious experience in general, most of their work was concerned with such questions as whether or not "pure thoughts" could occur without accompanying mental images. The early journals were replete with case studies of conscious experience that attempted to address such questions, together with the inevitable disagreements that are possible with such a data base. Clearly, each individual person or self was aware of his or her own apparently unique experience, and psychologists could not agree on a way in which these unique experiences could be studied. The rise of behaviorism in American psychology led to the study of public, objective events rather than inner, conscious experience. By 1930, behaviorism was the dominant approach in American psychology and interest in the self temporarily waned.

Within the past 20 years, there has been a resurgence of interest in the self. However, the nature of this more recent interest is rather different from that which predominated earlier in this century. William James (1892), one of America's earliest

LEONARD D. GOODSTEIN and DEBORAH LEE DOLLER • Department of Psychology, Arizona State University, Tempe, Arizona 85281.

and most influential philosopher-psychologists, initiated a distinction between the self as an active element in thinking and the self as an object. The former conceptualization of the self—the self as a thinking and emotional process—was the focus of interest for psychology at the turn of the century, as described above. The study of these inner states or the "stream of consciousness" was *the* subject matter of psychology. But, as we have noted, the difficulties involved in measuring and understanding this aspect of the self led psychology away from this focus. The second conceptualization of the self—the self as an object—is far more compatible with the demands for methodological rigor that typify contemporary psychology.

The intensity of interest in the self as an object or product, albeit an ever-changing and dynamic product, cannot be explained on methodological grounds. Rather, the rise of humanistic-existential philosophy and psychology apparently is at the heart of the resurgence of interest in the self. The importance given self-acceptance by Carl Rogers (1959) and the centrality of the self in the theories of Martin Buber, Rollo May, Gordon Allport, and others must be seen as major influences in this development.

Before we examine the several aspects of self as object, it would seem appropriate to point out that the work of George Herbert Mead, the American social psychologist, has been of considerable importance in moving the study of the self from that of process to that of product. As Mead himself asked, "How can an individual get outside of himself (experientially) in such a way as to become an object to himself?" (1934, p. 138). The answer provided by Mead beautifully exemplifies American pragmatism and the earlier insights of James. Mead notes that the self is never viewed directly but only by others. While it may be argued that it is possible for one to perceive one's self, the earliest experience of the self is through the evaluations of others, primarily parental figures. Initially, children are aware of the evaluations they receive from their parents, and, at a certain stage of their development, usually during the second or third year, they begin to make these evaluations of themselves, mimicking their parents. With age, children become more skillful and experienced in this evaluative role-playing activity, and their self-evaluations become internalized. Further, peers and others now begin to provide evaluations, and the myriad of evaluations that an individual receives through the course of his or her development creates a relatively constant although continually changing self-concept, primarily learned through one's interactions with others. What Mead provides is a developmental and dynamic focus to our understanding of the self as an object.

3. The Self as Object

It would appear that there are three different aspects of the self as an object or product: (1) identity, or how the person perceives him- or herself; (2) self-evaluation, or what the person thinks of him- or herself; and (3) self-esteem, or the subjective way in which the person values him- or herself. Let us examine each of these aspects of the self in turn before we deal with the issues involved in the measurement of these different aspects of the self.

3.1. Identity

There probably is no question asked more frequently, either implicitly or explicitly, of other people than "Who are you?" The early phases of the acquaintanceship process seemingly involve the individual in alternately asking and answering this question.

The response to the question "Who am I?" is typified by the response of then President Lyndon B. Johnson. "I am a free man, an American, a liberal, a conservative, a Texan, a taxpayer, a rancher, a businessman, a parent, a voter and not as young as I used to be nor as old as I expect to be—and I am all those things in no particular order" (from Gordon, 1968, p. 123). Gordon goes on to note that most people respond in a similar way to the instructions to list a number of answers to the question "Who am I?" Most people respond in terms of gender, age, roles (student, taxpayer, and so on), and personality traits, especially prevailing mood such as happy or sad, more or less in that order. It would appear that gender, age, and occupational roles as well as some personality characteristics are regarded by people at large as communicating a good deal of information about themselves to other people.

While personality characteristics do occur in the responses of most people, these are offered later rather than earlier in the response list. That people should regard such consistencies in their own behavior as central to their identity comes as no surprise, but that such characteristics are of lower priority than role determinants of behavior is an interesting although difficult-to-explain phenomenon. Also worthy of note is the typical failure to include one's goals, needs, and wants in responding to the query, especially since McDougall (1908) has argued that these lie at the core of the self. Either McDougall's ideas about the centrality of these factors need to be reconsidered, or, more likely, we need to reconsider our techniques for inquiring about the identity of others.

3.2. Self-Evaluation

In addition to the identity that is provided by the self-concept, each of the elements that may go into this identity can be evaluated. We may see ourselves as contributory citizens, or immature teenagers, or poor parents, or successful psychologists. Self-evaluation is used to designate the individual's evaluation of a specific ability, attribute, or material possession, each of which is part of the individual's identity. Thus we can evaluate our functioning as a bowler, a lover, a son or daughter, and so on—all of those characteristics which we have earlier identified as portions of our self-concept. These evaluations can be rather crude, as "I'm a pretty good bridge player," or rather precise, as "I was the top student in my law school graduating class."

What is important to note here is that the concept of self-evaluation is restricted to those evaluations of given aspects of the self, not the entire self. In principle, these evaluations can be measured against some objective standard that can be agreed on. Thus self-evaluations can be validated by comparing the person's self-evaluation to the objective evidence provided from the environment, including from other people.

3.3. Self-Esteem

While self-evaluation is concerned with particular attributes, self-esteem involves the global and subjective degree of positive regard which the individual has for her- or himself. Therefore, self-esteem is a measure of one's self-liking or self-regard. And, in contrast to self-evaluation, self-esteem is not open to external validation or comparison. While one can be checked as to one's self-evaluation as a tennis player, such a convenient basis of comparison is not available about generalized self-worth.

Self-esteem can range from pride or arrogance on the one hand to humility or despair on the other. We can see ourselves as a basically worthwhile person or as a worthless wretch, with all of the alternatives in between available to us as summary statements of our self-esteem.

At first glance, it would appear that one's self-esteem should be the simple summation of one's self-evaluations, but this is not the case. While an individual might have negative self-evaluations of a number of his or her attributes, these attributes may or may not be important attributes in his or her individualized self-esteem. Thus I may agree that I am a very poor tennis player and have very low mechanical aptitude, but, because these are attributes which have low salience in my model of a worthwhile or successful person, I may still have high self-esteem. On the one hand, it can be argued that individuals develop strong defenses against admitting that they have important deficiencies, and the low weights given to these attributes can be seen as a defense against perceived self-denigration. On the other hand, it can be argued that, developmentally, we tend to learn to regard highly those attributes which provide us with positive self-evaluations and to integrate these into our idealized self-concept—these become the attributes on which we base our self-esteem. While it is difficult to decide on the relative merits of these two positions, or some integration of both, it is clear that, because of the differential importance or salience of different attributes, the self-esteem of individuals is not the simple sum of their self-evaluations.

3.4. Self-Acceptance

To further complicate this matter, mature individuals may have learned to accept both their positive and negative self-evaluations. Indeed, such self-acceptance is often argued as the primary criterion of true self-esteem and psychological maturity. Thus I may agree that I am not financially successful when compared to nationwide income statistics, but, compared to other college professors, my income is quite reasonable and I accept a modest income because of the other rewards involved in being a college professor. Even though I know that my income is low, I refuse to think badly of myself because of it.

3.5. Ideal Self-Concept

Inferred in the previous discussion is the notion of an ideal self-concept—the individualized set of expectations of what kind of person I would like to be. These individual ideal self-concepts are certainly shaped by our culture, our individual learning histories, and a number of other factors. They are thus like some other ideals in some ways, unlike others in some other ways, and unique in still other ways. The discrepancy between our idealized self-concept and our actual self-concept becomes an important factor in determining our self-esteem. Large discrepancies lead to low self-esteem, small discrepancies to high self-esteem. While this is relatively straightforward, it overlooks a critical issue—the realism of the ideal self-concept.

If my ideal self-concept is unrealistic, then the discrepancy between my actual self-concept and this ideal will be positive or negative, depending on the direction of the unreality of my ideal. If the ideal self-concept is unrealistically high, then I can never reach it and there will always be a large discrepancy between my ideal and actual self-concepts. We all know individuals who appear quite successful to us, but who seem plagued by feelings of inferiority. Here, we would argue that an unrealistically high self-concept is at issue. Similarly, we know people who seem quite satisfied with rather modest successes and are difficult to motivate to further achievement. In this instance, it can be argued that an unrealistically low self-concept is a useful explanatory construct.

Finally, while we have discussed the self-concept in this section as though it were rather static, this is not the case. The work on level-of-aspiration over the past three decades (e.g., Lewin, Dembo, Festinger, & Sears, 1944) rather clearly demonstrates that, as our actual success varies, most of us modify our expectations of further success or failure accordingly, and that such changes in level-of-aspiration certainly are an integral and important part of our self-concept, especially our self-esteem. The dynamic and changing nature of the self-concept is another issue to be considered in its measurement.

4. The Development of the Self-Concept

We agree unanimously that adults have a self-concept, and, in contrast, that this concept is not present at birth. While we must infer the lack of a self-concept from infant behavior, the rather disjunctive and reflexive pattern of infant behavior does strongly support this inference.

Most child psychologists have tended to argue that individuals' first noteworthy experiences are with their own bodies. While the child's initial experiences are diffuse, such as pain or pleasure, and probably undifferentiated from the surrounding environment, over time the child learns greater differentiation of the world and its own physical self. Thus the mouth becomes a more specific source of pleasure, a wet or soiled diaper becomes a specific source of displeasure, and so on. The child begins to differentiate the boundaries of its own body and learns to identify the "I" or the "me." This learning is greatly facilitated by the parents as they begin to test the child's sense of identity as they question "Where is the baby?"

Most of us have observed infants as they seem to be endlessly fascinated by observing the movements of their own hands and feet, or as they seem to monitor their own early vocalizations. These behaviors seem to be an integral part of the development of an awareness of the body and its functioning as the beginnings of the self. Later, the child begins to learn about those external objects which belong to it, extending the concept of "me" to "mine." Learning that certain things are mine and defending them against others is a further step in the development of the self.

The child's early interactions with the environment, especially the interpersonal environment, are of primary importance in learning the boundaries of the physical self and of personal possession. Similarly, the child learns about the self from frustration and disappointment in not having its needs and wants met. As Freud (1911) and others have noted, the child whose needs were always met would have considerable difficulty in learning the psychological boundary conditions between self and environment. Because this theoretical situation can never occur in real life, there is little danger that this is possible, but the point does suggest the necessity of frustration in learning about the self, and, at the same time, producing a somewhat more realistic sense of self-esteem. It is interesting to note that identity can be attained only at the cost of frustration and reduced self-esteem.

In these early interactions with the environment, the child learns something about its importance, its potency in controlling the environment. While there is little direct evidence to support this contention, it is sensible to argue that the child learns whether or not its needs can be met on a regular basis, whether or not the environment is or is not flexible in meeting its changing needs, whether needs are met promptly or in some fixed time frame, whether modest or vigorous interactions are required to gain attention, and, in a myriad of other ways, some sense of self as compared to the environment in which it lives.

Later, there are direct parental evaluations of performance. While there is a dearth of research in this area, it would appear safe to argue that the initial self-evaluations are mirrors of parental evaluations, for the child has no other basis for deciding about the goodness or badness of its behavior. On the other hand, parents rather typically tell their children that their eating, toileting, sexuality, aggression, and so on make them a "good" or "bad" little boy or girl and, at the same time, provide strong reinforcers in terms of additional affection or the withdrawal of affection to underscore the points that they are making. Over time, the inescapable conclusion is that most children develop a sense of self-esteem that is largely shaped by their parents. In one of the few studies of this problem, Jourard and Remy (1955) found a high positive correlation (.70) between a measure of self-esteem and a measure of perceived parental regard for self. Of even more use would have been a direct parental measure of regard.

Such a study was reported by Coopersmith (1967), who studied 10- and 11-year-old boys. He compared two measures of these boys' self-esteem with parental evaluations obtained from depth interviews with the boys' mothers. Compared with boys with low self-esteem, boys with high self-esteem had mothers who expressed more affection, were more interested in their activities, and saw their sons in a generally more favorable light. It can be argued that, since the high-self-esteem boys were indeed more successful by societal standards, it was easier for the mothers to provide such positive evaluations. Nevertheless, Coopersmith's findings do suggest that there is an important parental role in the development of self-esteem.

However critical the parental role may be in the early development of self-esteem, evaluations by important others—peers, teachers, and other authority figures—quickly become equally if not more important in the shaping of one's self-esteem. For most of us in this society, peer relations and school work are particularly critical areas for evaluations by others. For school-age boys, athletic prowess is another, related area of evaluation. The bulk of the reported research shows a fairly clear-cut and positive relationship between success in school work, athletic skills, and social poise on the one hand and high self-esteem on the other.

What is difficult to determine from these reports, however, is the nature of the causal relationship between self-esteem and success. Does success cause high self-esteem, or vice versa? The answer to this question is even more complicated in the case of children whose parents may also encourage and support both their efforts at success and their self-esteem. While definitive studies are yet to be done, it would appear that there is a tightly linked, mutually causal relationship among behavior, self-esteem, and other evaluations. Although high self-esteem enhances the probability of success and the positive evaluations by others, success raises the positive evaluation by others and one's self-esteem, and so on. We understand very little about this mutually interdependent and often self-fulfilling process; however, there is little doubt that it can start at any phase of the cycle and rather quickly become self-renewing. And, of course, the reverse is equally true. Low self-esteem leads to failure and low evaluations by others in the same interlocking fashion. Clearly, nothing succeeds like the will to fail!

1. Issues in the Measurement of the Self-Concept

Earlier, we indicated that the rising interest in humanistic-existential psychology was probably the most important reason for the current resurgence of interest in the self-concept. The work of Carl Rogers is clearly paramount in this regard. For Rogers and his co-workers, the self-concept is the most important construct in any psychology of the individual. Rogers has proposed that the self-concept or self-structure is best regarded as an organized configuration of those perceptions of the self which are admissible to awareness. Such a self-concept is composed of such elements as the perceptions of one's characteristics and abilities, the percepts and concepts of the self in relation to others and to the environment, the values which are seen as associated with one's experiences and object, and the goals and ideals which the person perceives as having important positive or negative valences.

In his most current statement about the self, Rogers (1959) has defined the self-concept as "the organized consistent conceptual gestalt composed of perceptions of the characteristics of the 'I' or 'me' and the perceptions of the relationships of the 'I' or 'me' to others and to various aspects of life, together with the values attached to these perceptions. It is a gestalt which is available to awareness though not in awareness. It is a fluid and changing gestalt, a process, but at any given moment it is a specific entity" (p. 200).

Despite this fairly general statement which suggests all three elements of the self referred to earlier—identity, evaluation, and esteem—Rogers and his colleagues have been primarily interested only in the final one, self-esteem, and its collateral part, self-acceptance. Thus the Rogerian influence has led to the development of a variety of evaluative measures of the self-concept such as self-satisfaction, self-favorability, the congruence or discrepancy between the individual's ideal- and actual-self-concept, and so on, all stemming from the core concepts of self-esteem and self-acceptance.

While it is clear that there are some important differences between and among these terms—for instance, self-acceptance means respect for one's self, including one's limitations, while self-esteem means pride in one's self, perhaps overlooking or ignoring one's limitations—these terms are so overlapping and confounded that it is not possible to sort out these differences in any clear-cut way. As a consequence, Wylie (1968) has suggested that the general term "self-regard" be used for all these evaluative measures of the self.

While we initially argued that it was possible, and perhaps even worthwhile, to separate self-regard measures into those that involved separate attributes and those that were more global estimates of self-esteem, it is difficult to apply this distinction to the existing instruments and to the published literature. As we shall see, however, the questions of whether the particular instrument is a global one or a summative one and how a global instrument of self-esteem can be broken down into component elements are often encountered in the research literature.

While clinical and personality psychologists have been primarily interested in the evaluative measure of the self or self-regard, social psychologists and sociologists have been primarily concerned with the measurement of the identity aspects of the self, and there has been little overlap between these two approaches.

5.1. Identity

As noted above, self-identity is typically measured by a free-response "Who are you?" procedure initially developed by Bugenthal and Zelen (1950). They asked respondents to give three answers to this question and then categorize their answers by name, status, mood, and so on. More recent investigators have used the expanded version developed by Kuhn and McPartland (1954), who call their procedure the Twenty Statement Test because subjects are asked to give 20 responses to the question "Who am I?" in 12 min.

The major issue in using such free response involves the coding of the responses and interpreting the results. Kuhn and McPartland (1954) argue that the ordinal position of the response in the list is an important indicator of the importance of that construct in the identity of that individual. On the other hand, many psychologists would argue that many even more important aspects of one's identity would never be revealed early or easily in such a process. Obviously, how one decides on such a matter is a question of theoretical style rather than empirical data.

Gordon (1968) has surveyed and reported on a number of different coding systems for these free-response procedures. Gordon himself presents a 30-category coding system, together with some tentative data from several samples of college and high school students. While his coding system is obviously comprehensive, it also would appear to be laborious to use and present problems of interjudge reliability.

The data from these free-response "Who am I?" techniques are heavily descriptive of status and role categories such as gender, race, national origin, occupation, religion, and other dimensions that involve "ascribed characteristics" rather than direct descriptions. While being a Catholic, a teenager, or an American does permit the observer to make some inferences about the respondent, these are more indirect than if the person described him- or herself as industrious, intelligent, or blasé. These direct descriptions are, however, relatively less frequently given by respondents to the "Who am I?" query.

In an effort to obtain more direct personality descriptions, a number of psychologists have moved to using some form of an adjective checklist. Such lists provide a series of adjectives, often 200 or more, which the respondent is to check as "generally characteristic" or "generally noncharacteristic" of him- or herself. The adjectives are generally direct descriptions of personality traits, such as "happy-go-lucky," "lazy," or "intelligent." While such adjective checklists do provide more data on the respondent's self-perceptions, their social identity, the typical all-or-none response procedure limits the range of measurement, and there are serious difficulties involved in developing any organized view of the respondent when we face several hundred separate adjectives. While Gough and Heilbrun (1964) have provided some solution to this problem in providing a scoring scheme for their particular list of adjectives based on the Henry Murray Need System, there is little research support for this particular scheme.

5.2. Self-Regard

Perhaps the most significant approach to the measurement of overall self-regard involves the Q-sort, based on the work of William Stephenson of the University of Chicago. In such a Q-sort, the subject is given a packet or deck of cards, each containing a self-descriptive phrase or statement, such as "I am easy to talk with," "I am a submissive person," "I am likable," or "I am a hard worker." The subject is asked to read these statements and sort them into a prearranged distribution (typically 9 or 11 piles) along a continuum from those most characteristic to those least characteristic. The distribution approximates a normal distribution and, thus, for 100 cards, the subject would be asked to sort them into 11 piles as follows: 2-4-8-11-16-18-16-11-8-4-2. The subject keeps arranging the cards into the required piles until he or she is satisfied that the arrangement does represent the self-concept.

The subject typically is then asked to sort the cards according to the degree to which they are characteristic of his or her ideal self-concept, or how he or she would have sorted them when of a certain age, or how the subject's husband or wife would sort them, and so on. Each item in the sort may be assigned a value from 1 to 9 or 11 depending on the number of piles used, according to the pile in which the subject has placed the statement. If, for example, a subject placed the statement "I am a dominant person" in the least characteristic or eleventh pile, then that statement would have a value of "11" for that sort. For each subject, a Pearson correlation coefficient may be calculated for the scores obtained on the two sorts. Most typically, the subject's self-sort is correlated with his or her ideal-sort, and the obtained correlation coefficient is treated as a score for that person, and from that score the degree of his or her self-regard is estimated.

Most self-concept research includes repeated Q-sorts, with the changes in the self-ideal correlations used as the dependent measures, for example, in studies of the outcome of client-centered psychotherapy. Increases in these correlations are regarded as indicating greater congruence between the actual- and ideal-self-concept. These changes can occur either as a result of a change in the actual-self-concept in the direction of the ideal, or of a change in the ideal-self-concept in the direction of the actual, or of changes in both directions. The research findings thus far tend to support the last suggestion.

The most commonly used set of Q-sort items is that initially used by Butler and Haigh (1954). This set consists of 100 items "accidentally selected" from actual therapy protocols. Items included are "I usually feel driven" and "Self-control is no problem for me." Another widely used set was developed by Block (1961) and is sometimes referred to as the California Q-sort set. It consists of 70 adjectives such as "restless," "sarcastic," and "wise," which are to be sorted into seven categories along a forced normal distribution of "most like me" to "least like me." In addition to these readily available and widely used Q-sorts, there are over 100 other sets that have been developed and used in research projects of one kind or another.

How does the Q-sort differ from the typical self-report personality questionnaire, and how do these differences meet the methodological requirements of the phenomenologically oriented students of the self-concept? While the subject must sort the items into predetermined piles, the subject is free to distribute the items in terms of their relative applicability to him or her. Also, the comparison of the obtained sort is not with the culturally accepted view of the ideal person but with the subject's own view. Further, as we have just noted, it is possible to create a new set of items for whatever special purpose one has in mind, although for both the Butler-

Haigh and the Block sets, the items involved are acceptable for most potential subjects.

There are a number of yet-unanswered questions about the use of Q-sorts. The reliability of most of these Q-sort sets is still unknown. It is not known if combining the actual- and ideal-self-concept scores does anything more than increase the error variance. There is ample evidence that defensiveness—the desire of the subject to "look good"—and social desirability are important determinants of Q-sort responses. Finally, the question of how to assess the validity of the Q-sort is a thorny one because there is no acceptable operational definition of the self-concept. Thus, while the Q-sort was initially regarded as a methodological breakthrough in the measurement of the self-concept at the time it was introduced, its present status is much less clear.

In addition to these specially derived measures of the self-concept, there are a variety of more traditional tests that purport to measure the self-concept. Since these more usual procedures do not involve any special methodological advance or pose any new methodological problem, but are rather traditional personality questionnaires requiring either a true-false or Likert-type agreement response, these inventories will be surveyed in the later portions of this chapter. Each of the major instruments tapping the self-concept will be described and reviewed, first those intended for use with children and then those for use with adults. However, before we turn to these traditional instruments, we shall briefly focus our attention on one of the yet-unmentioned aspects of the self-concept—the unconscious self-concept.

5.3. Measurement of the Unconscious Self-Concept

While an unconscious self-concept may be regarded as a contradiction in terms, particularly if one accepts the phenomenological orientation of most of the work in this area, the concept has received some attention. After all, how can one have "an organized configuration of perceptions of the self" of which one is unaware? Yet Rogers, himself, in his 1959 definition (p. 200) recognizes that these perceptions may not be in awareness, although they should be "available to awareness." Clearly it can be argued that, at least for some persons, their very problem is that certain aspects of themselves are blocked from their own awareness. Also, the typically inadequate state of measurement in this field has led some psychologists to search for nonverbal, perhaps unconscious, indices of the self-concept.

From the early 1930s, there has been some involvement in expressive behavior as an approach to the measurement of the self. Gordon Allport, for example, has long insisted that the manner of style in which an act is performed, such as walking, writing, or talking—the personalized or idiosyncratic aspects—is a central clue to the nature of that person, including his or her self-concept. Allport (1965) analyzed a series of *Letters from Jenny*, demonstrating a new technique which he called "personal structure analysis" for uncovering the several underlying traits revealed by these letters. Wolff (1943), in an earlier set of studies, demonstrated that most persons could not recognize their own expressive products, such as samples of their own handwriting or voice, which had been collected some 6 months earlier. Such studies are very provocative in that they eliminate or substantially reduce the problems of deliberate faking which are inherent in all self-report tests of personality.

Projective techniques such as the Rorschach and the Thematic Apperception Test have also been regarded as sources for tapping the unconscious self-concept.

Unfortunately, however, there are no generally agreed-on procedures for using these instruments in this fashion, and space considerations preclude further discussion of these approaches at this juncture, although the chapters on these instruments elsewhere in the volume may provide the reader with additional notions about how to proceed along these lines.

In summary, there seems to be no clear agreement about the relative worth of measuring the unconscious self-concept. There is no clarity in the theoretical assumptions offered to support most of these attempts, and there has been no well-coordinated effort to cope with the issues involved in establishing the construct validity of this difficult-to-pin-down concept. There have been a wide range of hypotheses involved, a number of different instruments used, and a variety of findings reported, all of which make any clear generalization an impossibility.

Let us now turn our attention to the more typical approaches to the measurement of the self-concept, beginning with those instruments intended to measure the self-concepts of children.

6. Specific Measures of Children's Self-Concepts

6.1. Lipsitt's Self-Concept Rating Scale for Children

The Self-Concept Rating Scale for children contains 22 trait-descriptive adjectives designed to assess the self-concept of children (Lipsitt, 1958). Each adjective in the scale is prefaced by the phrase "I am . . . " and is followed by a 5-point rating scale with the alternatives "not at all," "not very often," "some of the time," "most of the time," and "all of the time." Of these adjectives, 19 are considered to reflect positive or socially desirable attributes, while the other three are considered to reflect negative attributes. An example of a positive item is "honest," and an example of a negative item is "jealous."

A subject receives a score of 1 if he or she checks the first point on the rating scale and a score of 5 if the last point on the scale is chosen. For the three negative adjectives, the scores are obtained in an inverse fashion. The total score for each subject is obtained by summing the ratings across all 22 adjectives, with lower scores supposedly reflecting some degree of self-disparagement.

Since Lipsitt believed that people often compared their own self-concepts with concepts of an ideal self, he also developed an ideal-self-concept scale to determine the discrepancy between a person's conception of him- or herself and his or her ideal. The Ideal Self-Rating Scale for Children consists of the same adjectives as does the Self-Concept Rating Scale, but in this scale each adjective is preceded by the phrase "I would like to be . . . ." The rating categories and scoring system previously described for the Self-Concept Rating Scale are also used for the Ideal Self-Rating Scale. To determine the discrepancy score, the total self-concept score on the Self-Concept Rating Scale for Children is subtracted from the total Ideal Self score.

6.1.1. Reliability

Lipsitt (1958) administered both of these scales to 300 fourth-, fifth-, and sixth-grade schoolchildren on the same day and also 2 weeks later. The distribution of scores was essentially normal, with no significant differences for grade or sex. The

2-week test-retest reliability coefficients for the Self-Concept measure alone ranged from .73 for boys in the fourth grade to .91 for girls in the fifth grade. All these correlations were significant at the .001 level. The test-retest reliability coefficients for the discrepancy scores, which ranged from .51 for girls in the sixth grade to .72 for boys in the fifth grade, were somewhat below those of the Self-Concept measure, but all were significant at the .01 level. Horowitz (1962) reported that, after 1 week, the test-retest reliability for the Self-Concept scale ranged from .54 to .89, with all correlations significant at less than the .025 level.

6.1.2. Validity

Lipsitt was interested in investigating the relationship between anxiety and self-concept. Significant negative correlations ranging from −.34 to −.63 were found between scores on the Self-Concept Rating Scale and the Children's Manifest Anxiety Scale (Castaneda, McCandless, & Palermo, 1956), with high anxious subjects producing low self-concept ratings. Similar results were also reported by Coopersmith (1959).

Horowitz (1962) hypothesized that high anxiety would be negatively correlated with overall self-concept and also with low sociometric status. To investigate this relationship, 111 elementary schoolchildren in the fourth, fifth, and sixth grades were given the Children's Manifest Anxiety Scale, Lipsitt's Self-Concept Rating Scale, and a sociometric ranking scale. The results of this study replicated the findings of Lipsitt; consistent negative correlations were found between anxiety and self-concept, with the high anxious child tending to have a poorer self-concept. Also, as predicted, negative correlations were found between anxiety and sociometric status, so that the high anxious child tended to have a poorer self-concept and also to be less popular on a ranking sociometric measure.

Reese (1961) reported findings which indicated the relationship between the self-concept and acceptance by others. Acceptance of others and acceptance by best friends is curvilinear, with moderately self-accepting children scoring high in sociometric status and low self-accepting children scoring low in sociometric studies. On the other hand, Mayer (1967) found no relationship between sociometric status and the scores on Lipsitt's Self-Concept Rating Scale in groups of mentally handicapped children.

Mann, Beaber, and Jacobson (1969) theorized that group counseling procedures would lead to a more positive self-concept for educable mentally handicapped boys. It was found that there were significant increases in scores on Lipsitt's Self-Concept Rating Scale after group counseling. No significant increases were reported for scores on the Piers-Harris Scale (see below).

Contrary to Mayer's (1966) hypothesis, mentally handicapped pupils placed in a special class early in their school lives did not develop more positive self-concepts, as determined by scores on the Piers-Harris Scale and the Lipsitt Scale, than those who were placed at a later time.

6.1.3. Summary

Individuals wishing to conduct self-concept research with children should be aware of some of the limitations of the Lipsitt Scale. The rationale for item choice is not explained. The scale does not include an equal number of positive and negative items to control for acquiescence-response set. Also, the scale has not been internally factor-analyzed, and few studies have been reported which are relevant to construct validity (Wylie, 1974). Further research and development are sorely needed to determine the utility of this instrument in self-concept research with children.

6.2. Coopersmith's Self-Esteem Inventory

Coopersmith (1959) used items from the Rogers and Dymond (1954) scale, reworded for use with children, in the development of his Self-Esteem Inventory (SEI). Expert judges decided if additional items were to be included or if certain original items were to be eliminated. Five psychologists sorted all the items into two groups, which were indicative of either high self-esteem or low self-esteem. Any items that appeared ambiguous or repetitious or that were not agreed on by the psychologists as adequate were eliminated. The items were next tested for comprehensibility with a group of 30 children. The final inventory consisted of 50 items, plus 8 Lie scale items, which concerned the child's perceptions in four areas: peers, parents, school, and self. The child checked one of two columns, either "like me" or "unlike me," which best described how he or she usually feels. An item checked in the "like me" column designates high self-esteem, while an item checked in the "unlike me" column designates low self-esteem.

6.2.1. Reliability

The test-retest reliability coefficient was found to be .88 after 5 weeks for a sample of 30 fifth-grade children (Coopersmith, 1959). There apparently are no other reliability estimates available for this scale.

6.2.2. Validity

The SEI was administered to two samples, 102 fifth and sixth graders in New York State and 1748 public schoolchildren in Connecticut. Wylie (1974) suggests that Coopersmith's use of highly restricted groups makes it difficult to evaluate construct validity. As an example, Coopersmith (1959) only used subjects in the New York sample who were high or low on SEI scores and also high or low in a Behavioral Rating Form. Wylie believes that this use of restricted groups limits the information about relationships between the SEI and other variables across the range of SEI scores.

Coopersmith (1959) also developed a Behavioral Rating Form (BRF) in which teachers or other persons closely associated with the child rated him or her on a 14-item, 5-point scale on behaviors presumed to be related to self-esteem. These ratings are based on how the person thinks the child feels about him- or herself, as evidenced by behavior. Coopersmith found substantial agreement between teachers' ratings of subjects and the subjects' own ratings of themselves in the New York sample. Coopersmith, however, never reports any interpretable statistical information to give the reader an idea of what "substantial" agreement indicates (Wylie, 1974).

With the fifth and sixth graders in the New York sample, Coopersmith found a significant correlation of .36 between scores on the SEI and Iowa Achievement Test scores. A significant partial correlation of .29 was found between self-esteem and sociometric status when achievement was held constant. Campbell's (1967) significant correlation of .31 provides further support for the hypothesis of a positive relationship between the Coopersmith Self-Esteem Inventory and Iowa Achievement Test scores.

Connell and Johnson (1970) hypothesized that subjects with high sex-role identification would have more positive feelings of self-esteem than subjects with low sex-role identification. Higher SEI scores were found for adolescent males who scored high on sex-role identification on Gough's Femininity Scale, thus supporting the theoretical prediction. No differences in self-esteem were found for adolescent females.

Boshier (1968) found significant correlations of .77 for girls and .81 for boys between SEI scores and liking one's first name. Trowbridge (1970) predicted that lower SEI scores would be found among children in a socioeconomically disadvantaged school district. Contrary to prediction, these children had higher mean SEI scores than more socioeconomically advantaged children.

6.2.3. Summary

Much of the available information and research about the SEI is reported in a book by Coopersmith (1967). Wylie (1974) concludes that much of Coopersmith's research is uninterpretable because of numerous limitations in his reporting of results. She concludes, "Altogether, the state of development of this inventory and the amount of available information about it do not make it an instrument of choice for self-concept research on child Ss. If further research and development were to be undertaken, this conclusion might be modified, depending on the results of such research" (p. 174).

6.3. Piers-Harris Children's Self-Concept Scale

The Piers-Harris Scale, an instrument designed to measure the way children feel about themselves, consists of 80 first-person simple declarative sentences which are answered "yes" or "no" by the child. The original pool of items was developed from Jersild's (1952) collection of children's statements about what they liked and disliked about themselves. Slightly more than half of the items are worded to indicate a negative self-concept, in order to reduce the effects of acquiescence. However, to reduce the confusion of a double negative to young children, negative terms such as "don't" are avoided, whenever possible. Sample items from the scale include "I am good in my schoolwork" and "I worry a lot." This instrument can be administered either individually or to classes and requires approximately 15–20 min to complete. The P-H Scale was designed to be used with children in grades 3–12. Although all statements are worded at the third-grade reading level, children below the third grade can take the test if the examiner reads the items.

The original item pool consisted of 164 statements which were administered in a pilot study to a sample of 90 third-, fourth-, and sixth-grade schoolchildren (Piers, 1969). Items were eliminated from the pool if they did not discriminate between subjects who were high and low on total scores or if they were not answered in the expected direction by at least half of the subjects with high total scores. Piers thought that the remaining 80 items would provide a good measure of general self-concept.

6.3.1. Reliability

The Kuder-Richardson Formula 21 was used to test internal consistency on an intermediate, 95-item form of the scale (Piers & Harris, 1964). The test was given to six groups of students in the third, sixth, and tenth grades, with results indicating no consistent sex or grade differences. The coefficients for the K-R 21 ranged from .78 for tenth-grade girls to .93 for third-grade boys. A retest conducted after 4 months on one-half of the sample resulted in coefficients ranging from .71 to .72.

6.3.2. Validity

A multiple factor analysis was conducted on the 80-item revised scale to investigate the structure of the scale (Piers & Harris, 1964; Piers, 1969). A sample of 457 sixth graders was used for this analysis. It was found that ten factors accounted for 42% of the variance, with the following six factors large enough to be interpretable: behavior, general and academic status, physical appearance and attributes, anxiety, popularity, and happiness and satisfaction.

Wylie (1974) points out that no evidence for a general factor was presumably found in this analysis, although the test was designed to be unidimensional and to reflect the "general self-concept" of a child. If the scale were six-dimensional, the single total score for the scale would lose considerable useful information.

However, in his review of the P-H Scale, Bentler (1972a) argues that the scale may be more unidimensional than would be suspected from the original factor analysis, because a common finding of a principal components analysis of binary items, which was used in this scale, tends to lead to several factors. Wylie (1974) suggests that further factor analytic work of the scale be done on subjects of the same and different ages to discover what factors would appear.

Michael and Smith (1975) gave the P-H Scale to three samples of 299 elementary school pupils, 302 junior high school students, and 300 senior high school students to determine the factorial dimensions of the P-H and to determine if they could replicate the six factors reported by Piers and Harris (1964). Factor analyses of the inter-correlations of the responses to the 80 items yielded the following three factors which appeared to be relatively invariant across each of the educational levels: physical appearance, socially unacceptable behavior, and academic confidence reflecting school and intellectual status. These findings replicate the first three constructs found by Piers and Harris. Within the domain of emotionality, a number of factors such as anxiety, abasement, self-contentment, and self-dissatisfaction were found, which were not invariant across the samples. These results were not consistent with the findings of Piers and Harris. Michael and Smith conclude that the items included under the domain of emotionality are interpreted more broadly and subjectively than are those items associated with physical appearance, academic status, and unacceptable behavior.

The following studies provide some support for the construct validity of the P-H Scale. It was predicted that the self-concept of institutionalized retardates

LEONARD D.
GOODSTEIN AND
DEBORAH LEE
DOLLER

would fall below that of normal children (Piers & Harris, 1964). The scale was given to 88 retardates with a mean age of 16.8 years. Piers and Harris found that the retardates obtained significantly lower scores on the 95-item version of the scale than did children in public school groups, indicating that the scale reflected the hypothesized lower self-concept or at least the level of self-report. Wylie (1974) notes that these results should be interpreted with caution because it is possible that the lower scores of retardates were due to unreliability of responding rather than low self-concept.

Guardo (1969) hypothesized that there would be a positive linear relationship between self-concept scores and peer nominations as "most popular" and "like the most" (positive sociometric status), while a negative linear relationship would be obtained between self-concept scores and peer nominations as "least popular" and "dislike the most" (negative sociometric status). The P-H Scale was given to 114 sixth graders in four different classes, who did not differ on mean self-concept scores. In general, the results supported the hypothesis, with total self-concept scores correlated in the predicted direction with the peer nominations. These results are congruent with those of Coopersmith (1959), who used a different measure of self-concept but the same type of sociometric measure as Guardo. Coopersmith found a significant correlation of .29 with his Self-Esteem Inventory and sociometric status. Bradley and Newhouse (1975) also investigated the relationship between self-concept and sociometric choice for 158 sixth graders. Each child completed the P-H Scale and listed three children in the class he or she liked best and three he or she liked least. Results were similar to those obtained by Guardo, indicating that self-concept was closely related to how children are perceived by their peers. However, similar results were not obtained by Mayer (1967), who found total P-H Self-Concept scores to be unrelated to sociometric status. Guardo believes that different correlations reported may be accounted for by the difference in the type of sociometric measure used. Wylie (1974) reaches a similar conclusion, stating the difficulty of reaching a synthesis of research findings when subjects and types of sociometric measures differ among studies. Nonetheless, she believes that the findings offer some support to the construct validity of total Self-Concept scores.

Very little information is available on the convergent and discriminant validity of the P-H. Mayer (1967) found a correlation of .68 with Lipsitt's (1958) Self-Concept Rating Scale for Children. Piers (1969) reported correlations ranging from −.04 to .48 between P-H scores and IQ scores on several different tests, with the majority of the correlations being nonsignificant. Wylie (1974) believes that additional research using the multitrait-multimethod matrix is required for evaluating the convergent and discriminant validity of the scale.

6.3.3. Summary

Of the available self-concept tests for children, the Piers-Harris appears to be the most satisfactory instrument for measuring the self-concept. Bentler (1972a) states that the authors have produced a psychometrically adequate scale which possesses sufficient reliability and validity to be used in research. Piers and Harris have presented a clear rationale for item choice and have attempted to control for acquiescence response set by including an approximately equal number of positive and negative items. In their manual, they stress the research use of the scale, in contrast to other applications for which the scale has not been validated. Wylie (1974) concludes that the P-H seems a worthy test for further research and development. For future research, Wylie suggests that studies of item stability be conducted among subjects with low, medium, and high total scores to investigate the possibility that random responding is confounded with low self-regard in low P-H scores. Also, she urges that further research be conducted to determine the convergent and discriminant validity of the scale.

7. The Measurement of Adult Self-Concepts

7.1. Butler and Haigh's Q-Sort

A general description of the Q-sort procedure was earlier discussed. The Q-sort developed by Butler and Haigh (1954) has been the most extensively used instrument of this procedure in self-concept research. This set consists of 100 items which are sorted into nine piles according to the degree to which they are "like me" or "I would most like within myself to be," or the degree to which they characterize the "ordinary person." In order to ensure a quasinormal distribution, subjects must assign a certain number of items to each of the piles.

Dymond (1953) obtained an Adjustment score for the 100 items. She gave the 100 items to two clinical psychologists, who sorted the statements into two piles which were either appropriately positive or negative for adjustment. Twenty-six items which were thought to be irrelevant to adjustment were eliminated, leaving 37 positive indicators and 37 negative indicators. An example of a negative item is "I am a failure," and an example of a positive item is "I am a responsible person." The final scale of 74 items was based on the reliability of classification by the two judges and also on agreement by five other judges. Many researchers use only the 74 items.

7.1.1. Reliability

As previously mentioned, the reliability of most Q-sort sets is still unknown, and the Butler and Haigh set is no exception. It is not known if the scores are able to discriminate significant individual differences at any testing time or if the rank ordering will remain stable over time. Livson and Nichols (1956) did present evidence that higher test-retest reliabilities would result if a prescribed forced distribution were used for the Q-sort procedure, rather than the use of quasinormal sorting. Stimson (1968) found a test-retest reliability coefficient of .74 for Dymond scores after 6 months. For a complete review of the numerous other questions and problems concerning reliability and consistency for this procedure, the reader should consult Wylie (1974). Wylie concludes that "reliability information concerning Q-sorts have been badly neglected" (p. 136).

7.1.2. Validity

Some evidence for convergent validity is found from correlations between the Butler and Haigh Q-sort scores and scores from other instruments measuring the self-concept. Shlien (1961) cited in Wylie (1974) correlated Self-Ideal r's from the following: the 100-item Butler and Haigh Q-sort; 80 items, mostly from the Butler and Haigh Q-sort; Q-sorts of the 49 adjectives from Bills' IAV; Q-sorts of 25 self-referent statements prepared by each subject as important to him- or herself; and Q-sorts from Hilden (1958). The correlations ranged from .82 between the 100-item and 80-item Butler and Haigh Q-sort to .50 between the 100-item Q-sort and the Q-sort from Bills' Index of Adjustment and Values.

Cartwright (1963) found a significant difference in scores on the Butler and Haigh Q-sort between students seeking counseling help and control subjects on a college campus. A significant correlation was reported between Self-Ideal r's on the Butler and Haigh Q-sort and adjustment, as measured by the California Test of Personality (Hanlon, Hofstaetter, & O'Connor, 1954). Winkler and Myers (1963) reported a significant negative relationship between scores on the Taylor Manifest Anxiety Scale and the Q-sort of Butler and Haigh, with high self-acceptance (congruence between the self and the ideal self) associated with low Anxiety scores.

Rogers and Dymond (1954) found significant increases in Self-Ideal r's after therapy, but no changes for a control group waiting to begin therapy. Shlien, Mosak, and Dreikurs (1962) reported a significant increase in Self-Ideal r's on an 80-item modified Butler and Haigh Q-sort as the consequence of psychotherapy, as compared to a control group. However, not all studies provide support for the view that Self-Ideal r's will increase after therapy. Phillips, Raiford, and El-Batrawi (1965) found no increase in Self-Ideal r's after therapy for 79 high school and college students.

7.1.3. Summary

The Q-sort procedure has been extensively used in self-concept research, often with little attention paid to the serious problems associated with this technique. As previously mentioned, questions concerning the role of reliability and validity remain to be answered. For the Butler and Haigh Q-sort, additional problems concern the question of social desirability influences on the subject's responses and the forced-choice format of the Q-sort, which might not accurately represent the subject's self-concept.

7.2. Bills' Index of Adjustment and Values, Adult Form (IAV)

The IAV was designed to measure variables of importance to client-centered therapists and to self-concept theorists (Bills, Vance, & McLean, 1951). A sample of 124 words was taken from Allport's list of 17,953 traits, with an effort being made to select items occurring frequently in client-centered interviews and also representing clear examples of self-concept definitions. Forty-four subjects were given the original 124 trait adjectives. Any items found to be unreliable by an item analysis were eliminated from the final form of the instrument. Of the 49 remaining items, 40 are "desirable" and 9 are "undesirable." Items include "calm," "mature," "cruel," and "stubborn."

On the IAV, words are arranged in a vertical list, followed by three blank columns. Subjects use each of the words to complete the sentence "I am a(an) _____ person" and to indicate on a 5-point scale how often this statement is like them. Ratings ranging from 1 ("seldom") to 5 ("most of the time") are placed in column 1. In column 2, subjects are asked to rate how they feel about being the way described in the first column. Ratings range from 1 ("I very much dislike being as I am in this respect") to 5 ("I very much like being as I am in this respect"). In column 3, the concept of the ideal self is measured. The subjects use each of the words to complete the sentence "I would like to be a(an) _____ person" and use the same ratings as used in column 1 to indicate how often they would like this trait to be characteristic of them. Columns 1–3 thus sample the concept of self, acceptance of self, and ideal self, respectively.

7.2.1. Reliability

Corrected split-half reliabilities for Self-scores (column 1) ranged from .53 for college students (Bills, undated manual) to .92 for factory workers (Lefkowitz, 1967). After a 6-week interval, test-retest coefficients for 160 college students were .90 (Bills, undated manual).

A corrected split-half r of .91 was obtained for Acceptance of Self scores (column 2) with 237 college students (Bills et al., 1951). The test was readministered after 6 weeks to 175 of the 237 subjects, with a test-retest r of .83 for the acceptance of Self scores. After 16 weeks, test-retest r's were .68 and .79 (Bills' undated manual).

For the discrepancy between self and ideal self (column 3), the corrected split-half r was .88 for 237 college students (Bills et al., 1951), while the test-retest r's were .87 after 6 weeks (Bills et al., 1951) and .69 and .52 after 16 weeks (Bills, undated manual).

7.2.2. Validity

Mitchell (1962) conducted an internal factor analysis on the self-ratings of the IAV, which yielded the following seven factors: freedom from anxiety, motivation for intellectual achievement, offensive social conduct, social poise and confidence, warm-hearted attitude toward others, impersonal efficiency, and dependability. Mitchell concluded that the use of a single Self-Concept score was unjustified in view of the results of the factorial analysis. Mitchell did not report how much of the variance was accounted for by the seven factors, and he also used a small number of subjects for the factor analysis (Wylie, 1974).

Bills reported the results of separate factor analyses of Self, Self-Acceptance, Ideal, and discrepancy scores (personal communication, 1971, cited in Wylie, 1974). The first factor accounted for 60–62% of the variance; a second factor accounted for 9–13% of the variance. Bills concluded that one general factor accounted for the majority of the variance, because no factor after the second one accounted for more than 6% of the variance.

Convergent validity of the IAV has been investigated by obtaining correlations between IAV scores and scores from other instruments which also supposedly measure self-regard, and by obtaining correlations among the various IAV scores. The reader interested in the results and correlations of the numerous studies investigating convergent validity should consult Wylie (1974). To summarize, moderate correlations have been found between the Self-Regard scores of the IAV and a variety of other instruments also claiming to measure self-regard. High correlations were also found among the IAV scores, which was expected because all three scores supposedly measure self-regard.

Some support for the construct validity of the IAV is provided by the following studies. In the Bills et al. (1951) study, subjects were asked to explain why they were unhappy. It was predicted that subjects with low Self-Acceptance scores would blame themselves for unhappiness in life, whereas subjects with high scores would blame others for their unhappiness. As expected, Bills et al. found that low scores were significantly related to threat from self, and high scores were significantly related to threat from others. Bills et al. also gave the IAV and the Rorschach to 20 female college students. These subjects were divided into two groups on the basis of the presence of neurotic or psychotic signs on their Rorschach protocols. Bills et al. found that the mean of the Self-Acceptance scores appeared to differentiate the groups, with 14 of the 15 subjects in the neurotic group having scores falling below the mean found for 482 college students. The scores for those five subjects having psychotic signs were all above the mean. Bills (1953a) reported that the IAV could separate groups with different personality characteristics. He found that Rorschach personality characteristics could distinguish between subjects with high and low scores on Self-Acceptance, with low scorers showing more perceptual accuracy and less degree of affect. Bills (1954) hypothesized that individuals with a small discrepancy between the Self and the Ideal Self would show fewer signs of depression on the Rorschach than people with a large discrepancy. The results confirmed the experimental predictions for five out of six Rorschach depression signs.

Roberts (1952) reported that emotionality is involved in those traits in which there is a discrepancy between the Self and the Ideal Self. On a free-association test, he found significantly longer reaction times to words on which the subject had a low Self-Acceptance score and also on which there was a discrepancy between the Self and the Ideal Self. Similar results were obtained in a replication study by Bills (1953b), who concluded that the IAV is a valid measure of changes in emotionality.

7.2.3. Summary

Despite the early popularity of Bills' IAV, there have been few recent studies in which the test has been used. More recent research is needed to determine the present status of the instrument. However, from the previous research, it appears that evidence for reliability is quite good. Wylie (1974) reports that the evidence for convergent validity is as good as that for other instruments measuring the self-concept. One question which remains unanswered about Bills' IAV concerns the role of social desirability. At least two studies have indicated that the test measures social desirability (Cowen & Tongas, 1959; Spilka, 1961). Future research on this issue is needed to determine if the construct validity of IAV scores has been lowered by the role of social desirability. Nevertheless, Bills' IAV does present a promising direction for self-concept measurement.

7.3. The Tennessee Self-Concept Scale

One of the most widely used instruments to measure the self-concept has been the Tennessee Self-Concept Scale (Fitts, 1964), which is a self-administering instrument consisting of 100 self-descriptive statements such as "I have a healthy body" and "I am a member of a happy family." Ninety of the items assess the self-concept, while the other ten are from the MMPI Lie scale and assess self-criticism. The items were selected from the literature on the self-concept and also from patient self-reports. The scale is suitable for subjects age 12 or older who have at least a sixth-grade reading level. The 90 items are phrased half positively and half negatively in order to control for acquiescence response set. Each item has five response alternatives, ranging from "completely true of me" to "completely false of me." The responses are scored according to a two-dimensional classification scheme, one dimension representing five aspects of the self, which are physical self, moral-ethical self, personal self, family self, and social self. The other dimension represents an internal frame of reference associated with each of the self-concepts, which are identity, what the person is; self-satisfaction, how the person accepts him- or herself; and behavior, how he or she acts. The total positive score for the 90 self-concept items is the overall self-esteem measure, but there are a number of subscores that can be derived. The scale provides scores for up to 29 variables, which furnishes the examiner with a rather complete and complex self-concept profile.

7.3.1. Reliability

The 2-week test-retest reliability coefficient for the total Self-Concept score was found to be .92 for 60 college students (Fitts, 1965). There appear to be no published reports on the internal consistency of the Tennessee Self-Concept Scale.

7.3.2. Validity

Conflicting results have been reported on the factor analytic work conducted on the TSCS. Rentz and White (1967) factor-analyzed a matrix of intercorrelations of 12 TSCS scales and found that the five major dimensions of the self in the scale were aspects of only two independent factors. Vacchiano and Strauss (1968) identified 20 interpretable factors from their factor analysis of the scale, but failed to find support for the three theorized measures of an internal frame of reference in the self.

Evidence for convergent validity has been provided by Vincent (1968), who hypothesized that Self-Satisfaction and Personal Satisfaction scores on the TSCS would be significantly intercorrelated with similar scores from different inventories. Nonsignificant correlations were found between TSCS scores and Self-Acceptance and Self-Control scores on the California Psychological Inventory, but significant correlations were found between the TSCS scores and Maslow's Security S-II scores and also between 16 PF Emotional Stability and Confident Adequacy scores. Bentler (1972b) states that correlations between the TSCS and various scales of the MMPI are frequently in the .50's and .60's.

The TSCS has been somewhat successful in differentiating normals from non-normals, such as psychiatric patients and alcoholics, thus providing some support for the construct validity of the scale. Crites (1965) reported that the test tends to discriminate psychiatric groups from normals and also different psychiatric groups from each other. Havener and Izard (1962) found that paranoid schizophrenics tended to rate themselves in a more favorable light than nonparanoid schizophrenics. Gross and Adler (1970) found that 140 male alcoholics differed significantly in a negative direction from a normal group on ten scales of the TSCS. The alcoholics viewed themselves as inadequate and unworthy of respect, and were also more self-critical than the normal group. Hebert (1968) found that individuals with low reading comprehension generally had low self-concept scores on the TSCS.

Suinn (1972) states that validation data for the TSCS must also determine the test's capability of measuring self-concept variables. Using Self-Concept scores as the criterion variable, it has been assumed that certain significant experiences or membership in certain groups would lead to changes in Self-Concept scores. Suinn reports that the results of different studies have generally, although not always, supported the assumption, with psychotherapy, hospitalization, and group membership, e.g., delinquency, appearing to affect TSCS scores. As an example, Ashcraft and Fitts (1964) found that total Self-Concept scores increased significantly for therapy patients, as compared to no change in a group of patients waiting for therapy.

7.3.3. Summary

The TSCS has generally received unfavorable reviews, although it is one of the most frequently used instruments for research and clinical purposes. Wylie (1974) believes the test has been used with little attention to the scarcity of methodologically adequate published research. She indicates that it would be unlikely to establish any kind of discriminant validity for the different scales, although it is usually assumed that the separate scores can be discriminantly interpreted. She also thinks that random responding rather than differences in self-regard might lead to differences in groups being compared. Wylie concludes that it would be difficult to justify using the TSCS because of the methodological limitations and she recommends the usage of other available instruments.

In his review, Bentler (1972b) describes numerous difficulties with the TSCS. One limitation he finds is the lack of information on the internal consistency of the scale, or on any of the scale subscores. Bentler also believes that Fitts has made too many overinterpretations regarding the scale relative to the available data. Bentler cites an example in the manual in which the TSCS was used to predict changes in therapy. It was predicted that there would be 88 scale changes after therapy for only six patients. In addition, Bentler indicates the scoring procedure is cumbersome.

Crites has the following to say in his review of the TSCS:

> If any questions are raised about the Scale at this stage of its development, they most likely will pertain to its rationale instead of its construction. Thus, it can be asked: What are the particular advantages of this instrument over its long line of precursors, e.g., the Bills Index of Adjustment and Values, the various published Q-sorts, etc. It is incumbent upon the author to demonstrate that his Scale is "simpler for the subject, more widely applicable, better standardized, etc." than other similar measuring devices. (Crites, 1965, p. 331)

7.4. The Personal Orientation Inventory

The Personal Orientation Inventory (POI) is a self-report instrument designed to measure attitudes, values, and behaviors based on Maslow's theory of self-actualization (Shostrom, 1964). Although self-actualization is a different concept from that of self-concept, the POI has been frequently used in recent years by phenomenologically and humanistically oriented psychologists, often in research attempting to measure the outcome of their therapeutic efforts. For this reason and also because there is a subscale on the POI which measures self-regard, it was decided to include the POI in this chapter.

The POI consists of 150 paired-choice items in which each concept is presented in terms of a positive and a negative statement, such as "I am afraid to be myself—I am not afraid to be myself." The subject selects the one statement in each pair that is most self-descriptive. The POI has two major scales, Time Competence to assess living in the present and Support to assess inner-directedness, each of which yields a ratio score. There are also ten subscales designed to measure values important in the development of the self-actualizing individual.

7.4.1. Reliability

Test-retest reliability coefficients ranging from .91 to .93 were found on a sample of 48 college students given the test twice, 1 week apart. The reliability coefficients for the 12 scales ranged from .55 to .85, with a median of .74 (Shostrom, 1964). Only three of the subscales had coefficients less than .70. No information is reported in the manual on the internal consistency of the subscales. Wise and Davis (1975) reported test-retest reliability coefficients of .75 and .88 for the Time Competence and Support scales, respectively, for an interval of 2 weeks.

7.4.2. Validity

Shostrom (1964) found that the POI discriminated between a sample of individuals nominated as self-actualizing and a sample of non-self-actualizing individuals. Certified clinical psychologists made the nominations for the two groups. Fox, Knapp, and Michael (1968) demonstrated that 100 hospitalized psychiatric patients had significantly lower scores on all POI scales than a self-actualizing group and a normal adult group. The hospitalized group was described in terms of inadequate self-realization, relatively nonautonomous functioning, and lower self-esteem. Shostrom and Knapp (1966) found that all 12 POI scales could differentiate a sample of outpatients just beginning therapy from those advanced in therapy (mean time in therapy was 2.2 years). It seems that the predictive validity of the POI is fairly well established when its ability to differentiate relatively healthy and normal groups from less well-functioning groups is considered.

A number of recent studies have related POI scores to concepts of adjustment measured by other instruments. Knapp (1965) found that POI scores were negatively related to the concept of neuroticism as measured by the Eysenck Personality Inventory (Eysenck & Eysenck, 1963). In addition, the subscale of Self-Regard on the POI was found to be significantly related to emotional stability. Shostrom and Knapp (1966) found the POI to be negatively related to measures of pathology on several scales of the MMPI. Knapp and Comrey (1973) found the major scales of Time Competence and Support to be significantly related to a measure of emotional stability on the Comrey Personality Scales (Comrey, 1970). The scale of Self-Regard on the POI demonstrated the highest subscale relationship to emotional stability. Mattocks and Jew (1974) investigated the relationship between POI scores and Q-sort scores and found that high scores on POI self-actualization were positively correlated with the concept of the "well-adjusted person" as defined by the Q-sort Adjustment Scale developed by Dymond (1953). The preceding studies provide support for the view that self-actualization is positively related to emotional stability or health.

Factorial studies have been conducted on the POI. However, the pervasive item overlap among the subscales precludes any meaningful factor analytic investigations. Since most of these studies have been confounded by this methodological difficulty, they will not be discussed here.

7.4.3. Summary

Bloxom (1972) believes the content validity of the scales on the POI is good and that the items in each scale are appropriately varied. Knapp (1976) believes the POI has contributed greatly to research involving values and behaviors important for the actualizing person. However, Coan (1972) gives a generally unfavorable review of the POI, stating that there appear to be no construct validity data for the subscales and that the selection of variables for inclusion in the questionnaire was arbitrary and theoretically biased. He also criticizes the wording of the statements in an absolute form, which forces the subject to choose between two extremes, which might not accurately describe his or her attitudes. A major problem with the POI is a rather pervasive item overlap among its subscales which leads to a very high level of intercorrelation among these subscales. Bloxom suggests that this problem could be alleviated if the two major scales of Time Competence and Support (Inner-Directedness) were used by themselves. Further research into the relationship between self-actualization and various measures of the self-concept should prove interesting to our understanding of both concepts.

7.5. Some Concluding Comments

A wide variety of instruments have been used to measure various aspects of the self-concept. However, most of these instruments have been used only in their author's dissertation work or very few other studies. Most of these tests have inadequate reliability or validity information, and the descriptions of the tests are often incomplete. It was not the purpose of this chapter to list and describe all the varoius tests that have been used to measure the self-concept. Only those tests that have received widespread application have been discussed. It is difficult to establish rigorous criteria for inclusion or exclusion of self-concept measures in a survey of this kind. Thus the writers' choice of instruments to be discussed may appear arbitrary to the reader.

8. Theoretical and Conceptual Issues

There seems to be widespread agreement on the need for self-concept measures with adequate reliability and validity. But most of the instruments currently available do not meet the minimal criteria for either reliability or validity, especially the latter. While the brief review of the current instruments above does provide some interesting leads for further research, none of the instruments included in the earlier review would appear to be psychometrically adequate for clinical use. Clearly, one caveat emerging from even the most cursory reading of this chapter should be that there is no instrument that can be used for the measurement of a self-concept/ of a client or patient in a clinical situation.

Problems of reliability can probably be handled in a relatively straightforward manner. Psychologists with adequate training in psychometrics could develop adequate indices of internal consistency, test-retest reliability, and so on, for most of the available measures, and modify these instruments so as to achieve the necessary minimal psychometric standards. However, even this kind of modification is expensive in both time and money. Clearly, what we do not need is additional theses or dissertations that attempt to produce new and still untried measures. The development effort involved in producing psychometrically sophisticated and sound instruments virtually precludes success within the time and money constraints typical of student research. Rather, what seems to be needed is the serious and continual effort of a major research laboratory with the necessary staff and other resources available.

The problem of validity, however, is a more difficult one to resolve. While the concept of the self has almost immediate subjective validity, this validity is much more difficult to establish on an objective, measurable level. As we noted earlier in this chapter, there is no clarity about the nature of the self. There are at least three general classes of self-concepts—identity, evaluation, and esteem. And there is even less clarity about which of these three should be included in a measure of the self-concept. To be more specific, should a self-concept measure permit the respondent to describe him- or herself, to dimensionalize his or her phenomenal world, and does this need to be done in the respondent's own words or can the test developer provide the words in some structured fashion? While there is always a problem of how important is the reduction in the freedom of the respondent's response (with the consequent problems of categorizing and coding these responses in some reliable and orderly fashion), one can argue that nowhere is this restriction of freedom more important than in describing the self-concept. "I am what I am," and no one can provide the words that adequately invoke one's personal sense of identity and uniqueness. But at the same time our science requires that we organize and systematize this uniqueness and produce some order of a fairly generalized sort.

To what degree should our measure of the self-concept involve a series of evaluations of the salient elements of the self? Who should provide the series of elements, and, if we as psychologists provide them, to what extent has our questioning directly changed the very concept that we intend to measure? While this problem analogous to the Heisenberg uncertainty principle pervades all of psychological measurement in the personality area, it is nowhere more critical than in the measurement of the self-concept.

Whether the elements are to be obtained or provided, how do we ascertain the relative weight of each of these elements in the evaluative schema of the self that the respondent has been using in his or her unique fashion? Even if we were able to develop a list or categorization of such attributes, would such a list adequately represent the configuration of those attributes that already exists in the self-concept of the respondent?

Finally, if we are to concentrate on the overall self-esteem of the respondent as the primary focus of our measure of the self-concept, can we develop a unitary measure of such self-acceptance? Seeking the answer to this question has been the focus of factor analytic studies of the existing instruments. If we conceptualize self-esteem or self-acceptance as a unitary construct, then factor analytic research is necessary to demonstrate a single, general factor that accounts for most of the interitem variance, with most of the remaining variance ascribable to several minor, interpretable factors and to measurement error. It can be noted that the development of such an instrument is a time-consuming and expensive procedure that requires a good bit of psychometric sophistication. As we noted earlier, work of this caliber requires the facilities of a major research laboratory.

Even if these facilities were available to us, how would we proceed to establish the validity of any of these three kinds of self-concept measures? Validity studies require investigating the relationship of our measures of self-concept to some behavioral indices that should be clearly related to our measures. But this is a good bit more difficult than it appears at first glance. In order to have clearly predictable relationships between a test measure of self-concept and other behavioral indices, there needs to be a more clearly articulated self-concept theory that enables such predictions to be more accurate and relevant. Even the most superficial reading of self-concept theorizing will quickly show that such specific theorizing has not yet been attempted. While some primitive predictions can and have been made, e.g., persons with high self-concepts should be less anxious than those with low self-concepts, these notions tend to involve relationships about rather simplistic trait concepts of personality, and reflect neither the more recent theorizing about the importance of situational factors in the genesis of behavior nor the trait-situation interaction influence in behavior. For example, does high self-esteem make a person more or less responsive to anxiety-producing cues in evaluative situations, and thus more anxious? Clearly, personality theory is moving into a heavy reliance on such interactive relationships in order to explain human behavior, and there is little work along these lines being done by self-concept theorists.

What we are arguing here is that the development of adequate measures of the self-concept requires a more careful and thorough development of self theory. Without such theoretical developments, self-concept research will remain a rather unending series of correlational studies between inadequate self-concept instruments and poorly articulated behavioral indices, typically inadequate measures of other poorly defined psychological attributes.

9. Conclusions

Although psychologists have long been interested in the self, the rise of existential and phenomenological psychology has given renewed vigor and a different emphasis to work in this area. The principal focus of this renewed interest is in the self as an object or product of experience.

We have suggested that there are three primary, different aspects of the self as an object: (1) identity, or how the person is self-perceived; (2) self-evaluation, or how the person evaluates the various elements of the self; and (3) self-esteem, or the subjective way in which the person values him- or herself as a totality. While there are some psychologists who would include the unconscious self-concept as a fourth aspect of the self, our review argues that there is little evidence to support this practice.

After briefly reviewing some of the critical factors in the development of the self in a social-learning theory context, we reviewed the several attempts to measure each of the three elements of the self described in this chapter. Identity has primarily been measured by "Who am I?" free-response questionnaire procedures, with the attendent problems of categorizing and coding the responses. Self-regard, including the evaluation of both elements of the self and overall self-esteem, has been measured by more typical questionnaire procedures, with either true-false or Likert-type response alternatives. The primary exception to such questionnaires has been the Q-sort, where decks of cards, each containing self-descriptive items, are sorted into a series of piles that cover the dimension of how descriptive each statement is of the respondent.

Finally, each of the major instruments that have been reported in the literature for the measuring of the self-concept was reviewed, first those intended for use with children and then those for use with adults. Most of these instruments were found to have both theoretical and methodological limitations that raise serious questions about their clinical use and even reduce their potential research effectiveness.

Despite the increase of interest of the self-concept in the last few years, very little progress has been made in either theorizing about the self-concept or developing of instruments designed to measure the self-concept. The instruments that have been developed for self-concept research frequently fail to meet the methodological expectations of good psychometric instruments. Many of these measures have been used in only one or very few other studies, often with little attention paid to reliability and validity. A more thorough development of the self theory is required before adequate measures of the self-concept can be developed.

10. References

Allport, G. W. *Letters from Jenny.* New York: Harcourt, Brace, and World, 1965.

Ashcraft, C., & Fitts, W. H. Self-concept change in psychotherapy. *Psychotherapy: Theory, Research and Practice,* 1964, *1,* 115–118.

Bentler, P. M. Review of the Piers-Harris Children's Self-Concept Scale. In O. K. Buros (Ed.), *The seventh mental measurements yearbook.* Highland Park, N.J.: Gryphon Press, 1972. (a)

Bentler, P. M. Review of the Tennessee Self Concept Scale. In O. K. Buros (Ed.), *The seventh mental measurements yearbook.* Highland Park, N.J.: Gryphon Press, 1972, 366–367. (b)

Bills, R. E. Index of adjustment and values. Manual. University, Alabama: Mimeographed, n.d.

Bills, R. E. Rorschach characteristics of persons scoring high and low in acceptance of self. *Journal of Consulting Psychology,* 1953, *17,* 36–38. (a)

Bills, R. E. A validation of changes in scores on the Index of Adjustment and Values as measures of changes in emotionality. *Journal of Consulting Psychology,* 1953, *17,* 135–138. (b)

Bills, R. E. Self-concepts and Rorschach signs of depression. *Journal of Consulting Psychology,* 1954, *18,* 135–137.

Bills, R. E., Vance, E. L., & McLean, O. S. An index of adjustment and values. *Journal of Consulting Psychology,* 1951, *15,* 257–261.

Block, J. *The Q-sort method in personality assessment and psychiatric research.* Springfield, Ill.: Thomas, 1961.

Bloxom, B. Review of the Personal Orientation Inventory. In O. K. Buros (Ed.), *The seventh mental measurements yearbook.* Highland Park, N.J.: Gryphon Press, 1972, 290–292.

Boshier, R. Self-esteem and first names in children. *Psychological Reports,* 1968, *22,* 762.

Bradley, F. O., & Newhouse, R. C. Sociometric choice and self-perceptions of upper elementary school children. *Psychology in the Schools,* 1975, *12,* 219–222.

Bugenthal, J. T., & Zelen, S. L. Investigations into the self-concept. *Journal of Personality,* 1950, *18,* 483–498.

Butler, J. M., & Haigh, G. V. Changes in the relation between self-concepts and ideal concepts consequent upon client-centered therapy. In C. R. Rogers & R. F. Dymond (Eds.), *Psychotherapy and personality change.* Chicago: University of Chicago Press, 1954.

Campbell, P. B. School and self-concept. *Educational Leadership,* 1967, *24,* 510–515.

Cartwright, R. D. Self-conception patterns of college students, and adjustment to college life. *Journal of Counseling Psychology,* 1963, *10,* 47–52.

Castenada, A., McCandless, B. R., & Palermo, D. S. The children's form of the Manifest Anxiety Scale. *Child Development,* 1956, *27,* 317–326.

Coan, R. W. Review of the Personal Orientation Inventory. In O. K. Buros (Ed.), *The seventh mental measurements yearbook*. Highland Park, N.J.: Gryphon Press, 1972, 292–294.

Comrey, A. L. *Comrey Personality Scales*. San Diego: Educational and Industrial Testing Service, 1970.

Connell, D. M., & Johnson, J. E. Relationship between sex-role identification and self-esteem in early adolescents. *Developmental Psychology*, 1970, *3*, 268.

Coopersmith, S. A method for determining types of self-esteem. *Journal of Abnormal and Social Psychology*, 1959, *59*, 87–94.

Coopersmith, S. *The antecedents of self-esteem*. San Francisco: Freeman, 1967.

Cowen, E. L., & Tongas, P. N. The social desirability of trait descriptive terms: Applications to a self-concept inventory. *Journal of Consulting Psychology*, 1959, *23*, 361–365.

Crites, J. O. Test reviews: Tennessee Self-Concept Scale. *Journal of Counseling Psychology*, 1965, *12*, 330–331.

Dymond, R. F. An adjustment score for Q-sorts. *Journal of Consulting Psychology*, 1953, *17*, 339–342.

Eysenck, H. J., & Eysenck, S. B. *The Eysenck Personality Inventory*. London: University of London Press, 1963.

Fitts, W. H. *Tennessee Self-Concept Scale: Test booklet*. Nashville, Tenn.: Counselor Recordings and Tests, Department of Mental Health, 1964.

Fitts, W. H. *Tennessee Self-Concept Scale: Manual*. Nashville, Tenn.: Counselor Recordings and Tests, Department of Mental Health, 1965.

Fox, J., Knapp, R. R., & Michael, W. B. Assessment of self-actualization of psychiatric patients: Validity of the Personal Orientation Inventory. *Educational and Psychological Measurement*, 1968, *28*, 565–569.

Freud, S. Formulations regarding the two principles in mental functioning. In P. Rieff (Ed.), *General psychological theory*. New York: Collier Books, 1963 (original 1911).

Gordon, C. Self-conceptions: Configurations of content. In Gordon & K. Gergen (Eds.), *The self in social interaction*. New York: Wiley, 1968.

Gough, H. G., & Heilbrun, A. B., Jr. *Manual for the Adjective Check List*. Palo Alto, Calif.: Consulting Psychologists Press, 1964.

Gross, W. F., & Adler, L. O. Aspects of alcoholics' self-concepts as measured by the Tennessee Self-Concept Scale. *Psychological Reports*, 1970, *27*, 431–434.

Guardo, C. Sociometric status and self-concept in sixth graders. *Journal of Educational Research*, 1969, *62*, 319–322.

Hanlon, T. E., Hofstaetter, P., & O'Connor, J. Congruence of self and ideal self in relation to personality adjustment. *Journal of Consulting Psychology*, 1954, *18*, 215–218.

Havener, P. H., & Izard, C. E. Unrealistic self-enhancement in paranoid schizophrenics. *Journal of Consulting Psychology*, 1962, *26*, 65–68.

Hebert, D. J. Reading comprehension as a function of self-concept. *Perceptual and Motor Skills*, 1968, *27*, 78.

Hilden, A. H. Q-sort correlation: Stability and random choice of statements. *Journal of Consulting Psychology*, 1958, *22*, 45–50.

Horowitz, F. D. The relationship of anxiety, self-concept, and sociometric status among fourth, fifth, and sixth grade children. *Journal of Abnormal and Social Psychology*, 1962, *65*, 212–214.

James, W. *Psychology: The briefer course*. New York: Holt, 1892.

Jersild, A. T. *In search of self: An exploration of the role of the school in promoting self-understanding*. New York: Teachers College, 1952.

Jourard, S. M., & Remy, R. M. Perceived parental attitudes, the self, and security. *Journal of Counseling Psychology*, 1955, *19*, 364–366.

Knapp, R. R. Relationship of a measure of self-actualization to neuroticism and extraversion. *Journal of Consulting Psychology*, 1965, *29*, 168–172.

Knapp, R. R. *Handbook for the Personal Orientation Inventory*. San Diego: Ed Its, 1976.

Knapp, R. R., & Comrey, A. L. Further construct validation of a measure of self-actualization. *Educational and Psychological Measurement*, 1973, *33*, 419–425.

Kuhn, M. H., & McPartland, T. S. An empirical investigation of self-attitudes. *American Sociological Review*, 1954, *19*, 68–76.

Lefkowitz, J. Self-esteem of industrial workers. *Journal of Applied Psychology*, 1967, *51*, 521–528.

Lewin, K., Dembo, T., Festinger, L., & Sears, P. Level of aspiration. In J. McV. Hunt (Ed.), *Personality and the behavior disorders*. New York: Ronald, 1944.

Lipsitt, L. P. A self-concept scale for children and its relationship to the children's form of the Manifest Anxiety Scale. *Child Development*, 1958, *29*, 463–472.

Livson, N. H., & Nichols, T. F. Discrimination and reliability in Q-sort personality descriptions. *Journal of Abnormal and Social Psychology*, 1956, *52*, 159–165.

Mann, P. H., Beaber, J. D., & Jacobson, M. D. The effect of group counseling on educable mentally retarded boys' self-concepts. *Exceptional Children*, 1969, *35*, 359–366.

Mattocks, A. L., & Jew, C. C. Comparison of self-actualization levels and adjustment scores of incarcerated male felons. *Educational and Psychological Measurement*, 1974, *34*, 69–74.

Mayer, C. L. The relationship of early special class placement and the self-concepts of mentally handicapped children. *Exceptional Children*, 1966, *33*, 77–81.

Mayer, C. L. Relationships of self-concepts and social variables in retarded children. *American Journal of Mental Deficiency*, 1967, *72*, 267–271.

McDougall, W. *Introduction to social psychology*. London: Methuen, 1908.

Mead, G. H. *Mind, self, and society*. Chicago: University of Chicago Press, 1934.

Michael, W. B., & Smith, R. A. The factorial validity of the Piers-Harris Children's Self-Concept Scale for each of three samples of elementary, junior high, and senior high school students in a large metropolitan school district. *Educational and Psychological Measurement*, 1975, *35*, 405–414.

Mitchell, J. V., Jr. An analysis of the factorial dimensions of the Bills' Index of Adjustment and Values. *Journal of Social Psychology*, 1962, *58*, 331–337.

Phillips, E. L., Raiford, A., & El-Batrawi, S. The Q-sort reevaluated. *Journal of Consulting Psychology*, 1965, *29*, 422–425.

Piers, E. V. *Manual for the Piers-Harris Children's Self-Concept Scale (The way I feel about myself)*. Nashville, Tenn.: Counselor Recordings and Tests, 1969.

Piers, E. V., & Harris, D. B. Age and other correlates of self-concept in children. *Journal of Educational Psychology*, 1964, *55*, 91–95.

Reese, H. W. Relationships between self-acceptance and sociometric choices. *Journal of Abnormal and Social Psychology*, 1961, *62*, 472–474.

Rentz, R. R., & White, W. F. Factors of self-perception in the Tennessee Self-Concept Scale. *Perceptual and Motor Skills*, 1967, *24*, 118.

Roberts, G. E. A study of the validity of the Index of Adjustment and Values. *Journal of Consulting Psychology*, 1952, *16*, 302–304.

Rogers, C. R. A theory of therapy, personality, and interpersonal relations, as developed in the client-centered framework. In S. Koch (Ed.), *Psychology: A study of a science. Volume III. Formulations of the person and the social context*. New York: McGraw-Hill, 1959, 184–258.

Rogers, C. R., & Dymond, R. F. (Eds.). *Psychotherapy and personality change*. Chicago: University of Chicago Press, 1954.

Shlien, J. M. Toward what level of abstraction in criteria? *University of Chicago Counseling Center Discussion Papers*, 1961, *6*, No. 16.

Shlien, J. M., Mosak, H. H., & Dreikurs, R. Effect of time limits: A comparison of two psychotherapies. *Journal of Counseling Psychology*, 1962, *9*, 31–34.

Shostrom, E. L. An inventory for the measurement of self-actualization. *Educational and Psychological Measurement*, 1964, *24*, 207–218.

Shostrom, E. L., & Knapp, R. R. The relationship of a measure of self-actualization (POI) to a measure of pathology (MMPI) and to therapeutic growth. *American Journal of Psychotherapy*, 1966, *20*, 193–202.

Spilka, B. Social desirability: A problem of operational definition. *Psychological Reports*, 1961, *8*, 149–150.

Stimson, R. C. Factor analytic approach to the structural differentiation of description. *Journal of Counseling Psychology*, 1968, *15*, 301–307.

Suinn, R. M. Review of the Tennessee Self-Concept Scale. In O. K. Buros (Ed.), *The seventh mental measurements yearbook*. Highland Park, N.J.: Gryphon Press, 1972, 367–369.

Trowbridge, N. Effects of socio-economic class on self-concept of children. *Psychology in the Schools*, 1970, *7*, 304–306.

Vacchiano, R. B., & Strauss, P. S. The construct validity of the Tennessee Self-Concept Scale. *Journal of Clinical Psychology*, 1968, *24*, 323–326.

Vincent, J. An exploratory factor analysis relating to the construct validity of self-concept labels. *Educational and Psychological Measurement*, 1968, *28*, 915–921.

Winkler, R. C., & Myers, R. A. Some concomitants of self-ideal discrepancy measures of self-acceptance. *Journal of Counseling Psychology*, 1963, *10*, 83–86.

Wise, G. W., & Davis, J. E. The Personal Orientation Inventory: Internal consistency, stability, and sex differences. *Psychological Reports*, 1975, *36*, 847–855.

Wolff, W. W. *The expression of personality*. New York: Harpers, 1943.

Wylie, R. C. The present status of self-theory. In E. F. Borgatta & W. W. Lambert (Eds.), *Handbook of personality theory and research*. Chicago: Rand McNally, 1968.

Wylie, R. C. *The self-concept*. Lincoln: University of Nebraska Press, 1974.

15

Objective Personality Inventories: Recent Research and Some Contemporary Issues

JAMES N. BUTCHER AND
PATRICIA L. OWEN

1. Introduction

The use of objective personality inventories to aid in clinical diagnosis and personality assessment has increased greatly in the past 40 years. In the face of a great deal of initial opposition and continual rejection by some professionals in both psychoanalytic and behavioral camps, some inventories like the Minnesota Multiphasic Personality Inventory (MMPI) have gained wide acceptance. As a matter of fact, many researchers place such confidence in the MMPI that they employ the scales as criteria for clinical research studies. How has the objective personality assessment approach that was originally viewed as an unwanted stepchild been elevated to the role of a messiah in clinical research? This has come about both through the strengths of the objective inventory approach and through weaknesses in the clinical research field—particularly the frustrating search for dependable external criteria.

The strengths of personality inventories in the clinical setting stand out: they are an efficient means of obtaining a large amount of self-report information; they are objective in that they have standard scoring formats, scales, or indices which summarize behavioral patterns; and there is an established system of generating reliable psychological interpretations from test indices which can be automatically applied by clinicians or even electronic computers. Most important to the success of personality inventories is the favorable cost/benefit ratio: personality inventories such as the MMPI provide a great deal of useful, valid personality/diagnostic informa-

JAMES N. BUTCHER and PATRICIA L. OWEN • Psychology Department, University of Minnesota, Minneapolis, Minnesota 55455.

tion for a minimum expenditure of professional clinical time. An experienced MMPI interpreter can generate a highly accurate clinical picture of a patient in minutes (a well-written interpretive computer program can do the same thing in seconds) that an experienced interviewer would need hours of interview time to duplicate. Moreover, the clinical interview is less reliable and valid than are results obtained by questionnaire.

The extensive literature on personality inventories defies summary in the confines of a review chapter. Dahlstrom, Welsh, and Dahlstrom (1975) published over 6000 references for the MMPI, and the magnitude of published sources on this instrument alone increases about 200 books, articles, and doctoral theses annually (Buros, 1971). The goal of this review is to focus on some of the broader issues that surround the use of several personality inventories, and not to focus on clinical applications since these are covered in another chapter of this volume (see Graham, Chapter 10). We limited our survey to four clinical assessment devices: the MMPI, the Sixteen Personality Factor Inventory (16PF), the unpublished Differential Personality Inventory (DPI), and the Millon Multiaxial Clinical Inventory (MMCI).* The choice of instruments to be included in this review was made on the basis of not only extensive use but also the test author's stated focus and the applicability of each inventory for clinical diagnosis and assessment. In order to gain a perspective on recent research developments with these instruments, we conducted a literature search (using published journal articles from 1972 to 1977) that used the MMPI, the 16PF, or the DPI. The MMCI is a newly published inventory; thus we have available for review only the test manual (Millon, 1977).

The bibliographical sources classified in Table 1† provide a perspective on the range of research in the personality inventory domain and give some idea of the relative use of the three clinical inventories. An inspection of the table suggests that

1. There is an abundance of research. In the brief time span and source coverage of this review (limited to published articles), there is a wide array of research into clinical problems, crime and delinquency, diagnostic procedures, relationships among measures, test characteristics, treatment outcome research, and employment screening, as well as research concerning many special problem areas or with special populations.
2. The bulk of research, about 84%, has been with the MMPI. Consequently, the concerns of this chapter will be tilted mainly in that direction.
3. Any classification of research according to title runs the risk of being too broad, too specific, too detailed, or too inexact. In spite of the classification

---

*A list of general guides and manuals for the MMPI is given in a separate reference section (Section 10.2) at the end of this chapter. The basic reference for the 16PF is Cattell, R. B., Eber, H. W., and Tatsuoka, M. M. *Handbook for the 16PF.* Champaign, Ill.: Institute for Ability Testing, 1970. No general comprehensive guide exists for the DPI. The MMCI is described in Millon, T. *Millon Multiaxial Clinical Inventory.* Minneapolis: National Computer Systems, 1977.

†All studies cited in Table 1 can be located by number in the reference section at the end of this chapter. Number 1–742 include MMPI studies, 743–879 include 16PF studies, and 880–888 include DPI studies. Articles cited in this chapter but not categorized in Table 1, because of their date of publication, are listed separately after the references for Table 1. References for Table 1 were obtained from a computer search (ERIC and PSYCH ABSTRACTS) from January 1972 to April 1977. (Because of the delay between publication and listing in *Psychological Abstracts*, many 1977 articles are not included.) Although our aim was to categorize all published journal articles on the MMPI, 16PF, and DPI for a 5-year period, we recognize that some publications may have been inadvertently missed.

477

OBJECTIVE
PERSONALITY
INVENTORIES:
RECENT RESEARCH
AND SOME
CONTEMPORARY
ISSUES

Table 1. Classification of Published Research on the MMPI, 16PF, and DPI for 1972–1977 (see Section 10.1)

	MMPI	16PF	DPI
Alcohol and drug abuse: detection and treatment	16, 17, 18, 30, 33, 34, 35, 41, 44, 63, 64, 102, 114, 125, 127, 130, 151, 158, 159, 183, 191, 194, 200, 209, 211, 232, 250, 253, 259, 260, 278, 279, 282, 284, 285, 286, 287, 298, 303, 305, 308, 309, 313, 320, 329, 331, 333, 344, 346, 349, 358, 367, 378, 381, 387, 400, 404, 405, 410, 419, 421, 422, 447, 449, 450, 451, 485, 489, 491, 497, 505, 507, 514, 521, 532, 533, 534, 554, 558, 561, 562, 563, 567, 574, 589, 609, 610, 611, 612, 613, 624, 655, 656, 657, 665, 742	760, 790, 821, 824, 826, 840, 841, 872	283, 284, 884, 886, 887
Automated interpretation	8, 13, 14, 57, 86, 88, 101, 149, 189, 193, 224, 231, 239, 240, 241, 242, 243, 244, 247, 248, 261, 340, 359, 361, 390, 701	810, 843	
Short forms	51, 95, 98, 124, 152, 156, 160, 165, 166, 167, 172, 173, 174, 175, 200, 206, 207, 208, 216, 228, 233, 251, 260, 262, 267, 276, 277, 288, 299, 303, 424, 425, 440, 442, 454, 457, 458, 459, 460, 461, 463, 465, 466, 468, 469, 470, 471, 482, 492, 493, 495, 496, 499, 516, 526, 570, 595, 602, 622, 649, 668, 669, 671, 678, 683, 684		
Brain damage or mental retardation	22, 42, 43, 115, 136, 137, 199, 218, 291, 299, 376, 386, 456, 537, 568, 575, 646, 704, 705	745, 836	
Crime and delinquency	9, 28, 45, 46, 83, 85, 116, 128, 133, 157, 162, 185, 201, 210, 213, 219, 257, 274, 275, 289, 290, 316, 319, 320, 332, 343, 368, 369, 371, 392, 415, 416, 427, 443, 501, 502, 503, 504, 515, 526, 536, 602, 621, 628, 658, 659, 660, 661, 678, 679, 690, 710 713, 719, 721, 741	750, 758, 800, 802, 847, 871	880

(Continued)

Table 1. (*Continued*)

JAMES N. BUTCHER
AND PATRICIA L.
OWEN

	MMPI	16PF	DPI
Depression and suicide	40, 66, 80, 87, 89, 139, 140, 141, 142, 143, 144, 145, 236, 252, 280, 297, 318, 336, 356, 357, 366, 374, 375, 431, 435, 498, 506, 519, 527, 583, 616, 635, 667, 673, 716, 717, 727, 728	784	
Anxiety and stress	52, 69, 97, 129, 188, 236, 342, 431, 433, 462, 467, 473, 509, 527, 564, 674, 685, 714	772, 746, 747, 825	
Medical patients, physical disorders, and symptoms	4, 49, 60, 78, 147, 160, 193, 195, 224, 268, 281, 323, 325, 327, 335, 350, 351, 354, 362, 365, 393, 396, 426, 442, 471, 481, 523, 524, 525, 538, 541, 584, 586, 587, 596, 597, 598, 605, 606, 617, 632, 639, 640, 684, 691, 709, 714, 736	752, 757, 773, 803, 815, 820, 850	
Drug therapy: choice and effect	39, 58, 74, 192, 252, 269, 297, 326, 337, 338, 339, 356, 357, 364, 401, 402, 411, 418, 455, 539, 546, 551, 552, 604, 631, 724, 725, 727, 728		
Psychometric characteristics (e.g., items, factor analysis, scales, response sets)	1, 2, 3, 15, 26, 59, 65, 96, 104, 105, 117, 178, 213, 220, 229, 237, 294, 300, 304, 322, 324, 352, 353, 379, 389, 403, 428, 437, 438, 444, 569, 573, 580, 591, 592, 599, 638, 642, 670, 674, 686, 688, 689, 693, 694, 697, 698, 700, 718	763, 764, 768, 769, 770, 782, 787, 798, 799, 800, 811, 814, 827, 861, 867, 876	885, 888
Diagnostic considerations: rules, profiles, and code types	48, 55, 70, 82, 84, 93, 100, 119, 123, 134, 177, 184, 190, 221, 225, 245, 301, 347, 373, 377, 383, 384, 388, 434, 448, 464, 472, 474, 478, 488, 490, 494, 540, 542, 548, 553, 578, 581, 582, 620, 625, 637, 650, 652, 666, 699, 706, 730, 734, 735	765, 766, 767, 771, 833, 856	
Sleep	75, 76, 110, 256, 328, 417, 565, 696, 708, 711	788, 796	
Parents, couples, and families	11, 20, 54, 61, 71, 99, 126, 173, 174, 175, 197,	751, 759, 795, 808, 823, 860	

Table 1. *(Continued)*

479

**OBJECTIVE
PERSONALITY
INVENTORIES:
RECENT RESEARCH
AND SOME
CONTEMPORARY
ISSUES**

	MMPI	16PF	DPI
	205, 233, 264, 272, 273, 295, 407, 408, 409, 429, 436, 439, 475, 506, 510, 511, 512, 551, 692, 731, 739, 740		
Sexual problems	38, 116, 180, 296, 522, 556, 560, 663, 664	866	
Women	12, 60, 85, 90, 93, 97, 147, 168, 182, 187, 207, 235, 293, 316, 330, 336, 356, 357, 412, 413, 420, 453, 486, 502, 517, 521, 534, 551, 562, 563, 580, 586, 602, 603, 629, 654, 662, 665, 679, 732, 737, 738	748, 749, 758, 852, 873	
Aging	12, 119, 123, 192, 252, 376, 604	776, 786, 868	
College students and adolescents	24, 25, 79, 81, 82, 90, 148, 150, 168, 169, 170, 265, 321, 330, 341, 361, 406, 439, 440, 441, 457, 466, 476, 487, 500, 517, 545, 547, 571, 585, 590, 593, 629, 634	744, 772, 793, 800, 803, 809, 822, 827, 838, 844, 845, 851, 852, 853, 858, 859, 869, 873, 877, 879	881
Use with other tests or rating scales	1, 7, 19, 27, 36, 47, 56, 77, 91, 94, 116, 129, 132, 133, 141, 143, 146, 147, 148, 164, 176, 212, 230, 234, 265, 271, 274, 283, 284, 317, 318, 348, 385, 386, 414, 443, 445, 446, 477, 480, 483, 484, 513, 518, 528, 543, 544, 555, 577, 600, 627, 633, 636, 641, 660, 672, 681, 687, 705, 716, 717, 720, 722, 723, 733, 798, 799	116, 146, 147, 484, 722, 762, 781, 783, 794, 797, 798, 801, 805, 806, 813, 818, 819, 828, 829, 831, 847, 849, 855, 865, 866, 870, 871, 875	681, 881
Correlation with diverse criteria	6, 10, 12, 31, 67, 72, 103, 118, 131, 138, 146, 153, 161, 181, 196, 198, 222, 223, 266, 270, 292, 302, 310, 312, 345, 376, 382, 394, 423, 432, 508, 520, 535, 550, 559, 566, 608, 615, 619, 647, 675, 695, 702, 703, 715, 729	753, 754, 756, 774, 775, 777, 778, 779, 780, 791, 816, 817, 830, 832, 835, 862, 863, 874	
Treatment variables and outcome studies	5, 32, 37, 50, 53, 92, 106, 113, 135, 179, 203, 217, 226, 227, 263, 311, 314, 315, 355, 370, 372, 380, 397, 398, 399, 430, 479,	785, 792, 807, 837, 839, 864	

(Continued)

Table 1. (*Continued*)

	MMPI	16PF	DPI
	531, 549, 557, 588, 594, 607, 614, 626, 651, 680, 682		
Race, cross-cultural, and ethnic	29, 68, 107, 108, 109, 111, 120, 121, 122, 154, 155, 172, 214, 215, 238, 246, 249, 363, 395, 454, 500, 529, 530, 576, 586, 601, 618, 648, 653, 677, 726	743, 744, 755, 759, 761, 773, 774, 783, 787, 797, 798, 812, 822, 823, 825, 827, 829, 834, 838, 839, 842, 844, 846, 854, 858, 859, 860, 869, 877, 879	882
Employment screening and job performance	21, 23, 62, 73, 112, 163, 171, 202, 204, 254, 255, 258, 306, 307, 334, 360, 391, 452, 484, 572, 579, 630, 643, 644, 645	761, 789, 804, 812, 848, 857, 878	

problems, we decided that the great advantages to having such a table would outweigh the possible problems.

In this chapter, we will focus on areas that have received the most research attention in recent years, and will attempt to highlight some of the issues which we believe are important in the future of the personality inventory domain.

2. Detection of Alcohol and Drug Problems with the MMPI

Miller (1976) reviewed studies aimed at detecting the addiction-prone personality, using psychological measures. His conclusion that objective personality assessment methods fail to predict well was arrived at *after* he reviewed a number of successful MMPI prediction studies. Certainly, the results of early alcoholism-detection studies with the MMPI were often equivocal and probably inspired a high degree of wariness on the part of psychologists. However, the more recently developed MMPI-based addiction measures have shown impressive accuracy and deserve to be given a balanced consideration.

The classification of personality test studies in Table 1 indicates that the area of addiction has been a very widely researched one. Studies aimed at predicting alcohol or drug abuse have generally followed two lines: One approach has been focused on devising separate MMPI scales that empirically differentiate alcoholics or drug addicts from other groups. The other approach involves using established MMPI measures as a basis for devising a cluster-discriminant analytic typology. Both of these approaches have met with success. We will highlight some of the studies in these areas to give you an overview of the work that has been done.

2.1. MMPI Alcoholism and Addiction Scales

For almost 25 years, researchers have attempted to devise a new, separate MMPI scale that would identify alcoholics (see Table 2). In one sense, all of these scales are similar; each was empirically constructed from existing MMPI items which were

481

OBJECTIVE
PERSONALITY
INVENTORIES:
RECENT RESEARCH
AND SOME
CONTEMPORARY
ISSUES

Table 2. Comparison of MMPI Alcoholism and Addiction Scales

Studies	Scale name	Composition of scale	Target population
Hampton (1953)	*Al*	125 items	Alcoholics
Button (1956) (based on an earlier study by Holmes)	*Am*	59 items	Alcoholics
Hoyt and Sedlacek (1958)	*Ah*	68 items	Alcoholics
MacAndrew (1965)	*Mac*	49 items	Alcoholics
Cavior et al. (1967)	*He*	57 items	Heroin addicts
Haertzen et al. (1968)	*AAF*	87 items	Alcoholics/addicts
Rich and Davis (1969)	*A Rev*	40 items: a combination of *Al*, *Am*, and *Ah*	Alcoholics
Finney et al. (1971)	*ALF*	85 items: a combination of *Al*, *Am*, *Ah*, *Mac*, and *AAF*	Alcoholics
Rosenberg (1972)	*A Ros*	27 items: a combination of *Ah*, *Am*, and *Mac*	Alcoholics

answered differently by alcoholics than by nonalcoholics. Why have so many different alcoholism scales been constructed?

The first scales (*Al*, *Am*, and *Ah*) proved to be inadequate because they only differentiated alcoholics from normals. The result was a general scale of maladjustment on which alcoholic patients' scores were highly similar to those of general psychiatric patients. In fact, the correlation between the *Al* scale and Welsh's factor *A* was shown to be 0.83 (Rosenberg, 1972), and, in one study, scale *F* alone did a better job of differentiating alcoholics from nonalcoholics than the *Al* scale (Apfeldorf & Huntley, 1976). Many other studies have shown the general inadequacy of all three of these first MMPI alcoholism scales (e.g., MacAndrew & Geertsma, 1974; Rotman & Vestre, 1964; Hoffmann, Loper, & Kammeier, 1974).

MacAndrew (1965) recognized that the success of an MMPI alcoholism scale would depend on its accuracy to detect alcoholics in a clinical setting. MacAndrew compared the MMPI responses of alcoholics with those of nonalcoholic psychiatric patients; the total sample of 600 consisted of male outpatients who varied greatly in age, income, and level of education. The result was a 49-item scale which, with a cutoff score of 24, accurately classified 81.75% of the sample, with 8.75% false negatives and 9.5% false positives. Cross-validation achieved similar results. MacAndrew's alcoholism scale (*Mac*) has since demonstrated impressive accuracy in other studies (see Table 3).

Further developmental work has been done on MacAndrew's alcoholism scale. Originally, MacAndrew found 51 items which differentiated his sample of alcoholics and nonalcoholics, but deleted two (No. 215, "I have used alcohol excessively," and No. 460, "I have used alcohol moderately or not at all") for two reasons: (1) the scale was intended to measure a variable other than amount of alcohol consumption (addiction proneness), and (2) both are obvious items, vulnerable to "faking." Although MacAndrew found that inclusion of these items increased the scale's accuracy somewhat, he felt that this was not as likely to happen in a clinical setting where people may feel inclined to deny their alcohol problems. Researchers vary as to whether they use the 49- or 51-item scale, and it is not yet known to what extent clinical accuracy is affected.

Further work has also been done to determine the most adequate cutoff score. Most people use 24, as MacAndrew recommends. Changing the cutoff score can in-

JAMES N. BUTCHER
AND PATRICIA L.
OWEN

Table 3.   Validation of MacAndrew's Alcoholism Scale

Study	Cutoff score	Overall accuracy	False negatives	False positives	Composition of study
MacAndrew (1965) (cross-validation)	24	81.5%	8.5%	10%	Alcoholics and psychiatric patients; male outpatients
Wisler and Cantor (1966)[a]	24	55%	7.9%	37.1%	Alcoholics and normals; male inpatients
	28	61.5%	17.8%	20.7%	
Rhodes (1969)	24	76%	10%	14%	Alcoholics and psychiatric patients; male outpatients
Uecker (1970)	24	69.5%	(not reported)		Alcoholics and psychiatric patients; male inpatients
Rich and Davis (1969)	Not reported; different for males & females	73–77%	(not reported)		Alcoholics, psychiatric patients, and normals; male and female inpatients
Vega (1971)	26	71%	9.6%	19%	Alcoholics, psychiatric patients, and normals; male inpatients
DeGroot and Adamson (1973)	26	73.5%	8.5%	18%	Alcoholics and psychiatric patients; male inpatients
Apfeldorf and Huntley (1975)	24	62%	7%	30%	Alcoholics and offenders; male inpatients
Schwartz (1977)	28	76%	(not reported)		Alcoholics, antisocial personalities, and normals; female inpatients (no cutoff score accurately separated similar male groups)
Burke and Marcus (1977)	24	74%	10%	16%	Alcoholics, psychiatric patients, and normals; male inpatients

[a]Results of this study may be inaccurate because of the possibility that individuals in the nonalcoholic group had alcohol-related problems.

crease the overall accuracy, but usually at the cost of achieving unacceptable levels of false negatives (e.g., Wisler & Cantor, 1966). One exception bears mention: women tend to score lower on the *Mac* than men, and adjusting their cutoff score appears appropriate (Schwartz, 1977; Rich & Davis, 1969).

A third concern has been whether or not to exclude MMPIs with F scale scores equal to or greater than 16, as did MacAndrew. Apfeldorf and Huntley (1975) suggest that high F profiles provide useful data, and found that their inclusion does little harm to overall accuracy.

Most of the validation work on MacAndrew's alcoholism scale has been to determine its range of utility. Although it was derived from a sample of male outpatients, it has shown comparable accuracy in samples of females, and in inpatient settings (see Table 3). MacAndrew's alcoholism scale appears to measure enduring qualities of alcoholic personalities. Prealcoholics score significantly higher on the MacAndrew than do their nonalcoholic peers (Hoffmann, Loper, & Kammeier, 1974), and even after treatment their *Mac* scores remain high (Rohan, Tatro, & Rotman, 1969; Chang, Caldwell, & Moss, 1973). This characteristic is important to recognize in using the *Mac* in a clinical setting (as well as in research). A high *Mac* score may not reflect current alcohol abuse; instead, either it may reflect a history of alcoholism which may no longer be a problem, or it may predict future alcoholism.

483

OBJECTIVE
PERSONALITY
INVENTORIES:
RECENT RESEARCH
AND SOME
CONTEMPORARY
ISSUES

Validation of MacAndrew's scale in populations which include antisocial personalities has met with varied results. Apfeldorf and Huntley (1975) found that disciplinary offenders in a domiciliary setting achieved *Mac* scores similar to those of alcoholics. Ruff, Ayers, and Templer (1976) obtained similar results with their sample of felons. It must be pointed out, however, that the felons were not screened for alcoholism. Schwartz (1977) compared *Mac* scores of alcoholics with those of psychiatric patients diagnosed as antisocial personalities, and, although he was able to find no significant difference in the males' scores, he found significant differences among the females. The psychopathic character trait may be a confounding variable, but in light of the above findings it is premature to state the true extent of its effect.

MacAndrew's alcoholism scale has not shown accuracy in differentiating alcoholics from drug abusers. Studies have shown that opiate addicts and polydrug abusers achieve *Mac* scores in the same elevated range as alcoholics (Burke & Marcus, 1977; Kranitz, 1972; Fowler, 1975; Lachar et al., 1976). In Burke and Marcus's study, MacAndrew's alcoholism scale correctly identified 85% of the alcoholics and 69% of the drug abusers. It is interesting to note that it correctly identified 94% of those with a history of both alcoholism and drug abuse.

MMPI scales have been devised which detect drug abuse, specifically. In 1967, Cavior, Kurtzberg, and Lipton constructed a 57-item scale (*He*) which identified 80% of their sample of male heroin addicts from incarcerated nonaddicts. Burke and Marcus (1977) found that the Cavior *He* scale correctly identified 77% of drug abusers in their sample of drug abusers, alcoholics, and psychiatric patients; it did not significantly differentiate alcoholics from drug abusers.

In an attempt to differentiate addicts from alcoholics, Haertzen, Hill, and Monroe (1968) devised an 87-item scale (*AAF*) on which addicts and alcoholics showed small but significant differences. On this scale, high scores indicate alcoholism; low scores indicate addiction. In a later study (Finney et al., 1971) factor-analyzed the *AAF* (along with four other alcoholism scales) and found that high and low scores on the *AAF* do reflect different personality characteristics. This scale has not undergone much validation work, so comments on its utility must be withheld.

2.2. MMPI Profile Similarities in Alcoholism and Drug Abuse

Early in MMPI history, an elevation on scale 4 (*Pd*) was recognized to be a frequent component in the profiles of alcoholics (Hewitt, 1943). Further studies have refined the picture. A most important contribution was made by Goldstein and Linden (1969); by using cluster analysis they delineated four profile types which accounted for 45% of their original sample of alcoholics and 42% of their replication sample. The two largest groups were those with spike 4 profiles (termed personality trait disturbance), and those with elevations on scales 2, 7, and 4 (psychoneurosis with anxiety or depressive reaction). The third group was a normal-limits profile with elevations on 4-9-2 (alcoholism with psychopathic personality, mixed type), and the last group had elevations on 4-9, with a low point on scale 2 (alcoholism with secondary problems of drug addiction and paranoid features). Similar subgroups of alcoholics have been found in later studies (Whitelock, Overall, & Patrick, 1971; Glen, Royer, & Custer, 1973). The importance of secondary elevations in distinguishing alcoholic profiles has been stressed by many researchers. Typical findings are demonstrated by Goss and Morosko (1969); in their sample of 200 male alcoholics, over half had secondary elevations on scale 2, and the most common three-point code was 4-2-7. Elevation on scale 7 has been suggested to indicate severity of alcohol abuse (Patrick, Connolly, & Overall, 1970).

From studies such as those described above, it can be seen that, while alcoholics are not a homogeneous population, their profiles are similar in that they usually reflect some degree of anxiety and depression, along with the psychopathic character traits measured by scale 4.

The profiles of drug abusers are not the same as profiles of alcoholics. Overall (1973) examined MMPIs of narcotic addicts and alcoholics, and found that only 15% of the profiles of the two groups overlapped. Although both groups achieved elevations on scale 4, secondary elevations reflected markedly different personalities; alcoholics had secondary elevations on scales 2, 3, 7, and 8, while addicts had secondary elevations on scales K and 9. It appears that the addicts' profiles present a picture of psychopathic traits of hostility and impulsivity, whereas the alcoholics' profiles present a more neurotic personality structure.

MMPIs of narcotic addicts may also differ from those of people who abuse other substances. Smart and Jones (1970) found that abusers of soft drugs (e.g., LSD, stimulants, barbiturates) achieved elevations on 8-9 more often than on 4-9.

In considering the accuracy of comparing addicts' and alcoholics' profiles, several confounding variables must be recognized. Alcoholics tend to be older than drug abusers, and heroin addicts tend to be older than soft drug abusers. Indeed, Fitzgibbon, Berry, and Shearn (1973) found that profiles of drug abusers (ages 14–25) did not differ significantly from profiles of same-age psychiatric patients who denied drug abuse. They concluded that the traits associated with drug abuse in this age group actually reflect general disturbance not specific to drug use.

Another confounding variable is the effect of the substance itself. Do profile elevations indicate stable traits, or do they merely reflect reactions to drug-use experience? Zuckerman and Sola (1975) addressed this question and found that, although overall elevations of soft and hard drug users decreased after residence in an addiction treatment program, a residual 4-9 profile remained.

Profiles of alcoholics also appear to have stable elements. Loper, Kammeier, and Hoffmann (1973) examined the MMPIs of men admitted to an alcoholic treatment center which were taken, on the average, 13 years prior to treatment. These men, as prealcoholics, had a modal 4-2 profile, significantly different from that of their nonalcoholic peers.

In summarizing the research in the area of detection of alcoholism and drug abuse by analysis of MMPI profiles, it appears that there are indeed significant group differences among alcoholics, drug abusers, and nonabusers. While a clinician can use this information to suggest whether addiction or alcoholism may be a problem, predicting the substance of choice may lead to false interpretations.

A most promising measure to differentiate alcoholics from addicts has been devised by Overall (1973). Using a discriminant function analysis, he determined weights to be accorded to each MMPI validity and clinical scale (except 5 and 0). Applying the formula $DF = (.0917)L + (.0602)F - (.0939)K - (.0367)Hs + (.0300)D +$

$(.1180)Hy - (.0317)Pd + (.0388)Pa + (.1266)Pt + (.0327)Sc - (.0950)Ma$ to the group means of alcoholics and addicts resulted in an 85% correct separation of the two groups. McLachlan (1975) used the discriminant function in a similar sample, and achieved an accuracy level of 65%; he noted, however, that when normal profiles were first excluded (using Goldberg's first rule), the accuracy rate rose to 80%.

From our survey of the MMPI's utility in the detection of alcoholism and addiction, we conclude that, although there is need for further research, there is substantial evidence to demonstrate that objective measures derived from the MMPI are capable of achieving impressive levels of accuracy.

485

OBJECTIVE
PERSONALITY
INVENTORIES:
RECENT RESEARCH
AND SOME
CONTEMPORARY
ISSUES

3. Use of the MMPI with Medical Patients

The MMPI has been used extensively in research with medical patients. Historically, these studies have comprised three main areas: (1) differentiation between patients with psychosomatic disorders and those with organic diseases, (2) delineation of psychological factors associated with psychosomatic disorders, such as ulcers and asthma, and (3) prediction of surgery outcome and rapidity of recovery from physical illness. The intention of this discussion is not to provide a literature review of these areas (see references in Table 1, and Dahlstrom, Welsh, and Dahlstrom, 1975), but to highlight some of the major findings.

It has long been recognized that certain profiles, particularly those with elevations on scales 1 and 3, indicate that the patient may be protesting too much, and can serve as a warning flag to a physician attempting to make a diagnosis on essentially unremarkable physical findings. (The 1-3/3-1 code type is the most common code type in medical settings.) But how confidently can the clinician suggest that a patient's disease is functional when confronted with a 1-3/3-1 profile? With psychiatric patients, the 1-3 code type has repeatedly been found to reflect denial of social anxiety and expression of psychological discomfort through numerous somatic complaints of little (medical) consequence. Recent studies have indicated that the same may not hold true for medical patients; while there may be a large neurotic overlay to the overall symptom picture, a 1-3 profile by no means precludes a diagnosis of organic disease. Schwartz, Osborne, and Krupp (1972), in their survey of the MMPIs of 50,000 medical patients, examined the medical records of a large sample of male and female patients who achieved elevations on scales 1 and 3, and found that this code type, no matter how elevated, "does not appear significantly related to the likelihood of receiving a functional diagnosis."

Confounding the picture are findings that, although MMPI profiles tend to remain within normal limits during physical distress of short duration, patients with *chronic* medical disease often achieve elevations on the neurotic triad—scales 1, 2, and 3 (Fracchia, Sheppard, Ricca, & Merlis, 1973; Goldstein, & Reznikoff, 1972). Here the elevations on 1 and 3 may reflect an adaptive reaction to the hospital regime, a cheerful front while dutifully reporting diverse physical changes in minute detail. The elevation on scale 2 may simply reflect a normal response to prolonged hospitalization.

When the MMPI profile does describe a documented psychosomatic illness, it does not appear to differentiate among "asthma personalities," "ulcer personalities," and other hypothesized psychosomatic personalities; all groups seem to present the familiar 1-3/3-1 profile or minute variations thereof. This suggests either that the

MMPI is not sensitive to psychological factors which distinguish between the groups or that the factors are too variable within the psychosomatic group itself.

The above studies all share one common flaw: coexisting rather than preexisting MMPI profiles are correlated with somatic complaints. This allows us only to speculate as to whether the patient's psychological state is a cause of, or a reaction to, medical illness.

Perhaps the most intriguing area of medicine which could benefit from MMPI research is that of examining subtle emotional changes which may influence the body's resistance to disease. Schmale and Iker (1966) found that elevations on scale 2 of MMPIs taken *before* diagnosis of cancer correlated with later findings of malignancy. Most other research in this area has been based on "life events" checklists and laboratory animal studies. Stein, Schiavi, and Camerino (1976) provide an excellent review of extensive animal research which indicates that psychological factors do indeed influence the effectiveness of the immunological system. It seems only sensible, at this point, for MMPI researchers to turn away from continually rediscovering that psychological disturbance is associated with real or imagined somatic distress, and instead turn to exploring just how state of mind affects the appearance of disease. As Schmale and Iker's study indicates, creative research with the MMPI can provide some of the missing links.

4. Cross-Cultural and Subcultural Applications of the MMPI

In recent years the MMPI has been used with populations that differ greatly from the original standardization sample—lower-class urban dwellers, black and Latino groups, and a wide range of national groups from Australia to Japan to Switzerland. The application of any psychological test in populations that differ in important respects from the original standardization sample is questionable. A transplanted test cannot be assumed to have the same meaning and validity in the target culture or subculture as it had in the developmental domain. Why do psychologists working with ethnically or nationally diverse groups use the MMPI? Do the MMPI scales and factors operate in the new culture as they do in the original? Does the MMPI have validity generalization in the target population?

These questions cannot be answered fully in this brief section. The extent of MMPI use in other countries is great—there have been over 40 different translations of the items, and a recent handbook (Butcher & Pancheri, 1976) cited over 600 MMPI references with a cross-cultural focus. Why the MMPI? Psychology, as a profession, is in its infancy in many countries, and their resources for developing psychological measuring techniques are not available. Many psychologists have explored the MMPI literature and consider the MMPI constructs to be relevant for use in their country.* Once the items are translated and the scales are applied in clinical contexts, the translator finds that the inventory seems to be measuring the same constructs as well in the target country as in the United States. Butcher and Pancheri (1976) reviewed many of the problems of test translation and restandardization. They reported on a cross-national validation of the MMPI that shows the robustness of many of the MMPI scales for detecting psychopathology in several countries. A

---

*One psychologist from Spain reported that he ran across an MMPI booklet. He decided to translate the inventory because the content appeared to be very relevant to psychopathology in Spain.

recent study by Merbaum and Hefez (1976) with an Israeli sample further supports the validity generalization of the MMPI in other countries.

487

OBJECTIVE
PERSONALITY
INVENTORIES:
RECENT RESEARCH
AND SOME
CONTEMPORARY
ISSUES

It appears that, although there are translation and standardization problems that require resolution, the MMPI works sufficiently well to warrant use in other countries. The MMPI works with only slight modification in Western, industrialized nations, but it requires some modification of the structure of the instrument itself and some alteration in the interpretation of the scales when used with non-Western people.

Are there problems with using the MMPI in the assessment of subcultural samples within the United States? Gynther (1972) reviewed the literature on use of the MMPI with blacks and more recently (Gynther, 1977) with blacks and other minority groups. He noted a number of problems with applying essentially white norms to nonwhite populations. Readers interested in these issues should become familiar with his work. There is some recent evidence to indicate that when the MMPI is applied to populations for which it was intended, i.e., psychiatric patients, the MMPI profiles for various diagnostic groups do not differ for black and white samples (Marks, Bertelson, & May, 1977). This evidence supports the use of the MMPI in clinical diagnosis regardless of the ethnic population from which the profile is obtained.

Further study is needed to determine if special norms for ethnic or other national populations are required.

5. MMPI Short Forms

One frequent complaint from people required to answer the 566 questions of the MMPI is that it is too long and tedious to fill out. Is the MMPI administration too time-consuming? Does the inventory ask too many questions? Can it be shortened to a more "reasonable" length and still provide enough information to serve as a reliable diagnostic indicator of psychopathology?

The length of the MMPI has been a concern of researchers and clinicians since the inventory was published in the early 1940s. Hathaway attempted to develop a short form of the instrument but gave it up when he became disappointed with its utility. Butcher (1972), reviewing some of the problems with the MMPI, discussed a paradoxical situation in which the MMPI was both too long and too short (too short in that the item pool is not broad enough to sample many clinically relevant domains). However, recent years have witnessed the development of a number of shortened versions of the MMPI which have been published for use with different populations, for different purposes, and following different statistical procedures.

In evaluating the need for and value of a particular short form, several factors or characteristics of the MMPI should be kept in mind:

1. It usually takes only about $1\frac{1}{2}$ hr in a single sitting to administer the full MMPI.
2. Many facilities administer the full MMPI to patients while they are waiting for appointments or medical tests; thus "useful" clinical time is often not wasted in MMPI administration.
3. The actual professional time for MMPI administration and scoring is little. Actually, many facilities use clerks to administer, score, and draw up the profile.

4. All the MMPI items do not need to be administered in order to score the standard clinical and validity scales. Only about 400 items are required. Thus the MMPI administration can be abbreviated by quite a bit without loss of any of the usual information.

5. If an MMPI answersheet is incomplete (but at least 200 items have been answered), there are tables available for prorating the scores to obtain full scale estimates. This information may be found in Appendix K of Dahlstrom, Welsh, and Dahlstrom (1972).

6. The MMPI, at best, is an imperfect predictor and serves only as a gross screening measure of some psychopathological factors. Drastically abbreviating the scales may further reduce scale reliability and validity below an acceptable level.

7. The responsibility of demonstrating the validity of the alleged alternate "form" falls on the short-form developer because it cannot be assumed that just because the same scale names are used (and a few of its items) that it is the same instrument.

There is not sufficient space in this review to discuss all the research on the many MMPI short forms that has been published in recent years (see Table 1). Most of the research has been focused on developing new abbreviated scales and showing how the shortened scales correlate with the longer version in different settings or with different populations. Very little empirical research has been directed toward external validation.

The first formal short form of the MMPI, published by Olson in 1954, received little attention in the literature. The most widely researched MMPI short form is the Mini-Mult developed by Kincannon (1968). It is a 71-item questionnaire that provides scale score estimates for all the standard clinical scales except the *Mf* and *Si*. The questions were originally placed in the interrogative form and could be administered orally in a brief interview. The Midi-Mult, a "lengthened" short form, published by Dean (1972), contained the 71 Mini-Mult items plus an additional 15 items. A third variation on the theme is the Maxi-Mult (Spera & Robertson, 1974), which is the Mini-Mult plus the Grayson critical items.

Another approach to shortening the MMPI was taken by Faschingbauer (1974). He used a substitution and regression model to develop a 166-item short form called the FAM.

Overall and Gomez-Mont (1974) developed an abbreviated version of the MMPI by using simply the first 168 items in the booklet. (Item 168 is the last item on page 7 of the Form R booklet.) They then used least squares regression equations to estimate conventional *K*-corrected raw scores from the raw scores obtained in the first 168 items.*

Two additional short versions that have been developed will be mentioned, although they are fairly lengthy and may not be considered as short enough by some people. Hugo (1972) published a 173-item form, and Blaser and Gehring (1973) developed a 221-item form in conjunction with their translation and adaptation of the MMPI in Switzerland.

---

*This strategy for short-form development actually had an additional advantage in that it avoided criticism from The Psychological Corporation, lessee of the MMPI copyright, which has taken a dim view of short-form development and voiced concern over copyright violation in some cases of item reorganization.

489

OBJECTIVE
PERSONALITY
INVENTORIES:
RECENT RESEARCH
AND SOME
CONTEMPORARY
ISSUES

How well do the short forms of the MMPI perform? Many studies have presented correlations with the long-version MMPI scales as evidence for the value of the short form. In most cases, there is a respectable correlation (usually ranging from the low 50s to the mid 80s). In most cases, this moderate-to-high degree of positive association between two measures would be considered an acceptable relationship. However, two measures with a correlation of +.50 actually have an overlap of only .25. Thus the prediction error for individuals would be high. When one considers the already imperfect relationship between the longer version of the MMPI and external criteria, use of a short form does not appear justified for prediction in a clinical context when correct assessment of the individual is important. This difficulty is highlighted in studies that have examined classification hit rates for short form scales. Hoffmann and Butcher (1975) evaluated the question of how well three short forms (the Mini-Mult, the FAM, and MMPI-168) classified the patient according to code type, which is one of the most frequently used interpretive indices. They examined 58 code types in a psychiatric population. The classification performance of all three short forms was generally poor—36.7% for the Mini-Mult, 40.4% for the MMPI-168, and 49.4% for the FAM. The problem of poor classification success of short forms has also been noted by other investigators (Fillenbaum and Pfeiffer, 1976; Hedlund, Won Cho, & Powell, 1975).

It appears that coverage of MMPI-based concepts and accuracy of individual prediction may be greatly sacrificed if the clinician decides to use an abbreviated scale. Can anything be done about the problem of scale length and loss of information resulting from deleting items?

One possible solution to the dilemma of length vs. coverage in personality inventories may be to tailor-make tests for each individual, using an adaptive testing approach. Individual assessment would begin with a large comprehensive pool of items, and each subject would be administered a limited subset of items, as necessary, to obtain a full description of his or her personality. That is, the test administration would be tailor-made for each person through the use of branching strategies in a computer interactive administration. An adaptive testing approach could be developed with an array of personality measures that have different foci—for example, psychopathological states (MMPI, DPI), personality dimensions (16PF, PRF, CPI, etc.), specific behavioral or problem checklists, and special abilities. These items could be stored in a computer and administered to a subject, via a cathode ray tube (CRT) or television console, in a fixed order that is determined in advance, or, better yet, in a flexible order that is contingent on the previous response or pattern of answers. The former approach is presently being used with the MMPI at the Institute of Psychiatry in Rome (Butcher & Pancheri, 1976). In the latter approach, a specific subset of items would be administered to each person analogous to an interview situation, in which each question asked of the subject is based on his or her response to a previous question.

The main deterrents to flexible adaptive personality testing at this time are the scarcity of valid predictors for items or small groups of items and a lack of information about how to branch to other subdomains of items according to specific responses. For example, suppose a person answers "true" to the item "I believe I am being plotted against." Do we, knowing this, now branch to (1) a new symptom domain, (2) a more thorough evaluation of persecutory beliefs, e.g., relating to the extent of the individual's concerns about the CIA, FBI, police, Russians, etc., (3) a subdomain of other "paranoid"-like thoughts, or (4) an item array dealing with aggressive fantasies to determine if the person might be inclined to act on delusions, etc. Establishing a logic for contingent administration is a mammoth undertaking and has not been developed to the point that adaptive personality testing can be practically applied.

One recent study demonstrated the feasibility of an adaptive typological approach to psychiatric screening (Clavelle & Butcher, 1977). Following a sequential or multilevel strategy, the authors demonstrated that a possible "entry" into the branching process might be accomplished by first administering a limited but fixed subset of MMPI items to provide an estimate of the individual's personality type (MMPI code). With an idea of what general kinds of psychopathology one is dealing with, more specific branches into other item domains could be developed. Clavelle and Butcher selected nine MMPI code types as the target pathology groups, and obtained 100 psychiatric cases for a developmental sample and 50 cases for a cross-validation sample for each of the nine pathology groups [1-3/3-1 and 2-3/3-2 (neurotic), 2-4/4-2 and 4-9/9-4 (personality disorder), 6-8/8-6 and 8-9/9-8 (psychotic), 2-4-8 and 2-7-8 (borderline-schizoid), and a group of psychiatric patients with normal profiles] to be predicted. The study sought to determine whether a small group of MMPI items could be used to differentiate among the code types and then narrow down the range of clinical groups in which an individual might be classified. Using discriminant function analysis, they obtained the 69 items that had the most discriminating power in differentiating among the groups. The 69 items were then entered into the discriminant function analysis in groups of ten to determine the classification accuracy with the addition of more items. Classification accuracy reached 60% after only 30 items and rose to an asymptote of about 73% after 50 items. Shrinkage on cross-validation was not excessive, less than 4%. When the original code type groups were collapsed into five molar categories—neurotic, character disorder, psychotic, borderline, and "normal-range MMPI" patients—the classification rates were even higher, 81% with 50 items.

The classification results were impressive. Even with the simplest classification scheme and a small number of items (i.e., classify a person into that code type for which he or she obtains the highest probability), the hit rate was high. The classification into broader clinical, diagnostic categories was even higher. Moreover, a phenomenon of diminishing returns was obtained after relatively few items. That is, an asymptote of accuracy was reached well before 69 items, after which additional items did not improve the classification.

The implications of this study are that, in the first stage of an adaptive testing situation, patients could be given a small subset of items (e.g., 50 or 69, depending on the accuracy one desires) to provide a tentative classification which narrows down the range of clinical alternatives that need to be considered. When the preliminary discrimination is made, the testing focus could then be directed to other domains such as content scales, severity of disorder type items, or potential for change items. The adaptive testing model shows some promise in revolutionizing the application of personality inventories. A great deal of additional research on branching strategies is needed before a tailor-made system could be operative clinically. The technology of computer science on which a branched system could be based presently exists. It awaits the development of an empirical personality psychology to provide the content for assessment.

6. Content Interpretation

OBJECTIVE
PERSONALITY
INVENTORIES:
RECENT RESEARCH
AND SOME
CONTEMPORARY
ISSUES

The earliest personality inventories, such as Woodworth's Personal Data Sheet, were developed according to a rational scale-construction strategy. Items were devised according to a preconceived idea of the scale construct and how it would be measured by the items. A test author developed item content from the "armchair" and assumed that, if items had face validity, they actually would work in the way they were intended. In many cases, items did not relate to the construct in the way that the test constructor hypothesized, and often worked in the *opposite* direction. Empirical scale-construction methods were first developed by Strong, in the vocational interest domain, to improve the predictive power of scales. The success of empirical item selection led other test authors to follow the criterion validation approach. In their development of the MMPI, Hathaway and McKinley (Hathaway, 1965) employed a fairly strict empirical item-selection strategy to maximize the external validity of the MMPI scales.

The advantages of the empirical scale-construction method over the armchair approach was forcefully argued by Meehl (1945) in what has been referred to as the empiricist's manifesto. This now-classic paper presented the case for empirical validity of items and scales at the expense of ignoring item content. A generation of MMPI users was encouraged to consider only scale scores, or, better yet, profile configuration of the patients' responses, and ignore the actual content of the items in test interpretation.

Within the "multcult," however, there were occasional heretics of the dustbowl empiricism tradition who peeked at item content. Item content was viewed as an important source of MMPI information by several writers: Carson (1969) discussed MMPI item responses as communications between the patient and the clinician; Grayson (1951) published a set of "critical items" or items that were considered to have special importance as pathognomonic indications; and Harris and Lingoes (1968) published a set of MMPI subscales, based on a rational-content analysis, to aid the clinician in assessing MMPI scale meanings. A clinical example illustrates the importance of test item content. When the senior author of this paper was a psychology intern, he interviewed a patient, as part of a diagnostic evaluation, several days after the patient completed the MMPI. At one point, following a query about the patient's presenting complaints (some unusual physical symptoms), the patient adamantly pointed out that he had already answered that question—it was on the answer form that he had previously filled out—hadn't the interviewer even looked at his answers? It was clear that many patients respond to test item content with the expectation that the psychologist will evaluate it to better understand the patients' problems.

In recent years, psychometric practice has come full circle, and rational item selection and content analysis of self-report behavior have received a greater share of attention. Hase and Goldberg (1967) compared several strategies for constructing personality inventories and found essentially no differences in the relative success of empirical, rational, or factor analytic approaches. Jackson (1971) reviewed the issues of empirical vs. rational item selection raised by Meehl (1945) and made a strong case for developing test items using a rational strategy based on a theoretical model. Jackson, assuming that people adopt a strategy of more-or-less complete honesty when they respond to personality inventories, developed several scales—the

JAMES N. BUTCHER
AND PATRICIA L.
OWEN

Personality Research Form (PRF) and (with Messick) the *Differential Personality Inventory* (DPI). The PRF is a "normal-range" personality inventory focusing on needs, e.g., need for achievement and need for abasement. The DPI focuses on dimensions of psychopathology and overlaps to some extent with MMPI-based constructs.

Meehl (1972), in reevaluating his earlier position on item content, noted that

> One reason for the difficulties of psychometric personology, a reason that I did not appreciate adequately in my "dustbowl empiricist" paper of 1945, is the sad state of psychological theory. The superiority of mechanical, actuarial prediction and interpretation arises from several factors, one of which is theoretical inadequacy. The clinician who attempts to mediate predictions or other kinds of inferences, whether from test or history or interview raw data, by utilizing a psychodynamic causal model will, no matter how clever he is, almost never be able to meet the conditions which any undergraduate student of chemistry or physics knows are necessary in order to forecast the subsequent state of a physical system (or to infer to as yet unobserved aspects of its concurrent state) on the basis of scientific theory. In order to mediate predictions (using the word epistemically rather than with a time reference as to the state of nature) by theoretical constructs, one must satisfy two epistemic conditions:
> 1. One must have a powerful (high-verisimilitude) theory, that is, he must "know" how the system works.
> 2. One must have reasonably accurate knowledge of the initial and boundary conditions of the system, that is, he must have an accurate measurement technology.
> Now it is perfectly obvious that the clinical psychologist, for the most part, does not satisfy either of these two conditions for powerful theory-mediated prediction, whereas, it is necessary in making predictions on this basis that one should satisfy both. That this is an obvious limitation, admitted by all competent scholars, gives me continued faith in the general line of empirical-actuarial predictive and interpretative methods—despite my recognition that such a monolithically "criterion-statistical" view on item analysis as that of my 1945 paper is too strong. (p. 150)

The balanced position of recognizing the importance of item content and the need to use more advanced psychological "theories" to guide item selection is important in the development of new personality scales. Nevertheless, we consider external validation of personality scales as the most important criterion of the ultimate worth of a personality scale. If it does not predict what it is supposed to, no matter how interesting and "relevant" the content, it is worthless.

Two approaches to evaluating item content in the MMPI have been given wide attention or use in recent years, largely through inclusion in computerized personality testing. The most systematic approach to summarizing item content involves the development of content scales or subsets of homogeneous content items that, when summed, give the clinician an idea of how many items of a similar nature the patient has endorsed. The second approach involves isolating individual items which have special importance, that is, items which are considered to be pathognomonic or "critical" for signaling certain problem areas.

The most adequate treatment of content dimensions of the MMPI was done by Wiggins (1969), who developed a set of homogeneous content scales in order to measure the main self-report dimensions in the MMPI item pool. The 13 mutually exclusive scales (see Table 4) are internally consistent, are moderately independent, and represent the major substantive content cluster in the MMPI item pool.

The second approach to evaluating the content of a patient's responses involves the use of pathognomonic or "critical" items. The subset of items devices by Grayson (1951) has been most widely used. Another rationally devised item list deemed

Table 4. Description of MMPI Content Scales[a]

493

**OBJECTIVE
PERSONALITY
INVENTORIES:
RECENT RESEARCH
AND SOME
CONTEMPORARY
ISSUES**

SOC	Social Maladjustment	High SOC is socially bashful, shy, embarrassed, reticent, self-conscious, and extremely reserved. Low SOC is gregarious, confident, assertive, and relates quickly and easily to others. He is fun-loving, the life of a party, a joiner who experiences no difficulty in speaking before a group. This scale would correspond roughly with the popular concept of "introversion-extraversion."
DEP	Depression	High DEP experiences guilt, regret, worry, unhappiness, and a feeling that life has lost its zest. He experiences difficulty in concentrating and has little motivation to pursue things. His self-esteem is low, and he is anxious and apprehensive about the future. He is sensitive to slight, feels misunderstood, and is convinced that he is unworthy and deserves punishment. In short, he is classically depressed.
FEM	Feminine Interests	High FEM admits to liking feminine games, hobbies, and vocations. He denies liking masculine games, hobbies, and vocations. Here there is almost complete contamination of content and form, which has been noted in other contexts by several writers. Individuals may score high on this scale by presenting themselves as *liking* many things, since this item stem is present in almost all items. They may also score high by endorsing interests that, although possibly feminine, are also *socially desirable*, such as an interest in poetry, dramatics, news of the theater, and artistic pursuits. This has been noted in the case of Wiggins's *Sd* scale. Finally, of course, individuals with a genuine preference for activities that are conceived by our culture as "feminine" will achieve high scores on this scale.
MOR	Poor Morale	High MOR is lacking in self-confidence, feels that he has failed in life, and is given to despair and a tendency to give up hope. He is extremely sensitive to the feelings and reactions of others and feels misunderstood by them, while at the same time being concerned about offending them. He feels useless and is socially suggestible. There is a substantive overlap here between the Depression and Social Maladjustment scales and the Poor Morale scale. The Social Maladjustment scale seems to emphasize a lack of social ascendance and poise, the Depression scale feelings of guilt and apprehension, while the present scale seems to emphasize a lack of self-confidence and hypersensitivity to the opinions of others.
REL	Religious Fundamentalism	High scorers on this scale see themselves as religious, church-going people who accept as true a number of fundamentalist religious convictions. They also tend to view their faith as the true one.
AUT	Authority Conflict	High AUT sees life as a jungle and is convinced that others are unscrupulous, dishonest, hypocritical, and motivated only by personal profit. He distrusts others, has little respect for experts, is competitive, and believes that everyone should get away with whatever he can.
PSY	Psychoticism	High PSY admits to a number of class psychotic symptoms of a primarily paranoid nature. He admits to hallucinations, strange experiences, loss of control, and classic paranoid delusions of grandeur and persecution. He admits to feelings of unreality, daydreaming, and a sense that things are wrong, while feeling misunderstood by others.

(Continued)

Table 4. *(Continued)*

ORG	Organic Symptoms	High ORG admits to symptoms that are often indicative of organic involvement. These include headaches, nausea, dizziness, loss of motility and coordination, loss of consciousness, poor concentration and memory, speaking and reading difficulty, poor muscular control, tingling skin sensations, and disturbances in hearing and smelling.
FAM	Family Problems	High FAM feels that he had an unpleasant home life characterized by a lack of love in the family and parents who were unnecessarily critical, nervous, quarrelsome, and quick-tempered. Although some items are ambiguous, most are phrased with reference to the parental home rather than the individual's current home.
HOS	Manifest Hostility	High HOS admits to sadistic impulses and a tendency to be cross, grouchy, competitive, argumentative, uncooperative, and retaliatory in his interpersonal relationships. He is often competitive and socially aggressive.
PHO	Phobias	High PHO has admitted to a number of fears, many of them of the classically phobic variety such as heights, darkness, and closed spaces.
HYP	Hypomania	High HYP is characterized by feelings of excitement, well-being, restlessness, and tension. His is enthusiastic, high-strung, cheerful, full of energy, and apt to be hotheaded. He has broad interests, seeks change, and is apt to take on more than he can handle.
HEA	Poor Health	High HEA is concerned about his health and has admitted to a variety of gastrointestinal complaints centering around an upset stomach and difficulty in elimination.

[a]Wiggins, 1969, p. 145–146.

as critical, or of particular importance, is the set of eight Caldwell (1969) critical items, which is an extension of the Grayson list and includes some neurotic-type items.

The MMPI "critical" items (Grayson & Caldwell), which are considered to have special importance when answered in a particular direction, have been widely accepted as an important source of information about the patient, in spite of the fact that they were complete "armchair products" or had never been subjected to wide empirical validation. The unquestioned acceptance of any subset of MMPI items as more important than the remainder of the item pool has been criticized in a recent paper by Koss, Butcher, and Hoffman (1976). They noted the importance of empirical evaluation of the so-called critical items, because these items are being widely accepted and used in automated (computerized) systems as though they have been thoroughly validated. Koss et al. classified 1023 patients into six "crisis situation" groups according to presenting problems and examined the success of the Grayson and Caldwell items at detecting the patients' specific psychological problems at the time of admission. They found that some of the Grayson items appeared to be prominent among those that identified mental confusion and persecutory crises (the two most disturbed groups); however, this item subset made virtually no contribution in identifying any of the other crises: acute anxiety, depressed-suicidal, threatened assault, and alcoholism. The Caldwell items were more prominent among all crisis groups, but were also found to sample predominantly in the psychotic realm.

495

OBJECTIVE
PERSONALITY
INVENTORIES:
RECENT RESEARCH
AND SOME
CONTEMPORARY
ISSUES

The crisis situations studied by Koss et al. (1976) had been suggested by experienced clinicians as those most frequently occurring in clinical settings. Therefore, since the "critical items" seem to identify only a small subset of people experiencing psychotic symptoms, their application in general clinical or medical settings appears quite limited.

It is possible to develop subsets of pathognomonic items that have both content relevance and validity. Koss and Butcher (1973) examined the relationship of the content of patients' item responses and empirical descriptions of their behavior as reflected in diagnosis and MMPI code type information. They grouped patients according to presenting symptoms, as described above, into one of six crisis groups or a sample of "noncrisis" psychiatric control patients. Psychiatric patients who were classified in a particular crisis group tended to be described by other sources of clinical information, diagnosis, and MMPI code type in a consistent and meaningful way. For example, individuals experiencing an "anxiety" or "depressive" crisis tended to be diagnosed as neurotic and have MMPI profiles that would be classified as neurotic. Patients experiencing a "persecutory ideas" crisis were more often diagnosed as "psychotic" and had MMPI code types generally considered psychotic.

The major focus of this study, the relationship of item content to experienced crisis, was impressive. Many of the items significantly differentiating the groups clearly reflected the pathology manifested by individuals in those crisis situations. For example, many of the items differentiating the "depressed-suicidal" crisis clearly reflect depression—"Most of the time I feel blue," "The future seems hopeless to me," etc.

Koss and Butcher conclude:

> The results of the study suggest that in a large number of instances item responses communicate information which was in agreement with what was known about the S's behavior from other sources. The information contained in the S's item responses was found to be in agreement with various independent observations of their behavior such as the admitting physician's notes, or the psychiatrist's diagnosis. Likewise, the content of the item responses was found to be consistent with several empirical measures of the S's test performance such as code type or the patterning of scores on the major MMPI scales and factors. The ability of item responses to convey valid data was found to be consistent across a wide range of patients with varying diagnoses, MMPI code types and major problems, complaints and symptoms. Thus, the view that an item response represents veridically the behavior described by the item content was supported by this study. These patients were both willing and able to reveal useful information about themselves. (Koss and Butcher, 1973, p. 235)

7. Automated Personality Assessment

Personality inventories, with their objective scoring format, are particularly well suited to machine-scoring approaches. Additionally, when personality characteristics have been established for personality scales or scale patterns, the task of test interpretation can also readily be automated. In his classic monograph comparing clinical and statistical prediction methods, Meehl (1954) argued convincingly that actuarial prediction was superior to clinical methods. In a later paper (Meehl, 1955), he demonstrated that empirical descriptors developed on one sample of patients with various MMPI code types could be automatically applied to new cases with the same MMPI code with great accuracy. Following Meehl's suggestion for developing an actuarial system of MMPI interpretation, Gilberstadt and Duker

(1965), Marks and Seeman (1963), and Marks, Seeman, and Haller (1974) published extensive, practical diagnostic systems for actuarial interpretation of MMPI code types (Gilberstadt and Duker MMPI code types containing 19 code types and Marks, Seeman, and Haller code types containing 16 code types for adult populations and 29 code types for adolescents). These two systems classify approximately 20–55% of new cases in clinical settings. Additional MMPI code type descriptors have been carefully studied by Gynther and his colleagues (Gynther, Altman, & Sletten, 1973; Lewandowski & Graham, 1972). These studies focused on establishing replicable empirical correlates for MMPI codes and scale scores, and show the robust nature of many MMPI descriptors on cross-validation. Some investigators have not been content with the fairly rudimentary classification approach of considering only the first two or three scale elevations and have developed classification systems based on different MMPI information. Sines (1964) used a measure of profile similarity to classify profiles of the 4-3 type with good results. Goldberg (1965) used linear predictions methods to classify profiles as neurotic or psychotic. Overall (1976) employed multivariate statistical methods to examine the relative contribution of several sources of information (MMPI, behavior ratings, and history) to the classification of psychiatric disorders. Pancheri (reported in Butcher & Pancheri, 1976) developed an actuarial diagnostic system in which patients are classified according to a multivariate discriminant function model. Patients' MMPI profiles are assigned probability values of being correctly classified into one of the known patient groups on which the model was developed. All of these diverse approaches have demonstrated utility for diagnostic classification and warrant use in future actuarial diagnostic research studies as well as in clinical application.

Interest in the objective classification of patient self-report coincided with rapid technological growth in the electronic computer industry. The storage capacity and computational accuracy and speed of the electronic computer made automated test interpretation on a large scale feasible. Thus, in spite of the fact that MMPI actuarial research was in its infancy, the technology for a fully automated clinician became available. The first computerized MMPI system was developed by Pearson and Swenson at the Mayo Clinic in the early 1960s. This system, later distributed by The Psychological Corporation and sold commercially by National Computer Systems listed out several descriptive statements based on single score elevation and code type correlates. A number of MMPI-based computer interpretation systems have become available commercially. Most of these systems print out a narrative report along with the scale scores, a profile plotting, and "critical item" list that purportedly clue the clinician about particularly important item responses.

The narrative report is based generally on available empirical code type information. However, a large amount of unvalidated "clinical" information is usually included. Consequently, most systems should be referred to as automated clinicians rather than actuaries. A description of several systems is provided in Table 5 to give an idea of the nature and extent of automated interpretation systems available.

The extensive development of different computer assessment systems may give the impression that we have finally reached Meehl's promised land of empirical psychology described in his "Wanted: a good cookbook" article in 1955. Do we presently have the ultimate in objective actuarial prediction systems? Many zealous computer system advocates might like to create the impression that we do (a few of the systems publish flashy commercial advertisements that strongly imply this). However, it

497

OBJECTIVE
PERSONALITY
INVENTORIES:
RECENT RESEARCH
AND SOME
CONTEMPORARY
ISSUES

should be recognized that these systems primarily underscore the great advances in computer technology, and not the scientific status of the classification and description of personality by actuarial methods. Most MMPI computer systems rely on clinically generated interpretation of profile elements, because the actuarial base of MMPI interpretation is still rather limited. Gynther observed:

> The current MMPI interpreter must be quite sophisticated. He must be aware that the actuarial approach will eventually replace him because machines possess near perfect reliability. Yet he must recognize that the time has not yet arrived, since the rules and code books currently available are not comprehensive enough to handle even a majority of his cases. Furthermore, the task of cross validation of profile types already at hand has barely begun; what evidence is available suggests that local rules based on local data may be essential to achieve predictive accuracy in a given setting. (Gynther, 1972, pp. 242–243)

Although many of the computer-generated reports are creative, astute, and possibly very accurate sets of clinical hunches, they are not fully based on established actuarial data systems. Butcher and Tellegen (1976) noted that computerized interpretation using psychological test based information is little more than an art or craft disguised as a science.

A recent view of several commercially available automated MMPI systems (Butcher, 1978) disclosed a number of problems.

1. Although the use of the computer creates an aura of objectivity, most computer interpretation systems are based on "clinical guesses" rather than on actuarial systems.
2. Some systems rely on P.T. Barnum-type statements (glittering generalities) in the narrative reports as a substitute for actual data. Some systems include inferences derived from essentially unvalidated scales or indices. These interpretations may appear highly descriptive and informative; however, they are often not based on known test-behavior connections.
3. Blind, computerized interpretations that make specific predictions or personality descriptions may generate a great deal of misinformation (on a grand scale) about persons, because local norms, base rates, and various demographic situations are not built into the system.
4. The grandeur of a computerized report may give a clinician the idea that this is the "final" word about the patient and thus close off further inquiry. Actually, computer reports are no better than a source of hypotheses, and are not substitutes for clinical judgment.
5. Complex computer programs, once written, are often difficult and costly to modify. Thus many existing assessment systems use only part of the interpretive information available and do not incorporate new information. (It is interesting that these same criticisms are leveled by advocates of computer assessment against clinicians as the primary justification for using computer approaches over "old-fashioned clinical" interpretations.) The computer systems' nonsensitivity to change can be illustrated:
   a. One computer system (Psychological Corporation/NCS) prints out the old circa 1961 version of the Mayo Clinic MMPI Program, although the program designers (Swenson, 1976) consider this program obsolete and have modified the original Mayo Program for their own use at Mayo.

**JAMES N. BUTCHER
AND PATRICIA L.
OWEN**

Table 5. Listing of Computerized Personality Systems

System	System developer	Address of company or institution	Inventory	Target population	Description of output
Automated Psychological Assessment (APA)	David Lachar Lafayette Clinic Detroit, MI 48207	Division of Psychology 1270 Doris Road Pontiac, MI 48057	MMPI	Psychiatric	Computer scoring and interpretation of MMPI for adults and adolescents. Output includes scale and raw scores, critical items, profile sheet (including special norms for adolescents). Narrative reports based on traditional code type information.
Behaviordyne Psycho-diagnostic Laboratory Service	Joseph Finney Department of Educational Psychology and Counseling College of Education University of Kentucky Lexington, KY 40506	Behaviordyne 599 College Avenue Palo Alto, CA	MMPI CPI	Psychiatric Industrial Corrections Medical	Provides seven basic types of reports for different settings and purposes including one type of report for the subject's own information. The system provides scoring of basic MMPI and CPI scales plus scores for many scales developed by Finney. The reports are long and often include psychoanalytically oriented phrasing. Reports are often redundant and contradictory. Some conclusions are found that are inconsistent with regular MMPI scores since a large "correction factor" is applied (for "response sets"), thereby altering the MMPI profile.
Brussels Automated MMPI (BAMMPI)	J. P. DeWaele D. DeSchamphleire G. Van deMosselaer Laboratory of Social Pathology University of Brussels Johannalaan 44 Brussels, Belgium	Laboratory of Social Pathology University of Brussels Johannalaan 44 Brussels, Belgium	MMPI	Corrections	MMPIs are administered in French and Flemish but all printouts are in English. Scores for 129 scales, subscales, and indices are printed in tabular form (raw and K-corrected scores). The printout includes a profile, a classification following Diamond's scheme, a "critical item" listing, and a diagnosis. The narrative report is based on code type information and Wiggins content scale

499

**OBJECTIVE
PERSONALITY
INVENTORIES:
RECENT RESEARCH
AND SOME
CONTEMPORARY
ISSUES**

The Caldwell Report	Alex B. Caldwell 3122 Santa Monica Blvd. Penthouse West Los Angeles, CA 90404	MMPI	Psychiatric Industrial Corrections Medical	Provides MMPI scale scores for a number of special scales, extended critical item list, profile sheet, and lengthy narrative report. Remote terminals in other states may input into system and receive reports by data phone.
Gilberstadt-VA Automated System	Harold Gilberstadt Minneapolis Veterans Administration Hospital 54th St. and 48th Avenue South Minneapolis, MN 55417	MMPI	Psychiatric	Available only in the Veterans Administration Hospital system. A four-page printout is provided. Page 1 gives a profile plot. Page 2 includes a narrative report with sections devoted to validity scales, two-point scale configurations, Hovey's code system, three-point code interpretations. (These are actuarially derived statements.) Page 3 provides hypotheses related to trait and diagnostic possibilities based on 83 scales, including standard scales, special scales indices, Wiggins content scales, and Grayson items. Page 4 gives item responses.
Institute of Clinical Analysis MMPI Report	Edwin Dunlop Valentine C. Birds 1000 East Broadway Glendale, CA 91205	MMPI	Primarily medical Psychiatric	Provides scale scores and some unexplained indices ("MI" and "probability of significant disturbance"), profile sheets, and a review of problems rather than a full narrative report. The interpretations are generally superficial and out of date.
Institute of Psychiatry University of Rome (IPUR)	Paolo Pancheri Istituto di Psichiatria Viale Universita 30 Rome, Italy	MMPI	Psychiatric	Prints out standard MMPI scale scores, some additional scales, profile sheet, Grayson items, and narrative report based on code type interpretations. The language is Italian, but the system has

Table 5. (*Continued*)

System	System developer	Address of company or institution	Inventory	Target population	Description of output
					been translated into English and Spanish. System includes a discriminant function based approach to clinical diagnosis which prints out probability estimates of three most likely diagnoses. The system has been tied to a CRT self-administration format in which items are computer-administered in a fixed format.
Interpretative Scoring Systems (Millon Multiaxial Clinical Inventory)	Theodore Millon University of Miami Miami, Florida	Interpretative Scoring Systems (A Division of National Computer Systems, Inc.) 4401 West 76th St. Minneapolis, MN 55435	MMCI	Psychiatric	Scoring system is controlled by NCS. Keys and interpretative system are not available for individual use. Scoring is provided for 20 scales. Interpretations are based on quantitative studies and theory-based behavioral inferences. Narrative reports provide a paragraph noting limitations and restriction of use, and indication of test validity and a series of interpretations on the major features of the patient's personality and impairment. A symptom summary and "noteworthy responses" to items suggesting (a) health preoccupation, (b) interpersonal alienation, (c) emotional dyscontrol, and (d) self-destructive potential are provided.
Multiphasic Data Analysis Corporation	Frank J. Connolly Eugene C. Levitt Wm. George McAdoo N-604 University Hospital	N-604 University Hospital Indiana University Medical Center Indianapolis, IN 46202	MMPI	Psychiatric	Provides scoring and interpretation that can be accessed by answer sheets (by mail) or remote terminal. The MMPI report is based on the standard clinical scales, special scales, and several indices,

501

OBJECTIVE
PERSONALITY
INVENTORIES:
RECENT RESEARCH
AND SOME
CONTEMPORARY
ISSUES

Organization	Contact	Address	Test	Application	Description
		Medical Center Indianapolis, IN 46202			signed. A list of critical item content (46 items of which only 18 overlap with Grayson's) covering the following areas: Anxiety, Anger, Depression, Health Concern, Reality Distortion, Obsessive Personality, Hysterical Personality, and Special Behavioral Problem.
Psychological Assessment Services	Raymond D. Fowler Department of Psychology University of Alabama Tuscaloosa, Alabama	Department of Psychology University of Alabama Box 2968 University, AL 35486	MMPI	Corrections	Similar format to Roche Psychiatric Program. Scales relevant to correctional settings are included. Narrative reports are written for corrections personnel as an aid in making decisions about detention, bail, housing, rehabilitation, work release, and predictions about prison adjustment.
Psychological Corporation/National Computer Systems	John Pearson Wendell Swenson Department of Psychiatry Mayo Clinic Rochester, MN	Psychological Measurement Division The Psychological Corporation 757 Third Avenue New York, NY 10010 National Computer Systems, Inc. 4401 West 76th St. Minneapolis, MN 55435	MMPI	Medical Diagnostic	A scoring service which provides a one-page MMPI report: scores for 4 validity scales, ten clinical scales, 12 research scales, a profile, and a listing of 8–15 of the 72 or so possible personality descriptors contained in the statement library. Interpretations are based mostly on single scale elevations, but a few configural rules are included. The system is the original 1961 Mayo Clinic version and has not been recently updated.
Psychological Resources	Herbert Eber 1430 West Peachtree Street N.W. Atlanta, GA 30709	1430 West Peachtree Street N.W. Atlanta, GA 30709	16PF CAQ MAT SVIB Bender-Gestalt Culture-fair IQ test DAT GATB	Counseling Clinical Correctional	Scores, plots, profiles, and interprets several tests and combines them into a narrative report. Assesses general and specific abilities; life-styles, habits, and temperament; clinical or counseling problems; motivational and interest patterns.

Table 5. (*Continued*)

System	System developer	Address of company or institution	Inventory	Target population	Description of output
Roche-Hans Huber System	Peter Blaser Anna Maria Gehring Hoffman-LaRoche Company Basel, Switzerland	Hans Huber Company Länggabstr. 76 CH-3000 Bern 9, Switzerland	MMPI	Psychiatric	The Roche-Fowler system has been translated and adapted for use in Europe in German, Spanish, Italian, Dutch, and French. The output provides raw scores K-corrected scores for standard scales and 44 other scales, Welsh code, profile, "critical item" list, and a narrative report. The report is a conservative interpretation of code types, Si and Mf. There are 213 statements in the library. There is one version for males and one for females.
The Roche Psychiatric Institute: MMPI Interpretation System	Raymond D. Fowler Department of Psychology University of Alabama Tuscaloosa, Alabama	Roche Psychiatric Service Institute Nutley, NJ 07110	MMPI SVIB	Psychiatric Medical	Provides scoring service as well as narrative clinical report. The narrative report is based on MMPI code type descriptors and interpretations of Mf, Si, and special scales. Additional information is provided by interpretations of Wiggins's content scales. The MMPI profile is plotted with 4 validity scales, the standard scales and 14 special scales. The Welsh code type is printed out. The score on the MacAndrew addiction proneness scale is interpreted. The subject's responses are printed out in an answer matrix.

503

OBJECTIVE
PERSONALITY
INVENTORIES:
RECENT RESEARCH
AND SOME
CONTEMPORARY
ISSUES

   b. Most MMPI-based systems routinely print out the Grayson items as though they are direct pipelines to the patient's critical problem. This practice continues in spite of the fact that they have no demonstrated validity (Koss & Butcher, 1973). Newer, empirically based "critical items" have not been included in any computer system to date.

6. Interpretive statements in narrative reports have not been sufficiently validated. Several studies aimed at validating computer-based narrative statements have been published—Fowler and Miller (1969); Webb, Miller, and Fowler (1969); Webb (1970); Luschene and Gilberstadt (1972); Lachar (1974); Fowler (1975); Adams and Shore (1976); Lachar, Klinge, and Grisell (1976); and Millon (1977). However, these approaches have generally not used a very stringent research design. These studies have validated the reports by showing a clinician, who is familiar with the case, the report and asked him or her if the report matches the patient. System validation is a formidable task but one that deserves much greater attention than it has received in the past.

7. There have been instances in which computer interpretation systems have fallen in the hands of "caretakers" who are not qualified clinical assessment psychologists. In fact, one commercial system presently seems to be operating without a psychologist on the staff. The potential abuses in this situation are great. Although there have been guidelines developed by the American Psychological Association for automated personality assessment, these do not appear sufficient for monitoring such large-scale and still relatively unproven psychological evaluation enterprises.

These criticisms of the automated assessment field are not meant to condemn the enterprise, but are offered with an eye toward improving the scientific basis of the operations and toward increasing the quality of the product. Concern for the individual being evaluated has also been an important consideration in our desire to make the computer evaluation system companies accountable for their evaluations. The profession needs to develop more adequate self-monitoring techniques for these procedures, or public consumer advocacy groups will become involved in self-protection. Some of the abuses we have seen suggest that this may indeed be in order.

8. Future Development of Self-Report Diagnostic Measures

Criticism of the MMPI is a perennial activity. Complaints about specific aspects of the inventory, or what it fails to do, may be found extensively in the literature. Many attacks on the MMPI have been unfounded, or later (after filling numerous journal pages) proved to be relatively unimportant (see Dahlstrom, 1969). However, a number of criticisms of the present MMPI are justified. A volume by Butcher (1972) highlighted the problems with the MMPI at the item, scale, and interpretive levels, and discussed a number of issues surrounding a possible revision of the inventory. In the years since this volume was published, no concrete steps have been taken by the test publishers to alleviate the problems. The reluctance to revise the MMPI is based on several factors:

1. MMPI researchers do not unanimously agree that it needs to be revised. Some people have taken the position that, although it is somewhat archaic and limited as a screening measure, the validity coefficients would probably not increase in magnitude with a revision. Thus the final product would not be worth the effort required to revise it. The MMPI may be as good an instrument as can be expected in self-report measurement.
2. There is much reluctance on the part of the test publishers to tinker with a product that is selling well and has no visible competition at this time.
3. There is some concern that a revision, if done well and extensively, would change the MMPI is such a drastic way as to frustrate the present consumers.

What are some of the problems with the present MMPI? Are these problems serious enough to warrant a revision? Are there other diagnostic instruments on the scene that might quietly (or otherwise) replace the MMPI? What concrete steps might be followed for a revision if one were to be undertaken? These are some questions that require serious consideration at this time. The interested reader is referred to the informative chapters by Hathaway, Loevinger, Norman, Dahlstrom, Meehl, and Campbell in the volume edited by Butcher (1972) and to Chapter 9 of Block's monograph (1965). The viewpoints presented here serve as a requisite background for the problem. We will not have space in this chapter to review the topic comprehensively. However, a summary of some of the problems is given in Table 6.

Funeral bells have been tolling for the MMPI for some time. One of the earliest came from Ellis (1946), and one of the more recent from Goldberg (1974), who noted:

> Whatever one thinks of the present status of the MMPI, virtually no one will deny its extraordinary historical influence upon assessment research and upon psychodiagnostic practice. Eventually, however, old inventories, like old soldiers, must slowly fade away. Hopefully the next decade will bring the MMPI's successor, perhaps the new *Differential Personality Inventory*, if it can be lured out of hiding.

One of the major early contenders as a replacement for the diagnostic function of the MMPI was Cattell's Sixteen Personality Factor scale (16PF). The 16PF was published in 1949 and is composed of a number of factor analytic scales that relate to the general personality domain as defined by Cattell (1964). The publications relating the 16PF to the psychopathology domain are somewhat more limited in scope and quantity than the MMPI (see Table 1). Although there is some overlap of constructs in the 16PF and the MMPI, there is a sufficient uniqueness associated with each instrument to serve as a caution to anyone tempting to substitute one for the other.

The second and perhaps more serious challenger to the MMPI is the Differential Personality Inventory developed by Jackson and Messick. This Psychopathology-related inventory was heralded by Goldberg (1974) as the replacement for the MMPI. The inventory contains a number of scales such as Headache Proneness, Sadism, Insomnia, Psychotic Tendencies, and Neurotic Disorganization, which would provide a clinician with a great deal of information about the patient's problem situation. These scales, developed primarily by a rational scale construction strategy (Jackson, 1971), are homogeneous content scales. There are important advantages to using homogeneous content scales, particularly if one views item responding as a source of patient communication. The most severe limitation to the DPI at this time, as shown in the categorized references given in Table 1, is the lack of substantial external validation of the inventory. It appears that Goldberg's (1974) projection

505

OBJECTIVE
PERSONALITY
INVENTORIES:
RECENT RESEARCH
AND SOME
CONTEMPORARY
ISSUES

Table 6. Some Criticism of the MMPI

Item problems	Scale problems	Interpretational problems	Profile sheet	General
Some item content is out of date, awkward wording, offensive, useless, redundant. Limited item pool does not measure important problem areas: personal strengths, motivation, change potential. Not sufficient attention is paid to gender-related symptom review. Too long (too many items) for quick screening purposes. Item importance should be considered. Items could be given weight according to their power to predict.	Some are too long and cumbersome. Contain heterogeneous content. Contain items that overlap heavily with other scales. Scale norms are out of date. Original normative data are not readily available to researchers. Scales are not clearly trait, state dispositioned. They are hodgepodgy. More clearly defined scales could be developed, perhaps reflecting several types of information about subject. Separate scales for personality disposition and emotional status. Many "additional" or experimental scales are not sufficiently validated to be considered useful scales. Too much scale proliferation without quality control. Many empirical scales contain "dead weight" items. These items could be deleted or replaced.	The scales and norms are misused—use for adolescents, industrial screening; and other populations is questionable. The MMPI is not sufficient for many types of clinical decisions being made with it. Prediction and description accuracy is less than optimal. Code type interpretation is rudimentary. More sophisticated procedures using all information could be developed. Code types are often unstable, and interpretation would change dramatically with a small raw point change. Valid content measures not systematically incorporated in interpretation. Not a simple measure of change due to item qualities, although many people apply it this way. Actuarial information has not been accumulated sufficiently to serve as a basis for fully automated interpretation. Proliferation of computer interpretations of systems of variable quality.	Incomplete. Does not include convenient conversion format for newer, useful scales, e.g., *A, R, ES, Mac.* *K*-corrected weights need revision. These are routinely applied across all settings in spite of the lack of empirical justification.	The MMPI publishers seem reluctant to initiate change. Needed changes have been recommended for years, but there has been virtually no change in MMPI itself since it was published.

for a new standard for psychopathology measurement was overly optimistic. The DPI has not, as yet, caught on to the degree that would enable it to supplant the MMPI. An examination of the published research over the past few years (see Table 1) does not show much validational information on the DPI. It also appears that the domain of item content for the DPI may only partly cover the MMPI construct domain (Trott & Morf, 1972).

The most recent challenger to the MMPI monopoly on clinical assessment is the Millon Multiaxial Clinical Inventory (MMCI). Millon (1977), with an acknowledged debt to the MMPI, took as one starting point the weakness of the MMPI. The MMCI represents an attempt at constructing a clinical inventory that utilizes the strengths in the rational, factorial, and empirical scale-construction methods and avoids some of the problems other scales have encountered. The MMCI is presented in such a way as to maximize the transfer of conceptual and interpretive skills of the MMPI user to the new test. Many of the pathology scales have a familiar ring, configural scoring is recommended, code types are employed, and an automated (computerized) interpretation system is available.

Will the MMCI replace the MMPI as the "standard" clinical diagnostic instrument? It would be premature to form any conclusion since at this writing (1978) only the test manual has been published and the inventory has not had the testing-ground scrutiny that other instruments have had. Extensive review of the MMCI cannot be attempted in this chapter. However, many features of the inventory are attractive, and much prepublication test development work was done. The MMCI scale concepts are appropriate, and the format is familiar and contains elements that have been widely accepted in clinical application. The inventory is reasonably brief (175 items) and requires a minimum amount of time to complete. The test format is somewhat atypical. Rather than using reusable booklets and answer sheets, the test publisher provides a place to mark the item on the booklet itself. The booklet is then returned to NCS for scoring. This nonreusable format may be a more expensive operation for consumers who are accustomed to hand scoring. The NCS does not make available the scoring templates; thus the user must rely on the test publisher (although item classification is provided in the manual). This situation may discourage test use because time delays due to mail problems, etc., defeat the purpose of rapid assessment techniques.

The 20 MMCI scales are fairly long—about 16–47 items each. Thus there is a great deal of item overlap between scales—a feature criticized by some researchers, but actually built into the MMCI. Some test users may blink at the relatively small number and type of normal people (college student and industrial workers) used in the normative sample (a total of 297; 144 were males). However, the test construction sample of psychiatric patients was larger, 1591 subjects (699 females). A cross-validation sample of 256 patients (111 females) was used.

The items were selected from a large pool of around 3500 and reduced to the final set by rational, internal consistency and external empirical methods. The final pool of items has some characteristics that make it distinctive as an assessment instrument. The "pathological" direction of scoring of an item is usually in the "true" direction. It is unclear how this feature might be susceptible to response sets. Rating procedures were used to assure that items were obviously related to constructs being measured. This makes the honesty of the self-report an important situation to take into account. For example, in situations where an individual is being screened for a purpose where a "good" picture is important and he or she wishes to deny pathology, the desired pattern may be easy to produce.

507

OBJECTIVE
PERSONALITY
INVENTORIES:
RECENT RESEARCH
AND SOME
CONTEMPORARY
ISSUES

The scales are base rate scales rather than the more usual "continuous distribution" scales. This could serve to maximize classification. It is not clear how such scales would apply in local settings, because base rates vary on factors such as population and presenting problems. Future research will need to address the question of validity generalization.

Millon has approached the issues of scale validation in a serious way. Prior to publication of the test, a number of validation studies (involving the internal structure and external correlates) were done. In addition, the computerized reporting service available through the National Computer Systems, Inc. (NCS) has been subjected to a validity study comparing the adequacy of reports with two MMPI computer services.

Could the MMPI be improved by a revision? The answer to this question is definitely affirmative. But the difficulty comes in deciding how much, or to what degree, changes should be made. In order to make the MMPI more useful, changes should be more than just cosmetic. However, if modifications are too drastic, the instrument may be unacceptable to present users. If changes require great effort on the part of users to "relearn" a new instrument, they may continue to use the present MMPI because it is a known entity. This outcome would be undesirable since great confusion would result from having two MMPIs.

There are several levels on which a possible MMPI revision might be focused:

1. The first (and least drastic) approach might involve changes at the interpretive level. These alterations would not involve changes in the items or scales but would center on changes in the profile sheet and test manual to make interpretation easier. For example, changes in the profile sheet might include display of additional scales, or the manual might include established interpretation material for the additional scales, etc. A revision at this surface level might also include an official short form for quick screening purposes.
2. A second level of revision would include the type of changes described in level 1 but would go further to redevelop the present MMPI scales. This revision might leave the MMPI items intact, but would focus on strengthening the present scales by altering the scoring keys by deleting weaker items, etc. Some renorming on more recent populations (both normal and clinical samples) would be necessary.
3. The third and more drastic approach would include the changes in both of the previous revision levels but would also involve major changes at the item level. The item pool would be expanded to sample from a wider range of problems and to include more items that dealt with personality factors, such as positive attributes and change potential. Some present items might be deleted or placed at the end of an extended booklet. New normative data would need to be collected and updated norms developed.

The MMPI has made a substantial contribution to personality psychology and clinical practice. However, in spite of its strengths, a number of problems and weaknesses exist with the present MMPI. With sufficient attention, these problems could be lessened or eliminated, and the MMPI could be substantially improved. We believe that an MMPI revision is long overdue. An instrument so widely used and so important for objective personality assessment should not be allowed to lie in a state of evident disrepair.

9. Conclusion

In spite of early resistance against the use of personality inventories, instruments like the MMPI and 16PF have attained widespread use as measures of psychopathology. In this chapter, we examined the research on some personality inventories over the past 5 years and pointed out the areas of greatest research focus for the MMPI, 16PF, and the DPI. The greatest amount of clinical research with personality inventories has been done with the MMPI; thus a greater emphasis is given to it in this review. The most active research involving personality inventories is the study of alcoholism and drug abuse. Methods of detecting alcoholism and addiction, using the MMPI, in a clinical population were discussed. Alcoholics and drug addicts can often be identified both by their profile similarities and by their scores on special separate scales that have been constructed. MacAndrew's alcoholism scale appears to offer the most promise as an MMPI-based measure for addiction proneness.

Another clinical research area of great productivity involving personality inventories concerns the assessment of medical patients. In our review of the use of the MMPI with medical patients, we saw that the 1-3/3-1 profile is ubiquitous. Both chronically ill medical patients and psychosomatic patients often achieve these elevations. This provides us with little new information. More intriguing areas in medical research such as immunological response to stress could greatly benefit from careful and creative research with personality inventories like the MMPI.

In recent years, the MMPI and 16PF have been widely used with populations that differ greatly from the standardization samples, for example, with ethnic groups in the United States and with diverse national populations. The application of psychological tests in cross-cultural settings raises a number of questions ranging from possible translation problems to the unknown effects cultural differences might have on validity generalization. Research has shown that clinical measures, particularly the MMPI, have a great deal of robustness in other cultural settings. Thus it is likely that they will enjoy an even more expanded use in the future. The importance of determining transplant validity for target populations has been highlighted.

A great deal of recent research has been aimed at developing brief personality scales—particularly short forms of the MMPI. The relative value of short MMPI forms over the standard-length MMPI were considered. Several MMPI short forms were described. The clinical utility of MMPI short forms has been questioned because no short form appears to result in very accurate predictions of the full-scale profile type. Nevertheless, the search for a means of reducing the number of items goes on. One approach to reduced item administration that offers promise is the computer-administered, tailor-made inventory for personality assessment. One preliminary study of the feasibility of using an "adaptive" branched diagnostic approach was discussed.

The importance of examining the content of a subject's response to personality items was discussed. Two approaches to evaluation of this important aspect of personality test responding in the MMPI were discussed—content-homogeneous scales and the use of pathognomonic items such as "critical" items are unusually important information in understanding the patient's problems. Some recent research on these approaches to content interpretation was highlighted.

The current status of computerized personality assessment was evaluated. A summary description of 14 computerized personality systems (12 for the MMPI) was given. We noted that, although this is an important development for future personality assessment approaches to take, we are concerned with some current practices. We are particularly concerned that the scientific base for automated test interpretation has not kept stride with computer technology or with the consumer demand for quick computer-based psychological reports.

Finally, we examined the present status of personality assessment and clinical diagnosis with personality inventories and pointed out some of the problems with the leading instrument, the MMPI. The question of whether other instruments on the scene (16PF, DPI, MMCI) will replace the MMPI was considered. We noted that, while the MMPI has a great deal of strength and utility, at present there are a number of problems that limit its usefulness. We concluded that the MMPI should and could undergo some revision that would substantially improve its field performance.

10. References

10.1. List of Classified References for 1972–1977

10.1.1. MMPI References

1. Abbott, R. D. Improving the validity of affective self-report measures through constructing personality scales unconfounded with social desirability: A study of the Personality Research Form. *Educational and Psychological Measurement*, 1975, *35*, 371–377.
2. Abbott, R. D., Fry, R. M., & Abbott, S. K. The R scale of the MMPI as a measure of acquiescence: Replication for non-pathological content trait adjectives. *Psychological Reports*, 1972, *31*, 806.
3. Abbott, R. D., Fry, R. M., & Kiem-Abbott, S. Tests of an alternative explanation of data supporting the R scale of the MMPI as a measure of acquiescence. *Psychological Reports*, 1973, *32*, 1243–1246.
4. Abram, H. S., Meixel, S. A., Webb, W. W., & Scott, H. W. Psychological adaptation to jejunoileal bypass for morbid obesity. *Journal of Nervous and Mental Disease*, 1976, *62*, 151–157.
5. Abramowitz, C. V., Abramowitz, S. I., Roback, H. B., & Jackson, C. Differential effectiveness of directive and nondirective group therapies as a function of client internal-external control. *Journal of Consulting and Clinical Psychology*, 1974, *42*, 849–853.
6. Adams, H. B., Cooper, G. D., & Carrera, R. N. Individual differences in behavioral reactions of psychiatric patients to brief partial sensory deprivation. *Perceptual and Motor Skills*, 1972, *34*, 199–217.
7. Adams, J., Rothstein, W., & McCarter, R. E. A canonical-correlation analysis of 16 fear factors and the MMPI. *Journal of Personality Assessment*, 1973, *37*, 156–164.
8. Adams, K. M., & Shore, D. L. The accuracy of an automated MMPI interpretation system in a psychiatric setting. *Journal of Clinical Psychology*, 1976, *32*, 80–82.
9. Adams, T. C. Some MMPI differences between first and multiple admissions with a state prison population. *Journal of Clinical Psychology*, 1976, *32*, 555–558.
10. Adams, T. C., & West, J. E. Another look at the use of the MMPI as an index to "escapism." *Journal of Clinical Psychology*, 1976, *32*, 580–582.
11. Alley, G. R., Snider, B., Forsyth, R. A., & Opitz, E. Comparative parental MMPI protocols of children evaluated at a child development clinic. *Psychological Reports*, 1974, *35*, 1147–1154.

509

OBJECTIVE
PERSONALITY
INVENTORIES:
RECENT RESEARCH
AND SOME
CONTEMPORARY
ISSUES

12. Alpaugh, P. K., & Birren, J. E. Are there sex differences in creativity across the adult life span? *Human Development*, 1975, *18*, 461–465.

13. Altman, H., Gynther, M. D., Warbin, R. W., & Sletten, I. W. A new empirical automated MMPI interpretive program: The 6-8/8-6 code type. *Journal of Clinical Psychology*, 1972, *28*, 495–498.

14. Altman, H., Warbin, R. W., Sletten, I. W., & Gynther, M. D. Replicated empirical correlates of the MMPI 8-9/9-8 code type. *Journal of Personality Assessment*, 1973, *37*, 369–371.

15. Anthony, N. Malingering as role-taking. *Journal of Clinical Psychology*, 1976, *32*, 32–41.

16. Apfeldorf, M. Contrasting assumptions and directions in MMPI research on alcoholism. *Quarterly Journal of Studies on Alcoholism*, 1974, *35*, 1375–1379.

17. Apfeldorf, M., & Huntly, P. J. Application of MMPI alcoholism scales to older alcoholics and problem drinkers. *Journal of Studies on Alcohol*, 1975, *36*, 645–653.

18. Apfeldorf, M., & Huntly, P.J. Exclusion of subjects with *F* scores at or above 16 in MMPI research on alcoholism. *Journal of Clinical Psychology*, 1976, *32*, 498–500.

19. Apfeldorf, M., Smith, W. J., Peixotto, H. E., & Huntly, P. J. Is the representation of the objective body-image in figure drawings related to the personality characteristics of the drawer? *Psychological Reports*, 1974, *34*, 1015–1020.

20. Armentrout, J. A. Repression-sensitization and MMPI correlates of retrospective reports of parental child-rearing behaviors. *Journal of Clinical Psychology*, 1975, *31*, 444–448.

21. Arvey, R. D., Mussio, S. J., & Payne, G. Relationships between MMPI scores and job performance measures of fire fighters. *Psychological Reports*, 1972, *31*, 199–202.

22. Ayers, J., Templer, D. I., & Ruff, C. F. The MMPI in the differential diagnosis of organicity vs. schizophrenia: Empirical findings and a somewhat different perspective. *Journal of Clinical Psychology*, 1975, *31*, 685–686.

23. Azen, S. P., Snibbe, H. M., & Montgomery, H. R. A longitudinal predictive study of success and performance of law enforcement officers. *Journal of Applied Psychology*, 1973, *57*, 190–192.

24. Banreti-Fuchs, K. M. Attitudinal, situational and mental health correlates of academic achievement at the undergraduate university level. *British Journal of Educational Psychology*, 1975, *45*, 227–231.

25. Banreti-Fuchs, K. M., & Meadows, W. M. Interest, mental health, and attitudinal correlates of academic achievement among university students. *British Journal of Educational Psychology*, 1976, *46*, 212–219.

26. Barna, J. D. Invasion of privacy as a function of test set and anonymity. *Perceptual and Motor Skills*, 1974, *38*, 1028–1030.

27. Bartlett, F. E. & Cooke, P. E. A correlational study of the Community Adaptation Schedule and the MMPI. *Community Mental Health Journal*, 1972, *8*, 189–195.

28. Bauer, G. E., & Clark, J. A. Personality deviancy and prison incarceration. *Journal of Clinical Psychology*, 1976, *32*, 279–283.

29. Baughman, E. E., & Dahlstrom, W. G. Racial differences on the MMPI. In S. S. Guterman (Ed.), *Black psyche: The modal personality patterns of black Americans*. Berkeley, Calif.: Glendessary Press, 1972.

30. Bean, K. L., & Karasievich, G. O. Psychological test results at three stages of inpatient alcoholism treatment. *Journal of Studies on Alcohol*, 1975, *36*, 838–852.

31. Bergquist, W. H., & Klemm, H. D. Acquisition of verbal concepts as a function of explicit and implicit experimental demands and repression-sensitization. *Journal of General Psychology*, 1973, *89*, 67–80.

32. Berzins, J. I., Bednar, R. L., & Severy, L. J. The problems of intersource consensus in measuring therapeutic outcomes: New data and multivariate perspectives. *Journal of Abnormal Psychology*, 1975, *84*, 10–19.

33. Berzins, J. I., & Ross, W. F. Experimental assessment of the responsiveness of addict patients to the "influence" of professionals versus other addicts. *Journal of Abnormal Psychology*, 1972, *80*, 141–148.

34. Berzins, J. I., Ross, W. F., English, G. E., & Haley, J. V. Subgroups among opiate addicts: A typological investigation. *Journal of Abnormal Psychology*, 1974, *83*, 65–73.

35. Bess, B., Janus, S., & Rifkin, A. Factors in successful narcotics renunciation. *American Journal of Psychiatry*, 1972, *128*, 861–865.

36. Beutler, L. E., Karacan, I., Anch, A. M., Salis, P. J., Scott, F. B., & Williams, R. L. MMPI and MIT discriminators of biogenic and psychogenic impotence. *Journal of Consulting and Clinical Psychology*, 1975, *43*, 899–903.

511

OBJECTIVE
PERSONALITY
INVENTORIES:
RECENT RESEARCH
AND SOME
CONTEMPORARY
ISSUES

37. Bierenbaum, H., Nichols, M. P., & Schwartz, A. J. Effects of varying session length and frequency in brief emotive psychotherapy. *Journal of Consulting and Clinical Psychology*, 1976, *44*, 790–798.

38. Birk, L., Huddleston, W., Miller, E., & Cohler, B. Avoidance conditioning for homosexuality. *Archives of General Psychiatry*, 1971, *25*, 314–323.

39. Biro, M. Evaluation by means of the MMPI of residual syndromes in antidepressive drug therapy. *Revija Za Psihologiju*, 1975, *5*, 3–14.

40. Birtchnell, J. The personality characteristics of early-bereaved psychiatric patients. *Social Psychiatry*, 1975, *10*, 97–103.

41. Black, F. W. Personality characteristics of Viet Nam veterans identified as heroin abusers. *American Journal of Psychiatry*, 1975, *132*, 748–749.

42. Black, F. W. Use of the MMPI with patients with recent war-related head injuries. *Journal of Clinical Psychology*, 1974, *30*, 571–573.

43. Black, F. W. Unilateral brain lesions and MMPI performance: A preliminary study. *Perceptual and Motor Skills*, 1975, *40*, 87–93.

44. Black, F. W., & Heald, A. MMPI characteristics of alcohol- and illicit drug-abusers enrolled in a rehabilitative program. *Journal of Clinical Psychology*, 1975, *31*, 572–575.

45. Blackburn, R. Dimensions of hostility and aggression in abnormal offenders. *Journal of Consulting and Clinical Psychology*, 1972, *38*, 20–26.

46. Blackburn, R. An empirical classification of psychopathic personality. *British Journal of Psychiatry*, 1975, *127*, 456–460.

47. Bloom, R. B., & Entin, A. D. Intellectual functioning and psychopathology: A canonical analysis of WAIS and MMPI relationships. *Journal of Clinical Psychology*, 1975, *31*, 697–698.

48. Boerger, A. R., Graham, J. R., & Lilly, R. S. Behavioral correlates of single-scale MMPI code types. *Journal of Consulting and Clinical Psychology*, 1974, *42*, 398–402.

49. Boll, T. J., Heaton, R., & Reitan, R. M. Neurophysiological and emotional correlates of Huntington's chorea. *Journal of Nervous and Mental Disease*, 1974, *158*, 61–69.

50. Bolton, B. A factor analysis of personal adjustment and vocational measures of client change. *Rehabilitation Counselor Bulletin*, 1974, *18*, 99–104.

51. Bolton, B. Homogeneous subscales for the Mini-Mult. *Journal of Consulting and Clinical Psychology*, 1976, *44*, 684–685.

52. Boudewyns, P. A., & Levis, D. J. Autonomic reactivity of high and low ego-strength subjects to repeated anxiety eliciting scenes. *Journal of Abnormal Psychology*, 1975, *84*, 682–692.

53. Boudewyns, P. A., & Wilson, A. E. Implosive therapy and desensitization therapy using free association in the treatment of inpatients. *Journal of Abnormal Psychology*, 1972, *79*, 259–268.

54. Bradley, P. E., Wakefield, J. A., Jr., Yom, B. L., Doughtie, E. B., Cox, J. A., & Kraft, I. A. Parental MMPIs and certain pathological behaviors in children. *Journal of Clinical Psychology*, 1974, *30*, 379–382.

55. Brandsma, J. M., & Ludwig, A. M. A case of multiple personality: Diagnosis and therapy. *International Journal of Clinical and Experimental Hypnosis*, 1974, *22*, 216–233.

56. Briggs, P. F., Rouzer, D. L., Hamberg, R. L., & Holman, T. R. Seven scales for the Minnesota-Briggs History Record with reference group data. *Journal of Clinical Psychology*, 1972, *28*, 431–448.

57. Bringmann, W. G., Balance, W. D. G., & Giesbrecht, C. A. The computer vs. the technologist: Comparison of psychological reports on normal and elevated MMPI profiles. *Psychological Reports*, 1972, *31*, 211–217.

58. Brodsky, L., & Zuniga, J. Nitrous oxide: A psychotogenic agent. *Comprehensive Psychiatry*, 1975, *16*, 185–188.

59. Brown, P. M. The congruence between moral judgment and selected scales of the MMPI. *Journal of Clinical Psychology*, 1976, *32*, 627–630.

60. Brown, R. S., Haddox, V., Posada, A., & Rubio, A. Social and psychological adjustment following pelvic exenteration. *American Journal of Obstetrics and Gynecology*, 1972, *114*, 162–171.

61. Burger, G. K., Armentrout, J. A., & Rapfogel, R. G. Recalled parental behavior and objective personality measures: A canonical analysis. *Journal of Personality Assessment*, 1975, *39*, 514–522.

62. Burgess, M. M., Duffey, M., & Temple, F. G. Two studies of prediction of success in a collegiate program of nursing. *Nursing Research*, 1972, *21*, 357–366.

63. Burke, E. L., & Eichberg, R. H. Personality characteristics of adolescent users of dangerous drugs as indicated by the MMPI. *Journal of Nervous and Mental Disease*, 1972, *154*, 291–298.

64. Burke, H. R., & Marcus, R. MacAndrews MMPI alcoholism scale: Alcoholism and drug addictiveness. *The Journal of Psychology*, 1977, *96*, 141–148.

65. Burish, T. G., & Houston, B. K. Construct validity of the Lie scale as a measure of defensiveness. *Journal of Clinical Psychology*, 1976, *32*, 310–314.

66. Burns, B. H., & Nichols, M. A. Factors related to the localization of symptoms to the chest in depression. *British Journal of Psychiatry*, 1972, *121*, 405–409.

67. Bush, M. Relationship between color-word test interference and MMPI indices of psychoticism and defensive rigidity in normal males and females. *Journal of Consulting and Clinical Psychology*, 1975, *43*, 926.

68. Butcher, J. N., & Gur, R. Hebrew translation of the MMPI: An assessment of translation adequacy and preliminary validation. *Journal of Cross-Cultural Psychology*, 1974, *5*, 220–227.

69. Butcher, J. N., & Ryan, M. Personality stability and adjustment to an extreme environment. *Journal of Applied Psychology*, 1974, *59*, 107–109.

70. Button, J. H., & Reivich, R. S. Obsessions of infanticide: A review of 42 cases. *Archives of General Psychiatry*, 1972, *27*, 235–240.

71. Byong-Hee, L. Y., Bradley, P. E., Wakefield, J. A., Jr., Kraft, I. A., Doughtie, E. B., & Cox, J. A. A common factor in the MMPI scales of married couples. *Journal of Personality Assessment*, 1975, *39*, 64–69.

72. Calhoun, L. G., & Selby, J. W. Help-seeking attitudes and severity of psychological distress. *Journal of Clinical Psychology*, 1974, *30*, 247–248.

73. Callan, J. P. An attempt to use the MMPI as a predictor of failure in military training. *British Journal of Psychiatry*, 1972, *121*, 553–557.

74. Capone, T., Brahen, L. S., & Wiechert, V. Personality factors and drug effects in a controlled study of cyclazocine. *Journal of Clinical Psychology*, 1976, *32*, 489–495.

75. Cartwright, R. D. Sleep fantasy in normal and schizophrenic persons. *Journal of Abnormal Psychology*, 1972, *80*, 275–279.

76. Cartwright, R. D., & Ratzel, R. W. Effects of dream loss on waking behaviors. *Archives of General Psychiatry*, 1972, *27*, 277–280.

77. Cash, T. F., & Stack, J. J. Locus of control among schizophrenics and other hospitalized psychiatric patients. *Genetic Psychology Monographs*, 1973, *87*, 105–122.

78. Caslyn, D. A., Louks, J., & Freeman, C. W. The use of the MMPI with chronic low back pain patients with a mixed diagnosis. *Journal of Clinical Psychology*, 1976, *32*, 532–536.

79. Catlin, N., Croake, J. W., & Keller, J. F. MMPI profiles of cohabiting college students. *Psychological Reports*, 1976, *38*, 407–410.

80. Cerbus, G., & Dallara, R. F., Jr. Seasonal differences of depression in mental hospital admissions as measured by the MMPI. *Psychological Reports*, 1975, *36*, 737–738.

81. Cerbus, G., & Travis, R. J. Seasonal variation of personality of college students as measured by the MMPI. *Psychological Reports*, 1973, *33*, 665–666.

82. Chase, T. V., Chaffin, S., & Morrison, S. D. False positive adolescent MMPI profiles. *Adolescence*, 1975, *40*, 507–519.

83. Christensen, L., & Le Unes, A. Discriminating criminal types and recidivism by means of the MMPI. *Journal of Clinical Psychology*, 1974, *30*, 192–193.

84. Clavelle, P. R., & Butcher, J. N. An adaptive typological approach to psychiatric screening. *Journal of Consulting and Clinical Psychology*, 1977, *45*, 851–859.

85. Climent, C. E., Rollins, A., Ervin, F. R., & Plutchik, R. Epidemiological studies of women prisoners: 1. Medical and psychiatric variables related to violent behavior. *American Journal of Psychiatry*, 1973, *130*, 985–990.

86. Clopton, J. R. A computer program for MMPI scale development with contrasted groups. *Educational and Psychological Measurement*, 1974, *34*, 161–163.

87. Clopton, J. R. Suicidal risk assessment via the MMPI. In C. Neuringer (Ed.), *Psychological assessment of suicide risk*. Springfield, Ill.: Thomas, 1974.

88. Clopton, J. R. Automated MMPI interpretation based on a modification of Gilberstadt's codebook. *Journal of Clinical Psychology*, 1975, *31*, 648–651.

89. Clopton, J. R., & Jones, W. C. Use of the MMPI in the prediction of suicide. *Journal of Clinical Psychology*, 1975, *31*, 52–54.

90. Clopton, J. R., & Neuringer, C. An MMPI scale to measure scholastic personality in women. *Perceptual and Motor Skills*, 1973, *37*, 963–966.

513

OBJECTIVE
PERSONALITY
INVENTORIES:
RECENT RESEARCH
AND SOME
CONTEMPORARY
ISSUES

91. Clum, G. A. Relations between biographical data and patient symptomatology. *Journal of Abnormal Psychology*, 1975, *84*, 80–83.

92. Coché, E., & Flick, A. Problem-solving training groups for hospitalized psychiatric patients. *Journal of Psychology*, 1975, *91*, 19–29.

93. Coché, E., & Steer, R. A. The MMPI response consistencies of normal, neurotic, and psychotic women. *Journal of Clinical Psychology*, 1974, *30*, 194–195.

94. Coché, E., & Taylor, S. Correlations between the Offer Self-image Personality Inventory in a psychiatric hospital population. *Journal of Youth and Adolescence*, 1974, *3*, 145–152.

95. Cochran, M. L. Abbreviated MMPI booklet forms: The 300- and 366-item scales with *K*-correction. *Journal of Clinical Psychology*, 1975, *31*, 298–300.

96. Cohen, J., & Lefkowitz, J. Development of a biographical inventory blank to predict faking on personality tests. *Journal of Applied Psychology*, 1974, *59*, 404–405.

97. Cohler, B. J., Grunebaum, H. U., Weiss, J. L., Robbins, D. M., Shader, R. I., Gallant, D., & Hartman, C. R. Social role performance and psychopathology among recently hospitalized and nonhospitalized mothers: 2. Correlates with life stress and life-reported psychopathology. *Journal of Nervous and Mental Disease*, 1974, *159*, 81–90.

98. Cohler, B. J., Weiss, J. L., & Grunebaum, H. U. "Short-form" content scales for the MMPI. *Journal of Personality Assessment*, 1974, *38*, 563–572.

99. Cohler, B. J., Weiss, J. L., Grunebaum, H. U., Lidz, C., & Wynne, L. C. MMPI profiles in hospitalized psychiatric patients and their families. *Archives of General Psychiatry*, 1972, *26*, 71–78.

100. Coie, J. D., Costanzo, P. R., & Cox, G. Behavioral determinants of mental illness concerns: A comparison of gatekeeper professions. *Journal of Consulting and Clinical Psychology*, 1975, *43*, 626–636.

101. Colligan, R. C. Atypical response sets and the automated MMPI. *Journal of Clinical Psychology*, 1976, *32*, 76–78.

102. Collins, H. A., Burger, G. K., & Taylor, G. A. An empirical typology of heroin abusers. *Journal of Clinical Psychology*, 1976, *32*, 473–476.

103. Collins, J. F., Newman, P. A., & Hutson, S. P. Personality correlates of visual perceptual responses. *Perceptual and Motor Skills*, 1974, *38*, 1183–1187.

104. Conger, A. J., & Jackson, D. N. Suppressor variables, prediction, and the interpretation of psychological relationships. *Educational and Psychological Measurement*, 1972, *32*, 579–599.

105. Constantinople, A. Masculinity-femininity: An exception to a famous dictum? *Psychological Bulletin*, 1973, *80*, 389–407.

106. Cooper, E. B., Eggertson, S. A., & Galbraith, S. A. Clinician personality factors and effectiveness: A three-study report. *Journal of Communication Disorders*, 1972, *5*, 270–274.

107. Costello, R. M. Item level racial differences on the MMPI. *Journal of Social Psychology*, 1973, *91*, 161–162.

108. Costello, R. M., Fine, H. J., & Blau, B. I. Racial comparisons on the MMPI. *Journal of Clinical Psychology*, 1973, *29*, 63–65.

109. Costello, R. M., Tiffany, D. W., & Gier, R. H. Methodological issues and racial (black-white) comparisons on the MMPI. *Journal of Consulting and Clinical Psychology*, 1972, *38*, 161–168.

110. Coursey, R. D., Buchsbaum, M., & Frankel, B. L. Personality measures and evoked responses in chronic insomniacs. *Journal of Abnormal Psychology*, 1975, *84*, 239–249.

111. Cowan, M. A., Watkins, B. A., & Davis, W. E. Level of education, diagnosis and race-related differences in MMPI performance. *Journal of Clinical Psychology*, 1975, *31*, 442–444.

112. Crovitz, E., Huse, M. N., & Lewis, D. E. Selection of physician's assistants. *Journal of Medical Education*, 1973, *48*, 551–555.

113. Crawder, J. E. Relationship between therapist and client interpersonal behaviors and psychotherapy outcome. *Journal of Counseling Psychology*, 1972, *19*, 68–75.

114. Crowley, T. J., Chesluk, D., Dilts, S., & Hart, R. Drug and alcohol abuse among psychiatric admissions: A multidrug clinical-toxicologic study. *Archives of General Psychiatry*, 1974, *30*, 13–20.

115. Crumpton, E., & Mutalipassi, L. R. The veteran NP patient: Past and present. *Journal of Clinical Psychology*, 1972, *28*, 94–101.

116. Cubitt, G. H., & Gendreau, P. Assessing the diagnostic utility of MMPI and 16PF indexes of homosexuality in a prison sample. *Journal of Consulting and Clinical Psychology*, 1972, *39*, 342.

117. Davis, H. What does the *P* scale measure? *British Journal of Psychiatry*, 1974, *125*, 161–167.

118. Davis, H. M. Psychometric prediction of institutional adjustment: A validation study. *British Journal of Social and Clinical Psychology*, 1974, *13*, 269–276.

119. Davis, W. E. Age and the discriminative "power" of the MMPI with schizophrenic and nonschizophrenic patients. *Journal of Consulting and Clinical Psychology*, 1972, *38*, 151.

120. Davis, W. E. Race and differential "power" of the MMPI. *Journal of Personality Assessment*, 1975, *39*, 138–140.

121. Davis, W. E., Beck, S. J., & Ryan, T. A. Race-related and educationally-related MMPI profile differences among hospitalized schizophrenics. *Journal of Clinical Psychology*, 1973, *29*, 478–479.

122. Davis, W. E., & Jones, M. H. Negro versus Caucasian test performance revisited. *Journal of Consulting and Clinical Psychology*, 1974, *42*, 675–679.

123. Davis, W. E., Mozdzierz, G. J., & Macchitelli, F. J. Loss of discriminative "power" of the MMPI with older psychiatric patients. *Journal of Personality Assessment*, 1973, *37*, 555–558.

124. Dean, E. F. A lengthened Mini: The Midi-Mult. *Journal of Clinical Psychology*, 1972, *28*, 68–71.

125. DeCourcy, P., & Duerfeldt, P. H. The impact of number and type of models on claimed success rate and mood of adult alcoholics. *Journal of Genetic Psychology*, 1973, *122*, 63–79.

126. Dee, C., & Dee, H. L. MMPIs of parents of emotionally disturbed, motor dysfunctioned, and normal children. *Journal of Consulting and Clinical Psychology*, 1972, *38*, 464.

127. DeGroot, W. G., & Adamson, J. D. Responses of psychiatric inpatients to the MacAndrew alcoholism scale. *Quarterly Journal of Studies on Alcohol*, 1973, *34*, 1133–1139.

128. Deiker, T. E. A cross-validation of MMPI scales of aggression on male criminal criterion groups. *Journal of Consulting and Clinical Psychology*, 1974, *42*, 196–202.

129. Dekker, D. J., & Webb, J. T. Relationships of the Social Readjustment Rating scale to psychiatric patient status, anxiety, and social desirability. *Journal of Psychosomatic Research*, 1974, *18*, 125–130.

130. De Leon, G., Skodol, A., & Rosenthal, M. S. Phoenix House: Changes in psychopathological signs of resident drug addicts. *Archives of General Psychiatry*, 1973, *28*, 131–135.

131. Delk, J. L. Some personality characteristics of skydivers. *Life-Threatening Behavior*, 1973, *3*, 51–57.

132. Derogatis, L. R., Rickels, K., & Rock, A. F. The SCL-90 and the MMPI: A step in the validation of a new self-report scale. *British Journal of Psychiatry*, 1976, *128*, 280–289.

133. Devore, J. E., & Fryrear, J. L. Analysis of juvenile delinquents' hole drawing responses on the tree figure of the House-Tree-Person technique. *Journal of Clinical Psychology*, 1976, *32*, 731–736.

134. DeWolfe, A. S., & Davis, W. E. Pattern analysis and deviation scores in clinical research: Mean scatter revisited. *Journal of Personality Assessment*, 1972, *36*, 307–313.

135. Dietzel, C. S., & Abeles, N. Client-therapist complementarity and therapeutic outcome. *Journal of Counseling Psychology*, 1975, *22*, 264–272.

136. Dikman, S., & Reitan, R. M. MMPI correlates of dysphasic language disturbances. *Journal of Abnormal Psychology*, 1974, *83*, 675–679.

137. Dikman, S., & Reitan, R. M. MMPI correlates of localized cerebral lesions. *Perceptual and Motor Skills*, 1974, *39*, 831–840.

138. Doherty, E. G. Labeling effects in psychiatric hospitalization: A study of diverging patterns of inpatient self-labeling processes. *Archives of General Psychiatry*, 1975, *32*, 562–568.

139. Donnelly, E. F., & Murphy, D. L. Primary affective disorder: Delineation of a unipolar depressive subtype. *Psychological Reports*, 1973, *32*, 744–746.

140. Donnelly, E. F., & Murphy, D. L. Primary affective disorder: MMPI differences between unipolar and bipolar depressed subjects. *Journal of Clinical Psychology*, 1973, *29*, 303–306.

141. Donnelly, E. F., & Murphy, D. L. Primary affective disorder: Bender-Gestalt sequence of placement as an indicator of impulse control. *Perceptual and Motor Skills*, 1974, *38*, 1079–1082.

142. Donnelly, E. F., Murphy, D. L., & Goodwin, F. K. Cross-sectional and longitudinal comparisons of bipolar and unipolar depressed groups on the MMPI. *Journal of Consulting and Clinical Psychology*, 1976, *44*, 233–237.

143. Donnelly, E. F., Murphy, D. L., & Scott, W. H. Perception and cognition in patients with bipolar and unipolar depressive disorders: A study in Rorschach responding. *Archives of General Psychiatry*, 1975, *32*, 1128–1131.

144. Donnelly, E. F., Murphy, D. L., Waldman, I. N., & Reynolds, T. D. MMPI difference between unipolar and bipolar depressed subjects: A replication. *Journal of Clinical Psychology*, 1976, *32*, 610–612.

145. Donovan, D. M., & O'Leary, M. R. Relationship between distortions in self-perception of depression and psychopathology. *Journal of Clinical Psychology*, 1976, *32*, 16–19.

146. Dreger, R. M., & Johnson, W. E., Jr. Characteristics of volunteers, nonvolunteers, and no shows in a clinical follow-up. *Journal of Consulting and Clinical Psychology*, 1974, *42*, 746–747.

515

OBJECTIVE
PERSONALITY
INVENTORIES:
RECENT RESEARCH
AND SOME
CONTEMPORARY
ISSUES

147. Drunkenmolle, C. Psychological investigations of patients with breast carcinoma: A pilot study. *Psychiatria Clinica*, 1975, *8*, 127–139.

148. Dudley, H. K., Ellis, M. C., Mason, M., & Hirsch, S. M. Drawings of the opposite sex: Continued use of the Draw-A-Person test and young state hospital patients. *Journal of Youth and Adolescence*, 1976, *5*, 201–219.

149. Dunn, T. G., Lushene, R. E., & O'Neil, H. F., Jr. Complete automation of the MMPI and a study of its response latencies. *Journal of Consulting and Clinical Psychology*, 1972, *39*, 381–387.

150. Eddy, G. L., & Sinnett, E. R. Behavior setting utilization by emotionally disturbed college students. *Journal of Consulting and Clinical Psychology*, 1973, *40*, 210–216.

151. Edinger, J. D., Bogan, J. B., Harrigan, P. H., & Ellis, M. F. Altitude and quotient-IQ discrepancy as an index of personality disorganization among drug offenders. *Journal of Clinical Psychology*, 1975, *31*, 575–578.

152. Edinger, J. D., Kendall, P. C., Hooke, J. F., & Bogan, J. B. The predictive efficacy of three MMPI short forms. *Journal of Personality Assessment*, 1976, *40*, 259–265.

153. Edwards, A. E., & Husted, J. R. Penile sensitivity, age, and sexual behavior. *Journal of Clinical Psychology*, 1976, *32*, 697–700.

154. Elion, V. H. The validity of the MMPI as a discriminator of social deviance among black males. *FCI Research Reports*, Vol. 6, No. 3. Tallahassee, Fla.: Federal Correctional Institution, 1974.

155. Elion, V. H., & Megargee, E. I. Validity of the MMPI *Pd* scale among black males. *Journal of Consulting and Clinical Psychology*, 1975, *43*, 166–172.

156. Elsie, R. D., & McLachlan, J. F. Reliability of the Maxi-Mult and scale equivalence with the MMPI. *Journal of Clinical Psychology*, 1976, *32*, 67–70.

157. Emmons, T. D., & Webb, W. W. Subjective correlates of emotional responsivity and stimulation seeking in psychopaths, normals, and acting-out neurotics. *Journal of Consulting and Clinical Psychology*, 1974, *42*, 620.

158. English, G. E., & Ton, C. A. Psychological characteristics of drug abuse clients seen in a community mental health center. *Journal of Community Psychology*, 1973, *1*, 403–407.

159. Equi, P. J., & Jabara, R. F. Validation of the self-rating depression scale in an alcoholic population. *Journal of Clinical Psychology*, 1976, *32*, 504–507.

160. Erickson, R. C., & Freeman, C. Using the MMPI-168 with medical inpatients. *Journal of Clinical Psychology*, 1976, *32*, 803–806.

161. Erickson, R. C., Post, R. D., & Paige, A. B. Hope as a psychiatric variable. *Journal of Clinical Psychology*, 1975, *31*, 324–330.

162. Eron, L. D., Huesmann, L. R., Lefkowitz, M. M., & Walder, L. O. Does television violence cause aggression? *American Psychologist*, 1972, *27*, 253–263.

163. Evans, D. R. The use of the MMPI to predict conscientious hotline workers. *Journal of Clinical Psychology*, 1976, *32*, 684–686.

164. Ewing, D. R., & Thelen, M. H. Psychiatric patient self-description via self-report and the MMPI. *Journal of Clinical Psychology*, 1972, *28*, 510–514.

165. Faschingbauer, T. R. A 166-item short form of the group MMPI: The FAM. *Journal of Consulting and Clinical Psychology*, 1974, *42*, 645–655.

166. Faschingbauer, T. R. Some clinical considerations in selecting a short form of the MMPI. *Professional Psychology*, 1976, *7*, 177–184.

167. Faschingbauer, T. R. Substitution and regression models, base rates, and the clinical validity of the Mini-Mult. *Journal of Clinical Psychology*, 1976, *32*, 70–74.

168. Faunce, P. S., & Loper, R. G. Personality characteristics of high ability college women and college women-in-general. *Journal of College Student Personnel*, 1972, *13*, 499–504.

169. Feinberg, L. Faculty-student interaction: How students differ. *Journal of College Student Personnel*, 1972, *13*, 24–27.

170. Felton, G. S. Use of the MMPI Underachievement Scale as an aid in counseling academic low achievers in college. *Psychological Reports*, 1973, *32*, 151–157.

171. Fenster, C. A., & Locke, B. Patterns of masculinity-femininity among college- and noncollege-oriented police officers: An empirical approach. *Journal of Clinical Psychology*, 1973, *29*, 27–28.

172. Fillenbaum, G. G., & Pfeiffer, E. The Mini-Mult: A cautionary note. *Journal of Consulting and Clinical Psychology*, 1976, *44*, 698–703.

173. Finch, A. J., Jr., Edwards, G. L., & Griffin, J. L., Jr. Utility of the Mini-Mult with parents of emotionally disturbed children. *Journal of Personality Assessment*, 1975, *39*, 146–150.

174. Finch, A. J., Jr., Griffin, J. L., Jr., & Edwards, G. L. Abbreviated *Mf* and *Si* scales: Efficacy with parents of emotionally disturbed children. *Journal of Clinical Psychology*, 1974, *30*, 80.

175. Finch, A. J., Jr., Kendall, P. C., Nelson, W. M., & Newmark, C. S. Application of Fauschingbauer's abbreviated MMPI to parents of emotionally disturbed children. *Psychological Reports*, 1975, *37*, 571–574.

176. Fine, B. J. Field-dependent introvert and neuroticism: Eysenck and Witkin united. *Psychological Reports*, 1972, *31*, 939–959.

177. Fine, H. K. Studying schizophrenia outside the psychiatric setting. *Journal of Youth and Adolescence*, 1973, *2*, 291–301.

178. Fink, A. M., & Butcher, J. N. Reducing objections to personality inventories with special instructions. *Educational and Psychological Measurement*, 1972, *32*, 631–639.

179. Finney, J. C. Therapist and patient after hours. *American Journal of Psychotherapy*, 1975, *29*, 593–602.

180. Finney, J. C., Brandsma, J. M., Tondow, M., & LeMaistre, G. A study of transsexuals seeking gender reassignment. *American Journal of Psychiatry*, 1975, *132*, 962–964.

181. Finney, J. C., Skeeters, D. E., Auvenshine, C. D., & Smith, D. F. Phases of psychopathology after assassination. *American Journal of Psychiatry*, 1973, *130*, 1379–1380.

182. Fisher, S., & Greenberg, R. P. Selective effects upon women of exciting and calm music. *Perceptual and Motor Skills*, 1972, *34*, 987–990.

183. Fitzgibbons, D. J., Berry, D. F., & Shearn, C. R. MMPI and diagnosis among hospitalized drug abusers. *Journal of Community Psychology*, 1973, *1*, 79–81.

184. Fitzgibbons, D. J., & Hokanson, D. T. The diagnostic decision-making process: Factors influencing diagnosis and changes in diagnosis. *American Journal of Psychiatry*, 1973, *130*, 972–975.

185. Flanagan, J. J., & Lewis, G. R. First prison admissions with juvenile histories and absolute first offenders: Frequencies and MMPI profiles. *Journal of Clinical Psychology*, 1974, *30*, 358–360.

186. Ford, C. V., Bray, G. A., & Swerdloff, R. S. A psychiatric study of patients referred with a diagnosis of hypoglycemia. *American Journal of Psychiatry*, 1976, *133*, 290–294.

187. Ford, C. V., Castelnuovo-Tedesco, P., & Long, K. D. Women who seek therapeutic abortion: A comparison with women who complete their pregnancies. *American Journal of Psychiatry*, 1972, *129*, 546–552.

188. Ford, C. V., & Spaulding, R. C. The Pueblo Incident: A comparison of factors related to coping with extreme stress. *Archives of General Psychiatry*, 1973, *29*, 340–343.

189. Fowler, R. D. Automated psychological test interpretation: The status in 1972. *Psychiatric Annual*, 1972, *2*, 10–17.

190. Fowler, R. D., & Hodo, G. L. A comparison of classification rates of the original and revised Marks and Seeman rules. *Journal of Clinical Psychology*, 1975, *31*, 665–667.

191. Fracchia, J., Sheppard, C., & Merlis, S. Some comments about the personality comparison of incarcerated and street heroin addicts. *Psychological Reports*, 1973, *33*, 413–414.

192. Fracchia, J., Sheppard, C., & Merlis, S. Treatment patterns in psychiatry: Clinical and personality features of elderly hospitalized patients during milieu, single-drug and multiple-drug programs. *Journal of American Geriatrics Society*, 1974, *22*, 212–216.

193. Fracchia, J., Sheppard, C., Ricca, E., & Merlis, S. MMPI performance in chronic medical illness: The use of computer-derived interpretations. *British Journal of Psychiatry*, 1973, *122*, 242–243.

194. Frankel, A., & Murphy, J. Physical fitness and personality in alcoholism: Canonical analysis of measures before and after treatment. *Quarterly Journal of Studies on Alcohol*, 1974, *35*, 1272–1278.

195. Freeman, C., Caslyn, D., & Louks, J. The use of the MMPI with low back pain patients. *Journal of Clinical Psychology*, 1976, *32*, 294–298.

196. French, A. P., Russell, T. L., & Tupin, J. P. Subjective changes with the Sentic Cycles of Clynes: A preliminary psychometric study. *Diseases of the Nervous System*, 1972, *33*, 598–602.

197. Friedman, R. J. MMPI characteristics of mothers of pre-school children who are emotionally disturbed or have behavior problems. *Psychological Reports*, 1974, *34*, 1159–1162.

198. Fromme, D. K., & Schmidt, C. K. Affective role enactment and expressive behavior. *Journal of Personality and Social Psychology*, 1972, *24*, 413–419.

199. Fruhauf, K. Psychometric determination of behavioral maturity in the brain-damaged. *Zeitschrift fur Psychologie*, 1975, *183*, 279–293.

200. Gaines, L. S., Abrams, M. H., Toel, P., & Miller, L. M. Comparison of the MMPI and the Mini-Mult with alcoholics. *Journal of Consulting and Clinical Psychology*, 1974, *42*, 619.

517

OBJECTIVE
PERSONALITY
INVENTORIES:
RECENT RESEARCH
AND SOME
CONTEMPORARY
ISSUES

201. Gallemore, J. L., Jr., & Panton, J. H. Inmate responses to lengthy death row confinement. *American Journal of Psychiatry*, 1972, *129*, 167–172.

202. Garetz, F. K., & Anderson, R. W. Patterns of professional activities of psychiatrists: A follow-up of 100 psychiatric residents. *American Journal of Psychiatry*, 1973, *130*, 981–984.

203. Garfield, S. L., Prager, R. A., & Bergin, A. E. Some further comments on evaluation of outcome in psychotherapy. *Journal of Counseling and Clinical Psychology*, 1974, *42*, 296–297.

204. Garrard, J., & Weber, R. G. Comparison of three- and four-year medical school graduates. *Journal of Medical Education*, 1974, *49*, 547–553.

205. Gartner, D., & Goldstein, H. S. Some characteristics of mothers of severely disturbed children in a therapeutic nursery. *Psychological Reports*, 1972, *30*, 901–902.

206. Gayton, W. F., Bishop, J. S., Citrin, M. M., & Bassett, J. S. An investigation of the Mini-Mult validity scales. *Journal of Personality Assessment*, 1975, *39*, 511–513.

207. Gayton, W. F., Fogg, M. E., Tavorimina, J., Bishop, J. S., Citrin, M. M., & Bassett, J. F. Comparison of the MMPI and Mini-Mult with women who request abortion. *Journal of Clinical Psychology*, 1976, *32*, 648–650.

208. Gayton, W. F., Ozman, K. L., & Wilson, W. T. Investigation of a written form of the Mini-Mult. *Psychological Reports*, 1972, *30*, 275–278.

209. Gellens, H. K., Gottheil, E., & Alterman, A. I. Drinking outcome of specific alcoholic subgroups. *Journal of Studies on Alcohol*, 1976, *37*, 986–989.

210. Gendreau, P. Psychological test usage in corrections in English-speaking Canada: 1972–1973. *Canadian Journal of Criminology and Corrections*, 1975, *17*, 215–220.

211. Gendreau, P., & Gendreau, L. P. A theoretical note on personality characteristic of heroin addicts. *Journal of Abnormal Psychology*, 1973, *82*, 139–140.

212. Gendreau, P., Gibson, M., Surridge, C. T., & Hug, J. J. The application of self-esteem measures in corrections: A further report on the SEI. *Journal of Community Psychology*, 1973, *1*, 423–425.

213. Gendreau, P., Irvine, M., & Knight, S. Evaluating response set styles on the MMPI with prisoners: Faking good adjustment and maladjustment. *Canadian Journal of Behavioral Science*, 1973, *5*, 183–194.

214. Genther, R. W., & Graham, J. R. Effects of short-term public psychiatric hospitalization for both black and white patients. *Journal of Consulting and Clinical Psychology*, 1976, *44*, 118–124.

215. Ghei, S. N. A cross-culture comparison of the social desirability variable. *Journal of Cross-Cultural Psychology*, 1973, *4*, 493–500.

216. Gilroy, F. D., & Steinbacher, R. Extension of the Mini-Mult to a college population. *Journal of Personality Assessment*, 1973, *37*, 263–266.

217. Ginsburg, A. B., & Goldstein, S. G. Age bias in referral for psychological consultation. *Journal of Gerontology*, 1974, *29*, 410–415.

218. Gocka, E. F. MMPI item responses for male neuropsychiatric patients. *Catalog of Selected Documents in Psychology*, 1976, *6*, 12.

219. Godfrey, E. A., & Schulman, R. E. Age and a group test battery as predictors of type of crime. *Journal of Clinical Psychology*, 1972, *28*, 339–342.

220. Gold, E. M., & Hoffman, P. J. Flange detection cluster analysis. *Multivariate Behavioral Research*, 1976, *11*, 217–235.

221. Goldberg, L. R. Man versus mean: The exploitation of group profiles for the construction of diagnostic classification systems. *Journal of Abnormal Psychology*, 1972, *79*, 121–131.

222. Golden, C. J., & Golden, E. E. Resistance to cognitive interference as a function of MMPI profile. *Journal of Consulting and Clinical Psychology*, 1975, *43*, 749.

223. Golden, C. J., & Golden, E. E. A note on self-reported behavioral correlates of resistance to interference. *Journal of Genetic Psychology*, 1976, *128*, 299–300.

224. Goldstein, A. M., & Reznikoff, M. MMPI performance in chronic medical illness: The use of computer-derived interpretations. *British Journal of Psychiatry*, 1972, *120*, 157–158.

225. Goodson, J. H., & King, G. D. A clinical and actuarial study on the validity of the Goldberg Index for the MMPI. *Journal of Clinical Psychology*, 1976, *32*, 328–335.

226. Graham, J. R., Friedman, I., Paolino, A. F., & Lilly, R. S. An appraisal of the therapeutic value of the mental hospital milieu. *Journal of Community Psychology*, 1974, *2*, 153–160.

227. Graham, J. R., Lilly, R. S., Konick, D. S., Paolino, A. F., & Friedman, I. MMPI changes associated with short-term psychiatric hospitalization. *Journal of Clinical Psychology*, 1973, *29*, 69–73.

228. Graham, J. R., & Schroeder, H. E. Abbreviated *Mf* and *Si* scales for the MMPI. *Journal of Personality Assessment*, 1972, *36*, 436–439.

229. Gravitz, M. A., & Gerton, M. I. An empirical study of internal consistency in the MMPI. *Journal of Clinical Psychology*, 1976, *32*, 567–568.

230. Gray-Little, B. Attitudes toward conflict with authority as a function of sex, I-E, and dogmatism. *Psychological Reports*, 1974, *34*, 375–381.

231. Grayson, H. M., & Backer, T. E. Scoring accuracy of four automated MMPI interpretation report agencies. *Journal of Clinical Psychology*, 1972, *28*, 366–370.

232. Greer, R. M., & Callis, R. The use of videotape models in an alcohol rehabilitation program. *Rehabilitation Counseling Bulletin*, 1975, *18*, 154–159.

233. Griffin, J. L., Finch, A. J., Edwards, G. L., & Kendall, P. C. MMPI Midi-Mult correspondence with parents of emotionally disturbed children. *Journal of Clinical Psychology*, 1976, *32*, 54–56.

234. Griffiths, R. D. The accuracy and correlates of psychiatric patients' self-assessment of their work behavior. *British Journal of Social and Clinical Psychology*, 1975, *14*, 181–189.

235. Gruba, G. H., & Rohrbaugh, M. MMPI correlates of menstrual distress. *Psychosomatic Medicine*, 1975, *37*, 265–273.

236. Gurney, C., Roth, M., Garside, R. F., Kerr, T. A., & Schapira, K. Studies in the classification of affective disorders: The relationship between anxiety states and depressive illnesses. II. *British Journal of Psychiatry*, 1972, *121*, 162–166.

237. Gynther, M. D. MMPI items for invasion of privacy studies. *Journal of Clinical Psychology*, 1972, *28*, 76–77.

238. Gynther, M. D. White norms and black MMPIs: A prescription for discrimination? *Psychological Bulletin*, 1972, *78*, 386–402.

239. Gynther, M. D., Altman, H., & Sletten, I. W. Development of an empirical interpretive system for the MMPI: Some after-the-fact observations. *Journal of Clinical Psychology*, 1973, *29*, 232–234.

240. Gynther, M. D., Altman, H., & Sletten, I. W. Replicated correlates of MMPI two-point code types: The Missouri actuarial system. *Journal of Clinical Psychology*, 1973, *29*, 263–289.

241. Gynther, M. D., Altman, H., & Warbin, R. W. A new empirical automated MMPI interpretive program: The 2-4/4-2 code type. *Journal of Clinical Psychology*, 1972, *28*, 498–501.

242. Gynther, M. D., Altman, H., & Warbin, R. W. A new empirical automated MMPI interpretive program: The 2-7/7-2 code type. *Journal of Clinical Psychology*, 1973, *29*, 58–59.

243. Gynther, M. D., Altman, H., & Warbin, R. W. A new actuarial-empirical automated MMPI interpretive program: The 4-3/3-4 code type. *Journal of Clinical Psychology*, 1973, *29*, 229–231.

244. Gynther, M. D., Altman, H., & Warbin, R. W. A new empirical automated MMPI interpretive program: The 6-9/9-6 code type. *Journal of Clinical Psychology*, 1973, *29*, 60–61.

245. Gynther, M. D., Altman, H., & Warbin, R. W. Behavioral correlates for the MMPI 4-9/9-4 code types: A case of the emperor's new clothes? *Journal of Consulting and Clinical Psychology*, 1973, *40*, 259–263.

246. Gynther, M. D., Altman, H., & Warbin, R. Interpretation of uninterpretable MMPI profiles. *Journal of Consulting and Clinical Psychology*, 1973, *40*, 78–83.

247. Gynther, M. D., Altman, H., Warbin, R. W., & Sletten, I. W. A new actuarial system for MMPI interpretation: Rationale and methodology. *Journal of Clinical Psychology*, 1972, *28*, 173–179.

248. Gynther, M. D., Altman, H., Warbin, R. W., & Sletten, I. W. A new empirical automated MMPI interpretive program: the 1-2/2-1 code type. *Journal of Clinical Psychology*, 1973, *29*, 54–57.

249. Gynther, M. D., & Witt, P. H. Windstorms and important persons: Personality characteristics of black educators. *Journal of Clinical Psychology*, 1976, *32*, 613–616.

250. Hampton, P. T., & Vogel, D. B. Personality characteristics of servicemen returned from Viet Nam identified as heroin abusers. *American Journal of Psychiatry*, 1973, *130*, 1031–1032.

251. Harford, T., Lubetkin, B., & Alpert, G. Comparison of the standard MMPI and the Mini-Mult in a psychiatric outpatient clinic. *Journal of Consulting and Clinical Psychology*, 1972, *39*, 243–245.

252. Harmatz, J. S., & Shader, R. I. Psychopharmacologic investigations in healthy elder volunteers: MMPI depression scale. *Journal of the American Geriatrics Society*, 1975, *23*, 350–354.

253. Harmatz, J. S., Shader, R. I., & Salzman, C. Marijuana users and nonusers: Personality test differences. *Archives of General Psychiatry*, 1972, *26*, 108–112.

254. Harrell, T. W. High earning MBA's. *Personnel Psychology*, 1972, *25*, 523–530.

255. Harrell, T. W., & Harrell, M. S. The personality of MBA's who reach general management early. *Personnel Psychology*, 1973, *26*, 127–134.

256. Hartmann, E., Baekeland, F., & Zwilling, G. R. Psychological differences between long and short sleepers. *Archives of General Psychiatry*, 1972, *26*, 463–468.

519

OBJECTIVE
PERSONALITY
INVENTORIES:
RECENT RESEARCH
AND SOME
CONTEMPORARY
ISSUES

257. Hawk, S., & Peterson, R. A. Do MMPI psychopathic deviancy scores reflect psychopathic deviancy or just deviance? *Journal of Personality Assessment*, 1974, *38*, 362–368.

258. Heath, D. H. Adolescent and adult predictors of vocational adaptation. *Journal of Vocational Behavior*, 1976, *9*, 1–19.

259. Heaton, R. K., & Victor, R. G. Personality characteristics associated with psychedelic flashbacks in natural and experimental settings. *Journal of Abnormal Psychology*, 1976, *85*, 83–90.

260. Hedberg, A. G., Campbell, L. M., Weeks, S. R., & Powell, J. A. The use of the MMPI (Mini-Mult) to predict alcoholics' response to a behavioral treatment program. *Journal of Clinical Psychology*, 1975, *31*, 271–274.

261. Hedlund, J. L., Morgan, D. W., & Master, F. D. The Mayo Clinic automated MMPI program: Cross-validation with psychiatric patients in an Army hospital. *Journal of Clinical Psychology*, 1972, *28*, 505–510.

262. Hedlund, J. L., Won Cho, D., & Powell, B. J. Use of MMPI short forms with psychiatric patients. *Journal of Consulting and Clinical Psychology*, 1975, *43*, 924.

263. Heikkinen, C. A., & Wegner, K. W. MMPI studies of counselors: A review. *Journal of Counseling Psychology*, 1973, *20*, 275–279.

264. Heilbrun, A. B., Jr., & Norbert, N. Style of adaptation to aversive maternal control and paranoid behavior. *Journal of Genetic Psychology*, 1972, *120*, 145–153.

265. Held, M. L., & Snow, D. L. MMPI, internal-external control, and Problem Checklist scores of obese adolescent females. *Journal of Clinical Psychology*, 1972, *28*, 523–525.

266. Hendrie, H. C., Lachar, D., & Lennox, K. Personality trait and symptom correlates of life change in a psychiatric population. *Journal of Psychosomatic Research*, 1975, *19*, 203–208.

267. Henning, J. J., Levy, R. H., & Aderman, M. Reliability of MMPI tape recorded and booklet administrations. *Journal of Clinical Psychology*, 1972, *28*, 372–373.

268. Henrichs, T. F., & Waters, W. F. Psychological adjustment and response to open-heart surgery: Some methodological considerations. *British Journal of Psychiatry*, 1972, *120*, 491–496.

269. Henry, B. W., Overall, J. E., & Woodward, J. A. Actuarial justification for choice of drug treatment for psychiatric patients. *Diseases of the Nervous System*, 1976, *37*, 555–557.

270. Herzberg, F., Mathapo, J., Wierner, Y., & Wieson, L. E. Motivation-hygiene correlates of mental health: An examination of motivational inversion in a clinical population. *Journal of Consulting and Clinical Psychology*, 1974, *42*, 411–419.

271. Higdon, J. F., & Brodsky, S. L. Validating Hand Test acting out ratios for overt and experimentally induced aggression. *Journal of Personality Assessment*, 1973, *37*, 363–368.

272. Hill, M. S. Heredity influence on the normal personality using the MMPI: 2. prospective assortative mating. *Behavior Genetics*, 1973, *3*, 225–232.

273. Hill, M. S., & Hill, R. N. Heredity influence on the normal personality using the MMPI. I. Age-corrected parent-offspring resemblances. *Behavior Genetics*, 1973, *3*, 133–144.

274. Hindelang, M. J. The relationship of self-reported delinquency to scales of the CPI and MMPI. *Journal of Criminal Law, Criminology, and Police Science*, 1972, *63*, 75–81.

275. Hindelang, M. J. Variations in personality attributes of social and solitary self-reported delinquents. *Journal of Consulting and Clinical Psychology*, 1973, *40*, 452–454.

276. Hobbs, T. R. Scale equivalence and profile similarity of the Mini-Mult and MMPI in an outpatient clinic. *Journal of Clinical Psychology*, 1974, *30*, 349–350.

277. Hobbs, T. R., & Fowler, R. D. Reliability and scale equivalence of the Mini-Mult and MMPI. *Journal of Consulting and Clinical Psychology*, 1974, *42*, 89–92.

278. Hodo, G. L., & Barker, H. R. Discriminating alcoholic and nonalcoholic patients with conventional and factored MMPI scales: A comparison. *Journal of Clinical Psychology*, 1976, *32*, 495–497.

279. Hodo, G. L., & Fowler, R. D. Frequency of MMPI two-point codes in a large alcoholic sample. *Journal of Clinical Psychology*, 1976, *32*, 487–489.

280. Hoey, H. P. Lethality of suicidal behavior and the MMPI. *Psychological Reports*, 1974, *35*, 942.

281. Hoffman, A. L. Psychological factors associated with rheumatoid arthritis: Review of the literature. *Nursing Research*, 1974, *23*, 218–234.

282. Hoffmann, H. MMPI changes for a male alcoholic state hospital population—1959–1971. *Psychological Reports*, 1973, *33*, 139–142.

283. Hoffmann, H., & Jackson, D. N. Substantive dimensions of psychopathology derived from MMPI content scales and the Differential Personality Inventory. *Journal of Consulting and Clinical Psychology*, 1976, *44*, 862.

284. Hoffmann, H., Jackson, D. N., & Skinner, H. A. Dimensions of psychopathology among alcoholic patients. *Journal of Studies on Alcohol*, 1975, *36*, 825–837.

285. Hoffmann, H., & Jansen, D. G. Relationships among discharge variables and MMPI scale scores of hospitalized alcoholics. *Journal of Clinical Psychology*, 1973, *29*, 475–477.

286. Hoffmann, H., Jansen, D. G., & Wefring, L. R. Relationships between admission variables and MMPI scale scores of hospitalized alcoholics. *Psychological Reports*, 1972, *31*, 659–662.

287. Hoffmann, H., Loper, R. G., & Kammeier, M. L. Identifying future alcoholics with MMPI alcoholism scales. *Quarterly Journal of Studies on Alcohol*, 1974, *35*, 490–498.

288. Hoffmann, N. G., & Butcher, J. N. Clinical limitations of three MMPI short forms. *Journal of Consulting and Clinical Psychology*, 1975, *43*, 32–39.

289. Holland, T. R., & Holt, N. Personality patterns among short-term prisoners undergoing presentence evaluations. *Psychological Reports*, 1975, *37*, 827–836.

290. Holland, T. R., & Holt, N. Prisoner intellectual and personality correlates of offense severity and recidivism probability. *Journal of Clinical Psychology*, 1975, *31*, 667–672.

291. Holland, T. R., Lowenfeld, J., & Wadsworth, H. M. MMPI indices in the discrimination of brain-damaged and schizophrenic groups. *Journal of Consulting and Clinical Psychology*, 1975, *43*, 426.

292. Hood, R. W. The construction and preliminary validation of a measure of reported mystical experience. *Journal for the Scientific Study of Religion*, 1975, *14*, 29–41.

293. Horn, J. H., & Turner, R. G. MMPI profiles among subgroups of unwed mothers. *Journal of Consulting and Clinical Psychology*, 1976, *44*, 25–33.

294. Horn, J. L., Wanberg, K. W., & Appel, M. On the internal structure of the MMPI. *Multivariate Behavioral Research*, 1973, *8*, 131–171.

295. Horn, J. M., Green, M., Carney, R., & Erickson, M. T. Bias against genetic hypotheses in adoption studies. *Archives of General Psychiatry*, 1975, *32*, 1365–1367.

296. Horstman, W. R. MMPI responses of homosexual and heterosexual male college students. *Homosexual Counseling Journal*, 1975, *2*, 68–76.

297. House, K. M., & Martin, R. L. MMPI delineation of a subgroup of depressed patients refractory to lithium carbonate therapy. *American Journal of Psychiatry*, 1975, *132*, 644–646.

298. Huber, N. A., & Danahy, S. Use of the MMPI in predicting completion and evaluating changes in a long-term alcoholism treatment program. *Journal of Studies on Alcohol*, 1975, *36*, 1230–1237.

299. Huisman, R. E. Correspondence between Mini-Mult and standard MMPI scale scores in patients with neurological disease. *Journal of Consulting and Clinical Psychology*, 1974, *42*, 149.

300. Hunt, H. The differentiation of malingering, dissimulation and pathology. In M. Hammer, K. Salzinger, & S. Sutton (Eds.), *Psychopathology: Contributions from the social, behavioral, and biological sciences*. New York: Wiley, 1973.

301. Hunter, S., Overall, J. E., & Butcher, J. N. Factor structure of the MMPI in a psychiatric population. *Multivariate Behavioral Research*, 1974, *9*, 283–302.

302. Husted, J. R., & Edwards, A. E. Personality correlates of male sexual arousal and behavior. *Archives of Sexual Behavior*, 1976, *5*, 149–156.

303. Jabara, R. F., & Curran, S. F. Comparison of the MMPI and Mini-Mult with drug users. *Journal of Consulting and Clinical Psychology*, 1974, *42*, 739–740.

304. Jackson, D. N., & Messick, S. Judged frequency of endorsement and frequency of occurrence scale values and dispersions for MMPI items. *Psychological Reports*, 1973, *33*, 183–191.

305. Jansen, D. G. Use of the psychological screening inventory with hospitalized alcoholics. *Journal of Consulting and Clinical Psychology*, 1972, *39*, 170.

306. Jansen, D. G., Bonk, E. C., & Garvey, F. J. MMPI characteristics of clergymen in counseling training and their relationship to supervisor's and peers' ratings of counseling effectiveness. *Psychological Reports*, 1973, *33*, 695–698.

307. Jansen, D. G., & Garvey, F. J. High-, average- and low-rated clergymen in a state hospital clinical program. *Journal of Clinical Psychology*, 1973, *29*, 89–92.

308. Jansen, D. G., & Hoffmann, H. Demographic and MMPI characteristics of male and female state hospital alcoholic patients. *Psychological Reports*, 1973, *33*, 561–562.

309. Jansen, D. G., & Hoffmann, H. MMPI scores of counselors on alcoholism prior to and after training. *Journal of Consulting and Clinical Psychology*, 1975, *43*, 271.

310. Jansen, D. G., & Johnson, L. E. Patients who schedule meetings with a state hospital review board. *Psychological Reports*, 1975, *36*, 283–286.

521

OBJECTIVE
PERSONALITY
INVENTORIES:
RECENT RESEARCH
AND SOME
CONTEMPORARY
ISSUES

311. Jansen, D. G., & Nickles, L. A. Variables that differentiate between single- and multiple-admission psychiatric patients at a state hospital over a 5-year period. *Journal of Clinical Psychology*, 1973, *29*, 83–85.

312. Jansen, D. S. Personality characteristics of state hospital patients' rights office visitors. *Journal of Clinical Psychology*, 1974, *30*, 347–349.

313. Jarvis, L. G., Simnegar, R. R., & Traweek, A. R. An MMPI comparison of U.S.A.F. groups identified as drug users. *Psychological Reports*, 1975, *37*, 1339–1345.

314. Jeske, J. O. Identification and therapeutic effectiveness in group therapy. *Journal of Counseling Psychology*, 1973, *20*, 528–530.

315. Joanning, H. Behavioral rehearsal in group treatment of socially nonassertive individuals. *Journal of College Student Personnel*, 1976, *17*, 313–318.

316. Joesting, J., Jones, N., & Joesting, R. Male and female prison inmates' differences on MMPI scales and revised beta IQ. *Psychological Reports*, 1975, *37*, 471–474.

317. Johnson, D. T., Workman, S. N., Neville, C. W., Jr., & Beutler, L. E. MMPI and 16PF correlates and the A-B Therapy Scale in psychiatric inpatients. *Psychotherapy: Theory Research and Practice*, 1973, *10*, 270–272.

318. Johnson, J. H. Bender-Gestalt constriction as an indicator of depression in psychiatric patients. *Journal of Personality Assessment*, 1973, *37*, 53–55.

319. Johnson, J. H. A cross validation of seventeen experimental MMPI scales related to antisocial behavior. *Journal of Clinical Psychology*, 1974, *30*, 564–565.

320. Johnston, N., & Cooke, G. Relationship of MMPI alcoholism, prison escape, hostility control, and recidivism scales to clinical judgments. *Journal of Clinical Psychology*, 1973, *29*, 32–34.

321. Jones, F. H. A 4-year follow-up of vulnerable adolescents: The prediction of outcome in early adulthood from measures of social competence, coping style, and overall level of psychopathology. *Journal of Nervous and Mental Disease*, 1974, *159*, 20–39.

322. Jones, F. W., Neuringer, C., & Patterson, T. W. An evaluation of an MMPI response consistency measure. *Journal of Personality Assessment*, 1976, *40*, 419–421.

323. Jones, N. F., Kinsman, R. A., Schum, R., & Resnikoff, P. Personality profiles in asthma. *Journal of Clinical Psychology*, 1976, *32*, 285–291.

324. Jones, R. R., & Rorer, L. G. Response biases and trait descriptive adjectives. *Multivariate Behavioral Research*, 1973, *8*, 313–330.

325. Jordan, J. M., & Whitleer, R. A. Atopic dermatitis anxiety and conditioned scratch responses. *Journal of Psychosomatic Research*, 1974, *18*, 297–299.

326. Judd, L. L., & Grant, I. Brain dysfunction in chronic sedative users. *Journal of Psychedelic Drugs*, 1975, *7*, 143–149.

327. Jurko, M. F., Andy, O. J., & Giurintano, L. P. Changes in the MMPI as a function of thalamotomy. *Journal of Clinical Psychology*, 1974, *30*, 569–570.

328. Kales, A., Caldwell, A. B., Preston, T. A., Healey, S., & Kales, J. D. Personality patterns in insomnia: Theoretical implications. *Archives of General Psychiatry*, 1976, *33*, 1128–1134.

329. Kammeier, M. L., Hoffmann, H., & Loper, R. G. Personality characteristics of alcoholics as college freshmen and at time of treatment. *Quarterly Journal of Studies on Alcohol*, 1973, *34*, 390–399.

330. Kane, F. J., Jr., Moan, C. A., & Bolling, B. Motivation factors in pregnant adolescents. *Diseases of the Nervous System*, 1974, *35*, 131–134.

331. Kaplan, R., Blume, S., Rosenberg, S., Pitrelli, J., & Turner, W. J. Phenytoin, metronidazole and multivitamins in the treatment of alcoholism. *Quarterly Journal of Studies on Alcohol*, 1972, *33*, 97–104.

332. Karacan, I., Williams, R. L., Guerrero, M. W., Salis, P. J., Thornby, J. I., & Hursch, C. J. Nocturnal penile tumescence and sleep of convicted rapists and other prisoners. *Archives of Sexual Behavior*, 1974, *3*, 19–26.

333. Keller, J., & Redfering, D. L. Comparison between the personalities of LSD users and nonusers as measured by the MMPI. *Journal of Nervous and Mental Disease*, 1973, *156*, 271–277.

334. Kelly, W. L. Psychological prediction of leadership in nursing. *Nursing Research*, 1974, *23*, 38–42.

335. Kilpatrick, D. G., Miller, W. C., Allain, N., Huggins, M. B., & Lee, W. H., Jr. The use of psychological test data to predict open-heart surgery outcome: A prospective study. *Psychosomatic Medicine*, 1975, *37*, 62–73.

336. Kissinger, J. R. Women who threaten suicide: Evidence for an identifiable personality type. *Omega*, 1973, *4*, 73–84.

337. Klapper, J. A., & McColloch, M. A. Personality and reactivity to stimulants and depressants. *Journal of Nervous and Mental Disease*, 1972, *154*, 439–444.

338. Klapper, J. A., McColloch, M. A., & Merkey, R. P. The relationship of personality to tolerance of an irritant compound. *Journal of Personality and Social Psychology*, 1973, *26*, 110–112.

339. Klapper, J. A., McColloch, M. A., & Sidell, F. R. The effect on personality of reactivity to 1,2-dimethyl-heptyl-tetrahydrocannabinol. *Archives of General Psychiatry*, 1972, *26*, 483–485.

340. Kleinmuntz, B. The computer as clinician. *American Psychologist*, 1975, *30*, 379–387.

341. Klinge, V., & Strauss, M. Effects of scoring norms on adolescent psychiatric patients' MMPI profiles. *Journal of Personality Assessment*, 1976, *40*, 13–17.

342. Klonoff, H., Clark, C., Horgan, J., Kramer, P., & McDougall, G. The MMPI profile of prisoners of war. *Journal of Clinical Psychology*, 1976, *32*, 623–627.

343. Knott, P. D., Lasater, L., & Shuman, R. Aggression-guilt and conditionability for aggressiveness. *Journal of Personality*, 1974, *42*, 332–344.

344. Kochansky, G. E., Hemenway, T. S., Salzman, C., & Shader, R. I. Methaqualone abusers: A preliminary survey of college students. *Diseases of the Nervous System*, 1975, *36*, 348–351.

345. Koh, S. D., & Peterson, R. A. Perceptual memory for numerousness in "nonpsychotic schizophrenics." *Journal of Abnormal Psychology*, 1974, *83*, 215–226.

346. Kojak, G., Jr., & Canby, J. P. Personality and behavior patterns of heroin-dependent American servicemen in Thailand. *American Journal of Psychiatry*, 1975, *132*, 246–250.

347. Kolton, M. S., & Dwarshuis, L. A clinical factor analytic method for inferring construct meaning. *Educational and Psychological Measurement*, 1973, *33*, 653–661.

348. Koss, M. P., & Butcher, J. N. A comparison of psychiatric patients' self-report with other sources of clinical information. *Journal of Research in Personality*, 1973, *7*, 225–236.

349. Kranitz, L. Alcoholics, heroin addicts and nonaddicts: Comparisons on the MacAndrew alcoholism scale of the MMPI. *Quarterly Journal of Studies on Alcohol*, 1972, *33*, 807–809.

350. Kristianson, P. A comparison between the personality changes in certain forms of psychomotor and grand mal epilepsy. *British Journal of Psychiatry*, 1974, *125*, 34–35.

351. Kristianson, P. The personality in psychomotor epilepsy compared with the explosive and aggressive personality. *British Journal of Psychiatry*, 1974, *125*, 221–229.

352. Kroger, R. O. Faking in interest measurement: A social-psychological perspective. *Measurement and Evaluation Guide*, 1974, *7*, 130–134.

353. Kroger, R. O., & Turnbull, W. Invalidity of validity scales: The case of the MMPI. *Journal of Consulting and Clinical Psychology*, 1975, *43*, 48–55.

354. Kuha, S., Moilanen, P., & Kampman, R. The effect of social class on psychiatric psychological evaluations in patients with pulmonary tuberculosis. *Acta Psychiatrica Scandinavica*, 1975, *51*, 249–256.

355. Kurtz, R. R., & Grummon, D. L. Different approaches to the measurement of therapist empathy and their relationship to therapy outcomes. *Journal of Consulting and Clinical Psychology*, 1972, *39*, 106–115.

356. Kutner, S. J., & Brown, W. L. Types of oral contraceptives, depression, and premenstrual symptoms. *Journal of Nervous and Mental Disease*, 1972, *155*, 153–162.

357. Kutner, S. J., & Brown, W. L. History of depression as a risk factor for depression with oral contraceptives and discontinuance. *Journal of Nervous and Mental Disease*, 1972, *155*, 163–169.

358. Kwant, F., Rice, J. A., & Hays, J. R. Use of Heroin Addiction Scale to differentiate addicts from rehabilitation clients. *Psychological Reports*, 1976, *38*, 547–553.

359. Lachar, D. Accuracy and generalizability of an automated MMPI interpretation system. *Journal of Consulting and Clinical Psychology*, 1974, *42*, 267–273.

360. Lachar, D. Prediction of early U.S. Air Force freshman cadet adaptation with the MMPI. *Journal of Counseling Psychology*, 1974, *21*, 404–408.

361. Lachar, D., Klinge, V., & Grisell, J. L. Relative accuracy of automated MMPI narratives generated from adult norm and adolescent norm profiles. *Journal of Consulting and Clinical Psychology*, 1976, *44*, 20–24.

362. Lair, C. V., & King, G. D. MMPI profile predictors for successful and expired open heart surgery patients. *Journal of Clinical Psychology*, 1976, *32*, 51–54.

363. Lamont, J., & Tyler, C. Racial differences in rate of depression. *Journal of Clinical Psychology*, 1973, *29*, 428–432.

364. Lauer, J. W. The effect of tricyclic antidepressant compounds on patients with passive-dependent personality traits. *Current Therapeutic Research*, 1976, *19*, 495–505.

523

OBJECTIVE
PERSONALITY
INVENTORIES:
RECENT RESEARCH
AND SOME
CONTEMPORARY
ISSUES

365. Lebovits, B., Licher, E., & Moses, V. K. Personality correlates of coronary heart disease: A re-examination of the MMPI. *Social Science and Medicine*, 1975, *9*, 207–219.

366. Leonard, C. V. Self-ratings of alienation in suicidal patients. *Journal of Clinical Psychology*, 1973, *29*, 423–428.

367. Lester, D., & Narkunski, A. An exploratory study of correlates of success in a vocational training program for ex-addicts. *Psychological Reports*, 1975, *37*, 1212–1214.

368. Lester, D., Perdue, W. C., & Brookhart, D. Murder and the control of aggression. *Psychological Reports*, 1974, *34*, 706.

369. Leunes, A., & Christensen, L. A comparison of forgers with other criminals. *Journal of Community Psychology*, 1975, *3*, 285–288.

370. Leve, R. M. A comment on Garfield, Prager, and Bergin's evaluation of outcome in psychotherapy. *Journal of Consulting and Clinical Psychology*, 1974, *42*, 293–295.

371. Levine, R. V., & Megargee, E. I. Prediction of academic success with the MMPI and Beta Intelligence Test in a correctional institution. *Catalog of Selected Documents in Psychology*, 1975, *5*, 343.

372. Levitt, E. A. Procedural issues in the systematic desensitization of air-travel phobia. *New Zealand Psychologist*, 1975, *4*, 2–9.

373. Lewandowski, D., & Graham, J. R. Empirical correlates of frequently occurring two-point MMPI code types: A replicated study. *Journal of Consulting and Clinical Psychology*, 1972, *39*, 467–472.

374. Lewinson, P. M., & Graf, M. Pleasant activities and depression. *Journal of Consulting and Clinical Psychology*, 1973, *41*, 261–268.

375. Lewinson, P. M., Lobitz, W. C., & Wilson, S. "Sensitivity" of depressed individuals to aversive stimuli. *Journal of Abnormal Psychology*, 1973, *81*, 259–263.

376. Lewinson, P. M., & MacPhillamy, D. J. The relationship between age and engagement in pleasant activities. *Journal of Gerontology*, 1974, *29*, 290–294.

377. Lichtenstein, S. Conditional non-independence of data in a practical Bayesian decision task. *Organizational Behavior and Human Performance*, 1972, *8*, 21–25.

378. Lin, T. Use of demographic variables, WRAT, and MMPI scores to predict addicts' types of discharge from a community-like hospital setting. *Journal of Clinical Psychology*, 1975, *31*, 148–151.

379. Listiak, R. L., Stone, L. A., & Coles, G. J. Clinicians' multidimensional perceptions of MMPI scales. *Journal of Clinical Psychology*, 1973, *29*, 29–32.

380. Longabaugh, R., & Eldred, S. H. Pre-morbid adjustments, schizoid personality and onset of illness as predictors of post-hospitalization functioning. *Journal of Psychiatric Research*, 1973, *10*, 19–29.

381. Loper, R. G., Kammeier, M. L., & Hoffmann, H. MMPI characteristics of college freshman males who later become alcoholics. *Journal of Abnormal Psychology*, 1973, *82*, 159–162.

382. Lopiccolo, J., & Blatt, S. J. Cognitive style and sexual identity. *Journal of Clinical Psychology*, 1972, *28*, 148–151.

383. Loro, B., & Woodward, J. A. The dependence of psychiatric diagnosis on psychological assessment. *Journal of Clinical Psychology*, 1975, *31*, 635–639.

384. Lorr, M., & Gilberstadt, H. A comparison of two typologies for psychotics. *Journal of Nervous and Mental Disease*, 1972, *155*, 144–148.

385. Lottman, T. J., Davis, W. E., and Gustafson, R. C. MMPI correlates with locus of control in a psychiatric population. *Journal of Personality Assessment*, 1973, *37*, 78–82.

386. Louks, J., Caslyn, D., & Lindsay, F. Personality dysfunction and lateralized deficits in cerebral functions as measured by the MMPI and Reitan-Halstead Battery. *Perceptual and Motor Skills*, 1976, *43*, 655–659.

387. Lowe, W. C., & Thomas, S. D. Assessing alcoholism treatment effectiveness: A comparison of three evaluation measures. *Journal of Studies on Alcohol*, 1976, *37*, 883–889.

388. Ludwig, A. M., Brandsma, J. M., Wilbur, C. B., Bendfeldt, F., & Jameson, D. N. The objective study of a multiple personality: Or, are four heads better than one? *Archives of General Psychiatry*, 1972, *26*, 298–310.

389. Lunneborg, P. W. Dimensionality of MF. *Journal of Clinical Psychology*, 1972, *28*, 313–317.

390. Lushene, R. E., O'Neil, H. F., Jr., & Dunn, T. Equivalent validity of a completely computerized MMPI. *Journal of Personality Assessment*, 1974, *38*, 353–361.

391. Machota, P., Ott, J. E., Moore, V., Dungy, C., & Fine, L. Predictors of clinical performance of child health associates. *Journal of Allied Health*, 1975, *4*, 25–31.

392. Mallory, C. H., & Walker, C. E. MMPI O-H Scale responses of assaultive and nonassaultive pris-

oners and associated life history variables. *Educational and Psychological Measurement*, 1972, *32*, 1125–1128.

393. Malmquist, A., Kopfstein, J. H., Frank, E. T., Picklesimer, K., Clements, G., Ginn, E., Cromwell, R. L. Factors in psychiatric prediction of patients beginning hemodialysis: A follow-up of 13 patients. *Journal of Psychosomatic Research*, 1972, *16*, 19.

394. Markel, N. N., Phillis, J. A., Vargas, R., & Howard, K. Personality traits associafed with voice types. *Journal of Psycholinguistic Research*, 1972, *1*, 249–255.

395. Marsella, A. J., Sanborn, K. O., Kameoka, V., Shizuru, L., & Brennan, J. Cross-validation of depression among normal populations of Japanese, Chinese, and Caucasian ancestry. *Journal of Clinical Psychology*, 1975, *31*, 281–287.

396. Marsh, G. G. Parkinsonian patients' scores on Hovey's MMPI scale for CNS disorder. *Journal of Clinical Psychology*, 1972, *28*, 529–530.

397. Martin, P. J., & Sterne, A. L. Prognostic expectations and treatment outcome. *Journal of Consulting and Clinical Psychology*, 1975, *43*, 572–576.

398. Martin, P. J., & Sterne, A. L. Subjective objectivity: Therapists' affection and psychotherapy. *Psychological Reports*, 1976, *38*, 1163–1169.

399. Martin, P. J., Sterne, A. L., Moore, J. E., & Friedmeyer, M. H. Patient's and therapists' expectancies and treatment outcome: An elusive relationship reexamined. *Research Communications in Psychology, Psychiatry and Behavior*, 1976, *1*, 301–314.

400. Martin, W. R., Jasinski, D. R., Haertzen, C. A., Kay, D. C., Jones, B. E., Mansky, P. A., & Carpenter, R. W. Methadone—A reevaluation. *Archives of General Psychiatry*, 1973, *28*, 286–295.

401. Maskin, M. B., Riklan, M., & Chabot, D. A preliminary study of selected emotional changes in Parkinsonians on L-dopa therapy. *Journal of Clinical Psychology*, 1972, *28*, 604–605.

402. Maskin, M. B., Riklan, M., & Chabot, D. Emotional functions in short-term vs. long-term L-dopa therapy in Parkinsonism. *Journal of Clinical Psychology*, 1973, *29*, 493–495.

403. Match, J., & Wiggins, N. Individual viewpoints of social desirability related to faking good and desirability estimation. *Educational and Psychological Measurement*, 1974, *34*, 591–606.

404. Matefy, R. E., & Krall, R. G. An initial investigation of the psychedelic drug flashback phenomena. *Journal of Consulting and Clinical Psychology*, 1974, *42*, 854–860.

405. Matefy, R. E., & Krall, R. Psychedelic drug flashbacks: Psychotic manifestation or imaginative role playing? *Journal of Consulting and Clinical Psychology*, 1975, *43*, 434.

406. Maudal, G. R., Butcher, J. N., & Mauger, P. A. A multivariate study of personality and academic factors in college attrition. *Journal of Counseling Psychology*, 1974, *21*, 560–567.

407. McAdoo, W. G. The application of Goldberg's classification rules to parents in a child guidance clinic and in an adult psychiatric clinic. *Journal of Community Psychology*, 1974, *2*, 174–175.

408. McAdoo, W. G., & Connolly, F. J. MMPIs of parents in dysfunctional families. *Journal of Consulting and Clinical Psychology*, 1975, *43*, 270.

409. McAdoo, W. G., & Roeske, N. A. A comparison of defectors and continuers in a child guidance clinic. *Journal of Consulting and Clinical Psychology*, 1973, *40*, 328–334.

410. McAree, C. P., Steffenhagen, R. A., & Zheutlin, L. S. Personality factors and patterns of drug usage in college students. *American Journal of Psychiatry*, 1972, *128*, 890–893.

411. McCabe, O. L., Savage, C., Karland, A., & Unger, S. Psychedelic (LSD) therapy of neurotic disorders: Short term effects. *Journal of Psychedelic Drugs*, 1972, *5*, 19–28.

412. McCall, R. J. MMPI factors that differentiate remediably from irremediably obese women. *Journal of Community Psychology*, 1973, *1*, 34–36.

413. McCall, R. J. Group therapy with obese women of varying MMPI profiles. *Journal of Clinical Psychology*, 1974, *30*, 466–470.

414. McCraw, R. K., & White, R. B., Jr. Social introversion-extraversion and Rorschach human responses in adult psychiatric patients. *Psychological Reports*, 1974, *35*, 932–934.

415. McCreary, C. P. Personality differences among child molesters. *Journal of Personality Assessment*, 1975, *39*, 591–593.

416. McCreary, C. P. Personality profiles of persons convicted of indecent exposure. *Journal of Clinical Psychology*, 1975, *31*, 260–262.

417. McDonald, D. G., Shallenberger, H. D., Koresko, R. L., & Kinzy, B. G. Studies of spontaneous electrodermal responses in sleep. *Psychophysiology*, 1976, *13*, 128–134.

418. McGlothlin, W., Cohen, S., & McGlothlin, M. S. Long lasting effects of LSD on normals. *Archives of General Psychiatry*, 1967, *17*, 521–532.

525

OBJECTIVE
PERSONALITY
INVENTORIES:
RECENT RESEARCH
AND SOME
CONTEMPORARY
ISSUES

419. McGuire, J. S., & Megargee, E. J. Personality correlates of marijuana use among youthful offenders. *Journal of Consulting and Clinical Psychology*, 1974, *42*, 124–133.

420. McKay, M. J., & Richardson, H. Personality differences between one-time and recidivist unwed mothers. *Journal of Genetic Psychology*, 1973, *122*, 207–210.

421. McLachlan, J. F. Classification of alcoholics by an MMPI actuarial system. *Journal of Clinical Psychology*, 1975, *31*, 145–147.

422. McLachlan, J. F. An MMPI discriminant function to distinguish alcoholics from narcotic addicts: Effects of age, sex, and psychopathology. *Journal of Clinical Psychology*, 1975, *31*, 163–165.

423. McLachlan, J. F. C. Revised scale for estimating ability to judge complex behavior. *Perceptual and Motor Skills*, 1972, *35*, 250.

424. McLachlan, J. F. C. A hostility scale for Form R of the MMPI. *Journal of Clinical Psychology*, 1974, *30*, 369–371.

425. McLachlan, J. F. C. Test-retest stability of long and short MMPI scales over two years. *Journal of Clinical Psychology*, 1974, *30*, 189–191.

426. McMahon, A. W., Schmitt, P., Patterson, J. F., & Rothman, E. Personality differences between inflammatory bowel disease patients and their healthy siblings. *Psychosomatic Medicine*, 1973, *35*, 91–103.

427. Megargee, E. I. Recent research on overcontrolled and undercontrolled personality patterns among violent offenders. *Sociological Symposium*, 1973, No. 9, 37–50.

428. Megargee, E. I., & Cook, P. E. Negative response bias and the MMPI overcontrolled-hostility scale: A response to Deiker. *Journal of Consulting and Clinical Psychology*, 1975, *43*, 725–729.

429. Meikle, S., & Gerritse, R. A comparison of husband-wife responses to pregnancy. *Journal of Psychology*, 1973, *83*, 17–23.

430. Melnick, B. Patient-therapist identification in relation to both patient and therapist variables and therapy outcome. *Journal of Consulting and Clinical Psychology*, 1972, *38*, 97–104.

431. Mendels, J., Weinstein, N., & Cochrane, C. The relationship between depression and anxiety. *Archives of General Psychiatry*, 1972, *27*, 649–653.

432. Mendelsohn, G. A., & Lindholm, E. P. Individual differences and the role of attention in the use of cues in verbal problem solving. *Journal of Personality*, 1972, *40*, 226–241.

433. Merbaum, M., & Hefez, A. Some personality characteristics of soldiers exposed to extreme war stress. *Journal of Consulting and Clinical Psychology*, 1976, *44*, 1–6.

434. Messick, S., & Jackson, D. N. Judgmental dimensions of psychopathology. *Journal of Consulting and Clinical Psychology*, 1972, *38*, 418–427.

435. Mezzich, J. E., Damarin, F. L., & Erickson, J. R. Comparative validity of strategies and indices for differential diagnosis of depressive states from other psychiatric conditions using the MMPI. *Journal of Consulting and Clinical Psychology*, 1974, *42*, 691–698.

436. Miller, W. H., & Gottlieb, F. Predicting behavioral treatment outcome in disturbed children: A preliminary report on the Responsibility Index of Parents (RIP). *Behavior Therapy*, 1974, *5*, 210–214.

437. Merbaum, M. Simulation of normal MMPI profiles by repressors and sensitizers. *Journal of Consulting and Clinical Psychology*, 1972, *39*, 171.

438. Millimet, C. R., & Cohen, H. J. A test of the homogeneous versus heterogeneous categorization of the repression-sensitization dimension. *Educational and Psychological Measurement*, 1973, *33*, 773–785.

439. Mlott, S. R. Some significant relationships between adolescents and their parents as revealed by the MMPI. *Adolescence*, 1972, *7*, 169–182.

440. Mlott, S. R. The Mini-Mult and its use with adolescents. *Journal of Clinical Psychology*, 1973, *29*, 376–377.

441. Mlott, S. R. Degree of agreement among MMPI scores, self-ratings, and staff ratings of inpatient adolescents. *Journal of Clinical Psychology*, 1973, *29*, 480–481.

442. Mlott, S. R., & Mason, R. L. The practicability of using an abbreviated form of the MMPI with chronic renal dialysis patients. *Journal of Clinical Psychology*, 1975, *31*, 65–68.

443. Montague, D. J., & Prytula, R. E. Human figure drawing characteristics related to juvenile delinquents. *Perceptual and Motor Skills*, 1975, *40*, 623–630.

444. Morf, M. E. & Jackson, D. N. An analysis of two response styles: True responding and item endorsement. *Educational and Psychological Measurement*, 1972, *32*, 329–353.

445. Morgan, D. W., Weitzel, W. D., Guyden, T. E., Robinson, J. A., & Hedlund, J. L. Comparing MMPI statements and mental status items. *American Journal of Psychiatry*, 1972, *129*, 693–697.

446. Morris, L. A., & Shapiro, A. K. MMPI scores for field-dependent and field-independent psychiatric outpatients. *Journal of Consulting and Clinical Psychology*, 1974, *42*, 364–369.

447. Mott, J. The psychological basis of drug dependence: The intellectual and personality characteristics of opiate users. *British Journal of Addiction*, 1972, *67*, 89–100.

448. Moxley, A. W. Clinical judgment: The effects of statistical information. *Journal of Personality Assessment*, 1973, *37*, 86–91.

449. Mozdzierz, G. J., Macchitelli, F. J., & Lottman, T. J. Personality correlates of coffee consumption in an alcoholic population. *Psychological Reports*, 1973, *32*, 550.

450. Mozdzierz, G. J., Macchitelli, F. J., Conway, J. A., & Krauss, H. H. Personality characteristic differences between alcoholics who leave treatment against medical advice and those who don't. *Journal of Clinical Psychology*, 1973, *29*, 78–82.

451. Mozdzierz, G. J., Macchitelli, F. J., Planek, T. W., & Lottman, T. J. Personality and temperament differences between alcoholics with high and low records of traffic accidents and violations. *Journal of Studies on Alcohol*, 1975, *36*, 395–399.

452. Muha, T. M., & May, J. R. An employment index for identifying unfit job applicants. *Journal of Community Psychology*, 1973, *1*, 362–365.

453. Munjack, D. J., & Staples, F. R. Psychological characteristics of women with sexual inhibition (frigidity) in sex clinics. *Journal of Nervous and Mental Disease*, 1976, *163*, 117–123.

454. Murray, L., Heritage, J., & Holmes, W. Black-white comparisons of the MMPI Mini-Mult. *Southern Journal of Educational Research*, 1976, *10*, 105–114.

455. Naditch, M. P. Ego functioning and acute adverse reactions to psychoactive drugs. *Journal of Personality*, 1975, *43*, 305–320.

456. Neuringer, C., Dombrowski, P. S., & Goldstein, G. Cross-validation of an MMPI scale of differential diagnosis of brain damage from schizophrenia. *Journal of Clinical Psychology*, 1975, *31*, 268–271.

457. Newmark, C. S., Boas, B., & Messervy, T. An abbreviated MMPI for use with college students. *Psychological Reports*, 1974, *34*, 631–634.

458. Newmark, C. S., Conger, A. J., & Faschingbauer, T. R. The interpretive validity and effective test length functioning of an abbreviated MMPI relative to the standard MMPI. *Journal of Clinical Psychology*, 1976, *32*, 27–32.

459. Newmark, C. S., Cook, L., Clarke, M., & Faschingbauer, T. R. Application of Faschingbauer's abbreviated MMPI to psychiatric inpatients. *Journal of Consulting and Clinical Psychology*, 1973, *41*, 416–421.

460. Newmark, C. S., Cook, L., & Greer, W. Application of the Midi-Mult to psychiatric inpatients. *Journal of Clinical Psychology*, 1973, *29*, 481–484.

461. Newmark, C. S., Falk, R., & Finch, A. J. Interpretive accuracy of abbreviated MMPIs. *Journal of Personality Assessment*, 1976, *40*, 10–12.

462. Newmark, C. S., Faschingbauer, T. R., Finch, A. J., & Kendall, P. C. Factor analysis of the MMPI-STAI. *Journal of Clinical Psychology*, 1975, *31*, 449–452.

463. Newmark, C. S., & Finch, A. J. Comparing the diagnostic validity of an abbreviated and standard MMPI. *Journal of Personality Assessment*, 1976, *40*, 10–12.

464. Newmark, C. S., & Finkelstein, M. Maximizing classification rates of Marks and Seeman code types. *Journal of Clinical Psychology*, 1973, *29*, 61–62.

465. Newmark, C. S., Galen, R., & Gold, K. Efficacy of an abbreviated MMPI as a function of type of administration. *Journal of Clinical Psychology*, 1975, *31*, 639–642.

466. Newmark, C. S., & Glenn, L. Sensitivity of the Faschingbauer Abbreviated MMPI to hospitalized adolescents. *Journal of Abnormal Child Psychology*, 1974, *2*, 299–306.

467. Newmark, C. S., Hetzel, W., & Frerking, R. A. The effects of personality tests on state and trait anxiety. *Journal of Personality Assessment*, 1974, *38*, 17–20.

468. Newmark, C. S., Newmark, L., & Cook, L. The MMPI-168 with psychiatric patients. *Journal of Clinical Psychology*, 1975, *31*, 61–64.

469. Newmark, C. S., Newmark, L., & Faschingbauer, T. R. Utility of three abbreviated MMPIs with psychiatric out-patients. *Journal of Nervous and Mental Disease*, 1974, *159*, 438–443.

470. Newmark, C. S., Owen, M., Newmark, L., & Faschingbauer, T. R. Comparison of three abbreviated MMPIs for psychiatric patients and normals. *Journal of Personality Assessment*, 1975, *39*, 261–270.

471. Newmark, C. S., & Raft, D. Using an abbreviated MMPI as a screening device for medical patients. *Psychosomatics*, 1976, *17*, 45–48.

472. Newmark, C. S., Raft, D., Toomey, T., Hunter, W., & Mazzaglia, J. Diagnosis of schizophrenia: Pathognomic signs or symptom clusters. *Comprehensive Psychiatry*, 1975, *16*, 155–163.

473. Newmark, C. S., Ray, J., Lyman, R. A. F., & Paine, R. D. Test-induced anxiety as a function of psychopathology. *Journal of Clinical Psychology*, 1974, *30*, 261–264.

474. Newmark, C. S., & Sines, L. K. Characteristics of hospitalized patients who produce "floating" MMPI profiles. *Journal of Clinical Psychology*, 1972, *28*, 74–76.

475. Newmark, C. S., & Toomey, T. The MF scale as an index of disturbed marital interaction: A replication. *Psychological Reports*, 1972, *31*, 590.

476. Newton, M., & Krauss, H. H. The health-engenderingness of resident assistants as related to student achievement and adjustment. *Journal of College Student Personnel*, 1973, *14*, 321–325.

477. Neziroglu, F. The relationships among the Hoffer-Osmond Diagnostic Test, the MMPI, and independent clinical diagnoses. *Journal of Clinical Psychology*, 1975, *31*, 430–433.

478. Nichols, D. S. The Goldberg Rules in the detection of MMPI codebook modal diagnoses. *Journal of Clinical Psychology*, 1974, *30*, 186–188.

479. Nichols, M. P. Outcome of brief cathartic psychotherapy. *Journal of Consulting and Clinical Psychotherapy*, 1974, *42*, 403–410.

480. Nichols, M. P., Gordon, T. P., & Levine, M. D. Development and validation of the Life Style Questionnaire. *Journal of Social Psychology*, 1972, *86*, 121–125.

481. Norton, J. C. Patterns of neuropsychological test performance in Huntington's disease. *Journal of Nervous and Mental Disease*, 1975, *161*, 276–279.

482. Ogilvie, L. P., Kotin, J., & Stanley, D. H. Comparison of the MMPI and the Mini-Mult in a psychiatric outpatient clinic. *Journal of Consulting and Clinical Psychology*, 1976, *44*, 497–498.

483. Oldroyd, R. J. A principle components analysis of the BPI and MMPI. *Criminal Justice and Behavior*, 1975, *2*, 85–90.

484. Oldroyd, R. J., Pappas, J. P., & Hart, D. A comparison of three personality inventories as screening instruments to select effective teachers. *Journal of Student Personnel Association and Teaching Education*, 1973, *12*, 45–53.

485. O'Leary, M. R., Donovan, D. M., & Hague, W. H. Relationships between locus of control and MMPI scales among alcoholics: A replication and extension. *Journal of Clinical Psychology*, 1974, *30*, 312–314.

486. O'Neil, H. F., Teague, M., Lushene, R. E., & Davenport, S. Personality characteristics of women's liberation activists as measured by the MMPI. *Psychological Reports*, 1975, *37*, 355–361.

487. Oshman, H., & Manosevitz, M. The impact of the identity crisis on the adjustment of late adolescent males. *Journal of Youth and Adolescence*, 1974, *3*, 207–216.

488. Overall, J. E. Comparison of error rates associated with alternative MMPI profile classification schemes. *Educational and Psychological Measurement*, 1973, *33*, 255–266.

489. Overall, J. E. MMPI personality patterns of alcoholics and narcotic addicts. *Quarterly Journal of Studies on Alcohol*, 1973, *34*, 104–111.

490. Overall, J. E. Actuarial methods in the diagnosis of schizophrenia. *Phenomenology and Treatment of Schizophrenia*, in press.

491. Overall, J. E., Brown, D., Williams, J. D., & Neill, L. T. Drug treatment of anxiety and depression in detoxified alcoholic patients. *Archives of General Psychiatry*, 1973, *29*, 218–221.

492. Overall, J. E., Butcher, J. N., & Hunter, S. Validity of the MMPI-168 for psychiatric screening. *Educational and Psychological Measurement*, 1975, *35*, 393–400.

493. Overall, J. E., & Gomez-Mont, F. The MMPI-168 for psychiatric screening. *Educational and Psychological Measurement*, 1974, *34*, 315–319.

494. Overall, J. E., & Higgins, C. W. An application of actuarial methods in psychiatric diagnosis. *Journal of Clinical Psychology*, in press.

495. Overall, J. E., Higgins, C. W., & De Schweinitz, A. Comparison of differential diagnostic discrimination for abbreviated and standard MMPI. *Journal of Clinical Psychology*, 1976, *32*, 237–245.

496. Overall, J. E., Hunter, S., & Butcher, J. N. Factor structure of the MMPI-168 in a psychiatric population. *Journal of Consulting and Clinical Psychology*, 1973, *41*, 284–286.

497. Overall, J. E., & Patrick, J. H. Unitary alcoholism factor and its personality correlates. *Journal of Abnormal Psychology*, 1972, *79*, 303–309.

498. Pallis, D. J., & Birtchnell, J. Personality and suicidal history in psychiatric patients. *Journal of Clinical Psychology*, 1976, *32*, 246–253.

499. Palmer, A. B. A comparison of the MMPI and Mini-Mult in a sample of state mental hospital patients. *Journal of Clinical Psychology*, 1973, *29*, 484–485.

500. Pandey, R. E. Personality characteristics of successful, dropout, and probationary black and white university students. *Journal of Counseling Psychology*, 1972, *19*, 382–386.

527

OBJECTIVE
PERSONALITY
INVENTORIES:
RECENT RESEARCH
AND SOME
CONTEMPORARY
ISSUES

501. Panton, J. H. Personality characteristics of management problem prison inmates. *Journal of Community Psychology*, 1973, *1*, 185-191.

502. Panton, J. H. Personality differences between male and female prison inmates measured by the MMPI. *Criminal Justice and Behavior*, 1974, *1*, 332–339.

503. Panton, J. H. Personality characteristics of death-row prison inmates. *Journal of Clinical Psychology*, 1976, *32*, 306–309.

504. Panton, J. H. Significant increase in MMPI Mf scores within a state prison population. *Journal of Clinical Psychology*, 1976, *32*, 604–606.

505. Panton, J. H., & Behre, C. Characteristics associated with drug addiction within a state prison population. *Journal of Community Psychology*, 1973, *1*, 411–416.

506. Pardue, L. H. Familial unipolar depressive illness: A pedigree study. *American Journal of Psychiatry*, 1975, *132*, 970–972.

507. Paredes, A., Gregory, D., & Jones, B. M. Induced drinking and social adjustment in alcoholics: Development of a therapeutic model. *Quarterly Journal of Studies on Alcohol*, 1974, *35*, 1279–1293.

508. Pattison, E. M., Lapins, N. A., & Doerr, H. A. Faith healing: A study of personality and function. *Journal of Nervous and Mental Disease*, 1973, *157*, 397–409.

509. Patton, G. W. R., & Kotrick, C. A. Visual exploratory behavior as a function of manifest anxiety. *Journal of Psychology*, 1972, *82*, 349–353.

510. Paulson, M. J., Afifi, A., Chaleff, A., Thomason, M., & Lui, V. An MMPI scale for identifying at risk abusive parents. *Journal of Clinical Child Psychology*, 1975, *4*, 22–24.

511. Paulson, M. J., Afifi, A., Thomason, M. L., & Chaleff, A. The MMPI: A descriptive measure of psychopathology in abusive parents. *Journal of Clinical Psychology*, 1974, *30*, 387–390.

512. Paulson, M. J., Schwemer, G. T., & Bendel, R. B. Clinical application of the *Pd*, *Ma*, and (OH) experimental MMPI scales to further understanding of abusive parents. *Journal of Clinical Psychology*, 1976, *32*, 558–564.

513. Payne, F. D., & Wiggins, J. S. MMPI profile types and the self-report of psychiatric patients. *Journal of Abnormal Psychology*, 1972, *79*, 1–8.

514. Penk, W. E., & Robinowitz, R. Personality differences of volunteer and nonvolunteer heroin and nonheroin drug users. *Journal of Abnormal Psychology*, 1976, *85*, 91–100.

515. Penner, L. A., Summers, L. S., Brookmire, D. A., & Dertke, M. S. The lost dollar: Situational and personality determinants of a pro- and antisocial behavior. *Journal of Personality*, 1976, *44*, 274–293.

516. Percell, L. P., & Delk, J. L. Relative usefulness of three forms of the Mini-Mult with college students. *Journal of Consulting and Clinical Psychology*, 1973, *40*, 487.

517. Perez-Reyes, M. G., & Falk, R. Follow-up after therapeutic abortion in early adolescence. *Archives of General Psychiatry*, 1973, *28*, 120–126.

518. Perkins, C. W. Some correlates of Category Test scores for nonorganic psychiatric patients. *Journal of Clinical Psychology*, 1974, *30*, 176–178.

519. Persky, H. Tetrahydrocortisol/tetrahydrocortisone ratio (H-sub-4F/H-sub-4E) as an indicator of depressive feelings. *Psychosomatic Medicine*, 1976, *38*, 13–18.

520. Petroni, F. A. Correlates of the psychiatric sick role. *Journal of Health and Social Behavior*, 1972, *13*, 47–54.

521. Phillips, B. J., Phillips, I. F., & Davidson, E. E. Juvenile delinquent drug abuse in females: A clinical study. *Australian and New Zealand Journal of Psychiatry*, 1975, *9*, 281-286.

522. Pierce, D. M. Test and nontest correlates of active and situational homosexuality. *Psychology*, 1973, *10*, 23–26.

523. Pierce, D. M., Freeman, R., Lawton, R., & Fearing, M. Psychological correlates of chronic hemodialysis estimated by MMPI scores. *Psychology*, 1973, *10*, 53–57.

524. Pierce, D. M. Freeman, R., Lawton, R., & Fearing, M. Longitudinal stability of psychological status of hemodialysis patients. *Psychology*, 1973, *10*, 66–69.

525. Pierloot, R. A., Wellens, W., & Houben, M. E. Elements of resistance to a combined medical and psychotherapeutic program in anorexia nervosa: An overview. *Psychotherapy and Psychosomatics*, 1975, *26*, 101–117.

526. Platt, J. J., & Scura, W. C. Validity of the Mini-Mult with male reformatory inmates. *Journal of Clinical Psychology*, 1972, *28*, 528–529.

527. Poeldinger, W. J., Gehring, A., & Blaser, P. Suicide risk and MMPI scores, especially as related to anxiety and depression. *Life-Threatening Behavior*, 1973, *3*, 147–153.

528. Powell, A., & Gable, P. Adult locus of control and self-righteous attitudes. *Psychological Reports*, 1973, *32*, 302.

529. Powell, L., Cameron, H. K., Asbury, C. A., & Johnson, E. H. Some characteristics of a special urban educational program. *Journal of Negro Education*, 1975, *44*, 361–367.

530. Powell, L., & Johnson, E. H. The black MMPI profile: Interpretive problems. *Journal of Negro Education*, 1976, *45*, 27–36.

531. Prager, R. A., & Garfield, S. L. Client initial disturbance and outcome in psychotherapy. *Journal of Consulting and Clinical Psychology*, 1972, *38*, 112–117.

532. Price, R. H., & Curlee-Salisbury, J. Patient-treatment interaction among alcoholics. *Journal of Studies on Alcohol*, 1975, *36*, 659–669.

533. Pugliese, A. C. A study of methadone maintenance patients with the MMPI. *British Journal of Addiction*, 1975, *70*, 198–204.

534. Rae, J. B. The influence of the wives on the treatment outcome of alcoholics: A follow-up study at two years. *British Journal of Psychiatry*, 1972, *120*, 601–613.

535. Rapfogel, R. G., & Armentrout, J. A. Inner- versus other-directedness and hypomanic tendencies in a nonpsychiatric population. *Journal of Clinical Psychology*, 1972, *28*, 526–527.

536. Rawlings, M. L. Self-control and interpersonal violence: A study of Scottish adolescent male severe offenders. *Criminology*, 1973, *11*, 23–48.

537. Reitan, R. M. MMPI studies in brain damage. *Annual Review of Psychology*, 1976, *27*, 204–208.

538. Rennick, P. M. Psychosocial evaluation of individuals with epilepsy. In G. N. Wright (Ed.), *Epilepsy rehabilitation*. Boston: Little, Brown, 1975.

539. Resnick, R., Orlin, L., Geyer, G., Schuyten-Resnick, E., Kestenbaum, R. S., & Freedman, A. M. L-Alpha-acetylmethadol (LAAM): Prognostic considerations. *American Journal of Psychiatry*, 1976, *133*, 814–819.

540. Reynolds, W. M., & Sundberg, N. D. Recent research trends in testing. *Journal of Personality Assessment*, 1976, *40*, 228–233.

541. Rhodes, R. J. Failure to validate an MMPI headache scale. *Journal of Clinical Psychology*, 1973, *29*, 237–238.

542. Rice, J. A. The psychodiagnostic profile. *Journal of Special Education*, 1974, *8*, 193–203.

543. Rice, L. N., & Gaylin, N. L. Personality processes reflected in client vocal style and Rorschach performance. *Journal of Consulting and Clinical Psychology*, 1973, *40*, 133–138.

544. Rice, R. G., & Narus, L. R., Jr. The WAIS vocabulary subscale as a reading test. *Newsletter of Research in Mental Health and Behavioral Science*, 1975, *17*, 12–13.

545. Richards, J. M., Jr., Calkins, E. V., McCanse, A., & Burgess, M. M. Predicting performance in a combined undergraduate and medical education program. *Educational and Psychological Measurement*, 1974, *34*, 923–931.

546. Riklan, M., Halgin, R., Maskin, M., & Weissman, D. Psychological studies of longer range L-dopa therapy in Parkinsonism. *Journal of Nervous and Mental Disease*, 1973, *157*, 452–464.

547. Rios-Garcia, L. R., & Cook, P. E. Self-derogation and defense style in college students. *Journal of Personality Assessment*, 1975, *39*, 273–281.

548. Ritter, D. R. Concurrence of psychiatric diagnosis and psychological diagnosis on the MMPI. *Journal of Personality Assessment*, 1974, *38*, 52–54.

549. Roback, H. B., & Strassberg, D. S. Relationship between perceived therapist-offered conditions and therapeutic movement in group psychotherapy. *Small Group Behavior*, 1975, *6*, 345–352.

550. Roback, H. B., Webb, W. W., & Strassberg, D. Personality differences between fee-paying and non-fee-paying patients seen for psychological testing. *Journal of Consulting and Clinical Psychology*, 1974, *42*, 734.

551. Rodgers, D. A., & Ziegler, F. J. Social role theory, the marital relationship, and the use of ovulation suppressors. *Journal of Marriage and Family*, 1968, *30*, 584–591.

552. Rodin, E. A., Rim, C. S., Kitano, H., Lewis, R., & Rennick, P. M. A comparison of the effectiveness of primadone versus carbamazepine in epileptic outpatient. *Journal of Nervous and Mental Disease*, 1976, *163*, 41–46.

553. Rogers, R., & Wright, E. W. Behavioral rigidity and its relationship to authoritarianism and obsessive-compulsiveness. *Perceptual and Motor Skills*, 1975, *40*, 802.

554. Rohan, W. P. MMPI changes in hospitalized alcoholics: A second study. *Quarterly Journal of Studies on Alcohol*, 1972, *33*, 65–76.

555. Roll, S., & Hertel, P. Arrow-dot measures of impulse, ego, and superego functions in noncheaters, cheaters, and super cheaters. *Perceptual and Motor Skills*, 1974, *39*, 1035–1038.

556. Rosen, A. C. Brief report of MMPI characteristics of sexual deviation. *Psychological Reports*, 1974, *35*, 73–74.

529

OBJECTIVE
PERSONALITY
INVENTORIES:
RECENT RESEARCH
AND SOME
CONTEMPORARY
ISSUES

557. Rosen, A. C., & Golden, J. S. The encounter-sensitivity training group as an adjunct to medical education. *International Review of Applied Psychology*, 1975, *24*, 61–70.

558. Rosenberg, N. MMPI alcoholism scales. *Journal of Clinical Psychology*, 1972, *28*, 515–522.

559. Rosenbluh, E. S., Owens, G. B., & Pohler, M. J. Art preference and personality. *British Journal of Psychology*, 1972, *63*, 441–443.

560. Ross, M. W. Relationship between sex role and sex orientation in homosexual men. *New Zealand Psychologist*, 1975, *4*, 25–29.

561. Ross, S. M. Fear, reinforcing activities and degree of alcoholism: A correlational analysis. *Quarterly Journal of Studies on Alcohol*, 1973, *34*, 823–828.

562. Ross, W. F., & Berzins, J. I. Personality characteristics of female narcotic addicts on the MMPI. *Psychological Reports*, 1974, *35*, 779–784.

563. Ross, W. F., McReynolds, W. T., & Berzins, J. I. Effectiveness of marathon group psychotherapy with hospitalized female narcotic addicts. *Psychological Reports*, 1974, *34*, 611–616.

564. Roth, M., Gurney, C., Garside, R. F., & Kerr, T. A. Studies in the classification of affective disorders: The relationship between anxiety states and depressive illnesses—I. *British Journal of Psychiatry*, 1972, *121*, 147–161.

565. Roth, T., Kramer, M., & Lutz, T. The nature of insomnia: A descriptive summary of a sleep clinic population. *Comprehensive Psychiatry*, 1976, *17*, 217–220.

566. Routh, D. K., & Keller, W. Instructions, word association, and the hospitalized psychiatric patient. *Psychological Reports*, 1973, *32*, 579–585.

567. Ruff, C. F., Ayers, J., & Templer, D. I. Alcoholics' and criminals' similarity of scores on the Mac-Andrew alcoholism scale. *Psychological Reports*, 1975, *36*, 921–922.

568. Russell, E. W. Validation of a brain damage vs. schizophrenia MMPI key. *Journal of Clinical Psychology*, 1975, *31*, 659–661.

569. Ryan, D. V., & Neale, J. M. Test-taking sets and the performance of schizophrenics on laboratory tests. *Journal of Abnormal Psychology*, 1973, *82*, 207–211.

570. Rybolt, G. A., & Lambert, J. A. Correspondence of the MMPI and Mini-Mult with psychiatric inpatients. *Journal of Clinical Psychology*, 1975, *31*, 279–281.

571. Rychlak, J. F. Time orientation in the positive and negative free phantasies of mildly abnormal versus normal high school males. *Journal of Consulting and Clinical Psychology*, 1973, *41*, 175–180.

572. Saccuzzo, D. P., Higgins, G., & Lewandowski, D. Program for psychological assessment of law enforcement officers: Initial evaluation. *Psychological Reports*, 1974, *35*, 651–654.

573. Sacks, J. M., & Kirtley, D. D. Some personality characteristics related to response to subtle and obvious items on the MMPI. *Journal of Consulting and Clinical Psychology*, 1972, *38*, 66–69.

574. Salzman, C., Lieff, J., Kochansky, G. E., & Shader, R. I. The psychology of hallucinogenic drug discontinuers. *American Journal of Psychiatry*, 1972, *129*, 755–761.

575. Sand, P. L. Performance of medical patient groups with and without brain damage on the Hovey (O) and Watson (Sc-O) MMPI scales. *Journal of Clinical Psychology*, 1973, *29*, 235–237.

576. Sappington, A., & Grizzard, R. Self-discrimination responses in black school children. *Journal of Personality and Social Psychology*, 1975, *31*, 224–231.

577. Sappington, A. A., & Michaux, M. H. Prognostic patterns in self-report, relative report, and professional evaluation measures for hospitalized and day-care patients. *Journal of Consulting and Clinical Psychology*, 1975, *43*, 904–910.

578. Sappington, J. Psychometric correlates of defensive style in process and reactive schizophrenics. *Journal of Consulting and Clinical Psychology*, 1975, *43*, 154–156.

579. Saunders, B. T., & Fenton, T. MMPI profiles of child care applicants at a children's residential treatment center. *Devereux Forum*, 1975, *10*, 16–19.

580. Saunders, T. R., Jr., & Gravitz, M. A. Sex differences in the endorsement of MMPI critical items. *Journal of Clinical Psychology*, 1974, *30*, 557–558.

581. Scagnelli, J. The significance of dependency in the paranoid syndrome. *Journal of Clinical Psychology*, 1975, *31*, 29–34.

582. Schinka, J. A., & Sines, J. O. Correlates of accuracy in personality assessment. *Journal of Clinical Psychology*, 1974, *30*, 374–377.

583. Schless, A. P., Mendels, J., Kipperman, A., & Cochrane, C. Depression and hostility. *Journal of Nervous and Mental Disease*, 1974, *159*, 91–100.

584. Schmidt, R. T. Personality and fainting. *Journal of Psychosomatic Research*, 1975, *19*, 21–25.

585. Schneider, L. J., & Cherry, P. MMPI patterns of college males from 1969 to 1973. *Journal of College Student Personnel*, 1976, *17*, 417–419.

531

OBJECTIVE
PERSONALITY
INVENTORIES:
RECENT RESEARCH
AND SOME
CONTEMPORARY
ISSUES

586. Schonfield, J. Psychological and life-experience differences between Israeli women with benign and cancerous breast lesions. *Journal of Psychosomatic Research*, 1975, *19*, 229–234.

587. Schonfield, J. Psychological factors related to delayed return to an earlier life-style in successfully treated cancer patients. *Journal of Psychosomatic Research*, 1976, *20*, 41–46.

588. Schonfield, J., & Donner, L. The effect of serving as a psychologist on students with different specialty preferences. *Journal of Medical Education*, 1972, *47*, 203–209.

589. Schoolar, J. C., White, E. H., & Cohen, C. P. Drug abusers and their clinic-patient counterparts: A comparison of personality dimensions. *Journal of Consulting and Clinical Psychology*, 1972, *39*, 9–14.

590. Schubert, D. S. P. Increase of apparent adjustment in adolescence by further ego identity formation and age. *College Student Personnel Journal*, 1973, *7*, 3–5.

591. Schubert, D. S. P. Increase of personality consistency by prior response. *Journal of Clinical Psychology*, 1975, *31*, 651–658.

592. Schubert, D. S. P., & Fiske, D. W. Increase of item response consistency by prior item response. *Educational and Psychological Measurement*, 1973, *33*, 113–121.

593. Schubert, D. S. P., & Wagner, M. E. A subcultural change of MMPI norms in the 1960s due to adolescent role confusion and glamorization of alienation. *Journal of Abnormal Psychology*, 1975, *84*, 406–411.

594. Schubert, D. S. P., & Wagner, M. E. "A" therapists as creative and personally involved with other people. *Journal of Consulting and Clinical Psychology*, 1975, *43*, 266.

595. Schwartz, M. S. Separate versus full MMPI method: Reliability of the pseudoneurologic scale. *Journal of Clinical Psychology*, 1974, *30*, 79.

596. Schwartz, M. S. The Repression-Sensitization Scale: Normative, age, and sex data on 30,000 medical patients. *Journal of Clinical Psychology*, 1972, *28*, 72–73.

597. Schwartz, M. S., & Brown, J. R. MMPI differentiation of multiple sclerosis vs. pseudoneurologic patients. *Journal of Clinical Psychology*, 1973, *29*, 471–474.

598. Schwartz, M. S., Osborne, D., & Krupp, N. E. Moderating effects of age and sex on the association of medical diagnoses and 1-3/3-1 MMPI profiles. *Journal of Clinical Psychology*, 1972, *28*, 502–505.

599. Schwartz, S., & Giacoman, S. Convergent and discriminant validity of three measures of adjustment and three measures of social desirability. *Journal of Consulting and Clinical Psychology*, 1972, *39*, 239–242.

600. Scott, D. P., & Severance, L. J. Relationship between the CPI, MMPI, and locus of control in a non-academic environment. *Journal of Personality Assessment*, 1975, *39*, 141–145.

601. Scott, J., & Gaitz, C. Ethnic and age differences in mental health measurement. *Diseases of the Nervous System*, 1975, *36*, 389–393.

602. Scott, N. A., Mount, M. K., & Kosters, S. A. Correspondence of the MMPI and the Mini-Mult among female reformatory inmates. *Journal of Clinical Psychology*, 1976, *32*, 792–794.

603. Shader, R. I., & Harmatz, J. S. Molindone: A pilot evaluation during the premenstruum. *Current Therapeutic Research*, 1975, *17*, 403–406.

604. Shader, R. I., Harmatz, J. S., Kochansky, G. E., & Cole, J. O. Psychopharmacologic investigations in healthy elderly volunteers: Effects of pipradol-vitamin (Alertonic) elixir and placebo in relation to research design. *Journal of the American Geriatric Society*, 1975, *23*, 277–279.

605. Shaffer, J. W., Nussbaum, K., & Little, J. M. MMPI profiles of disability insurance claimants. *American Journal of Psychiatry*, 1972, *129*, 403–407.

606. Shapiro, A. K., Shapiro, E., Wayne, H., & Clarkin, J. The psychopathology of Gilles de la Tourette's syndrome. *American Journal of Psychiatry*, 1972, *129*, 427–434.

607. Shapiro, A. K., Struening, E., Shapiro, E., & Barten, H. Prognostic correlates of psychotherapy in psychiatric outpatients. *American Journal of Psychiatry*, 1976, *133*, 802–808.

608. Sharp, M. W., & Reilley, R. R. The relationship of aerobic physical fitness to selected personality traits. *Journal of Clinical Psychology*, 1975, *31*, 428–430.

609. Shaw, J. A., Donley, P., Morgan, D. W., & Robinson, J. A. Treatment of depression in alcoholics. *American Journal of Psychiatry*, 1975, *132*, 641–644.

610. Sheppard, C., Fracchia, J., Ricca, E., & Merlis, S. Indications of psychopathology in male narcotic abusers, their effects and relation to treatment effectiveness. *Journal of Psychology*, 1972, *81*, 351–360.

611. Sheppard, C., Ricca, E., Fracchia, J., & Merlis, S. Indications of psychopathology in applicants to a county methadone maintenance program. *Psychological Reports*, 1973, *33*, 535–540.

612. Sheppard, C., Ricca, E., Fracchia, J., & Merlis, S. Personality characteristics of urban and sub-urban heroin abusers: More data and another reply to Sutker and Allain. *Psychological Reports*, 1973, *33*, 999–1008.

613. Sheppard, C., Ricca, E., Fracchia, J., Rosenberg, N., & Merlis, S. Cross-validation of a heroin addiction scale from the MMPI. *Journal of Psychology*, 1972, *81*, 263–281.

614. Sherman, A. R. Real life exposure as a primary therapeutic factor in the desensitization treatment of fear. *Journal of Abnormal Psychology*, 1972, *79*, 19–28.

615. Shershow, J. C., King, A., & Robinson, S. Carbon dioxide sensitivity and personality. *Psychosomatic Medicine*, 1973, *35*, 155–160.

616. Shipley, C. R., & Fazio, A. F. Pilot study of a treatment for psychological depression. *Journal of Abnormal Psychology*, 1973, *82*, 372–376.

617. Shipman, W. G., Greene, C. S., & Laskin, D. M. Correlation of placebo responses and personality characteristics in myofascial pain-dysfunction (MPD) patients. *Journal of Psychosomatic Research*, 1974, *18*, 475–483.

618. Shore, R. E. A statistical note on "differential misdiagnosis of blacks and whites by the MMPI." *Journal of Personality Assessment*, 1976, *40*, 21–23.

619. Shows, W. D., Gentry, W. D., & Wyrick, L. C. Social constriction in psychiatric patients: A normative study. *American Journal of Psychiatry*, 1974, *131*, 1287–1288.

620. Shweder, R. A. How relevant is an individual difference theory of personality? *Journal of Personality*, 1975, *43*, 455–484.

621. Silver, S. N. Outpatient treatment for sexual offenders. *Social Work*, 1976, *21*, 134–140.

622. Simono, R. B. Comparison of the standard MMPI and the Mini-Mult in a university counseling center. *Educational and Psychological Measurement*, 1975, *35*, 401–404.

623. Siskind, G. Hovey's 5-item MMPI scale and psychiatric patients. *Journal of Clinical Psychology*, 1976, *32*, 50.

624. Skinner, H. A., Jackson, D. N., & Hoffmann, H. Alcoholic personality types: Identification and correlates. *Journal of Abnormal Psychology*, 1974, *83*, 658-666.

625. Slavney, P. R., & McHugh, P. R. The hysterical personality: An attempt at validation with the MMPI. *Archives of General Psychiatry*, 1975, *32*, 186–190.

626. Sloan, R. B., Staples, F. R., Cristol, A. H., Yorkston, N. J., & Whipple, K. Patient characteristics and outcome in psychotherapy and behavior therapy. *Journal of Consulting and Clinical Psychology*, 1976, *44*, 330–339.

627. Smith, R. C. Item ambiguity in the 16PF and MMPI: An assessment and comparison. *Journal of Consulting and Clinical Psychology*, 1972, *38*, 460.

628. Smukler, A. J., & Schiebel, D. Personality characteristics of exhibitionists. *Diseases of the Nervous System*, 1975, *36*, 600–603.

629. Snow, D. L., & Held, M. L. Relation between locus of control and the MMPI with obese female adolescents. *Journal of Clinical Psychology*, 1973, *29*, 24–25.

630. Solway, K. S., Hays, J. R., & Zieben, M. Personality characteristics of juvenile probation officers. *Journal of Community Psychology*, 1976, *4*, 152–156.

631. Soskin, R. A. The use of LSD in time-limited psychotherapy. *Journal of Nervous and Mental Disease*, 1973, *157*, 410–419.

632. Spielberger, C. D., Auerbach, S. M., Wadsworth, A. P., Dunn, T. M., & Taulbee, E. S. Emotional reactions to surgery. *Journal of Consulting and Clinical Psychology*, 1973, *40*, 33–38.

633. Stansell, V., Beutler, L. E., Neville, C. W., & Johnson, D. T. MMPI correlates of extreme field independence and field dependence in a psychiatric population. *Perceptual and Motor Skills*, 1975, *40*, 539–544.

634. Starbird, D. H., & Biller, H. B. An exploratory study of the interaction of cognitive complexity, dogmatism, and repression-sensitization among college students. *Journal of Genetic Psychology*, 1976, *128*, 227–232.

635. Steinmeyer, E. M. An experimental evaluation of self-descriptions of depressive symptoms by psychopathological groups. *Zeitschrift für experimentelle und angewandte Psychologie*, 1975, *22*, 290–315.

636. Steinmeyer, E. M. Investigation on the automatic taxonomy (cluster analysis) of FPI-test values within psychiatric practice. *Zeitschrift für experimentelle und angewandte Psychologie*, 1976, *23*, 140–150.

637. Stenson, H., Kleinmuntz, B., & Scott, B. Personality assessment as a signal detection task. *Journal of Consulting and Clinical Psychology*, 1975, *43*, 794–799.

638. Stephans, J. H., Harris, A. H., Brady, J. V., & Shaffer, J. W. Psychological and physiological variables associated with large magnitude voluntary heart rate changes. *Psychophysiology*, 1975, *12*, 381–387.

533

OBJECTIVE
PERSONALITY
INVENTORIES:
RECENT RESEARCH
AND SOME
CONTEMPORARY
ISSUES

639. Stephens, F. G., & Valentine, M. MMPI and clinical scales compared. *British Journal of Psychiatry*, 1974, *125*, 42–43.

640. Stevens, J. R., Milstein, V., & Goldstein, S. Psychometric test performance in relation to the psychopathology of epilepsy. *Archives of General Psychiatry*, 1972, *26*, 532–538.

641. Stewart, D. J., Powers, J., & Gouaux, C. The Wechsler in personality assessment: Object Assembly subtest as predictive of bodily concerns. *Journal of Consulting and Clinical Psychology*, 1973, *40*, 488.

642. Stewart, R. A. C. Factor analysis and rotation of the 566 MPI items. *Social Behavior and Personality*, 1974, *2*, 147–154.

643. Stone, L. A., Bassett, G. R., Brosseau, J. D., DeMers, J., & Stiening, J. A. Psychological test scores for a group of MEDEX trainees. *Psychological Reports*, 1972, *31*, 827–831.

644. Stone, L. A., Bassett, G. R., Brosseau, J. D., DeMers, J., & Stiening, J. A. Psychological test characteristics associated with training-success in a Medex (physician's extension) training program. *Psychological Reports*, 1973, *32*, 231–234.

645. Stone, L. A., & Brosseau, J. D. Cross-validation of a system for predicting training success of Medex trainees. *Psychological Reports*, 1973, *33*, 917–918.

646. Storms, L. H. Relationships among patients' emotional problems, neurologists' judgments, and psychological tests of brain dysfunction. *Journal of Clinical Psychology*, 1972, *38*, 54–60.

647. Storms, L. H., & Acosta, F. X. Effects of dynamometer tension on stimulus generalization in schizophrenic and nonschizophrenic patients. *Journal of Abnormal Psychology*, 1974, *83*, 204–207.

648. Strauss, M. E., Gynther, M. D., & Wallhermfechtel, J. Differential misdiagnosis of blacks and whites by the MMPI. *Journal of Personality Assessment*, 1974, *38*, 55–60.

649. Streiner, D. L., Woodward, C. A., Goodman, J. T., & McLean, A. Comparison of the MMPI and Mini-Mult. *Canadian Journal of Behavioral Science*, 1973, *5*, 76–82.

650. Stricker, L. J., Jacobs, P. I., & Kogan, N. Trait interrelations in implicit personality theories and questionnaire data. *Journal of Personality and Social Psychology*, 1974, *30*, 198–207.

651. Strupp, H. H., & Bloxom, A. L. An approach to defining a patient population in psychotherapy research. *Journal of Counseling Psychology*, 1975, *22*, 231–237.

652. Subotnik, L. "Spontaneous remission" of deviant MMPI profiles among college students. *Journal of Consulting and Clinical Psychology*, 1972, *38*, 191–201.

653. Sue, S., & Sue, D. W. MMPI comparisons between Asian-American and non-Asian students utilizing a student health psychiatric clinic. *Journal of Counseling Psychology*, 1974, *21*, 423–427.

654. Suter, B., & Domino, G. Masculinity-femininity in creative college women. *Journal of Personality Assessment*, 1975, *39*, 414–420.

655. Sutker, P. B. Personality characteristics of heroin addicts: A response to Gendreau and Gendreau. *Journal of Abnormal Psychology*, 1974, *83*, 463–464.

656. Sutker, P. B., & Allain, A. N. Incarcerated and street heroin addicts: A personality comparison. *Psychological Reports*, 1973, *32*, 243–246.

657. Sutker, P. B., Allain, A. N., & Cohen, G. H. MMPI indices of personality change following short- and long-term hospitalization of heroin addicts. *Psychological Reports*, 1974, *34*, 495–500.

658. Sutker, P. B., & Moan, C. E. A psychosocial description of penitentiary inmates. *Archives of General Psychiatry*, 1973, *29*, 663–667.

659. Sutker, P. B., & Moan, C. E. Prediction of socially maladaptive behavior within a state prison system. *Journal of Community Psychology*, 1973, *1*, 74–78.

660. Sutker, P. B., Moan, C. E., & Swanson, W. C. Porteus Maze Test qualitative performance in pure sociopaths, prison normals, and antisocial psychotics. *Journal of Clinical Psychology*, 1972, *28*, 349–353.

661. Syndulko, K., Parker, D. A., Jens, R., Maltzman, I., & Ziskind, E. Psychophysiology of sociopathy: Electrocortical measures. *Biological Psychology*, 1975, *3*, 185–200.

662. Tancredi, F. N., & Wagner, M. E. Women volunteers for dormitory coeducational living. *College Student Journal*, 1975, *9*, 19–22.

663. Tanner, B. A. A comparison of automated aversive conditioning and a waiting list control in the modification of homosexual behavior in males. *Behavior Therapy*, 1974, *5*, 29–32.

664. Tanner, B. A. Avoidance training with and without booster sessions to modify homosexual behavior in males. *Behavior Therapy*, 1975, *6*, 649–653.

665. Tarter, R. E. Personality of wives of alcoholics. *Journal of Clinical Psychology*, 1976, *32*, 741–743.

666. Tarter, R. E., & Perley, R. N. Clinical and perceptual characteristics of paranoids and paranoid schizophrenics. *Journal of Clinical Psychology*, 1975, *31*, 42–44.

667. Tarter, R. E., Templer, D. I., & Perley, R. L. Social role orientation and pathological factors in suicide attempts of varying lethality. *Journal of Community Psychology*, 1975, *3*, 295–299.

668. Taulbee, E. S. Mini-Mult vs. MMPI. *Journal of Personality Assessment*, 1974, *38*, 479.

669. Taulbee, E. S., & Samelson, J. Mini-Mult vs. MMPI. *Journal of Personality Assessment*, 1972, *36*, 590.

670. Taylor, J. B., Carithers, M., & Coyne, L. MMPI performance, response set, and the "self-concept hypothesis." *Journal of Consulting and Clinical Psychology*, 1976, *44*, 351–362.

671. Taylor, J. B., Ptacek, M., Carithers, M., Griffin, C., & Coyne, L. Rating scales as measures of clinical judgment. III: Judgments of the self on personality inventory scales and direct ratings. *Educational and Psychological Measurement*, 1972, *32*, 543–557.

672. Taylor, J. F., & Graham, J. R. A simplified MMPI form with reduced reading difficulty level. *Journal of Clinical Psychology*, 1974, *30*, 182–185.

673. Templer, D. I., & Connolly, W. Affective vs. thinking disturbance related to left- vs. right-sided brain functioning. *Psychological Reports*, 1976, *38*, 141-142.

674. Templer, D. I., & Lester, D. An MMPI scale for assessing death anxiety. *Psychological Reports*, 1974, *34*, 238.

675. Templer, D. I., Ruff, C. F., & Armstrong, G. Cognitive functioning and degree of psychosis in schizophrenics given many electroconvulsive treatments. *British Journal of Psychiatry*, 1973, *123*, 441–443.

676. Tharp, R. G., Watson, D., & Kaya, J. Self-modification of depression. *Journal of Consulting and Clinical Psychology*, 1974, *42*, 624.

677. Thomas, J. E. A cross validation study of the Hy scale of the MMPI in India. *Psychological Studies*, 1973, *18*, 50–52.

678. Thornton, L. S., Finch, A. J., & Griffin, J. L. The Mini-Mult with criminal psychiatric patients. *Journal of Personality Assessment*, 1975, *39*, 394–396.

679. Tortorella, W. M. Personality and intellectual changes in delinquent girls following long-term institutional placement. *Journal of Community Psychology*, 1973, *1*, 288–291.

680. Treppa, J. A., & Fricke, L. Effects of a marathon group experience. *Journal of Counseling Psychology*, 1972, *19*, 466–467.

681. Trott, D. M., & Morf, M. E. A multimethod factor analysis of the Differential Personality Inventory, Personality Research Form, and MMPI. *Journal of Counseling Psychology*, 1972, *19*, 94–103.

682. Truax, C. B., Altmann, H., & Wittmer, J. Self-disclosure as a function of personal adjustment and the facilitative conditions offered by the target person. *Journal of Community Psychology*, 1973, *1*, 319–322.

583. Trybus, R. J., & Hewitt, C. W. The Mini-Mult in a non-psychiatric population. *Journal of Clinical Psychology*, 1972, *28*, 371.

684. Tsushima, W. T. Relationship between the Mini-Mult and the MMPI with medical patients. *Journal of Clinical Psychology*, 1975, *31*, 673–675.

685. Tudor, T. G., & Holmes, D. S. Differential recall of successes and failures: Its relationship to defensiveness, achievement motivation, and anxiety. *Journal of Research in Personality*, 1973, *7*, 208–234.

686. Turner, R. G., & Horn, J. M. Effects of employing Goldberg's Ambdex statistic in the development of personality scales. *Psychological Reports*, 1976, *39*, 527–530.

687. Turner, R. G., & Horn, J. M. MMPI correlates of WAIS subtest performance. *Journal of Clinical Psychology*, 1976, *32*, 583–594.

688. Vanderbeck, D. J. A construct validity study of the O-H (Overcontrolled-Hostility) scale of the MMPI, using a social learning approach to the catharsis effect. *FCI Research Reports*, 1973, *5*, 1–18.

689. VanDeventer, J., & Webb, J. T. Manifest hostility as modified by the *K* and SO-R scales of the MMPI. *Journal of Psychology*, 1974, *87*, 209–211.

690. Verberne, T. J. P. Blackburn's typology of abnormal homicides: Additional data and a critique. *British Journal of Criminology*, 1972, *12*, 88–89.

691. Verberne, T. J. P. MMPI performance in chronic medical illness. *British Journal of Psychiatry*, 1972, *121*, 235.

692. Verinis, J. S. Maternal and child pathology in an urban ghetto. *Journal of Clinical Psychology*, 1976, *32*, 13-15.

693. Vesprani, G. J., & Seeman, W. MMPI *X* and zero items in a psychiatric outpatient group. *Journal of Personality Assessment*, 1974, *38*, 61–64.

535

OBJECTIVE
PERSONALITY
INVENTORIES:
RECENT RESEARCH
AND SOME
CONTEMPORARY
ISSUES

694. Vestre, N. D., & Watson, C. G. Behavioral correlates of the MMPI paranoia scale. *Psychological Reports*, 1972, *31*, 851–854.

695. Wagner, M. E., & Schubert, D. S. Increasing volunteer representativeness by recruiting for credit or pay. *Journal of General Psychology*, 1976, *94*, 85–91.

696. Wagner, M. K., & Mooney, D. K. Personality characteristics of long and short sleepers. *Journal of Clinical Psychology*, 1975, *31*, 434–436.

697. Wakefield, J. A., Bradley, P. E., Doughtie, E. B., & Kraft, I. A. Influence of overlapping and non-overlapping items on the theoretical interrelationships of MMPI scales. *Journal of Consulting and Clinical Psychology*, 1975, *43*, 851–857.

698. Wakefield, J. A., Sasek, J., Friedman, A. F., & Bowden, J. D. Androgeny and other measures of masculinity-femininity. *Journal of Consulting and Clinical Psychology*, 1976, *44*, 766–770.

699. Wakefield, J. A., Jr., Yom, B. L., Bradley, P. E., Doughtie, E. B., Cox, J. A., & Kraft, I. A. Eysenck's personality dimensions: A model for the MMPI. *British Journal of Social and Clinical Psychology*, 1974, *13*, 413–420.

700. Wales, B., & Seeman, W. Instructional sets and MMPI items. *Journal of Personality Assessment*, 1972, *36*, 282–286.

701. Warbin, R. W., Altman, H., Gynther, M. D., & Sletten, I. W. A new empirical automated MMPI interpretive program: 2-8 and 8-2 code types. *Journal of Personality Assessment*, 1972, *36*, 581–584.

702. Watson, C. G. Psychopathological correlates of anthropometric types in male schizophrenics. *Journal of Clinical Psychology*, 1972, *28*, 474–478.

703. Watson, C. G. Roles of impression management in the interview, self-report and cognitive behavior of schizophrenics. *Journal of Consulting and Clinical Psychology*, 1972, *38*, 452–456.

704. Watson, C. G. A simple bivariate screening technique to separate NP hospital organics from other psychiatric groups. *Journal of Clinical Psychology*, 1973, *29*, 448–450.

705. Watson, C. G., Davis, W. E., & McDermott, M. T. MMPI-WAIS relationships in organic and schizophrenic patients. *Journal of Clinical Psychology*, 1976, *32*, 539–540.

706. Watson, C. G., & Klett, W. G. A validation of the psychotic inpatient profile. *Journal of Clinical Psychology*, 1972, *28*, 102–109.

707. Waxer, P. Nonverbal cues for depth of depression: Set versus no set. *Journal of Consulting and Clinical Psychology*, 1976, *44*, 493.

708. Webb, W. B., Bonnet, M. H., & White, R. M. State and trait correlates of sleep stages. *Psychological Reports*, 1976, *38*, 1181–1182.

709. Weisman, A. D., & Worden, J. W. The existential plight in cancer: Significance of the first 100 days. *International Journal of Psychiatry in Medicine*, 1976–77, *7*, 1-15.

710. Weiss, J. M. A. The natural history of antisocial attitudes: What happens to psychopaths? *Journal of Geriatric Psychiatry*, 1973, *6*, 236–242.

711. Weiss, M. F. The treatment of insomnia through the use of electrosleep: An EEG study. *Journal of Nervous and Mental Disease*, 1973, *157*, 108–120.

712. Wener, A. E., & Rehm, L. P. Depressive affect: A test of behavioral hypothesis. *Journal of Abnormal Psychology*, 1975, *84*, 221–227.

713. Wenk, E. A., & Emrich, R. B. Assaultive youth: An exploratory study of the assaultive experience and assaultive potential of California Youth Authority wards. *Journal of Research on Crime and Delinquency*, 1972, *9*, 171–196.

714. Wennerholm, M. A., & Zarle, T. H. Internal-external control, defensiveness, and anxiety in hypertensive patients. *Journal of Clinical Psychology*, 1976, *32*, 644–648.

715. Wessman, A. E. Personality and the subjective experience of time. *Journal of Personality Assessment*, 1973, *37*, 103–114.

716. White, R. B. Variations of Bender-Gestalt constriction and depression in adult psychiatric patients. *Perceptual and Motor Skills*, 1976, *42*, 221–222.

717. White, R. B., & McCraw, R. K. Note on the relationship between downward slant of Bender figures 1 and 2 and depression in adult psychiatric patients. *Perceptual and Motor Skills*, 1975, *40*, 152.

718. White, W. C., Jr. Validity of the overcontrolled-hostility (O-H) scale: A brief report. *Journal of Personality Assessment*, 1975, *39*, 587–590.

719. White, W. C., Jr., McAdoo, W. G., & Megargee, E. I. Personality factors associated with over- and undercontrolled offenders. *Journal of Personality Assessment*, 1973, *37*, 473–478.

720. Wildman, R. W., & Wildman, R. W., II. An investigation into the comparative validity of several diagnostic tests and test batteries. *Journal of Clinical Psychology*, 1975, *31*, 455–458.

721. Wilkins, J. L., Scharff, W. H., & Schlottmann, R. S. Personality type, reports of violence and aggressive behavior. *Journal of Personality and Social Psychology*, 1974, *30*, 243–247.

722. Williams, J. D., Dudley, H. K., Jr., & Overall, J. E. Validity of the 16PF and the MMPI in a mental hospital setting. *Journal of Abnormal Psychology*, 1972, *80*, 261–270.

723. Wilson, J. P., & Aronoff, J. A sentence completion test assessing safety and esteem motives. *Journal of Personality Assessment*, 1973, *37*, 351–354.

724. Winstead, D. K., Anderson, A., Eilers, M. K., Blackwell, B., & Zaremba, A. L. Diazepam on demand: Drug-seeking behavior in psychiatric inpatients. *Archives of General Psychiatry*, 1974, *30*, 349–351.

725. Winstead, D. K., Lawson, T., & Abbott, D. Diazepam use in military sick call. *Military Medicine*, 1976, *141*, 180–181.

726. Witt, P. H., & Gynther, M. D. Another explanation for black-white MMPI differences. *Journal of Clinical Psychology*, 1975, *31*, 69–70.

727. Wittenborn, J. R., & Kiremitci, N. A comparison of antidepressant medications in neurotic and psychotic patients. *Archives of General Psychiatry*, 1975, *32*, 1172–1176.

728. Wittenborn, J. R., Kiremitci, N., & Weber, E. S. P. The choice of alternative antidepressants. *Journal of Nervous and Mental Disease*, 1973, *156*, 97–108.

729. Woerner, M. G., & Klein, D. F. 14 and 6 per second positive spiking. *Journal of Nervous and Mental Disease*, 1974, *159*, 356–361.

730. Woodward, C. A., & Armentrout, J. A. MMPI profile characteristics of psychiatric patients in an urban Canadian setting. *Canadian Journal of Behavioral Science*, 1974, *6*, 192–198.

731. Wright, L. The sick but slick syndrome as a personality component of parents of battered children. *Journal of Clinical Psychology*, 1976, *32*, 41–45.

732. Yamamoto, K. J., & Kinney, D. K. Pregnant women's ratings of different factors influencing psychological stress during pregnancy. *Psychological Reports*, 1976, *39*, 203–214.

733. Yarnell, T. Validation of the Seeking of Noetic Goals Test with schizophrenic and normal *Ss*. *Psychological Reports*, 1972, *30*, 79–82.

734. Young, R. C. Clinical judgment as a means of improving actuarial prediction from the MMPI. *Journal of Consulting and Clinical Psychology*, 1972, *38*, 457–459.

735. Young, R. C. Profile generalizability in the use of the MMPI with psychiatric inpatients. *Journal of Clinical Psychology*, 1974, *30*, 552–557.

736. Zaretsky, H. H., Lee, M. H., & Rubin, M. Psychological factors and clinical observations in acupuncture analgesia and pain abatement. *Journal of Psychology*, 1976, *93*, 113–120.

737. Zeldow, P. B. Clinical judgment: A search for sex difference. *Psychological Reports*, 1975, *37*, 1135–1142.

738. Zeldow, P. B. Effects of nonpathological sex role stereotypes on student evaluations of psychiatric patients. *Journal of Consulting and Clinical Psychology*, 1976, *44*, 304.

739. Zimmerman, R. L., Vestre, N. D., & Hunter, S. H. Validity of family informants ratings of psychiatric patients: General validity. *Psychological Reports*, 1975, *37*, 619–630.

740. Zimmerman, R. L., Vestre, N. D., & Hunter, S. H. Validity of family informants ratings of psychiatric patients: Differential validity. *Psychological Reports*, 1976, *38*, 555–564.

741. Zuckerman, M., Bone, R. N., Neary, R., Mangelsdorff, D., & Brustman, B. What is the sensation seeker? Personality trait and experience correlates of the sensation-seeking scales. *Journal of Consulting and Clinical Psychology*, 1972, *39*, 308–321.

742. Zuckerman, M., Sola, S., Masterson, J., & Angelovie, J. V. MMPI patterns in drug abuse before and after treatment in therapeutic communities. *Journal of Consulting and Clinical Psychology*, 1975, *43*, 286–296.

10.1.2. Sixteen Personality Factor (16PF) References

743. Adcock, C. J. Review of Peter Saville, the British standardization of the 16PF. *New Zealand Psychologist*, 1973, *2*, 43–44.

744. Adcock, N. V. Testing the test: How adequate is the 16PF with a N.Z. student sample? *New Zealand Psychologist*, 1974, *3*, 2–10.

745. Alcorn, C. L., & Nicholson, C. L. A vocational assessment battery for the educable mentally retarded. *Education and Training of the Mentally Retarded*, 1975, *10*, 78–83.

746. Ashton, H., Savage, R. D., Telford, R., Thompson, J. W., & Watson, D. W. The effects of cigarette

537

OBJECTIVE
PERSONALITY
INVENTORIES:
RECENT RESEARCH
AND SOME
CONTEMPORARY
ISSUES

smoking on the response to stress in a driving simulator. *British Journal of Pharmacology*, 1972, *45*, 546–556.

747. Ashton, H., Savage, R. D., Thompson, J. W., & Watson, D. W. A method for measuring human behavioral and physiological responses at different stress levels in a driving simulator. *British Journal of Pharmacology*, 1972, *45*, 532–545.

748. Bachtold, L. M. Personality characteristics of women of distinction. *Psychology of Women Quarterly*, 1976, *1*, 70–78.

749. Bachtold, L. M., & Werner, E. E. Personality characteristics of creative women. *Perceptual and Motor Skills*, 1973, *36*, 311–319.

750. Banister, P. A., Heskin, K. J., Bolton, N., & Smith, F. V. A study of variables related to the selection of long-term prisoners for parole. *British Journal of Criminology*, 1974, *14*, 359–368.

751. Barton, K., & Cattell, R. B. Marriage dimensions and personality. *Journal of Personality and Social Psychology*, 1972, *21*, 369–375.

752. Barton, K., & Cattell, R. B. Personality before and after a chronic illness. *Journal of Clinical Psychology*, 1972, *28*, 464–467.

753. Barton, K., Cattell, R. B., & Silverman, W. Personality Correlates of verbal and spatial ability. *Social Behavior and Personality*, 1974, *2*, 113–118.

754. Barton, K., & Vaughan, G. M. Church membership and personality: A longitudinal study. *Social Behavior and Personality*, 1976, *4*, 11–16.

755. Bartussek, D. Note on the reliability and factorial validity of the German 16PF. *Diagnostica*, 1974, *20*, 49–55.

756. Bell, C. R. Accurate performance of a time-estimation task in relation to sex, age, and personality variables. *Perceptual and Motor Skills*, 1972, *35*, 175–178.

757. Boleloucky, Z. Cattell's personality factors in ulcerative colitis male patients. *Activitas Nervosa Superior*, 1974, *16*, 116–117.

758. Bowman, J. T., Cook, S. D., & Whitehead, G. Pre-release training of female public offenders. *Psychological Reports*, 1974, *35*, 1193–1194.

759. Braun-Galkowska, M. Features of personality conditioning family authority. *Roczniki Filozoficzne: Annales de Philosophie*, 1972, *20*, 59–74.

760. Brien, R. L., Kleiman, J., & Eisenman, R. Personality and drug use: Heroin, alcohol, methadrine, mixed drug dependency and the 16PF. *Corrective Psychiatry and Journal of Social Therapy*, 1972, *18*, 22–23.

761. Bull, P. E. Should the 16PF be used in personnel selection? *New Zealand Psychologist*, 1974, *3*, 11–15.

762. Burdsal, C. A., & Schwartz, S. A. The relationship of personality traits as measured in the questionnaire medium and by self-ratings. *Journal of Psychology*, 1975, *91*, 173–182.

763. Burdsal, C. A., & Vaughn, D. S. A contrast of the personality structure of college students found in the questionnaire medium by items as compared to parcels. *Journal of Genetic Psychology*, 1974, *125*, 219–224.

764. Campus, N. Transituational consistency as a dimension of personality. *Journal of Personality and Social Psychology*, 1974, *29*, 593–600.

765. Cattell, R. B. The 16PF and basic personality structure: A reply to Eysenck. *Journal of Behavioral Science*, 1972, *1*, 169–187.

766. Cattell, R. B. Personality pinned down. *Psychology Today*, 1973, *7*, 40–46.

767. Cattell, R. B. *Personality and mood by questionnaire*. San Francisco: Jossey-Bass, 1973.

768. Cattell, R. B. A large sample cross-check on 16PF: Primary structure by parcelled factoring. *Multivariate Experimental Clinical Research*, 1974, *1*, 79–95.

769. Cattell, R. B. Third order personality structure in Q-data: Evidence from eleven experiments. *Journal of Multivariate Experimental Personality and Clinical Psychology*, 1975, *1*, 118–149.

770. Cattell, R. B., & Delhees, K. H. Seven missing normal personality factors in the questionnaire primaries. *Multivariate Behavioral Research*, 1973, *8*, 173–194.

771. Cattell, R. B., Pierson, G., Finkbeiner, C., Willes, P., Brim, B., & Robertson, J. Proof of alignment of personality source trait factors in questionnaires and observer ratings: The theory of instrument-free patterns. Advance publication No. 38. Boulder, Colo.: Institute for Research on Morality and Self-Realization, 1974.

772. Cattell, R. B., Shrader, R. R., & Barton, K. The definition and measurement of anxiety as a trait and a state in the 12- to 17-year range. *British Journal of Social and Clinical Psychology*, 1974, *13*, 173–182.

773. Chynoweth, R. Psychological complications of hysterectomy. *Australian and New Zealand Journal of Psychiatry*, 1973, *7*, 102–104.

774. Codol, J. P. Degree of value attributed to a social situation and the phenomenon of self-acceptance. *Bulletin de Psychologie*, 1974–1975, *28*, 321–327.

775. Cooper, C. L., & Bowles, D. Structured exercise-based groups and the psychological conditions of learning. *Interpersonal Development*, 1974–1975, *5*, 203–212.

776. Costa, P. T., Jr., & McCrae, R. R. Age differences in personality structure: A cluster analytic approach. *Journal of Gerontology*, 1976, *31*, 564–570.

777. Curran, J. P. Differential effects of stated preferences and questionnaire role performance on interpersonal attraction in the dating situation. *Journal of Psychology*, 1972, *82*, 313–327.

778. Darden, E. 16PF profiles of competitive bodybuilders and weightlifters. *Research Quarterly*, 1972, *43*, 142–147.

779. Deabler, H. L., Hartl, E. M., & Willis, C. A. Physique and personality: Somatotype and the 16PF. *Perceptual and Motor Skills*, 1973, *36*, 927–933.

780. Duffy, J. C., & Kanak, N. J. Ego strength and confidence thresholds in two methods of paired-associate learning. *American Journal of Psychology*, 1975, *88*, 245–252.

781. Edwards, A. L., & Abbott, R. D. Relationship between the EPI scales and the 16PF, CPI, and EPPS scales. *Educational and Psychological Measurement*, 1973, *33*, 231–238.

782. Eysenck, H. J. Primaries of second-order factors: A critical consideration of Cattell's 16PF battery. *British Journal of Social and Clinical Psychology*, 1972, *11*, 265–269.

783. Feij, J. A. An investigation into the meaning of the Achievement Motivation Test. I. Questionnaire correlates. *Nederlands Tijdschrift Voor de Psychologie en Haar Grensgebieden*, 1974, *29*, 171–190.

784. Forbes, A. R. Some differences between neurotic and psychotic depressives. *British Journal of Social and Clinical Psychology*, 1972, *11*, 270–275.

785. Forster, J. R., & Hamburg, R. L. Further exploration of the 16PF and counselor effectiveness. *Counselor Education and Supervision*, 1976, *15*, 184–187.

786. Fozard, J. L. Predicting age in the adult years from psychological assessments of abilities and personality. *Aging and Human Development*, 1972, *3*, 175–182.

787. Gaensslen, H., & Mandl, H. The constancy of personality traits and attitudes exemplified by repeating tests after 15 months. *Zeitschrift für experimentelle und angewandte Psychologie*, 1974, *21*, 367–377.

788. Gershman, L., & Clouser, R. A. Treating insomnia with relaxation and desensitization in a group setting by an automated approach. *Journal of Behavior Therapy and Experimental Psychiatry*, 1974, *5*, 31–35.

789. Goodman, G., & McKinnon, A. J. Personality characteristics of student teachers of the emotionally disturbed. *Journal of the Student Personnel Association for Teacher Education*, 1975, *13*, 107–112.

790. Gross, W. F., & Nerviano, V. J. The prediction of dropouts from an inpatient alcoholism program by objective personality inventories. *Quarterly Journal of Studies on Alcohol*, 1973, *34*, 514–515.

791. Gupta, V. P. The relationship between physical fitness and personality characteristics as measured by 16PF inventory. *Journal of Psychological Researches*, 1972, *16*, 94–95.

792. Gutsch, K. U., & Holmes, W. R. Training counselors using an attitudinal group-centered approach. *Small Group Behavior*, 1974, *5*, 93–104.

793. Halpin, G., Payne, D. A., & Ellett, C. D. Life history antecedents of current personality traits of gifted adolescents. *Measurement and Evaluation in Guidance*, 1975, *8*, 29–36.

794. Hammer, W. M., & Tutko, T. A. Validation of the Athletic Motivation Inventory. *International Journal of Sport Psychology*, 1974, *5*, 3–12.

795. Heritage, J. G., & Daniels, J. L. Postdivorce adjustment. *Journal of Family Counseling*, 1974, *2*, 44–49.

796. Hill, A. B. Personality correlates of dream recall. *Journal of Consulting and Clinical Psychology*, 1974, *42*, 766–773.

797. Hobi, V. A comparison of MMPI, 16PF, and FPI in small sample tests. *Zeitschrift für Klinische Psychologie und Psychotherapie*, 1973, *21*, 129–139.

798. Hobi, V., & Klar, A. A combined factor analysis of the MMPI, FPI, and 16PF. *Zeitschrift für Klinische Psychologie*, 1973, *1*, 27–48.

799. Howarth, E. Were Cattell's personality sphere factors correctly identified in the first instance? *British Journal of Psychology*, 1976, *67*, 213–230.

800. Irvine, M. J., & Gendreau, P. Detection of the fake "good" and "bad" response on the 16PF in prisoners and college students. *Journal of Consulting and Clinical Psychology*, 1974, *42*, 465–466.

539

OBJECTIVE
PERSONALITY
INVENTORIES:
RECENT RESEARCH
AND SOME
CONTEMPORARY
ISSUES

801. Jacobs, K. W. 16PF correlates of locus of control. *Psychological Reports*, 1976, *38*, 1170.
802. Jacobs, K. W. 16PF correlates of sensation-seeking: An expansion and validation. *Psychological Reports*, 1975, *37*, 1215–1218.
803. Jensema, C. Reliability of the 16PF Form E for hearing impaired college students. *Journal of Rehabilitation of the Deaf*, 1975, *8*, 14–18.
804. Jeske, J. O., & Whitten, M. R. Motivational distortion of the 16PF questionnaire by persons in job applicants' roles. *Psychological Reports*, 1975, *37*, 379–383.
805. Johnson, D. T., Workman, S. N., Neville, C. W., & Beutler, L. E. MMPI and 16PF correlates of the A-B Therapy Scale in psychiatric inpatients. *Psychotherapy: Theory, Research and Practice*, 1973, *10*, 270–272.
806. Jones, H. L., Sasek, J., & Wakefield, J. A. Maslow's need hierarchy and Cattell's 16PF. *Journal of Clinical Psychology*, 1976, *32*, 74–76.
807. Jones, L. K. The Counselor Evaluation Rating Scale: A valid criterion of counselor effectiveness. *Counselor Education and Supervision*, 1974, *14*, 112–116.
808. Jones, W. P. Some implications of the 16PF questionnaire for marital guidance. *Family Coordinator*, 1976, *25*, 189–192.
809. Josephs, A. P., & Smithers, A. G. Personality characteristics of syllabus-bound and syllabus-free sixth-formers. *British Journal of Educational Psychology*, 1975, *45*, 29–38.
810. Karson, S., & O'Dell, J. W. A new automated interpretation system for the 16PF. *Journal of Personality Assessment*, 1975, *39*, 256–268.
811. Karson, S., & O'Dell, J. W. Is the 16PF factorially valid? *Journal of Personality Assessment*, 1974, *38*, 104–114.
812. Kaul, L. A factorial study of the personality traits of popular teachers. *Indian Educational Review*, 1974, *9*, 66–78.
813. Kear-Colwell, J. J. The factor structure of the 16PF and the Edwards Personal Preference Schedule in acute psychiatric patients. *Journal of Clinical Psychology*, 1973, *29*, 225–228.
814. Kear-Colwell, J. J. Second stratum personality factors found in psychiatric patients' response to the 16PF. *Journal of Clinical Psychology*, 1972, *28*, 362–365.
815. Kidson, M. A. Personality and hypertension. *Journal of Psychosomatic Research*, 1973, *17*, 35–41.
816. King, J. P., & Chi, P. S. Personality and the athletic social structure: A case study. *Human Relations*, 1974, *27*, 179–193.
817. Kirchner, J. H., & Lemke, E. A. I-dots in the handwriting of a clinical sample. *Perceptual and Motor Skills*, 1973, *36*, 548–550.
818. Kirchner, J. H., & Marzolf, S. S. Personality of alcoholics as measured by 16PF questionnaire and House-Tree-Person color-choice characteristics. *Psychological Reports*, 1974, *35*, 627–642.
819. Kirchner, J. H., & Marzolf, S. S. The HTP weeping willow and personality traits. *Perceptual and Motor Skills*, 1974, *38*, 25–26.
820. Kornfeld, D. S., Heller, S. S., Frank, K. A., & Moskowitz, R. Personality and psychological factors in postcardiotomy delirium. *Archives of General Psychiatry*, 1974, *31*, 249–253.
821. Koslowsky, M., & Deren, S. A comparison of three procedures for classifying addicts. *Journal of Consulting and Clinical Psychology*, 1975, *43*, 433.
822. Kostrzewski, J. The level of mental development and personality traits of country and town children. *Roczniki Filozoficzne: Annales de Philosophie*, 1972, *20*, 33–58.
823. Kotaskova, J. Models of interaction between mother and child obtained by means of factor analysis. *Ceskoslovenska Psychologie*, 1973, *17*, 293–305.
824. Krug, S. E., & Henry, T. J. Personality, motivation, and adolescent drug use patterns. *Journal of Counseling Psychology*, 1974, *21*, 440–445.
825. Lader, M. H., & Marks, I. M. The rating of clinical anxiety. *Acta Psychiatrica Scandinavica*, 1974, *50*, 112–137.
826. Lind, C. W. 16PF screening instrument for alcoholics. *Journal of Clinical Psychology*, 1972, *28*, 548–549.
827. Lin, Y. A validity study of Factor B Scale of Cattell 16PF in a college sample. *Acta Psychologica Taiwanica*, 1973, *15*, 1–5.
828. Mann, W. R., & Rizzo, J. L. Composition of the Achiever Personality Scale of the OAIS. *Psychological Reports*, 1972, *31*, 218.
829. Marko, J. Self-evaluation and personality profile in Cattell's 16PF test. *Psychologia a Patopsychologia Dietata*, 1973, *8*, 19–28.
830. Marzolf, S. S. Common sayings and 16PF traits. *Journal of Clinical Psychology*, 1974, *30*, 202–204.

831. Marzolf, S. S., & Kirchner, J. H. House-Tree-Person drawings and personality traits. *Journal of Personality Assessment*, 1972, *36*, 148–165.

832. McCutcheon, L. E. Personality and speed of handwriting. *Perceptual and Motor Skills*, 1974, *38*, 1154.

833. McIver, D., & Presly, A. S. Towards the investigation of personality deviance. *British Journal of Social and Clinical Psychology*, 1974, *13*, 397–404.

834. Mehryar, A. H. Personality patterns of Iranian boys and girls on Cattell's 16PF test. *British Journal of Social and Clinical Psychology*, 1972, *11*, 257–264.

835. Moffett, L. A., & Dreger, R. M. Sculpture preferences and personality traits. *Journal of Personality Assessment*, 1975, *39*, 70–76.

836. Muhiern, T. J. Use of the 16PF with mentally retarded adults. *Measurement and Evaluation in Guidance*, 1975, *8*, 26–28.

837. Myrick, R. D., Kelly, F. D., & Wittmer, J. The 16PF questionnaire as a predictor of counselor effectiveness. *Counselor Education and Supervision*, 1972, *11*, 293–301.

838. Nakamura, M. The validity and underlying factors of scholastic traits. *Japanese Journal of Psychology*, 1974, *45*, 9–20.

839. Nellesen, L., & Svensson, A. A factor analytical description of the T-group. *Gruppendynamik Forschung und Praxis*, 1972, *1*, 92–110.

840. Nerviano, V. J. The second stratum factor structure of the 16PF for alcoholic males. *Journal of Clinical Psychology*, 1974, *30*, 83–85.

841. Nerviano, V. J., & Gross, W. F. A multivariate delineation of two alcoholic profile types of the 16PF. *Journal of Clinical Psychology*, 1973, *29*, 371–374.

842. Nowakowska, M. Polish adaptation of the 16PF questionnaire of R. B. Cattell, as a source of cross-cultural comparisons. *Polish Psychological Bulletin*, 1974, *5*, 25–33.

843. Paitich, D. Computers in behavioral science: A comprehensive automated psychological examination and report (CAPER), *Behavioral Science*, 1973, *18*, 131–136.

844. Pandey, R. E. A comparative study of dropout at an integrated university: The 16PF test. *Journal of Negro Education*, 1973, *42*, 447–452.

845. Payne, D. A., Halpin, W. G., Ellett, C. D., & Dale, J. B. General personality correlates of creative personality in academically and artistically gifted youth. *Journal of Special Education*, 1975, *9*, 105–108.

846. Philip, A. E. Cross-cultural stability of second-order factors in the 16PF. *British Journal of Social and Clinical Psychology*, 1972, *11*, 276–283.

847. Roessler, R. T., & Bolton, B. Behavior rating correlates of the 16PF. *Psychological Reports*, 1974, *35*, 1160.

848. Rose, L. D., & Lawlis, G. F. The nurse: A helping personality. *Journal of Multivariate Experimental Personality and Clinical Psychology*, 1975, *1*, 165–175.

849. Roseman, M. F., & Albergottie, G. J. Personality scales of the Bender-Gestalt Test. *Catalog of Selected Documents in Psychology*, 1973, *3*, 10.

850. Rosenthal, S. V., Aitken, R. C., & Zealley, A. K. The Cattell 16PF personality profile of asthmatics. *Journal of Psychosomatic Research*, 1973, *17*, 9–14.

851. Ruffer, W. A. Two studies of personality: Male graduates in physical education. *Perceptual and Motor Skills*, 1975, *41*, 187–191.

852. Ruffer, W. A. Two studies of personality: Female graduate students in physical education. *Perceptual and Motor Skills*, 1976, *42*, 1268–1270.

853. Ruffer, W. A. Three studies of personality: Undergraduate students in physical education. *Perceptual and Motor Skills*, 1976, *43*, 671–677.

854. Saville, P. The standardization of an adult personality inventory on the British population. *Bulletin of the British Psychological Society*, 1973, *26*, 25–29.

855. Schwartz, S. Multimethod analysis of three measures of six common personality traits. *Journal of Personality Assessment*, 1973, *37*, 559–567.

856. Serban, G., & Katz, G. Schizophrenic performance on Form E of Cattell's 16PF test. *Journal of Personality Assessment*, 1975, *39*, 169–177.

857. Shiflett, S. C. Stereotyping and esteem for one's least preferred co-worker. *Journal of Social Psychology*, 1974, *93*, 55–65.

858. Stewart, R. A. The concept of personality: A symposium. Personality change: The effects on New Zealand adolescents of a scholarship exchange year in the U.S.A. *Journal of Psychological Researches*, 1973, *17*, 28–46.

541

OBJECTIVE
PERSONALITY
INVENTORIES:
RECENT RESEARCH
AND SOME
CONTEMPORARY
ISSUES

859. Singh, S. B., & Nigam, A. A comparative study of the personality profile of the male and female medical students. *Indian Journal of Psychometry and Education*, 1973, *4*, 30–33.

860. Singh, S. B., Nigam, A., & Saxena, N. K. 16PF study in the cases of marital disharmony. *Indian Journal of Clinical Psychology*, 1976, *3*, 47–52.

861. Stricker, L. J. Response styles and 16PF higher order factors. *Educational and Psychological Measurement*, 1974, *34*, 295–313.

862. Sweney, A. B., Fiechtner, L. A., & Samores, R. J. An integrative factor analysis of leadership measures and theories. *Journal of Psychology*, 1975, *90*, 75–85.

863. Terry, R. L., & Ertel, S. L. Exploration of individual differences in preferences for humor. *Psychological Reports*, 1974, *34*, 1031–1037.

864. Turner, E. V., Helper, M. M., & Kriska, S. D. Predictors of clinical performance. *Journal of Medical Education*, 1974, *49*, 338–342.

865. Turner, R. G., Willerman, L., & Horn, J. M. A test of some predictions from the Personality Assessment System. *Journal of Clinical Psychology*, 1976, *32*, 631–643.

866. Turner, R. K., Pielmaier, H., James, S., & Orwin, A. Personality characteristics of male homosexuals referred for aversive therapy: A comparative study. *British Journal of Psychiatry*, 1974, *125*, 447–449.

867. Vagg, P. R., & Hammond, S. B. The number and kind of invariant personality (Q) factors: A partial replication of Eysenck and Eysenck. *British Journal of Social and Clinical Psychology*, 1976, *15*, 121–129.

868. Vanderplate, C., & Fitzgerald, J. M. Personality factors and perceived peer personality as predictors of social role variables in the aged. *Human Development*, 1976, *19*, 40–48.

869. Vaughn, G. M., & Cattell, R. B. Personality differences between young New Zealanders and Americans. *Journal of Social Psychology*, 1976, *99*, 3–12.

870. Wakefield, J. A., Jr., & Cunningham, C. H. Related factors of the MTAI and the 16PF. *Psychology in the Schools*, 1976, *13*, 149–151.

871. Ward, G. R., Cunningham, C. H., & Wakefield, J. A. Relationships between Holland's VPI and Cattell's 16PF. *Journal of Vocational Behavior*, 1976, *8*, 307–312.

872. Wardell, D., & Mehra, N. Prediction of marijuana usage among students in a university residence. *Journal of College Student Personnel*, 1974, *15*, 31–33.

873. Widdop, J. H., & Widdop, V. A. Comparison of the personality traits of female teacher education and physical education students. *Research Quarterly*, 1975, *46*, 274–281.

874. Williams, C. L., Henderson, A. S., & Mills, J. M. An epidemiological study of serious traffic offenders. *Social Psychiatry*, 1974, *9*, 99–109.

875. Williams, J. D., & Williams, C. M., Canonical analysis of the Vocational Preference Inventory and the 16PF questionnaire. *Psychological Reports*, 1973, *32*, 211–214.

876. Winder, R., O'Dell, J. W., & Karson, S. New motivational distortion scales for the 16PF. *Journal of Personality Assessment*, 1975, *39*, 532–537.

877. Witte, H., & Witte, E. H. Self-descriptions of actual and ideal personality by juveniles from different social strata and by juvenile delinquents. *Zeitschrift für Sozial Psychologie*, 1974, *5*, 219–232.

878. Wood, C. L. The practitioner's guide to research: Teacher morale and the principal. *National Association of Secondary School Principals Bulletin*, 1973, *57*, 113–117.

879. Yang, P. L. Some personality correlates of individual modernity in Chinese college students. *Acta Psychologica Taiwanica*, 1973, *15*, 46–53.

10.1.3. Differential Personality Inventory (DPI) References

880. Carlson, K. A. Classes of adult offenders: A multivariate approach. *Journal of Abnormal Psychology*, 1972, *79*, 84–93.

881. Constantini, A. F., Braun, J. R., Davis, J. E., & Iervolino, A. The Life Change Inventory: A device for quantifying psychological magnitude of changes by college students. *Psychological Reports*, 1974, *34*, 991–1000.

882. Hoffmann, H., & Jackson, D. Comparison of measured psychopathology in Indian and non-Indian alcoholics. *Psychological Reports*, 1973, *33*, 793–794.

883. Hoffmann, H., & Jackson, D. N. DPI for male and female alcoholics. *Psychological Reports*, 1974, *34*, 21–22.

884. Hoffmann, H., Nelson, P. C., & Jackson, D. N. The effects of detoxification on psychopathology for alcoholics as measured by the DPI. *Journal of Clinical Psychology*, 1974, *30*, 89–93.
885. Jackson, D. N., & Carlson, K. A. Convergent and discriminant validation of the DPI. *Journal of Clinical Psychology*, 1973, *29*, 214–219.
886. Nelson, P. C., & Hoffmann, H. Effect of long-term treatment on personality change on high-risk alcoholics. *Psychological Reports*, 1972, *31*, 799–802.
887. Nelson, P. C., & Hoffmann, H. Personalities of alcoholics who leave and seek treatment. *Psychological Reports*, 1972, *30*, 949–950.
888. Morf, M. E., Miller, C. M., & Syrotuik, J. M. A comparison of cluster analysis and Q-factor analysis. *Journal of Clinical Psychology*, 1976, *32*, 59–64.

10.2. General Guides and Manuals

Block, J. *The challenge of response sets: Unconfounding meaning, acquiescence, and social desirability in the MMPI.* New York: Appleton-Century-Crofts, 1965.

Butcher, J. N. (Ed.). *MMPI: Research developments and clinical applications.* New York: McGraw-Hill, 1969.

Butcher, J. N. *Objective personality assessment.* Morristown, N.J.: General Learning Press, 1971.

Butcher, J. N. (Ed.). *Objective personality assessment: Changing perspectives.* New York: Academic Press, 1972.

Butcher, J. N., & Pancheri, P. *Handbook of cross-national MMPI research.* Minneapolis: University of Minnesota Press, 1976.

Carkhuff, R. R. *The MMPI: An outline for general clinical and counseling use.* Buffalo: State University of New York, 1961.

Carkhuff, R. R., Barnett, L., Jr., & McCall, J. N. *The counselor's handbook: Scale and profile interpretation of the MMPI.* Urbana, Ill.: R. W. Parkinson, 1965.

Carson, R. C. Interpretative manual to the MMPI. In J. N. Butcher (Ed.), *MMPI: Research developments and clinical applications.* New York: McGraw-Hill, 1969, pp. 279–296.

Dahlstrom, W. G., Welsh, G. S., & Dahlstrom, L. E. *An MMPI handbook, Volume I: Clinical interpretation.* Minneapolis: University of Minnesota Press, 1972.

Dahlstrom, W. G., Welsh, G. S., & Dahlstrom, L. E. *An MMPI handbook, Volume II: Research applications.* Minneapolis: University of Minnesota Press, 1975.

Drake, L. E., & Oetting, E. R. *An MMPI codebook for counselors.* Minneapolis: University of Minnesota Press, 1959.

Duckworth, J., & Duckworth, E. *MMPI interpretation manual for counselors and clinicians.* Muncie, Ind.: Accelerated Development, Inc., 1975.

Eichman, W. J. Factored scales for the MMPI: A clinical and statistical manual. *Journal of Clinical Psychology* (monogr. suppl.), 1962, *18*, 363–396.

Faschingbauer, T. R., and Newmark, C. S. *Short forms of the MMPI.* Lexington, Mass.: Heath, 1977.

Gilberstadt, H., & Duker, J. *A handbook for clinical and actuarial MMPI interpretation.* Philadelphia: Saunders, 1965.

Good, P. K.-E., & Brantner, J. P. *The physician's guide to the MMPI.* Minneapolis: University of Minnesota Press, 1961.

Good, P. K.-E., & Brantner, J. P. *A practical guide to the MMPI.* Minneapolis: University of Minnesota Press, 1974.

Graham, J. R. *The MMPI: A practical guide.* New York: Oxford University Press, 1977.

Hathaway, S. R. MMPI: Professional use by professional people. *American Psychologist*, 1964, *19*, 204–210.

Hathaway, S. R., & McKinley, J. C. *The Minnesota Multiphasic Personality Inventory manual.* New York: The Psychological Corporation, 1951; revised 1967.

Hathaway, S. R. & Meehl, P. E. *An atlas for the clinical use of the MMPI.* Minneapolis: University of Minnesota Press, 1951.

Hathaway, S. R., & Monachesi, E. D. *An atlas of juvenile MMPI profiles.* Minneapolis: University of Minnesota Press, 1961.

Hathaway, S. R., & Monachesi, E. D. *Adolescent personality and behavior: MMPI patterns of normal, delinquent, dropout, and other outcomes.* Minneapolis: University of Minnesota Press, 1963.

Hedlund, D. E. A review of the MMPI in industry. *Psychological Reports*, 1965, *17*, 875–889.

543

OBJECTIVE
PERSONALITY
INVENTORIES:
RECENT RESEARCH
AND SOME
CONTEMPORARY
ISSUES

Kleinmuntz, B. Annotated bibliography of MMPI research among college populations. *Journal of Counseling Psychology*, 1962, *9*, 373–396.

Lachar, D. *The MMPI: Clinical assessment and automated interpretation*. Los Angeles: Western Psychological Services, 1974.

Lanyon, R. I. *A handbook of MMPI group profiles*. Minneapolis: University of Minnesota Press, 1968.

Marks, P. A., & Seeman, W. *The actuarial description of abnormal personality: An atlas for use with the MMPI*. Baltimore: Williams and Wilkins, 1963.

Marks, P. A., Seeman, W., & Haller, D. L. *The actuarial use of the MMPI with adolescents and adults*. Baltimore: Williams and Wilkins, 1974.

Pearson, J. S., & Swenson, W. M. *A user's guide to the Mayo Clinic automated MMPI program*. New York: The Psychological Corporation, 1967.

Swenson, W. M., Pearson, J. S., & Osborne, D. *An MMPI source book: Basic item, scale, and pattern data on 50,000 medical patients*. Minneapolis: University of Minnesota Press, 1973.

Tellegen, A. The MMPI. In L. E. Abt & B. F. Riess (Eds.), *Progress in clinical psychology* (Vol. 6). New York: Grune and Stratton, 1964.

Welsh, G. S., & Dahlstrom, W. G. (Eds.). *Basic readings on the MMPI in psychology and medicine*. Minneapolis: University of Minnesota Press, 1956.

10.3. Additional References Cited in This Chapter

Burke, H. R. & Marcus, R. MacAndrew MMPI alcoholism scale: Alcoholism and drug addictiveness. *The Journal of Psychology*, 1977, *96*, 141–148.

Buros, O. K. (Ed.). *The seventh annual mental measurements yearbook*. Highland Park, N.J.: Gryphon Press, 1972.

Butcher, J. N., & Tellegen, A. Haunting problems with the use of the MMPI in actuarial and automated assessment. Paper presented at the Eleventh Annual Symposium on Recent Developments in the Use of the MMPI, Minneapolis, 1976.

Button, A. D. A study of alcoholics with the MMPI. *Quarterly Journal of Studies on Alcohol*, 1956, *17*, 263–281.

Caldwell, A. B. MMPI critical items. Mimeo, 1969.

Carson, R. C. Issues in the teaching of clinical MMPI interpretation. In J. N. Butcher (Ed.), *MMPI: Research developments and clinical applications*. New York: McGraw-Hill, 1969.

Cattell, R. B. Beyond validity and reliability: Some further concepts and coefficients for evaluating tests. *Journal of Experimental Education*, 1964, *33*, 133–143.

Cavior, N., Kurtzberg, R. L., & Lipton, D. S. The development and validation of a heroin addiction scale with the MMPI. *International Journal of Addictions*, 1967, *2*, 129–137.

Chang, A., Caldwell, A., & Moss, T. Stability in personality traits in alcoholics during and after treatment as measured by the MMPI: A one year follow-up study. *Proceedings of the 81st Annual Convention of the American Psychological Association*, 1973, *8*, 387–388.

Clavelle, P. R., & Butcher, J. N. An adaptive typological approach to psychiatric screening. *Journal of Consulting and Clinical Psychology*, 1977, *45*, 851–859.

Dahlstrom, W. G. Recurrent issues in the development of the MMPI. In J. N. Butcher (Ed.), *MMPI: Research developments and clinical applications*. New York: McGraw-Hill, 1969.

Ellis, A. The validity of personality questionnaires. *Psychological Bulletin*, 1946, *43*, 385–440.

Finney, J., Smith, D., Skeeters, D., & Auvenshine, C. MMPI alcoholism scales, factor structure and content analysis. *Quarterly Journal of Studies on Alcohol*, 1971, *32*, 1055–1060.

Fowler, R. A method for the evaluation of the abuse prone patient. Scientific exhibit at the American Academy of Family Physicians, Chicago, 1975.

Fowler, R. D., Jr., & Miller, M. L. Computer interpretation of the MMPI: Its use in clinical practice. *Archives of General Psychiatry*, 1969, *21*, 505–508.

Gehring, A., & Blaser, P. MMPI-computer-service: Design and validation of an abridged version of the MMPI. Mimeographed materials, 1973.

Glen, A., Royer, F., & Custer, R. A study of MMPI profile types of hospitalized alcoholic veterans. *Newsletter for Research in Mental Health and Behavioral Sciences*, 1973, *15*, 53–56.

Goldberg, L. R. Diagnosticians vs. diagnostic signs: The diagnosis of psychosis vs. neurosis from the MMPI. *Psychological Monographs*, 1965, *79* (9; whole No. 602), 1–28.

Goldberg, L. R. Objective diagnostic tests and measures. In M. R. Rosenzweig & L. W. Porter (Eds.), *Annual Review of Psychology*, 1974, *25*, 343–367.

Goldstein, S. G., & Linden, J. D. Multivariate classification of alcoholics by means of the MMPI. *Journal of Abnormal Psychology*, 1969, *74*, 661–669.

Goss, A., & Morosko, T. Alcoholism and clinical symptoms. *Journal of Abnormal Psychology*, 1969, *74*, 682–684.

Grayson, H. M. *A psychological admissions testing program and manual.* Los Angeles: Veterans Administration Center, Neuropsychiatric Hospital, 1951.

Gynther, M. D. Review of the MMPI. In O. Buros (Ed.), *Seventh mental measurements yearbook.* Highland Park, N.J.: Gryphon Press, 1972.

Gynther, M. D. Ethnicity and personality: Recent findings. Paper presented at the Twelfth Annual MMPI Symposium, St. Petersburg, Fla., February 3, 1977.

Haertzen, C. A., Hill, H. E., & Monroe, J. J. MMPI scales for differentiating and predicting relapse in alcoholics, opiate addicts, and criminals. *International Journal of Addiction*, 1968, *3*, 91–106.

Hampton, P. J. The development of a personality questionnaire for drinkers. *Genetic Psychology Monograph*, 1953, *48*, 55–115.

Harris, J. G., & Lingoes, J. C. Subscales for the MMPI: An aid to profile interpretation. Mimeographed materials. Department of Psychiatry, University of California, 1955 (corrected version, 1968).

Hase, H. D., & Goldberg, L. R. Comparative validity of different strategies of constructing personality inventory scales. *Psychological Bulletin*, 1967, *67*, 231–248.

Hathaway, S. R. Personality inventories. In B. B. Wolman (Ed.), *Handbook of clinical psychology.* New York: McGraw-Hill, 1965.

Hedlund, J. L., Powell, B. J., & Cho, D. W. The use of MMPI short forms with psychiatric patients. Paper presented at the annual American Psychological Association meeting, New Orleans, 1974.

Hewitt, C. C. A personality study of alcohol addiction. *Quarterly Journal of Studies on Alcohol*, 1943, *4*, 368–386.

Hoyt, D. P., & Sedlacek, G. M. Differentiating alcoholics from normals and abnormals with the MMPI. *Journal of Clinical Psychology*, 1958, *14*, 69–74.

Hugo, J. Abbreviation of the MMPI through multiple regression. Unpublished doctoral dissertation, University of Alabama, 1972.

Jackson, D. N. The dynamics of structured personality tests: 1971. *Psychological Review*, 1971, *78*, 229–248.

Kincannon, J. C. Prediction of the standard MMPI scale scores from 71 items: The Mini-Mult. *Journal of Consulting and Clinical Psychology*, 1968, *32*, 319–325.

Koss, M. P., Butcher, J. N., & Hoffman, N. G. The MMPI critical items: How well do they work? *Journal of Consulting and Clinical Psychology*, 1976, *44*, 921–928.

Lushene, R. E., & Gilberstadt, H. Validation of VA MMPI computer-generated reports. Paper presented at the Veterans Administration Cooperative Studies Conference, St. Louis, March 1972.

MacAndrew, C. The differentiation of male alcoholic outpatients from nonalcoholic psychiatric outpatients by means of the MMPI. *Quarterly Journal of Studies on Alcohol*, 1965, *26*, 238–246.

MacAndrew, C., & Geertsma, R. H. A critique of alcoholism scales derived from the MMPI. *Quarterly Journal of Studies on Alcohol*, 1964, *25*, 68–76.

Marks, P. A., Bertelson, A., & May, G. Race and MMPI: Some new findings and considerations. Paper presented at the 85th annual convention of the American Psychological Association, San Francisco, 1977.

Meehl, P. E. The dynamics of structured personality tests. *Journal of Clinical Psychology*, 1945, *1*, 296–303.

Meehl, P. E. Wanted—a good cookbook. Presidential address, Midwestern Psychological Association, Chicago, April, 1955. *American Psychologist*, 1956, *11*, 263–272.

Meehl, P. E. Reactions, reflections, projections. In J. N. Butcher (Ed.), *Objective personality assessment: Changing perspectives.* New York: Academic Press, 1972.

Miller, W. R. Alcoholism scales and objective assessment methods: A review. *Psychological Bulletin*, 1976, *83*, 649–674.

Millon, T. *Millon Multiaxial Clinical Inventory manual.* Minneapolis: National Computer Systems, Inc., 1977.

Olson, G. The Hastings short form of the group MMPI. *Journal of Clinical Psychology*, 1954, *10*, 386–388.

Overall, J. E. MMPI personality patterns of alcoholics and narcotic addicts. *Quarterly Journal of Studies on Alcohol*, 1973, *34*, 104–111.

545

OBJECTIVE
PERSONALITY
INVENTORIES:
RECENT RESEARCH
AND SOME
CONTEMPORARY
ISSUES

Overall, J. E. Implementation of an actuarial diagnostic program in a clinic setting. Paper presented at the Eleventh Annual Symposium on Recent Developments in the Use of the MMPI, Minneapolis, 1976.

Patrick, J., Connolly, A., & Overall, J. Personality correlates of alcohol abuse among new admissions to a state hospital. *Proceedings of the 78th Annual Convention of the American Psychological Association*, 1970, *5*, 321–322.

Rich, C. C., & Davis, H. G. Concurrent validity of MMPI alcoholism scales. *Journal of Clinical Psychology*, 1969, *25*, 425–426.

Rohan, W., Tatro, R., & Rotman, S. MMPI changes in alcoholics during hospitalization. *Quarterly Journal of Studies on Alcohol*, 1969, *30*, 389–400.

Rotman, S. R., & Vestre, N. D. The use of the MMPI in identifying problem drinkers among psychiatric hospital admissions. *Journal of Clinical Psychology*, 1964, *20*, 526–530.

Schmale, A. H., & Iker, H. P. The affect of hopelessness and the development of cancer. *Psychosomatic Medicine*, 1966, *28*, 714–721.

Schwartz, M. F. The MacAndrews alcoholism scale: A construct validity study. Unpublished doctoral dissertation, 1977.

Sines, J. O. Actuarial methods as appropriate strategy for the validation of diagnostic tests. *Psychological Review*, 1964, *71*, 517–523.

Smart, R. G., & Jones, D. Illicit LSD users: Their personality characteristics and psychopathology. *Journal of Abnormal Psychology*, 1970, *75*, 286–292.

Spera, J., & Robertson, M. A 104-item MMPI: The Maxi-Mult. Paper presented at the annual meeting of the American Psychological Association, New Orleans, 1974.

Stein, M., Schiavi, R. C., & Camerino, M. Influence of brain and behavior on the immune system. *Science*, 1976, *191*, 435–439.

Swenson, W. M. Directions in actuarial and automated assessment. Paper presented at the Eleventh Annual Symposium on Recent Developments in the Use of the MMPI, Minneapolis, 1976.

Uecker, A. E. Differentiating male alcoholics from other psychiatric patients. *Quarterly Journal of Studies on Alcohol*, 1970, *31*, 379–383.

Webb, J. T. Validity and utility of computer-produced MMPI reports with Veterans Administration psychiatric populations. *Proceedings of the 78th Annual Convention of the American Psychological Association*, 1970.

Webb, J. T., Miller, M. L., & Fowler, R. D., Jr. Validation of a computerized MMPI interpretation system. *Proceedings of the 77th Annual Convention of the American Psychological Association*, 1969.

Whitelock, P. R., Overall, J. E., & Patrick, J. H. Personality patterns and alcohol abuse in a state hospital population. *Journal of Abnormal Psychology*, 1971, *78*, 9–16.

Wiggins, J. S. Content dimensions in the MMPI. In J. N. Butcher (Ed.), *MMPI: Research developments and clinical applications*. New York: McGraw-Hill, 1969.

Wisler, R. H., & Cantor, J. N. The MacAndrew alcoholism scale: A cross-validation in a domiciliary setting. *Journal of Clinical Psychology*, 1966, *22*, 311–312.

16

Wolman's Sociodiagnostic Interview

BENJAMIN B. WOLMAN, ANDREA ALPER,
AND STEVE DeBERRY

1. Introduction

Wolman's sociodiagnostic interviewing technique is an outgrowth of experimental studies in social psychology and group dynamics and clinical studies in psychopathology. The first sociopsychological studies, inspired by J. L. Moreno's (1953) sociometric theory and technique, were conducted in Israel in 1948 at the time of the War of Independence. Wolman (1953) reported that the group morale in Israel is only partly related to Moreno's acceptance-rejection categories, and it is far more dependent on devotion to an ideal. This desire to give oneself to a beloved person, idea, or country was christened by Wolman with the name "vectorialism," indicative of going out from oneself toward others. In the same paper, Wolman suggested three types of social interaction based on participants' motivation. When an individual's aim is to have his needs satisfied, to get, his attitude is called instrumental; when his intention is to give whatever he can, expecting the same from others, his attitude is mutual; when he is ready to give without expecting anything in return, the attitude is vectorial. Detailed theoretical, clinical, and experimental studies are described as follows.

2. Power and Acceptance

The observable behavior of living organisms is directed toward the universal goal of survival. C. Darwin, T. Huxley, I. P. Pavlov, K. Goldstein, and scores of

BENJAMIN B. WOLMAN • 10 West 66th Street, New York, New York 10023. ANDREA ALPER and STEVE DeBERRY • Doctoral Program in Clinical Psychology, Long Island University, Brooklyn, New York 11201. Bernice Hoffman, Rosalie Hirschfeld, and Linda Pasternak, students in the Doctoral Program of Clinical Psychology at the Long Island University, also took part in this research.

other research workers indicated that survival was the main and universal motive in the entire animal world. All living organisms take in air, food, and water, and all of them resist the danger of destruction by flight or fight.

Let us define "power" as the ability to protect life. A "strong" organism is an organism that is able to provide whatever is necessary for its survival and to resist danger. A "weak" organism is unable to do so. Survival depends on several factors such as the intake of air, water, and food, and protection from harsh temperature and hostile animals. Usually we describe these factors as necessary for survival in terms of "needs." Instead of saying "Food is a necessary prerequisite for our survival," one can say "We have the 'need' for food." Accordingly, one can define power as the ability to satisfy needs.

The term "satisfaction of needs" is used here in a nonhedonistic connotation. We do not discuss here the question of whether the intake of food is "satisfying" in the sense of producing subjective, pleasurable feelings. The objective fact is that without food the dog will not survive, whether the food tastes good, is enjoyable, or is not.

The protection of life can be divided into a series of distinct functions of the living organism, such as breathing, eating, and fighting. The term "protection of life" should also include improvement of vital functioning and increased chances for survival. Some needs are direct and immediate, and must be satisfied instantly, e.g., mammals cannot delay breathing. Other functions of the organism are less directly connected with the main goal of survival and can be postponed, e.g., the need for sleep or rest. In a lethal danger, even the sleepy or tired animal will run for life. As Pavlov's (1928, p. 188ff.) experiments have shown, in dogs the need for food is stronger than the need to protect the skin from burns but less strong than the need to protect the bones. Sexual needs apparently become inhibited in animals fleeing a mortal danger. Of course, a mild food stimulant cannot compete with a powerful skin stimulant; however, Pavlov's experiments have shown that certain "nerve centers" are stronger than others; accordingly, certain "needs" are more pronounced, and not all needs have the same chances in case of an inner conflict.

2.1. Omnipotence

Let us imagine someone who is absolutely powerful. Obviously, all his needs are satisfied and he has no needs. If he is omnipotent, he can go on living forever. Omnipotence includes immortality, that is, the ability of eternal survival or unlimited protection of life. Protection of life has been defined as power; an omnipotent being has, by definition, all the power, and therefore the ability to survive forever. To be mortal means not to be able to protect life and not to be omnipotent.

Men have always dreamed about such a superb, immortal, omnipotent being. They have called it God. Primitive religions ascribed their absolute power to natural forces such as wind, sun, and earth. The ancient Greeks had many gods. Their gods were immortal, though not omnipotent. The omnipotent force was called *Moira* or *fatum*, which was the force of historical necessity and the inescapable sequence of events. Monotheistic religions have believed that the omnipotent being was the Creator, the omnipotent Father of the world. Judaism called him "Father in Heaven," and, after Judaism, Christianity and Islam used this term. The Father is good, for what else can He be? Since He has no needs (all His needs are, by definition of His unlimited power, already satisfied), how can He be hostile? What for? He has no enemies, for no one can contest His power or disobey His laws. Only punitive gods were warriors, but the omnipotent monotheistic God does not need to fight. To be omnipotent implies being *necessarily good* (cf. Spinoza, 1911, part I).

Poor souls want to get. Mediocrities want to keep what they possess; they are afraid they may lose whatever they have and become poorer. But those who possess an unlimited wealth do not need to get or to keep. The only thing for them to do is to be generous and to give. Hence, giving away, generosity, and creativeness are the privilege of those who do not need to get and are not afraid to lose. Unlimited resources cannot be exhausted. The stronger one feels, the less he cares about possession (Wolman, in preparation).

Hence creativity is the most profound symbol and sign of power. Lord, says the scripture, created the world out of nothing. We comment on it and say that he didn't need to take anything from outside. He did not need to destroy anything to live; gods and angels do not need food and they do not need to fight for survival.

Consider the parallels between ethics (being good) and creativeness (being strong). Love means protection of life and creation of new life. The stronger one is, the more he is inclined to give to others, to be good to those who are weak. Ethics is the law of absolute power; the more power, the stronger the desire to give, to create, to protect others. Poor, insecure, frightened animals have to fight. The more power to mankind, the less need to fight. Hence the prophesy of Isaiah about men of the future who do not fight each other but plow together.

Ethics is not a philosophical whim or invention. It is the necessity of God, i.e., Nature. Survival is the supreme law of nature, and protection of life is the supreme law of ethics. Hence the Jewish commandment "Thou shalt not kill." This is the law of the omnipotent God, creator of life, provider and protector of men. This principle of protection of human life, the sanctity of life, became the fundamental ethical principle of the Western civilization. All ethics, secular or religious, affirm life, the life of all.

2.2 Power as Seen by Oneself

Men have always desired to accumulate power, be it by storing food, clothing, or arms, or by developing physical strength, skills, shrewd strategies, etc. Not always has this accumulation been rational or offered a real protection of life; for instance, amulets and charms do not necessarily increase one's power.

One must distinguish between the power one possesses and one's perception of one's own power. These two differ frequently; the feelings of inferiority or superiority reflect what one thinks about himself in terms of power. People may perceive themselves as strong or weak, or they may be inconsistent in that perception of self, and their estimate of own power may not correspond to truth.

No man can live alone. Man is born so weak, that unless others will use their power for his protection, he will not survive. The newborn infant is at the mercy of its parents or other individuals who are in control of it. It seems that the higher the species, the longer the road from the start of life to adulthood, i.e., to the point when one has power.

People may acquire the feeling of power through alliance with powerful individuals. An infant may feel cramps in its stomach; it may feel cold and hungry, or wet and uncomfortable; it has no power and cannot satisfy its needs. It is, therefore, weak. Infants get panicky when food is not forthcoming or when they are hit, hurt, or thrown. We may hypothesize about infants' feelings by comparison with other beings in stress. Most probably, infants feel weak (perceive themselves as weak) when their needs are not taken care of; when their needs are taken care of, they may see themselves as strong or, as Ferenczi (1926) suggested, they "hallucinate" omnipotence. Actually, their true power, i.e., their ability to satisfy needs, was the same in both cases. Yet their moods fluctuated from elation (feeling strong) to depression (feeling weak). The urge to feel strong is obviously a derivative of the most fundamental urge to survive.

The more realistic the evaluation of one's own power in comparison to friends and foes, the greater are his chances to act realistically, to take the proper precautions, and to overcome the dangers.

Depression is the feeling of one's own weakness, helplessness, and inability for self-protection and survival. When one perceives himself as being weak, i.e., unable to satisfy needs, he feels angry, unhappy, apprehensive; that is, depressed. However, it is one thing to be weak, and quite another to feel weak. Well-balanced individuals usually perceive themselves and their environment correctly. They are neither extremely depressed nor extremely elated. They are happy in victory and afraid in danger, they try to cope with threatening situations by fight or flight. Depressed individuals do not see things in proportion and are less capable to protect themselves because they magnify the dangers. Elated individuals underestimate the dangers.

There are undoubtedly many chemical, social, and psychological factors that influence the perception of one's own power. Some drugs (stimulants) make people feel great, while others (depressants) make people shrink in their own eyes. Hunger, thirst, and pain are undoubtedly depressing.

Human relations seem to be of great importance in the self-rating of one's own power. Children are much influenced by parental judgment of their power, and their depressive moods are usually sociogenic. The internalized voice of parents, the superego, is the source of one's self-evaluation; when a hypercritical superego turns against one's ego, the individual experiences depression. Parental criticism, internalized in the superego, is the source of depression. In cases of a very cruel superego, the individual will experience agitated depression.

A maniac, at the peak of his elated mood, apparently believes that he possesses unlimited powers. He is joyous and outgoing, industrious and friendly. His superego has merged with his ego; there is no self-criticism, no limit to the feeling of power. However, when contradicted or challenged in his feeling of power, he may become furious and assaultive. The myth of his own power has been destroyed, and he must fight.

This distinction between one's power as it is and his own estimate of his power is of great importance in psychopathology. It is not the same to be strong and to feel strong, to be weak and to feel weak. In well-balanced individuals, these two things are closely correlated and individuals have a fairly objective picture of their abilities and disabilities. Their feelings of strength and elation and their feelings of inadequacy and defeat both correspond to reality.

Pathological elation and depression stem from within. They represent the attitude of the superego to the ego and a failure on the part of the ego to do reality testing. When this reality testing or the ability to distinguish between inner and outer stimuli fails, the individual may hallucinate.

2.3. Impressing Others

The more one has power, the greater is his safety and the better his protection of life. When one's enemies know his power, his safety increases, because they wouldn't dare to attack or resist him. This may be why lions roar, gorillas hit their chests, dogs bark, and little cats hiss and arch their backs; presumably, each tries to look stronger, more impressive, more threatening. Ancient warriors and contemporary youngsters boast about their own strength and ridicule that of their adversaries before the actual combat begins. Joshua's warriors enhanced their own courage and reduced the courage of their enemies by marching and shouting around the walls of Jericho; no wonder Jericho's hearts fell and the walls collapsed. So-called modern psychological warfare undermines the courage of enemies and enhances one's own courage by emphasizing one's own strength and underscoring the enemies' weakness. "Morale" is ultimately nothing but the high rating of one's own power or ability to survive or to satisfy certain needs.

An individual can "impress" others or make them believe in his power in more than one way. The less one is sure of his own power, the more important it is to convince others; the more one is afraid, the greater the need to scare away his enemies. Little boys show off their physical strength. A nouveau riche is inclined to show his newly acquired wealth; "conspicuous consumption" is typical in such a case. Insecure individuals are frequently boastful; some boast of their own wealth, some boast of wisdom, some boast of friendliness, connections, good taste, clothing, land of origin, school marks, sex, or anything else.

2.4. Destructive Power

Power can be used in two directions: to support life, i.e., to satisfy needs, and/or to destroy life, i.e., to prevent the satisfaction of needs. Accordingly, our definition of power reads: *Power is the ability to satisfy needs of oneself and/or of others or to prevent their satisfaction.*

Both building and destroying require some amount of power. A weak person can neither help nor hurt. Destruction requires less power than construction. Compare the erection of a house to its destruction, the making of a car to the breaking of it, healing to wounding, creating life to killing. A child cannot build a house, but can set it on fire. It takes time and effort to plant an orchard, but in no time it can be devastated.

Even weak individuals may acquire the feeling of power by being malicious. Hence the widespread but erroneous belief that bad people are necessarily strong and good ones are weak. Because all men wish to be strong, evil power, destruction, and violence attract so many. Some children and teenagers are susceptible to this enhancement.

Hostile and destructive power can be more impressive than friendly power. When one is friendly, his good intentions are not always conspicuous. Hostility seems to be more expressive than friendliness; hostile animals bark, hiss, roar. Newspapers usually pay more attention to one murderer than to a thousand constructive workers. One can easily understand why little children play cowboys and Indians and other war games, and why almost all of them want to be on the winning side.

All observers of living organisms have observed that most general and universal phenomenon, fight for survival. P. Kropotkin's (1902) idea of mutual aid does not contradict this universal tendency. The only conclusion one may draw from Kropotkin's beautiful and humane book is that cooperation among members of the same species or group improves their chances in their fight against other species. Group cohesiveness helps in peace and in war.

One can distinguish four types of hostility. We shall, for lack of better terminology, attach a name to each type: "defense," "aggression," "panic," and "terror." These four names will help us to recognize, later, each type of hostility. The first type is the most universal, defensive fight, let us say of a sheep against the attacking wolf. The wolf does not "hate" the sheep; the wolf "loves" to eat it up. But the sheep hates the wolf and fights for survival. No wonder minority groups and persecuted individuals are accused of being "aggressive." The wolves are usually the accusers.

The second type of hostile action is the aggressive behavior of the wolf. As mentioned, the wolf does not necessarily hate the sheep. The wolf wants to eat, and it, too, fights for survival. The only fault of the sheep or of Jews, Armenians, Blacks, and other minority groups is their weakness. No wonder wolves and others try to destroy them and take away their life and property. Whenever victims defend themselves, the wolves become frustrated and infuriated. One may say that frustration often elicits or intensifies hostile action, but there has been plenty of hostility in the animal and human society started by victorious wolves.

The third type of hostility occurs in a group panic and can best be characterized by herd behavior in an escape from danger. Wild goats are not gentle to each other when they run for life. On a narrow passage, the stronger will push the weak one.

All three types of hostile action can be magnified by frustration, can be turned away from the main target and displaced on a substitute target (scapegoat), can be shared by a group as chauvinism, can be acted out against innocent bystanders, can be combined with sexual pleasure (sadism), can become a disguised cruelty in the name of a worthy cause (fanaticism, "holy" wars, etc.), can be put in a subtle fashion of criticism and ridicule, undermining the adversary's self-esteem and self-confidence, etc., can be a show-off of brutality, and can be also sublimated into fight for justice and freedom.

The fourth type of hostility is the blind rage of a wounded animal that fights desperately against anyone who comes near it. It is the hostility in a mortal danger, it is the most profound combination of fear and hate, of panic and rage. These two feelings stem from the same source of threat to life and merge into one feeling or terror in face of death. The aggressive and defensive hostility is directed toward a definite person, animal, or object; panic and terror are not object-directed. Aggression and panic may be free of hostile feelings; defense and terror are always accompanied by intense hate.

3. Fear and Hate

Since the connection between fear and hate is of greatest importance for the understanding of the etiology and symptomatology of schizophrenia, we shall examine it more closely. Threat elicits fear and rage; both are hostile feelings that represent the wish to get rid of the source of threat by fight or flight. We do not fear friends. Enemies we fear and hate. When they are weak, we fight; when they are strong, we tend to escape.

A threat that comes from without produces fear and elicits fight or flight. Children who believe in parental omnipotence are often shocked when they see their parents in fight or flight. Children usually believe in parental omnipotence. Parents who have temper tantrums or run away from home have a great share in the development of mental disorder in their children.

Human beings learn not to act immediately but to control and postpone their actions. In many situations, we control fear and anger. Sometimes we express our fear and anger in words, but we do not act it out. Well-balanced individuals control their feelings and act on them in a rational way, i.e., the way that brings the best possible solutions. Disturbed individuals fall prey to their emotions of fear and anger even when these emotions do not correspond to real threats.

4. Social Perception

One may say that all of us act on our correct or incorrect perception of the world. We view the power of self and others; we may overestimate or underestimate, but our actions are guided by our estimates. The interindividual relations depend on power and acceptance as perceived by us and by others. We do not relate in the same way to those we believe to be able to satisfy our needs, i.e., strong ones, and to those we believe to be weak. This social perception plays an important role in interindividual relations.

It is easy to show that power as it is and power as perceived by others are frequently two different things. A magician has no real power, yet his co-tribesmen believe in his power. Furthermore, if power is defined as the ability to satisfy needs, the socially perceived power of an individual depends on the needs of the group. In a classroom, the teacher is strong; in a sickroom, the physician; on a job, the employer. Each group perceives power differently, depending on its specific needs; even the strongest athlete or best bridge player is perceived as weak on a broken, stranded bus unless he also happens to be an auto mechanic. Social relations are a function of power and acceptance as perceived by the group in accordance with the needs of that group.

One may impress others by verbal or nonverbal communication. "Conspicuous consumption" aims apparently at the impression on others of one's financial power. Claiming poverty aims at impressing others as to one's financial weakness. Normally we strive at a correct estimate of our own power and that of others. However, it seems to be relatively easy to mislead others, as commercial advertising, political propaganda, and mental disorder prove. The needs or motivation on one hand and the social perception on the other are obviously weighty factors in social relations.

Friendliness and hostility are not easily recognized. Humans act on perceived situations; they do not react to things as they are but to stimuli as perceived. This basic fact relates the entire human behavior to the problems of cognition. Children may feel more love for the candy-buying aunt than for the bread-buying mother. One would like to believe that humans are rational beings and that their behavior is controlled by a realistic perception and logic. One would like to believe that humans perceive themselves and their environment correctly. However, it has frequently been observed that people act not necessarily on what is absolutely necessary for their survival but on what they perceive as needs and believe to be necessary for their self-preservation; sometimes they act even in violation of their own judgment. Our reaction to a stimulus depends on how that stimulus was perceived. The perceptions of well-adjusted adults correspond more or less to the stimuli. The perceptions of children, as Piaget, Freud, Abraham, Sullivan, and others found, do not correspond very closely to the external stimuli. Our perceptions are colored by our experiences and present emotions. Our "psychological field" is not a photograph of reality, but reality as perceived by the individual, and, in accordance with the above-said, each individual pursues his "needs" inasmuch as he is aware or dimly aware of them (Wolman, 1956, 1958a).

5. Statogram

Whatever exists, exists in a certain quantity. We may not be able to measure something today, but we may tomorrow find out how to measure it. Power can be presented in a linear scale starting from a zero point that indicates no power and going up in plus numbers. The higher the plus number, the more power. Power cannot have negative numbers.

In interindividual relations, power can be used either for protection or for destruction of life. Power is the ability to satisfy needs, i.e., to protect life, or to prevent their satisfaction, i.e., to hurt and destroy. This interindividual relation must be presented not only in one dimension of amount of power but also in another dimension of the use of it. Whenever power is used to support life, it is friendly; whenever it is used for destruction, it is hostile. Thus the entire relationship can be presented on truncated Cartesian ordinates, as shown in Figure 1. The vertical S-W (strong-weak) line represents power, while the horizontal F-H (friendly-hostile) line represents acceptance or the direction in which the power is used.

A study of social relations in classroom situations (Wolman, 1949) pointed to four different types of reactions between students and teachers related to these two dimensions of power and acceptance. Four categories or relationships developed. Teachers perceived by students as weak and hostile were openly defied and could not control their classes. Those perceived as weak and friendly had very unstable discipline; students obeyed only those instructions that they liked; whenever they disliked the teachers' suggestions they disobeyed. Teachers regarded as strong and hostile controlled their classes, but the discipline was involuntary and based on fear and suppressed hatred. Teachers perceived as strong and friendly were willingly obeyed by their students; the interviewed students explained that they wouldn't dare

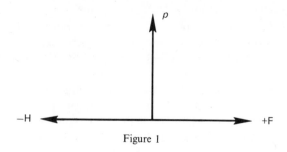

Figure 1

alienate a "strong" teacher or want to hurt the feelings of a "friendly" one. Strong and friendly teachers were true leaders; the children willingly accepted their leadership and followed instructions (cf. Wolman, 1958b).

This study has led to the development of a statometric technique, called "statogram," which measures one's social position in the two dimensions of power (strongweak) and acceptance (friendly-hostile).

The two-dimensional perception of people in interpersonal relations is decisive in establishing one's social status. Hyman (1942) has distinguished three types of status; the first related to subjective evaluation by a person of comparable status, the second to "real" power relations, the third to evaluation by others. The present writers think that an individual's position or status in a group depends on the attitude of other people toward this particular individual. More precisely, a person's status is a function of his power, as seen by others, and of his being accepted by others. Power is defined as the ability to satisfy needs (or to deny such satisfaction); acceptance is defined as the readiness to do so. Thus

$$S = f(P, A) \tag{1}$$

where status (S) is a function (f) of power (P) and acceptance (A).

Leadership has been defined here as a relationship in which the leader stimulates, instigates, and sometimes controls and determines the functions of others, called followers. Obviously, leadership is a function of power, and no one can be a leader unless people recognize his power.

In an undemocratic group, an unpopular bully or a tyrant can lead by power alone, either by satisfying the needs of others or by deprivation. He is regarded by his followers as a very strong although not necessarily friendly person.

In a democratic group, no one can be a leader unless he is regarded as a friendly person. Of course, he must be both friendly and strong; otherwise, he could not be chosen and accepted as a leader. This can be summarized in a mathematical function valid for groups in which followers are free to follow the leader of their choice (democratic groups):

$$L = f(P, A) \tag{2}$$

where leadership (L) is a function (f) of power (P) and acceptance (A), in accordance with the former definitions of P and A.

This is a general formula for leadership which requires a breakdown with respect to various types of groups. In some groups, A can be more or less important than P.

In contradistinction to Moreno's (1953) sociogram, which deals with attraction vs. repulsion, the statogram adds a second dimension, of strength vs. weakness (Wolman, 1956). The statogram is a research tool which rates group members on strongweak, friendly-hostile, chosen-rejected, and leadership scales. The statogram was administered to group members, and the results of the statogram were compared with the estimates of the observers. While Bales's (1950) interaction analysis describes a person's status as seen by observers, statogram analysis gives direct assessment of status by the rating of the participants in a group.

The members of groups score each other. The power quotients represent the group's estimate of power of each individual. Then acceptance quotients are computed for each group member indicating what the group thinks about the person's friendliness or hostility. Obviously, the status of each group member depends on how he is perceived by others in terms of power and acceptance.

These experimental studies have shed some light on the nature of status, leadership, and cohesiveness in face-to-face groups and have emphasized the importance of social perception. Interindividual relations seem to be a function of power and acceptance as perceived by the participating individuals.

5.1. Self-Statogram

Preliminary studies with self-statogram have been conducted. The individuals were asked to note themselves in terms of power and acceptance, and their ratings of themselves were compared with their rating by others.

Striking differences in self-ratings as compared to the rating by others were checked in individual interviews. Some individuals, rated by others as strong, i.e., competent on the task presented to their group, rated themselves as very weak, and vice versa. The same happened with the friendly-hostile (acceptance) dimension.

The implications of these studies for assessment of personality are obvious. We are rated not only by others; we tend to rate ourselves. Our own estimate of our friendliness or hostility can be as easily influenced as our estimate of our strength or weakness. Well-balanced individuals usually evaluate themselves correctly and know when they are friendly ("good") or hostile ("bad"), and how strong they are.

A serious deviation from reality in the estimate of one's own power and acceptance inevitably interferes with one's adjustment. As mentioned, the feeling of elation indicates a serious overestimation of one's own power typical of maniacs. It is usually accompanied by the feeling of one's own immense friendliness. On the other hand, the feeling of depression indicates an underestimation of one's own power and/or own friendliness.

This idea has led to the development of a system of classification of mental disorders (Krauss & Krauss, 1977; Wolman, 1973) and the Sociodiagnostic Interview (Wolman, 1965b).

Wolman attempted to solve the problem of classification by taking into consideration the overt symptoms, etiology, and therapeutic considerations. The classificatory system has been described in detail in the book *Call No Man Normal* (1973) and in Chapter 2 in the present volume.

This classificatory system (Wolman, 1965a, 1973) leans heavily on Freud's topographic model (the concept of unconscious), dynamics (balance of cathexes), and structural theory (id, ego, and superego), with several far-reaching modifications. The main emphasis, however, is on interindividual relations in terms of power and acceptance.

It has been observed in psychotherapeutic work, especially in the setting of group therapy, that these attitudes dominate the total pattern of overt behavior of the patients. The psychopathic individuals are hyperinstrumental; they always ask something for nothing; they show no consideration of others and demand incessant attention; in group therapy, they try to monopolize the conversation; in individual therapy, they demand immediate gain; in relationships with the outer world, they try to loot; they seem to believe that the world owes them everything; they are dishonest whenever they can be.

The latent schizophrenics are hypervectorial. They are loving, devoted, affectionate, shy, hyperethical, hyperaltruistic individuals; as insecure as they are, they always know best what is good for their love object; they are always ready for self-sacrifice; in group therapy, they are usually quiet and believe that the others have priority; in individual therapy, they often express worries about the therapist; they seem to believe that they owe the world everything; they are absolutely honest.

The manic-depressives are dysmutual. They are masters of inconsistency; they may overdo in loving others and hating others; when they love, they expect the others to return even more love to them; they demand that the others appreciate how nice they are; they may be as brutal as psychopaths, and as sensitive as the schizophrenics. Their inconsistency in human relations makes them appear phony; their affectionate and self-sacrificing attitude easily turns into a selfish tactlessness; they easily shift from honesty to dishonesty.

In social relations, the psychopaths strive to have others serve them; the latent schizophrenics desire their services to be accepted; the manic-depressives swing from one to the other. The psychopaths hate whoever does not serve them; the latent schizophrenics are afraid to hate; the manic-depressives swing from one extreme to the other.

5.2. Division along Vertical Lines

Psychopathic individuals act on an insufficient reality principle and often yield to the pleasure principle. Their superego is practically nonexistent; their ego is primitive. Their libido is narcissistic with very little if any object relation, usually on the oral-cannibalistic level.

The economy of intra- and interpersonal cathexes shows a definite abundance of self-cathexis and no or very limited object-cathexis. Their destrudo is powerfully object-cathected, and the psychopaths hate intensely. The hyperinstrumentalism translated into the conceptual framework of psychoanalysis means secondary narcissism, oral-cannibalistic love, destrudo directed to others, ego yielding to the id, and a very weak superego.

The latent schizophrenics are the opposite of the psychopaths. Their superego is overdeveloped, domineering, self-righteous, demanding, and moralistic. Their ego is overmobilized, their id severely overcontrolled. Their libido is lavishly object-hypercathected, with an insufficient, if any, self-cathexis. Destrudo is repressed. No wonder such an impoverishment of the system may lead to mental catastrophy and to a most severe regression. It is indeed a vectoriasis praecox or a hypervectorialism developed too much, too early, and at too costly a price.

The manic-depressives stand between the two. Their superego is inconsistent, sometimes furiously attacking the ego in depression, sometimes embracing it in elation. The ego is disoriented, demoralized, demobilized, often in a daze. The libido swings from self-cathexis to object-cathexis; the same holds true of the destrudo.

According to the proposed division along vertical lines, the so-called psychopathic personality disorders belong to the hyperinstrumental group, the schizophrenias and obsessive-compulsive neuroses to the hypervectorial group, and hysteria and manic-depressive disorders to the dysmutual group.

5.3. Division along Horizontal Lines

Division along horizontal lines is based on interpersonal relations and on the economy of the interindividual and intraindividual cathexes of the libido and destrudo. It is not the only possible classification. A full classification of mental disorder should take into consideration also the topographical aspects of personality, i.e., the unconscious, preconscious, and conscious, and the relative position of the mental apparatus, i.e., the id, ego, and superego.

Such a classification will go along horizontal lines, classifying all mental disorder in accordance to the two abovementioned criteria, topography and apparatus. Five levels can be distinguished, starting from neurosis, through character disorder, latent psychosis, manifest psychosis, to complete dementia or collapse of the mental structure.

The neuroses are characterized by repression of the unconscious material and the struggle of the ego against the pressures stemming from the id and superego. A profound feeling of anxiety accompanies the mounting tensions, and severe symptoms may develop. Yet, in neurosis, the ego clings to reality in warding off the inner pressures.

In character disorders, the neurotic symptoms "take over." The ego does not fight anymore; it comes to terms with the symptoms. Primary and secondary gains dominate the picture. A "character armor" serves as a protective shell. The neurosis forms the essence of one's personality.

In psychosis, the ego fails. It fails in its tasks of reality testing and of countercathexis. At the latent phase of psychosis, the ego is still engaged in a losing battle. It develops, as Hoch found, pseudoneurotic symptoms. When these fail to protect the ego, a full-blown psychosis develops. In neurosis, the individual suffers anxieties; the person with a character disorder often is in a state of fright; the psychotic is in a panic.

According to Freud, in neurosis the ego renounces the gratification of instinctual desires; according to Federn (1952), in neurosis the ego is on the defensive, but in psychosis it has already collapsed. It may be further added that, in character disorders, the ego accepts the neurotic symptoms as if they were the best protective shell against further deterioration and eventual breakdown.

The differential diagnosis should take into consideration both the vertical and horizontal lines of division. The vertical lines discern three types of mental disorder, namely the hyperinstrumental, the dysmutual, and the hypervectorial, or, respectively, the self-hypercathected, the cyclic-cathected, and the object-hypercathected types. Then the five levels are added, 15 different clinical pictures emerge, representing the five levels of each type. Accordingly, the self-hypercathected instrumentalism can be divided into the (1) psychopathic neurosis, in which the neurotic personality structure (topography and mental apparatus) is geared to the struggle of the ego against powerful instinctual forces which violate the reality principle. The fear of external danger leads to symptom formation and escape into illness; apparently, many cases of so-called anxiety neurosis and traumatic neurosis fall into this category. The second level of the hyperinstrumentalism is represented by the (2) psychopathic character; in this case, the individual has accepted his extreme selfishness and neurotic symptoms and derives out of them primary and secondary gains. On the third level, the "armor" does not help, and the (3) latent psychopathic psychotics act out their primitive impulses. The ego is shattered and the instinctual forces exercise decisive influence. It is the uncontrollable *haltlose* type of behavior, failing with little if any inhibitions, leading to a manifest antisocial behavior. The fourth level is described as (4) moral insanity, or a total victory of secondary narcissism and object-directed destrudo. It seems that some patients described in the literature

Table 1. Classification of Psychosociogenic Mental Disorders

	Narcissistic hyperinstrumental type (I)	Depressive dysmutual type (M)	Schizohypervectorial type (V)
Neurotic level	Hyperinstrumental neurosis (narcissistic neurosis)	Dysmutual neurosis (dissociations, hysterias, and depressions)	Hypervectorial neurosis (obsessional, phobic, and neurasthenic neuroses)
Character neurotic level	Hyperinstrumental character neurosis (narcissistic character)	Dysmutual character neurosis (depressive and hysteric character)	Hypervectorial character neurosis (schizoid and obsessional character)
Latent psychotic level	Latent hyperinstrumental psychosis (psychopathic narcissism bordering on psychosis)	Latent dysmutual psychosis (borderline depressive psychosis)	Latent vectoriasis praecox (borderline and latent schizophrenia)
Manifest psychotic level	Hyperinstrumental psychosis (psychotic psychopathy and moral insanity)	Dysmutual psychosis (manifest depressive psychosis)	Vectoriasis praecox (manifest schizophrenia)
Dementia level	Collapse of personality structure		

as criminal schizophrenics belong rather to this category. Then a complete dementia takes place; in cases of social upheavals such as war and famine, the cyclic type can be presented in a similar five-level scheme. The first is a neurotic level; it is the (1) hysteria with its inconsistencies, changing moods, and dramatic personality dissociations in the style of Dr. Jekyll and Mr. Hyde. Next comes the (2) cycloid (or hysteroid) character; then (3) latent manic-depressive disorder; then comes (4) manifest manic-depressive psychosis; last (5) is the dementive stages of a deep regression into a prenatal type of behavior.

The hypervectorial type can also be divided into five levels, starting with (1) obsessive-compulsive neurosis characterized by severe superego and guilt feelings; (2) schizoid character, which uses compulsion as the protective shell; (3) latent schizophrenic character whose ego loses the battle; (4) manifest schizophrenic whose ego lost the battle and regressed; last (5) the dementive stages. On the level of dementia, the differences among the three types are less pronounced.

The entire system can be presented as shown in Table 1.

6. Interview as a Diagnostic Tool

For the entire 40 years of clinical practice, the senior author has been, as have all other clinicians, much concerned with and often perturbed by diagnostic difficulties. For years, he has used mental measurements and projective techniques in hospital and clinic practice, and less often in private practice with his own patients and when colleagues referred a patient for diagnostic purposes.

However, in the last 15–20 years, he has most frequently used the diagnostic interview (Matarazzo, 1965; Goodman, 1972; Wolman, 1965b). He has worked with the assumption that symptoms are a result of certain noxious causes, and etiology and symptomatology represent a cause-and-effect chain. In other words, when a patient adequately describes his symptoms, the therapist should be able to deduce their underlying causes. Following Tolman's (1932) principles, the patient's past history should be viewed as the independent variable, the theoretical assumptions of psychopathology as the intervening variable, and the present symptoms as the dependent variable. Ideally, the therapist should be able to proceed from either end, but it is usually easier to assess present symptoms.

It is necessary to stress that this method has been applied exclusively to sociogenic disorders, that is, disorders believed to be produced by morbid interindividual relationships. There is no reason to assume that noxious interaction always starts at birth and always ends at the school age, but a damage caused earlier in life usually is more severe than one done later. It is sort of an anvil-hammer relationship. The same blow of a hammer causes more damage to a weaker surface than to a more sturdy one, and a very young child is usually more susceptible and more vulnerable than an older one. Wolman's monograph on childhood schizophrenia, called *Children without Childhood* (1970), has adduced proof that the earlier a child is hurt, the more severe is his disorder.

The question is, however, to what extent the interviewed patients are capable and willing to produce an adequate description of their symptoms. A detailed discussion of this problem is offered by Dr. Matarazzo in the present volume. Here suffice it to say that many patients are neither capable nor willing to describe their symptoms. Quite often, they come to therapy complaining about irrelevant issues which, unwittingly, serve as a cover-up for their real problems.

In constructing a diagnostic interview, one must, therefore, select issues that seem to be relevant and word them in such a manner that reduces the fear of patients to say things they are afraid to say.

7. Diagnostic Criteria

Several authors stressed the importance of social relations as the main, or at least a highly significant, diagnostic clue (Foulds, 1965; Phillips & Draguns, 1971; Sullivan, 1953; and many others). In fact, Freud himself related etiology to parent-child interaction. He assumed that every child goes through biologically determined stages of psychosexual development, namely the oral, anal, urethral, and phallic phases. Together with K. Abraham, Freud developed a timetable of fixation at and/or regression to a particular phase (Fenichel, 1945). Freud believed that the time period of traumatic events is the main determinant of a certain type of disorder.

Although it seems rather rigid to link every clinical type to an etiological timetable, Freud's system left enough room for flexibility and variability dependent on patterns of social interaction within a family unit. Although children were believed to go through certain phases of psychosexual development, how they went through was largely determined by a particular parent-child interaction. The degrees of severity of fixation and regression were clearly linked to the patterns of family life and intrafamilial interaction.

Alfred Adler, Karen Horney, Harry Stack Sullivan, Erich Fromm, and Erik Erikson went further than Freud in stressing the importance of *interactional patterns* in early childhood. It seems quite feasible that the abovementioned theories have inspired a growing interest in the family unit and its role in producing mental disorder in the offspring. The etiology of schizophrenia has attracted a great deal of interest. After decades of research in genetics and biochemistry, psychological and psychiatric journals witnessed an upsurge of research directed to intrafamilial dynamics. In the mid-1950's, at almost the same time and without knowing of each other's work, Gregory Bateson, Theodore Lidz, and Wolman published their studies describing the "sick family" which produced schizophrenic children. Bateson, Jackson, Haley, and Weakland (1956) described the "double-bind" communication in schizophrenic families, Lidz, Fleck, and Cornelison (1955) described striking peculiarities in those families, and Wolman (1957, 1961, 1967) came out with his sociopsychogenic theory of schizophrenia based on his study of disturbed interactional patterns related to his above-described power and acceptance theory of social relations. At the same time, Ackerman (1958) published his influential work on family therapy.

8. The Rationale of Wolman's Technique

There have been three assumptions underlying this technique: (1) that most mental disorders are sociopsychogenic, or that, with the exception of organic cases, all mental disorders are caused by mismanagement of people (children) by people (parents); (2) that interindividual relations offer a highly significant diagnostic clue; and (3) that interviewing technique is one of the best assessment methods.

The rationale of Wolman's technique was described in detail in the *Handbook of Clinical Psychology* (1965) as follows:

> The Socio-Psychological Diagnostic Inventory of Observation and the Socio-psychological-Diagnostic Interview roughly correspond to the techniques of statogram and self-statogram, respectively. In the Inventory of Observations the observer or observers record carefully the overt patterns of behavior of the subject and categorize them in terms of power and acceptance. The observers register empirical data, record them carefully and tabulate. To increase the objectivity of observations one can employ several observers, as reported in one experimental study (Wolman, 1956), and correlate their ratings. This observation includes actions (eating, sleeping, working, entertainment) and interaction and communication with other individuals.
>
> The Socio-Psychological Diagnostic Interview reflects the subject's perception of himself and his environment in terms of power and acceptance. The interviewer conducts an open-end, focused-type interview. The subject is requested to tell his life history, dwell on his childhood memories, describe his past experiences, etc. The interviewer avoids asking any direct questions; he encourages a free flow of communication and whenever necessary tries to bring out a point by asking a question such as "And what happened next? What have you done? How did you feel about it? And what was the reaction of others?" etc.
>
> The foremost diagnostic problem is to find out the type of disorder; the problem of level of disorder comes next. The following description of sociodiagnostic clues is devoted mainly to the types, especially in the neurotic and latent psychotic levels.

8.1. Behavioral Clues

> The diagnostic clues described below are not precise, rigid patterns but descriptive hints not to be taken literally. They are meaningful only in the context of a total personality picture.
> 1. Observations in terms of power may start with a general activity and vitality. Hypervectorials (schizophrenic type) display as a rule less vitality, less energy, and an overall reduced initiative and activity as compared to average normal subjects. They are more precise and pay more attention to detail but are usually much slower than other people are. The hyperinstrumentals (psychopathic type) are active whenever it serves the satisfaction of their needs; otherwise they do not make much effort. The dysmutuals (manic-depressive type) are either sense-

lessly hyperactive, doing things no one needs and being loud, verbose, and full of energy, or senselessly passive even when passivity jeopardizes their well-being.

2. In intellectual functioning the hypervectorials display certain peculiarities. While they may be especially keen, attentive, and alert in one area, they often display lack of interest and apathy in many others. When involved in something, they are exceptionally perceptive, their judgment sharp and logical. The hyperinstrumentals seldom show such an acuity of mind; rarely are they seriously involved in anything outside their own immediate, usually material or sexual, needs. The dysmutuals can be exceedingly alert in one moment and go entirely blank and oblivious in another.

3. The three types differ also in the patterns of *thinking*. Intelligence is not correlated with mental disorder, and one may find mental disorders associated with any degree of innate intellectual abilities; there are intellectually inferior and superior individuals in all three types. However, certain peculiarities in the thought process are distinguishable by psychological tests and, in extreme cases, even in a simple observation. The hypervectorials overlook gross detail; they are logical (unless deteriorated) but not empirically minded. They are prone to indulge in abstract thinking and deep speculation with little regard to reality and overemphasis on minute detail. Their fantasy is rich but often unrealistic, leading to autistic thinking and bizarre reasoning.

The hyperinstrumentals sleep well and like to sleep many hours, unless under threat. Dysning, more plagiarists than inventors. Their thinking lacks depth, and their ideas are narrow. The dysmutuals are rarely as shrewd as hyperinstrumentals or as deep as hypervectorials; they are, as a rule, more practical than the hypervectorials and more profound than the hyperinstrumentals. When deteriorated, their mind goes blank and dull as in the hyperinstrumentals.

4. The three types differ also in the *intake of food*. Food is highly important to hyperinstrumentals, who can barely stand any food deprivation. Hypervectorials are usually finicky eaters; eating is a problem to many schizophrenics. They either refuse to eat or overeat (to reduce anxiety) or toy with food. Dysmutuals eat quickly and often overeat. At meals in the hospital, schizophrenics are usually the slowest and manic-depressives the fastest eaters.

5. The rhythm of *waking* and *sleeping* states is frequently disturbed in hypervectorials. Whenever disturbed, they have difficulties in falling asleep and cannot sleep the night through. On the neurotic level, sleep difficulties are often the outstanding symptom that brings the patient to the consultation room. In latent and manifest schizophrenics sleep disorders may become tantamount to the inability to fall asleep.

The hyperinstrumentals sleep well and like to sleep many hours, unless under threat. Dysmutuals are either sleepy, falling asleep whenever perturbed by inner or outer threats, or unable to sleep when excited. In manifest, manic-depressive psychosis, they frequently go to bed early, being unable to stay up late in the evening. In depressive moods they wake up very early in the morning hating themselves and the world; in these the danger of suicide is quite high.

6. Personal care offers another clue in differential diagnosis. Hypervectorials do not care much for themselves but worry what other people will think about them. On the neurotic, character neurotic, and latent psychotic levels they are meticulously neat. Neglect in personal cleanliness and appearance is usually a sign of serious deterioration. On manifest, and even more on dementive, levels all personal care may disappear entirely.

The hyperinstrumentals take good care of themselves but are not too particular about cleanliness. They are quite concerned with their external appearance whenever they meet strangers whom they would like to impress. The dysmutuals swing from an extreme show-off care to a complete self-neglect.

7. There are definite differences between the three types in regard to property and money. Hyperinstrumentals are greedy and acquisitive, hypervectorials are retentive, dysmutuals are inconsistent. Hyperinstrumentals grab what they can and are unwilling to share. Hypervectorials cannot part with their possessions and sometimes would rather spend money on others than on themselves.

8. At work, hyperinstrumentals are inclined to work hard only when driven by fear or reward; they cheat whenever they can. The hypervectorials are, as a rule, highly conscientious workers. Dysmutuals depend on their fluctuating moods.

In success, hypervectorials tend to worry; in failure they blame themselves. Hyperinstrumentals in success act as victorious beasts, greedy and triumphant; in defeat they become subservient. Dysmutuals exaggerate in a joyful self-praise at a slight success and exaggerate in blaming themselves and others whenever defeated.

10. In regard to pain one can say that hypervectorials are usually masochistically inclined, hyperinstrumentals sadistically, and dysmutuals sadomasochistically. Hypervectorials frequently neglect their own health, notwithstanding pain. Hyperinstrumentals are highly sensitive to pain and overdo in demanding medical care. Dysmutuals go from one extreme to the other.

11. The hypervectorials fear mostly their own hostile impulses that will prove to the world how bad they are. Hyperinstrumentalists distrust and fear people. Dysmutuals in elation have no fear, in depression fear everything.

12. Self-esteem is usually low in all three types. Feelings of inadequacy and dissatisfaction with oneself accompany all mental disorders. yet the hypervectorials feel most dissatisfied with themselves because they believe they are bad. They perceive themselves as hostile and worry lest others may feel the same way and blame them. The hyperinstrumentals are little concerned with what others think about their moral standards. They themselves worry about their own power only—power to get what they need and destroy whatever is in their way. As one psychopathic patient put it, "I feel either as a tiger that can tear the world apart or as a vegetable, anyone can step over me." Their self-esteem depends on tangible achievements.

Manic-depressives combine the power and acceptance dimensions. They swing, in their own eyes, from giants to dwarfs. When they feel accepted, they feel strong and friendly; when rejected, they feel weak and hostile to themselves and the outer world. Self-esteem in hypervectorials depends on whether their love has been accepted, that is, whether parental figures or another significant person whom they love has accepted the love. Dysmutuals need to receive love from everywhere and are never satiated; occasionally they may believe they are loved and enjoy short periods of elation.

8.2. Interactional Clues

There are distinct differences in the way the three types relate to and interact with other people.

1. Hypervectorials display a great deal of empathy; i.e., they sense the feelings of others. Instrumentals have very little empathy, if any. Dysmutuals have less empathy than hypervectorials and more than hyperinstrumentals. Schizophrenics are not always friendly, but they are usually understanding; psychopaths do not care about others; manic-depressives go from one extreme to the other.

2. Hypervectorials excel also in sympathy. Hyperinstrumentals have no sympathy and no mercy, but they expect sympathy from others. Dysmutuals go to extremes; occasionally they are hypersympathetic and self-sacrificing and swing back to an almost psychopathic cruelty. Hypervectorials are cruel when furious; hyperinstrumentals are cruel when it pays to be; dysmutuals are cruel when agitated.

3. Hypervectorials in neurotic, latent psychotic, and remissive phases are usually tactful and considerate; they are often cold and cruel in schizotype character neuroses and manifest schizophrenia. Psychopathic hyperinstrumentals are tactful toward those they perceive a strong and tactless and brutal toward those they perceive as weak. Dysmutuals are oversentimental toward those whose love they wish to get and brutal toward those they do not care for; they are rarely tactful.

4. Moral rigidity characterizes hypervectorials; lack of morality is typical of hyperinstrumentals; moral inconsistency is the sign of dysmutualism. Hypervectorials cling to principles, are dogmatic and self-righteous. Hyperinstrumentals have no moral principles whatsoever; they are radical opportunists. Dysmutuals are highly idealistic and moralistic in one situation and the reverse in another. Hyperinstrumentals try hard to be godlike angels and fear they are devils; when defenses fail, their destrudo erupts in a wild violence. Hyperinstrumentals are overtly selfish and unfair and believe they are within their rights. The whole world seems to be one lebensraum for their ever-hungry wolf jaws, while they believe themselves to be

innocent sheep. Dysmutuals are Dr. Jekyll and Mr. Hyde. When they feel rejected, they become brutal and aggressive.

5.   Hypervectorials tend to blame themselves; hyperinstrumentals blame others; dysmutuals do both.

6.   All disturbed individuals are prone to tell lies. Hyperinstrumentals lie whenever it is profitable. Hypervectorials rarely lie but may do so if their self-esteem is in jeopardy; they lie when they are afraid people will think they are bad or stupid. Dysmutuals lie frequently, usually for self-aggrandizement. Their lies are fantastic, often nonsensical; sometimes they say things that do not make sense even to themselves. Dysmutuals often sound insincere even when they are sincere.

7.   The picture that hypervectorials have of other people is highly confused. They usually perceive others as better, stronger, smarter than themselves and the members of their family. Their feeling of inferiority spreads to those for whom they feel responsible.

Hyperinstrumentals divide the world into those to fear and those to exploit. Dysmutuals divide the world into those who love and those who reject.

8.   Hypervectorials are slow to form friendship, get lastingly overinvolved, and are unable to break off an attachment. Hyperinstrumentals have no friends on a give-and-take basis; a friend to them is someone to be exploited. Their friendships are formed for practical reasons and accordingly are either dropped or conveniently preserved. Dysmutuals easily develop profound attachments, but their feelings are rarely lasting.

9.   Hypervectorials are more persistent and involved in love. When their love is not accepted, it turns into hate. Dysmutuals are never deeply in love, but they hate those who refuse to give love to them. Dysmutuals are "love addicts," constantly in search of new love objects. Their love is always ambivalent, and when it is not returned, it becomes hate.

10.   Sexual deviations accompany all mental disorders. Psychopaths are most frequently polymorphous perverts, capable of and willing to participate in any type of sexual activity. Schizophrenics are frequently torn by the conflict of sex identification and fear of homosexuality. Manic-depressives frequently display impotence, frigidity, and other sexual disturbances.

11.   The hypervectorials try to control hostility; they display hostility whenever rejected, offended, or unable to bear inner hostility and when their defense mechanisms fail. Hyperinstrumentals are hostile whenever their needs are frustrated; that is, whenever their victims protest or anyone gets in their way. Their basic attitude is the defensive-aggressive hostility. The dysmutuals frequently show ambivalent hostility, hating friends who do not love them enough. A schizophrenic fights because he cannot control hostile impulses; a psychopath fights to win; the manic-depressive vents his hostility whenever he is not loved. While the hypervectorial schizophrenics are often hostile, they cannot take hostility. Blame or criticism sets off hostile reactions in hypervectorials. Hyperinstrumentals will accept criticism from those they perceive as strong and retaliate for criticism coming from weak individuals. Dysmutuals are not very sensitive to criticism coming from strangers but become aggressive-depressive (i.e., hostile toward others and themselves) when criticized by those who are expected to love.

In deep regression, the hyperinstrumental psychopaths wish to bite and regress to bestiality, cannibalism, and ruthless murder. The dysmutual manic-depressives wish to sleep and regress into a sleepy intrauterine, parasitic life. The hypervectorial schizophrenics do not wish anything. They withdraw from life, and if not taken care of, will die.

Similar diagnostic clues can be obtained from the Psycho-socio-diagnostic Interview. The main difference between the Interview and the Observation Inventory is the observer. In the Inventory, the descriptive data are obtained by one or more observers, while in the Interview the interviewed individual reports his observations.

The observations of the interviewed subject, whether patient or a member of his family, contain facts as seen by an interested and interesting party. The evaluation of the observed facts by the one being interviewed has great psychological significance. What actually happened can be found by interviewing several members of the same family unit, but how they see and evaluate what happened offers highly important sociopsychological clues.

While the interviewed subjects describe themselves and others, these descriptions can be tabulated in accordance with the power and acceptance categories. What does the subject think of himself? Does he believe himself to be active, alert, efficient? Or, outside these clues, does he believe himself to be intelligent, good-looking, successful, etc.?

These self-ratings are not objective measurements of personality. They are merely patterns of self-rating that will go up in hyperinstrumentals whenever they experience tangible success, will fluctuate rapidly in dysmutuals, and will be persistently low in hypervectorials.

In describing others, hyperinstrumentals will give scanty, rather mechanized descriptions such as "the girl in the office," "the supervisor," etc., while hypervectorials will spend a great deal of time talking about others and describing their feelings. Dysmutuals will most often resemble the hyperinstrumentals in their egocentric talk but will pay more attention to the feelings of others.

In the dimension of acceptance, the differences are even more pronounced. Hypervectorials criticize themselves and avoid criticizing others; when they hate, they tend to develop projective mechanisms and claim that others hate them. When they talk about parents and other relatives, they use a great deal of caution. Hyperinstrumentals speak frankly and critically about all whom they dislike. They find their hostility justified and give a frank though often distorted picture of interaction with others. Dysmutuals are more critical than the other two types. They blame everyone, including themselves, are highly opinionated, and label others. They either praise or condemn, and their story is full of value judgment. When they repeat the same detail in a subsequent interview, the two accounts rarely resemble each other.

In summary, the way people interact with others offers highly important diagnostic clues. The peculiar patterns of interaction as represented by the four above-mentioned categories of hostility, instrumentalism, mutualism, and vectorialism, and their combinations, over-, and underemphases are both etiologically and symptomatologically significant.

9. Pilot Studies

The first draft proposal of the Sociodiagnostic Interview was published in the *Handbook of Clinical Psychology* (Wolman, 1965a), parts of which were quoted above. This has been followed by a series of pilot studies conducted by students in

BENJAMIN B.
WOLMAN, ANDREA
ALPER, AND
STEVE DeBERRY

the Doctoral Program in Clinical Psychology of Long Island University, monitored by Wolman.

The initial, exploratory research was conducted in the form of an open-end interview aimed at diagnosing schizophrenics. The choice of schizophrenia was based on the abundance of diagnostic studies of this disorder (Carpenter, Strauss, & Bartko, 1973; Feighner, Robins, Guize, Woodruff, Winokur, & Munoz, 1972; Wolman, 1961, 1966, 1967; Woodruff, 1974; and others).

The interviewers were students of advanced standing in the Doctoral Program in Clinical Psychology at Long Island University, Brooklyn, New York. The interviewees were inmates, chosen at random, in public mental hospitals in Greater New York. The interviewers did not obtain any information concerning the patients they interviewed, and only at the completion of the project were their data compared to those obtained by the hospital.

The interviewers received the following guidelines:

9.1. The Sociodiagnostic Interview (Pilot Study No. 1): Guidelines

I. Motivation and Perception

1. Motivation and perception are the chief determinants of behavior.

2. The main motive is survival; almost all human needs are derivatives of the urge to survive.

3. The basic needs, such as food, shelter, rest, etc., are direct derivatives.

4. The acquired needs (so-needs) such as possessions, prestige, security, are learned behavioral patterns based on the fundamental need for survival.

5. The ability to satisfy needs is called *power*. The most primitive power is related to muscles.

6. People do not necessarily act on the basis of power they have, but power *as perceived* by them. A strong man may see himself as being weak, and vice versa.

7. People may have power and be willing to satisfy the needs of others (be friendly) or use their power to prevent the needs of others (be hostile).

8. People perceive *themselves* and *others* in the two dimensions of *power* (that is, ability to satisfy needs) and *acceptance* (that is, willingness to do so or to do the opposite). Sexuality is a most significant area of interaction, through the estimate of one's own and partner's power and acceptance.

9. The *statogram* is a research tool that serves the assessment of interindividual relations viewed as strong-weak (power) and friendly-hostile (acceptance).

II. Mental Disorders

1. Mental disorders affect the total personality, especially the motivation for survival, the willingness to protect one's life or to renounce it or even destroy it, and the attitude to other people.

2. The attitude towards oneself and towards others offers most significant disposition clues, according to the classificatory system based on hostile (H), instrumental (I), mutual (M), and vectorial (V) types of interactional behavior.

3. All sociogenic mental disorders can be divided into three types and five levels.

4. This classificatory system is somewhat isomorphic to psychoanalytic concepts. The balance of libido and destrudo cathexes determines the *types* (hyperinstrumental, dysmutual, and hypervectorial) and the five *levels* (neurosis, character neurosis, latent psychosis, manifest psychosis, and dementive stage), are related to the strength of the ego.

III. Interviewing Technique

1. The interview must be conducted in a free conversational atmosphere bordering on free association. The subject must feel free to say whatever he pleases.

2. The interviewer must have a skeleton-plan aimed at covering the subject's total estimate of his own Power and Acceptance, and his estimate of what others think of him in terms of Power and Acceptance.

3. The interview should continue over several sessions, one hour each.

4. Some questions can be straight and open, some must be veiled. All questions must be open-ended.

5. Tape record the interview.

6. Tabulate (P, A)

7. Content analysis: Topic
                     Frequency
                     Degree (1–5)
                     Profile

IV.   Introductory Questions

1. Name
2. Age, education
3. Occupation
4. Parents' names, ages, occupation
5. Siblings
6. Other relatives
7. Friends, colleagues, associates
8. Daily life, routines concerning food, rest
9. Sleep and dream
10. Hobbies
11. Overall description of childhood
12. Main wishes and hopes
13. Main fears and worries

V.   Subject's Estimate of His Own Power

1. His opinions of himself, in terms of power in general.
2. His estimate of his looks, appearance.
3. His estimate of his health.
4. His estimate of his physical force, physical prowess, agility, motor coordination.
5. His estimate of his intelligence, reasoning powers, memory, learning speed, and special abilities.
6. His estimate of his wealth, possessions.
7. His estimate of his standing in his occupation, business, or profession. How successful he is, how does he compare to others.
8. Assessment of his (or her) own sexual charm, attractiveness, prowess and success.
9. His evaluation of his own difficulties, fears, failure, frustrations.
10. Outlook to future: optimistic, pessimistic.

VI.   Subject's Estimate of His Social Attitudes (Acceptance)

1. What does he think of himself: is he (she) basically friendly or hostile?
2. Is he strong and friendly?
3. Is he strong and hostile?
4. Is he weak and friendly?
5. Is he weak and hostile?
6. His attitude toward his father. Explain in detail.
7. His attitude toward his mother. Explain in detail.
8. His attitude toward his siblings. Explain in detail.
9. His attitude toward his children. Exlain in detail.
10. His attitude toward his superiors. Explain in detail.
11. His attitude toward his dependents and subordinates. Explain in detail.
12. His attitude toward other people. Explain in detail.
13. His attitude toward people in general. Explain in detail.
14. His estimate of his social attitudes: submissive–ascendent?
                                         outgoing–withdrawn?
                                         trusting–suspicious?
                                         aggressive–peaceful?
                                         fearful–bold?

BENJAMIN B.
WOLMAN, ANDREA
ALPER, AND
STEVE DeBERRY

VII. What Others Think of Him in Terms of Power & Acceptance

1. The interviewer asks the same questions as in V and VI, related to what the subject thinks people think of him. Presently, the interviewer hears who are the significant figures in his environment.
2. What does subject's father think of him? Why does he think so?
3. Mother?
4. Siblings?
5. Other significant figures?
6. People in general?

The interviews were taped and served as a basis for future studies. Although the results seemed to be encouraging, the technique was open to criticism on at least two counts. First, more disturbed patients did not respond too well to the interview. Some of them simply agreed to everything, some answered in monosyllables, and still others were defiant and negativistic. Obviously, it takes time and patience to develop adequate rapport.

The interviews were open-end type, and the patients who were willing to respond to the interviewers took 2–3 hr. The typewritten report covered a great number of pages, and content analysis and tabulation of every single interview required an enormous expenditure of time.

After several months of work, the idea of the open-end interview was abandoned, and a more structured form was introduced. The following 70 questions were given to hundreds of hospitalized patients in a few public hospitals. The patients were chosen at random, and the interviewers were another team of doctoral candidates in clinical psychology at Long Island University. The patients were required to give "yes" or "no" answers to the 70 questions.

9.2. Structured Interview (Pilot Study No. 2)

I. Self-Esteem

1. I believe that I can work out most of my problems.
2. I don't think that I am particularly smart.
3. I am basically a very able person.
4. I often worry that something is wrong with the way I look.
5. I can never do things as well as they should be done.
6. Most people I meet like me very much.
7. I try to be fair but I'll stick up for my rights.
8. I enjoy being the center of attention.
9. I feel terrible when people disagree with me.
10. Criticism doesn't bother me.

II. Work: Success, Failure, Blame

1. I don't like to be around when things go wrong because I am usually blamed for it.
2. When I have made a mistake it's usually been my own fault.
3. I don't feel bad when I am criticized.
4. A person has only himself to blame or praise for what he has accomplished.
5. I always finish what I start.
6. I enjoy taking risks and trying new things.
7. Just when things are going well you can expect trouble.
8. I make decisions easily.
9. I blame myself when I don't succeed at something.
10. I must do my work perfectly.

III. Bodily Care and Functioning

1. Many times I lay awake and am unable to fall asleep.
2. I feel uneasy about the way I look.

3. I usually eat quickly.
4. I find it difficult to sleep and wake up frequently during the night.
5. I often feel aches and pains but they don't bother me.
6. I rarely worry that food I eat may be spoiled.
7. I feel sick more often than most people.
8. I enjoy having my picture taken.
9. I rarely worry about my health.
10. I hate to go to doctors.

IV.   Morality and Relatedness

1. I go out of my way to be careful not to hurt other people.
2. People should learn to mind their own business.
3. In every case it is better to tell the truth than to lie.
4. It is unfair to blame people for their mistakes.
5. When I see some injustice that does not concern me, I try not to get involved.
6. The problem with the world is that people do not know right from wrong.
7. I don't believe that people should be punished for their crimes.
8. There is always an answer to people's problems if they just try hard enough.
9. I have always tried to do the right thing.
10. When two people argue, both could be right.

V.   Friendship and Love

1. I am usually friendly to others but other people are rarely friendly to me.
2. Love is a wonderful feeling.
3. I wish I could see some of my childhood friends again.
4. Whenever I get close to someone, I end up getting hurt.
5. You can't always trust the ones you love.
6. It takes me a long time to really trust somebody.
7. When I have a friend it is a friend for life.
8. A good friend is one of the most important things in life.
9. Love is fine but you have to worry about yourself.
10. People let you down in the end.

VI.   Hostility

1. Sometimes I am afraid that I may hurt people I like.
2. I try not to argue with people.
3. I don't like to be critical of people.
4. When I get angry I try to control it.
5. When someone is annoying me I worry that I may hurt that person.
6. If I see two people fighting, I leave right away.
7. Once a friend disappoints me, that's it.
8. If someone makes me angry I tell that person.
9. It's better not to fight.
10. I will stick up for my rights, even if everyone disagrees with me.

VII.   Family Interaction

1. I was given a lot of responsibility as a child.
2. In my house, my mother was the boss.
3. Both my parents have had it rough.
4. When I was young, I could never do anything right.
5. My parents always tried to do their best.
6. I never had any long conversations with my mother.
7. My father was not very strong.
8. My parents used to fight a lot.
9. My family was always on good terms with relatives and neighbors.
10. I used to worry a lot about my parents.

The Structured Interview (second pilot study) was easier to administer and to score, but a close analysis discovered that some of the questions were too obvious and some were rather too general and, therefore, not too helpful. Differential diagnosis apparently required additional tightening of the interview.

A great deal of work was done in order to eliminate the too broad and not too discriminating questions. In a follow-up of the second pilot study a small number of patients carefully diagnosed by the hospital psychologists were chosen. Unfortunately, in a vast majority of cases the diagnostic workup is not too dependable (Beck, 1962; Feighner et al., 1972; Hunt, Herrmann, & Noble, 1957; Woodruff, 1974; Zubin, 1967). Classification should serve as the basis for diagnostic procedures, but there is not much order in that field, and the looseness and often inconsistency of the classificatory system make diagnostic procedures resemble *Waiting for Godot* (see Chapter 2 in this volume).

In the third pilot study, the questions were chosen on the basis of the follow-up study. A small number of patients already diagnosed by the hospitals as schizophrenics were pretested, and 68 questions were chosen in the belief that they offered significant diagnostic clues. This second structured interview again was based on "yes" or "no" answers.

9.3. The Second Structured Interview (Pilot Study No. 3)

1. When I have made a mistake it's usually been my own fault.
2. I don't feel bad when I am criticized.
3. A person has only himself to blame or praise for what he has accomplished.
4. I always finish what I start.
5. Just when things are going well you can expect trouble.
6. I make decisions easily.
7. I blame myself when I don't succeed at something.
8. I find it difficult to sleep and wake up frequently during the night.
9. I rarely worry about my health.
10. I go out of my way to be careful not to hurt other people.
11. In every case it is better to tell the truth than to lie.
12. I don't believe that people should be punished for their crimes.
13. There is always an answer to people's problems if they just try hard enough.
14. I have always tried to do the right thing.
15. Love is a wonderful feeling.
16. I wish I could see some of my childhood friends again.
17. You can't always trust the ones you love.
18. When I have a friend it is a friend for life.
19. A good friend is one of the most important things in life.
20. Sometimes I am afraid that I may hurt people I like.
21. I try not to argue with people.
22. I don't like to be critical of people.
23. When I get angry I try to control it.
24. When someone is annoying me I worry that I may hurt that person.
25. If someone makes me angry I tell that person.
26. It's better not to fight.
27. In my house my mother was the boss.
28. Both my parents have had it rough.
29. My parents always tried to do their best.
30. I never had any long conversations with my mother.
31. My parents used to fight a lot.
32. I used to worry a lot about my parents.
33. It is better to stay away from people so they won't hurt you.
34. I would never do anything unfair.
35. I would rather be hurt than hurt others.

36. My parents always blamed me when things went wrong.
37. There is satisfaction in doing what is right even if no one cares.
38. I hesitate to try new things.
39. There is much truth to the saying, "it is better to give than to receive."
40. I am always ready to learn from my mistakes.
41. It is better not to get involved in other people's problems.
42. My body does not function as well as it should.
43. It is better not to fall in love.
44. I often wish I was someone else.
45. I don't believe in love at first sight.
46. When I see people in love I feel jealous.
47. My mother rarely if ever praised me for my school work.
48. Most people are dishonest.
49. Friendship is not important to me.
50. People are often hostile to me.
51. Friends or lovers usually desert you in the end.
52. One should not hope for too much.
53. Sometimes I feel as if my anger will get out of control.
54. I usually trust people.
55. I know that I am a very good person.
56. A person should make an effort not to appear angry.
57. I resent my parents.
58. I believe that most people have good intentions.
59. I would like to find someone very strong to take care of me.
60. Most people like me.
61. I don't get angry easily but when I do it's like an explosion.
62. I feel sorry for my parents.
63. I am suspicious when people ask me to help them.
64. I easily get angry.
65. When I was a child, I tried hard to please my parents.
66. In my school years I easily made friends with everybody.
67. My mother never asked for my help.
68. My parents were always kind to each other.

9.4. Results of Pilot Study No. 3

The results were rank-ordered according to the number of questions answered in the predicted direction. The diagnosis listed in Table 2 is the diagnosis according to the hospital records.

9.5. Discussion of Pilot Study No. 3 (Second Structured Interview)

Examination of the results shown in Tables 2 and 3 reveals that the study failed to support the hypothesis that patients diagnosed schizophrenic by the hospital would significantly answer more questions in the direction predicted by the theory. For the inpatient group, only five out of the 20 patient sample were diagnosed as schizophrenic. Their distribution tends to be toward the lower rather than the upper range of the sample. If one examines Table 2, it appears that patients diagnosed as depressive or obsessive-compulsive answered more questions in the direction predicted for schizophrenics than did the reputed schizophrenics.

Equally unsubstantiating were the results obtained for the sample of 23 outpatients (Table 3). Of the total sample, 11 patients were diagnosed as schizophrenic by the hospital. In this case, their distribution is equally scattered throughout the

Table 2. Rank-Ordered Questions Answered as Predicted by Diagnosis for 21 Inpatients

	Number correctly answered	Diagnosis
1.	29	Antisocial personality
2.	30	Adult adjustment reaction
3.	31	Depressive neurosis
4.	32	Paranoid schizophrenia
5.	33	Depressive neurosis
6.	33	Antisocial personality
7.	34	Simple schizophrenia
8.	34	Acute schizophrenic episode
9.	35	Antisocial personality
10.	36	Paranoid schizophrenia
11.	37	Narcissistic personality
12.	37	Paranoid personality
13.	39	Masochistic personality
14.	39	Phobic neurosis
15.	39	Depressive neurosis
16.	40	Manic-depressive circular
17.	41	Obsessive-compulsive neurosis
18.	45	Anorexia nervosa
19.	46	Psychotic depressive neurosis
20.	46	Paranoid schizophrenia
21.	51	?

Table 3. Rank-Ordered Questions Answered as Predicted by Diagnosis for 23 Outpatients

	Number correctly answered	Diagnosis
1.	25	Paranoid schizophrenia
2.	25	Undifferentiated schizophrenia
3.	26	Paranoid schizophrenia
4.	28	Obsessive personality with phobic features
5.	28	Senile dementia
6.	31	Paranoid schizophrenia
7.	31	Phobic neurosis
8.	32	Chronic undifferentiated schizophrenia
9.	32	Obsessive personality
10.	33	Obsessive personality
11.	35	Obsessive personality
12.	36	Schizophrenia
13.	37	Paranoid schizophrenia
14.	38	Organic brain syndrome
15.	41	Schizophrenia in remission
16.	41	Obsessive personality
17.	42	Undifferentiated schizophrenia
18.	46	Schizoid with phobic features
19.	47	Hysterical neurosis
20.	48	Reaction of adult life
21.	49	Paranoid schizophrenia
22.	50	Hysterical personality
23.	50	Paranoid schizophrenia

range of scores, with three schizophrenics having the lowest scores, two the highest, and the remaining approximately equally distributed among the sample.

The results lend themselves to three possible explanations: (1) that the theory from which the hypotheses and questionnaire were generated was wrong; (2) that the screening questionnaire was wrong; or (3) that the hospital-assigned diagnosis was wrong.

The possibility that the theory is wrong cannot be concluded from this study alone. According to Wolman (1970, 1973), schizophrenics should consistently maintain a hypervectorial cathexis toward some people and be hypocathected toward the self. Generically, they are docile, are fearful of their own anger and imagined power, and suffer from an overly sadistic superego. However, a theory of schizophrenia, or any theory for that matter, is postulated in order to better understand and perhaps predict certain phenomena. That is, the ultimate value of a theory is utilitarian. In this sense, the value of an interindividual cathexis or sociopsychosomatic theory of schizophrenia still remains to be proven. Observations, formulated in a clinical manner, have to be cross-checked through empirical validation. This is usually a time-consuming process because one must be certain that clinical data are not epiphenomena or idiographic behavior of a specific subpopulation. Additional studies employing clinically diverse patient populations must be conducted before any conclusion regarding the theory can be drawn. In this sense, the present study is best considered a pilot that could be the basis for future research. The possibility remains that the sample was biased or, more likely, that the questionnaire was not optimally designed to tap the desired behavioral variables as predicted by the theory. It seems parsimonious to consider the methodology and sample in error.

However, the results also raise the possibility that explanation 3 is true, i.e., that the hospital diagnoses were in error (Beck, 1962; Zubin, 1967). This seems plausible for several reasons. First, there were no uniform criteria or controls for any of the diagnoses. For the study, the diagnoses used were the ones taken from the patients' charts and usually represented intake or admission diagnoses. Therefore, there were no common or control criteria under which these diagnostic judgments were made. It is possible that the diagnosis of paranoid schizophrenia (outpatient No. 3) could have been made on the basis of clinical impression while the same diagnosis for patient No. 23 was made after a series of diagnostic workups including projective tests such as the Rorschach. Likewise, little information can be found in such diagnoses as obsessive personalities, phobic neurosis, or reaction of adult life. An obsessive personality can be the precursor of a schizophrenic state just as a hysterical or antisocial reaction could mask an underlying schizophrenic process. Further complications arise because no one symptom is pathognomonic to any single syndrome. Thus diagnoses such as phobic neuroses (No. 7), paranoia (No. 12), and anorexia (No. 18) could be symptoms of a more complex disease entity rather than entities in themselves. Likewise, the diagnoses of narcissistic (no. 11) or masochistic (No. 13) personality may represent behavioral observations which do not preclude an underlying thought disorder. It is possible, therefore, that failure to obtain significant results was due to the lack of clarity and validity of the assigned diagnoses.

Thus the problem becomes one of trying to validate a theory on the basis of diagnostic categories that are of questionable validity themselves. Future research should attempt to have diagnoses made on the basis of extensive common control criteria, including nomothetic parameters. A standard assessment of ego functions and the use of several experienced diagnostic raters would be a step toward improving the reliability of the diagnoses and the studies. Once a common basis for diagnosing patients is established, a control would exist for the use of the present or a new questionnaire. Using the "validated" diagnoses as a standard sample, the hypothesis that the questionnaire could correctly identify schizophrenics could be adequately tested.

10. References

Ackerman, N. W. *The psychodynamics of family life.* New York: Basic Books, 1958.
Bales, R. F. *Interaction process analysis.* Reading, Mass.: Addison-Wesley, 1950.
Bateson, G., Jackson, D. D., Haley, J., & Weakland, J. Toward a theory of schizophrenia. *Behavioral Science,* 1956, *1,* 251–264.
Beck, A. T. Reliability of psychiatric diagnosis: A critique of systematic studies. *American Journal of Psychiatry,* 1962, *119,* 210–216.
Carpenter, W. T. Jr., Strauss, J. S., & Bartko, J. J. Flexible system for the diagnosis of schizophrenia. Report from the WHO International Pilot Study of Schizophrenia. *Science,* 1973, *182,* 1275–1278.
Federn, P. *Ego psychology and the psychoses.* New York: Basic Books, 1952.
Feighner, J. P., Robins, E., Guize, S. B., Woodruff, R. A., Winokur, G., & Munoz, R. Diagnostic criteria for use in psychiatric research. *Archives of General Psychiatry,* 1972, *26,* 57–68.
Fenichel, O. *The psychoanalytic theory of neurosis.* New York: Norton, 1945.
Ferenczi, S. *Further contributions to the theory and technique of psychoanalysis.* London: Hogarth Press, 1926.
Ferster, C. B. Classification of behavioral psychology. In L. Krasner & L. P. Ullman (Eds.), *Research in behavior modification.* New York: Holt, Rinehart, 1966, pp. 6–26.
Foulds, G. A. *Personality and personal illness.* London: Tavistock, 1965.
Gibb, C. The principles and traits of leadership. *Journal of Abnormal and Social Psychology,* 1947, *42,* 267–294.
Goodman, J. D. The psychiatric interview. In B. B. Wolman (Ed.), *Manual of child psychopathology.* New York: McGraw-Hill, 1972, pp. 743–766.
Hunt, W. A., Herrmann, R. S., & Noble, H. The specificity of the psychiatric interview. *Journal of Clinical Psychology,* 1957, *13,* 49–53.
Hyman, H. H. The psychology of status. *Archives of Psychology,* 1942, *269.*
Krauss, H. H., & Krauss, B. J. Nosology: Wolman's system. In B. B. Wolman (Ed.), *International encyclopedia of psychiatry, psychology, psychoanalysis, and neurology.* New York: Van Nostrand Reinhold/Aesculapius, 1977.
Kropotkin, P. *Mutual aid: A factor in evolution.* London: Allen and Unwin, 1902.
Lidz, T., Fleck, S., & Cornelison, A. *Schizophrenia and the family.* New York: International Universities Press, 1955.
Matarazzo, J. D. The interview. In B. B. Wolman (Ed.), *Handbook of clinical psychology.* New York: McGraw-Hill, 1965, pp. 403–450.
Moreno, J. L. *Who shall survive?* New York: Beacon House, 1953.
Pavlov, I. P. *Lectures on conditioned reflexes.* New York: Liveright, 1928.
Phillips, L. & Draguns, J. G. Classification of the behavior disorders. *Annual Review of Psychology,* 1971, *22,* 447–482.
Sanford, F. H. Research in military leadership. In W. Dennis (Ed.), *Psychology in world emergency.* Pittsburgh: University of Pittsburgh Press, 1952.
Spinoza, B. *Ethics.* London: Bell, 1911.
Sullivan, H. S. *Interpersonal theory of psychiatry.* New York: Norton, 1953.
Tolman, E. C. *Purposive behavior in animals and man.* New York: Appleton-Century-Crofts, 1932.
Wolman, B. B. *Freedom and discipline in education* (Hebrew). Tel Aviv: Massadah, 1949.
Wolman, B. B. Sociological analysis of Israel. In M. M. Davis (Ed.), *M. M. Kaplan jubilee volume.* New York: Jewish Theological Seminary, 1953, pp. 531–549.
Wolman, B. B. Leadership and group dynamics. *Journal of Social Psychology,* 1956, *43,* 11–25.
Wolman, B. B. Explorations in latent schizophrenia. *American Journal of Psychotherapy,* 1957, *11,* 560–588.

Wolman, B. B. Instrumental, mutual acceptance and vectorial groups. *Acta Sociologica*, 1958, *3*, 19–28. (a)

Wolman, B. B. Education and leadership. *Teachers College Record*. 1958, *59*, 465–473 (b)

Wolman, B. B. *Contemporary theories and systems in psychology*. New York: Harper & Row, 1960. (a)

Wolman, B. B. The impact of failure on group cohesiveness. *Journal of Social Psychology*, 1960, *51*, 409–418. (b)

Wolman, B. B. Fathers of schizophrenic patients. *Acta Psychologica*, 1961, *9*, 193–210.

Wolman, B. B. Mental health and mental disorders. In B. B. Wolman (Ed.), *Handbook of clinical psychology*. New York: McGraw-Hill, 1965, pp. 1119–1139. (a)

Wolman, B. B. Schizophrenia and related disorders. In B. B. Wolman (Ed.), *Handbook of clinical psychology*. New York: McGraw-Hill, 1965, pp. 976–1029. (b)

Wolman, B. B. *Vectoriasis praecox or the group of schizophrenias*. Springfield, Ill.: Thomas, 1966.

Wolman, B. B. The socio-psycho-somatic theory of schizophrenia. *Psychotherapy and Psychosomatics*, 1967, *15*, 373–387.

Wolman, B. B. *Children without childhood: A study in childhood schizophrenia*. New York: Grune & Stratton, 1970.

Wolman, B. B. *Call no man normal*. New York: International Universities Press, 1973.

Wolman, B. B. *Courage to live*. In preparation.

Woodruff, R. A. Jr., Goodwin, D. W., & Guze, S. B. *Psychiatric diagnosis*. New York: Oxford University Press, 1974.

Zubin, J. Classification of mental disorders. *Annual Review of Psychology*, 1967, *18*, 373–406.

II
Differential Diagnosis

17

Concerning the Rationale of Diagnostic Testing

ALBERT I. RABIN AND DAVID L. HAYES

1. Introduction

Early in the history of clinical psychology, the use of tests for the purposes of diagnosis and classification was self-evident. It was readily understood that the diagnostic enterprise was an indispensable part of the functioning of the clinical psychologist. In more recent years, the diagnostic function in general and that of testing in particular is no longer self-evident. Consequently, it has become necessary to review the reasons for the diagnostic activity and to present a convincing rationale for it.

During the last couple of decades, the functions of classification and diagnosis in mental disorder have been placed under question. Critics have questioned the very existence of mental disorders or mental "illness" (Szasz, 1961). If such an entity does not exist as a class, classifications within that meaningless entity make no sense. If the diagnostic undertaking is denied relevance, then the use of psychological tests for the purposes of aiding in this diagnosis is equally senseless.

As it happens, this radical view of mental disorders is not universally accepted, and psychodiagnosis is considered by many as a highly important activity preliminary to psychotherapy and other modes of intervention. It would, perhaps, be most useful to review the purposes of diagnosis in general and then concentrate on a discussion of diagnostic testing as part of this overall process in dealing with patients who are mentally disturbed and disordered. We also need to pay attention to the relationship between the two closely allied concepts of classification and diagnosis. They are often employed interchangeably but, for the purposes of more precise analysis, need to be distinguished from each other.

ALBERT I. RABIN and DAVID L. HAYES • Department of Psychology, Michigan State University, East Lansing, Michigan 48824.

ALBERT I. RABIN
AND DAVID L. HAYES

2. Definition and the Scope of Diagnosis

Diagnosis is an integral part of the problem-solving process. Diagnosis, viewed as a general process of gathering information about the nature and causes of a problem or a situation, permits conceptualization, encourages understanding, and facilitates appropriate action. People typically make informal assessment of the likely outcome of various courses of action when faced with alternatives, and they evaluate the environment or context within which a decision is to be made. Diagnosis in this informal sense is no less a part of the practice of medicine or of clinical psychology. With this narrowing of scope to focus on medicine and clinical psychology, however, a more specific and exact meaning of diagnosis can be formulated (Korchin, 1976).

As an aid to developing a clearer formulation, we will first look at the use of diagnosis in medicine, then examine its role in traditional psychiatry, the interface between medicine and psychology, and finally discuss classification and diagnosis in a general way.

2.1. Diagnosis and Medicine

The historical function of diagnosis in medicine has been to identify disease so that appropriate remedial steps can be taken. This view has changed but little over the years, save for increasing sophistication in understanding etiologies and planning interventions (Altschule, 1970). But the essential character of diagnosis remains; as defined by medical men themselves, diagnosis is "the art, science, or act of recognizing disease from signs, symptoms, or laboratory data" (Engle & Davis, 1963). Whether art or science, however, diagnosis is clearly an established part of medical practice, and most physicians would argue that it is a prerequisite for proper case management.

The conception of disease, including onset, course, and outcome, identified with particular syndromes and caused by a particular disease agent, is most accurate when talking about infectious diseases such as those described by Sydenham (Engle, 1963a). With the advent of sophisticated knowledge about heredity and genetics, it has become possible for disease to be conceptualized as a result of many factors aside from infectious agents, including mutation due to mechanical difficulties in miosis and mitosis, chemicals, irradiation, nutrients, psychosomatic stress, and many others (Engle, 1963b). With this increasing sophistication of understanding etiology of various diseases and disease processes, the concept of diagnosis in medicine has moved away from the simple identification of a symptom complex. However, diagnosis has retained its place of importance in medical practice. Its function has been described as follows:

1. To demonstrate the etiological factors [however conceptualized].
2. To differentiate between organic and functional disorders.
3. To discover the . . . reaction of the organism to its disability.
4. To discover the extent of organic damage with resulting functional disability.
5. To estimate the extensity or intensity of the morbid process in relation to actuarial data concerning type and severity.
6. To determine the prognosis or probable course.
7. To provide a rational basis for specific [therapy].
8. To provide a rational basis for discussing the case with the patient and relatives.
9. To provide a scientific basis for classification and statistical analysis of data. (Thorne, 1947, pp. 161–162)

Because of the changing understanding of disease already described, the "medical model" to be described below may be something of an anachronism within the field of medicine itself. However, at the time that psychiatry was developing, the infectious disease model was in ascendance. Therefore, we turn next to traditional psychiatry, where we will search for the impact of medicine.

2.2. Diagnosis in Traditional Psychiatry

Traditional psychiatry offers the opportunity to examine the recent evolution of mental health care and to judge the magnitude and importance of the contribution which medicine has made to current mental health practices. This consideration is particularly important in discussing diagnosis, because "diagnosis" is essentially a medical term appropriated for slightly different uses by psychiatry and psychology, but retaining nonetheless certain medical connotations as excess baggage. In fact, the too-ready acceptance of the notion of diagnosis as used by medicine, without consideration of some of the ideas implicit in its use, has led to major criticism both of traditional psychiatry (and psychology) and of diagnosis, as we shall see (e.g., Goldfried & Kent, 1972; Kanfer & Saslow, 1969; Stuart, 1970).

One way to gain a sense of these implicit ideas is to view psychiatry from a historical perspective. The rejection of the notion that disordered behavior is caused by possession by demons, by the power of the moon, or by changes in the stars, at least by dissatisfied scientists or medical practitioners, was accompanied by attempts to formulate alternative explanations. Starting with Pinel, efforts were made to observe, describe, and classify. There was a strong consensus that mental illness was a disease of the brain and central nervous system, and that its cause would be found there. This was in accord with prevailing medical opinion and practice, which favored looking to changes in body tissues and conditions to explain illness and disease. This somatogenic hypothesis received immense support in the nineteenth century with the discovery of the organic basis of general paresis.

Initial observation and description isolated a particular syndrome, which had a typical beginning, course, and outcome and which possessed a characteristic symptom complex. The succeeding years allowed more detailed study of the onset of paresis and the organic damage which accompanied it. Understanding of the etiology became clear with the discovery of the relationship between syphilis and general paresis, and finally with the demonstration of the presence of the syphilitic infectious agent in the brains of general paretics (White & Watt, 1973). The enthusiasm generated by this and other similar accomplishments of medicine and psychiatry eventually resulted in a victory for the somatogenic hypothesis. It is also responsible for defining mental disorder in terms of what became known as the "medical model."

The medical or disease model of mental illness has been attacked by psychiatrists as well as by psychologists, sociologists, and social critics (e.g., Szasz, 1961). The arguments usually contend that the use of medical metaphors does not enhance, and may interfere with, understanding people and how their lives can be afflicted with psychosocial difficulties. Korchin (1976) has summarized some of the elements usually ascribed to the medical approach to understanding psychological difficulties:

1. There are disease entities, which have etiology, course, and outcome.
2. These diseases are of organic origin.
3. Even if conceived as psychological diseases, they are viewed in analogy with physical

ailments. There is an underlying state which is manifested in surface symptoms. Disease is to be inferred from symptoms; changing symptoms will not cure the disease.

4. People get these diseases through no fault of their own.

5. Cure depends on professional intervention, preferably by people with medical training.

6. The diseases are in the person and, although they may have culturally distinct manifestations, the essential disease process is universal and not culturally specific. (Korchin, 1976, p. 90)

Korchin notes a potential overemphasis on searching for specific etiologies, therapies, and prognoses, the danger of labeling and stigmatizing, and the emphasis on the pathological themes in life to the neglect of sources of strength and competence.

The approach to diagnosis of the prototypical traditional psychiatrist is no more clear than in the *Diagnostic and Statistical Manual of Mental Disorders* (DSM II, 1968) of the American Psychiatric Association. The DSM II has been roundly criticized for having inadequate theoretical underpinnings, possessing principles of classification which are not consistent and which vary widely, insufficiently characterizing distinguishing features of different classes, and unreliably diagnosing and inadequately representing the full range of problems which clinicians encounter, to name a few (e.g., Kanfer & Saslow, 1969; Korchin, 1976; Stuart, 1970; Zigler & Phillips, 1961). Although the DSM II (1968) does not represent the traditional medical model, vestiges of this earlier way of looking at psychological problems clearly still exist.

3. On Diagnosis and Classification

The issue of diagnostic classification and the broader area of classification in general demand attention in any detailed consideration of the assessment process. In order to be clear about classification, we need first to look at the relationship between classification and assessment. Although the assignment of a diagnostic label is frequently although not always a part of diagnostic testing, it should be clear that the two are not identical. The contribution of diagnostic testing to an assessment is generally sufficient to make classification possible. However, a good assessment provides much more information than is implied by the nomothetic notion of class membership. Indeed, many arguments for assessment by clinicians, as opposed to actuaries (Meehl, 1954), are based on the potential idiographic qualities of competent clinical assessment. We would say, with Korchin (1976), that "Clinical assessment is the process by which clinicians gain understanding of the patient necessary for making informed decisions" (p. 174). Basically, the distinction which must be kept in mind is that, while classification can be a part of diagnostic testing, it is not all of diagnostic testing. As will be noted below, identifying classification alone as assessment is a major logical mistake which plagues many arguments against the usefulness of diagnostic testing.

It is traditional, and probably important, to begin a discussion of classification by recognizing that humans seem to have a predilection for classifying things (e.g., Borofsky, 1974; Menninger, 1963). Classification inheres in language. Classification is our way of ordering our experience, of making sense of what would otherwise remain an endless chain of unrelated events. Classification recognizes and gives importance to constancies across experiences, to similarities between events. Classification is one of the tools of science by which knowledge is advanced. Yet these statements imply neither that classification is useful in every instance nor that diagnostic classification in particular is inevitably a practical approach to the assessment and description of personality. Before considering the issue of personality classification, however, there are some other attributes of classification in general which merit attention.

One characteristic of classification, pointed out by Zigler and Phillips (1961), is that when something is assigned to a class, certain individual features of that something are irretrievably lost. Because there are no pure types, because members of a class differ from each other in some irrelevant aspects, the uniqueness of each class member cannot be preserved after it is classified. However, on the other side of the coin, classification potentially offers a gain which more than makes up for this loss of information. This gain is represented in the attributes and correlates of class membership. To the extent that classificatory principles can be chosen to include relevant dimensions and exclude irrelevant ones (this is, of course, the dilemma), classification is an abstracting procedure, one that allows a look beyond the obvious and below the surface. At the same time, however, when a specific classificatory schema does not produce useful information, it is not an indictment of classification per se. It merely indicates that the categories may not be the best ones for that particular purpose. The magnitude of the potential gains and losses of information inherent in classifying anything are clearly dependent on the choice of categories which throw away as little important information as possible.

Moving to the specific instance of diagnosing and classifying personality, another distinction becomes necessary. Classification in personality assessment serves two related but distinct functions. On the one hand, classification is substantially involved in the clinical procedures of diagnostic testing and decision making. That is, classification is employed because of its presumed, or at least potential, clinical utility. (That classification is sometimes achieved by diagnostic testing is certainly also true.) At the same time, classification of personality is a part of the practice of taxonomy which is common to all science. As Zigler and Phillips (1961) note, to argue against the entire classificatory enterprise because, for example, it fails to predict some other interesting variable accurately, is to confuse diagnosis as an act of scientific classification with the clinical practice of diagnosis. The error here lies in confusing diagnosis as basic science with the application of specific diagnostic techniques in practice.

Diagnostic categories have been criticized as being unreliable and invalid (e.g., Kanfer & Saslow, 1969; Stuart, 1970). This criticism seems to weaken somewhat when the assessment process is considered in terms of decision theory, as opposed to classical measurement theory (Cronbach & Gleser, 1957; Levine, 1968). This point will be elaborated further below, but briefly the argument is that if tests can be usefully employed to help make decisions it is not important whether or not they are reliable or valid by classical standards.

The charge that the classes now in use are not homogeneous with respect to symptoms or etiology or prognosis or some other variable has been considered by Zigler and Phillips (1961). Their observation that classes need only be homogeneous with respect to the classificatory principle is clearly correct at the epistemological level, but it does not address the practical difficulties implied by heterogeneity.

The problems which exist when the classificatory scheme which is used is a psychiatric nosology have been succinctly described by Szasz (1957). He asserts that the very words "psychiatric nosology" suggest at the same time an interest in disease and a medical approach to its conceptualization (e.g., general paresis) and an interest in psychological and behavioral phenomena with no apparent organic basis (e.g., schizophrenia, homosexuality). The current categories do not clearly define the scope and subject matter to be designated as psychiatric (i.e., brain, mind, or behavior), the techniques which characterize treatment (i.e., physicochemical or psychological), or the nature of the phenomena to be described (i.e., changes in the brain, social behavior, or behavior toward specific individuals). As a solution to these problems, Szasz proposes what he calls operational definitions of categories.

Diagnostic classification is used in many different settings, e.g., mental hospitals, psychological or psychiatric outpatient clinics, child guidance clinics, schools, military service, and courts of law, yet the methods employed and the purpose for which diagnoses are made differ. The concept of operational diagnosis recognizes that these differences exist. A diagnosis made for a mental hospital may be most concerned with whether or not an individual is psychotic; a court of law wants to know about whether someone was legally sane; an employer may want to know if an employee can work or not. What is here being stressed is the necessity of being flexible when approaching an assessment and being ready to answer a question which perhaps the assignment of a DSM II label would not answer. It is an alternative statement of Levine's (1968) position that an adequate assessment demands careful consideration of the referral question to be answered.

A recent critical look at the field by Borofsky (1974) provides a general approach. He outlines five broad areas as issues relating to the structure and content of a system of personality classification. His analysis and theoretical predilections result in his describing an adequate classification as embodying the following aspects in those five areas. Psychological functioning should be viewed as ranging along a continuum rather than being classified into discrete and discontinuous types. Classification should utilize the same variables, mechanisms, and logic for explaining both adaptive and maladaptive functioning. It should recognize the overdetermined quality of behavior and therefore rely mainly on intrapsychic factors. Heuristic considerations should take precedence over short-range clinical utility, so that science is not given short shrift. Finally, personality should be described in terms of variables that are observable and measurable both clinically and from psychological test data. Although this is but one analysis of the classification question, it nonetheless shows the range of problems which must be considered in describing the psychological functioning of any individual.

In conclusion, we have drawn a distinction between classification and the broader procedure of assessment or diagnosis, and between classification as scientific taxonomy and classification as pragmatic clinical utilization of knowledge. It would seem that classification is not useless; neither is it without problem. However, to abandon assessment because of difficulties in the present classification schema, or to cease in the taxonomic task as a result of some particularly practical difficulty which becomes apparent, would be to make a serious mistake.

4. Decision Making and the Diagnostic Process

Up to this point, although we have been considering questions which are germane to the study of diagnostic testing, the focus has been on more abstract issues. While these have certainly been substantive issues, they tend nonetheless to be more conceptual than pragmatic. But when we begin to consider making decisions based on assessment, we really begin to enter the practical world of the tester; elegant theoretical exposition frequently must give way to the actual demands of the situation in this practical world. For this section, we will take up the pragmatic issues that arise when assessment is carried out.

Prior to 1957, an enlightened view of assessment, as represented for example by Rapaport and associates (Rapaport, 1945), was that assessment is the process of constructing individualized models of personality, bringing together information obtained from the careful administration of a battery of psychological tests. A battery is necessary because no one test provides all of the information needed for developing such an integrated picture of personality functioning. At the same time, such a multimethod approach makes it possible to generate hypotheses and then test them against other data, an important safeguard of this type of approach. Given this orientation, the model of personality is derived from the test data by inference, and this model of personality subsequently forms the basis for any decisions which need to be made. The reasoning behind using a multitest battery in assessment is sound, and is as applicable today as when Rapaport (1945) was originally writing about it or Murray (1938) was developing it. It is in thinking about the decision-making process that things have changed.

The turning point in this thinking seems to have occurred with the publication of a book relating decision-making theory and game theory to psychological testing (Cronbach & Gleser, 1957). The emphasis of this new approach was on the decision-making process per se as opposed to the tests, and it evaluated tests (or any other part of the assessment procedure for that matter) in terms of what they contributed to the decision-making process. This value of tests for decision making was to be balanced by the cost of giving any particular test, measured in money, professional time, or whatever. This way of conceptualizing psychological testing led to a reorientation of thinking about assessment, reflected in the twofold definition of assessment as the formulation of a working model of the person-situation and the process of making decisions (Sundberg & Tyler, 1962; see also Levy, 1963).

The important aspects of decision theory presented by Cronbach and Gleser as relevant to the process of psychological testing and assessment have been summarized as follows:

1. Emphasis should be on *payoff* or outcomes, not on specific techniques.
2. Questions of the validity of tests or other assessment activities should be considered as problems of *improving on existing procedures*, rather than improving on chance.
3. *Strategies of assessment* or whole sequences should be the object of concern; one asks about the contribution of both test and nontest procedures to the ultimate outcome.
4. Examination of values is fundamental to assessment; decisions are made that will maximize movement toward goals. (Sundberg & Tyler, 1962, p. 84, authors' italics)

These points clearly suggest a particular approach to assessment.

In the first place, it is important to precisely formulate the decisions which are to be made. We will return to the examination of referral questions below, but at this point it may be noted that the situation in which the psychologist or tester works is typically complex, and not infrequently has inherent but subtle ambiguities and contradictions. (On this point Schafer's, 1954, analysis of the testing situation is cogent.)

A second implication of decision theory is that the multitest battery remains the choice approach. A tangential but related point is that, in this formulation, the use of projective techniques finds a theoretical rebuttal to the abundance of research demonstrating low reliability and predictive validity for these tests. The vindication of projectives is achieved by thinking of projectives as one part of a battery, as wideband instruments to direct attention to areas of difficulty which might otherwise be overlooked or which are not tapped by more objective tests. This manner of using projectives considers that the criteria of classical measurement theory regarding reliability and validity are beside the point, and that the projective techniques are a helpful part of a decision-making strategy.

A recent survey of clinical psychologists regarding their use of psychological tests (Wade & Baker, 1977) reports that when a sample of clinical psychologists was asked to rank the importance of various reasons for using tests, the information which tests provide about personality structure was given the highest rating, significantly higher than any other reason, including accurate behavioral prediction. The psychometric properties of reliability and validity were accorded only moderate importance by these same respondents. As the authors point out, such data contain implicit criticism of much of the testing research in the literature, because it typically employs reliability, validity, and accuracy of prediction as outcome measures. These qualities of tests are viewed as rather unimportant by practicing clinicians; this may also help to explain why testing, particularly projective testing, remains so popular despite the many negative research outcomes which have appeared in the literature (cf. Meehl, 1960).

The emphasis on an assessment strategy comprising a sequence of procedures does more than reaffirm the multitest battery; it places the psychologist or tester squarely in the middle of the assessment process. The role of the clinician, initially, on being asked to do some testing, is to formulate a strategy which seems likely to provide help in making whatever decision is required, or in answering whatever questions have been raised. Yet this formulation of strategy represents the end point of a series of actions already undertaken by the tester. Faced with a problem (the referral question or a request for testing), the clinician gathers information. This information may be gathered from case notes already provided with the testing request, from a description of the situation by a caseworker, from demographic data about the person to be tested, or only from the referral itself. The clinician's judgment of what techniques and procedures will test hypotheses and generate additional ideas is the first visible result—the decision of which battery of test and nontest procedures to employ. Depending on the specificity of the referral question, the time available for testing, and the potential consequences of a bad decision, among other things, the clinician chooses between structured and unstructured tests or interviews, between wideband and narrowband instruments (Levine, 1968), between objective and projective tests, between a need to know certain facts very accurately and a need to get a broad view of the situation in a manner suggestive of additional hypotheses.

Following the assembling of a test battery, the testing itself begins. During the administration of the tests, the clinician is constantly observing and "processing" the test and nontest behavior of the person being tested. This processing may consist of the generation of further hypotheses to be tested, perhaps by additional tests not yet included in the battery. The assessment process curves back on itself in this way, formulating hypotheses, testing them in a way that often generates more questions, and trying to answer the questions raised by the assessment.

This procedure must end at some point. That point is reached when the additional benefit (i.e., information) which would accrue from giving an additional test or asking an additional question no longer outweighs the cost incurred by continuing. Then the clinician scores the tests, evaluates them relative to published norms where applicable, generates more hypotheses based on various aspects of the data collected, tests the hypotheses against other parts of the data, and integrates the test and nontest findings into a considered judgment about whatever question or decision is to be reached.

Meehl (1954) has distinguished between actuarial and clinical predictions; clearly, the assessment procedure we are here describing includes aspects of both at almost every point in the assessment. However, the emphasis here is on the flexibility of a strategy when tests are viewed as adding increments of information in a sequential decision-making process, and on the importance of the clinician as a generator of hypotheses and modifier of the strategy. The assessment procedure is determined at any point by what has already been discovered and by what else might therefore be necessary to ultimately facilitate an adequate answer or decision.

5. Possible Decisions

Raising the question of what decisions may be made as a result of diagnostic testing directs attention to the issue of referral questions. Diagnostic psychological testing is done in public and private clinics, in public and private mental hospitals and general hospitals, in the schools, in industry, in the courts, in the military, and in other settings as well. It is used to decide whether or not someone ought to receive psychotherapy, and, if so, individual or group, supportive or uncovering, long term or time limited, whether or not someone ought to be hospitalized, whether or not someone ought to be hired or promoted or admitted to a program, whether or not someone should be held legally responsible for his actions, or whether disturbances in behavior or school performance are functional or the result of organic impairment, to name but a few. It is precisely because of the extensive, wide-ranging list of uses of assessment that it is necessary in any given case to formulate as clearly as possible the reason why testing is required and the question which needs to be answered. Only in that way is it possible to tailor-make the assessment procedure to the situation, thus avoiding an inefficient and potentially ineffective approach to testing.

Levine (1968) has undertaken an analysis of five different situations in which psychological testing is frequently requested. He discusses the use of psychological testing in the psychiatric clinic, the general medical setting, the legal context, the educational system and the psychological clinic. He concludes that these situations differ in many salient respects and that it is consequently a crucial part of the psychologist-tester's job to be aware of the complex context within which he tests and to determine the essential referral question and the available alternatives. It is unrealistic to think that the decision maker will always formulate a clear concise referral question. If we choose to consider assessment within a decision-making theory, it is incumbent on those who assess to provide information which aids the decision-making process.

In the context of outpatient psychiatric or psychological treatment, the first decision to be made is whether treatment is indicated. The next decision is what kind of treatment is appropriate and in what setting. These two questions actually encompass many alternatives, including inpatient vs. outpatient treatment vs. referral to another agency, long-term vs. time-limited therapy, individual vs. group therapy, as well as various theoretical options.

The kind of information which a decision maker requires to make determinations of appropriate case dispositions will vary according to the theoretical predilections of that person. It is possible, however, to sketch broadly the kind of information which tests do provide. A competently administered, scored, and interpreted battery of tests can indicate interpersonal style, intelligence, ego strength, cognitive style, preferred defenses including adaptiveness and flexibility, psychological mindedness, motivation, areas of interpersonal and intrapsychic conflict, and other factors which suggest that one or another kind of intervention is most appropriate. The uses of testing will be discussed in greater detail in a later section.

Testing has additional applications. For example, during the course of treatment, testing can provide personality evaluation while intervention proceeds, can be used to evaluate therapeutic progress, or can help in evaluating the intervention process itself. Some of the same information used to plan intervention procedures can also be used to aid personnel decisions in industry (Williams & Kellman, 1956; Snowden, 1956). The court relies on diagnostic testing to help make determinations of legal sanity and culpability.

6. Diagnostic Testing

For many years, diagnostic testing was the major if not the sole activity of psychologists employed in clinical settings. Gradually, especially beginning with the post-World War II years, the horizons of clinical psychology have broadened to include other functions, chiefly the previously proscribed psychotherapy. During the past two decades, psychotherapy in all its variations and ramifications has taken a place of prominence and is on the top of the list of functions in the job description of clinical psychologists. Diagnostic testing has taken a back seat and has become, as Shakow (1965) put it, an "infra-dig" activity of the clinical psychologist; it is no longer a primary or major function. In some settings, it has become a very minor aspect of the clinical operation indeed; in others, it has been entirely eliminated (Fein, 1977).

The question arises, of course, Why this turn of events? Why is diagnostic testing no longer a major activity of the clinical psychologist? What are some of the cardinal causes that underlie this decline?

Some of the reasons are due to certain attitudes of the scientific psychology community, which has been severely critical of the entire clinical enterprise, and especially of the various testing instruments that have not met the rigorous statistical standards of validity and reliability. Holt wrote:

> Indeed, I believe that psychology as a whole will be much poorer without psychodiagnosis and clinical assessment. There are powerful forces within psychology working to bring about this impoverishment in the name of science. The final irony comes when the enemies of clinical psychology try to use the tallies of published successes and failures of what they call clinical and statistical predictions as evidence from which to generalize about the inadequacies of clinical methods. For in doing so they forsake scientific standards of evaluating evidence and generalizing results, and let their prejudices blind them to the irrelevancy of the published surveys to the judgment they wish to make. (Holt, 1970, pp. 338–339)

Although the above quote indicates that the scientific criticism of the use of tests was influential, a recent survey of clinical psychologists on the use of psychological tests points to a weakening effect of the indictment (Wade & Baker, 1977). The authors point out that "While a sizable proportion of clinicians were cognizant of the poor reliability of many tests, such awareness was apparently not important in their decision to use them." They further attempt to explain the reason clinical psychologists are not persuaded to abandon diagnostic testing altogether:

> They feel that the relevant research is inadequate; they do not view behavioral prediction or accurate diagnostic assignment (common criterion measures in testing research) as the most important goals of test usage; they adhere to therapeutic models that value intrapsychic assessment over other assessment procedures with greater face validity (e.g., behavioral observation); they believe testing is too subjective or complex to objectify and examine in an analytic fashion; they depend upon personal experience with tests to determine the utility of testing. . . . (Wade & Baker, 1977, p. 881)

With the possible exception of the criticism regarding the failure of clinicians to analytically examine their instruments, the foregoing statement portrays fairly accurately the present attitudes and state of affairs in diagnostic testing. In a sense, it highlights the "two cultures" of psychology: the strict psychometric-nomothetic approach that is concerned with the traditional issues of validity and reliability, defined in statistical terms, and the context-oriented, clinical-idiographic approach concerned with the decision-making process in the individual and unique case.

These political and social changes in our society have accentuated a certain sensitivity to procedures that involve comparisons between individuals and between people in general. Such comparisons are in the very nature of any test. The testing movement at its inception was concerned with the study of individual differences and with classification or group differences. However, in recent years, tests, especially intelligence tests, which have often been employed in making decisions regarding educational placement and advancement, have come under fire from many quarters. Tests have been viewed as biased against minorities, lower socioeconomic groups, bilingual persons, etc., and have been alleged to aid in the perpetuation of class restrictions, racial segregation, and a variety of other social ills. There has been little distinction made between the tests themselves and the decisions that decision makers base on them. That is, the tests have been confused with the decision-making process. Often, tests have been employed mechanically, without relation to other sources of information, without context. It is this confusion of instrument with user that impelled many negative reactions to the application of psychological tests in the decision-making processes in a variety of settings—educational, industrial, clinical, and others. One might proceed with a listing of the whole plethora of complaints that have been leveled against the testing movement which have weakened the position of diagnostic testing as a professional activity of the clinical psychologist. However, the presentation of further details would be redundant and unproductive. At this point, it would be more useful to concern ourselves with the withdrawal of many psychologists from diagnostic testing more for professional than for political and social-pressure reasons.

Historically, there was, perhaps, a major professional reason for psychologists to turn away from diagnostic testing. As we mentioned, testing was at one time the major function of clinical psychologists. They were co-diagnosticians with the psychiatrist, or in an ancillary status, and had not yet penetrated into the field of therapy to any extent. Thus the "strivings of psychologists for autonomous professional roles versus the traditional role ancillary to medicine" (Fein, 1977) led away from psychodiagnostic function.

One might also mention a variety of other reasons. That the routine testing customary in many institutional settings scarcely made a difference in the disposition of the patients hardly contributed to the psychologists' self-esteem. Moreover, testing "in a vacuum" where the examiner knows nothing about the examinee outside of the testing situation has led to further discouragement, because the examiner lacks sufficient opportunity to "check reality" in relation to his results and interpretations. There was no "feedback," which resulted in isolation, alienation (Fein, 1977), and insufficient advancement of diagnostic skills and sophistication.

A corollary of some of these points is the subsequent status of training in the clinical programs at the universities. The training in psychodiagnostic testing has been poor or indifferent at best. Teachers have been ambivalent or insufficiently trained themselves (Fein, 1977; Holt, 1967). Thus a vicious circle results, of incompetence causing lack of success in the diagnostic enterprise, bringing about denigration of the activity as unreliable, unscientific, etc., and, in turn, perfunctory teaching of a new generation of clinicians.

Finally, the process of interpretation in diagnostic testing and the integration of the disparate strands of information into a meaningful and unique personality portrait and clinical formulation is a highly complex cognitive achievement. It requires, in addition to knowledge of psychopathology and personality dynamics, a capacity for organizing a great deal of complex data, garnished with clinical acumen. Such operations are difficult to teach and taxing to undertake. Many clinicians prefer to take the easy way out and proceed with decision making based on limited information and understanding. Interacting with clients in the psychotherapeutic relationship and being involved in the "process" is much less demanding intellectually and conceptually than the psychodiagnostic operation in reporting and consultation. The past trend away from diagnostic testing is part of the recent trend of "irrationality and the erosion of the excellence" in the training of clinical psychologists decried by Strupp (1976).

7. Concerning the Rationale

More than 30 years ago, a number of important suggestions were presented in the pioneering work on *Diagnostic Psychological Testing* (Rapaport, 1945). Working in a psychiatric setting, Rapaport and his associates viewed diagnostic testing as complementary to the case history and to the psychiatric clinical observations. They also pointed out the unique aspects and contributions of the test battery. Whereas the clinician who takes the history and makes the clinical observations (usually a psychiatrist in those days) is idiosyncratically selective in the areas covered, the testing battery affords a more complete and encompassing study of the patient's personality. Testing provides for systematic sampling of the patient's perceptual, verbal, and motor behavior with much less subjectivity involved in securing the data.

Furthermore, there is a considerable difference at the next stage following the obtaining of the data; it is the point at which the material obtained is evaluated. The organization of the interview and observational material by the psychiatrist (or other interviewer and behavior observer) is liable to be quite subjective. The evaluation pertains "uniquely" to a specific individual. The psychological testing, on the other hand, compares the person's performance with that of others, with standards, and yields a diagnostic statement concerning a particular individual. By comparing scores and patterns of other cases, the psychologist gives some information regarding interindividual comparisons. Thus, as Rapaport (1945) suggests, there is a certain complementarity between the two types of information. Ideally, he advocates the parallel and independent generation of clinical and testing data and their subsequent integration into a complete diagnostic formulation.

Reference was made above to the more objective characteristics of tests as compared with other kinds of clinical data. This is not to deny, however, that there is a good deal of subjectivity in the testing situation as well. It was pointed out by many authors that this is an interpersonal situation, and the sex, personality characteristics of the examiner, and his attitude and general mien have an influence on the nature of the responses given by the testee. On the other hand, there is a great deal of what has been called "extratest behavior" on the part of the person being tested that is very informative to the observing and sensitive clinician. This matter in the context of Rorschach testing was treated in detail some time ago by Schafer (1954). This author has analyzed in painstaking detail and with a great deal of empathy the multifarious reactions of patients to the unstructured testing situation and how this standardized setting can yield rich observational material as well as personality inferences from the test responses themselves.

Schafer (1954) concerns himself with numerous characteristic modes of coping which come to expression in the typical Rorschach testing situation. How the individual may deal with the requirement of "self-exposure in the absence of trust," with anxiety over possible loss of control in the interpersonal situation, and with "regressive temptations" is very revealing and offers important clues to the understanding of personality in addition to the test findings proper. Furthermore, the patterns of defense mechanisms as well as coping mechanisms that come into play in the testing situation enrich and increase the amount of clinical data to be utilized in the ultimate achievement of the diagnostic formulation.

Some have called diagnostic testing, and especially the Rorschach, "a standardized or controlled interview." Considering the above, there is a great deal to support this notion. However, the testing reduces the subjectivity of the ordinary interview, and, as was stated before, supplies objective interpersonal comparison as well. Yet there is the influence of the testing situation and the interpersonal interaction process which add some subjectivity. However, as Hutt (1968) states, we need not be concerned about it; on the contrary, we should "utilize it."

7.1. In Psychotherapy

Reference was made earlier to the decision-making process to which diagnostic testing contributes. What, then, are the kinds of decision that need to be made?

First and foremost is the decision whether to undertake psychotherapy. "If psychotherapy is to be undertaken, it is with the expectation that some change for the better in behavioral functioning will occur. Hence it would be useful if we could predict which individual would be most likely to profit from a particular form of psychotherapy" (Hutt, 1968). Generally speaking, persons with less severe psychopathology are likely to show greater improvement within a relatively shorter period of time than those with severe pathology who may require protracted therapy and prolonged attention. Thus the determination of level of psychopathology, which can be aided markedly by the diagnostic testing, is an important objective and supplies the activity with a reasonable rationale. However, as Hutt points out, measures of health and ego strength are not the only criteria that can be used in prediction of success in psychotherapy. "For example, if the therapeutic method involves prolonged exposure to anxiety laden experiences in therapy, as psychoanalysis and other forms of 'uncovering' therapy do, those individuals who are low in anxiety tolerance (no matter what the general level of psychopathology is) or who are poorly motivated for prolonged and sometimes painful therapeutic experience may fare badly in such programs" (Hutt, 1968).

On the other hand, the assessment of the presence of anxiety as an important motive for entering therapy must also be recognized. "Anxiety of a chronic nature and other ego-dystonic experiences bring the patient to the therapist. The patient's capacity to enter the therapeutic relationship and benefit from it is not assured by this initial step. He must possess a capacity for partial regression in the therapeutic situation, and at the very same time maintain control over the regressive process. This regression in the service of the ego, of 'adaptive regression,' in some measure is a prerequisite for psychotherapy and personality reintegration" (Rabin, 1965).

It must be recognized, however, that not every patient who seeks help can withstand the extensive probing and uncovering of the analytic type of therapy. Moreover, not every patient can allow himself the adaptive regression for fear of an inability to oscillate-regress and readily achieve control again. In many instances, supportive therapy or conditioning procedures may be more suitable and may achieve more limited objectives than radical or fundamental personality changes.

Among the numerous pretherapy situations when diagnostic testing can be of use is that of "time-limited psychotherapy" (Mann, 1973). In this type of treatment, which involves the contract between patient and therapist as to the total number of sessions that are to be undertaken in pursuit of desirable changes in the patient's condition, a definitely targeted psychodiagnostic enterprise is indicated. Central to this approach in the psychotherapeutic process is the identification of a specific and relatively circumscribed problem area which is to be the therapist's major concern. There is a realistic disclaimer not to deal with or modify the "total personality," but to direct one's efforts at a core problem and a significant deficit in personality functioning. Diagnostic testing in such situations may assist markedly to identify that problem area, either during the intake interviews or during the first few preliminary sessions. The psychodynamic bases of the problem, when uncovered, would give direction to the thrust of the time-limited psychotherapeutic effort. Diagnostic testing may clearly help pinpoint the target area.

Holt suggested that

> changes occur in the prevailing ways of dealing with "mental patients" . . . the values of diagnostic testing will change accordingly. Conceivably psychotherapy and psychoanalysis may be entirely supplanted by some new form of chemotherapy or behavior shaping, but I find it inconceivable that any such advances will change one basic fact about people, on which the values of diagnostic testing squarely rests; "*there are stable and pervasive personality characteristics in personality . . . which enable us to predict that people will respond differently to the same stimuli, press or treatment.*" (Holt, 1967, p. 457)

Along with this stability which facilitates prediction of response to treatment, there must be a consideration of changes that occur naturally as well as a consequence of intervention. There are "enduring sentiments" (Rabin, 1977), but the vicissitudes of life and the efforts of the clinician are often directed toward change in personality.

Here, we enter another area of testing and evaluation of a diagnostic nature.

During the series of psychotherapeutic contacts, it is often desirable to check on the status of the case in a more objective way than is possible for the therapist himself. In case an impasse is reached, diagnostic information can be useful in order to understand the underlying processes which are handicapping the further progress. Speaking of projective tests, Hutt (1968) states that "sometimes they are administered during the course of psychotherapy to assist the therapist to deal more effectively with the patient" (p. 79). He further points out their value in generating additional hypotheses and in furnishing evidence concerning individual dynamics.

Evaluation of therapeutic results has been and remains an objective of major concern in research as well as clinical practice. Criteria of "improvement" are hardly universally agreed on. A recent contribution to this problem in the form of "a tripartite model of mental health and therapeutic outcomes" (Strupp & Hadley, 1977) stresses three primary perspectives on mental health. These perspectives are from the viewpoint of society, the individual under treatment, and the mental health professional. While the "measures" used from the viewpoint of society are behavioral observations concerned with the individual's fulfillment of social expectations, and those used from the viewpoint of the individual are general feelings of self-esteem and well-being, the professional's evaluation is much more complex. They describe the measures of mental health and therapeutic outcomes from the professional's perspective as follows: "Clinical judgment, aided by behavioral observations and psychological tests of such variables as self-concept, sense of identity, balance of psychic forces, unified outlook on life, resistance to stress, self-regulation, ability to cope with reality, absence of mental and behavioral symptoms, adequacy in love, work, and play, adequacy in interpersonal relations" (p. 190). Strupp and Hadley conclude that it is rather inadequate to evaluate a person or the outcome of his treatment on the basis of one criterion or from a single perspective, and that "*a truly adequate, comprehensive picture of an individual's mental health is possible only if the three facets of the tripartite model of functioning—behavior, affect, and inferred psychological structure—are evaluated and integrated*" (p. 196). We noted above that for a complete presentation and understanding of the third facet of the model, diagnostic testing is paramount. The "inferred psychological structure" which is most fundamental to the professional's understanding and evaluation can hardly be accomplished successfully without the use of diagnostic psychological testing that addresses itself to the numerous components of that structure.

Diagnosis goes on all the time—at the beginning, during, and at the conclusion of the therapeutic relationship. Strupp expresses it as follows: "it is a simple fact that no therapist or any other human being can listen to someone without reflecting about that person's experience and without almost instantaneously trying to order, divine, and comprehend it" (Strupp, 1976, p. 564). He further elaborates in noting that "thinking, reflecting, and diagnosing (in a broad sense) are integral parts of one's organismic functioning." As mentioned, similar sentiments with respect to classification are expressed by Borofsky (1974), who observes that "The tendency to classify experience appears to be an innate function of the human brain. Classification enables us to make order out of various (and seemingly chaotic) elements of human experience" (p. 24). We note, therefore, that diagnosis and classification are informally engaged in by people involved in interaction with alters. Diagnostic testing adds a new and formal dimension to the process and subjects it to more disciplined procedures of evaluation and classification.

7.2.   Diagnostic Operations as a Facilitator of Psychotherapy

ALBERT I. RABIN
AND DAVID L. HAYES

Another aspect of the rationale of diagnostic testing involves its direct facilitation of the therapeutic process itself. This applies especially to the use of the so-called expressive projective techniques. These techniques represent a bridge between, and, often, a combination of, the diagnostic and therapeutic (Rabin, 1960). Such methods as doll play, free artistic productions, puppetry, etc., are classifiable as both diagnostic and therapeutic; on the one hand they are investigatory and diagnostic, while on the other they may also be described as cathartic and abreactive.

An interesting example is that of the Pickford Pictures (1963), which consist of 120 line drawings that represent a wide variety of situations encountered by children in their everyday life; TAT-type stories are requested from the children. Six selected pictures, based on the presenting problem(s), are used per session. Thus 20 sessions may be based on this series, which is recommended as a facilitator in the child's self-expression. In addition to the diagnostic information obtained by these means, several aspects of a therapeutic nature are involved in this procedure. First, there is the abreactive experience, which permits the child to "share his disturbing and dangerous fantasy." Second, there is the participation of the clinician in the reflection of the content to the child, which facilitates some self-understanding; and, third, there is the employment of direct interpretation to the child, which represents still further exploitation of the testing materials.

A sophisticated approach to psychotherapy via the utilization of diagnostic testing with college students has been reported by Holzberg (1963). Conventional projective techniques (TAT) were employed as a first step in an effort to overcome resistance to change in psychotherapy. The author reported the use of projective technique interviews with students who refused therapy but who in the course of discussing their interviews and test results "actively accepted the idea of treatment."

An attempt was made in Holzberg's report to explain the "softening" process and the breaking down of the initial resistance to (and anxiety about) self-revelation. The question as to what caused a shift in attitudes is considered at length by Holzberg. "The thesis here advanced is that the lowering of the level of psychic functioning inherent in the process of psychotherapy has associated with it considerable anxiety. . . ." If this hypothesis of regression and anxiety about it is acceptable, then the projective test experience provides an opportunity for experiencing adaptive regression. It is an opportunity to learn about regression under conditions sufficiently controlled so as to minimize the potential anxiety associated with the process. Hence projective testing permits the "practice of regression"; the experience becomes more acceptable, and the prospect of therapy is less threatening. The projective testing situation allows relief from the anxiety and guilt which would be experienced when entering therapy directly and permits the prospective patient to externalize responsibility. Moreover, spaced administration of testing may also be a critical factor in this operation, for it does not expose the patient to "massive doses of anxiety."

The publication on "the creative variations in the projective techniques" (Harrower, Vorhaus, & Bauman, 1960) offered several innovative applications of diagnostic testing. Harrower, who was concerned with "projective counseling," illustrates the counselee's confrontation with his own productions on the tests and opportunity to compare them with those of others. It is a sort of reality-testing procedure which is conducive to the gaining of insight, which, in turn, may be an important step on the way to modification of behavior. Much of current diagnostic testing is based on this paradigm in which the patient, with the aid of the clinician, confronts his own productions. Here, too, we may readily note the bridge between diagnosis and treatment.

Bauman's "interaction testing" is another diagnostic innovation and a contribution to the therapeutic endeavor undertaken with small groups. This method involves two administrations of a particular technique. First, the test is administered individually to each member of the group or family. Then responses to the test material based on group decisions are obtained. Although the interaction process itself during the decision-making session is of interest, the inferential data involving reinforcement of some individual responses, selection of responses, and the emergence of new responses not given in the individual administration are all contributory to the diagnostic and treatment process of couples, families, or small groups under consideration.

7.3. More Circumscribed Goals in Diagnostic Testing

The implicit assumption in the preceding pages was that diagnostic testing contributes substantially to the overall diagnostic-clinical operation in order to facilitate decisions about psychotherapy, aid in directing its course, and evaluate the outcome. However, many of the decisions that need to be made (Levine, 1968) are in response to specific questions asked in a variety of clinical and social contexts. It is true that the purpose of psychological assessment is to understand the whole person, but, as Korchin (1976) remarks, "in actual practice assessment necessarily has to serve more modest ends." In the case of the "undifferentiated clinical usefulness of diagnostic testing in a hospital or clinic . . . the psychodiagnostician first of all contributes to the understanding of etiology. He weighs the relative contribution of organic and functional factors . . . ego structure . . . abilities and the degree of their functional and organic impairment" (Holt, 1967, p. 456).

There emerge two major trends in the practice of diagnostic testing—the general and the specific. The general approach refers to the comprehensive evaluation by means of a large battery of tests of the "total personality." There are no specific questions asked by the referring agents, and the result is "a more or less complex statement of the psychopathology of a psychiatric patient," which is Rycroft's (1968) definition of a "diagnostic formulation."

The other major trend refers to a targeted diagnostic statement in response to a specific request by the referring agent. Often, the diagnosis requested is that of a statement of classification to aid in the decision-making process. Is this patient mentally retarded to the degree that he is unable to live independently and requires supervision? Should this person be hospitalized because he is psychotic? These and many other determinations of this kind demand an understanding of psychopathology and testing techniques as well as of the social and institutional context in which the decisions have to be made.

An illustration of the more limited objectives and predictions of diagnostic testing is represented by the volume on clinical and research applications of the Rorschach (Goldfried, Stricker, & Weiner, 1971). The several chapters of this book address themselves to the use of the Rorschach technique in identifying particular pathological or deviant conditions. The application of the Rorschach in the prediction of suicide, prognosis in therapy, and the diagnosis of neurosis, schizophrenia, organicity, and other disorders is illustrated clinically and buttressed by research data. It demonstrates the use of the testing primarily in classification. However, much decision making is based on this aspect of the diagnosis and not much more. Shakow points up the importance of classification as follows: "I do not understand how a psychologist can adopt a professional orientation which does not acknowledge classification as fundamental in dealing with the multiplicity of phenomena involved in the diagnosis of mental disorder" (Katz, Cole, & Barton, 1965, p. 117).

We pointed out earlier that classification is not identical with diagnosis; rather, "it implies and involves the possibilities of diagnosis" (Engel, 1972). In instances where intelligence tests are a major part of diagnostic testing, classification as to retardation or no retardation, as well as level of retardation if such is identified, is the primary contribution. Since the objective and comparative nature of such tests is paramount in the classificatory operation, because observation and clinical impression are much less accurate, then their contribution to the diagnosis is of primary importance. The usefulness of the intelligence tests in the assessment of abnormalities in mental development has been amply documented (e.g., Rabin, 1967).

Another area in which the goals of testing are rather circumscribed is that of behavioral therapy or modification. It is difficult to ascertain exactly the rationale for assessment used by behavior therapists because their writings rarely address this issue directly. Instead, their contributions to the assessment literature generally have taken the form of pronouncements that assessment is "a most crucial and significant step in . . . behavior therapy" (Goldfried & Pomeranz, 1968, p. 76), vigorous, almost polemical, arguments against "traditional" assessment techniques as based on problematical conceptions of personality (Goldfried & Kent, 1972) or diagnosis (Kanfer & Saslow, 1969; Stuart, 1970), or a "how to" description of assessment, with little or no attention to presentation of underlying rationale (e.g., Goodkin, 1967; Cautela, 1968; Tharp & Wetzel, 1969).

However, clear statements of rationale do exist, standing as exceptions to the foregoing. For example, Kanfer and Phillips (1970) describe the necessity of locating the problem to be exposed to therapeutic attention and translating the initial complaint into a form to which available behavioral technology is applicable. Mischel (1968) suggests that the purpose of behavioral assessment is to identify the problem behaviors, determine the conditions maintaining them, and implement and evaluate techniques to change them. Peterson (1968) writes that the competent practice of behavior therapy demands knowledge of the external and internal conditions arousing maladaptive responses, of the reinforcing consequences which sustain these behaviors, and of stimulus changes which might elicit and sustain more acceptable behavior.

Whether a rationale for assessment in behavior therapy is stated explicitly or must be inferred from a consideration of the techniques of behavior assessment, the methods of such an approach have been thoroughly described (e.g., Cautela, 1968; Kanfer & Phillips, 1970; Kanfer & Saslow, 1969; Mischel, 1968; Peterson, 1968; Stuart, 1970; Tharp & Wetzel, 1969). These authors stress the necessity of (1) identifying the problem, (2) identifying the eliciting conditions and maintaining consequences, (3) implementing procedures to effect a change, and (4) evaluating the effectiveness of the change procedures; implicit in these descriptions is the assumption, suggested by the word "necessity," that behavior therapy without behavior assessment is ineffective, does not work well. From that point of view, the rationale for doing behavior assessment is clearly to enhance the potency of behavior therapy to make changes in maladaptive behavior.

Goldfried and Kent (1972) have compared traditional and behavioral approaches to personality assessment, listing several theoretical and methodological assumptions which they feel distinguish the two. They describe traditional assessment methods as based on a conception of personality structure which underlies behavior, and traditional instruments as composed of items selected on the basis of the test constructor's assumptions regarding the (underlying) personality variable(s) in question. Behaviorally oriented testers, on the other hand, conceive of personality as based on previous social learning history and current environmental antecedents and/or consequences of the behavior. They select test items in an attempt to adequately represent the stimulus conditions which they want to predict. Goldfried and Kent go on to characterize the alternative approaches: "Traditional assessment . . . has been directed primarily toward an understanding of the individual's underlying personality characteristics or traits as a means of predicting behavior; . . . behavior assessment . . . is more of a direct measurement of the individual's response to various life situations" (p. 4).

Behavior therapists recognize the importance of adequate assessment to allow their techniques to function effectively, and, being behavior therapists, they show a predilection for behavioral types of assessment. They seem in essential agreement with a statement made in a slightly different context: "What is done about a problem depends on how it is defined. The way a . . . problem is defined determines the focus, the techniques for intervention, and the criteria for evaluation" (Zifferblatt & Hendricks, 1974, p. 750).

In a review of assessment techniques and instruments currently in use in behavior therapy, Dickson (1975) describes three main categories. Most widely used and most adequately validated are a variety of paper and pencil Fear Survey Schedules for use in assessing areas of phobic behavior and designed to lead to specific behavioral intervention. An allied but separate type of instrument is the Reinforcement Survey Schedule. This type of test is used to formulate interventions based on operant conditioning theory, and is given in situations ranging from individual behavior problems to marital difficulties to token economies in mental hospitals. Finally, such specialized techniques as vividness scales for mental imagery and assertiveness measures are mentioned, although these measures are considered less well developed than the previous two types. In conjunction with direct observation, these techniques form the armamentarium of the tester with a behavior modifier's orientation.

In the context of behavior therapy and behaviorally oriented clinical work, the diagnostic (testing) methods described in this volume are largely irrelevant. Classification and underlying personality structure are of little or no concern in the context of behavior therapy intervention. The assessment methods that are used are closely tied to the identification of specific symptoms which are to be eliminated. Herein lies the main rationale for this type of "diagnostic testing."

8. Conclusion

We have attempted to indicate the usefulness of ordering information about people (classification) and of understanding the unique multilevel functioning of the individual (diagnosis). Classification is an important aspect of diagnosis; its relationship to the decision-making processes in clinical work has been stressed. Although diagnostic testing has been neglected for a variety of professional and social reasons in recent years, there is ample evidence that it remains an important function of the clinical psychologist. In addition to clinical and behavioral history and observational data, it contributes more detailed information concerning personality structure and dynamics, which is useful in case management in psychotherapy, counseling, and environmental design. Diagnostic testing is especially useful in targeting treatment and, in some instances, as part of the treatment process itself. Most important is the function of testing in checking critically the data and observations obtained from other sources and its use in integrating them in the final diagnostic formulation.

9. References

Altschule, M. D. Disease entity, syndrome, state of mind, or figment? In R. Cancro (Ed.), *The schizophrenic reactions*. New York: Bruner/Mazel, 1970.

Borofsky, G. Issues in diagnosis and classification of personality functioning. In A. I. Rabin (Ed.), *Clinical psychology: Issues of the seventies*. East Lansing: Michigan State University Press, 1974.

Cautela, J. R. Behavioral type and the need for behavior assessment. *Psychotherapy; Theory, Research and Practice*, 1968, *5(3)*, 175–179.

Cronbach, L. E., & Gleser, G. L. *Psychological tests and personnel decisions*. Urbana, Ill.: University of Illinois Press, 1957.

Dickson, C. R. Role of assessment in behavior therapy. In P. McReynolds (Ed.), *Advances in psychological assessment* (Vol. 3). San Francisco: Jossey-Bass, 1975.

DSM II: Diagnostic and statistical manual of mental disorders (2nd ed.). Washington, D.C.: American Psychiatric Association, 1968.

Engel, M. *Psychopathology in childhood*. New York: Harcourt Brace Jovanovich, 1972.

Engle, R. Medical diagnosis: Present, past, and future II. *Archives of Internal Medicine*, 1963a, *112*, 520–529.

Engle, R. Medical diagnosis: Present, past and future III. *Archives of Internal Medicine*, 1963b, *112*, 530–543.

Engle, R., & Davis, B. J. Medical Dx: Present, past and future I. *Archives of Internal Medicine*, 1963, *112*, 512–519.

Fein, L. G. Current status of psychological testing among practitioners. Papers read at the Annual Meetings of the American Psychological Association, San Francisco, August 1977.

Goldfried, M. R., & Kent, R. W. Traditional versus behavioral personality assessment: A comparison of methodological and theoretical assumptions. *Psyhcological Bulletin*, 1972, *77(6)*, 409–420.

Goldfried, M., & Pomeranz, D. Role of assessment in behavior modification. *Psychological Reports*, 1968, *23*, 75–87.

Goldfried, M. R., Stricker, G., & Weiner, I. B. *Rorschach handbook of clinical and research applications*. Englewood Cliffs, N.J.: Prentice-Hall, 1971.

Goodkin, R. Some neglected issues in the literature of behavioral treatment. *Psychological Reports*, 1967, *20*, 415–420.

Greenspoon, J., & Giersten, C. A new look at psychological testing: Psychological testing from the standpoint of a behaviorist. *American Psychologist*, 1967, *22*, 848–853.

Harrower, M., Vorhaus, P., & Bauman, G. *Creative variations in the projective techniques*. Springfield, Ill.: Thomas, 1960.

Holt, R. R. Diagnostic testing: Present status and future prospects. *The Journal of Nervous and Mental Disease*, 1967, *144(6)*, 444–465.

Holt. R. R. (Ed.). *Diagnostic psychological testing by Rapaport, Gill & Schafer* (rev. ed.). New York: International Universities Press, 1968.

Holt, R. R. Yet another look at clinical and statistical prediction: Or, is clinical psychology worthwhile? *American Psychologist*, 1970, *25(4)*, 337–349.

Holzberg, J. D. Projective techniques and resistance to change in psychotherapy as viewed through a communication model. *Journal of Projective and Personality Assessment*, 1963, *27*, 430–435.

Hutt, M. L. Psychopathology, assessment, and psychotherapy. In A. I. Rabin (Ed.), *Projective techniques in personality assessment*. New York: Springer, 1968.

Kanfer, F., & Phillips, J. S. *Learning foundations of behavior therapy*. New York: Wiley, 1970.

Kanfer, F. H., & Saslow, G. Behavioral diagnosis. In C. M. Franks (Ed.), *Behavior therapy: Appraisal and status*. New York: McGraw-Hill, Inc., 1969.

Katz, M. M., Cole, J. O., & Barton, W. E. (Eds.). *Classification in psychiatry and psychopathology*. Chevy Chase, Md.: National Institute of Mental Health, 1965.

Korchin, S. J. *Modern clinical psychology*. New York: Basic Books, 1976.

Levine, D. Why and when to test: The social context of psychological testing. In A. I. Rabin (Ed.), *Projective techniques in personality assessment*. New York: Springer, 1968.

Levy, L. H. *Psychological interpretation*. New York: Holt, Rinehart and Winston, 1963.

Mann, J. *Time-limited psychotherapy*. Cambridge, Mass.: Harvard University Press, 1973.

Meehl, P. E. *Clinical versus statistical prediction: A theoretical analysis and a review of the evidence*. Minneapolis: University of Minnesota Press, 1954.

Meehl, P. The cognitive activity of the clinician. *American Psychologist*, 1960, *15*, 19–27.

Menninger, K. *The vital balance*. New York: Viking Press, 1963.

Mischel, W. *Personality and assessment*. New York: Wiley, 1968.

Murray, H. A., et al. *Explorations in personality*. New York: Oxford University Press, 1938.

Peterson, D. R. *The clinical study of social behavior*. New York: Appleton-Century-Crofts, 1968.

Rabin, A. I. Projective methods and projection in children. In A. I. Rabin & M. R. Haworth (Eds.), *Projective techniques with children*. New York: Grune & Stratton, 1960.

Rabin, A. I. Projective test research and its applications to therapeutic practice. Paper presented at the Postgraduate Center for Mental Health, New York City, May 1965.

Rabin, A. I. Adapting and devising projective methods for special purposes. (See Hutt, 1968.)

Rabin, A. I. Assessment of abnormalities in intellectual development. In J. Zubin & G. A. Jervis (Eds.), *Psychopathology of mental development*. New York: Grune & Stratton, 1967.

Rabin, A. I. Enduring sentiments: The continuity of personality over time. *Journal of Personality Assessment*, 1977, *41(6)*, 563–572.

Rapaport, D. *Diagnostic psychological testing*. Chicago: The Year Book Publishers, 1945.

Rycroft, C. *A critical dictionary of psychoanalysis*. New York: Basic Books, 1968.

Schafer, R. *Psychoanalytic interpretation in Rorschach testing*. New York: Grune & Stratton, 1954.

Shakow, D. Seventeen years later: Clinical psychology in the light of the 1947 committee on training in clinical psychology report. *American Psychologist*, 1965, *20*, 353–362.

Snowden, R. F. Top management and the Rorschach technique. In B. Klopfer (Ed.), *Developments in the Rorschach technique*. New York: Harcourt, Brace & World, 1956.

Strupp, H. H. Clinical psychology, irrationalism, and the erosion of excellence. *American Psychologist*, 1976, *31(3)*, 561–571.

Strupp, H. H., & Hadley, S. W. A tripartite model of mental health and therapeutic outcomes; with special reference to negative effects in psychotherapy. *American Psychologist*, 1977, *32(3)*, 187–196.

Stuart, R. B. *Trick or treatment: How and when psychotherapy fails*. Champaign, Ill.: Research Press, 1970.

Szasz, T. S. The problem of psychiatric nosology. *American Journal of Psychiatry*, 1957, *114*, 405–413.

Szasz, T. S. *The myth of mental illness*. New York: Harper & Row, 1961.

Sundberg, N. D., & Tyler, L. E. *Clinical psychology*. New York: Appleton-Century-Crofts, 1962.

Tharp, R., & Wetzel, R. *Behavior modification in the natural environment*. New York: Academic Press, 1969.

Thorne, F. The clinical method in science. *American Psychologist*, 1947, *2*, 159–166.

Wade, T. C. & Baker, T. B. Opinions and use of psychological tests: A survey of clinical psychologists. *American Psychologist*, 1977, *32(10)*, 874–882.

White, W., & Watt, N. F. *The abnormal personality*. New York: Ronald Press, 1973.

Williams, G., & Kellmen, S. The Rorschach technique in industrial psychology. In B. Klopfer (Ed.), *Developments in the Rorschach technique*. New York: Harcourt, Brace & World, 1956.

Zifferblatt, S., & Hendricks, L. Applied behavioral analysis of societal problems. *American Psychologist*, 1974, *29(2)*, 250–276.

Zigler, E., & Phillips, L. Psychiatric diagnosis: A critique. *Journal of Abnormal and Social Psychology*, 1961, *3*, 607–618.

18

Diagnosing Brain Impairment

THOMAS J. BOLL

1. Introduction

> While the brain has long been recognized as the organ of behavior, subserving intelligence, cognition, and emotional responses, specific attempts to elucidate brain-behavior relationships with measurements based on formal psychological testing represent a relatively recent effort. Until recently these efforts have not made great contributions, principally because so many factors over and beyond recognized brain damage are significant determinants of psychological status. As a consequence, it has been difficult to devise an approach and psychological evaluation that would have specific significance with regard to the condition of the human brain. The problems in making progress in this area have related principally to the complexity of human behavior on one hand and the complexity of the pathological conditions that involve the human brain on the other. Finally, procedural requirements in correlating brain and behavioral findings have contributed another problem. (Reitan, 1973)

Two principal approaches to the psychological examination, diagnosis, and understanding of the relationship between the organic integrity of the brain and human abilities can be identified. The first, which is most similar to the medical or neurological model, might be described as diagnostic in goal, dichotomous in approach, and closed-ended in result. This approach has characterized much of what appears in our scientific literature and is taught in training programs. This approach appears to assume that the brain is a unitary organ or that impairment of this organ will have a unitary or at least a single overriding effect. It further assumes that, despite the complexity of the brain itself, the variety of difficulties which can befall the brain (including location, lateralization, size, rate of growth, age at onset, and pathological types of disorder) will have but a single behavioral effect. It fails to take into account the biopsychosocial complexity of the human person which results in thousands of possible combinations of behavioral characteristics which may be subject to assessment

THOMAS J. BOLL • Division of Child and Adolescent Psychiatry, University of Virginia Medical Center, Charlottesville, Virginia 22901. This work was partially supported by National Institutes of Neurological and Communicative Disorders and Stroke Contract No. 1-NS-5-2329, Biopsychosocial Aspects of Epilepsy-Comprehensive Epilepsy Program.

by means of psychological tests. Finally, an approach designed to produce binary decisions (brain damage vs. no brain damage) suggests that this type of classification has inherent meaning or usefulness and could represent the sole reason for the use of these procedures. It also assumes that this is an appropriate area of investigation for behavioral clinicians and scientists.

Despite the clinical inadequacy of the above-mentioned approach, validity can be demonstrated for binary-type behavioral measures. Diagnosis of brain damage can indeed have clinical utility, and use of such procedures for such purposes by psychologists and psychiatrists is in some settings the only available means to obtain such data.

The second approach can be characterized as the neuropsychological model and has the goal of understanding, as broadly as possible, the individual patient's abilities, strengths, and weaknesses. This approach is developmental or normative rather than dichotomous. Its result is open-ended. It provides a description of current functioning relevant to treatment and daily performance rather than simply a diagnostic label. The first approach, which most closely approximates the medical and neurological model, depends on the occurrence of symptoms or instances of deviant or impaired performances. It depends primarily on pathognomonic signs which are unidirectional (presence means problems but absence does not mean health). It is selective, too, in its emphasis on areas of complaint and tends only to obtain those data necessary to reach a diagnostic conclusion. The neuropsychological model, while sharing some of the same interests, goes beyond the search for pathology. The use of normative data allows for inference of degrees of health as well as deficiency. The neuropsychological model has as its philosophical purpose understanding of the interaction of a range of human functions sufficient to do justice to the complexity of the organ of behavior as well as to the behavioral repertoire it subserves. It is through this more comprehensive evaluative effort that information pertinent to the appropriate behavioral intervention techniques can be obtained.

Lashley pointed out: "It should be a fundamental principle of neural interpretation of psychological functions that the nervous activities are as complex as psychological activities which they constitute" (Cobb, 1960, p. xx). Reitan (1966a) in turn suggested that our methods for assessing behavioral change should be as complex as the brain which subserves these behaviors and behavioral changes. Certainly, the neurological and neuropsychological models have common antecedents, overlapping goals, and the purpose of aiding the patient and advancing our knowledge. Rather than becoming lost in debate over which model should be adopted and which to deplore, the requirements of the real-life situation from which neuropsychological questions arise recommends the adoption alternately or concurrently of both models. "Anyone who feels that a single model or theory can be proposed which will be sufficient to meet all needs should be gently encouraged to recognize that his thinking is involved in a crippling state of bias and prejudice" (Reitan, 1968). Agreement on use of one or several models or approaches assumes the appropriateness of the use of psychological tests for neurological diagnosis. Several subissues that contribute to this overall consideration include (1) the value of making such a diagnosis, (2) the uniqueness or redundancy of psychological measures in the effort, (3) the validity of the result, and (4) the areas of measurement and the tools necessary to embark on neuropsychological practice.

1.1. Value of Diagnosis

It is becoming generally recognized that concepts such as "organicity" or brain damage imply the presence of a unitary entity with no basis in scientific or clinical reality. With this recognition has come the parallel awareness that any test purporting to "diagnose" brain damage or organicity is likewise meaningless. Diagnostic efforts based on this type of an understanding could quite easily result in a serious disservice to the patient examined. A condition of brain damage can exist on a lifelong basis without medical significance or recognized behavioral effect. A clinical example is a patient with static damage in the right parietal lobe caused by a perinatal event. The patient, while never very good in art class, completed college and functioned successfully both socially and occupationally. Suddenly, two close family members became ill and died, leaving him with significant additional financial and personal responsibilities. His loss-produced grief and increased life stress led to a prolonged depression for which he sought help. As part of his evaluation, a test to "rule out organicity" was administered and his performance placed him in the brain-damaged category. Is the diagnosis correct? Yes. Did his perinatal lesion contribute to his depression? No connection has ever been documented. This diagnosis could represent at best a gratuitous label in his chart and at worst convince some therapists that his treatment prognosis is poor because he is brain damaged. Such an examination has certainly done no good and reflects the inherent limitation of an approach to human behavior limited to dichotomous classification rather than behavioral understanding.

Behavioral approaches to neurological diagnosis have been seen as unproductive because many types of brain damage represent static conditions which do not require medical attention. Behavioral consequences of such damage can be evaluated and remediated without reference to neurological substrates. Such an argument contends that unless there is a question of a medically significant disorder, identification of which would lead to medical or surgical intervention, the behavior speaks for itself and there is no need to open the black box. All psychological behavioral examinations should focus on providing recommendations for treatment and not on attempting to establish etiology of the behavioral problem. While such an argument, like any call to action, is attractive, it may be quite inefficient. Without a valid understanding of the nature of the problem, intervention is reduced to trial and error and the discovery of a successful approach may be needlessly delayed. Therapeutic approaches are enhanced by increased knowledge of the disorder at hand.

1.2. Uniqueness and Redundancy of Neuropsychological Examination

It has been suggested that attempts to assess impairment of brain function and/or structure on the basis of psychological tests can only hope to confirm what other sources of information have already discovered, thus rendering them redundant. However, neurological diagnoses are rarely, if ever, made on the basis of a single type of examination. Neurologists progress in stepwise fashion through a series of procedures designed to provide information from several independent sources. The initial data obtained are the patient's complaints and a careful history. Direct physical examination assesses reflexes, muscles, and cranial nerves through direct visual and tactile inspection. X-rays and electroencephalographic examination are commonly included.

The examination procedures with the highest specificity and validity (pneumoencephalogram, angiogram, direct surgical inspection) carry the greatest risk of morbidity (pain or disability) and mortality (death). These procedures are therefore utilized only when results of other less risky procedures indicate their necessity. The neuropsychological examination, far from being redundant, fits the overall design of maximizing data from diverse sources and represents a contribution of considerable uniqueness. In addition to its diagnostic validity, it is physically noninvasive and without risk. Such an examination taps areas, or at least types, of dysfunction not available to even the most heroic procedures. As Luria states, "The restricted limits of regular, neurological symptoms is a result of some very important facts: lesions of the *highest* (secondary or tertiary) zones of the cortex—which are considered as specifically human parts of hemispheres—do not result, as a rule in any elementary sensory or motor defects and remain inaccessible for classical neurological examination. They are associated with alterations of very complex behavioral processes (cognitive processes, elaboration of complex programs of behavior and their control), and that is why one has to establish new complex methods that could be used to study dysfunctional disorders evoked by their injuries. It is thus necessary to apply methods of *neuropsychology* for local diagnosis of lesions of these complex cortical zones" (Luria, 1973). Finally, as discussed earlier, another distinguishing feature of neuropsychological examination is its ability to go beyond diagnosis as an endpoint. It provides a comprehensive evaluation of the patient which can be repeatedly updated. Such an examination produces recommendations for rehabilitation. The information has practical value to the patient and his family in aiding them to understand the patient's cognitive situation, which aids in adaptation to change in ability. By preventing misinterpretation of changed behavioral capacity and its resultant fear and anger, a major roadblock to successful coping with neurological disorder can be avoided. There are, however, certain types of impairment which, while known to be present, are quite unavailable to routine neurological examination procedures. We have seen many patients following head injury who appear normal to electroencephalographic and physical neurological examinations but who continue to demonstrate a cognitive deficit not demonstrable on physical or mental status examination. This deficit is often of sufficient severity to preclude returning to school or work. Such patients typically show excellent recovery in time. Failure to recognize the presence of these clinically subtle deficits can result in a too-soon return to cognitive competition, which has resulted in failure, anxiety, and reduced self-concept for many patients. This develops into a downward spiral, with negative consequences for adjustment in excess of the brain injury itself. These avoidable psychosocial consequences often persist long after cognitive recovery has taken place. While such a phenomenon is well documented (Smith, 1975; Hook, 1969; Reitan, 1973), it cannot be prevented without identification of the areas of impairment. Such identification requires comprehensive neuropsychological examination.

1.3. Neuropsychological Validity

The validity of a neuropsychological examination will be considered in detail in another section. Batteries of procedures such as those developed by Halstead but significantly expanded structurally and conceptually by Reitan and further modified in various ways by Boll, Klonoff, Matthews, Russell, Kløve, and Meier (Reitan &

Davison, 1974) have been shown to have validity comparable to that of most or all standard neurological diagnostic procedures considered individually (Filskov & Goldstein, 1974). Batteries employing somewhat different tasks but with similar underlying neuropsychological conceptualizations have enjoyed similar success (Milner, 1958; Satz, 1966b; Parsons, 1970; Smith, 1975; Hartlage & Hartlage, 1977). Detailed examination of this issue will be taken up in a later section.

1.4. Tools and Areas of Neuropsychological Investigation

A neuropsychological examination must be able to sample broadly from the large range of brain-related disorders on the one hand and the enormously extensive and varied array of human abilities and functions on the other. To do this, such a battery would include tests of stored information and experience, receptive and expressive language, attention and concentration, memory, motor skills, perceptual ability, learning, problem solving, abstraction, and concept formation, as well as tests that combine these skills and modalities. This provides the opportunity to tap similar mental functions involving different modalities and different mental functions across similar modalities. Practical considerations such as cost and patient and examiner time must be attended to. More importantly, we must keep in mind that simple answers to complex questions may be far more extravagant than would be a serious attempt to provide an adequate response to the clinical problem. Many current neurological texts recommend psychological examination as an integral part of the mental status segment of the neurological exam. There is also a growing recognition that a serious professional effort deserves the time required. I. S. Wechsler indicated: "No neurological status is complete without a mental examination" and "a complete mental examination takes several hours" (Wechsler, 1963). DeJong (1967) recommended a battery of psychological tests as part of the mental evaluation and as essential for neurological diagnosis.

The selection of procedures can be approached in many ways. Theoretical models of brain function or brain damage such as that espoused by Goldstein (1952) or Halstead (1947) have certainly been responsible for knowledge advancement. They have also produced some useful techniques. An approach guided by theory, however incomplete, has the advantage of spelling out areas of search which can be approached systematically. These are subject to cross-validation and evaluation by any interested investigator-clinician. However, they have consistently been found to be inadequate due to an underestimation of the complexity of brain behavior relationships. Eschewing all theory, Reitan (1966a) stated, "it would appear that the limitations of our present investigational method may well be so severe that presently available results hardly form a proper basis for building or rejecting theories of psychological effects of brain lesions. We might do far better to recognize the complexity of the problems and to continue to struggle with them rather than anxiously to submit to the need for closure." A second approach can be described as a selective pursuit of leads and interests. "I'll give a few tests and then see what else is needed" characterizes this style of examination. An appropriate question here would appear to be "needed for what?" Such an approach typically focuses selectively on pathology and tends to ignore countervailing strengths. Further, because each patient is treated as a totally unique case, no basis can be developed for scientific generalization. Certainly, depending largely on the brilliance of the clinician, interesting and valid insights can be derived from purely idiographic approaches, as witness the work of Luria (1973). Unfortunately, when it is recommended not as a style of selective experimentation but as a basis for test choice in clinical settings (Lezack, 1976), it leaves the practitioner without a framework for development of interpretations. Unless a commonality of approach is developed (be it psychological tests or placement of EEG leads), all hope for scientific generalization must be abandoned.

The approach which seems to have borne the most fruit can be characterized as an experimental or, more humbly, "best guess" approach to instrument selection (Reitan, 1974a). Such an approach begins with an effort to cover the array of human abilities as broadly as possible within practical limits. The second step is to validate these procedures by controlled investigation prior to their recommendation for clinical use. Such an approach, using differing individual tests, has been followed by Reitan (1974b), Smith (1975), Parsons (1970), Russell (1975a), Satz, Fennell, and Reilly (1970), Hartlage and Hartlage (1977), Klonoff and Low (1974), Knights (1973), Rourke, (1975), Matthews (1974), and Boll (1974a). Additional requirements specific to individual laboratories included choosing tests which (1) are available in alternate forms, (2) are narrowband, i.e., measure a single ability, (3) are broadband, i.e., require integration of several abilities such as visual and motor skills, (4) assess similar functions across several different modalities and vice versa, (5) are portable, (6) are objectively scored, (7) maximize the complementary use of more than a single method of interpretive inference, and (8) are standardized, valid, and reliable. This list pertains to psychological procedures which generate clinical information that is scientifically communicable, subject to empirical cross-validation, and likely to allow generalization on the basis of data obtained. The organization of a battery of tests will directly influence its clinical utility.

2. Methods of Clinical Inference

One factor in test selection, the maximization of several methods of clinical inference, deserves additional discussion. Most traditional clinical data are predicated on and restricted to a single inferential method for their evaluation. Scientific publications are almost totally restricted in this regard. It is possible that many pseudoissues surrounding validity and reliability and an even greater number of incorrect conclusions have emerged because of this limitation to which very few exceptions exist (Boll and Reitan, 1972c).

2.1. Level of Performance

The most scientifically acceptable and commonly clinically employed method of inference is level of performance. Attention is directed entirely toward how well or poorly a person performs. Comparisons can be against an absolute standard or against a set of representative performances by others referred to as norms. In the scientific literature, this approach is utilized to determine whether one group of individuals differs from another in terms of central tendency taking into account the group's variability. Such data rely on comparisons of group data and may fail to reveal the clinical utility or lack thereof of a set of scores for the characterization of a single individual's performance. Many studies have used this approach to demonstrate that brain-damaged and non-brain-damaged patients differ in various areas in human ability (Benton, 1968; McManis, 1974; Heilbrun, 1958; Bender, 1946; Reitan, 1955c; Boll, 1974a). The uniqueness and major advantage of this method are in its ability to document health and ability strength rather than simply to identify pathology or deficit. Most psychological tests, with their emphasis on quantified scoring, standardization, normative performances, reliability, and cutoff scores, are designed to be evaluated in a level of performance manner. Such an approach yields much valuable and valid information. A person with a Wechsler Verbal IQ or 120 can be described as able in many ways on the basis of this datum alone. Similarly, a person with a Verbal IQ of 60 can be predicted to perform quite poorly in certain situations. Neither of these scores tells us if the person has always been at this level, if he used to be much brighter, or if he has just shown a gain of 20 points. Even less can be learned about the etiology of these behaviors.

It is especially important to keep in mind the large number of factors which can influence level of performance. Because a specified level of performance is necessary to categorize a person as "in the brain-damaged range," it in no way implies that it is sufficient for such a categorization. Equally, a person with evidence of brain damage may demonstrate performances well within the normal range and yet reveal from other aspects of his performance that he indeed has neurologically based ability deficits. The level of one's performance can be affected by motivation, emotional reactions such as anxiety or depression, medication, impaired energy level due to poor health, lack of sleep, or other causes, situational factors such as patient-examiner incompatibility, noise and distractions, sociocultural linguistic background differences, peripheral sensory handicaps such as blindness and deafness, peripheral motor dysfunction, speech disorder, and examiner style and competence. This list represents only a sample of factors that must be considered along with the effect of the condition of the brain when interpreting data tied solely to level of performance.

Two studies employing the Halstead-Reitan neuropsychological procedures demonstrate the limitation to scientific communication presented by reliance on level of performance. Reitan (1964) performed an analysis of variance to determine whether a large battery of behavioral measures could distinguish among patients with different types of brain damage. These neuropathological types included intracerebral tumor, extracerebral tumor, cerebrovascular lesions, and traumatic head injury. He then performed a similar analysis to determine differences among the groups on the basis of location of this damage in either the right anterior, right posterior, left anterior, or left posterior quadrant of the brain. Prior to this statistical analysis, however, Reitan had, on the basis of utilization of multiple inferential methods, produced correct classifications of individual subjects by neuropathological type and lateralization which far exceed those which would occur by chance alone. Yet, on the basis of traditional analysis of level of performance alone, he concluded that "the small number of significant differences, however, was almost sufficient to make one who is especially faithful to our conventional statistical models ask if it must not have been extrasensory perception which was responsible . . ." for the correct clinical classifications. A more likely explanation is that the averaging and canceling of individual peaks and valleys that occur when individuals are grouped served to obscure the inter- and intraindividual characteristics necessary for correct classification. An identical problem was encountered when Reitan and Boll (1973) applied standard statistical procedures to four groups of children. There were one normal group, one group with brain damage, and two groups classified as having minimal brain dysfunction. Few differences emerged between the two MBD and the normal groups. However, when individual analyses of the data were applied to affect categorization, the accuracy which resulted produced a highly significant χ^2. We must conclude that level of performance alone, either for individuals or for groups, is inadequate for obtaining an understanding of the relationship between the integrity of brain functions and human abilities.

2.2. Pattern of Intra- and Intertest Performance

A second method of inference frequently used, although often without explicit recognition, is pattern of performance. If a patient completes two tasks, three pieces of data are available: performance on task 1, performance on task 2, and the actual vs. the expected relationship between these performances. This method recognizes that some abilities may be impaired by brain damage while others remain intact. Obviously, those abilities impaired and those spared vary depending on many characteristics of the brain damage. Initially, attempts were made to find tasks which were impervious to brain impairment (Hold Tests, Wechsler, 1958) and others which were especially sensitive to the effects of generalized impairing conditions of the brain (Don't Hold Tests). This particular scheme, while addressing the need to go beyond level of performance, underestimated the diversity of behavioral deficits produced by different types and locations of brain damage. A more recent and successful use of pattern involves the comparison of Verbal vs. Performance Scale abilities. Comparison of Verbal with Performance Scale IQ scores has shown differences related to right and left cerebral hemisphere damage (Andersen, 1950, 1951; Reitan, 1955a; Vega and Parsons, 1967; Fields and Whitmyre, 1969). It should be noted, however, that this generalization, as with most others, requires considerable qualification prior to clinical application. Pattern analysis can be carried out among subsections of a single test or across several tests tapping different types of ability. Many conditions of neurological impairment are in fact characterized by far greater impairment in some abilities than in others. Disorders such as Huntington's chorea and Parkinson's disease have been shown to produce significant motor deficit while IQs may appear quite average (Boll, Heaton, & Reitan, 1974; Reitan & Boll, 1971). Closed head injuries frequently produce little motor impairment yet cause significant decrease in complex mental processes (Smith, 1975). However, factors other than the differential efficiency of various areas of the brain can produce unusual patterns of performance. By itself, this inferential method is no more sufficient than any other and is, instead, designed to be interpreted in the context of careful ability assessment and concurrent use of several other inferential approaches.

2.3. Specific Behavioral Deficits

Specific or pathognomonic signs can provide valid indication of impairment of brain functions. Certain behaviors, while not present in all persons with brain damage, are almost incompatible with abnormality. These behavioral signs are conceptually similar to the type of signs of central nervous system disorder examined for during the physical neurological examination. Certain abnormal responses are not scored but are simply recorded as present or absent as indications of evidence of dysfunction. Examples of such signs include language disorders such as the inability to name simple objects or form written letters. Inability to copy or draw geometric designs or to recognize such shapes by touch is included in this category. While most data obtained from neuropsychological examination are objective and subject to quantified scoring, this is not the case for pathognomonic sign data. These behaviors are observed as present or absent and are, therefore, somewhat more dependent on subjective or clinical judgment. Because there is no range of normality but only presence or absence, and because the presence of a sign implies impairment, a conservative stance requiring that the sign be obvious must be adopted to avoid false positives. This is done with the recognition that the number of false negatives will be elevated and require separation in other ways. Few formal studies have specifically included this method of inference in addition to consideration of level of performance. Boll and Reitan (1972c) compared 35 brain-damaged children with 35 normally functioning children without evidence of nervous system impairment. Among the signs identified was failure to complete any of the three motor tasks. Of the nine children who demonstrated this sign, 100% were brain damaged. While no false positives were noted, 27 brain-damaged children were not identified by this approach. This method, like all others, was not designed to stand alone.

2.4. Comparative Performance of the Two Sides of the Body

The fourth method of inference involves comparison of the efficiency of the two sides of the body. Measures of simple and complex motor performance, tests of sensory sensitivity, including tactile, auditory, and visual modalities, and measures of tactile perception are included. We know that, in global terms, the right side of the body is controlled by the left or contralateral cerebral hemisphere. The left side of the body is controlled by the right cerebral hemisphere. Damage restricted to one cerebral hemisphere could alter motor or sensory performance on one side of the body while the other side remained unaffected. An advantage of this method is its use of the patient as his own control. While depression, anxiety, or laziness can lower overall motor speed, it is unlikely that such would have a strictly unilateral effect. Patients who may be motivated to appear impaired due to their involvement in litigation or claims for compensation rarely have enough knowledge to know the type of pattern required to bring their motor and sensory performances in line with other data.

This method of inference is particularly helpful in the examination of children. In addition to all of the previously mentioned qualifiers as to meaning of level, pattern, and sign, children add another to the list. Unlike adults, who come to the examination with a reasonably well-established baseline of characteristic functioning, children are operating with a constantly changing baseline. Normal developmental progress allows for wide variation in level, changes in level each year, uneven rate of development across areas, and the presence of deficits today that are gone tomorrow. The one reasonably constant factor in all of this is the relationship of the child to himself with respect to functions of the right and left sides of the body. The previously mentioned study by Boll and Reitan (1972c) also included comparison of right-left differences. A significantly more deviant relationship between the two sides of the body was noted in the brain-damaged than in the non-brain-damaged children.

Above all, it must be remembered that nothing is either simple or absolute or sufficient by itself. Some patients with lateralized cerebral lesions fail to show lateralized motor or sensory deficits. Some patients classified as having generalized impairment nevertheless do show significant right-left differences. These four methods of inference and a battery of tests designed to enhance their complementary use expand in both quality and quantity the information one can obtain from a fixed number of examinations and procedures.

Two additional methods of inference can be mentioned. These do not influence the types of tests used as much as they influence the types of uses of the tests. The fifth method is pre- and post-brain-damage comparison. Few examples of adequate use of this approach exist. A series of studies of patients who were examined on the Army General Classification Test prior to injury and on this and other tests following their injury have been reported by Teuber and his associates (Teuber, 1962). The very limited nature of the AGCT represents a recognized restriction on the use of this inferential method. The obvious practical difficulties of carrying out a truly adequate prospective study suggest that this method will always play a small role.

The sixth method of inference relies on examinations over time of patients who have already sustained brain damage. In contrast to pre- and post-damage examination, this procedure is commonly employed and has been exceptionally valuable both as a clinical and as an investigational procedure. Perhaps the most frequent instance of repeat examination occurs following head injury. Total recovery, and particularly recovery of higher-level cognitive functions, occurs gradually. During much of that recovery time, the patient is physically healthy. He may need guidance as to rehabilitational efforts. Even more likely, he and his family will require aid in understanding the significance of these subtle cognitive deficits and their likely behavioral consequences. Litigation efforts often include evaluation of the psychological losses sustained. Repeat evaluation can contribute to predictions of degree of permanent loss and disability. Significant recovery as seen on second examination serves to document that the first examination did indeed reflect reduction in function and not merely premorbidly low ability levels.

Quality of survival is an issue receiving greater attention each year. As medical-neurological and neurosurgical procedures advance and change, there is an increased need to evaluate the implications of such procedures for the quality of the life that has been saved. Burkland and Smith (1975) have shown that follow-up can demonstrate improvement during the third postoperative year in deficits which had, to that time, appeared quite static and fixed. Meier and his colleagues (Meier & Resch, 1967; Meier, 1974) have demonstrated the usefulness of a battery of psychological measures in monitoring and even predicting rate and degree of recovery following cerebrovascular accident. They report that the effect of cerebrovascular lesions on psychological test performances serves as a better predictor of eventual outcome (including mortality) than does the presence of aphasia, hemiplegia, or sensory loss. Perhaps this is because the neuropsychological battery is inclusive in assessing brain-related behaviors and does not focus selectively on apparent deficits which may represent only one of many variables contributing to the outcome.

3. Neuroanatomical Organization and Causes of Impairment

A brief review of neuroanatomy followed by a discussion of the major neuropathological types of impairment will precede discussion of use of specific tests and batteries in the understanding of the brain and its disorders. Clinical attempts to understand the relationship between impairment of brain functions and human behavior are far from a recent activity. Nevertheless, systematic advancement of knowledge about specific relationships based on scientific method of investigation is far more recent. As recently as 1835, Gall was suggesting that topographical irregularities in the skull could be used to assess "underlying" human faculties. The identification of the relationship of the left cerebral hemisphere damage to the occurrence of language impairment by Broca in 1861 and the identification of the precentral motor area by Fritsch and Hitzig in 1870 indicates our state of knowledge barely one century ago. Since then, an enormous burgeoning of neuroscience research has produced spectacular advances (Pines, 1977). Despite the wide availability of such knowledge and its increasing presence in the popular and scientific press, its inclusion as part of the formal training of clinical practitioners of behavioral science has lagged far behind (Matthews, 1976). The "man on the street" is well aware that the brain plays an all-pervasive role in day-to-day life. Damage to the brain is viewed as endangering one's memory, intelligence, personality, and emotional stability. Yet many attempts to utilize formal psychological measurement devices to determine the presence or assess the effect of brain damage on behavior reflect a far more limited conceptualization of its role. Behavioral analysis of the most common practice in this area suggests that many behavioral clinicians feel brain damage can be expected to result in a deficiency in one's ability to produce quasigeometric designs. Furthermore, it would appear that this deficit is felt to provide an adequate representation of the behavioral effects of brain damage. The hopeless inadequacy of any single behavior as a reflection of brain-behavior relationships will be a major theme of this chapter.

3.1. Description of the Brain

The human brain is encased in a bony skull, floats in liquid, and is girdled by several elastic and inelastic membranes. Its consistency is gelatinous. The human brain-to-body weight ratio is approximately 1:50. The brain is made up of 10 billion neurons and 100 billion glial cells. There are two cerebral hemispheres (left and right) of equal size and almost identical appearance. These centers of highest human behavior overlie control centers for all bodily functions. Cerebrospinal fluid circulates around the brain and into cavities (ventricles) within the brain. The brain's blood supply is provided by two vertebral and two internal carotid arteries. The vertebral arteries form the basilar artery at the base of the brain. The basilar and internal carotid arteries join with communicating arteries to form the circle of Willis. From this circle of arteries rise the anterior, middle, and posterior cerebral arteries nourishing the two cerebral hemispheres.

Each cerebral hemisphere is divided into four lobes: frontal, parietal, temporal, and occipital. The entire surface of the hemispheres is characterized by multiple convolutions forming hills and valleys called gyri and sulci. The central sulcus (Rolandic fissure) separates the frontal from the parietal lobe. The area forward (anterior) of this sulcus (the back of the frontal lobe) is referred to as the motor area or motor strip. The area just behind (posterior to) the central sulcus is referred to as the somato-sensory area. The functions and locations characterizing the role of these two areas of the brain are described graphically in Figures 8 and 9 by the homunculus hanging by his knees over the lateral surface of the brain.

Cerebral organization in man is better characterized as a complex of integrations than as a set of specific and independent locations of function. Certain generalizations can be offered, with the warning that exceptions and qualifications are the

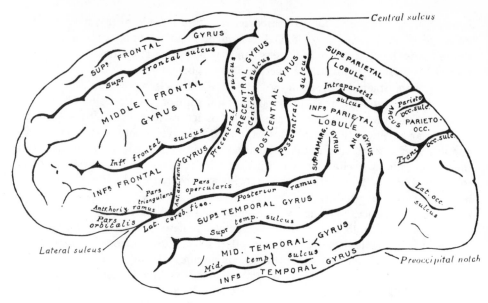

Figure 1. Lateral surface of left cerebral hemisphere, viewed from the side. Reprinted with permission of the publisher of *Gray's Anatomy*, 29th edition, Lea and Febiger, 1973.

rule. The left cerebral hemisphere is the symbolic or verbal hemisphere. Impairment here can produce receptive and expressive language deficit and right-sided motor and sensory loss. Right hemisphere damage may produce spatial-constructional deficits, nonverbal auditory perceptual impairment, and reduction in sensitivity or recognition of tactile and kinesthetic cues, in addition to left-sided sensory and motor problems. The frontal lobes, despite their status as the largest and most frequently

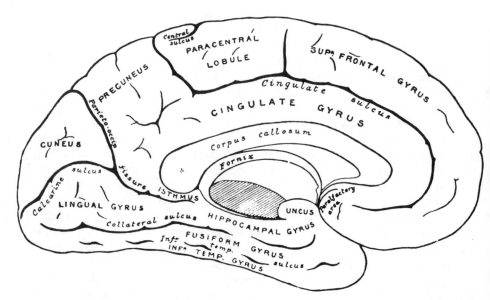

Figure 2. Medial surface of left cerebral hemisphere. Reprinted with permission of the publisher of *Gray's Anatomy*, 29th edition, Lea and Febiger, 1973.

discussed portion of the brain, remain the least well understood. Early notions about their special role in human cognition have failed of validation. Disorders involving lack of initiative and ambition and lack of planning and foresight, even with unimpaired psychometric and verbal abilities, have been reported following frontal damage. Such persons function reasonably well in structured contexts when the require-

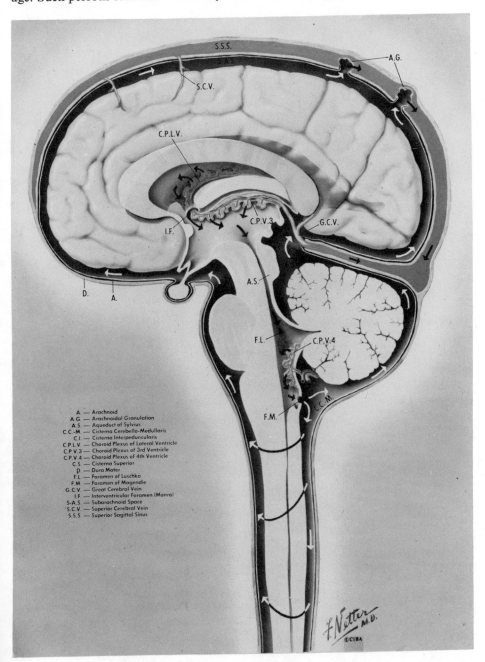

Figure 3.   Cerebrospinal fluid circulation. Reprinted with permission of the publisher from *Ciba Collection of Medical Illustrations*, Volume I: *Nervous System*, Frank H. Netter, 1962.

ments are clear, but do poorly when left to their own devices (Lezack, 1976). The left temporal lobe plays a central role in expressive and receptive language functions, including activities such as reading, writing, and arithmetic. Damage to the right temporal lobe impairs ability to recognize nonverbal sounds (music, environmental noises). When temporal lobe damage extends to the hippocampus, memory deficits

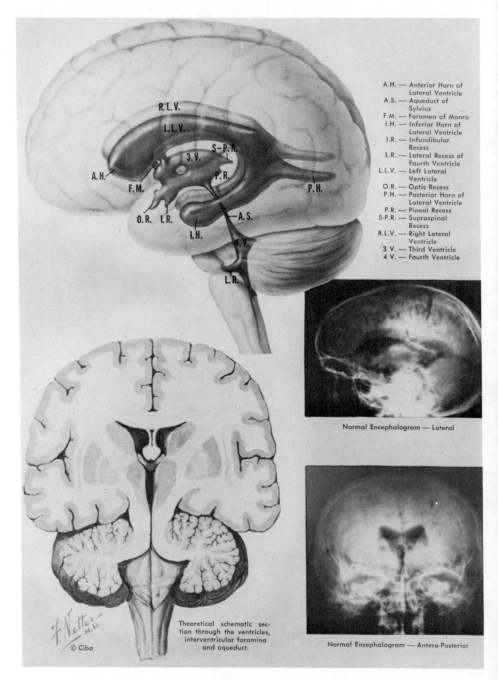

A.H. — Anterior Horn of Lateral Ventricle
A.S. — Aqueduct of Sylvius
F.M. — Foramen of Monro
I.H. — Inferior Horn of Lateral Ventricle
I.R. — Infundibular Recess
L.R. — Lateral Recess of Fourth Ventricle
L.L.V. — Left Lateral Ventricle
O.R. — Optic Recess
P.H. — Posterior Horn of Lateral Ventricle
P.R. — Pineal Recess
S-P.R. — Supraspinal Recess
R.L.V. — Right Lateral Ventricle
3 V. — Third Ventricle
4 V. — Fourth Ventricle

Theoretical schematic section through the ventricles, interventricular foramina and aqueduct.

Normal Encephalogram — Lateral

Normal Encephalogram — Antero-Posterior

Figure 4. Ventricles of the brain. Reprinted with permission of the publisher from *Ciba Collection of Medical Illustrations*, Volume I: *Nervous System*, Frank H. Netter, 1962.

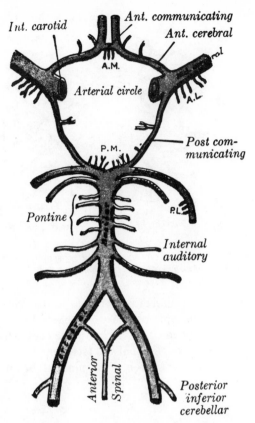

Figure 5.   Arterial circulation at the base of the brain. A.L., anterolateral; A.M., anteromedial; P.L., posterolateral; P.M., posteromedial ganglionic branches. Reprinted with permission of the publisher of *Gray's Anatomy*, 29th edition, Lea and Febiger, 1973.

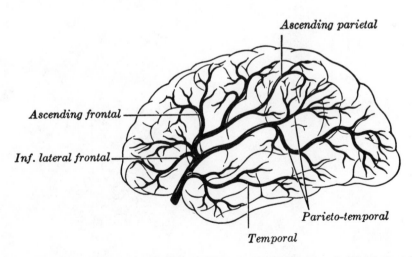

Figure 6.   Branches of the middle cerebral artery to the lateral surface of the cerebral hemisphere. Modified after Foix. Reprinted with permission of the publisher of *Gray's Anatomy*, 29th edition, Lea and Febiger, 1973.

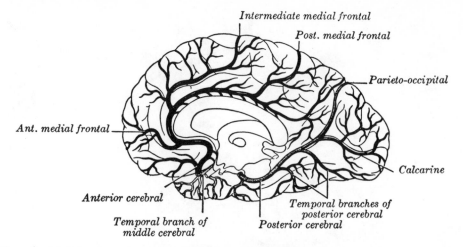

Figure 7. Medial surface of cerebral hemisphere, showing areas supplied by cerebral arteries. Reprinted with permission of the publisher of *Gray's Anatomy*, 29th edition, Lea and Febiger, 1973.

affecting learning and consolidation of verbal or nonverbal material occur. The parietal lobes play a special role in somatosensory awareness. Damage in these areas produces deficits in utilization of tactile and kinesthetic cues. Misrecognition of body parts and shapes presented through visual and tactile modalities is often noted. Deficits in body awareness and recognition predominate following right parietal lobe

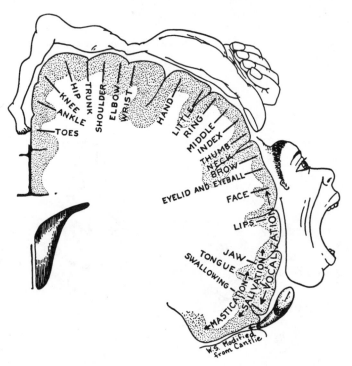

Figure 8. Motor homunculus illustrating motor representation in area 4 (anterior central gyrus). After Penfield and Rasmussen, *Cerebral Cortex of Man*, Macmillan. Reprinted with permission of the publisher of *Gray's Anatomy*, 29th edition, Lea and Febiger, 1973.

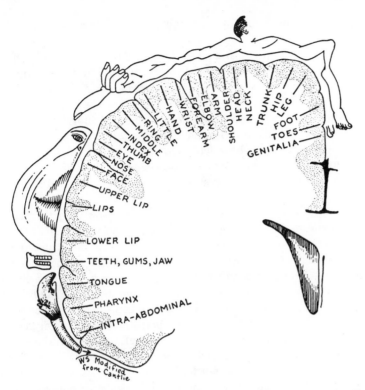

Figure 9. Sensory homunculus showing representation in the sensory cortex. After Penfield and Rasmussen, *Cerebral Cortex of Man*, Macmillan. Reprinted with permission of the publisher of *Gray's Anatomy*, 29th edition, Lea and Febiger, 1973.

lesions, as do visual spatial constructive deficits. Misrecognition of familiar faces (prosopagnosia) and apraxias or disorders of voluntary movement for such familiar actions as dressing are also seen following right parietal lobe damage. Right-left disorientation arises from left hemisphere deficit. The occipital lobes are primarily concerned with mediation of vision, including some aspects of visual memory. Even this partial and cautious recounting of location-related behavioral disorders must be qualified by the knowledge that brain lesions are produced by Mother Nature and not by experimenters' scalpels. The damage occurs in a total organism in which variables such as age, general health, lesion size, growth rate, pathological type, progressive or static character, and duration must be considered. A brief description of the more frequently occuring causes of brain impairment or damage will make more clear the importance of appreciating this complexity.

3.2. Types of Brain Damage

3.2.1. Head Injury

Most head injuries result from vehicular or work-related accidents. In an accident, brain tissue can be injured by compression, tension, and/or shearing. Any or all of these may occur simultaneously or in succession. The most common terms used to describe the physical effects of head injury are "concussion," "contusion," and "laceration."

Concussion is a widespread and immediate paralysis of brain functions following a blow to the head. This is typically brief, reversible, and not necessarily associated with visible changes in brain substance. The patient may be dazed or unconscious for a few seconds. Higher-level mental functions may be impaired while at the same time the patient seems, both to himself and to others, perfectly normal. It is not unusual for a patient to go about his routine quite normally for several hours and then afterward have no recollection of these activities. This is called posttraumatic amnesia. The loss of memory for events occurring before the accident is called retrograde amnesia. If a patient is unable to recall events for a considerable period of time after the accident, this is referred to as anterograde amnesia.

Cerebral contusion is a focal or diffuse brain disruption characterized by edema, capillary hemorrhage, and disintegration of cortical nerve cells. Headache is common and often made worse by strenuous activity, i.e., stooping, sneezing, and even emotional excitement. Motor instability and brief vertigo frequently occur, as do signs of disruption in higher cognitive processes often clinically described as memory and concentration problems. The term "cerebral laceration" indicates that the contusion was severe enough to cause visible change in the substance of the brain.

The pattern of neuropsychological test performance following head injury is characterized by considerable intra- as well as interindividual variation. A patient may show mild motor deficit on the right hand in one task and on the left in another. Closed head injuries may, but tend not to, produce focal behavioral or neurological deficits. Verbal-Performance splits on the Wechsler Scale are not characteristic, nor are significant sensory or tactile perceptual losses. Even very serious head injuries frequently show amazingly rapid and complete recovery over a 6- to 12-month period. The most common area of difficulty is that least obvious to routine clinical inspection. Higher-level problem solving, concept formation, new learning, and mental flexibility tend to be the most impaired and the slowest to recover. Such deficits may be present in persons whose appearance, conversation, and even IQ scores suggest good abilities, and it is this type of mental ability which seems to recover most slowly. This discrepancy between subtle and obvious deficits may result in a person's returning to a high-demand position which he temporarily cannot handle. The consequences of such too-rapid return to competition far outweigh the disadvantages of delaying that return. The role of the neuropsychological evaluation following head injury is to provide understanding of the presence and type of psychological deficit. This is the first step toward assuring a proper rate of return to normal preinjury activities.

Head injury without complications is a disorder for which recovery is the natural course. Psychological examinations are frequently requested to contribute to the determination of deficit and aid with prognosis. The relationship between neuropsychological examination and other prognostic indicators underwent careful study by Kløve and Cleeland (1972). Psychological measurements have been shown to be more effective than duration of unconsciousness in predicting recovery following head injury (Reynell, 1944). In fact, the importance of length of unconsciousness as an indicant of quality of recovery continues to be debated. Early investigators felt that great differences in duration of unconsciousness signified little of prognostic value (Dencker, 1958; Ruesch, 1944). Others found both duration of unconsciousness and length of posttraumatic amnesia related to mental changes. This applied to closed head injuries. Penetrating head injuries, which may cause little or even no period of unconsciousness but result in significant brain damage, also often result in significant psychological sequellae (Smith, 1961). Varying degrees of unconsciousness (1 hr, 3–24 hr, 3–5 days, or 2–3 weeks) were not found to produce behavioral differences on tests of motor functioning, language or perceptual functions, or complex problem-solving skills. For patients unconscious 3–4 weeks, mental functions were found to be impaired. Moreover, this impairment was present when testing occurred 7–18 months after injury (Kløve & Cleeland, 1972). Persistence of abnormality on the physical neurological exam following head injury has also been reported to predict poor psychological recovery (Tooth, 1947). The physical neurological exam is only slightly related to cognitive functions in mixed neurology patients (Kløve, 1963). Patients with persisting abnormalities on the physical exam after head injury, however, were consistently poorer on all types of ability measures than were those with normal physical exams (Kløve and Cleeland 1972). These differences reflected a weak relationship, achieving statistical significance in only four of 15 instances. In this same study, patients with persisting abnormality on EEG recordings were also more impaired on behavioral examination than those with normal EEGs. A subdural hematoma which must be surgically evacuated is a post-head-injury complication which is associated with less satisfying behavioral recovery. A skull fracture sounds like, and can indeed be, the signal of a very serious injury. In the Kløve and Cleeland study, however, when skull fracture was considered as the independent variable, its occurrence did not suggest that the patient was likely to suffer a greater amount of psychological deficit. As an additional comparison, patients with a combination of persisting abnormalities on EEG and physical neurological exam were separated into groups with and without skull fracture. Patients in this comparison who had sustained a skull fracture actually demonstrated less neuropsychological impairment than those who had not. These results are consistent with the thesis that the fracture itself dissipates some of the force that might otherwise have been absorbed by the brain. Differences in direction of force and movement of the head in fracturing vs. nonfracturing injuries may also contribute to these findings.

3.2.2. Intracranial Neoplasm

The symptoms of intracranial tumor fall into two categories. Focal symptoms vary with each tumor and depend on the area of brain affected. General symptoms due to increase intracranial pressure include headache, papilledema, and vomiting. Headache is often throbbing and bursting. It typically occurs on awakening and may last a brief period and then disappear. Papilledema is edema of the optic disk. Vomiting occurs at night or early in the morning, often with a headache.

Glioma. Glioma constitutes 40–50% of all brain tumors and originates from the supporting structures of the brain. The most frequent type of gliomas are (1) astrocytomas, which compose 40% of the gliomas and are relatively slowly growing; (2) glioblastoma multiformae, which make up 35–40% of all gliomas and are extremely malignant, usually occurring between ages 40 and 55; and (3) medulloblastomas, which occur most frequently in the cerebellum of children, arising from the roof of the fourth ventrical, and are relatively rapidly growing.

Meningioma. Meningiomas compose 25% of intracranial tumors. They are usually extracerebral, because they do not infiltrate brain tissue.

Metastatic Tumors. Metastatic tumors are secondary to primary tumors elsewhere, most commonly in the lung, breast, stomach, and kidney, and make up 5% of intracranial neoplasms. These tumors vary in size, location, and number and can involve both cerebral hemispheres simultaneously.

Effects of Intracranial Tumors. Tumors produce behavioral effects in three ways. They destroy tissue at their site, producing focal effects. Their size causes distortion of the rest of the brain, producing distance effects of a generalized nature. Tumors also invade the corpus callosum, which can produce its own mental effects (Geschwind, 1963) or serve as a path to direct invasion of the opposite hemisphere. The behavioral expression of tumors depends on rapidity of growth, on location, and on whether they are intracerebral or extracerebral. Primary intracerebral tumors produce focal signs specific to the hemisphere involved, such as Verbal-Performance splits, mild to moderate motor impairment, and tactile perceptual impairment. These deficits may indeed be quite focal and the uninvolved side of the brain may appear reasonably unimpaired. However, nonlateralized higher-level cognitive functions as reflected by measures of memory, learning, attention, and mental flexibility, and tasks requiring hypothesis testing, planning, and judgment, and those requiring solution of unfamiliar problems often indicate significant impairment even when IQ scores are at or above the average range. Extracerebral tumors may also produce relatively focal and lateralized deficits, but Verbal-Performance discrepancy is less common.

Supratentorial lesions involving the cerebral hemispheres on an intracerebral or extracerebral basis are generally found to be accompanied by some form of mental change. Subtentorial lesions are far less well understood behaviorally. The general clinical impression is of relatively mild, later-occurring cognitive problems, often combined with signs of cerebellar or brain stem impairment. These types of impairment include disorders of movement such as ataxia, difficulty with rapidity of alternating movements (dysdiadochokinesis), stagger, and at times jerky and even explosive speech patterns. Norton and Matthews (1972) discovered that patients with subtentorial lesions (35% of whom had subtentorial tumors) were more impaired on simple and complex motor performances than were patients with lesions involving the cerebral hemispheres. However, they showed essentially average IQs and only mildly impaired memory and concentrating skills. On cognitive tasks, however, the patients with supratentorial damage were consistently more impaired than those with subtentorial damage.

3.2.3. Cerebrovascular Disorder

Occlusion of vessels supplying blood to the brain can be partial or complete, gradual or sudden. The two common causes of occlusion are thrombus and embolus. A thrombus is a plug in a blood vessel formed at the site of the occlusion. Arteriosclerosis is the most common cause of cerebral thrombus, although many other diseases and disorders can produce this result. "Cerebral embolism" is a term used to describe the occlusion of a cerebral vessel due to the movement of fat, air, tumor, bacteria, or clotted blood, to a point where its size prohibits further passage. The result of an occlusion is cerebral infarction or softening of brain tissue. The most frequent area for vascular infarct is the distribution of the middle cerebral artery. Cerebral vascular lesions are the most frequent cause of general and focal brain impairment.

Warning symptoms prior to a cerebrovascular accident are not necessary and, if they occur, may seem quite ordinary. Among the most common are headache, dizziness, and transitory behavioral symptoms such as aphasia, confusion, or motor and sensory dysfunction. These are due to ischemia, which is a reduction in the blood flow due to constriction or some degree of obstruction of the vessel. Behavioral effects of a cerebrovascular accident depend on the general condition of the vasculature and the area of brain to which the vessel supplies blood. Disruption of the blood flow to the anterior cerebral artery may produce contralateral lower limb paralysis, language disorder, and cognitive impairment of a generalized nature. Middle cerebral artery occlusion can affect the motor and sensory areas, producing contralateral generalized impairment, aphasia, or visual constructive deficits and generalized cognitive defect. A posterior artery occlusion may produce significant motor impairment and sensory disruption ranging from loss of sensation to significant pain. The middle cerebral artery and its branches are the most commonly affected of the three cerebral arteries.

A condition in the vascular system not produced by clogging of vessels is that of intracranial aneurysm. Intracranial aneurysms are dilatations in the blood vessel wall, often found at points of bifurcation such as the circle of Willis. Aneurysms are usually considered to be due to congenital weakness of the vessel. These bulges may vary in size from a pea to a peach. Aneurysms may be asymptomatic throughout life and are found in 2% of autopsied adult cases. While aneurysms can occur anywhere along the vessel path, the majority occur near the basilar surface of the skull, with the internal carotid and middle cerebral arteries being involved in 50% of the cases (Merritt, 1967). Rupture, often associated with physical exertion, is accompanied by headache, mental impairment, and motor, sensory, and language deficit. Unconsciousness occurs in about 30% of such cases and is a poor prognostic sign. Among those patients who survive (35% die immediately and 15% more die from a second rupture within a month), recovery is exceedingly variable. Behavioral deficits include generalized effects of significant cerebral insult and focal deficits depending on the site of the aneurysm and amount of damage to brain tissue.

Cerebral arteriosclerosis is a commonly mentioned condition implying degenerative changes in the arteries of the brain. It is associated with aging and a generalized decline in higher-level mental processes. The diagnosis of cerebral arteriosclerosis may be based on age and mental decline alone. Many elderly and demented patients, however, at autopsy have been found to possess unimpaired vasculatures. In contrast, cognitively able persons of advanced age may demonstrate significant arteriosclerotic changes. The inevitability of the connection between cerebral arteriosclerosis and mental decline has yet to be documented. The occurrence of this triad (age, dementia, and cerebrovascular disease) and their causal connections seem greatly overreported. While such a relationship certainly exists in some cases, we must also be aware that other age-connected disorders are also associated with dementia.

Many types of cerebrovascular impairment produce dramatic physical symptoms such as unconsciousness, seizure, and profound motor and sensory loss. Higher cognitive dysfunctions such as aphasia and visuoconstructive dyspraxias are also seen. Patients may show excellent conversational ability and may perform in an apparently normal (average) manner on routine tests of psychometric intelligence. These same patients, however, may show signs of loss of judgment, memory, abstractions, and mental efficiency and learning ability, all of which are poorly examined in traditional IQ tests and mental status exams (Meier, 1970; Benton, 1970; Smith, 1975).

THOMAS J. BOLL

3.2.4. Degenerative and Demyelinating Disease

Any textbook of clinical neurology provides a long list of disorders under the headings of degenerative and demyelinating disease or similar ones. Of these, the three most commonly discussed are Parkinson's disease, Huntington's chorea, and multiple sclerosis.

Parkinson's Disease. Parkinson's disease produces lesions involving the basal ganglia and cerebral cortex. Behavioral symptoms may occur following (sometimes many years later) encephalitis, manganese or other metallic poisoning, or carbon monoxide intoxication, or they may occur in association with cerebral arteriosclerosis. However, the most common form is idiopathic, with typical onset between ages 40 and 60. Motor signs such as stooped posture, muscular rigidity, shuffling, small-stepped gait, reduction in associated movements (e.g., reduced arm swing when walking), masklike facies, and tremor are the most visible manifestations. Early mention has been made of dementia associated with Parkinson's disease (Ball, 1882, cited by Mjones, 1949; Critchley, 1929). Clinical reports which either did not use controls or did not match subjects for education suggested that patients with Parkinson's disease showed normal cognitive performance. A study employing a control group matched for age and education, however, confirmed the presence of significant cognitive as well as motor deficit in patients with Parkinson's disease (Reitan & Boll, 1971). Nevertheless, these seriously impaired patients did obtain essentially average IQ scores. This study provides a bridge for understanding what might be seen as contradictory findings. Reitan and Boll (1971) found that Parkinson's patients experienced greatest relative deficit on tasks with a heavy motor requirement. They also found, however, serious problems in the Parkinson group on tasks of memory, attention, learning, and abstraction. Nevertheless, the Parkinson's group obtained an average Wechsler Scale FSIQ of 105.76. However, matched non-Parkinson controls were more able not only on motor and complex cognitive tasks but also on IQ. These subjects equated for age and education (average of 1 year of college) obtained FSIQs of 122.28. This is a demonstration of the difference between normal and average. It also points out the limitation of level of performance when used as a solitary method of inference. Any single test or inferential method can suggest normality when additional data may reveal serious decline from a previously more adequate level. The fact that these patients appear average yet often act intellectually disabled becomes understandable. Their need for increased clarity and redundancy in a rehabilitation program and the futility of an approach based on motivational techniques become apparent only when strengths and weaknesses across a range of human performances are available.

Huntington's Chorea. Huntington's disease (chorea) is a hereditary disease which, like Parkinson's disease, involves both the basal ganglia and the cerebral cortex. Onset is typically between ages 30 and 50, although cases with onset in very early childhood have been reported. The two predominant features of this disease are the disorders of movement and mental decline. Movements of the upper and lower extremities are abrupt and jerky, and seem restless and jittery. Such difficulties are increased by emotional tension or stress, which is the case with other neurological disorders as well. Despite general agreement concerning the presence of cognitive decline, the first study to provide controlled and comprehensive documentation of the relative degree of motor and cognitive deficits was reported by Boll et al. in 1974. These investigators found that as with Parkinson's disease, motor deficits were not only the most visible but also the problem of relatively greatest magnitude. Here too, however, cognitive disability was rated as serious in areas of new learning, concept formation, auditory verbal and nonverbal perception, attention, concentration, and general memory functions. The only area which at first blush appeared relatively unimpaired was psychometric intelligence (FSIQ 92.81). Control subjects matched for age and education (high school level) attained FSIQs of 118.5 ($p < .001$).

Emotional disruption has been associated with Huntington's chorea (Merritt, 1967). The special relationship, if any, between this disease and degree or type of psychopathology was identified almost exclusively from uncontrolled and subjective clinical impressions. Boll et al. (1974) controlled the degree of cognitive impairment due to brain damage and employed objective and empirical techniques to identify special types or degrees of such emotional disturbance. They found that "personality changes noted in Huntington's chorea are probably little different from those seen in patients experiencing a similar decline in adaptive abilities due to other types of cerebral damage or disease." In fact, this study went on to point out that responses which would be highly unusual in a physically healthy group may reflect little more than a reaction to the stress of possessing a physical disrupting disease with a very poor prognosis.

Multiple Sclerosis.   Multiple sclerosis is a disorder of unknown etiology characterized by multiple areas of demyelination in the central nervous system. This disorder occurs most commonly in colder climates and is rare in the tropics. Race and socioeconomic status appear unrelated to incidence. Sex ratios have been reported to favor both males and females depending on the study cited. Two-thirds of initial symptom identification occurs between ages 18 and 40. Onset frequently follows flu, trauma, or vaccination, or occurs during pregnancy. Nevertheless, the role of these supposed precipitants is poorly established. While some neurologists consider pregnancy contraindicated after diagnosis is made, others report remission of symptoms during pregnancy. Reports on the long-range relationship between childbearing and disease course are equally inconsistent. This may be in part due to the considerable inconsistency within and between people with respect to the course of the disease itself. The course can vary from fairly steady deterioration to periods of 20 years of total lack of symptoms following an initial symptomatic episode. Symptoms of motor weakness in one or more limbs, visual defects such as double vision, blindness in one eye or field defect, diminished sensation, or tremor are often the first to be noted, with onset over several hours or 1 or 2 days. Because lesions may occur at any place in the nervous system, symptoms may be equally diverse. Remissions following subsequent exacerbations are rarely as complete on each subsequent occasion.

Wide variation exists among estimates of mental impairment associated with this disorder. These range from 2% (Cottrell and Wilson, 1926) to 72% (Ombredane, 1929). More recent controlled and comprehensive investigations have found that multiple sclerosis patients do not differ in cognitive or affective terms from other brain-damaged patients with equal IQs (Matthews, Cleeland, & Hopper, 1970). Multiple sclerosis patients experience particular deficit in motor functions. Mixed brain-damaged and multiple sclerosis groups with average IQs fell just within the impaired range on the Halstead Neuropsychological Test Battery. This study found no support for the particular significance of depression in multiple sclerosis patients as measured by the Minnesota Multiphasic Personality Inventory. Again, many items contributing to categorization of these patients as "abnormal" described the actual physical symptoms of multiple sclerosis. Comparison with carefully matched non-brain-damaged controls also provides evidence for a much less severe form of mental decline in multiple sclerosis than was noted for Parkinson's disease or Huntington's chorea. In a study by Reitan, Reed, and Dyken (1971), patients with multiple sclerosis performed significantly more poorly not only on motor tests but also on measures of complex cognitive functioning than did matched controls. This was also true for psychometric IQ. However, despite their impairment relative to normal controls, the degree of deficit seen in multiple sclerosis patients tended to fall consistently in the mild range. Patients with Huntington's chorea and Parkinson's disease were routinely found to be in the range of moderate or severe impairment. The inconsistent early literature is understandable because it was based on a selective and limited rather than a comprehensive type of assessment. Good performance in a single area is not a guarantee of cognitive integrity. Isolated deficit does not necessarily signal a more encompassing difficulty. The inconsistency that is represented neuropathologically and clinically in multiple sclerosis also characterizes the behavioral concomitants of this disorder.

3.2.5. Intoxications

Alcohol. Alcoholism is the single most frequent form of abuse of toxins and has been subject to many behavioral studies. Recent reviews of the behavioral consequences are available, so only a summary of the most consistent findings will be presented here (Kleinknecht & Goldstein, 1972; Butters & Cermak, 1976; Parsons, 1977). One of the results of excessive long-term alcohol ingestion is the impairment of certain psychological abilities. This is due to general neurological deficit among chronic alcoholics and additional specific nutritionally related neurological deficits in Korsakoff's syndrome patients. Several studies have demonstrated the presence of cortical atrophy, usually on a bilateral basis, in alcoholic patients (Ferrer, 1970; Brewer & Perrett, 1971). These investigators utilized pneumoencephalographic data to document the presence of brain changes. This, of course, does not prove that alcohol caused the brain damage. Alcoholics suffer increased incidence of other brain-impairing conditions such as brain trauma and liver disorder, so the connection remains correlational and thus inferential. Patients with Korsakoff's syndrome have been found to suffer from a chronic thiamine deficiency. This has been postulated to produce atrophy of the dorsal medial nucleus of the thalamus and mammillary bodies (Victor, Adams, & Collins, 1971). The behavioral result is extreme deficit in new learning and generalized significant decline in current cognitive processing. Such patients may not show deficient motor skill and may earn average IQ levels (Butters, Cermak, Montgomery, & Adinolfi, 1977).

Chronic alcoholic patients, even with reasonable dietary habits, have been shown to experience mental deficits. Here too, it is not uncommon to find average IQ levels coexisting with these deficits. Deficits particularly in abstraction, spatial and temporal organization, and concentration are common (Tarter, 1975). Memory problems, so predominant in Korsakoff's syndrome patients, are not a regular or necessary feature of chronic alcoholism. Tarter and Jones (1971) demonstrated reversibility of some of these deficits, with amount of recovery depending on length of sobriety. Diagnostically, despite multiple attempts, no pattern of psychological test performance specific and exclusive to alcoholism has been identified. Wechsler (1958) and Rapaport, Gill, and Schafer (1945) attempted to develop such profiles. These profiles relied heavily on the Wechsler Scales of Intelligence. A careful review by Kleinknecht and Goldstein (1972) of studies utilizing the Wechsler Scales demonstrated that no single subtest or pattern of subtests was found consistently to be impaired, and only the Information scale was uniformly found to be unimpaired. Likewise, neither the Bender-Gestalt Test nor the Rorschach was found helpful in identifying behavioral traits pathognomonic of alcoholism (Kaldegg, 1956).

Psychoactive Drugs. Drugs from marijuana to LSD have been reported to cause brain damage and grave permanent psychological deficits (Kolansky & Moore, 1972; Accord & Barker, 1973; McGlothlin, Arnold, & Freedman, 1969). Other investigators have reported little harmful behavioral effects secondary to long use of marijuana (Culver & King, 1974), heroin (Fields & Fullerton, 1975), and LSD (Wright & Hogan, 1972). A series of careful longitudinal studies by Igor Grant and his colleagues (Grant & Judd, 1976) have attempted to assess the effect of multiple, mixed, and prolonged drug use on a broad range of simple and complex human abilities. Initial examination of persons routinely using several drugs on a daily basis revealed that 45% showed neuropsychological impairment and 43% demonstrated abnormalities on electroencephalographic examination. Behavioral deficits were in areas of abstraction and current mental problem solving, while general IQ and verbal skills remained intact. There appeared to be greatest deficit in persons who included alcohol, sedatives, or four or more drugs simultaneously in their routine of drug usage. The pattern found was not dissimilar to the nonspecific, generalized higher mental decline without serious sensory, motor, or verbal deficit reported for chronic alcoholism. While a definite link between alcoholic deficit and neurological impairment exists, data beyond corresponding EEG abnormalities are necessary before a similar link between chronic polydrug abuse and brain dysfunction can be said to be proven.

Epilepsy. "Epilepsy is paroxysmal and transitory disturbance of the functions of the brain which develops suddenly, ceases spontaneously and exhibits a conspicuous tendency to recurrence" (Brain, 1969, p. 919). Epilepsy is in fact not a disease but a symptom. Many types of neurological disorder may be accompanied by a seizure. For at least half of the patients with epilepsy, however, no etiology can be determined. Many patients with epilepsy do not have convulsions. The causes of epilepsy, the types of brain impairment involved, and the behavioral manifestations of this disorder are as diverse as the nervous system itself. Even the terminology for describing and the criteria for diagnosis of epilepsy are in flux. The recent International Classification of Epilepsy system lists four types of epilepsy: partial, generalized, unilateral, and unclassified. The two most familiar types of epilepsy (grand mal and petit mal) are listed under generalized seizures and are now referred to as "tonic-clonic" and "absence," respectively.

Epilepsy may begin at any age, with or without independent neurological disorder or identifiable precipitating factor. It may pass off with time or remain for life. The type of seizure may change over time within an individual, and one person may manifest more than one seizure type simultaneously. While no precipitant is necessary, neurological damage due to disease or trauma may produce seizures. High fever or extended hyperthermia, metabolic disturbance, and, of course, direct electrical current to the brain can produce seizures. Emotional stress may produce increased seizure frequency in patients with lowered seizure thresholds. While some persons do fake the occurrence of seizures (including some patients with a real seizure disorder), a real seizure produced by emotional distress in no way diminishes the neurological significance of the event. Both the emotional precipitant and the seizure disorder usually require treatment. Except in the case of faking, a question as to whether a seizure is psychogenic or real should be answered "yes." The role of both factors must be understood and not "ruled out."

It it not surprising that no specific pattern or type of psychological deficit is diagnostic of epilepsy. In fact, like the term "brain damage" or "organicity," the term "epilepsy" provides no psychological information that would be found to characterize all persons so diagnosed. In an excellent review, Kløve and Matthews (1974) addressed several major variables influencing the behavioral status of adult epileptic patients. They found that within a brain-damaged population, the addition of epilepsy is not associated with a significant increment in behavioral deficit. Adults with epilepsy, regardless of etiology, tend to perform in a manner somewhat inferior to that of matched non-brain-damaged controls. Nevertheless, many epileptics perform quite normally on psychological tests, and many more perform well in some areas while showing one or more circumscribed behavioral deficits.

Epileptics with known etiology tend to be more cognitively impaired than do those with idiopathic epilepsy. Type of seizure has also been studied. Patients with major motor or mixed (major motor and psychomotor) seizures perform generally more poorly than patients with psychomotor seizures alone. Within a single seizure type, Dikmen and Matthews (1977) have shown that greater frequency of seizures is associated with increased psychological deficit. Age at onset has also been shown to interact with type of seizure in ordering mental functions. Early onset of epilepsy has been consistently associated with greater mental impairment, while onset after 17 years of age is associated with lesser cognitive difficulty. Among patients with lateralized seizure disorders, behavioral deficits typically associated with the implicated area or hemisphere have been found. However, Verbal-Performance differences associated with lateralized brain damage have not typically been found among patients with chronic conditions such as long-standing seizure disorder. It is not surprising, in light of the many variables which interact to influence behavioral correlates of epilepsy, that no specific psychological sign or pattern of performance has been identified as diagnostic.

3.2.6. Schizophrenia

The inclusion of a section on schizophrenia in this chapter is not intended to characterize schizophrenia as a neurological disease or disorder. Neither, however, is it possible to rule this out as a possibility. After all, epilepsy used to belong to psychiatry, and autism is showing considerable interest in defection. Many biochemists seem to think that schizophrenia is biological and resides in the brain. Pneumoencephalographic data on adults (Haug, 1963) have indicated evidence of cortical atrophy in 61% of schizophrenic patients. Abnormal EEG findings among adult schizophrenics (Mirsky, 1969) and abnormal neurological organization among adolescent patients have also been reported (Hertzig & Birch, 1966, 1968). Mirsky (1969), in a review of studies reporting brain changes among schizophrenics, suggested that these patients possessed no special immunity to independently existing brain damage. Neurological disease, pre- or postdating onset of schizophrenia or even as a result of treatment (leukotomy), does occur with unknown frequency. Certainly, the possibility of brain impairment associated with alcoholism, trauma, infection, and poor diet resulting from deviant life-styles of schizophrenic patients make them no less likely candidates for brain impairment than nonschizophrenics. None of these data demonstrates that schizophrenia is neurological or that schizophrenics are brain damaged. They do, however, suggest that attempts at clear distinction between some form of generalized brain damage and schizophrenia may be artificial and even biologically inaccurate.

The preceding paragraph provides background for attempts to answer or at least deal with the question "Is the patient schizophrenic or brain damaged?" All questions contain at least one assumption of fact. Some assumptions are universally correct and allow a direct and accurate response. The assumption that all persons have been alive for a measurable period of time allows a sensible answer to the question "How old are you?" Other questions contain assumptions that are not or at least may not be correct. In order to answer a question, one must accept its assumptions. If one has never beaten his wife, the question "Have you stopped beating your wife?" has no sensible answer. The ability of an individual to convey meaningful information through answers is limited by the conceptualizations of the questioner. When knowledge in an area appears particularly deficient or unsatisfactory, it may be worthwhile to look not at the answers but at the questions. Szasz (1972) has referred to questions with particularly impossible assumptions as "semantic leukotomes." Such questions have the effect of frontal lobotomy, rendering the person toward whom they are directed incapable of further useful thought on that issue. The choices are to accept the question or to redefine the issue until answerable questions can be found. The formation of increasingly sophisticated and answerable questions is the manner in which all knowledge advances.

In order to address the question of schizophrenia vs. brain damage, several assumptions must be made: (1) schizophrenia is not itself a neurological disorder; (2) a schizophrenic person will not independently acquire brain damage; (3) brain-damaged persons will not become schizophrenic. No data exist to confirm any of these three assumptions. Unfortunately, many investigators have failed to recognize this difficulty, and the results of their studies have been predictably unhelpful. A number of studies have found that neuropsychological examination would not separate schizophrenic from brain-damaged patients (Watson, Thomas, Anderson, & Felling, 1968; Watson, Thomas, Felling, & Anderson, 1968, 1969). There are many areas for possible criticism of these and similar studies, including lack of adequate neurological examination for the schizophrenic patients, generalized and often poorly documented nature of the neurological defect in the brain-damaged group, failure to account for chronicity, length of hospitalization, or medication effects in either group, and the continuing difficulty in attaining agreement as to what constitutes schizophrenia itself. These problems are ably discussed by Zimet and Fishman (1970), Heaton (1976), and Goldstein and Halperin (1977). One issue not resolved in these discussions is whether the absence of separation should be viewed as a validation of the ability of neuropsychological tests to tap subtle neurological impairment among schizophrenics or as a reflection of their failure to distinguish between a brain-damaged and a non-brain-damaged but poorly socially adjusted group of patients. Klonoff, Fibiger, and Hutton (1970), in a characteristically thorough and well-designed study, also found little difference between schizophrenic and brain-damaged patients. However, they pointed out that the basis for the well-known cognitive deficits of schizophrenic patients, while subject to many theoretical speculations (Zimet & Fishman, 1970), has not been established. They postulate that degree of psychopathology and nature of neurological deficit may need specific control in future studies. It appears no longer satisfactory to treat either of these conditions as representing a homogeneous entity.

One reason for interest in this area is the clinically relevant concern that some patients may behave bizarrely on the basis of a treatable neurological disorder. Presence of brain damage may have no behavioral significance. Identification of its presence may not be helpful and could imply a problem where none exists. Identification of a medically significant neurological disorder, however, is essential, and psychological identification of such a disorder in behaviorally disturbed patients would be exceptionally valuable. On the other hand, ability to identify as not brain damaged those patients whose presenting problems suggest serious medical neurological illness would also be a contribution to clinical care fully justifying the time and effort required. Boll (1974b) attempted to separate schizophrenics from patients requiring medical-neurological treatment. He showed that patients with acute schizophrenia did not differ significantly from patients with static brain damage requiring no medical attention. However, the schizophrenic group was quite different from two groups of patients with neurological disorders (stroke and tumor) requiring active medical intervention and management. Matthews, Shaw, and Kløve (1966) attempted to separate two groups of patients presenting with medical-neurological rather than behavioral-psychiatric complaints. They found significant differences between these groups of patients both presenting with complications and symptoms suggestive of particularly serious neurological disorders. The performance of those patients eventually found to not have neurological disorder was significantly superior to that of patients with similar presenting complaints who were found to be neurologically impaired.

In an attempt to provide a clinically useful as well as empirically defensible approach to understanding patients who are schizophrenic and those with an identifiable neurological disorder, Russell (1975b) proposed the combined, sequential use of neuropsychological and personality assessment to more completely describe the behavior of these possibly different groups. He found that neuropsychological tests could separate brain-damaged and schizophrenic patients from normals. The Minnesota Multiphasic Personality Inventory could identify those patients who were schizophrenic. Thus the combination seemed to provide a more complete assessment than utilization of ability or personality measures alone. In a follow-up, Russell (1977) reviewed the traditional MMPI indicators of brain damage. These are combinations of the 2–9 and the 1–3–9 profiles. His study confirmed earlier findings by Schwartz (1969) that these profile types occurred rarely in patients with brain damage and could not be validated for such diagnostic purposes.

As long as schizophrenia remains a construct described by a poorly agreed on set of behaviors, our basic problem will remain. No field can move ahead of its criterion. The questions here await identification of the biological or other nature of schizophrenia. When we know what it is, we will have a better idea of those conditions from which it should or should not be distinguished.

With this background, it is now possible to discuss specific tests and batteries and their use in assessing conditions of brain impairment. In addition, the relationship of major areas of human ability to normal or impaired brain function will be considered.

4. General Intelligence and Generalized Brain Damage

The terms "psychometry" and "psychometrics" refer to the formal quantitative measurement of mental processes. Early formal IQ tests relied heavily on various aspects of verbal ability such as vocabulary, analogies, and verbal memory. Hebb

(1949) postulated that there were in fact two types of intellectual ability. One type referred to current ability to learn and solve problems and was labeled "Intelligence A." A second type reflected the possession of knowledge and skill previously learned and was called "Intelligence B." Hebb recognized that most intellectual measures with their emphasis on recall and manipulation of stored or verbal data relied almost entirely on Intelligence B. Hebb postulated that Intelligence A would be more vulnerable to brain damage. He further postulated (correctly, as will be seen in the section on children) that children rely far more heavily on Intelligence A for daily living, including the taking of intelligence tests. Therefore, the effect of brain damage is likely to be much different depending on whether it occurs during childhood or in adulthood. Hebb's position is consistent with the distinction between psychometric and biological intelligence developed by Halstead (1947). It also corresponds in general terms with Goldstein's (1952) position that, following brain damage, one's capacity for new learning will be diminished.

Intellectual assessment via cognitive tasks in the area of mental retardation and inability to learn was developed by Binet and Simon (1905) for application in the Paris school system. The next major step forward occurred when David Wechsler introduced his procedure for the examination of adults (Wechsler, 1939) and, 10 years later, a similar set of procedures for children (Wechsler, 1949). The Wechsler Intelligence Scales (Wechsler-Bellevue I and II), the Wechsler Adult Intelligence Scale (WAIS), and the Wechsler Intelligence Scale for Children (WISC) have been and continue to be the most commonly utilized tests for IQ (Lubin, Wallis, & Paine, 1971). The WAIS is appropriate for persons age 16 and older. It has three summary scores: Verbal IQ, Performance IQ, and Full Scale IQ. Its 11 subtests are divided into the Verbal and Performance scales. The Verbal scale includes tests of information, comprehension, digit span, similarities, arithmetic, and vocabulary. The Performance scale includes tests of picture completion, picture arrangement, block design, object assembly, and digit symbol. Matarazzo (1972), in a technically excellent, highly readable and comprehensive revision of *Wechsler's Measurement and Appraisal of Adult Intelligence*, provides the most complete and current information on the content and technical characteristics of this test. In many clinical settings, IQ tests are used to help understand the behavioral changes resulting from brain lesions. However, a range of standard intelligence tests, including the Wechsler Scales, demonstrated an insensitivity to even relatively major destruction of brain tissue (Hebb, 1949; Yates, 1954). Such major brain insults as lobotomy and even hemispherectomy were reported to be without significant intellectual sequellae (Gardner, 1932; Rowe, 1937; Bruell & Albee, 1962). Despite these apparent failures, Wechsler (1958) maintained his notion that selected patterns of tests would be differentially sensitive to brain damage or impairment as a general entity.

Reitan (1959a) compared 50 brain-damaged and 50 non-brain-damaged adults and found that the Wechsler Bellevue I was successful in separating the groups. In fact, the brain-damaged group performed significantly more poorly on the Verbal, Performance, and Full Scale IQ's and on each of the individual subtests except Digit Span. Clinical lore and Wechsler's hypotheses refer to patterns within the test rather than to the test as a total unit as specifically useful for identifying neurologically caused ability deficits. Therefore, Reitan identified various groupings claimed to have special significance with respect to diagnosis of brain damage and compared each with the Impairment Index derived from the Halstead Neuropsychological Test Battery.

Finally, he compared each of these measures with each other. Figure 10 presents the comparative ability of the Impairment Index vs. various Wechsler test groupings to separate groups of patients with and without brain damage. The Impairment Index produced a greater separation in 82% of the cases when compared against Verbal IQ, in 77% against Performance IQ, and in 71% against Full Scale IQ. The Impairment Index was more efficient in 80% of the cases when compared against Wechsler's Hold Tests and in 78% of the cases against the Don't Hold Tests. Wechsler's Deterioration Ratio, designed to be the single most sensitive indicator of cognitive defect, was less sensitive to brain damage than the Impairment Index in 94% of the cases. When

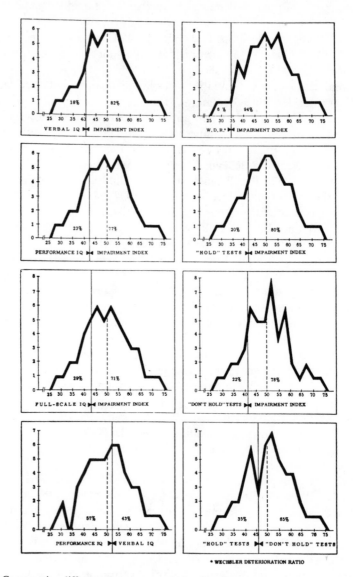

Figure 10.   Comparative difference between matched pairs with and without brain damage on various measures. Reprinted with permission of the publisher from Reitan, Ralph M. The comparative effects of brain damage on the Halstead Impairment Index and the Wechsler Bellevue Scale. *Journal of Clinical Psychology*, 1959, *15*, 281–285.

compared against the Performance IQ, the Verbal IQ produced a better separation of brain-damaged vs. non-brain-damaged groups in 43% of the cases. The Don't Hold Tests bested the Hold Tests in 65% of the cases. Superiority of the Impairment Index over the Wechsler groupings was statistically significant in each instance beyond the .001 level. Despite the general sensitivity of the Wechsler Scale to impairment from brain damage, no support was obtained for the notion that the effect of all brain damage could be characterized by a single pattern of performance on this Scale.

4.1. Lateralized Brain Impairment

Andersen (1950, 1951) was the first to report the relationship between right vs. left cerebral hemisphere damage and Verbal vs. Performance IQ levels on the Wechsler Scales. The finding that Verbal IQ will be lower than Performance IQ in patients with left hemisphere lesions and that Performance IQ will be lower than Verbal IQ in patients with right hemisphere lesions has been confirmed in numerous later studies (Reitan, 1955a; Kløve & Reitan, 1958; Satz, 1966; Satz, Richard, & Daniels, 1967; Parsons, Vega, & Burn, 1969; Zimmerman, Whitmyre, & Fields, 1970; Simpson & Vega, 1971). See Table 1 for raw scores.

A controversy has developed around what at first blush might appear to be failures to confirm this generalization. This controversy reflects the large number of variables that must be considered in understanding brain-behavior relationships. The major figure in this discussion appears to be Smith, whose excellent and wide-ranging studies have greatly aided our understanding of many of the complex issues in this field. In two studies, Smith (1965, 1966) described the results of examination of 211 patients with documented cerebral lesions. He found that only 12 of 64 nonaphasic

Table 1. Wechsler Verbal and Performance IQ Subgroups of Adult Patients with Lesions in Different Hemispheres of the Brain[a]

	Left	Right	Diffuse	Control	Investigator(s)
W–B I					
VIQ	79.7	91.1	80.7		Kløve and Reitan (1958)
PIQ	90.3	80.1	78.2		
VIQ	83.4	99.7	93.4	100.7	Kløve (1959)
PIQ	98.4	87.8	93.1	102.6	
VIQ	88.0	101.0	95.0	114.0	Doehring, Reitan, and Kløve (1961)
PIQ	97.0	84.0	93.0	117.0	
WAIS					
VIQ	94.9	107.2	90.2	100.0	Satz (1966)
PIQ	105.1	99.7	87.0	97.0	
VIQ	92.3	106.6	93.3	104.2	Satz, Richard, and Daniels (1967)
PIQ	104.9	96.1	95.3	99.3	
VIQ	90.3	98.8	92.0		Zimmerman, Whitmyre, and Fields (1970)
PIQ	91.3	93.4	81.5		
VIQ	78.8	89.1			Parsons, Vega, and Burn (1969)
PIQ	83.7	78.7			
VIQ	79.8	91.5	83.2		Simpson and Vega (1971)
PIQ	83.4	78.7	79.5		

[a] From *Wechsler's Measurement and Appraisal of Adult Intelligence* by Joseph D. Matarazzo. Copyright © 1972 by Williams and Wilkins Co. Reprinted by permission of Oxford University Press, Inc.

patients with acute left-sided lesions had lower Verbal than Performance scores. Levitt, Sindberg, Massert, and Albaum (1966) also reported that, although right-sided lesions produced lower Performance IQ, left-sided lesions did not lower Verbal IQ. Smith (1975) argued for the necessity of removal of aphasic patients from groups when assessing the sensitivity of Verbal IQ to left hemisphere damage. He did not, however, define how subtle or obvious the language deficit should be to qualify for exclusion, nor did he exclude patients with visual constructive defects from his right hemisphere group. Failure to find impairment in Performance IQ following right hemisphere lesion has also been reported (Vega & Parsons, 1969). Heilbrun (1956) found a similar failure, but his utilization of a different set of nonverbal tests makes direct comparison impossible. Nevertheless, these data, while in fact reflective of a larger truth, have often been misinterpreted because of each investigator's focus on the details of individual findings. Andersen is correct in indicating that lateralized brain lesions do produce selective Verbal or Performance IQ functions, while Smith is equally correct in indicating that this is not always the case. This seeming disagreement is basically the result of attempting a universal application of a generalization. It must be apparent that in any complex field there are myriad appropriate qualifications to each valid generalization. The issue revolves around the complexity of the relationship between the multiple parameters of impairment of brain function, of which lateralization is only one. These multiple parameters must be cast against the equally complex varieties of human ability. A Verbal-Performance difference of 10 points occurs in 30% of normals, and a split of 15 points occurs in 18% of normals (Matarazzo, 1972). It may occur in brain-damaged as well as normal persons for reasons other than brain damage. As we will see shortly, a major series of neurologically based qualifications such as acuteness of the lesion and neuropathological type are necessary in evaluating the presence or absence of a Verbal-Performance discrepancy. As Smith (1975), Matarazzo (1972), Kløve (1974), and Reitan (1974a) have correctly stressed, no single test, not even a generally valid and complex one such as the Wechsler Scales (much less any single index of performance derived from such a test), can provide sufficient information for an adequate evaluation of brain-behavior relationships.

4.2. Physical Neurological Signs and Wechsler Patterns

One method for determining the validity of a test is to determine its ability to match an independent criterion. Unequivocal evidence of brain damage is the desired criterion. However, less definite but more frequently available criteria can be investigated. Such investigation provides an opportunity for learning the relative sensitivity and interrelatedness of measurements using at least partially independent sources of data. Sensory imperception is a neurological sign which is manifested by a person's awareness of stimulation on only one side of the body when the stimulus was presented simultaneously to each side. Kløve (1959) examined a group of patients with right and a group with left sensory imperception. He also included a group demonstrating bilateral imperception and a group of patients who, while brain damaged, did not show sensory imperceptions. He found that patients with imperception on the right side of the body (suggesting left hemisphere damage) showed impairment of Verbal as compared with Performance IQ. Patients with left sensory imperception showed impairment of Performance IQ. Patients with bilateral or no sensory imperceptions did not show a discrepancy between Verbal and Performance scores.

Kløve and Reitan (1958) compared three groups of brain-damaged patients, demonstrating either aphasia, visuospatial construction deficit, or both. As Smith (1975) would predict, the patients with an aphasic disorder performed especially poorly on the items making up the Verbal IQ, without comparable deficit on visuospatial problem-solving tasks. Patients with constructional dyspraxia experienced greatest deficit on the Performance items and performed better on the Verbal section. Those patients with both perceptual and language disorders did not produce Verbal-Performance discrepancies but rather performed on each section in a manner most similar to the impaired performances shown by the other two groups. Doehring, Reitan, and Kløve (1961) examined groups of brain-damaged patients manifesting either right or left visual field defect (homonymous hemianopsia). A third group had brain damage but no visual field defect. The results were as would be predicted. The patients with the right visual field defect produced by a lesion in the left cerebral hemisphere showed lower Verbal IQ, while patients with left visual field defect showed a lower Performance IQ. The patients without visual field defect did not show a Verbal-Performance IQ discrepancy. Reed and Reitan (1963c) compared Wechsler Verbal and Performance IQ scores in groups with lateralized motor deficits resulting from brain damage to the contralateral cerebral hemispheres. They included a group of brain-damaged patients without lateralized motor problems. The patients with right motor impairment showed lower Verbal IQ and those with left motor problems showed lower Performance IQ. The group without lateralized motor problems failed to show Verbal-Performance differences.

It is quite common for a patient to be referred for neuropsychological evaluation while undergoing other examinations for suspected neurological disorder. Disorders such as intracerebral tumors and strokes are subject to definitive diagnosis through neurological and neuroradiological procedures. Neuropsychological aid for such patients is more often for baseline evaluations prior to surgery, for future monitoring of recovery, or for recommendations for a program of rehabilitation or environmental modification than it is for a documentation of aspects of the brain damage itself from a neurological viewpoint. However, patients with presenting complaints, signs, and symptoms of brain impairment but without definite evidence of brain damage are a population for whom neuropsychological diagnostic aid is most frequently sought. Matthews et al. (1966), having dealt with many such cases, identified 32 patients with well-documented evidence of brain damage. Compared with these were an equal number of patients admitted to their hospital for complaints that suggested the possibility of brain damage. These symptoms included nausea, weakness, sensory deficits, clumsiness, gait disturbance, headache, visual and auditory deficits, and episodes possibly consistent with seizures. Despite these worrisome complaints, each was determined not to have brain damage following a thorough physical and electroencephalographic examination as well as other procedures as indicated in individual instances. In all cases, psychiatric diagnoses were eventually applied to this latter group. Such patients represent a worthy test for any neuropsychological procedure. While Matthews and his colleagues at the University of Wisconsin Neuropsychology Laboratory used a complete battery of tests, only the results from the WAIS will be discussed here. The results indicated that the two groups were significantly different on IQ measures despite the careful matching of demographic data and the restriction of IQ to Full Scale scores above 80. These data suggest that a contribution to clinical care in difficult diagnoses can be made by careful psychological examination, including the WAIS. This is particularly impressive in light of the generalized as opposed to specific or focal nature of the disorders represented in each of these two groups.

4.3. Electroencephalographic Studies and Wechsler Results

Two studies demonstrate the correspondence shown between patterns of performance on the Wechsler Scales and electrical abnormalities in the brain as measured by the electroencephalogram. Kløve (1959) composed four groups of patients, each with well-documented evidence of brain damage. Group 1 consisted of 37 patients with EEG abnormalities maximized over the right cerebral hemisphere; group 2 had 42 patients with EEG abnormalities over the left cerebral hemisphere; group 3 had 45 patients with generalized EEG abnormality; group 4 had 61 patients with normal EEGs. As can be seen in Table 2, patients in group 1 were impaired on Performance IQ, while patients in group 2 were impaired on Verbal IQ. Patients with EEG abnormalities generalized over both hemispheres showed no Verbal-Performance discrepancy, nor did the patients with normal EEGs. It should be noted that this last group with proven brain damage and normal EEGs had IQs that were in the average range. Kløve's 1959 study, while carefully composing groups according to lateralized vs. generalized nature of the disorder, made no attempt to control for such variables as type of lesion or severity of the EEG abnormality. Obviously, no single study can control all relevant variables. The possibility that patients with brain damage but normal EEGs had less severe impairment than those with normal EEGs may be one factor in accounting for the average IQs. However, these IQs may in fact reflect significant decline from previous levels in these patients. This is a possibility one cannot verify when relying on level of performance alone. Therefore, to say that the Wechsler was or was not sensitive to brain damage in these patients is going beyond the data.

Any scientific effort must proceed in a sequential fashion, building on past data. It is unlikely that all the important questions will be known at the outset. Instead, they will be discovered and addressed as knowledge progresses. In a second EEG study, Kløve and White (1963) addressed the variable of severity of electroencephalographic abnormality. In this study, 179 patients with brain damage and 47 normal controls were divided into five groups. Group 1 was the normal control group; group 2 consisted of 50 brain-damaged patients with normal EEG records; group 3 had 28 brain-damaged patients whose records were classified as mildly abnormal; group 4

Table 2. Mean Values for Four Brain-Damaged Groups Who Differed with Regard to EEG Findings[a]

	EEG			
Item	Right (N = 37)	Left (N = 42)	Diffuse (N = 45)	Normal (N = 61)
Verbal IQ	99.79	88.43	93.46	100.75
Performance IQ	87.82	98.43	93.15	102.62
Full Scale IQ	93.88	92.69	92.61	101.88
Impairment Index	.65	.70	.63	.61

[a]Reprinted with permission of the publisher from Reitan, R. M., and Davison, L. (Eds.), *Clinical Neuropsychology: Current Status and Applications*, Hemisphere Publishing Corporation, 1974.

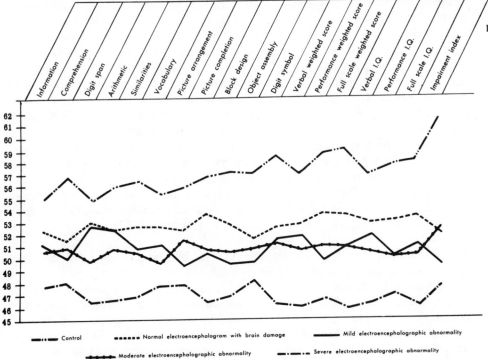

Figure 11. *T* score means, Wechsler-Bellevue and Impairment Index. Reprinted from *Neurology* © 1963 by Harcourt Brace Jovanovich, Inc.

had 42 brain-damaged patients who were classified as moderately abnormal; and group 5 contained 59 brain-damaged patients whose EEG records reflected severe abnormalities. Unfortunately, Kløve and White reported converted *T* scores instead of raw scores. The results seen in Figure 11 indicate that the normal control group obtained higher IQ scores than any of the brain-damaged groups. Groups 2 and 3 did not differ from each other, nor did groups 3 and 4, but groups 2, 3, and 4 performed better than group 5. In this study, EEG abnormalities represented the explicit organizing principle. Different EEG patterns and degrees of severity, however, typically reflect a variety of other underlying neurological factors such as type of lesion and its static vs. progressive nature. These are not experimentally manipulable independent variables because they occur in humans as the result of accidents of nature. They must be investigated as they naturally occur. The clear conclusion from this study is that degree of electroencephalographic abnormality has a rather striking ordering influence on psychological data reflecting underlying human abilities in adults.

4.4. Acute vs. Chronic Brain Damage

Two issues emerge when discussing the acuteness-chronicity dimension of brain damage. The first is whether the Wechsler Scales considered *in toto* or any set of patterns or ratios derived from its various subtest scores is effective in separating groups with acute vs. chronic brain damage. The second issue is whether the acuteness-chronicity dimension influences whether lateralized brain damage will be reflected in Verbal-Performance IQ differences. Direct evidence on the first issue was provided in a study by Fitzhugh, Fitzhugh, and Reitan (1961). These authors compared three groups of brain-damaged subjects and a control group. Group 1 was composed of patients with an acute neurological disorder. Group 2 patients were characterized as having a relatively static lesion. These patients either had recovered from an acute neurological disorder or had a slowly progressive disease. Group 3 patients were referred to as "chronic static" and consisted of those with epilepsy of long duration. Group 4 was a control group which included patients hospitalized for disorders not including brain damage. The performance of the control group was superior to that of the three brain-damaged groups. The acute brain-damaged group obtained IQ scores lower than those of the other two brain-damaged groups. Groups 2 and 3 did not differ from one another. These data indicate that the Wechsler is sensitive to presence or absence of brain impairment in both chronic and acute disorders. In addition, it is able to demonstrate sensitivity to behavioral differences produced by varying degrees of neurological acuteness.

The second issue was thoughtfully discussed by Smith (1962), who postulated that duration, age at onset, rate of growth, and type of lesion would influence psychological-behavioral performances. Three studies have addressed the relationship between lateralized brain damage and acuteness of the disorder as reflected by Wechsler results (Kløve & Fitzhugh, 1962; Fitzhugh, Fitzhugh, & Reitan, 1962; Russell, 1972). Kløve and Fitzhugh separated patients with long-standing epilepsy into three groups with EEG disorders characterized as reflecting right hemisphere abnormality, left hemisphere abnormality, or bilateral abnormality, and a fourth group having normal EEG. Unlike the results from a similarly organized study of patients with acute lesions (Kløve, 1959), the results from these chronically neurologically impaired groups failed to produce differential Verbal-Performance scores relating to lateralization of the EEG abnormalities. Fitzhugh, Fitzhugh, and Reitan composed three acute groups (right, left, and diffuse brain damage) and three similarly designated groups with chronic brain damage. Their results with the acute groups confirmed previous reports indicating that Verbal IQ is lowered following left hemisphere brain damage and that Performance IQ is lowered following damage to the right hemisphere. Such Verbal-Performance correspondence to lateralization of damage was not found for the patients with chronic brain damage. Russell compared 34 patients with static lateralized brain damage. These patients had a range of neurological disorders but were not epileptic. Russell reported that the results of this study were consistent with the previous findings which indicated the absence of Verbal-Performance IQ discrepancies in patients with lateralized but chronic brain damage. Thus the acuteness-chronicity dimension does, indeed, influence the finding of lateralized effects on Verbal-Performance IQ differences.

4.5. Type of Brain Damage

If all brain damage is not alike, then it is conceivable that behavioral correlates of one type will differ from those of another. Reed (1962) reported an interaction between type of lesion and effect of lateralization on the Verbal-Performance IQ split. This report analyzed results from patients with lateralized lesions of four different types including intracerebral tumor, extracerebral tumor, cerebrovascular disease, and head injury. Reed found that Verbal-Performance discrepancy in the expected direction occurred in the groups of patients with cerebrovascular accident and intracerebral brain tumor. No such Verbal-Performance split was seen in groups with lateralized extracerebral tumors or head injuries. Those conditions which have been found clinically to produce Verbal-Performance splits are those which involve tissue damage. Those which typically do not produce such structural brain changes, such as closed head injury, extracerebral tumors, and epilepsy, do not typically result in Verbal-Performance splits.

The Wechsler Scales have been shown to include a series of tasks which will validly reflect changes in human ability due to brain damage. The Scales are sensitive to the general impairment which occurs following many conditions of brain damage. It is also sensitive to aspects of lateralization and duration of such damage. It is at least equally true, however, that the Wechsler Scales alone are not adequate to make these distinctions. Many factors, including normal variation, can produce reduced levels of IQ and Verbal-Performance splits in persons with perfectly normal brain functions. The findings from the Wechsler Scales develop meaning for individual patients as they are compared with measures of other types of abilities and evaluated across multiple methods of inference.

5. The Halstead-Reitan Neuropsychological Test Battery

Within the field of neuropsychology, no set of procedures considered as a unit has received more careful investigation than that developed by Halstead and modified by Reitan. This set of procedures meets well-accepted criteria for usefulness of psychological techniques: (1) the technique should examine human behaviors broadly and use a number of tests; (2) the technique should show validated ability to discriminate between patients with and without impairment of brain functions; (3) the results of examinations with these techniques should be quantifiable and subject to scientific communication; and (4) the effects of factors such as age, sex, race, and education should be accounted for whenever appropriate. As documented in recent reviews (Matarazzo, 1972; Reitan & Davison, 1974; Smith, 1975; Hartlage & Hartlage, 1977), most neuropsychologists employ a wide range of tests of human ability. The two most frequently occurring points of overlap are the use of the Wechsler Scales and the Halstead Battery as part of a total neuropsychological examination. For this reason, we are focusing on research using these procedures. Some additional procedures such as grip strength and the Trail Making Test, which are frequently used in conjunction with the Halstead Battery, will be reported here to retain the integrated nature of the findings.

Halstead (1947) described the process of development and selection of his procedures for the study of brain behavior relationships in a book entitled *Brain and Intelligence: A Quantitative Study of the Frontal Lobes*. He pursued a field observational approach, seeing patients in his office but also spending time with them in activities of a more social nature. Such observations led to postulates as to the types of ability deficits being experienced by these individuals which he then sought to measure via new or modified tests and experimental procedures. Halstead recognized that here were many human abilities not sampled by traditional psychometric tests. He believed there was, in each person, a degree of biopsychological adaptiveness not well measured by IQ tests which he referred to as "biological intelligence."

This ability was directly related to the integrity of functioning of the human brain. He felt that this more basic intelligence was not dependent on acquired or formal knowledge or training and played a major role in "man's survival as an organism" (Halstead, 1947, p. 7). This ability allowed him to adapt to the world on a day-to-day basis.

Halstead employed factor analytic techniques to examine his tests to determine which best reflected this "biological intelligence." From a group of 27 tests, 13 were chosen. These 13 tests were used to examine 50 patients with brain damage, and these results produced four factors which Halstead identified and described:

1. A central integrative field factor C. This factor represents the organized experience of the individual. It is the ground function of the "familiar" in terms of which the psychologically "new" is tested and incorporated. It is a region of coalescence of learning and adaptive intelligence. Some of its parameters are probably reflected in measurements of psychometric intelligence which yield an intelligence quotient.
2. A factor abstraction A. This factor concerns basic capacity to group to a criterion as in the elaboration of categories, and involves the comprehension of essential similarities and differences. It is the fundamental growth principle of the ego.
3. A power factor P. This factor reflects the undistorted power factor of the brain. It operates to counterbalance or regulate the affective forces and thus frees the growth principle of the ego for further ego differentiation.
4. A directional factor D. This factor constitutes the medium through which the process factors, noted here, are exteriorized at any given moment. On the motor side, it specifies the "final common pathway," while on the sensory side, it specifies the avenue or modality of experience. (Halstead, 1947, p. 147)

Halstead then chose ten tests which had the highest t value in differentiating brain damage from controls and established a cutoff point for each test. For every test on which a patient performs beyond the cutoff point, a value of .1 is contributed to a summary score called the Impairment Index. The Impairment Index and the 13 tests used for the factor analysis shared eight tests in common. Two of these (Critical Flicker Fusion and Time Sense Test) have since been omitted because of the lack of clinical usefulness found in the case of the latter and because of failure of statistical validation of the former.

5.1. Description of Halstead's Tests

Three batteries of tests identified with the work of Halstead and Reitan have been developed. The battery for adults (ages 15 and older) is referred to as the Halstead Neuropsychological Test Battery. A modification by Reitan of several of these procedures made it applicable for children aged 9–14 years. This "intermediate" battery is referred to as the Halstead Neuropsychological Test Battery for Children. A battery for children aged 5–8 includes some of Halstead's tests in modified forms. These modifications as well as several new procedures were developed by Reitan. This set of procedures is referred to as the Reitan Indiana Neuropsychological Test Battery for Children. The more common term "Halstead-Reitan Battery" is generally used to refer to either of these batteries and certain associated procedures (Trail Making Test, Strength of Grip Test) not formally part of any of the three. In clinical and most research settings, the full neuropsychological examination also includes tests described elsewhere such as the Wechsler Scales, Aphasia Screening Battery, and the Sensory-Perceptual Examination. The Halstead battery tests are described briefly below.

5.1.1. Category Test

The Category Test uses a slide projector to present stimuli on a screen. The adult version has 208 items, the intermediate version 168, and the version for young children 80. The answer panel contains four levers numbered 1 to 4 (colors red, green, blue, and yellow for young children). The patient is told that something about the stimulus will suggest a number from 1 to 4 (or a color). If the patient depresses the correct lever (chooses the correct number or color), a bell sounds. If his choice was incorrect, a buzzer sounds. Only one response is allowed per item. The task is to determine, through trial-and-error hypothesis testing, the underlying principle which determines the correct response. The patient may be required to change his idea many times and remember why he was correct when the bell sounds. Each subtest contains only one principle, but each new subtest may have a different principle. The adult version has seven subtests, the intermediate has six subtests, and the version for children 5–8 has five subtests. There are no time limits or requirements for verbal response. Score is the number of errors made. This test requires considerable learning efficiency, mental flexibility, abstractive skill, and ability to identify critical from noncritical aspects of new and unfamiliar situations.

5.1.2. Tactual Performance Test (Time, Memory, and Localization Components

The Tactual Performance Test (TPT) uses a modification of the Seguin-Goddard form board. The patient is blindfolded and at no time is allowed to see the board and blocks. His task is to place the blocks into the board as quickly as possible. This task is performed three times: first with the dominant hand, then with the nondominant hand, and finally using both hands. After completion of the test trials and after the blocks and board have been removed, the patient is asked to draw a board and draw in as many blocks as he can. He is also asked to locate them correctly in relation to each other. This is done from memory with no forewarning of this requirement. The adult version has ten blocks in a vertical board, intermediate has six blocks in a vertical board, while the young children must fit six blocks in a horizontally placed board. This task requires reliance on tactile and kinesthetic feedback, rapid motor movements, some degree of learning and efficiency in the face of a new problem, as well as ability to remember without being specifically directed to do so.

5.1.3. Seashore Rhythm Test

The Seashore Rhythm Test is a subtest of Seashore's Tests of Musical Talent. Thirty pairs of rhythmic beats are presented by a taped recording. The patient must indicate which pairs of beats were the same and which were different. This task requires sustained attention and auditory nonverbal perceptual skill. This is included in the Adult and Intermediate batteries.

5.1.4. Speech Sounds Perception Test

The Speech Sounds Perception Test utilizes a tape recorder to present 60 spoken nonsense words which all include the "ee" sound, i.e., *theeg, zeets*. The patient must identify the "word" spoken by selecting it from four "words" on a written form (three choices in intermediate battery). This test requires sustained attention and concentration, verbal perception, and visual recognition of spoken "word."

5.1.5. Finger Oscillation Test

The Finger Oscillation Test (used in the same form for all the batteries) is a test of motor speed in which the patient depresses (taps) as rapidly as possible a key attached to a counting apparatus for a 10-sec period. The score is the average of five consecutive trials obtained for each hand.

5.1.6. Halstead Impairment Index

The Halstead Impairment Index (computed for adult battery only) is a summary score based on seven scores from the five tests listed above (Category errors, TPT Time, Memory, Localization, Rhythm items correct, Speech Test errors, and Finger Tapping speed-dominant hand). Criterion values for the Impairment Index are available only for adults.

5.1.7. Trail Making Test

The Trail Making Test consists of two parts, A and B. The patient's task is to connect circles distributed on a sheet of paper. In Part A, the circles are numbered 1–25 (1–15 for intermediate battery) and are to be connected in order. Part B consists of 25 circles numbered 1–13 and lettered A–L (1–8 and A–H for intermediate battery). The patient is to connect the circles alternating between numbers, i.e., 1, A, 2, B, 3, C, etc. This test measures number and letter recognition, visual scoring, motor speed, mental flexibility, and ability to deal with two separate requirements of a situation simultaneously.

5.1.8. Strength of Grip Test

In the Strength of Grip Test, the Smedley hand dynamometer is used in our laboratory because it has a grip which can be adjusted for use by patients in the age range of all three batteries. The patient squeezes as hard as possible with each hand and a measure in kilograms is obtained.

The following tests are exclusive to the Reitan-Indiana Neuropsychological Test Battery for Children.

5.1.9. Marching Test

The Marching Test employs a practice page and five legal-size test pages. On each page, there are one series of connected circles on the left and an identical series on the right which runs from bottom to top. Part 1 requires the patient to "march" up the page, first with the preferred and then the nonpreferred hand, hitting each circle with a crayon. Part 2 requires the patient to follow the examiner's fingers as they march up the page alternating movement from one hand to the other. This test requires speed, coordination, and concentration.

5.1.10. Color Form Test

The Color Form Test requires the patient to move his or her finger from a shape of one color to a figure with similar shape. Following that he moves to a figure of similar color and proceeds around the page alternating from color to form to color to form, etc.

5.1.11. Progressive Figures Test

In the Progressive Figures Test, the patient is asked to connect shapes on a page as rapidly as possible. Each shape has a smaller and different shape drawn inside of it. The patient moves to the large shape identical to the small shape inside the last large shape he touched until all shapes have been connected. Color Form and Progressive Figures are scored time to completion and are somewhat similar to the Trail Making Test. They were designed to provide additional data about mental flexibility and efficiency and have no verbal requirement.

5.1.12. Matching Pictures Test

The Matching Pictures Test requires the patient to match items on the top to items on the bottom of five pages. The relationship of the figures to be matched progresses from identical figures to those belonging to the same general category such as weapon or animal. The score is number of correct matches.

5.1.13. Target Test

The Target Test consists of nine dots arranged in a square. A sequence of dots is touched by the examiner. After a 5-sec delay, the patient must connect the dots in the order they were touched.

5.1.14. Matching V's and Matching Pictures

In the Matching V's Test and the Matching Pictures Test, the subject is presented with a board with seven different shapes (V's of varying acuteness or squares with varying amounts of internal design). Seven individual chips are presented, each containing a single shape. The task is to match the shape on a chip to the shape (Picture or V) on the card.

5.2. Validity of the Halstead Battery

The first cross-validation of Halstead's claim of the ability of his tests to distinguish between persons with and without brain damage was provided by Reitan in 1955 in Indianapolis. Despite the differences in examiners and location of the laboratory and the expectation for results of cross-validation to be less impressive than the original finding, the opposite result occurred in this study. Fifty patients with heterogeneous selection of types of brain damage were matched for age, sex, and education with 38 hospitalized persons and 12 nonpatients who showed no symptoms of cerebral damage or disorder. Each of Halstead's tests except for critical flicker fusion (no longer utilized) produced significant differences between the two groups. In the same year, Reitan (1955d) compared 27 brain-damaged patients on parts A and B of the Trail Making Test. He found that both Parts A and B produced a separation significant at the .001 level between the two groups. Reitan (1958b) composed a significantly larger sample of brain-damaged (200) and non-brain-damaged (84) patients for further evaluation of the Trail Making Test. He again found Parts A and B able to separate the two groups at the .001 level of significance. The data from this study served to establish the clinical criteria or cutoff scores most commonly employed for this test. Reitan found that a cutoff score of 38 sec or less on Part A correctly identified 75% of the control and 78.5% of the brain-damaged group. A cutoff score of 88 sec or less on Part B produced a correct classification of 81% of the controls and 88.5% of the brain-damaged patients. An attempt to develop a cutoff score for the combined Parts A and B times added little to the discriminative value of Part B alone.

A battery of tests of this complexity used with a wide variety of populations which attempts to tie its validity to biological reality cannot hope to attain wide acceptance until it has been demonstrated that investigators other than those responsible for its development can and do learn to apply it in a valid manner. Vega and Parsons (1967) compared the performance of a control group of mixed hospitalized and nonhospitalized subjects against that of a group of patients with brain damage. They found that, while the absolute level of test performances differed from that reported by Reitan, the ability of the test to discriminate between the brain-damaged and non-brain-damaged groups was substantiated. With the exception of the Time Sense Test memory component, all tests produced differences that attained the .001 level. Many other studies from various parts of the United States, Canada, and Europe have reported consistently similar findings, including Chapman and Wolff in New York (1959), Goldstein, Deysach, and Kleinknecht in Portland, Oregon (1973), Russell in Miami (1976), Schreiber, Goldman, Kleiman, Goldfader, and Snow in St. Louis (1976), Kløve and Lochen in Norway (Kløve, 1974), Klonoff et al. in Vancouver, British Columbia (1970), and Matthews and Booker in Madison, Wisconsin (1972).

An informative and unique study has come from the laboratory of Steven Goldstein, whose untimely death in 1977 deprives the field of one of its most creative and productive young leaders. Filskov and Goldstein (1974) examined 171 patients with

Table 3. Mean Hit Rate for Lateralization and Neuropathological Process [a]

Procedure	Uncorrected hit rate	
Neuropsychological battery	.89	(.85)
Brain scan	.36	(.32)
Flow	.69	(.67)
EEG	.52	(.35)
Angiogram	.85	(.85)
Pneumoencephalogram	.80	(.86)
X-ray	.16	(.16)

[a] Reprinted with permission of author and publisher from Filskov, S., and Goldstein, S. Diagnostic validity of the Halstead-Reitan neuropsychology battery. *Journal of Consulting and Clinical Psychology*, 1974, *42*, 383–388.

documented evidence of brain damage. They compared the ability of a clinical actuarial approach (a clinician interpreting validated tests) to the Halstead Battery with neurological examination procedures. These latter procedures included X-ray, EEG, angiogram, and pneumoencephalogram. Table 3 indicates that behavioral data (without risk of morbidity or mortality), when interpreted by adequately trained neuropsychologists, can produce information about the integrity of brain functions including lateralization and neuropathological type that compares favorably to other available medical procedures.

5.2.1. Reliability

Issues of reliability have not been raised formally until quite recently. Reliability, along with validity, serves as a traditional cornerstone (or hobgoblin) of the construction and use of psychological measurement procedures. Klonoff et al. (1970) demonstrated test-retest correlations for schizophrenic patients that range from .87 on the Trail Making Test, Part B, to .59 on the localization component of the Tactual Performance Test. The next lowest r was .63. Shaw (1966) reported split-half reliability on the Category Test of .98. The traditional question asks whether the test is or is not reliable. A better question would be to ask, "Reliable for what?" If a test produces the same or a similar score each time it is administered, it is reliable. That is good, unless the entity measured has changed; then that's not so good. Reliability can be thought of in at least three forms: score, rank, and category. Neurological conditions and the behavioral abilities affected by them can change for the better due to recovery such as that frequently seen following head injury. Such conditions can worsen, as is the case with a progressive intracerebral neoplasm, and our psychological tests should reflect that. It would seem that in many circumstances we would want scores to change significantly in relatively short periods of time.

It is possible for an individual's score to change and yet his rank in a group remain the same. In this way, effects of test familiarity (practice effects) may lead to equally improved performance among all individuals in a group. Changes in performance levels may occur and yet allow individuals to be ranked within a group in the same order over several testings. Finally, there is reliability of category. Neurologists and other physicians are quite familiar with the fact that numerical values from laboratory tests change with each sampling. Yet, as long as these values stay "within normal limits," a similar conclusion can be reached. If a patient is tested following head injury and makes 110 errors on the Category Test, he is categorized as impaired. Six months later, with Category Test errors down to 65, he is still in the impaired range, even though the improvement shown will have definite behavioral correlates. Joseph Matarazzo and his colleagues have recognized the complexity of this issue. In two well-written and thorough articles, they have demonstrated that (1) the Impairment Index computed from the Halstead Battery possesses the needed reliability (stability) for classifying an individual who is normal and (2) the Impairment Index is reliable for an older brain-damaged population. These findings added to those of Klonoff et al. (1970) with schizophrenics suggest that these procedures possess the necessary psychometric and clinical reliability (Matarazzo, Weins, Matarazzo, & Goldstein, 1974; Matarazzo, Matarazzo, Weins, Gallo, & Klonoff, 1976).

THOMAS J. BOLL

5.2.2. Effects of Age and Education

Yet another important technical consideration is the influence of education and age on test performance. Vega and Parsons (1967) reported that amount of education influenced performance in their non-brain-damaged patients but not in those with brain damage. Granick and Friedman (1967) found that the use of statistical techniques (partial correlations) to control for education reduced the correlation between Halstead Battery test performances and age. Prigatano and Parsons (1976) also employed statistical methods to investigate the influence of education on Halstead Test performance by brain-damaged and two groups of non-brain-damaged patients (a group of medical-surgical patients and a group of psychiatric patients). They found a high correlation between education and test performance for the medical-surgical patients but not for the psychiatric patients. They also confirmed that education was not significantly related to the performance of the brain-damaged group. Finlayson, Johnson, and Reitan (1977) compared three levels of education in a brain-damaged and a non-brain-damaged group. They divided their groups into those with educational levels of 0–10, 12, or 15 or more. For brain-damaged patients, low, medium, or high amounts of education did not significantly influence Halstead Battery performance. Among controls, the high-education group surpassed the other two on only two of ten Halstead neuropsychological variables, even though they had bested the other two groups on ten of 14 Wechsler variables. In fact, the most striking finding was the separation of brain-damaged and control subjects at all educational levels.

The effect of age and aging on Halstead tests has been outlined by Reitan (1955b) and confirmed in more detail by Reed and Reitan (1962, 1963a, 1963b). Reitan found a correlation of .54 between age and Impairment Index for non-brain-damaged controls but only .23 for brain-damaged subjects. He found that the results for controls were due primarily to the considerable decline in adaptive abilities noted in subjects 45 years of age and older. In an attempt to specify the type of deficit being observed, Reed and Reitan (1963a) organized their tests along a continuum of abstraction. This continuum ranged from tests totally dependent on past learning and experience to those which call heavily on new learning, problem solving, and mental flexibility, with a minimum of emphasis on past experiences. They found no difference between old (age 53) and young (age 28) normals on experience-dependent tasks. As the tasks increased in demand for complex problem solving, however, significant differences were consistently seen in favor of the younger group. Reitan (1967) and Vega and Parsons (1967) reported correlations between age and Impairment Index of between .57 and .60 for normals and .37 to .44 for brain-damaged patients. Prigatano and Parsons (1976) confirmed these findings for both a psychiatric and a general medical-surgical control group. A correlation between age and performance has also been seen on the Trail Making Test, as would be expected in recognition of its problem-solving, concentration, and speed requirements. Nevertheless, Boll and Reitan (1973) demonstrated that the ability of this test to separate persons with and without brain damage was retained across age ranges of 15–65 years. Overall, then, it would appear that persons whose abilities are already compromised due to brain damage show less decline due to aging than do normal non-brain-damaged individuals.

Neurological Diagnostic Criterion and Halstead Battery Performance

There are many ways to obtain evidence of brain damage or impairment. The most definitive is direct inspection of the lesion. Indirect inspection through computerized axial tomography, angiogram, or pneumoencephalogram is possible for certain conditions of brain damage. Many types of cerebral impairment, however, are not subject to such verification. Abnormalities reported in presenting complaints or through history, abnormalities on physical examination, EEG changes, and subtle deviations from expected patterns and shapes on neuroradiological procedures can suggest the presence of alterations in brain structure and accompanying biological function. It would be expected that these alterations would have corresponding and measurable behavioral correlates the identification and understanding of which would be aided by neuropsychological evaluation. This is true, however, only if neuropsychological procedures are specifically sensitive to cerebral conditions producing abnormalities on neurological examinations.

Kløve (1963) studied the relationship between findings on the physical neurological examination and neuropsychological performance. In addition to a control group, he identified 70 patients with brain damage. Thirty-five had positive findings and 35 had negative findings on the physical neurological examination, which included examination of reflexes, coordination, locomotion and sensation, ophthalmoscopy, auscultation of the head, and cranial nerve examination. The group did not differ in diagnostic category. Kløve's data as seen in Table 4 indicated that the Halstead Battery was sensitive to presence of brain damage whether or not evidence for such damage was forthcoming on the physical exam. This represents an impressive additional validation of the Halstead Battery. The important psychological message of this study should be underscored. Patients with normal physical

Table 4. Raw-Score Means and Probability Levels for Differences between Means on Selected Halstead Tests in Control Group and Two Brain-Damaged Groups Who Differed with Regard to Results Based on Physical Neurological Examination[a]

| Test | Control $(N = 35)$ | Neurological examination | | 1–2 | 1–3 | 2–3 |
		Negative $(N = 35)$	Positive $(N = 35)$			
Category Test	42.97	66.70	59.73	.001	.001	n.s.
Tactual Performance Test						
Total Time	16.10	26.48	29.99	.001	.001	n.s.
Memory Component	6.57	5.23	4.86	.05	.005	n.s.
Localization Component	3.34	1.91	2.03	.001	.005	n.s.
Seashore Rhythm Test (raw score)	24.23	20.43	20.03	.001	.005	n.s.
Speech Sounds Perception Test	8.94	13.49	15.14	.01	.005	n.s.
Finger Tapping Test, dominant hand	47.22	45.14	39.22	n.s.	.02	n.s.
Time Sense Test, memory component	272.89	557.46	540.33	.01	.001	n.s.
Impairment Index	0.44	0.69	0.71	.001	.001	n.s.

[a]Reprinted with permission of the publisher from Reitan, R. M., and Davison, L. (Eds), *Clinical Neuropsychology: Current Status and Applications*, Hemisphere Publishing Corporation, 1974.

neurological examination must not be assumed to be unlikely to benefit from neuropsychological examination.

Assessment of the behavioral correlates of degree of severity of impairment depends even more heavily on the precision of the neurological criteria than does the identification of presence or absence. Kløve (1959) showed that the Halstead Battery was able to describe impairments in the ability structure of brain-damaged patients even when IQ levels and EEG tracings were normal. Kløve and White (1963) sought to determine whether Halstead Battery variables would be sensitive to degree of severity of EEG abnormality. In addition to a control group, the brain-damaged patient groups had mild, moderate, or severe degrees of EEG abnormality. The Halstead Battery Impairment Index was significantly better for the control than for the brain-damaged groups. The Impairment Index for the brain-damaged group with normal EEGs fell in the impaired range, as did the Impairment Index for the other brain-damaged groups. While no Impairment Index differences occurred among groups with varying degrees of EEG abnormality, the Impairment Index was significantly higher (more impaired) for the group with severe EEG abnormalities than for the brain-damaged group whose EEG was normal, suggesting that the Halstead Battery is more sensitive to all degrees of impairment than is the test utilized as a criterion in this study.

Procedures such as the pneumoencephalogram represent, at least for some conditions, a source for considerable increase in criterion information and accuracy beyond the physical neurological exam or the EEG. This gain is obtained at small but very real increase in risk of morbidity and mortality. Matthews and Booker (1972) identified 50 patients who had had a pneumoencephalogram and the Halstead neuropsychological examination. From this sample, they chose 15 patients with the smallest and 15 with the largest lateral ventricles. The performance of these patients with the smallest lateral ventricles bested that of patients with the largest ventricles for each of the Halstead Battery variables.

Heilbrun (1962) complained that neuropsychological procedures were focusing mainly on differentiating brain-damaged patients from those without neurological complaints or disorder. He felt that psychologists' major contribution would be the ability to validly diagnose persons with more subtle and confusing complaints about whom neurologists might not find easy agreement. Heilbrun's notion that neurological diagnosis should be psychology's major contribution is an unfortunate one. Clearly, neurodiagnosis does not represent the area of major uniqueness for psychology. Psychology's greatest contribution is far more likely to be an ability to accurately describe the psychological ability makeup of individual patients and, in so doing, to greatly enhance an area of patient care not already provided. If we can validly describe the neurological condition that has resulted in a behavioral profile, it is unlikely that that profile is due to chance, poor environment, or deficient motivation. Such factors may coexist, and require serious attention as well. Nevertheless, the ability to understand the psychological sequellae specific to an individual neurological disorder represents the first necessary step in establishing the validity of efforts at intervention. Matthews et al. (1966) attempted to determine whether neurological evaluation could distinguish a group of patients eventually found to require neurological intervention from a group whose final diagnosis indicated no neurologically significant disorder. Both groups presented with symptoms and complaints that strongly suggested the possibility of need for neurological treatment. These

Table 5. Raw-Score Means and Standard Deviations for Selected Halstead Tests and Probability Levels Comparing the Brain-Damaged and Pseudoneurological Groups[a]

| Variable | Brain damaged | | Pseudo-neurological | | |
	Mean	SD	Mean	SD	p
Category Test	63.66	27.66	44.53	24.63	<.01
Tactual Performance Test					
Total Time	27.60	13.55	14.79	6.32	<.001
Memory Component	6.44	1.86	7.56	1.41	<.05
Localization Component	3.16	2.38	4.38	2.34	<.05
Finger Tapping Test, dominant hand	37.78	10.04	43.90	9.15	<.01
Seashore Rhythm Test (raw score)	22.53	4.44	25.94	2.76	<.001
Speech Sounds Perception Test	8.25	4.06	6.25	4.00	<.05
Impairment Index	.63	.21	.32	.18	<.001

[a] Reprinted with permission of the publisher from Reitan, R. M., and Davison, L. (Eds.), *Clinical Neuropsychology: Current Status and Applications*, Hemisphere Publishing Corporation, 1974.

complaints include nausea, dizziness, headache, motor weakness, and ictal episodes simulating epilepsy and visual difficulties. The data in Table 5 indicate that the Halstead Battery Impairment Index correctly separated these two groups at the .001 level. Each test in the Halstead Battery, including the Trail Making Test, produced differences that significantly separated these clinically similar groups of patients. The authors pointed out, however, that despite the significant levels of separation achieved by each test, none by itself would have been clinically acceptable. Single test cutoff scores able to correctly classify most brain-damaged patients would have produced an unacceptably high false-positive classification. These findings further emphasize our continuing point that the idea of a single test for "organicity" must be abandoned.

5.4 Effects of Lateralization of Brain Lesions

Most neuropsychological batteries include tests of motor and sensory function to provide data about the differential efficiency of the two sides of the body. In addition, tests of aphasia and constructional praxis, also sensitive to left and right hemisphere functions, are common elements of such an examination. Russell (1974) provided a careful analysis of the differential sensitivity of the Halstead Battery variables to left vs. right hemisphere impairment. The Category Test, which has been shown to be generally sensitive to the effects of brain damage, was not found to be strongly lateralized. This corresponds quite closely to clinical experience. The Tactual Performance Test was found strongly affected by right hemisphere damage despite its use of both the right and the left upper extremity. This may be due to its heavy reliance on kinesthetic feedback and the demand for tactile form recognition. The right hemisphere has been shown to play a predominant role in tactile perceptual activity of this nature (Boll, 1974c). Speech Perception is primarily a left hemisphere function, while Rhythm relates (weakly) to the right cerebral hemisphere. Clinical experience tends to confirm that the Memory and Localization components of the Tactual Performance Test are equally impaired by damage to either the right or left cerebral hemisphere.

5.5. Sensitivity to Type and Location of Lesion

The most comprehensive demonstration of the validity of the use of multiple inferential methods applied to a valid battery of behavioral tests in the measurement of the psychological correlates of type and location of brain damage was reported by Reitan (1964). Sixty-four patients representing four neuropathological types (intracerebral tumor, extracerebral tumor, cerebrovascular lesion, focal head injury) were identified. There were 16 patients of each type. Each lesion type was represented equally in each of four locations: left anterior, left posterior, right anterior, and right posterior. Such a distribution also provides 64 patients grouped by laterality (32 left and 32 right) and 64 grouped on an anterior-posterior axis as well. To these 64 patients with focal impairment were added additional groups of 16 patients, each with diffuse cerebral impairment due to either closed head injury, multiple sclerosis, or cerebral arteriosclerosis. Each patient was examined using the Halstead variables as well as other tests routinely included in a neuropsychological examination (Wechsler Scales, aphasia and sensory perceptual exam, Trail Making Test, and the Minnesota Multiphasic Personality Inventory). Of the 64 patients with focal lesions, 57 were so identified through clinical interpretation of behavioral data. Forty-six of the 48 patients with diffuse damage were correctly identified. With respect to laterality, left hemisphere locations were correctly identified in 20 of 32 cases, while 22 of 32 right hemisphere cases represented hits. An anterior location of a focal lesion was correctly identified in 16 out of 32 cases, while 26 out of 32 posterior lesions were identified. This finding underscores the actual elusiveness of frontal areas to quantitative behavioral analysis (Luria, 1966; Meier, 1974). Posterior lesions, by contrast, have been subject to far more quantified and descriptive efforts (Mountcastle, 1962). The hit rates out of 16 patients in each quadrant were left anterior, 9; left posterior, 11; right anterior, 7; and right posterior, 15. With respect to type of lesion with 16 in each focal category, hit rates were intracerebral tumor, 13; extracerebral tumor, 8; cerebrovascular lesion, 12; and focal head injury, 13. Among the diffuse lesion groups, the hit rates were multiple sclerosis, 15; arteriosclerosis, 14; and diffuse head injury, 14. These findings do far more than indicate the validity of the procedures for identifying presence or absence of brain damage. They point out the complexity of this area of clinical practice. The effect of a lesion depends on its neuropathological type. The effect of any type of lesion depends on whether it is focal, bilateral, or diffuse. The effect of any type of focal lesion depends on its lateralization. The effect of any type of lesion in the left or right cerebral hemisphere depends on where in the hemisphere it occurs. Further, the effect depends on the lesion's size (Chapman and Wolff, 1959), its rate of growth, the duration of its presence, and the patient's age when it began (Smith, 1975). Despite the enormous complexity involved, it is clear that neuropsychological tests can make a valid and independent contribution to patient care through advancement of our understanding of the effect of impairment in brain functions on human behavior.

5.6. Effects of Language Disorders: Aphasia

It was not until a paper by Marc Dax in 1836 that loss of speech became associated with damage to the left cerebral hemisphere. This discovery, however, was presented at a local meeting and went unrecognized. Only when his son, also a physician, presented the paper again in 1863 and had it published in 1865 did he receive recognition for his findings. At this same time, Broca cared for two patients with significant expressive language deficits who could understand and pantomime. He discovered following their deaths that each had a lesion in the area of the brain (now referred to as Broca's area or the area for expressive or motor speech) which includes the posterior-inferior aspects of the left frontal lobe. Wernicke (1874) found that a lesion in the superior portion of the temporal lobe would impair the understanding of speech. Marie (1906) criticized these and other clinical impressions of the day and indicated that the anatomical data on which the correlations for location of language disorders had been based were not adequate to support the conclusions. Further, he indicated that the clinical examination had not been sufficient to identify the type and range of language problems that the patient did or did not have. For example, despite Broca's emphasis on speech loss in his patients, they also could not write, were apparently limited in their understanding, and were not described as to presence or absence of reading disability. Marie also indicated that, while not necessarily demented, aphasic patients did indeed suffer a general lowering of intelligence.

Despite the many specific types of language disorder that have been identified and for which cerebral localizations have been attempted, it is rare that a focal cerebral lesion disrupts a single physiological function. The same psychological disorder may be caused by more than one kind of physiological disturbance. Gross categorizations of aphasia into expressive (Broca's) due to impairment of the anterior temporal and posterior frontal areas and receptive (Wernicke's) due to posterior temporal and parietal area, while still in use, underestimate the nature of the language disorder actually present and the complexity of its neural representation. Aphasia may develop along with other symptoms of a progressive structural lesion. It may develop as part of a generalized cortical degeneration or appear suddenly following an intracranial insult or penetrating head injury. A closed head injury producing no obvious structural damage can also result in significant aphasic deficits.

When recovery is part of the natural history of the disorder producing aphasia, i.e., head injury, the rate of recovery is typically a declining one from its beginning at the time of insult. Generally, the expectation is for 80–90% of total recovery to occur during the first 12 months of the recovery period, with additional improvement a possibility for many years. Smith has reported good recovery of language functions after 3 years during which no recovery was apparent. This recovery continued for 2 years until premorbid levels were obtained (Smith, 1975). Delay in onset of aphasia has been reported associated with some surgical procedures.

The majority of clinical evaluations of aphasia are accomplished by informal, brief, and nonsystematic questioning. Formal but nonquantified language assessments such as the Halstead Wepman Aphasia Screening Battery (Halstead and Wepman, 1949) or modifications by Reitan and Matthews are in common use by psychologists, psychiatrists, and neurologists (see Figure 12 and Table 6). This procedure provides examination of a range of language-dependent abilities. In addition, a sample of visuospatial constructional ability is included. This allows a brief yet valid examination of functions of the right and the left cerebral hemisphere (Heimburger & Reitan, 1961; Wheeler & Reitan, 1962). As can be seen in Table 7, a variety of specific but usually multiply present language disorders are dependably associated with left hemisphere lesions, while constructional dyspraxia is lateralized in the right cerebral hemisphere. It is possible to find proponents of the neuroanatomical specificity of aphasic disorders (Geschwind, 1963; Goodglass, Quadfasel, & Timberlake, 1964). It is

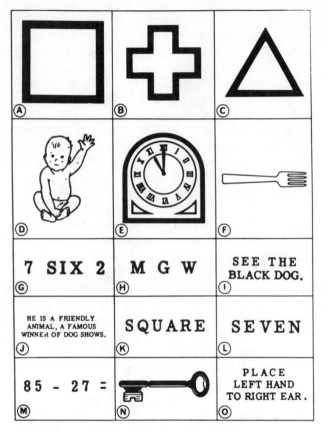

Figure 12. Stimulus figures for Reitan's modification of the Halstead Wepman Aphasia Screening Battery.

equally possible to discover backers of a more general representation of language functions (Schuell, Jenkins, & Jiminez-Pabon, 1965).

An issue as hotly argued as that of specific vs. general location of language deficits is the relationship between language and higher mental processes in man. This question has captured the interest of scientists and philosophers as being central to the understanding of the difference between human and nonhuman animals. Meyers (1948) has provided a review of historical interest. Watson (1924) drew the line sharply when he postulated that thinking was nothing more than subvocal speech. Lenneberg (1967) insisted that differences between man and other animals are qualitative and organizational, and not simply a function of enlarged association areas of the brain. He felt that language was an example of the qualitative rather than the quantitative differences in thinking ability demonstrated by man. Language and thinking are intimately connected in a manner suggesting that neither one is primary or causal to the other. Taking the other position, Furth (1966) held that the internal organization of intelligence does not depend on the current or even the past presence of a language system. He studied deaf children with and without language and found no differences in language, concept formation, and problem-solving tasks. He indicated that intelligence does not require a formal or socially recognizable symbol system.

Two issues are being combined in these arguments. The first is the necessity of language for the development of thought and vice versa. The second is the likelihood

Table 6. **Instructions for use of Reitan's modification of the Halstead Wepman Aphasia Screening Battery**

Patient's task	Examiner's instructions to the patient
1. Copy SQUARE (A)	FIRST, DRAW THIS ON YOUR PAPER. (Point to square, item A.) I WANT YOU TO DO IT WITHOUT LIFTING YOUR PENCIL FROM THE PAPER. MAKE IT ABOUT THIS SAME SIZE. (Point to square.) Elaborate on the requirement for a continuous line if necessary. If the patient is concerned about making a heavy or double line, point out that only a reproduction of the shape is required. If the patient has obvious difficulty in drawing any of the figures, encourage him to proceed until it is clear that he can make no further progress. If he does not accomplish the task reasonably well on his first try, ask him to try again, and instruct him to be particularly careful to do it as well as he can.
2. Name SQUARE	WHAT IS THAT SHAPE CALLED?
3. Spell SQUARE	WOULD YOU SPELL THAT WORD FOR ME?
4. Copy CROSS (B)	DRAW THIS ON YOUR PAPER. (Point to cross). GO AROUND THE OUTSIDE LIKE THIS UNTIL YOU GET BACK TO WHERE YOU STARTED. (Examiner draws a finger-line around the edge of the stimulus figure.) MAKE IT ABOUT THIS SAME SIZE. (Point to cross.) Additional instructions, if necessary, should be similar to those used with the square.
5. Name CROSS	WHAT IS THAT SHAPE CALLED?
6. Spell CROSS	WOULD YOU SPELL THAT WORD FOR ME?
7. Copy TRIANGLE (C)	Similar to 1 and 4 above.
8. Name TRIANGLE	WHAT IS THAT SHAPE CALLED?
9. Spell TRIANGLE	WOULD YOU SPELL THAT WORD FOR ME?
10. Name BABY (D)	WHAT IS THIS? (Show baby, item D).
11. Write CLOCK (E)	NOW I AM GOING TO SHOW YOU ANOTHER PICTURE BUT YOU DO *NOT* TELL ME THE NAME OF IT. I DON'T WANT YOU TO SAY ANYTHING OUT LOUD. JUST WRITE THE NAME OF THE PICTURE ON YOUR PAPER. (Show clock, item E.)
12. Name FORK (F)	WHAT IS THIS? (Show fork, item F.)
13. Read 7 SIX 2 (G)	I WANT YOU TO READ THIS. (Show item G.) If the subject has difficulty, attempt to determine whether he can read any part of the stimulus figure.
14. Read M G W (H)	READ THIS. (Show item H.)
15. Reading I (I)	NOW I WANT YOU TO READ THIS. (Show item I.)
16. Reading II (J)	CAN YOU READ THIS? (SHOW ITEM J.)
17. Repeat TRIANGLE	NOW I AM GOING TO SAY SOME WORDS. I WANT YOU TO LISTEN CAREFULLY AND SAY THEM AFTER ME AS CAREFULLY AS YOU CAN. SAY THIS WORD: TRIANGLE.
18. Repeat MASSACHUSETTS	THE NEXT ONE IS A LITTLE HARDER BUT DO YOUR BEST. SAY THIS WORD: MASSACHUSETTS.
19. Repeat METHODIST EPISCOPAL	NOW REPEAT THIS ONE: METHODIST EPISCOPAL.
20. Write SQUARE (K)	DON'T SAY THIS WORD OUT LOUD. (Point to stimulus word "square," item K.) JUST WRITE IT ON YOUR PAPER. If the patient prints the word, ask him to write it.
21. Read SEVEN (L)	CAN YOU READ THIS WORD OUT LOUD. (Show item L.)

(Continued)

Table 6. (*Continued*)

Patient's task	Examiner's instructions to the patient
22. Repeat SEVEN	NOW, I WANT YOU TO SAY THIS AFTER ME: SEVEN.
23. Repeat-explain HE SHOUTED THE WARNING	I AM GOING TO SAY SOMETHING THAT I WANT YOU TO SAY AFTER ME, SO LISTEN CAREFULLY: HE SHOUTED WARNING. NOW YOU SAY IT. WOULD YOU EXPLAIN WHAT THAT MEANS? Sometimes it is necessary to amplify by asking the kind of situation to which the sentence would refer. The patient's understanding is adequately demonstrated when he brings the concept of impending danger into his explanation.
24. Write: HE SHOUTED THE WARNING	NOW I WANT YOU TO WRITE THAT SENTENCE ON THE PAPER. Sometimes it is necessary to repeat the sentence so that the patient understands clearly what he is to write.
25. Compute 85 − 27 = (M)	HERE IS AN ARITHMETIC PROBLEM. COPY IT DOWN ON YOUR PAPER ANY WAY YOU LIKE AND TRY TO WORK IT OUT. (Show item M.)
26. Compute 17 × 3 =	NOW DO THIS ONE IN YOUR HEAD: 17 × 3
27. Name KEY (N)	WHAT IS THIS? (Show item N.)
28. Demonstrate use of KEY (N)	IF YOU HAD ONE OF THESE IN YOUR HAND, SHOW ME HOW YOU WOULD USE IT. (Show item N.)
29. Draw KEY (N)	NOW I WANT YOU TO DRAW A PICTURE THAT LOOKS JUST LIKE THIS. TRY TO MAKE YOUR KEY LOOK ENOUGH LIKE THIS ONE SO THAT I WOULD KNOW IT WAS THE SAME KEY FROM YOUR DRAWING. (Point to key, item N.)
30. Read (O)	WOULD YOU READ THIS? (Show item O.)
31. Place LEFT HAND TO RIGHT EAR	NOW, WOULD YOU DO WHAT IT SAID?
32. Place LEFT HAND TO LEFT ELBOW	NOW I WANT YOU TO PUT YOUR LEFT HAND TO YOUR LEFT ELBOW. The patient should quickly realize that it is impossible.

that with damage to one, the other will also be impaired. Findings have been reported on both sides of these issues. In a very carefully constructed experiment, Reitan (1960) compared brain-damaged patients with dysphasia to brain-damaged patients without language disorder. Impressive in this study was the careful matching of neuropathological types of disorders for the two groups. In this way, differences due to varying types of damage were minimized, and, therefore, within well-recognized limits, presence or absence of aphasia did indeed represent the independent variable. Although Reitan does not mention it, it seems likely in many instances that these carefully matched lesions were present in the left hemisphere for aphasics and in the right hemisphere for nonaphasics. His results demonstrate in which area aphasia makes a specific contribution and where it does not. Both aphasic and nonaphasic brain-damaged groups showed impairment on all tests. The aphasics demonstrated particular and significant additional problems on verbal measures, summarized by Verbal Intelligence Quotient, Speech Sounds Perception Test, and Part B of the Trail Making Test. On the other hand, tests most demanding of abstraction and complex problem solving and reflective of highest-level mental processes showed no differential impairment between the two groups when they could be performed on a nonverbal basis. Neither did aphasics do more poorly on tasks with a heavy visuospatial requirement. Archibald, Wepman, and Jones (1967) used Raven's Colored Matrices, the Elithorn Mazes, Sure-Wepman's Concept Shift Test, and the Grassi Block Substitution Test as measures of nonverbal concept formation. They concluded that "aphasia itself is specifically a defect of language and memory for language which may or may not be accompanied by impaired cognitive functioning." It appears that, for clinical purposes, the position of Marie in 1906 accurately reflects the situation. He held that all aphasics, in addition to their expressive problems, usually have some less severe defect in comprehension (receptive loss). They also show some decline in general cognitive and intellectual functions, albeit not necessarily a serious one. He further felt that, on careful examination, patients labeled as experiencing a specific language problem in one area would be found to be less able in related language areas as well. Whether it is an adult with a focal lesion recently acquired or a child with so-called specific dyslexia, the clinical rule of Marie to look more broadly before being satisfied with the limits of a problem has borne great fruit (Boll, 1972).

Table 7. Percentage of Each Criterion Group Showing a Positive Sign for Each Aphasia Test Variable: Left and Right Indicators Separated and Listed by Rank Order of Percentage Response in Appropriate Group [a]

	Criterion groups			
	Left	Right	Diffuse	Control
Test variable, left indicator				
Dyscalculia	55.32	14.04	20.37	00.00
Central dysarthria	55.32	10.53	37.04	08.65
Dysnomia	53.19	00.00	16.67	00.96
Dysgraphia	51.06	01.75	25.93	00.00
Spelling dyspraxia	48.94	05.26	16.67	06.73
Dyslexia	46.81	00.00	20.37	00.00
Right-left disorientation	42.55	05.26	29.63	09.62
Right Finger dysgnosia	36.17	01.75	25.93	00.96
Right dysstereognosis	29.79	01.75	09.26	00.00
Visual letter dysgnosia	25.53	00.00	07.41	00.00
Right tactile imperception	14.89	00.00	18.52	00.00
Auditory verbal dysgnosia	12.77	00.00	07.41	00.00
Visual number dysgnosia	10.64	00.00	01.85	00.00
Test variable, right indicator				
Construction dyspraxia	14.89	61.40	44.44	07.69
Left dysstereognosis	02.13	29.82	11.11	00.00
Left finger dysgnosia	00.00	28.07	16.67	02.88
Left tactile imperception	02.13	21.05	14.81	00.00
Left visual imperception	02.13	15.79	07.41	00.00
Left auditory imperception	02.13	14.04	18.52	00.00
Average % response of groups to sets of variables				
Left indicators	27.11	03.10	18.23	02.07
Right indicators	03.90	28.36	18.83	01.76
Total set	26.60	11.08	18.42	01.97

[a] Reprinted with permission of author and publisher from Wheeler, Lawrence, and Reitan, Ralph M. Presence and laterality of brain damage predicted from responses to a short aphasia screening test. *Perceptual and Motor Skills*, 1962, *15*, 783–799.

5.7. Effects of Sensory and Tactile-Perceptual Disorders

The history of mental measurement began with attempts to use motor and sensory skills as reflectors of higher-level processes. Galton (1893) employed auditory discrimination of pitch and visual estimation of length in addition to the direct measurement of parts of the body (anthropometrics). He was knighted for his contributions in using sensorimotor tasks to differentiate mentally defective people from those with normal abilities. Cattell (1890) used strength, speed, reaction time, and pain sensitivity in addition to memory and referred to each of these as mental tests. Binet and Henri (1895) criticized these psychological measures as being too sensory. In so doing, they began what became an almost total abandonment of such procedures. Most current mental tests rely exclusively on expressive and receptive language and visuospatial skill. The more recent interest in understanding the role of brain and human behavior has provided the impetus for a rediscovery of some of the original psychological test procedures.

6. Procedures for Sensory Perceptual Examination

6.1. Sensory Imperception

The purpose of the Sensory Imperception Procedure (all ages) is to determine whether patients can perceive stimuli to both sides of the body when they are presented in a bilateral simultaneous manner. Prior to this test, it must be determined that the patient can perceive unilateral stimuli accurately. This tests the tactile, visual, and auditory sensory modalities. For example, once it is determined that a patient can hear a relatively faint sound when it is presented to each ear one at a time, this stimulus is presented to both ears simultaneously. Normal persons, asked which ear received the stimulus, will respond "both." If the stimulus was perceived in only one ear, the deficit is not peripheral hearing loss, because this has already been ruled out by correct perception of unilateral stimuli. Such imperceptions during bilateral simultaneous stimulation may indicate a lesion in the cerebral hemisphere across from the side of the body on which the failure to perceive occurred.

6.2. Tactile Finger Recognition Test

The Tactile Finger Recognition Test (all ages) taps the patient's ability to recognize body parts when touched. Each finger is numbered, and when the examiner touches the fingers (predetermined order, four touches to each finger of each hand), the patient is to respond with the corresponding number of some other indication as to the finger touched. This test is done with eyes closed or hand placed through a board to prevent use of visual cues. Failure to correctly identify fingers touched is referred to as finger agnosia, and the score is the number of errors made by each hand.

6.3. Finger Tip Number Writing Perception Test

The Finger Tip Number Writing Perception Test (intermediate and adult batteries) assesses the patient's ability to recognize numbers written by the examiner on the patient's finger tips. (For children 5–8, X's and O's are substituted for numbers and the test is called Finger Tip Symbol Writing Perception Test.) This task is performed without visual cues. Numbers (or symbols) are written in predetermined order on each finger of each hand, and the score is the number of errors for each hand.

6.4. Tactile Form Recognition Test

In the Tactile Form Recognition Test (all ages), the patient places his hand through a board and a small plastic shape (square, cross, circle, triangle) is placed in his fingers. In front of the patient on a board is a strip containing a duplicate of each of these shapes. The patient's task is to feel the shape with one hand and point to its twin with the other hand. It is not necessary to name the shapes, and no verbal response is required. Each of the four shapes is placed in each hand twice. The score is the number of errors in identification for each hand and total time in seconds which has elapsed before identifications are made for each hand. These last two tests tap stereognostic ability, and each portion of the sensory perceptual examination provides for comparison of the performance of the two sides of the body.

6.5. Validity of Sensory Perceptual Procedures

Tests of bilateral simultaneous stimulation were recommended by Oppenheim in 1885 and introduced by Bender in 1945 as the Double Simultaneous Stimulation Test (DSS) (Smith, 1975). Bender (1970) found that, with hemiparetic patients, single sensory stimuli identified the presence of impairment of sensation in 29 persons, while the DSS found such problems in 44 of the 50 patients tested. However, as Table 7 indicates, the occurrence of these disorders, even in populations with well-documented brain lesions, is not high unless the damage is severe; therefore, the absence of such errors does not indicate the absence of impairment. Conversely, however, the presence of such deficits is rarely misleading in its suggestion of impairment of brain functions. Smith and his colleagues (Smith, Champoux, Leri, London, & Muraski, 1972) reported on the relationship between deficits on the DSS and performance on other neuropsychological tests. They found that patients with or without hemiplegia who showed presence of bilateral sensory errors were more impaired in language, reasoning, and memory than were similar patients demonstrating only unilateral sensory deficits. Those patients without errors on the DSS were less impaired in higher-level cognitive functions than were either of the sensory-impaired groups. This is a brief procedure which provides evidence of a sign nature indicating the presence of brain impairment. It also provides a comparison, through sensory channels on each side of the body, of the comparative efficiency of the two cerebral hemispheres.

There is general clinical agreement that tactile-perceptual and motor tasks are subserved primarily by the contralateral side of the brain. Semmes (1968) postulated differential organization in the two cerebral hemispheres for such functions. Sensory and motor abilities, according to Semmes, are represented diffusely in the right cerebral hemisphere. Therefore, a small lesion affecting only a part of this organization scheme need not lead to behavioral defect. The left cerebral hemisphere, on the other hand, is characterized by focal organization. Thus a small but unfortunately placed lesion could cause severe deficit. Such would apply for simple tasks. In the case of complex or multimodal tasks (requiring sensation, perception, movement, etc.), a lesion in the right hemisphere may lead to a relatively greater defect. This in turn may cause the right hemisphere to be viewed as "dominant" or "leading" for sensory-perceptual-motor tasks in the same way that the left hemisphere is viewed as "dominant" or "leading" for language functions. Direct evidence on this point, as well as a demonstration of the validity of tests of tactile perception in the assessment of the effects of brain impairment, was provided by Boll (1974c). He noted that, on tasks which varied from simple to multimodal, the patients with right hemisphere lesions made a larger total number of errors than did the left brain-damaged group. Patients with right hemisphere brain damage showed greater contralateral and ipsilateral tactile difficulties than did the left hemisphere group. It would appear that, while the rule of contralateral representation still holds, it is also true that the right hemisphere has a special role in tactile perceptual activities on both sides of the body. Two additional studies indicate that sensory-motor and perceptual functions may have a strong ordering effect on higher-level mental abilities consistent with that report by Smith et al. (1972) for the DSS Test. Reitan (1970) divided brain-damaged patients into upper and lower third of his total group on the basis of sensory-motor impairment or intactness. He found that patients with intact sensory-motor abilities surpassed the sensory-motor-impaired group on language, memory, problem solving, concentration, attention, and visual-perceptual abilities. Performance of the intact (but brain-damaged) group also reflected a tendency toward less severe degree of emotional pathology on the MMPI. Boll, Berent, and Richards (1977), using brain-damaged and normal children, found significant correlations between tactile-perceptual functioning and cognitive functions including academic progress. Subjects with best and those with poorest tactile perceptual performances were identified (independent of presence or absence of brain impairment). A significant separation (quite similar to that found between the brain-damaged and non-brain-damaged groups) occurred between these two groups on measures of learning, memory, attention, language, and spatial skill. These separations also occurred between the brain-damaged patients divided into good vs. poor tactile perceivers. This ordering influence of tactile perceptual ability on cognitive functions was also present for the normally functioning control subjects. It would appear important to include such human functions when attempting to provide a complete psychological description of a patient experiencing difficulty in academic or work settings.

6.6. Effects of Memory Disorders

Memory has been treated as a unitary concept in a manner similar to that of brain damage. Tests for memory were developed which reflect this unitary notion. In fact, several tests set out to evaluate the effect on memory of brain damage. Thanks largely to the excellent experimental-clinical investigations of the groups at McGill and at the Boston Veterans Administration Hospital, recognition of the great complexities subserved under the term "memory" is growing. There is now general agreement that verbal memory is the responsibility of the left side of the brain and pattern or design memory is represented on the right. Studies by Butters, Samuels, Goodglass, and Brody (1970) and Samuels, Butters, and Fedio (1972) suggest these additional variables must be considered: (1) modality—is the item to be remembered presented visually or auditorially; (2) material—is the item to be remembered verbal or patterned; and (3) level of memory—immediate, short-term, long-term, or distant. Russell (1975a) defines these four levels of memory as follows: immediate memory—

up to 60 sec; short-term memory—between 1 and 30 min (possible up to 60); long-term memory—at least 30 min; distant memory—stored memory of events in one's past life. Samuels et al. (1972) suggest different mechanisms for different levels of memory. Short-term memory is modality specific. This means that auditory material with or without a language content is processed by the temporal lobes. Visual material, either pattern or language, is processed by the parietal lobes. Milner (1962, 1967, 1968) found a relationship between verbal material and the left hemisphere and nonverbal material and the right hemisphere which would apply to the mechanism of long-term memory. When one realizes that individuals may employ different memory strategies for the same material, an additional degree of complexity is added. Patients with right temporal defects may attempt to remember a geometric design through application of verbal labels and descriptions. A patient with a left temporal lesion may process this form directly as a visual pattern. The elements of a test for memory must include consideration of these variables (modality, material, laterality of deficit, and length of memory). The Wechsler Memory Scale (Wechsler, 1945) was developed in an era when tests assumed that memory and brain damage were unitary concepts. The underlying assumption was that the brain performed as a single unit and not through integration and coordination of more localized functions (Luria, 1973). Russell (1975a) has developed and validated a scoring system for the WMS that greatly enhances its sophistication and recommends it for inclusion as part of the neuropsychological examination. The criteria set were (1) memory scales should be sensitive to lateralization issues with respect to verbal and figural memory; (2) the tests should measure immediate and long-term memory; (3) if the memory test is to be used to assess the effects of brain damage, it should be validated in that context. This validity should have two components. It should be sensitive to impairment due to brain damage and also to the differences in semantic vs. figural memory reflected in patients with left vs. right hemisphere lateralized lesions. It should also be relatable to other tests within a set of neuropsychological procedures. All six Wechsler Memory Scale measures adapted by Russell were found to be valid in these respects. He indicated that when a $\frac{1}{2}$-hr repeat testing on the logical memory and visual reproduction subtests was included, this scale provided assessment of immediate (digit span), short-term (logical memory and visual reproduction), and long-term (logical memory and visual reproduction retest) memory. Procedures for assessment of distant events (Williams, 1968) are not included in the Wechsler Memory Scale. This revision provides an assessment of multiple areas of content, modality, and length of memory using a readily available and newly validated, quantified procedure.

6.7. Individual Tests for Brain Damage

A large number of individual tests, either developed to diagnose brain damage or currently so used in spite of their original purpose, are in common use. It is, in light of the previous pages, naive to think of any measure as a test of brain damage or "organicity." It is likely, however, that a test of any human ability is sensitive to some aspect of brain functions. In fact, if it isn't, then one is left to postulate that the ability it does measure is represented some place outside of the brain. The majority of tests of brain damage measure some aspect of visuospatial perceptual skill. Despite the obvious inadequacies of limited behavioral samples, hundreds of studies have been published documenting the statistical validity of single tests for brain damage. This is possible for several reasons. Brain damage appears to have both a general and a specific effect. Any individual patient may show one or both of these effects to widely differing degrees. When patients with heterogeneous types of brain damage are combined into a group, the result is a group of patients who are, in effect, impaired on everything. Reitan (1974b) and Boll (1974a) reported comparisons between normals and brain-damaged patients whose neurological damage and consequent behavioral deficits were quite heterogeneous. They utilized over 40 separate tests. In each study, it was found that most of these tests significantly separated the two groups. This means that each could have been reported separately as a "validated" test for brain damage. The real challenge would be to find a psychological test that does not show this effect.

In addition to this general effect, brain damage can produce specific areas of dysfunction. Each test for brain damage, if it measures anything at all, may well be performed especially poorly by a few of the patients in a heterogeneous group who have the appropriate type of damage for that test. Only a very few very poor scores can be enough to separate an already generally compromised group from one with normal brain functions.

Of all tests for brain damage, none is so well known as the Bender Visual Motor Gestalt Test (Bender, 1938). This procedure was not originally developed to test for brain damage. However, the efforts of Pascal and Suttell (1951), Hutt (1969), and Koppitz (1964) to produce norms and an objective scoring system have led to its use as a test of presence or absence of brain damage in adults and children. A suggested modification by Canter (1968) increases the difficulty of the task. Despite rave reviews in the past (Benton, 1953) and a loyal following, evaluations by Bruell and Albee (1962), Korman and Blumberg (1963), and Russell (1976) make it clear that this excellent procedure for the assessment of visual perceptual abilities cannot be made to bear the weight of representing the entire human behavioral repertoire. Bruell and Albee (1962) report use of the Bender along with other tests to assess effects of removal of an entire right cerebral hemisphere (half of the brain). Evaluation of Bender drawings indicated that "organicity" was only a remote possibility. Russell compared the Bender with the Halstead Battery to evaluate a brain-damaged patient and found two problems with the former test. Despite the presence of serious brain damage resulting in aphasia and difficulty walking, results from the Bender-Gestalt were normal. In fact, results from other single tests from the Halstead Battery with high statistical sensitivity to brain damage (Category Test) were also normal. Nonetheless, complete neuropsychological evaluation was able to document the presence of brain damage. A second disadvantage is even more of a problem for psychologists. This is the limited psychological information provided by the Bender. Like the EEG, even if it tells you that someone is or is not brain damaged, that is about all it tells you. On the other hand, *despite* the normal Category Test score, the Halstead Battery still arrived at the correct diagnosis. More importantly, *because* of the normal Category Test score, an important area of cognitive strength was identified in addition to a catalogue of deficits. In addition, rather than contributing incorrect diagnostic data (as it would have if used alone), the good Category Test performance in the context of significant impairment in other areas greatly contributed to an understanding of the type (static vs. progressive) of brain damage that was being dealt with.

Other commonly used tests measuring primarily visuospatial-constructional skill include the Visual Retention Test (Benton, 1963), the Memory for Designs Test (Graham & Kendall, 1960; McManis, 1974), and the Block Rotation Test (Satz, 1966;

Satz, Fennell, & Reilly, 1970). Satz (1966) provided an excellent discussion of the need to consider base rates for occurrence of the target condition in a particular clinical population as part of the overall validity of the assessment of any psychological procedure. A hit rate of 80% may seem impressive unless it is accomplished in a setting where 90% of the patients have that condition. Further, Satz noted that a test may seem to represent a single function when, in fact, it requires several abilities. A test that requires visual perception, motor manipulation, problem solving, and verbal memory could well be affected by brain damage which impairs any one of these areas or functions. Such broadband tests represent only a partial solution to the measurement requirements in assessing brain-behavior relationships. It is true that even a single but very broadband instrument might well be sensitive to a broad spectrum of psychologically impairing conditions, locations, and degrees of severity. This would greatly enhance its chances of producing a high hit rate. Unfortunately, for each gain in breadth there is a corresponding loss in specificity. This specificity is both neurological and behavioral. If several types and locations of brain damage will lower scores on a single test, these scores contribute not at all to a description that goes beyond presence or absence. Because the test requires several different abilities for its successful performance, it is often impossible to tell which one is deficient. This precludes the making of recommendations for environmental adjustment to aid in compensation, and it also suggests little specific by way of appropriate rehabilitation. Spreen and Benton (1965) published a list of 38 common and not so common tests for cerebral damage and evaluated their hit rates. They conclude, as most others have, that "there is little doubt that composite and weighted scores predict more accurately than single measures."

7. Brain Damage in Children

The behavioral consequences of brain damage for children are of interest to diverse fields including education, neurology, psychology, and psychiatry. The major scientific effort has been a series of attempts to determine whether particular behavioral excesses or deficiencies were due to "organic" disorders. Unfortunately for science but fortunately for the individual patients, children with hyperactivity, learning disabilities, or EEG abnormalities rarely can be subjected to direct brain examination. This situation leaves us with a hypothesis that if children without definite neurological disorder behave similarly to children with proven brain damage they must then have some (*minimal* amount) of that type of damage. This hypothesis makes assumptions about facts not yet in evidence. It assumes an already existing knowledge about the behavioral correlates of documented brain damage. Many data are yet to be obtained, and those which we do possess represent work so recent as to come well after the development of this hypothesis. This hypothesis also assumes a predictable (quantitative) continuum among behavioral effects of brain dysfunction, brain impairment, and brain damage. It, in fact, initially assumes a quantitative rather than a qualitative difference in the brain-behavior relationships of brain-damaged and non-brain-damaged children. The issues which must be addressed in investigation of childhood brain-behavior relationships are, if anything, even more complex than those involved in obtaining the same type of information from adults. In addition to all of the variables relevant to brain-behavior relationships in adults, we must add age at onset for children. Further, the interpretation of the results of any study must take into account an important source of normal variation: development. While development is a lifelong process, it is clearly an extraordinary factor during childhood. There are many questions, at least partially answered for adults, which have not been adequately studied in children. Does structural brain damage produce the same type of behavioral disorder as does a focus of electrical abnormality in the brain? Is lateralized structural defect likely to produce the same pattern of behavior as lateralized impairment not damaging brain tissue? Do differing degrees of brain damage produce a behavioral continuum? Can this continuum, if it exists, be expected to explain disordered and even normal behavior as simply lesser degrees of that seen in patients with actual brain damage? Questions of this nature must be asked about children for whom definite neurological criterion information is obtainable before conditions frequently associated with neurological dysfunction but not subject to neurological verification (learning disabilities, hyperactivity) can be demonstrated to relate to brain disorder. For this reason, discussion will be primarily restricted to behavioral correlates of children with documented neurological damage or disorder.

A careful but seldom cited review by Herbert (1964) discussed many of the commonly used single tests either designed for or converted to use in the diagnosis of brain damage. He concluded that the unitary concept of brain damage has little if any clinical utility. Many individual procedures have successfully separated groups of children with brain damage from groups with normal brain functions. No single test, however, has demonstrated its validity for clinical application to individual children. Nothing in the more recent literature leads us to quarrel with Herbert's conclusions or to alter them. A more recent review (Davison, 1974) provides a detailed listing of 45 tests yielding 79 variables commonly incorporated into neuropsychological batteries for use with children between the ages of 5 and 15 years. Davison's evaluation of these procedures as contributors to a battery rather than as single tests for brain damage is both exceptionally comprehensive and unique. He provides a description of tests that indicates which areas of human functioning they measure, what strengths and weaknesses they possess, and how they compare to other similar and different approaches. Davison's chapter represents the best single source for test selection with accompanying critical evaluation.

Two studies published almost concurrently with Herbert's (1964) review represent the foundation on which a majority of the recent work in child neuropsychology has been built. Graham, Ernhart, Craft, and Berman (1963) and Ernhart, Graham, Eichman, Marshall, and Thurston (1963) set out to determine whether brain damage produced a characteristic cognitive or personality deficit, a lesser version of which might be found among children whose failure in some area of adjustment could then be explained as due to a neurological dysfunction. This two-part study produced several significant findings that have been supported in more recent research. They found that children with definite brain damage were, as a group, impaired in all areas of cognitive functioning. However, no single test in their battery selected a substantial number of brain-injured children correctly. The battery correctly identified 72.7% of the brain-damaged group, with 10.6% false positives. A second finding was the large increase in task variability for the brain-damaged group compared to normals. This should not be surprising in a group of patients with heterogeneous severity, duration, and location of damage. Variability results from the expression across group members of different areas of particular defect with or without more generalized impairment. Brain impairment may also produce a decrease in attention and concentration, further enhancing the likelihood of unstable and fluctuating performance on tasks requiring either persistence over time or the screening out of irrelevant environmental stimuli.

Reed, Reitan, and Kløve (1965) demonstrated the use of a modification for children of the Halstead-Reitan procedures. This study has been replicated for children aged 5–8 by Reitan (1974b) and for children aged 9–14 by Boll (1974a). The results are quite consistent in demonstrating generally significant superiority of normals over brain-damaged children across a broad range of psychological functions. Each of these authors again stressed the need for a comprehensive understanding of individual strengths and weaknesses in order to understand the effects of brain damage on any single patient. While most of the variables separated the two groups at significant levels, none by itself was impressive in avoiding false negatives and false positives. Within any group of brain-damaged persons, many normal and above-normal abilities will be present. So too within many brain-damaged persons individually. It is the total interrelationship of performances that allows development of correct diagnostic inference and, more important, correct behavioral description and intervention guidelines.

An issue basic to interpretation is the similarity of effect of brain damage between adults and children. By way of generalization, brain damage occurring in an adult is most likely to impair abstract thinking, problem solving, and mental flexibility. These are abilities typically examined for in neuropsychological batteries such as that developed by Halstead and Reitan. Abilities demonstrating past learning and experience such as those tapped by the Wechsler Verbal Scale may remain relatively intact. Far from producing similar results, the effect of brain damage on children appears to be almost entirely the opposite. The single most sensitive test in the Graham et al. (1963) study was Vocabulary. In studies by Reed et al. (1965), Reitan (1974b), and Boll (1974c), the Wechsler Scales produced the greatest group separations. This is consistent with Hebb's postulate that type A intelligence is more vulnerable to brain damage. Children rely more on (type A) current learning and problem-solving intelligence than on stored knowledge for the day-to-day performance. For adults, the Wechsler reflects knowledge (type B) acquired through use of type A abilities in the past without necessarily implying that these abilities are still available for future cognitive growth. While low IQs can result from many nonneurological factors in children and adults, very good IQs go farther to indicate adequate current functions in children than they do in adults. There is a serious limitation on our ability to generalize understandings obtained from adults to the behavioral defects and strengths which characterize brain damage in children.

Kurt Goldstein (1940), studying adult patients, came to the conclusion that brain damage resulted in a qualitative change in the organism. Such a change would do more than lower ability level. It would change the manner in which people perceive problems and thus how they approach a solution. Reitan (1958a, 1959b) demonstrated that for adults the interrelationships of tests were quite similar in brain-damaged and non-brain-damaged persons, suggesting the possibility of differences in level but not in quality of approach to the tasks in question. Graham et al. (1963) raised this question for children and found a different pattern of functioning in the brain-damaged than in the normal children. Boll and Reitan (1972a, 1972b) utilized the methodology of Reitan's adult studies specifically to address this issue with children. Again, in contrast to the adult data, these studies found significant differences in the test interrelationships of the brain-damaged and control groups. Many variables such as duration of damage, type of damage, and severity may have been responsible for these differing results. The significant differences in style of thought seen at different ages during childhood and described so elegantly by Piaget (Flavell, 1963) and the developmental disruption and delay produced by brain damage, however, may indeed render these children qualitatively as well as quantitatively different. The fact that pattern of impairment may be tied to developmental stage was suggested again when differences in deficits produced by brain damage were found to depend on age of the children tested (Teuber and Rudel, 1962).

Despite the obvious variability within and between brain-damaged children, it is sometimes mentioned that brain damage produces such serious overall impairment that specific types of patterns of deficit experienced by such a child cannot be determined. This argument is used to defend a limited behavioral assessment on the assumption that deficit in one ability suggests deficit everywhere for brain-damaged children. However, in other populations such as those labeled as having minimal brain dysfunction, the opposite clinical assumption has developed. Frequently, learning difficulties are attributed to one relatively specific deficit. The most common of these deficits is visuoperceptual-constructive immaturity. This in turn has developed in part from the common practice of using tests of visuoperceptive expression or reception as measures of "brain damage" in adults. If brain-damaged children have perceptual problems, then perhaps children with perceptual problems without other evidence of brain damage can be logically inferred to have something wrong with their brains as well. Boll (1972) designed a study that would address this issue. Tests were chosen to represent major ability areas including concept formation (Category Test), visual perception (Block Design Tests), auditory nonverbal perception (Seashore Rhythm Test), tactile perception (Reitan-Kløve Tactile Form Recognition Test), and motor function (Finger Oscillation Tests). Each of these tests was performed significantly more poorly by brain-damaged than by normal children in this study. Despite this context of demonstrated overall deficit, the relative sensitivity of these tests to brain damage was found to vary significantly in eight of ten comparisons. The popular belief that brain damage produces perceptual problems above all else was not confirmed. Concept formation ability was found to be more impaired in brain-damaged children than was visual, auditory, or tactile perception or motor functions. In order of descending sensitivity following conceptual skill were visual perception, auditory nonverbal perception, motor functioning, and tactile perception. This study also demonstrates that, even within a significantly impaired group of children, psychological measurement can distinguish relative degrees of deficit.

An as yet unsettled issue is the likelihood that lateralized brain damage in children will produce Verbal-Performance splits on the Wechsler Scales similar to those found for adults. It is also important to know the likelihood that a Verbal-Performance split, when present, can be interpreted as reflecting differential integrity of the two cerebral hemispheres and possibly even actual brain damage. Partly because lateralized lesions within the cerebral hemispheres occur even less frequently in children than adults, the reseach required to adequately answer these questions has not been completed. Several studies reporting performance of children with non-lateralized brain impairment, such as epilepsy (Black, 1976; Boll & Berent, 1977), head injury (Klonoff & Paris, 1974; Klonoff & Low, 1974), and cerebral palsy (Annett, 1973; Kohn & Dennis, 1974; Reed & Reitan, 1969), have, however, found a high incidence of occurrences of Verbal-Performance discrepancies. Boll & Berent (1977) found that 39.9% of their sample had Verbal-Performance splits of 14 or more points. In addition, 85% of these differences favored the Verbal IQ. This tendency toward higher Verbal than Performance IQ among children with nonlateralized brain impairment was also found by Reed and Reitan (70%) and Black (85%). Black's (1974) head injury study, while not reporting percentages, indicated that Verbal IQ was significantly higher than Performance IQ in his diffusely damaged group.

Fedio and Mirsky (1969) found agreement between lateralization of temporal lobe epilepsy and direction of Verbal-Performance discrepancies in children between the ages of 6 and 14. However, in two studies of patients suspected of neurological disorder, lateralized EEG abnormalities were not reflected in corresponding VIQ-PIQ discrepancies (Pennington, Galliani, & Voegele, 1965; Rourke, MacDonald, & Daly, 1970). Because neurological disorder was only suspected, and in light of the uncertain relationship between EEG findings and brain damage or behavioral deficit, the patients in these two studies may have had lesser or no brain impairment in contrast to the subjects in the study by Fedio and Mirsky who had a documented neurological disorder. The presence of EEG abnormality provides less information and is even less reliable and valid from a psychological-educational viewpoint than it is as a neurological diagnostic tool. Hughes (1968) reported that 50% of children with behavior or school problems showed abnormal EEGs. However, Tymchuk, Knights, and Hinton (1970) found that such children with EEG abnormalities performed better on psychological measures than did children with similar problems but normal EEGs. Such paradoxical findings relating to EEG abnormalities represent far from an isolated example. Hughes (1968) found that learning-disabled children with abnormal EEGs did better on psychological tests than those with normal EEGs. Better response to remedial efforts was also found among learning-disabled children with abnormal EEGs. Morin (1965) found that stutterers with EEG abnormalities did better in speech therapy than did those with normal EEGs. EEG abnormalities were found to carry no negative prognostic significance in a mentally retarded population (Vogel, Kun, Meshover, Broverman, & Klaiber, 1969). These data suggest that EEG is not a useful diagnostic tool for behavior or learning disabilities or as a predictor of human performance in incidences of suspected neurological deficit. Neurological criteria of a more definitive nature are necessary in any attempt to understand brain-behavior relationships among children.

Patients with clearly lateralized physical neurological abnormalities (but conceivably generalized brain damage) were examined by Reed and Reitan (1969), Annett (1973), and Kohn and Dennis (1974). Children with right- or left-sided hemiplegia following birth or infancy-onset brain damage failed to show corresponding VIQ-PIQ splits. In another study, children with learning disabilities but without evidence or symptoms of brain damage were grouped according to EEG classification: normal, right hemisphere, left hemisphere, or generalized abnormalities. No significant differences between Verbal and Performance IQ corresponding to lateralization of EEG were found (Levin, 1971). The results of these studies suggest the need for considerable caution when approaching the interpretation of Verbal-Performance IQ differences in children.

VIQ-PIQ splits of 14 points or more can and do occur in patients with generalized brain damage but also occur in 18% of the normal population (Matarazzo, 1972). Children with lateralized brain damage are most likely to have extracerebral and subtentorial lesions, found least likely to produce Verbal-Performance splits in adults. The types of brain damage most common among children, i.e., epilepsy, head injury, and cerebral palsy, are rarely purely lateralized, and this may account for the absence of Verbal-Performance splits in many such patients. It may still be the case, however, that once brain damage has been established as present through other psychological or neurological measures the direction of a Verbal-Performance split will reflect the differential integrity of the two cerebral hemispheres. This may be particularly likely as the size of the split increases. This, too, represents a hypothesis to be tested. There are currently no data to support "magic" numbers such as 15- or 20-point Verbal-Performance discrepancies as indicating brain damage. Verbal-Performance differences, if used to indicate presence or absence of brain impairment and/or to indicate lateralization of brain impairment, are at least as likely to be incorrect and misleading as they are to be correct and helpful.

A factor which looms large in understanding the behavioral effects of brain damage in children is age at onset of the lesion. Kløve and Matthews (1974) found adults with onset of epilepsy during childhood were more impaired than those with onset during or after adolescence. Those who postulate that the brain is a plastic organ in early childhood, on the other hand, point to children who have undergone surgical removal of an entire cerebral hemisphere (hemispherectomy) and yet developed a full repertoire of cognitive abilities (Smith, 1972). Most patients appearing in clinical settings, however, experience less severe and more generalized disorders such as that produced by anoxia, trauma, or infection. Teuber and Rudel (1962) found inconsistent results depending on the abilities tapped when age at onset was varied. This important study indicated that variability across time within and between patients must be considered. They noted that brain damage may produce immediate effects which pass off after months or even several years. It may also produce permanent defects. Certain behavioral deficits may not appear immediately but appear several years after injury, at the time the damaged area of the brain is required to express itself. Boll (1973) also investigated the ability of the brain to learn and develop behavioral competence following brain damage which occurred after specified lengths of normal development. Children were placed into three age-at-onset groups: (1) Damage at or before birth. This period was chosen because of the frequent occurrence of brain impairment during this time. (2) Age 2–4 years. During these years, language is learned and consolidated, and brain damage here may specifically affect this ability. (3) Age 5–7 years. This period was chosen to include children who have enjoyed normal development of basic motor, perceptual, and language functions but who have experienced little formal education. If the child's brain is sufficiently plastic to allow reorganization of functions to nondamaged areas, the children damaged at birth should have had sufficient time to demonstrate this by age $7\frac{1}{2}$, at which time all children were tested. If, on the other hand, one would be advised to experience as much of life and learning as possible prior to sustaining brain damage, the 5–7 year age-at-onset group should have the advantage.

The results clearly favored the later- over the early-onset group for those abilities on which differences were obtained. Analysis of variance yielded results ($p < .01$) indicating that the 5–7 year age-at-onset group performed best on the Wechsler Intelligence Scale for children. This group also outperformed the brain-damaged-at-birth group on four neuropsychological battery variables (Color Form, Matching Figures, Progressive Figures, and Matching Pictures), but bested the 2–4 year age-at-onset group only on Color Form. Although ordering of absolute values showed that the later the damage the better the performance, the number of these differences reaching statistical significance was relatively small and included no motor or tactile perceptual tests. The WISC variables and those tapping abstract thinking and problem solving produced the greatest separation in these groups. The general clinical impression that early-onset, generalized brain damage is most functionally impairing received considerable support from this study.

The effects of head injury have received more careful psychological study than any other source of brain damage during childhood. By far the most comprehensive detailed and complete study was that conducted by Harry Klonoff and colleagues at the University of British Columbia (Klonoff & Low, 1974; Klonoff & Paris, 1974). They found a generalized decrement in psychological functions following head injury in children from ages 2 to 15. In children suffering brief loss of consciousness, only 13% showed decline in school performance. This group showed good recovery in deficit areas 1 year after injury. Children with more severe injuries and longer periods of coma (1 week or more) included 33% with IQs less than 70 and only one-third above 80 at 1 year after injury (Brink, Garrett, Hale, Woo-Sam, & Nickel, 1970). Brink et al. found that those severely injured children who recovered best sustained their injury after 10 years of age. Alajouanine and Lhermitte (1965) found no difference in recovery from aphasia in patients 5–9 years of age or 10–15 years of age. Two-thirds recovered in 6 months, with all showing recovery at 1 year. Klonoff and Paris (1974) found that younger children have more skull fractures, while older children show greater anterograde amnesia. Skull fracture, length of unconsciousness (coma), posttraumatic amnesia, and brain stem damage have all been associated with more significant neuropsychological deficits in children (Russell & Smith, 1961; Klonoff & Paris, 1974; Heiskanen & Kaste, 1974; Levin & Grossman, 1976; Levin, Grossman, & Kelly, 1976). Certainly no single behavioral deficit is produced by head injury, nor is one single pattern obtainable on any battery of measures. In fact, this variability in higher-level function, including deficit in memory, perception, and concept formation with typically lesser motor and sensory deficit, is the hallmark of this condition. Considering the multitude of variables involved, including the variety of types and severities of head injury itself, this should not be surprising.

Despite the need for additional study of aspects of children's brain damage such as type, location, duration, and age at onset, we can point to considerable validity for current batteries in reflecting neurologically determined behavioral patterns and deficiencies in children. The 49 tests described in detail by Davison (1974) used in various combinations in test batteries include the WISC, academic measures, motor and sensory tests, language and perceptual tests, and tests of complex problem solving, abstraction, concentration, and memory. Studies already cited using these batteries reported high levels of statistical significance and impressive hit rates for anoxia in children (Graham et al., 1963), for mixed progressive and static neurological disorder in children aged 5–8 (Reitan, 1974b) and 9–14 (Reed et al., 1965; Boll, 1974a), for head injury (Klonoff & Paris, 1974; Klonoff & Low, 1974), and for epilepsy (Boll and Berent, 1977). Children with school learning or behavioral problems without evidence of brain damage have been accurately separated from children with brain damage and from normals (Reitan and Boll, 1973). Other potential sources of brain compromise such as maternal pelvic size (Willerman, 1970b) and position of head during the birth process (Willerman, 1970a; Rosenbaum, 1970) have produced dependable behavioral alterations even in ostensibly normally functioning children. Conditions with direct or indirect implications for brain function and integrity such as Turner's syndrome (Kolb & Heaton, 1975), neonatal respiratory problems (Lievens, 1974), viral encephalitis (Sabatino & Cramblatt, 1969), and highly suspicious medical histories without definite diagnosis or etiology for current "questionable brain disorder" (Tsushima & Towne, 1977) have produced neuropsychological test performances that allowed for correct identification of impairment even when nontest clinical impression did not suggest such deficits.

8. Concluding Comments

The psychological and neurological complexity involved in attempts to produce valid and responsible services in the area of neuropsychology is hard to overestimate. Whether that service is knowledge advancement, patient care, or both, one's preparation for work in this area requires, as a baseline, an excellent background in clinical psychology, in addition to, quoting Reed (1976), "formal training in neuroanatomy, neurophysiology, pharmacology and neurology . . ." to which must be added ". . . a one or two year internship . . . supervised by a senior neuropsychologist." Rourke (1976), with even more vigor, warns against the use of a single workshop or reading list as preparation for clinical activities. "The egregious oversimplifications and downright errors which result rather routinely from such ill-advised efforts are legion." He, too, calls for a minimum of 1 year of intensive didactic training in neurological science and careful clinical supervision for persons already well-prepared in areas of psychometrics, psychopathology, development, and clinical assessment and intervention. Goldstein et al. (1973) demonstrated significant development of diagnostic validity for clinical psychologists after 15 weeks of systematic training and supervision. They demonstrated that even this minimal amount of experience, in conjunction with utilization of a carefully validated neuropsychological battery, allowed clinicians to significantly surpass in diagnostic accuracy the judgments made by far more senior clinicians who utilized traditional but less appropriate procedures (MMPI, Bender, WAIS). They hastened to add, however, that "simple statements as to the presence or absence of organic impairment are often irrelevant." If one's goal is strictly diagnosis, it is quite likely that neither the battery of tests nor the training period need be so long or so carefully constructed. If, however, one's goal is the understanding of the behavioral correlates of normal and impaired brain function with an eye toward clinical description of the patient in areas not covered by medical procedures, the requirements go up. If, in addition, one seeks to be able to generate hypotheses for educational, rehabilitational, and environmental reintegration programs, the current batteries cannot be too complete or one's training too comprehensive. As with so many specialties which have developed from a felt need among general practitioners for more specific training in an area of service, so too is neuropsychology emerging as an identifiable subspecialty. As the cadre of well-trained human clinical neuropsychologists increases and exerts greater influence on graduate curricula, the understanding of these procedures, and their availability to the general clinician, will, of course, increase. However, this area will always, to at least a certain extent, represent a specialty or subspecialty type of practice, as do family therapy, biofeedback, and psychoanalysis. Despite the fact that training in these areas is shared, in part, by all clinicians, there will also be those professionals recognized as specially prepared and equipped for certain tasks not routinely performed by every well-trained general clinical psychologist.

ACKNOWLEDGMENT

The author wishes to express his gratitude to Dr. Randy Finger for her critical reading of the manuscript.

9. References

Accord, L. D., & Barker, D. D. Hallucinogenic drugs and cerebral deficits. *Journal of Nervous and Mental Disease*, 1973, *156*, 281–283.

Alajouanine, T., & Lhermitte, F. Acquired aphasia in children. *Brain*, 1965, *86*, 653–662.

Andersen, A. L. The effect of laterality localization of brain damage on Wechsler-Bellevue indices of deterioration. *Journal of Clinical Psychology*, 1950, *6*, 191–194.

Andersen, A. L. The effect of laterality localization of focal brain lesions on the Wechsler-Bellevue subtests. *Journal of Clinical Psychology*, 1951, *7*, 149–153.

Annett, M. Laterality of childhood hemiplegia and the growth of speech and intelligence. *Cortex*, 1973, *9*, 4–33.

Archibald, Y. M., Wepman, J. M., & Jones, L. V. Non-verbal cognitive performance in aphasic and non-aphasic brain-damaged patients. *Cortex*, 1967, *3*, 275–294.

Bender, L. Visual Motor Gestalt Test and its clinical use. *American Orthopsychiatric Research Monograph*, 1938.

Bender, L. *Instructions for the use of the Visual Motor Gestalt Test*. New York: American Orthopsychiatric Association, 1946.

Bender, M. D. Perceptual interactions. *Modern Trends in Neurology*, 1970.

Benton, A. L. Review of the Visual Motor Gestalt Test. In O. K. Burros (Ed.), *The fourth mental measurements yearbook*. Highland Park, N.J.: Gryphon Press, 1953.

Benton, A. L. *The Revised Visual Retention Test*. New York: Psychological Corporation, 1963.

Benton, A. L. Differential behavioral effects in frontal lobe disease. *Neuropsychologia*, 1968, *6*, 53–60.

Benton, A. L. Behavioral changes in cerebrovascular disease. In R. P. Siekert (Ed.), *Cerebrovascular survey report*. Washington D.C.: Joint Councils Subcommittee on Cerebrovascular Disease, 1970.

Binet, A., & Henri, V. La psychologie individuelle. *Année Psychologie*, 1895, *2*, 441–463.

Binet, A., & Simon, T. Méthodes nouvelles pour le diagnostic du niveau intéllectuel des anormaux. *Année Psychologie*, 1905, *11*, 191–244.

Black, F. W. Patterns of cognitive impairment in children with suspected and documented neurological dysfunction. *Perceptual and Motor Skills*, 1974, *39*, 115–120.

Black, F. W. Learning problems and seizure disorders. *Journal of Pediatric Psychology*, 1976, *1*, 32–35.

Boll, T. J. Correlation of WISC with motor speed and strength for brain-damaged and normal children. *Journal of Psychology*, 1971, *77*, 169–172.

Boll, T. J. Conceptual vs. perceptual vs. motor deficits in brain-damaged children. *Journal of Clinical Psychology*, 1972, *28*, 157–159.

Boll, T. J. The effect of age at onset of brain damage on adaptive abilities in children. Paper presented at American Psychological Association, Montreal, 1973.

Boll, T. J. Behavioral correlates of cerebral damage in children aged 9–14. In R. M. Reitan and L. A. Davison (Eds.), *Clinical neuropsychology: Current status and applications*. Washington, D.C.: V. H. Winston and Sons, 1974. (a)

Boll, T. J. Psychological differentiation of patients with schizophrenia versus lateralized cerebrovascular, neoplastic or traumatic brain damage. *Journal of Abnormal Psychology*, 1974, *83*, 456–458. (b)

Boll, T. J. Right and left cerebral hemisphere damage and tactile perception: Performance of the ipsilateral and contralateral sides of the body. *Neuropsychologia*, 1974, *12*, 235–238. (c)

Boll, T. J., & Berent, S. Psychosocial aspects of coping with epilepsy. Paper presented at American Psychological Association, San Francisco, August 1977.

Boll, T. J., Berent, S., & Richards, H. Tactile-perceptual functioning as a factor in general psychological abilities. *Perceptual and Motor Skills*, 1977, *44*, 535–539.

Boll, T. J., Heaton, R., & Reitan, R. M. Neuropsychological and emotional correlates of Huntington's chorea. *Journal of Nervous and Mental Disease*, 1974, *158*, 61–69.

Boll, T. J., & Reitan, R. M. Comparative ability interrelationships in normal and brain-damaged children. *Journal of Clinical Psychology*, 1972, *28*, 152–156. (a)

Boll, T. J., & Reitan, R. M. The comparative intercorrelations of brain-damaged and normal children on the Trail Making Test and the Wechsler-Bellevue Scale. *Journal of Clinical Psychology*, 1972, *28*, 491–493. (b)

Boll, T. J., & Reitan, R. M. Motor and tactile-perceptual deficits in brain-damaged children. *Perceptual and Motor Skills*, 1972, *34*, 343–350. (c)

Boll, T. J., & Reitan, R. M. Effect of age on performance on the Trail Making Test. *Perceptual and Motor Skills*, 1973, *36*, 691–694.

Brain, W. R., & Walton, J. N. *Brain's diseases of the nervous system*. London: Oxford University Press, 1969.

Brewer, C., & Perrett, L. Brain damage due to alcohol consumption: An air-encephalographic, psychometric and electroencephalographic study. *British Journal of Addiction*, 1971, *60*, 170–182.

Brink, J. D., Garrett, A. L., Hale, W. R., Woo-Sam, J., & Nickel, V. L. Recovery of motor and intellectual function in children sustaining severe head injuries. *Developmental Medicine and Child Neurology*, 1970, *12*, 565–571.

Broca, T. Sur la faculté du langage articulé. *Bulletin de la Société d'Anthropologie*, 1865, *6*, 493.

Bruell, J. H., & Albee, G. W. Higher intellectual functions in a patient with hemispherectomy for tumors. *Journal of Consulting Psychology*, 1962, *15*, 281–285.

Burkland, C. W., & Smith, A. Factors in prognosis following cerebral infarctions and long-term neuropsychological studies following surgical excisions of focal cerebral lesions, cited in Smith, A.: Neuropsychological testing in neurological disorders. *Advances in Neurology*, 1975, *7*, 52–110.

Butters, N., & Cermak, L. S. Neuropsychological studies of alcoholic Korsakoff patients. In G. Goldstein and C. Neuringer (Eds.), *Empirical studies in alcoholism*. Cambridge: Ballinger, 1976, pp. 153–193.

Butters, N., Cermak, L. S., Montgomery, K., & Adinolfi, A. Some comparisons of the memory and visuoperceptive deficits of chronic alcoholics and patients with Korsakoff's disease. *Alcoholism: Clinical and Experimental Research*, 1977, *1*, 73–80.

Butters, N., Samuels, I., Goodglass, H., & Brody, B. Short-term visual and auditory memory disorders after parietal and frontal lobe damage. *Cortex*, 1970, *6*, 440–459.

Canter, A. The BIP Bender Test for the detection of organic brain disorder: Modified scoring method and replication. *Journal of Consulting and Clinical Psychology*, 1968, *32*, 522–526.

Cattell, J. Mck. Mental tests and measurements. *Mind*, 1890, *15*, 373–380.

Chapman, L. F., & Wolff, H. G. The cerebral hemispheres and the highest integrative functions of man. *Archives of Neurology*, 1959, *1*, 357–424.

Cobb, S. A salute from neurologists. In F. A. Beech, D. O. Hebb, C. T. Morgan, & H. W. Nissen (Eds.), *The neuropsychology of Lashley*. New York: McGraw-Hill, 1960.

Cottrell, S. S., and Wilson, S. A. K. Affective symptomatology of disseminated sclerosis. *Journal of Neurology and Psychopathology*, 1926–1927, *7*, 1–30.

Critchley, M. Arterio-sclerotic parkinsonism. *Brain*, 1929, *52*, 23–83.

Culver, C. M., & King, F. W. Neuropsychological assessment of undergraduate marijuana and LSD users. *Archives of General Psychiatry*, 1974, *31*, 707–711.

Davison, L. A. Current status of clinical neuropsychology. In R. M. Reitan & L. A. Davison (Eds.) *Clinical neuropsychology: current status and applications*. Washington, D.C.: Winston, 1974, 325–362.

DeJong, R. N. *The neurologic examination*. New York: Hoeber, 1967.

Dencker, S. J. A follow-up study of 128 closed head injuries in twins using co-twins as controls. *Acta Psychiatrica et Neurologica*, 1958, *33*, Suppl. 123.

Dikmen, S., & Matthews, C. G. Effect of major motor seizure frequency upon cognitive-intellectual functions in adults. *Epilepsia*, 1977, *18*, 21–29.

Doehring, D. G., Reitan, R. M., & Kløve, H. Changes in patterns of intelligence test performance associated with homonymous visual field defects. *Journal of Nervous and Mental Disease*, 1961, *132*, 227–233.

Ernhart, C. B., Graham, F. K., Eichman, P. L., Marshall, J. M., & Thurston, D. Brain injury in the preschool child: Some developmental considerations: II. Comparison of brain-injured and normal children. *Psychological Monographs*, 1963, *77* (whole No. 574), 17–33.

Fedio, P., & Mirsky, A. F. Selective intellectual deficits in children with temporal lobe or centrancephalic epilepsy. *Neuropsychologia*, 1969, *7*, 287–300.

Ferrer, S. *Complicaciones neurologicas cronicas del alcoholismo*. Santiago: Editorial Universitaria, S.A., 1970.

Fields, F. R. J., & Fullerton, J. R. Influence of heroin addiction on neuropsychological functioning. *Journal of Consulting and Clinical Psychology*, 1975, *43*, 114.

Fields, F. R. J., & Whitmyre, J. W. Verbal and performance relationships with respect to laterality of cerebral involvement. *Diseases of the Nervous System*, 1969, *30*, 177-179.

Filskov, S. B., & Goldstein, S. G. Diagnostic validity of the Halstead-Reitan Neuropsychological Battery. *Journal of Consulting and Clinical Psychology*, 1974, *42*, 383-388.

Finlayson, M. A. J., Johnson, K. A., & Reitan, R. M. Relationship of level of education to neuropsychological measures in brain-damaged and non-brain-damaged adults. *Journal of Consulting and Clinical Psychology*, 1977, *45*, 536-543.

Fitzhugh, K. B., Fitzhugh, L. D., & Reitan, R. M. Psychological deficits in relation to acuteness of brain dysfunction. *Journal of Consulting and Clinical Psychology*, 1961, *25*, 61-66.

Fitzhugh, K. B., Fitzhugh, L. D., & Reitan, R. M. Wechsler-Bellevue comparisons in groups of "chronic" and "current" lateralized and diffuse brain lesions. *Journal of Consulting Psychology*, 1962, *26*, 306-310.

Flavell, J. *The developmental psychology of Jean Piaget*. Princeton, N.J.: Van Nostrand, 1963.

Fritsch, G., & Hitzig, E. On the electrical excitability of the cerebrum. In G. von Bonin (Ed.), *Some papers on the cerebral cortex*. Springfield, Ill.: Thomas, 1960 (translation of German paper, 1870).

Furth, H. G. *Thinking without language*. New York: Free Press, 1966.

Gall, F. J. *Critical review of some anatomical-physiological works, with an explanation of a new philosophy of the moral qualities and intellectual faculties* (Vol. 6). Boston: Marsh, Capen and Lyon, 1835.

Galton, F. *Inquiries into human faculty and its development*. London: Macmillan, 1893.

Gardner, W. J. Removal of the right hemisphere for infiltrating glioma. *Archives of Neurology and Psychiatry*, 1932, *28*, 470.

Geschwind, N. Disconnection syndromes in animals and man. *Brain*, 1963, *88*, 237-295.

Geschwind, N. The apraxias: neural mechanisms of disorders of learned movement. *American Scientist*, 1973, *53*, 188-195.

Goldstein, G. and Halperin, K. M. Neuropsychological differences among subtypes of schizophrenia. *Journal of Abnormal Psychology*, 1977, *86*, 34-40.

Goldstein, K. *Human nature*. Cambridge, Mass.: Harvard University Press, 1940.

Goldstein, K. The effects of brain damage and personality. *Psychiatry*, 1952, *15*, 245-260.

Goldstein, S. G., Deysach, R. E., & Kleinknecht, R. A. Effect of experience and amount of information on identification of cerebral impairment. *Journal of Consulting and Clinical Psychology*, 1973, *41*, 30-34.

Goodglass, H., Quadfasel, F. A., & Timberlake, W. H. Phrase length and the type of severity of aphasia. *Cortex*, 1964, *1*, 133-153.

Graham, F. K., Ernhart, C. B., Craft, M., & Berman, P. W. Brain injury in the preschool child: Some developmental considerations. I. Performance of normal children. *Psychological Monographs*, 1963, *77* (whole No. 573), 1-16.

Graham, F. K., & Kendall, B. S. Memory-for-Designs Test: Revised general manual. *Perceptual and Motor Skills Monograph Supplement*, No. 2-VII, 1960, *11*, 147-188.

Granick, S., & Friedman, A. S. The effect of education on the decline of psychometric test performance with age. *Journal of Gerontology*, 1967, *22*, 191-195.

Grant, I., & Judd, L. I. Neuropsychological and EEG disturbances in polydrug users. *American Journal of Psychiatry*, 1976, *133*, 1039-1042.

Halstead, W. C. *Brain and intelligence: A quantitative study of the frontal lobes*. Chicago: University of Chicago Press, 1947.

Halstead, W. C., & Wepman, J. M. The Halstead-Wepman Aphasia Screening Test. *Journal of Speech and Hearing Disorders*, 1949, *14*, 9-13.

Harris, J. Depression and hysteria as symptoms of brain tumor. *Henry Ford Hospital Medical Journal*, 1965, *13*, 457.

Hartlage, L. C., & Hartlage, P. L. Psychological testing in neurological diagnosis. In J. Youmans (Ed.), *Neurological surgery*. Philadelphia: Saunders, 1977.

Haug, J. O. *Pneumoencephalographic studies in mental disease*. Norway: Scandinavian University Books, 1963.

Heaton, R. K. The validity of neuropsychological evaluations in psychiatric settings. *The Clinical Psychologist*, 1976, *29*, 10-11.

Hebb, D. O. *The organization of behavior*. New York: Wiley, 1949.

Heilbrun, A. B. Psychological test performance as a function of lateral localization of cerebral lesions. *Journal of Comparative and Physiological Psychology*, 1956, *49*, 10–14.

Heilbrun, A. B. The Digit Span Test and the prediction of cerebral pathology. *AMA Archives of Neurology and Psychiatry*, 1958, *80*, 228–231.

Heilbrun, A. B. Issues in the assessment of organic brain damage. *Psychological Reports*, 1962, *10*, 511–515.

Heimburger, R. F., & Reitan, R. M. Easily administered written test for lateralizing brain lesions. *Journal of Neurosurgery*, 1961, *18*, 301–312.

Heiskanen, O., & Kaste, M. Late prognosis of severe brain injury in children. *Developmental Medicine Child Neurology*, 1974, *16*, 11–14.

Herbert, M. The concept and testing of brain damage in children: A review. *Journal of Child Psychology and Psychiatry*, 1964, *5*, 197–216.

Hertzig, M. E., & Birch, H. G. Neurologic organization in psychiatrically disturbed adolescent girls. *Archives of General Psychiatry*, 1966, *15*, 590–598.

Hertzig, M. E., & Birch, H. G. Neurologic organization in psychiatrically disturbed adolescents. *Archives of General Psychiatry*, 1968, *19*, 528–537.

Hook, O. Comments on rehabilitation of the brain-injured. In A. E. Walker, W. F. Caveness, & M. Critchley (Eds.), *Effects of Head Injury*. Springfield, Ill.: Thomas, 1969.

Hughes, J. Electroencephalography and learning. In H. Myklebust (Ed.), *Progress in learning disabilities*. New York: Grune & Stratton, 1968.

Hutt, M. *The Hutt Adaptation of the Bender-Gestalt Test* (2nd ed.). New York: Grune & Stratton, 1969.

Kaldegg, A. Psychological observation in a group of alcoholic patients with analysis of Rorschach, Wechsler-Bellevue and Bender Gestalt Test results. *Quarterly Journal for the Study of Alcoholism*, 1956, *17*, 608–628.

Kleinknecht, R. A., & Goldstein, S. G. Neuropsychological deficits associated with alcoholism. *Quarterly Journal of Studies in Alcoholism*, 1972, *33*, 999–1019.

Klonoff, H., Fibiger, C. H., & Hutton, G. H. Neuropsychological patterns in chronic schizophrenia. *Journal of Nervous and Mental Disease*, 1970, *150*, 291–300.

Klonoff, H., & Low, M. Disordered brain function in young children and early adolescents: Neuropsychological and electroencephalographic correlates. In R. M. Reitan & L. A. Davison (Eds.) *Clinical neuropsychology: Current status and applications*. Washington, D.C.: Winston, 1974, pp. 121–178.

Klonoff, H., & Paris, R. Immediate, short-term and residual effects of acute head injuries in children: Neuropsychological and neurological correlates. In R. M. Reitan and L. A. Davison (Eds.), *Clinical neuropsychology: Current status and applications*. Washington, D.C.: Winston, 1974, pp. 179–210.

Kløve, H. Relationship of differential electroencephalographic patterns to distribution of Wechsler-Bellevue scores. *Neurology*, 1959, *9*, 871–876.

Kløve, H. Relationship between neuropsychologic test performance and neurologic status. Paper presented at the American Academy of Neurology, Minneapolis, 1963.

Kløve, H. Validation studies in adult clinical neuropsychology. In R. M. Reitan & L. Davison (Eds.), *Clinical neuropsychology: Current status and applications*. Washington, D.C.: Winston, 1974, pp. 211–246.

Kløve, H., & Cleeland, C. S. The relationship of neuropsychological impairment to other indices of severity of head injury. *Scandinavian Journal of Rehabilitation Medicine*, 1972, *4*, 55–60.

Kløve, H., & Fitzhugh, K. B. The relationship of differential EEG patterns to the distribution of Wechsler-Bellevue scores in a chronic epileptic population. *Journal of Clinical Psychology*, 1962, *18*, 334–337.

Kløve, H., & Matthews, C. G. Neuropsychological studies of patients with epilepsy. In R. M. Reitan & L. Davison (Eds.), *Clinical Neuropsychology: Current Status and Applications*. Washington, D.C.: Winston, 1974, pp. 247–266.

Kløve, H., & Reitan, R. M. The effect of dysphasia and spatial distortion on Wechsler-Bellevue results. *Archives of Neurology and Psychiatry*, 1958, *80*, 708–713.

Kløve, H., & White, P. T. The relationship of degree of electroencephalographic abnormalities to the distribution of Wechsler-Bellevue scores. *Neurology*, 1963, *13*, 423–430.

Knights, R. M. Problems of criteria and diagnosis: A profile similarity approach. *Annals of the New York Academy of Sciences*, 1973, *205*, 124–131.

Kohn, B., & Dennis, M. Selective impairments of visuo-spatial abilities in infantile hemiplegics after right cerebral hemidecortication. *Neuropsychologia*, 1974, *12*, 505–512.

Kolansky, H., & Moore, W. T. Toxic affects of chronic marijuana use. *Journal of the American Medical Association*, 1972, *222*, 35–41.

Kolb, J. E., & Heaton, R. K. Lateralized neurologic deficits and psychopathology in a Turner syndrome patient. *Archives of General Psychiatry*, 1975, *32*, 1198–1200.

Koppitz, E. M. *The Bender-Gestalt Test for Young Children*. New York: Grune & Stratton, 1964.

Korman, M., & Blumberg, S. Comparative efficiency of some tests of cerebral damage. *Journal of Consulting Psychology*, 1963, *27*, 303–309.

Lenneberg, E. H. *Biological foundations of language*. New York: Wiley, 1967.

Levin, H. S., & Grossman, R. G. Storage and retrieval. *Journal of Pediatric Psychology*, 1976, *1*, 38–41.

Levin, H. S., Grossman, R. G., & Kelly, P. J. Short-term recognition memory in relation to severity of closed head injury. *Cortex*, 1976, *12*, 175–182.

Levin, J. The relationship between lateralized electroencephalographic abnormalities and selected measures of intelligence and academic achievement in children with learning disabilities. Unpublished Master's Major Paper, University of Windsor, 1971.

Levitt, H., Sindberg, R., Massert, B., & Albaum, A. The laterality hypothesis assessment of localized brain damage. *Journal of Consulting Psychology*, 1966, *30*, 180.

Lezack, M. D. *Neuropsychological assessment*. New York: Oxford University Press, 1976.

Lievens, P. The organic psychosyndrome of early childhood and its effects on learning. *Journal of Learning Disabilities*, 1974, *7*, 626–631.

Lubin, B., Wallis, R. S., & Paine, C. Patterns of psychological test usage in the United States: 1935–1969. *Professional Psychology*, 1971, *2*, 70–74.

Luria, A. R. *Higher cortical functions in man*. New York: Basic Science Books, 1966.

Luria, A. R. Neuropsychological Studies in the U.S.S.R., Part I. *Proceedings of the National Academy of Science*, 1973, *70*, 959.

Malamud, N. Psychiatric disorder with intracranial tumors of limbic system. *Archives of Neurology*, 1967, *17*, 113.

Marie, P. La troisième circumvolution frontale gauche ne joue aucun rôle spécial dans la fonction du langage. *Seminaires Medicale*, 1906, *26*, 241–247.

Matarazzo, J. D. *Wechsler's measurement and appraisal of adult intelligence, fifth and enlarged edition*. Baltimore: Williams and Wilkins, 1972.

Matarazzo, J. D., Matarazzo, R. G., Wiens, A. N., Gallo, A. E., & Klonoff, H. Retest reliability of the Halstead Impairment Index in a normal, a schizophrenic, and two samples of organic patients. *Journal of Clinical Psychology*, 1976, *32*, 338–349.

Matarazzo, J. D., Wiens, A. N., Matarazzo, R. G., & Goldstein, S. G. Psychometric and clinical test-retest reliability of the Halstead Impairment Index in a sample of healthy, young, normal men. *Journal of Nervous and Mental Disease*, 1974, *158*, 37–49.

Matthews, C. G. Applications of neuropsychological test methods in mentally retarded subjects. In R. M. Reitan & L. Davison (Eds.) *Clinical neuropsychology: Current status and applications*. Washington, D.C.: Winston, 1974, pp. 267–288.

Matthews, C. G. Problems in the training of neuropsychologists, *The Clinical Psychologist*, 1976, *29*, 11–13.

Matthews, C. G., & Booker, H. E. Pneumoencephalographic measurements and neuropsychological test performance in human adults. *Cortex*, 1972, *8*, 69–92.

Matthews, C. G., Cleeland, C. S., & Hopper, C. L. Neuropsychological patterns in multiple sclerosis. *Diseases of the Nervous System*, 1970, *31*, 161–170.

Matthews, C. G., Shaw, D. J., & Kløve, H. Psychological test performances in neurologic and "pseudo-neurologic" subjects. *Cortex*, 1966, *2*, 244–253.

McGlothlin, W. H., Arnold, D. O., & Freedman, D. X. Organicity measures following repeated LSD ingestion. *Archives of General Psychiatry*, 1969, *21*, 704–709.

McManis, D. L. Memory-For-Design performance of brain-damaged and non-damaged psychiatric patients. *Perceptual and Motor Skills*, 1974, *38*, 847–852.

Meier, M. J. Objective behavioral assessment in diagnosis and prediction. In A. L. Benton (Ed.), *Behavioral change in cerebrovascular disease*. New York: Hoeber, 1970, pp. 119–154.

Meier, M. J. Some challenges for clinical neuropsychology. In R. M. Reitan & L. Davison (Eds.), *Clinical neuropsychology: Current status and applications*. Washington, D.C.: Winston, 1974, pp. 289–324.

Meier, M. J., & Resch, J. A. Behavioral prediction of short-term neurologic change following acute onset of cerebrovascular symptoms. *Mayo Clinic Proceedings*, 1967, *46*, 641.

Merritt, H. H. *A textbook of neurology, fourth edition*. Philadelphia: Lea and Febiger, 1967.

Meyers, R. Relationship of "thinking" and language: An experimental approach using dysphasic patients. *Archives of Neurology and Psychiatry*, 1948, *60*, 119.

Milner, B. Psychological defects produced by temporal lobe excision. *Association for Research in Nervous and Mental Disease, Research Publications*, 1958, 36, 244–257.

Milner, B. Laterality effects in audition. In V. B. Mountcastle (Ed.), *Interhemispheric relations and cerebral dominance*. Baltimore: Johns Hopkins Press, 1962.

Milner, B. Brain mechanisms suggested by studies of temporal lobes. In F. L. Darley (Ed.), *Brain mechanisms underlying speech and language*. New York: Grune & Stratton, 1967.

Milner, B. Visual retention and recall after right temporal excision in man. *Neuropsychologia*, 1968, *6*, 191–210.

Mirsky, A. F. Neuropsychological bases of schizophrenia. *Annual Review of Psychology*, 1969, *20*, 321–348.

Mjones, H. *Paralysis agitans*. Copenhagen: Ejnar Munksgaard, 1949.

Morin, S. EEG correlates of stuttering. *EEG and Clinical Neurophysiology*, 1965, *18*, 425–430.

Mountcastle, V. B. *Interhemispheric relations and cerebral dominance*. Baltimore: Johns Hopkins University Press, 1962.

Norton, J. C., & Matthews, C. G. Psychological test performance in patients with subtentorial versus supratentorial CNS disease. *Diseases of the Nervous System*, 1972, *33*, 312–317.

Ombredane, A. *Les troubles mentaux de la sclerose in plaques*. Paris: Presses Universitaires de France, 1929.

Parsons, O. A. Neuropsychology. *Current topics in clinical and community psychology*. New York: Academic Press, 1970.

Parsons, O. A. Neuropsychological deficits in alcoholics: Facts and fancies. *Alcoholism: Clinical and Experimental Research*, 1977, *1*, 51–56.

Parsons, O. A., Vega, A., & Burn, J. Different psychological effects of lateralized brain damage. *Journal of Clinical and Consulting Psychology*, 1969, *33*, 551–557.

Pascal, G. R., & Suttell, B. J. *The Bender-Gestalt Test: Quantifications and validity for adults*. New York: Grune & Stratton, 1951.

Pennington, H., Galliani, C., & Voegele, G. Unilateral EEG dysrhythmia and children's intelligence. *Child Development*, 1965, *35*, 539–546.

Pines, M. A renaissance researcher tackles a vital problem: can the brain renew itself? *Psychology*, 1977, *1*, 16–19.

Prigatano, G. P., & Parsons, O. A. Relationship of age and education to Halstead Test performance in different patient populations. *Journal of Consulting and Clinical Psychology*, 1976, *44*, 527–533.

Rapaport, D., Gill, M., & Schafer, R. *Diagnostic psychological testing, volume 1*. Chicago: Yearbook Medical Publishers, 1945.

Reed, H. B. C. Differentiated impairment on the Wechsler-Bellevue Scale as a function of type and laterality of cerebral pathology. Paper presented at the Midwestern Psychological Association, Chicago, 1962.

Reed, H. B. C. Pediatric neuropsychology. *Journal of Pediatric Psychology*, 1976, *1*, 5–7.

Reed, H. B. C., & Reitan, R. M. The significance of age on the performance of a complex psychomotor task by brain-damaged and non-brain-damaged subjects. *Journal of Gerontology*, 1962, *17*, 193–196.

Reed, H. B. C., & Reitan, R. M. Changes in psychological test performances associated with normal aging process. *Journal of Gerontology*, 1963, *18*, 271–274. (a)

Reed, H. B. C., & Reitan, R. M. A comparison of the effects of the normal aging process with the effects of organic brain damage on adaptive abilities. *Journal of Gerontology*, 1963, *18*, 177–179. (b)

Reed, H. B. C., & Reitan, R. M. Intelligence test performances of brain-damaged subjects with lateralized motor deficits. *Journal of Consulting Psychology*, 1963, *27*, 102–106. (c)

Reed, H. B. C., Reitan, R. M., & Kløve, H. Influence of cerebral lesions on psychological test performances of older children. *Journal of Consulting Psychology*, 1965, *29*, 247–251.

Reed, J. C., & Reitan, R. M. Verbal and performance differences among brain-injured children with lateralized motor deficits. Perceptual and Motor Skills, 1969, *29*, 747–752.

Reitan, R. M. Certain differential effects of left and right cerebral lesions in human adults. *Journal of Comparative and Physiological Psychology*, 1955, *48*, 474–477. (a)

Reitan, R. M. The distribution according to age of a psychologic measure dependent upon organic brain functions. *Journal of Gerontology*, 1955, *10*, 330–340. (b)

Reitan, R. M. An investigation of the validity of Halstead's measures of biological intelligence. *Archives of Neurology and Psychiatry*, 1955, *73*, 28–35. (c)

Reitan, R. M. The relation of the Trail Making Test to organic brain damage. *Journal of Consulting Psychology*, 1955, *19*, 393–394. (d)

Reitan, R. M. Qualitative versus quantitative mental changes following brain damage. *Journal of Psychology*, 1958, *46*, 339–346. (a)

Reitan, R. M. Validity of the Trail Making Test as an indicator of brain damage. *Perceptual and Motor Skills*, 1958, *8*, 271–276. (b)

Reitan, R. M. The comparative effects of brain damage on the Halstead Impairment Index and the Wechsler-Bellevue scale. *Journal of Clinical Psychology*, 1959, *15*, 281–285. (a)

Reitan, R. M. Impairment of abstraction ability in brain damage: Quantitative versus qualitative changes. *Journal of Psychology*, 1959, *48*, 97–102 (b)

Reitan, R. M. The significance of dysphasia for intelligence and adaptive abilities. *Journal of Psychology*, 1960, *50*, 355–376.

Reitan, R. M. Psychological deficits resulting from cerebral lesions in man. In J. M. Warren & K. Akert (Eds.), *The Frontal Granular Cortex and Behavior*. New York: McGraw-Hill, 1964.

Reitan, R. M. Problems and prospects in studying the psychological correlates of brain lesions. *Cortex*, 1966, *2*, 127–154. (a)

Reitan, R. M. A research program on the psychological effects of brain lesions in human beings. In N. R. Ellis (Ed.), *International review of research in mental retardation*. New York: Academic Press, 1966, pp. 153–218. (b)

Reitan, R. M. Psychological changes associated with aging and with cerebral damage. *Mayo Clinic Proceedings*, 1967, *42*, 653–673.

Reitan, R. M. The role of models in clinical psychology: The neurological model. Paper presented at American Psychological Association, San Francisco, September 1968.

Reitan, R. M. Sensorimotor functions, intelligence and cognition, and emotional status in subjects with cerebral lesions. *Perceptual and Motor Skills*, 1970, *31*, 275–284.

Reitan, R. M. Psychological testing in neurological diagnosis. In J. R. Youmans (Ed.), *Neurosurgery: A comprehensive reference guide to the diagnosis and management of neurosurgical problems*. Philadelphia: Saunders, 1973, pp. 423–440.

Reitan, R. M. Methodological problems in clinical neuropsychology. In R. M. Reitan & L. Davison (Eds.), *Clinical neuropsychology: Current status and applications*. Washington, D.C.: Winston, 1974, pp. 19–46. (a)

Reitan, R. M. Psychological effects of cerebral lesions in children of early school age. In R. M. Reitan & L. A. Davison (Eds.) *Clinical neuropsychology: Current status and applications*. Washington, D.C.: Winston, 1974, pp. 53–90. (b)

Reitan, R. M., & Boll, T. J. Intellectual and cognitive functions in Parkinson's disease. *Journal of Consulting and Clinical Psychology*, 1971, *37*, 364–369.

Reitan, R. M., & Boll, T. J. Neuropsychological correlates of minimal brain dysfunction. *Annals of the New York Academy of Sciences*, 1973, *205*, 65–88.

Reitan, R. M., & Davison, L. *Clinical neuropsychology: Current status and applications*. Washington, D.C.: Winston, 1974.

Reitan, R. M., Reed, J. C., & Dyken, M. L. Cognitive, psychomotor, and motor correlates of multiple sclerosis. *Journal of Nervous and Mental Disease*, 1971, *153*, 218–224.

Reynell, W. R. A psychometric method of determining intellectual loss following head injury. *Journal of Mental Science*, 1944, *90*, 710.

Rosenbaum, A. L. Neuropsychologic outcome of children born via the occiput posterior position. In C. R. Angle & E. A. Bering (Eds.), *Physical trauma as an etiological agent in mental retardation*. Bethesda, Md.: U.S. Department of Health, Education and Welfare, 1970.

Rourke, B. P. Brain-behavior relationships in children with learning disabilities. *American Psychologist*, 1975, *30*, 911–920.

Rourke, B. P. Issues in the neuropsychological assessment of children with learning disabilities. *Canadian Psychological Review*, 1976, *17*, 89–102.

Rourke, B. P., MacDonald, G. W., & Daly, R. M. The relationship of lateralized electroencephalographic disturbance to selected neuropsychological abilities in children. Ontario Psychological Association, 1970.

Rowe, S. N. Mental changes following the removal of the right cerebral hemisphere for brain tumor. *American Journal of Psychiatry*, 1937, *94*, 604.

Ruesch, J. Intellectual impairment in head injury. *American Journal of Psychiatry*, 1944, *100*, 480.

Russell, E. W. WAIS factor analysis with brain-damaged subjects using criterion measures. *Journal of Consulting and Clinical Psychology*, 1972, *39*, 113–319.

Russell, E. W. The effect of acute lateralized brain damage on Halstead's biological intelligence factors. *Journal of General Psychology*, 1974, *90*, 101–107.

Russell, E. W. Multiple scoring method for assessment of complex memory functions. *Journal of Consulting and Clinical Psychology*, 1975, *43*, 800–809. (a)

Russell, E. W. Validation of a brain-damage versus schizophrenia MMPI. *Journal of Clinical Psychology*, 1975, *31*, 659–661. (b)

Russell, E. W. The Bender-Gestalt and the Halstead-Reitan Battery: A case study. *Journal of Clinical Psychology*, 1976, *32*, 355–361.

Russell, E. W. MMPI Profiles of brain-damaged and schizophrenic subjects. *Journal of Clinical Psychology*, 1977, *33*, 190–193.

Russell, E. W., Neuringer, C., & Goldstein, G. *Assessment of brain damage: A neuropsychological key approach*. New York: Wiley-Interscience, 1970.

Russell, W. R., & Smith, A. Post-traumatic amnesia in closed head injury. *Archives of Neurology*, 1961, *5*, 4–17.

Sabatino, D. A., & Cramblatt, H. A longitudinal study of children with learning disabilities subsequent to hospitalizations for viral encephalitis. II. *Journal of Learning Disabilities*, 1969, *2*, 124–135.

Samuels, I., Butters, N., & Fedio, P. Short-term memory disorders following temporal lobe removals in humans. *Cortex*, 1972, *8*, 283–298.

Satz, P. A block rotation task: The application of multi-variate and decision theory analysis for the prediction of brain disorder. *Psychological Monographs: General and Applied*, 1966, *80*, (whole No. 629), 1–29. (a)

Satz, P. Specific and non-specific effects of brain lesions in man. *Journal of Abnormal Psychology*, 1966, *71*, 65–70. (b)

Satz, P., Fennell, E., & Reilly, C. Predictive validity of six neurodiagnostic tests: a decision theory analysis. *Journal of Consulting and Clinical Psychology*, 1970, *34*, 357–381.

Satz, P., Richard, W., & Daniels, A. The alteration of intellectual performance after lateralized brain-injury in man. *Psychonomic Science*, 1967, *7*, 369–370.

Schreiber, D. J., Goldman, H., Kleinman, K. M., Goldfader, P. R., & Snow, M. Y. The relationship between independent neuropsychological and neurological detection and localization of cerebral impairment. *Journal of Nervous and Mental Disease*, 1976, *162*, 360–365.

Schuell, H., Jenkins, J. J., & Jiminez-Pabon, E. *Aphasia in adults*. New York: Harper & Row, 1965.

Schwartz, M. S. Organicity and the MMPI 1-3-9 and 2-9 codes. *Proceedings of the 77th Annual Convention of the American Psychological Association*, 1969, *4*, 519–520.

Semmes, J. Hemispheric specialization: A possible clue to mechanism. *Neuropsychologia*, 1968, *6*, 11–26.

Shaw, D. J. The reliability and validity of the Halstead Category Test. *Journal of Clinical Psychology*, 1966, *22*, 176–180.

Simpson, C. D., & Vega, A. Unilateral brain damage and patterns of age-corrected WAIS subtest scores. *Journal of Clinical Psychology*, 1971, *27*, 204–208.

Smith, A. Duration of impaired consciousness as an index of severity of closed head injuries. *Diseases of the Nervous System*, 1961, *22*, 69.

Smith, A. Psychodiagnosis of patients with brain tumors. *Journal of Nervous and Mental Disease*, 1962, *135*, 513–533.

Smith, A. Verbal and non-verbal test performances of patients with "acute" lateralized brain lesions (tumors). *Journal of Nervous and Mental Disease*, 1965, *141*, 517–523.

Smith, A. Certain hypothesized hemisphere differences in language and visual functioning in human adults. *Cortex*, 1966, *2*, 109–126.

Smith, A. Dominant and non-dominant hemispherectomy, In W. L. Smith (Ed.) *Drugs, development and cerebral function*. Springfield, Ill.: Thomas, 1972.

Smith, A. Neuropsychological testing in neurological disorders. *Advances in Neurology*, 1975, *7*, 49–110.

Smith, A., Champoux, R., Leri, J., London, R., & Muraski, A. *Diagnosis, intelligence and rehabilitation of chronic aphasics*. Ann Arbor: University of Michigan, 1972.

Spreen, O., & Benton, A. L. Comparative studies of some psychological test for cerebral damage. *Journal of Nervous and Mental Disease*, 1965, *140*, 323–333.

Szasz, T. Lecture at the University of Washington Child Development and Mental Retardation Center, Seattle, 1972.

Tarter, R. E. Psychological deficit in chronic alcoholics: A review. *International Journal of Addiction*, 1975, *10*, 327–368.

Tarter, R. E., & Jones, B. N. Motor impairment in chronic alcoholics. *Diseases of the Nervous System*, 1971, *32*, 632–636.

Teuber, H.-L. Effects of brain wounds implicating right or left hemisphere in man: Hemisphere differences and hemisphere interaction in vision, audition, and somesthesis. In E. B. Mountcastle (Ed.), *Interhemispheric relations and cerebral dominance*. Baltimore: Johns Hopkins University Press, 1962, pp. 131–157.

Teuber, H.-L. & Rudel, R. G. Behavior after cerebral lesions in children and adults. *Developmental Medicine and Child Neurology*, 1962, *4*, 3–20.

Tooth, G. On the use of mental tests for the measurement of disability after head injury. *Journal of Neurology, Neurosurgery and Psychiatry*, 1947, *10*, 1.

Tsushima, W. T., & Towne, W. S. Neuropsychological abilities of young children with questionable brain disorders. *Journal of Consulting and Clinical Psychology*, 1977, *45*, 757–762.

Tymchuk, A. J., Knights, R. M., & Hinton, G. C. Neuropsychological test results of children with brain lesions, abnormal EEG's and normal EEG's. *Canadian Journal of Behavioral Science*, 1970, *2*, 322–329.

Vega, A., & Parsons, O. Cross-validation of the Halstead-Reitan tests for brain damage. *Journal of Consulting Psychology*, 1967, *31*, 619–625.

Vega, A., & Parsons, O. A. Relationship between sensory-motor deficits and WAIS Verbal and Performance scores in unilateral brain damage. *Cortex*, 1969, *5*, 229–241.

Victor, M., Adams, R. E., & Collins, G. H. *The Wernicke-Korsakoff Syndrome*, Philadelphia: F. A. Davis, 1971.

Vogel, W., Kun, K. J., Meshover, E., Broverman, D. M., & Klaiber, E. L. The behavioral significance of EEG abnormality in mental defectives. *American Journal of Mental Deficiency*. 1969, *75*, 62–8.

Watson, C. G., Thomas, R. W., Anderson, D., & Felling, J. Differentiation of organics from schizophrenics at two chronicity levels by use of the Reitan-Halstead organic test battery. *Journal of Consulting and Clinical Psychology*, 1968, *32*, 679–684.

Watson, C. G., Thomas, R., Felling, J. & Anderson, D. Differentiation of organics from schizophrenics with Reitan's sensory-perceptual disturbance test. *Perceptual and Motor Skills*, 1968, *26*, 1191–1198.

Watson, C. G., Thomas, R. W., Felling, J., & Anderson, D. Differentiation of organics from schizophrenics with the Trail Making, dynamometer, critical flicker fusion and light-intensity matching tests. *Journal of Clinical Psychology*, 1969, *25*, 130–133.

Watson, J. B. *Behaviorism*. New York: People's Institute, 1924.

Wechsler, D. *The measurement of adult intelligence*. Baltimore: Williams and Wilkins, 1939.

Wechsler, D. *The measurement of adult intelligence, third edition*. Baltimore: Williams and Wilkins, 1944.

Wechsler, D. A standardized memory scale for clinical use. *Journal of Psychology*, 1945, *19*, 87–95.

Wechsler, D. *Wechsler Intelligence Scale for Children*. New York: Psychological Corporation, 1949.

Wechsler, D. *The measurement and appraisal of adult intelligence, fourth edition*. Baltimore: Williams and Wilkins, 1958.

Wechsler, I. S. *Clinical neurology*, Philadelphia: Strauss, 1963.

Wernicke, C. *Der aphasische Symptomencomplex*. Breslau: Max Cohn and Weigert, 1874.

Wheeler, L., & Reitan, R. M. The presence and laterality of brain damage predicted from responses to a short aphasia screening test. *Perceptual and Motor Skills*, 1962, *15*, 783–799.

Willerman, L. Fetal head position during delivery, and intelligence. In C. R. Angle & E. A. Bering (Eds.), *Physical trauma as an etiological agent in mental retardation*. Bethesda, Md.: U.S. Department of Health, Education and Welfare, 1970. (a)

Willerman, L. Maternal pelvic size and neuropsychological outcome. In C. R. Angle & E. A. Bering (Eds.), *Physical trauma as an etiological agent in mental retardation*. Bethesda, Md.: U.S. Department of Health, Education and Welfare, 1970. (b)

Williams, M. The measurement of memory in clinical practice. *British Journal of Social and Clinical Psychology*, 1968, *7*, 19–34.

Wright, M., & Hogan, T. P. Repeated LSD ingestion and performance on neuropsychological tests. *Journal of Nervous and Mental Disease*, 1972, *154*, 432–438.

Yates, A. J. The validity of some psychological tests of brain damage. *Psychological Bulletin*, 1954, *51*, 359.

Yates, A. J. Psychological deficit. *Annual Review of Psychology*, 1966, *17*, 111–144.

Zimet, C. N., & Fishman, D. B. Psychological deficit in schizophrenia and brain damage. *Annual Review of Psychology*, 1970, *21*, 113–154.

Zimmerman, S. F., Whitmyre, J. W., & Fields, F. R. J. Factor analytic structure of the Wechsler Adult Intelligence Scale in patients with diffuse and lateralized cerebral dysfunction. *Journal of Clinical Psychology*, 1970, *26*, 462–465.

19

Diagnosing Psychosomatic Situations

CHASE PATTERSON KIMBALL

1. Changing Concepts in Psychosomatic Medicine

Since Franz Alexander (1950) gave prominence to the Holy Seven Psychosomatic Diseases, the field of psychosomatic medicine has come a long way. While Alexander's emphasis on essential hypertension, thyrotoxicosis, bronchial asthma, rheumatoid arthritis, peptic ulcer, ulcerative colitis, and neurodermatitis may have been inadvertent, it nevertheless established in the minds of several generations of physicians that these were *the* psychosomatic diseases, while implying that other diseases were not so or less so. Their designation as diseases in which psychological determinants could be identified implied that they could be treated by psychotherapy. Although there are some studies suggesting that some of these diseases at some stages in some individuals in specific circumstances can be ameliorated if not cured with psychodynamically oriented psychotherapy, there has not been overwhelming success with this approach (Karush, Daniels, O'Connor, et al., 1969). Alexander's work is perhaps more notable in his identification of other factors involved in the precipitation of disease processes. His emphasis on the occurrence of an environmental event proximal to the disease onset has been an invaluable concept for those of us studying and treating disease. It is a hypothesis that motivates much of the research in psychosomatic medicine and psychiatry today (Holmes & Rahe, 1967; Paykel, Prusoff, & Uhlenhuth, 1971). His further suggestion that the environmental event serving to precipitate disease reevokes latent, unresolved conflicts derived from early infantile childhood experience remains an intriguing hypothesis. The idea that the nature of the conflict has specificity for the specific disease process is more difficult to substantiate. Nevertheless, this suggestion has continued to intrigue researchers over the past quarter century (Engel, 1956; Nemiah & Sifneos, 1964).

CHASE PATTERSON KIMBALL • Department of Psychiatry, University of Chicago, Chicago, Illinois 60637.

Alexander's third postulate of the vulnerable organ has survived largely because of its adaptiveness to several interpretations. It is not clear whether Alexander intended to invest it only with a psychogenic explanation (i.e., an organ sensitized by an early psychosexual trauma), a developmental conditioning explanation (i.e., an organ tuned by intrauterine or extrauterine environmental factors), a Mendelian genetic construct, or all of these. In the first situation, the postulate is at least partly redundant or implied in the conflict specificity concept, i.e., the organ system affected is the one undergoing development at the time of the psychosexual trauma. This hypothesis has been proferred also by Garma (1960) and Grinker (1967) as an explanation for the similarities in personality traits in different individuals with similar disease processes. Dunbar (1954) gave the greatest popularity to the idea of personality specificity as the basis for psychosomatic disease. Her theory gradually gave way to Alexander's. Ironically, to a large extent the idea of personality specificity has gained popularity through the extensive investigations of Friedman and Rosenman (1969) and others. Previously Ruesch (1948) and more recently Marty and d'Muzan (1963), Sifneos (1974), and Nemiah and Sifneos (1970) have suggested a core personality for patients with so-called psychosomatic disease. Whereas the definitions of specific personality types in themselves appear useful, critics suggest that the spectrum of psychosomatic disease in terms of psychosexual theory is a broad one, with some diseases correlating with earlier defensive patterns and others correlating with later ones. Throughout much of Alexander's work was the idea that a specific psychological predeterminant related to the development of a specific disease process, in line with earlier psychosomatic considerations.

Earlier speculations anticipated Alexander in postulating a psychogenic basis for illness. Groddeck (1961), in an early extrapolation from Freud's theory, cavalierly saw all disease as a product of one's psyche. Deutsche, Thompson, Pinderhughes, et al. (1962), in more abstract terms, viewed all illness as modified conversion reactions channeled through the autonomic as opposed to the voluntary nervous system. Engel (1968), in a later consideration, has postulated a neurophysiological mechanism as mediating the reaction. Experimental proof for this hypothesis remains to be performed. Miller and DiCara's (1969) work through instrumental conditioning of animals has demonstrated that learned responses can be obtained in the autonomic nervous system in the same manner as in the voluntary nervous system, thereby giving potential support to the ideas of the above researchers.

Mirsky (1958) and Weiner, Thaler, Reiser, et al. (1957), however, picked up on the vulnerable organ concept, interpreting it as suggesting that a biological-genetic construct was the predetermining factor in the development of a specific disease under the right circumstances. Their work, although not replicated, has been suggested by others in work with other diseases (Voth, Holzman, Katz, et al., 1970). Engel (1962) has suggested a broader somatic predisposition explaining individual reactivity to an environmental event. He sees an organism's reactivity as polarizing toward active arousal and engagement or withdrawal. This scheme is at variance with Freudian theory (Freud, 1959) on one hand, where the major reactivity is angst, and Cannon's (1920) fight-flight reaction on the other, where the underlying mechanism is also one of arousal. Engel is closer to Gellhorn's (1967) idea of the turning of the autonomic nervous system along the axis of the sympathetic (active)–parasympathetic (passive) component. Such conditioning may relate to biological, genetic, intrauterine, or extrauterine developmental influences. These are specific biological patterns that determine the behavior manifested. The work of some of these investigators has led to the suggestion of reversing the psychosomatic sequence to a somato-psychic sequence. Others would complex this with a somatopsychosomatic sequence, and still others would attempt to incorporate into this formula an environmental (social) component.

In addition to the stress-illness onset researchers mentioned previously, the attention to the environment in which disease is precipitated has been pursued by others. Groen (1967) noted that individuals with previous psychosomatic diseases ceased to experience these during incarceration in concentration camps but reexperienced them upon return to similar environments and life patterns. Hinkle, Whitney, Hehman, et al. (1968), Shekelle, Ostfeld, and Paul (1969), and Kasl and Cobb (1970) have noted specific social phenomena correlating with susceptibility to specific illnesses, including coronary artery disease, hypertension, rheumatoid arthritis, and peptic ulcer, among others. Their works have lent themselves to a theory of social incongruity as putting an individual at risk for an illness. Specific factors such as job loss, moving, and other social changes have been identified as correlating with specific diseases, as well as with general disease. Other social factors influencing the manifestation of disease appear to relate to family structure and interpersonal relationships, as in the work of Don Jackson (Jackson & Yalom, 1966) and S. Minuchin (Minuchin, Baker, Rosman, Liebman, Milman, & Todd, 1975). Gaddini (1970) has noted major developmental differences in children reared in different social environments, suggesting a correlation of disease risk with failure to develop a transitional object. Intercultural investigations identify that infants at birth vary from one ethnic group to another in terms of arousal and neurological development (Friedman, 1974). Later development in terms of the capacity for abstract thinking is affected by the culture. This, in turn, not only may affect how disease is viewed and responded to but also may relate to its occurrence (LeVine, 1973). Several studies have identified changing disease conditions in ethnic groups depending on environments; e.g., Japanese in Japan have higher incidences of gastric carcinoma and endometrial carcinoma than Japanese in Hawaii, who in turn have higher incidences of these cancers than Japanese in Seattle, even when dietary and other ethnic patterns remain the same (Kuller & Reisler, 1971; Manusco, Coulter, & MacDonald, 1973). In the United States, the incidence of cancer is different in blacks born in the North than in those born in the South (Manusco et al., 1973). On the other hand, the incidence of deaths from cerebrovascular accidents associated with hypertension has decreased as deaths from myocardial infarction have increased in Southern-born black men, now approaching the incidence of these diseases in white men (Cassell, Heyden, Bartel, et al., 1971). One explanation advanced is that this change has occurred simultaneously as social roles and related habits have become more similar. On the other hand, Harburg, Schull, Erfurt, et al. (1970) have identified that a black living in what is considered as a high-stress environment in Detroit is at greater risk for hypertension than his first-degree collateral relative living in a lower-stress suburb.

Thus, as times have changed, proponents for a predominantly psychological determinant in disease have come to share this with those who stress biological and/or social factors as the predominant ones in disease. Few today would take a stand supporting a unitary explanation of a disease. Controversy is more likely to revolve around the issue of the relationship of these to one another. Further compounding an explanation of the etiology of disease has been the large increase in what I have called the language systems addressing behavior (Kimball, 1977c). Whereas biology spawned a large number of sublanguage systems between the Middle Ages and the late nineteenth century, the languages of the psychological and social sciences have only recently evolved and only recently been applied to the concept of disease and medicine. In turn, both psychological and social science have each spawned derivative language systems that have attempted to explain the same aspect or different facets of the same disease. For example, psychology has gone further than just attempting to find explanation for the emotions; it also addresses itself to cognitive development, learning theory, and matters of perception, memory, and attention. Sociology has given rise to anthropology as well as a number of subsystems within itself. Both of these have acquired cross-linkages with other social sciences and with the humanities, e.g., the field of psycholinguistics. And both have flirted increasingly with such linkages with biology, e.g., sociobiology (Wilson, 1975), bioethics (Potter, 1971), and psychobiology (McGough, 1971). We have, in short, rather than coming full circle, been forced to develop an increasing number of language systems in order to address the complexity of handling a more complex social system in its efforts to understand a natural world whose horizons continue to expand through exploration (Gamow, 1953) advanced through a new technology.

The extent to which these language systems will be incorporated or utilized by medicine is problematic inasmuch as professions in general tend to hold tenaciously to past traditions. These newer disciplines are more likely to cluster around medicine as satellites moving closer or farther away, as instruments of society, applying their specific orientations to medicine as societal needs dictate. In their own right, they may tend to gain an identity as a legitimate discipline as the pure sciences have done in the past. Similar to these, although they may form a cluster worthy of the name, the basic behavioral sciences of medicine will also exist independently. The exception is psychosomatic medicine, whose integrity rests essentially on a philosophical approach to medicine, i.e., a holistic, comprehensive, and multidisciplinary one. Whether or not medicine will ever wholeheartedly accept this approach or will give the same credence to its scientific methodology as it does to the older and more unitary secular approaches of physiology, biochemistry, and immunology is doubtful. Psychosomatic medicine may be doomed to remain as a thread through the history of medicine, pursued by a small group of curious malcontents attempting to integrate the current seminal thoughts of physiology and biochemistry with those of a number of emerging psychological and social orientations. My thesis is that the survival of psychosomatic medicine as a forceful, discrete entity in and of itself will depend on the development of a more complex and synthetic theory that will prove useful in generating the necessary interdisciplinary activity to obtain the supporting empirical data necessary to guarantee the constant refinement of this approach. In the remainder of this chapter, I shall discuss several of the directions that this evolution of theory has taken and may take.

2. Toward New Theoretical Approaches to Psychosomatic Medicine

Among the difficulties with the present theories forming the basis of psychosomatic medicine is their fixation in nineteenth- and early twentieth-century scientific theory. These include a preoccupation with (1) causality, (2) linear relationships, (3) two-dimensional models, (4) fixed relationships over time between correlated systems, (5) unitary conceptual models between systems, (6) the Alexandrian septet,

(7) limited conceptual formulations, (8) the central nervous system as the final common pathway, and (9) solely psychodynamic formulations as the psychogenic component.

I suggest that we redress or replace the issues (1) causality with concurrence, (2) linearity with cyclicity and ordered sequence with disordered sequence, (3) two-dimensional relationships with three-dimensional ones, (4) fixed relationships with ones evolving over the disease course, (5) unitary models with pluralistic conceptual ones, (6) the Alexandrian septet with all disease, (7) the need for new hypotheses and theory, (8) the central nervous system as a final common pathway, with itself also as an end organ, and (9) solely psychodynamic formulations with a general systems approach.

2.1. Causal vs. Concurrent Relationships

Preoccupation with a unitary explanation for causality may have been the curse of earlier belief systems, despite the attempts of St. Anselm (McIntyre, 1954) and later Descartes (1724) to put this issue to rest once and for all in the eleventh and eighteenth centuries, respectively. Nineteenth-century science also was obsessively oriented toward identifying a unitary model for disease in terms of a single agent (cause)–single disease (effect) model perhaps best exemplified in Koch's (1882) formulation. Medicine as a whole and psychosomatic medicine especially is still preoccupied with specific causes, although in almost every instance the idea of a disease defies a unitary explanation. The presence of a tubercle bacillus does not cause tuberculosis, although it may be necessarily related to the disease. It is even possible that, in time, the pathological process known as tuberculosis may appear in the absence of a tubercle bacillus (*cf.* sarcoidosis). A passive-dependent personality does not cause peptic ulcer disease, although it may be related to it. Nor does a specific social situation cause a specific psychological reaction, although in a specific culture there may be a high correlation between the two. Even when this frequency is ascertained, a causal relationship has not been defined or explained in terms of specific processes. At best, these relationships are co-relations whose exact relationship is unknown. Rather than speak of causality, it is best to identify social, psychological, and physiological factors that concur with one another rather than to always place them in a temporal relationship that causality implies. Specificity may come in time to identify the specific concurrent clustering of factors identified as psychological, physiological, and social.

2.2. Linear vs. Cyclical Relationships: Sequential Ordered vs. Sequential Unordered

Even when a temporal relationship in a social, psychological, or physiological sequence is established, too often it is in terms of a stereotyped sequence. Presently, the most usual sequence is one of a social phenomenon occasioning a psychological reaction which ultimately gains expression physiologically. Less frequently among psychiatrists but more frequently among internists, the stereotype is a physiological process giving rise to social disruptions resulting in psychological distress. This sequence is easily transmuted to behavior, with or without physiological accompaniments, arising from psychological turmoil resulting in social upheaval. A cyclical as opposed to a linear sequencing would allow for entry at any site, especially if the directions of the sequences were identified as going in either direction.

2.3. Three Dimensional vs. Two Dimensional

A two-dimensional system allows for the examination of a variable or the interaction of two or three variables at a single point in time. A three-dimensional model implies both a historical and a future time period in terms of that schema. In other words, the psychological process has a developmental anlage, as do the physiological and the social processes. The interactions depend not only on the present but also on the past, and may be determined by a projected future. Three-dimensional Venn diagrams are useful in conceptualizing this (Feinstein, 1967). In addition, this schematization allows not only for looking at the interaction of the three variables but also for looking at the interaction of any two of the variables independently of the third. Thus the psychosocial, the sociobiological, and the psychobiological can be studied separately for the purpose of simplification. However, where the three overlap, we best approximate the organism whose existence is conceived in terms of its biological, social, and psychological temporal dimensions.

2.4. Fixed Relationships vs. Evolving Ones over Disease Course

The time dimension in psychosomatic medicine has been largely ignored. This is especially so in our tendency to identify fixed relationships for psychosomatic diseases over time. In doing this, we lose sight of the fact that the organism may be in a changed psychological and biological state and in a different social milieu over time. Reiser (1970) has described this nicely for essential hypertension. The individual at risk for essential hypertension may at first demonstrate liability of blood pressure ranging from hypotensive to hypertensive levels on specific types of stimulation (Williams, Kimball, & Willard, 1972). This correlates also with liability of arousal and affect. At a later stage, the blood pressure, especially the diastolic, becomes fixed. Concurrently, the previous lability of affect and arousal is less observable. Instead, one is struck by what seems to be a change in perception in these patients in which there develops a screening out of noxious stimuli (Sapira, Scheilp, Monaity, et al., 1971). In a third stage, there are cognitive changes which are directly attributable to the effects of hypertension on the cerebrovascular system and/or other organ systems. A similar analogy can be made for diabetes mellitus (Selzer, Fajans, & Conn, 1956). At sequential stages of illness, psychological, social, and biological approaches different from those previously used are more suited in understanding and attending to what is occurring at that time.

2.5. Unitary vs. Plural Conceptual Models between Systems: The Problem of Language

When we add the social dimension or perspective to the formula of the psychological and biological ones, we complete the sacred triangle of civilization and replicate the difficulties that triangular relationships have posed in religion and the nineteenth-century novel, as well as in psychoanalysis. We also fall deliberately into increasingly blurred areas that require definition and a logic in their own right apart from the parent disciplines from which they are derived. This difficulty is infinitely compounded by the multiple subsystem of languages that have developed in each of the three spheres. Whereas we are more comfortable with a sense of integrity within the biological spheres than in the social (cultural) or psychological ones, this complacency is deceptive. There is little similarity between taxonomic biology and physics or even between Newtonian and Einsteinian physics. The broad social or cultural aspects have split into two distinct camps, the social sciences and the humanities, and the latter distinguish the fine arts from supposedly nobler ones. Psychology has almost as many subgroups as it has followers. Yet common threads are identifiable that bind the individual spheres more closely together internally than with the whole of another sphere, although from time to time the outer electrons of one may temporarily move more closely into the orbit of the other discipline, if I may use this analogy. What I am suggesting here is that, whereas an organ-physiological explanation may be more useful in conceptualizing a disease state at a particular point in time than a molecular biological one for the biological component of the interaction, a behavioral model may be more useful than a psychoanalytic one for conceptualizing the psychological component. Similarly, an anthropological or an ethical model may be more useful for conceptualizing the social model than a sociological or historical one. Whereas all of these approaches may have heuristic value for the explanation of behavior at one time or another depending on the situation, at a particular point in time one will have greater practicality than the next in the specific situation. This demands that the student of behavior have a broad acquaintance with the multiple language systems available, even though few people will have mastery of all of these. What is important is that the analysis of a problem does not suffer from the constriction of the individual's expertise. The latter should at least be able to identify what disciplines outside of his own area would be most useful in further studying the problem. In this sense, the psychosomaticist is a user of many languages and a general systems analyst.

2.6. Alexandrian Septet vs. All Disease

The influence of Alexander's seminal work with seven diseases has unfortunately left the legacy for many physicians that some diseases are more psychosomatic than others. Whereas it may be true at specific times in the course of a disease that a biological, psychological, or social examination and/or approach may be most pragmatic in attending to the situation, the psychosomatic approach implies that there are always psychosocial aspects to a disease process. Sometimes these are useful in identifying the situation in which a disease process is precipitated; at other times, they may assist in looking at reactions to disease processes at various stages of illness. Sometimes the emphasis may be on the psychogenic component, at others on the socioenvironmental, and at still others on the somatopsychic. Again, the emphasis in psychosomatic medicine is less on single causation and more on the interaction of the psychological, social, and biological at a specific point in time. The revised hypothesis of disease is one of the timely clustering of significant factors conceptualized in these three spheres. In time, it may be possible to give one or more mathematical coefficients to each of these components which would be necessary to result in a particular disease at a single point in time.

CHASE PATTERSON
KIMBALL

2.7. The Need for New Hypothesis and Theory

Personality and behavioral patterns as correlates of disease have enjoyed an untimely demise and an uncertain resurrection. There is something in the observation that individuals with specific types of biological processes have specific personality characteristics in common. But the attempts to suggest that all individuals with a personality type or a particular biological process are at risk for the same biological process or the same personality are deceptive at best. Experience demonstrates that as soon as we define one personality–biological constellation, we can propose and observe the obverse personality associated with a similar biological constellation (Bahnson & Wardell, 1962). Attempts to define a single core personality for psychosomatic disease belie several precepts. One is that our present definition of psychosomatic medicine includes all disease. Another is that, even if we limit our formulations to the so-called classical psychosomatic diseases, we note (1) that many of these individuals manifest distinctly different personality traits during periods of remission and exacerbation (Engel, 1956), and (2) that there are, in general, few similarities in the sophistication of defenses, cognitive styles, or arousal states between individuals with different classical psychosomatic processes, e.g., asthma and essential hypertension. I suggest that what we need to propose as the common psychological factor in similar disease processes is more complex and more elusive than our present theories suggest. On the one hand, we may need to postulate an "x" factor that we will use until we have the methodological instruments for empirical findings, and, on the other, to attempt to distill from our present observations the single common element. Physics is often cited as having most success in postulating a phenomenon which has in time become a self-fulfilling prophecy. Likewise, Mendeleev's chemistry (Seubert, 1895) and many of the early formulations underlying modern-day pharmacology and immunology were based on the hypotheses that led to further discoveries, e.g., drug receptor sites and antigen-antibody relationships. Perhaps what we need most in psychosomatic medicine is a "quark" or a "nark" (Kokkedee, 1969).

2.8. The Central Nervous System as the Final Common Pathway

We have become as preoccupied with the brain as the final common pathway for things of the mind as the Greeks were with the heart and its control of emotions. We overlook that the brain is also an end organ. In development, its growth depends on the stimulus of the environment, processed first through the mother-child unity and subsequently through the child's body.

Perhaps because we emphasize thinking as opposed to the believing of an earlier time in history, we have given proof or sustenance to our existence (Descartes, 1724) and have accommodated a transition from the supremacy of a deity to that of the central nervous system. The increasingly common belief of the central nervous system as representing the final common pathway of behavior poses a number of questions. It ignores responses that look as if they take place entirely at the periphery even if they are subsequently duly recorded at some higher level. It suggests that feelings arise from the cognition as well as the perception of senses. It ignores the James-Lange (James, 1884) suggestion that peripheral feeling affects how we act as much as and perhaps more than our brain does. The hypothesis is that, whereas the integrative central nervous system can process and coordinate derivative behavior, at one time or another, organism responsivity is at the local level, independent of central nervous system interaction. At other times, the central nervous system might be viewed as an end organ itself, e.g., in some of the degenerative neurological diseases, and in mental illness in which disease might be conceptualized as the brain taking itself as object, e.g., via an autoimmunological process.

The concept of a brain as an end organ in and of itself subject to peripheral events is an interesting one not only in terms of James's and Lange's theory of emotion, but also in terms of our own present preoccupation with the neurochemistry of the central nervous system. There is still much merit in the observation that it is difficult to define an emotion without recourse to its biological components. The biological components may be secondary to the ideation of an emotion or the source of its cognition. In the well-functioning individual, we see these two aspects of emotion as temporally concurrent. When they are not, we usually have a clinical problem on our hands.

The central nervous system catecholamine imbalances that we hypothesize as the basis for some behavioral disturbances are not necessarily the driving force of the latter, but a reflection of them. At this point, we would probably keep our thinking clearer if we saw these as concurrent events, as opposed to having a cause-and-effect relationship. If we were to use a chemical model, we would view these as equations capable of going in either direction based on a third factor, the presence or absence of one or more catalysts.

On another level, the brain may be seen as much as an instrument of the milieu externa as of the milieu interna. To a considerable extent, according to the behaviorists, the reactions that it coordinates are directly the result of that milieu externa. As such, the central nervous system, to the extent that it has been conditioned, may be viewed as an extension of the social environment. The central nervous system then directs the organism to do the bidding of the environment.

2.9. The Phenomenological Dilemma

The above argument brings us full circle. The last or composite difficulty in present-day psychosomatic thinking derives from our emphasis on trying to relate three or more conceptual approaches to a phenomenon as though each one were a concrete object in and of itself. The only concrete objects in our system, I suppose, are the event, and ourselves as observer. All else is merely systems by which we view and approach the event from the basis of our specific orientations. For convenience, we have loosely clumped a large number of systems in the spheres of biological, psychological, and social, allowing multiple subsystems to each. These are artifacts. They exist only to the extent to which they are useful in our attempts to assure ourselves that there is an order in the universe. They are useful to the extent to which they facilitate the extension of the theory based on empirical observation, usually indirect, that a factual thing actually exists to support the theory. To a larger extent, our observations of an event rest on the biases of our approach. When we are viewing behavior, we use one approach or another to explain it. These approaches are directed at the same event. They are in essence a description of the event in the different terminology of a specific thought system. The correlations that we identify between these two thought systems are based on the new languages that we are developing and that attempt to give fuller and unitary explanation to the event under observation. While we are in this transitional process, we are caught in our correlations of correlating the two or more descriptions and explanations of a thing with one another. It is no startling fact, according to Euclidean geometry, that each of two things similar to a third thing is similar to each other. In other words, it seems to me that so many of our correlations mean little more than that we are describing the same event from different perspectives of different language systems. While this view does not denigrate the value of the correlation, it should at least cause us some humility in attempting to postulate causal relationships between the different aspects of an event viewed concurrently in time.

3. Diagnosing Psychosomatic Disease Disorders

3.1. The Environments of Illness

With the foregoing as background, we need for the moment to take stock of where we are in the psychosomatic field. We have identified that this is an approach to clinical medicine in the broadest sense. We have applied terms such as "holistic," "comprehensive," "total," "psychosomatic," "psychosocial," "somatopsychic," "sociopsychosomatic," and, if you would, more recently, "primary care"—all, I suppose, in an attempt to deemphasize the technological and mechanistic approaches of a "scientific," biophysiological and biochemical medicine rendered especially in the acute situation, namely the hospital, the cathedral of technological supremacy and excellence. This is the training place of our young, and, if we ignore the probable importance of early developmental processes on future practices, later attempts to counteract the earlier emphasis will go unheeded. What we do in these arenas, therefore, may be crucial in terms of our interest in proselytizing our young to at least a broader consideration of the dimensions of illness and to multiple language systems that may be applied in approaching and treating it (Kimball, 1977c).

From one standpoint at least, our task is improbable and perhaps insurmountable. We are on the scene at an untimely sequence in the spectrum of illness, the acute phase, the tip of the iceberg which, for the teaching hospital physician, is so much if not the whole practice of medicine. The acute phase may be seen as the dramatic center stage in which the clashes of pathophysiological processes occur. It is not that these are without their emotional correlates or antecedents and precedents of future emotional difficulties, but it is hardly the time for us to take front stage center as the major actor on the stage of life. In this setting, it is true, we have found lesser, albeit occasionally dramatic roles to play. This is especially so in terms of our skilled observational processes which help us assess from the wings the dramatic interactions of the leading players and the environments in which they perform. Our eyes are wide and our ears open. It is by working in these arenas, especially those of the coronary care, intensive care, burn, hemodialysis, substance abuse, and emergency units, that we have recorded so much of the process of illness in its most acute phase and with which we have filled the volumes composing the literature of consultation-liaison medicine and psychiatry over the past quarter century. It is true that, from time to time, we have played more of a role in terms of crises involving major alterations of consciousness and the behaviors associated with these interesting states. Especially our attention to the environment of care and the interactions between the staff and patients and their families have led in some places to greater understanding and some remedial attempts by our colleagues attending to these situations. This has been most satisfactory when one of us has joined such a unit for a major part of our professional activity as a full-fledged attending on the service, rubbing shoulders daily in the pits, so to speak. And to a considerable extent, if only because of their uniqueness and the drama that occurs in these arenas, they have become exciting locations, if not overwhelming, for sensitizing our younger colleagues to their social and psychological correlates.

Perhaps more should be said regarding teaching in these units, because the student's initial experience may not be unlike that of the patient. What is taken advantage of here for the student is the foreignness and uniqueness of this environment. It is something most students have never felt before, even if a television version has been imprinted over the years. They cannot help being overwhelmed, and while, in one sense, they are confused in their attempt to orient themselves, they necessarily record observations and offer explanations that are occasionally insightful and contributory to the more jaded eyes and ears of those of us familiar with these units. Occasionally, a student may structure these percepts in the form of a hypothesis and make more systematic observations in an attempt to support it. But more important may be the student's experience of his own emotion, beginning with the anxiety over this seemingly disordered environment and the confusion it communicates to him. Such a communicated experience may be used to suggest that this might be somewhat akin to the experience of the patient. Or, on the other hand, a blasé manifestation of imperturbability might be identified incredulously as denial by another student in the group, and thus discussed as one of the defenses by which patients may counter their overwhelming feelings of anxiety, sadness, anger, and despair. Another student may verbalize considerable criticism of the unit and identify a need to do something about it, perhaps too soon attempting to overcome and ignore his feelings for action, a frequent characteristic of the physician. Others may simply leave, unable to cope with unstated feelings. The student's uncertainty about the environment gradually extends to and includes his uncertainty about the patient and illness and, of course, his own sense of impotence to do anything. Again, there is a point in the transaction to wonder whether this might not be similar to what the patient feels, and may even explain some of the behavior we will subsequently identify in the patient.

Later, in the surveillance of rehabilitation units and their often chronic populations, we can help the student get in touch with his own feelings of pathos and despair, perhaps the very ones that he may be attempting to overcome by becoming a physician. In these units, the time frame is different. Change may be imperceptible. The qualities necessary are those of patience, a capacity for hope, endurance, constancy. There is also the need for new and vigorous interdisciplinary research around the problems of patients with chronic disabilities. Since the incapacities from these processes are markedly different, this research needs to be performed by individuals who take the time to become totally familiar with these conditions as well as with the individual patients. Several studies which were done some time ago are still good starting points for the clinician-therapist who would study new populations: Visotsky, Hamburg, Goss, and Lebovits's (1961) work with victims of poliomyelitis; Hamburg, Hamburg, and deGoza's (1953) work with severely burned patients; Pratt's (1906) work with tuberculosis patients; and the work of many individuals with patients undergoing chronic hemodialysis. But there are also new and more extensive investigations required for follow-up studies of patients with chronic cardiac, pulmonary, neurological, endocrine, orthopedic, and other problems where the assessment of the psychosocial parameters has been poorly or inadequately made in terms of the staggering morbidity figures available for these illnesses.

3.2. The Precursors of Illness

On the other end of the illness spectrum, it is surprising to what extent medicine in general continues to ignore investigation of the precursors of illness and the relationship of early developmental factors to these, despite the increasingly numerous correlations of stressful life situations with illness onset. Because specific mechanisms explaining these correlations are not immediately forthcoming, we remain suspicious and aloof from accepting these identifications. Despite the great impetus that psychoanalytic studies, cognitive psychology, and ethology have contributed to our understanding of derivative behavior, we pay little attention to even identifying factors of early development, physiologically or psychologically conceptualized, that may relate both to the development of a specific illness in later life and to patterns of behavioral reaction to that illness. True, such research is difficult and requires commitment and perseverance to longitudinal studies in difficult mobile populations in order to realize results (Kellam, Branch, Agrawal, & Ensminger, 1975). More important, the investment in such research needs to be attended by imaginative theoretical speculation and meticulously shaped hypotheses for which observational methodologies are available. Retrospective analyses obtained by detailed anamneses are still respectable approaches, especially as hypotheses-generating activities. This is a fundamental step that few clinical investigators experience in the course of their studies. Rather, they jump into the middle of someone else's research, in time taking off from there, without even getting involved with the evolution of the idea or their own primordial imperative "why" of pursuit. Without some subjectivity in this regard, it is problematic whether maximum objectivity can be attained.

At this point, I would remind the reader that the diagnosis and therapy of psychosomatic disorders lie first with approaches. Inherent to this approach is that there is no such thing as a psychosomatic disorder. All illness is psychosomatic inasmuch as it can be approached from the orientations of biology, psychology, and sociology.

Second, inherent in the idea of the psychosomatic approach is the process of finding out, of investigating. The psychosomatic approach is quite akin to good detective work. The work of the investigator is to accumulate the data, the pieces of the puzzle, until they fit together in a way that gives a satisfactory picture, a solution to the problem. This is in contradistinction to the idea that the same "psychosomatic" formula can be applied to every individual with the same problem. Each patient with a problem in which a psychosomatic approach is used becomes essentially a unique study in the factors and their relationships affecting that patient's illness. These facts obtained from the patient become and belong to an abstract view of the patient and as such are apart from the patient. Similarly, the pattern of interrelationships that are derived is also abstract. Their value for the patient lies only in their pragmatic worth in assisting the patient with his problem. Their value for the physician or other members of the health team lies in their ability to convey a sense of integration and synthesis, based on similarities (as opposed to identicalities), allowing us to develop hypotheses useful in approaching patients and their problems. Our theories are not formulas to be applied directly to a problem at hand. Our one-to-one correlations are specious, perhaps at most short-hand approaches to acknowledging sets of linkages and associations whose explanations may be forthcoming at a considerable period in the future. They are useful at the present only to suggest that patterns of relationships exist.

Third, closely allied to the investigational aspects of the psychosomatic approach is its communicative one, namely teaching (Kimball, 1973a, 1977d). The psychosomatic approach is a *way* of approaching health and illness, allowing in sequence but temporally at once, both analytic and synthetic functions in the process of understanding an illness experience. Thus we use analytic approaches to focus selectively on aspects of the illness problem and synthetic approaches to bring these selective approaches into an understandable correlation with one another. The difficulties that are inherent, especially in the synthetic aspects of this process, have been suggested in the second part of this discussion. Our teaching function is that of communicating both the analytic methods and the synthetic models utilized in viewing the illness of experience to our students and colleagues in the health research and caring sectors. As good teachers, we teach, not conclusions, but processes and hypotheses for our students to test out. Also, as teachers, it is incumbent on us to know that which we would teach. In medicine, that is the patient. There is no substitute for the consulting psychiatrist or medical-psychiatric liaison physician to know at first hand through clinical experience and research the patient population he consults on and teaches about. Knowing includes sophistication with the pathophysiological process, the specific diagnostic-therapeutic approaches, and the environments in which the patient is treated, as well as the psychological and other social dimensions related to the patient apart from the specific illness.

3.3. The Spectrum of Illness

Returning to the specific phenomena that characterize the newer approaches to psychosomatic medicine and the medical-psychiatric liaison activities, we can now focus more specifically on aspects of the illness experience. In this section, we shall address the spectrum of illness, early predilections, early illness experience, precursors of the present illness experience, the illness-onset situation, the phases of illness (acute, convalescent, rehabilitative), the aftermath of illness, the environments of illness, personality variables affecting illness, and aspects of coping and adaptation.

In Figure 1, we observe a schematic linear presentation of an individual's life and illness experiences. At the time we usually first see the patient, he or she is somewhere far along this spectrum, most usually in an acute process. It is around this process that we first relate with the patient. We then move back and forth along this linear schema, following the patient's lead, meanwhile filling in the pertinent factors as they emerge in terms of our relationship with the patient. Each ensuing interview will contribute more data which will add, amend, or emend previous information obtained for the different life stages. Ultimately, we shall have constructed a life chart for that individual which should contribute to an integrative understanding of the relationship of these various events in the patient's life, specifically to where he or she is at this point in time and may be at some subsequent point in time. In this chapter, it is convenient to present these data from the earlier to the present to the

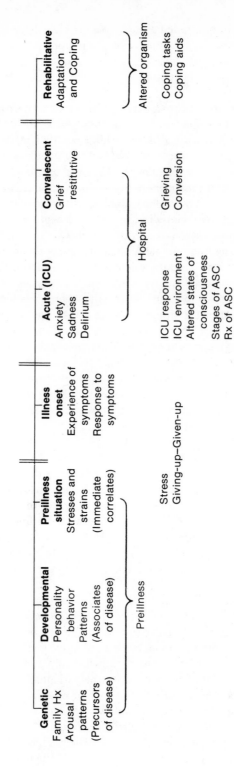

Figure 1. The stages of illness.

projected future, although obviously they cannot be optimally obtained in this manner.

3.4. Developmental Factors in Illness

We are interested in whatever genetic factors are known or may be suspected from descriptions of the patient's/family's past. I am using the term "genetic" in its broadest sense here to suggest that we cannot always be certain that this conforms to a Mendelian model of genetic inheritance or to some other basis of familial transmission such as the intrauterine conditioning of organ systems or postnatal learning experience. Specifically, we may find evidence for depressive illness, cardiovascular reactions, or ulcerative colitis that run through a family history and that certainly will orient us to look for this process in our patient. We will also take account of the generational family sequence in which our patient exists, e.g., in terms of migration and ascendency on a sociocultural ladder. This will give us some ideas as to the intrafamilial generational diatheses that may have occurred, affecting our patient's early development. We would assume that the child, particularly the first-born, of non-English-speaking parents adhering to another culture's way and unsophisticated in the ways of the new culture, would be exposed to situations for which he would have been less prepared than a child born of one or more generations familiar and secure with the cultural patterns of the contemporary culture. We would hypothesize that the presentation of novel situations for which the individual has not been exposed would be more stressful for that individual. Thus discontinuities and/or incongruities between generations on the basis of migration or rapid changes in culture (industrialization or war) or what might be identified as generational gaps (e.g., when a child is reared by grandparents as opposed to parents) may result in that child's being exposed to potentially more stress in development than his or her average contemporary. These differences will particularly affect the earliest years of growth and differentiation.

3.5. Cultural Aspects of Illness

Observational experience suggests that families at different stages of generational development within a culture may manifest and experience illness differently. For example, it appeared to those of us working with Puerto Rican families migrating to New York in the 1950s that classical conversion processes were common while, among their children, we became aware of the high prevalence of the psychosomatic processes of Franz Alexander, especially asthma and ulcerative colitis. It has been my similar experience in viewing Navaho Indians over a 10-year period of rapid acculturation that there is at least a changing manifestation of illness. For instance, among recently bereft widows, there appears a high incidence of clinic visits for complaints for which clear-cut pathophysiological processes are difficult to identify. An investigation of these individuals suggests that they have failed to go through what we would call a normal grieving period, but rather have endured an abortive one "legislated" by the Navaho way, traditional for an older generation that lived in different associations and patterns with one another. Although these observations and others need to be more fully documented and investigated, they suggest to the clinician-investigator possible factors to be sensitive to in exploring a patient's history. It is of interest to further reflect on the changing spectrum of illness that we have experienced in the University hospital during the past several decades. Not too long ago, when I wished to present one of Alexander's Holy Seven psychosomatic processes to students, I had no difficulty in finding several patients with thyrotoxicosis, gross hypothyroidism, or newly active peptic ulcer disease on any of several medical units in the University hospital. Such is no longer the case. Rather, we are relying more and more on the presentation of cardiovascular, arthritis, and chronic pulmonary processes to demonstrate clinical psychosomatic illness. The reality of this shift needs to be fully documented. We are, however, reminded of the shift that occurs in illness processes in some relatively intact ethnic groups as migration occurs and/or as major social changes happen. Japanese migrating from Japan to Hawaii have an incidence of several disease processes more like Western patterns. For example, the incidence of endometrial carcinoma decreases as the incidence of cervical carcinoma increases. This difference is even greater for Japanese who have migrated to the Seattle area. These differences exist despite an absence of change in many aspects of the dietary or other social forms. Within Japan itself, there has been a decrease in cerebrovascular disease, while there has been an almost compensatory increase in cardiovascular, specifically coronary artery, disease. A similar pattern has been observed in Southern blacks, who in recent years have come to show statistics in these processes more like those of Southern whites, i.e., a decrease in cerebrovascular disease with an increase in cardiovascular disease. Observational data suggest that this may relate to changes in behavioral activities and social codes other than dietary ones. These and other epidemiological findings suggest potentially rich areas for investigators to home in on and seek out specific psychosocial factors that may correlate with these shifts.

One further observation regarding conversion processes deserves mention. It is so rare to find "classical" conversion processes in our Northern hospitals that it is not unusual to find this phenomenon disavowed by neurologists and even by an increasing number of psychiatrists. A single visit to medical centers in Kentucky and Tennessee, at least, will rapidly convince the most reluctant and hesitant doubter of the existence of these processes. There, neurologists proudly display individuals afflicted with these paralyses. These are mostly individuals from the Appalachian hills who are members of clans in which incest and snake handling are common.

3.6. Organ Specificity and Illness

There are other early developmental factors that may be identified. One is struck by the investigations of several researchers involving seemingly fixed patterns of responses already present at birth (Bridger, 1962). Challenged by the sound of a bell, one neonate will show a response in a single organ system, such as increased or decreased heart rate, while in another the response may be increased or decreased respiration. A third may show a reaction in a different system. On subsequent ringing of the bell, not only does the reaction observed occur in the same organ system but also the increment or decrement of the response remains constant. While one may question to what extent a chance response is reinforced by the repeated challenge, it does not detract from the idea of specific patterns of responses to stimuli being present at birth and remaining constant thereafter. Further extrapolation from this observation raises the intriguing question as to what extent this specific organ system is "tuned" prenatally by Mendelian genetic factors and/or maternal behavior. In regard to the latter, we have learned that a variety of factors directly affect prenatal development and natal behavior, including maternal age, socioeconomic class, eating and smoking behavior, and specific illness.

Whatever the source of influences leading to the tuning of specific organ-system patterns, we can raise a number of suppositions regarding these influences and post-natal behavioral patterns. For instance, we may ask to what extent these patterns may be altered; to what extent a specific organ system is the organ system of response to a variety or possibly to all external stimuli; whether this responsive pattern, through wear and tear on an organ system, may in some way relate or predispose it to sub-sequent pathophysiological processes. Is this Alexander's (1950) vulnerable organ? In other words, does this become the target organ of disease later in life through a process of cumulative stress (Uhlenhuth & Paykel, 1973), a mechanism through which emotions are channeled and experienced (Deutsche et al., 1962) or in a some-what more complex way a manifestation of attempted adaptation by the organ system to repetitive stimulation, Selye's (1956) so-called diseases of adaptation?

Because there is some evidence for the constancy and consistency of an organ-system response to at least a specific stimulus, we may ask what effect or relation-ship this response has on other processes in the still-developing organism? To what extent does it influence other aspects of behavior? How does it relate to what we call personality development: the experience of emotions and the defenses fashioned to modulate these? How does the reactivity through this organ system affect inter-actions with others, especially the early mother-child relationship? To what extent is it compatible, similar, complementary, and/or incompatible and antagonistic? How much of the mother-child relationship is guided by the mutuality or lack of mutuality between dissimilar organ-response systems? To what extent does the mother's organ-response system program or modify, postnatally, the infant's develop-ment? These appear to be suitable questions for refinement into specific hypotheses for clinical research. In the interim, the ability to raise such questions on the part of the perceptive clinician may lead to observations that will be helpful in understand-ing developmental processes and the health states with which these correlate.

3.7. Psychological and Physiological Developmental Relationships

Regardless of the developing child-mother interaction, we seem to have an organism whose physiological responses to external stimuli have a baseline of re-sponse at birth. This response system not only *is* behavior in its own right but also will perpetuate present and shape future behavior of the individual. It is certainly one of the underpinnings of what we call personality inasmuch as it includes several of the characteristics of this elusive concept. Response includes not only direction in such terms as toward, away, or none but also quantity, much or little, and speed, slow or fast. It also, in time, comes to have specific characteristics in terms of the significant others in the environment, depending on the relationship of the respondent to these. The latter involves the concept of motivation, whose anlage may be based in protoplasmic drives. These characteristics underlie what comes to be identified as personality. In time, personality becomes increasingly individually embellished by the encrustment of attributes that are idiosyncratic for the individual. These are related to the development of increasingly sophisticated coping skills, commencing with the early defenses developed around the psychosexual stages of development and their renegotiation during subsequent stages of later development. Our interest is in how what we call personality is intimately related to physiological processes, i.e., how personality conditions organ-system responses, and how these responses, once fixed in time, contribute to changes in personality. In combination, we might call these *behavioral patterns*. It is on the basis of this interplay between initial organ-system responses, first to maternal and later to other environmental objects, that what we call personality-behavioral patterns are derived. These become increasingly tuned and refined in psychophysiological processes that, when repeatedly stressed, result in illness. Such a formulation is useful in explaining behavior pattern type A associated with coronary artery disease (Friedman & Rosenman, 1969) on the one hand and what has been identified as the lack of a specific behavior pattern or at best a pattern of ambivalence in some individuals who subsequently develop cancer (Thomas & Greenstreet, 1973).

The idea that trauma, unsuccessfully handled for whatever reason at specific stages of psychosexual development, leads to at least a partial fixation in terms of emotional development and also may affect other conceptualized developmental processes occurring at this time, including the physiological, is an intriguing one, especially when one considers the tuning or regulation of processes affecting the appetite and the large number of social restraints that need to be transmitted in order to accomplish the eventual socialization of the organism. Into this schema it is necessary to bring developmental concepts from other traditions, including the traditional and modified learning theories of Pavlov (1927), Skinner (1963), and Miller (Miller & DiCara, 1969), respectively; the cognitive theory of Piaget; the imprinting phenomena of Lorenz and the structuralism deriving from Levi-Strauss's dualism (Gardner, 1973); Erikson's (1963) more social development; and Kohlberg's (1972) attempt to define moral development. One or more of these developmental conceptual approaches may be useful in examining a specific behavior at a particular point in an individual's life. In a specific instance, one or more may be found to co-relate to a specific physiological process based on a coincidental concurrence with it during a specific phase in biological development.

Lastly, may I suggest that the emphasis that each of these approaches, led by Freudian psychoanalysis, places on early growth and development of the organism, while fundamental to our understanding of the health-illness continuum, is sadly and ironically ignored in our medical education at both the student and the resident level. Ironically, this is equally true in most of our educational programs in psychiatry. Rather, as adults, we are preoccupied with adult illness, whatever its anlage, perhaps because of our own loss of childhood, our own sense of vulnerability, and because adults are the ones who ultimately pay.

3.8. Early Illness Patterns and Illness Status

In our postnatal evolutionary approach to understanding the patient in health and illness, we next turn specifically to a retrospective review of the individual's early illness patterns and the times at which these occurred. Again, the time of occurrence, at what developmental stage, may suggest the fixations, emotionally at least, sometimes behaviorally and cognitively, and possibly physically, that have occurred. More likely, it may suggest the amount of regression that we may anticipate in our adolescent or adult patient during his present illness. To a large extent, reactions to illness in the adult may have similarities to the earlier illness experiences. This will depend on the similarity of circumstances available in the two situations, e.g., the presence of a responding and nurturing caretaker. The illness state (Mechanic, 1962; Parsons, 1951) is to a considerable extent a learned one, modeled after social institutions fostered by the family and society. It involves such concepts as permission to be ill, e.g., the sanctioning of the social structure-family, and of society via the physician, employers, and friends. There are also reinforcements for the individual to remain ill long enough to assure recovery to a productive capacity. While in the ill role, the individual is not only relieved of social responsibility but also to a large extent disenfranchised from his usual state as a family member, an agent of society, etc. Such a transition raises conflicts expressed as ambivalence in those called on to serve the role as caretaker (spouse, parents, children), the supporting casts (friends, neighbors), and employers. The regression allowed is a curious phenomenon because it is allowed by peers (spouse), authority figures (parents, surrogate parents, employers), or children, thereby distorting, often reversing, these complex relationships. It is no wonder then that many of us now speak of the ill family rather than the ill individual (Anthony, 1970). Indeed, the primary-care and general physician will learn that in illness he has never one patient but several; and his or her work is not complete until he has attended to each. For the pediatrician, the primary and sometimes only patient may be the mother, and only subsequently the child.

Concepts of the illness state reflect a cultural milieu and its interrelated social, cultural, political, economic, religious, and philosophical values. To a considerable extent, a society has to be wealthy enough to afford illness. Ultimately, it is a luxury at the expense of other members of the society, especially the young. The more complex a society, depending on the nature of the illness, the more intermediary roles between illness and health may be found; in less complex societies, only limited roles exist. In a technological society, where emphasis is placed on mass production by hourly paid wage earners, illness is most directly cost accountable and can be tolerated only to an economically determined extent, at which time its burdens are transferred to the state and its definition takes on an aspect of chronicity and with it further social alienation. Thus, in this same technological society, the challenge to medicine, an agent of society, and to the individual is directed at "short" illnesses, rapid effective treatment, short convalescence, little if any rehabilitation, and immediate reabsorption into the work force. This attitude, transmitted into concepts, is directly reflected in our diagnostic and therapeutic approaches. It is the basis on which we practice. Hence our approaches to illness are on the acute, rapidly treated, and rehabilitated processes. We look for the instant cure. We allow limited and incomplete regression. We exhort and provoke relatively rapid return to the marketplaces, to family, society, and work. Individuals failing to respond in this socially adaptable way soon find themselves left behind, increasingly ostracized and stigmatized. They form what might be called an internal third world, in which they enter a real or enforced dependency on the state, and relate to state-financed programs generally addressed to the maintenance of that status. The emphasis on gradual and complete recovery is virtually forgotten both by patient and certainly by medicine. The bed is needed, the work force suffers, the no longer extended family cannot manage. A paradigm is our present-day treatment of the behavior pattern-type A coronary artery disease-prone patient. In his rush to get to his infarct, he is equally rushed to get over it and get on with the business of living, jogging, fretting over diets, and living the full, productive, assertive life that possibly contributed to his downfall in the first place.

The expected patterns of illness in the adult will initially follow those of childhood. Usually, these childhood experiences are brief, episodic, and responded to with gentleness—maternal care is buttressed by an external figure, the physician, who may be fatherly or motherly to the mother. Regression is allowed, indeed encouraged. The child responds quickly, is in a hurry to get back to his tasks, and the episode in time becomes no more than the momentary ripple of a pebble tossed into a pond. Catastrophic illness in childhood is different, especially if it occasions residual disabilities and/or processes that require continued treatment, necessitating continued preoccupation on the part of parents and teachers, and repeated exposure to members of the health care delivery system. This reinforcement of the illness state obviously affects the victim and becomes a basis for his interaction with others for the rest of his life. Illness for him becomes a different phenomenon, with different expectations. Thus the experience of illness in childhood will shape at least initially the experience of illness in adulthood. For the adult with little individual experience of illness and no prolonged contact with the illness of others in childhood, the experience will be essentially unconditioned. He will have had no preparation for the ill role. His anxieties, fears, and emotional and cognitive expectations will be unprepared. This will be a new world, and an uncertain one. On the other hand, in the individual with a long and arduous chronic illness course, a new exacerbation or nuance may be met from an attitude of resignation and acceptance of yet another incident in a relentless progression of episodes or with a sense of the optimism of endurance—"this too shall be overcome." I suggest that this capacity for despair or hope comes from some early parent-child interaction, reinforced by challenging but not overburdening life situations. The study of such phenomena, while elusive, remains of fundamental importance in addressing the convalescent and rehabilitative phases of illness.

3.9. Separation and Illness

In a review of childhood-adolescence-early adult life, there are a number of life experiences which will acquaint us with our patient and suggest how he may react to, adjust to, or sustain the present illness experience. We might begin with separations. The earliest one is the gradual one from the mother. It may be useful, in our care of some patients, to learn not only about abrupt and catastrophic separations but also about that more gradual separation from the mother that is marked by transitional objects. For the moment, we might focus on the transitional object or objects and what they symbolized. Were there none? How long were these held onto? Do they remain? What of the variety of purposes they subserved over their lifetime? What can be recalled of the projective experiences of the child that were reflected off these? What can they tell us of attachments and alienations through growth and development, health and illness?

More gross separations, the loss through death, separation, or divorce of one or more parents or their surrogates, will characterize the past of more than a third of our patients. What we can recover of our patient's memories and negotiations with these processes will tell us something of how he may negotiate, at the time of illness, this potential loss of self or part of self. It will tell us something of how he will sustain the grieving experience that accompanies illness. At the same time, the primordial grief experience around loss may identify the residual learned capacities which the individual has developed and which he may utilize in coping with this latest assault on self.

Other separations worthy of note are those around absences of parents, of mothers for repeated childbirth, of fathers for war and/or business service. Regressive behaviors are frequently observed at such times, and it may be pertinent to learn through which organ systems they are manifested, e.g., thumbsucking, hair pulling, enuresis, encoporesis, tics, stuttering, school phobias, tantrums, asthma, eczema, cough, other illness. The first formal separations from parents and home to relatives or friends, nursery school, play school, or day care centers should be reviewed. Perhaps not enough attention has been focused on childhood behavior, including illness during the first full-time separation from mother that occurs with entrance to the first grade at age 6. Frequently, these illnesses are explained in epidemiological terms of exposure to strains of bacteria and viruses different from those to which the individual has developed immunity. We are less likely to consider whether the work of separation may relate to a reduction of immunological defenses as it may to the ego defenses around the transient loss of mother and home and the stresses of the alien environment of the classroom. Indeed, we might at least briefly consider the childhood illnesses and their manifestations as the illnesses of stress, at once reducing immunological defenses and giving stimulus to a rebuilding of these. This life phase would also be a time to investigate whether there are organ systems still in the process of maturation which might be more often the target organ for the reflection of stress. The musculoskeletal and cardiovascular systems (Kimball, 1973) come most readily to mind. Earlier, in a speculative review of his work on lymphomas, Greene (1954; Greene, Young, & Swisher, 1956) has hypothesized an umbilical phase of development that, when traumatized, might sensitize the organism for a subsequent lymphomatous process. Again, reaction to stress at these times would need to be addressed in a broad sense along the continuum of health and illness, including social, psychological, and physiological reactions. Whereas each one of these will always be present, the explanation that fits best at one time or another may be predominantly in terms of one approach. These reactions need not be addressed only in terms of pathology or decompensation, but should also be looked at in terms of their stimulus for growth and differentiation, again from each perspective. For most of us, social institutions seek to provide a stimulus for growth and differentiation, social, psychological, and biological. Without such forms, growth which occurs seems more likely to be aimless and distorted as viewed from these different approaches.

In this discussion of children and their subsequent growth as affected by stress, specifically the stress of loss, we need to include Brown's (1966) extensive studies relating to greater incidence of somatic, social, and psychological distress in the later life of children suffering the loss a parent under the age 15 as compared with controls. When this loss occurred prior to the age of 8 and/or included the loss of both parents, the resulting pathology was much greater than for controls as well as for losses between age 8 and 15.

Lesser stresses as seen by others may be major ones for the individual and may relate to how these are seen and sustained by other members of the family and the social system in which the individual lives. Moves, engaged in by 20% of the American population yearly, always provoke stress. When it is considered that this 20% figure includes families that move frequently, it suggests that provocation for some may be a repeated trauma. While these changes are frequently opportunities for growth and differentiation in terms of some families or some members of families, for others they may prove overwhelming and insurmountable, resulting in social breakdown as reflected in psychological, physical, or social morbidity.

Without such monumental potential for stress as moving or death, there are innumerable changes that may prove too much for easy coping for many individuals, depending on the time in the individual's or family's life that they occur and the social resources available. Some ages seem more vulnerable for negotiating with change than others. Adolescence may be a particularly difficult time for the removal from one group to another. If this is also a stressful move for the mother or father, the adolescent's ability to cope will be correspondingly less.

3.10. The Illness-Onset Situation

When an event or situation proves overwhelming, we can always expect that there will be a reaction in terms of the individual's self-perceptions. He will feel somewhat diminished. The environment will appear altered, perhaps distant, unfulfilling, hostile. There will be a distancing from others. In a very real sense, the distancing may be actually accompanied by a distortion of perception. Individuals will be seen as farther away; voices may sound distant. There develops a sense of alienation which accompanies an increased preoccupation with self, with one's own feelings, and frequently with bodily function. They may be especially so if one already is vulnerable to reflecting these feelings in one organ system or another, including the central nervous system. It is not unusual for the individual to feel discomfort in those systems that for whatever reason have previously been sensitized. Similar to the dog who lifts the once-injured paw and begins limping at a later time when scolded, we become aware of sensations in a long-forgotten scar, a migraine, a tightening over the left precordium, a pain in the neck when, because of fatigue, burdens that appear too much, intercurrent illness of another dimension, heap down around us. These are perhaps learned processes, communicative to ourselves and others with which we can no longer cope autonomously. We may need to stop, take stock, perhaps withdraw for the moment. They are signals and warnings. As behavior, they include not only the feeling and its perception but also the accompanying physiological mechanisms associated with the feeling, which may or may not include the changes of pathology. The perception and cognition of no longer being able to cope as well as usual, the sense of the usual supplies from without no longer being available or obtainable, the diminishing sense of self in a future and preoccupation of the sense of a hurt or injured self in the past, simultaneous with a sense of a withdrawal from previously cathected objects in the present, characterize the giving-up-given-up state that Engel and Schmale (1967) have identified as a potentially vulnerable one and the precursor of illness. The in-limbo state, described in psychological terms, concurrent with the perception of a social situation, can be assumed to have biological correlates yet to be identified. These biological processes, possibly in the vulnerable organ systems genetically predisposed, postnatally traumatized, or otherwise conditioned, may suggest the direction of a pathological process should this state be sustained. For example, in the individual likely to manifest a state of arousal through the cardiovascular system who has, because of repeated use of this system, sustained wear and tear, e.g., changes in blood vessels, the continued presence of this in-limbo state may lead to the pathophysiological decompensation resulting in a myocardial infarction. This does not preclude the possibility that another individual may react to stress with a different preconditioned tuning of the cardiovascular system, i.e., with a slowing of dynamics, resulting under a sustained giving-up-given-up state, in the same pathophysiologic process, a myocardial infarction. Whereas the sequence may be similar, the components of the formula may be different, dependent on the unique and individual psychosociobiological development of the patient.

The major difficulty in stress and illness research relationships is that of the definition of stress. Some, such as Selye (1956) and to an increasing extent Rahe (1976), emphasize the reaction as the definition of stress. Rahe calls this "strain." It would seem that the important link in this formulation is the individual's processing of an event. This will determine whether or not an event is perceived and/or felt as a stress, as well as how the individual experiencing it handles it. Each of these elements may be handled differently by different individuals. Whether an event is perceived as a stress will depend at least on the individual's state of cognition. It may also depend on the individual's style of processing the specific cognitive information. For instance, does he defend against it because it is too arousing, resulting in a denial of the percept? Or does he utilize some more sophisticated defensive process for coping with the percept? As the observer, we then need to assess whether these processes are adaptive or maladaptive in terms of a particular object. The basic objective will be taken by most of us as that of survival of the individual. This will be along a spectrum based on individual value systems. The important question is, adaptive for what? Whether perception and cognition, however processed, will lead to behavior adaptive for the individual's optimal functioning will depend on the apparatus responsible for effective coping, e.g., the intactness of the neuromuscular apparatus. These will also depend on the presence of resources external to the individual that can be utilized or mobilized.

3.11. The Acute Phase of Illness

Regardless of the exact mechanisms between stress and illness, the importance of identifying events concurrent with illness onset will be of potential value in attending to the patient and his concerns about these at the same time that he is contending with the added burden of illness. For example, the individual identified as having a behavior type-A pattern and sustaining a myocardial infarction may be as preoccupied about a recent business reversal or marital disharmony as he is about the infarct. In attempts to attend optimally to the latter, the physician may need to first identify and then attempt to attend to the former. Frequently, this is difficult to do. However, it is not always a matter of secondary priority. Patients may refuse treatment or in other ways demonstrate noncompliance with diagnostic and therapeutic procedures unless they are given an opportunity to talk of the concurrent life situation.

In patients with chronic pathophysiological processes, patterns of exacerbations and remissions may be identified. These will be useful to the physician in his management of the patient. Clinical experience and research repeatedly relate exacerbation of processes such as sickle cell crises, ulcerative colitis, asthma, and other illnesses to life situations in which stress factors may be identified. Most commonly, these relate to an actual, imminent, or fantasied loss of a meaningful object or relationship.

The event of illness becomes in and of itself a stress experience for the individual inasmuch as it is a potential loss of self. It is also always a partial loss of self, an experience of vulnerability and a reexperiencing of former vulnerabilities, i.e., the illnesses and other traumas of the past. It literally rocks the ego and calls on it to resort to emergency and reparative defenses if only to hold things together until further processing of the insult and its damages can be assessed.

A more or less usual immediate sequence of psychological processes may be identified for most victims of illness whether this is a bad cold, a myocardial infarction, or a major deformity. The difference may first be one of degree and only secondarily one of kind in terms of the specific trauma and of the specific psychological makeup of the individual. Essentially, the grief model of Lindemann (1944) serves as a useful one for anticipating an individual's reaction to illness. The earliest phase is that of shock, the shock of recognition, which most often is greeted with denial, however momentary. Since the word "denial" is a much-abused one, it is useful to clarify it with an object, i.e., denial of what—the event, feelings about the event, consequences of the event. In this way, we can more readily assess the adaptiveness or maladaptiveness of the denial. When the event itself is denied, while we expect that the underlying emotion may be potentially overwhelming, our first preoccupation as physicians is to do whatever is most pragmatic in sustaining life. For the patient, denial of symptoms frequently leads to a delay in the patient's receiving treatment (Olin & Hackett, 1964). Most frequently, the symptom may not be denied, but may be minimized or rationalized, again resulting in a delay in seeking help. Such processes may result in seeking assistance from less than appropriate resources, in the case of potentially catastrophic events, and/or the refusal to accept maximal assistance once available and proffered. When the latter is the case, the victim may need to be "shocked into a recognition of illness." This then becomes an emergency psychotherapeutic problem of some complexity. There is no single formula that will work for all physicians or with all patients. Confrontation tactics, while sometimes time-saving and effective, at other times will lead to an increase in defensive processes (Sifneos, 1967). Bargaining sometimes represents a temporarily intermediate position, whereby one accepts diagnostic procedures or initial treatment in order to appease another individual. The relatively slow and skillful precipitation of the feeling behind the denial may be costly in terms of time and extreme in its extent. Some observers feel that some denial of emotion at the time of the acute phase of illness is potentially adaptive, at least for some patients.

As emotions surface in some patients, the initial one is anxiety. The degree of anxiety correlates with the severity of discomfort rather than with some more distant concept, such as the loss of life. It is often the pain of living which floods the patient's concern. In its most manifest stage, anxiety is short-lived, peaking around the second day and giving way to what some investigators call depression, but what I prefer to call sadness, which peaks, at least initially, around the fourth day (Cassem & Hackett, 1971). Depression seems to accompany the dawn of awareness of the illness and some initial anticipation of the meaning of illness in terms of the future.

3.12. Altered States of Consciousness

Often overlooked and/or ignored in this early stage of illness are altered states of consciousness (Kimball, 1974). These are manifested initially by irritability and hypervigilance, and are quickly followed by minimal confusion as detected in orientation to time, place, and sometimes person; deficits in recent memory; difficulty in concentration and attending; sometimes changes in thinking, i.e., in making the kind of decisions usually expected of this individual; and emotional lability. The staff is usually so busy doing things to the patient that mild to moderate deficits in these areas go unattended. When those alterations are more severe, delusions and hallucinations, accompanied by increased restlessness and agitation, attract the attention of the staff. Such behavior will more acutely interfere with treatment as well as the organization in which care is rendered; i.e., it is potentially damaging to the patient and to the care of other patients. Efforts toward immediate calming of the manifestations of this behavior need to be undertaken. Unfortunately, had the anlage of this state been anticipated by attending to the earlier changes in cognition, emotion, and behavior, this part of the sequence might have been aborted. Instead, it may have been inadvertently fostered by the administration of hypnotics and analgesics that, together with other factors, have nurtured its development. Recognition of altered states of consciousness may be more deliberately accomplished by the use of a brief mental status examination at regular intervals during the day (Figure 2).

SCORE
(No. Errors)

NAME _____ UNIT NO. _____ DATE _____ EXAMINER _____

MENTAL STATUS QUESTIONNAIRE
(MSQ)

1. Where are you now? (What place is this? What is the name of this place? What kind of place is this?) _____

2. Where is it? (Address? Location?) _____

3. What is today's date? Day _____ (correct if + or - one day)
4.   Month _____
5.   Year _____
6. How old are you? _____
7. When were you born? Month _____
8.   Year _____
9. Who is the President of the United States? _____
10. Who was President before him? _____

    0–2 Errors = None or mild brain syndrome
    3–8 Errors = Moderate brain syndrome
    9–10 Errors = Severe brain syndrome

Reference: Kahn, R. L., Goldfarb, A. I., Pollack, M., and Peck, A. Brief Objective Measures for the Determination of Mental Status in the Aged. *Amer. Jour. Psychiat.* 117:326–328, 1960.

Figure 2. Mental status questionnaire.

Once this state is identified, depending on its severity, proper surveillance of the patient should be instituted (Kimball, 1974). When the deficits are severe, resulting in agitated behavior, a special attendant should be assigned to the patient until there is amelioration of these. Then, a search for specific etiological factors should be undertaken by a review of the medications. Hypnotics and other sedatives are always suspect; so too are analgesics. When one is suspected, attempts at substitution of another are advisable if cancellation is not possible. Withdrawal states from alcohol should always rank high on the suspect list. Failure to identify these may result in delirium tremens, which, once in progress, has a mortality rate of 15–30% even in the best of treatment centers. Untoward withdrawal from drugs may be associated with agitated states of behavior, putting the patient and others at risk. Other drugs used in the specific treatment of the illness may introduce iatrogenic effects. Cortisone and its derivatives are notorious for their effects, usually of heightened states of unconsciousness. The underlying illness will frequently result in metabolic changes which affect mood and cognitive processes, although the specific mechanisms responsible for these remain yet to be identified. A thorough review of systems will be helpful in identifying the responsible process or agent. Usually, it will take hours to several days for deranged functions to be restored to their usual state. If agitation, disorientation, delusions, and hallucinations are particularly disturbing to the care of the patient, reduction if not total amelioration can be effected by the use of small amounts of phenothiazines or butyrophenone. These are administered orally in low dosages, e.g., chlorpromazine, 25 mg. stat, followed by the same amount at 30–60 min intervals three or four times. Usually, this is sufficient to calm the agitation and is followed by a maintenance dosage given at 8-hr intervals based on the cumulative amount given. This is almost always below the cardiotoxic doses that have been identified. Orthostatic side-effects are not usually a problem for bedridden patients. Because the underlying metabolic alterations persist and patients remain concerned about the eruption of unconscious material into their conscious state, the maintenance dose is continued for 7–10 days. Hypnotics and sedatives frequently contribute to increased alterations in the state of consciousness and therefore are usually contraindicated.

Both anxiety and sadness may influence the degree of the altered state of consciousness. In order to be treated, these must be observed and/or heard. That they are to be expected is not sufficient reason for them not to be attended to. Attention is frequently antidotal in its own right. Giving a patient the opportunity to ventilate his anxiety neither increases it nor, so far as we know, contributes to further derangement of his physiological status. On the other hand, it may contribute to an alleviation of some of the inner stress on the patient occasioned by his held-back concern about himself for which he may gain some relief through the process of ventilation. We frequently observe that manifestations of anxiety may reappear at about the time of discharge from the acute care units. This is paradoxical, inasmuch as these units themselves are incriminated by patients as one of the causes for their anxiety (Klein, Kliner, Zipes, et al., 1968). This phenomenon has been explained by several patients on the basis that they were fearful of having to make it on their own in a less-well-attended care unit following leaving the acute one. It is also our impression that the sadness state observed in the acute units generally persists and oftentimes becomes of greater intensity during the convalescent state. This is attributed to a variety of factors. One is a residual fatigue state that has escalated from the illness-onset situation through the acute phase of illness. Our observations suggest that the majority of patients are deprived of sleep during this period. It may prove helpful to identify whether this deficit is specific for some stages of sleep as opposed to others. On return to the floor, some patients will enter a state which is best described as a conservation-withdrawal one (Engel, 1962b). Such patients will be observed to turn toward the wall, request not to see visitors, express irritation with doctors and other attendants seeking to minister to their needs, and may bluntly order away relatives, telling all who would listen that they are worn out and just wish to sleep. Others may continue to reveal a heightened state of anxiety until they become adjusted to the new environment and are assured that their needs will be met.

3.13. The Convalescent Phase of Illness

During the convalescent phase, many of the patterns of behavior observed will correlate with the individual's personality and behavioral patterns (Kimball, 1972). Patients with obsessive and compulsive traits will attempt mastery over the new environment by an exaggeration of these, frequently exhibiting demanding and plaintive behavior until assured as to routine and schedules. Patients with hysterical traits may act oblivious to any change in health and will annoy those in attendance with indiscreet actions unbecoming to their state of health. Patients with suspicious traits may look for evidence confirming their suspicions that something has been overlooked (a sponge), that they have been ill- or misinformed, that they have been improperly treated if not misdiagnosed. Patients with an impulsive disorder will exhibit short temper, demanding and provoking behavior. The more anxious they are, the more they will exhibit behavior that will become increasingly disruptive for other patients and the staff. Still other patients may exhibit greater regression during this stage of illness when their usual defenses either have been depleted or are less than adequate to meet the anxieties that have been evoked by the illness. This regression may result in more infantile patterns of behavior in which passivity and dependency are manifest. Most of these states can be managed and addressed by those in attendance if they keep in mind that the underlying emotion is usually anxiety, sadness, or anger. These cannot be attended to until they are heard. This frequently requires the permission of those in attendance. To hear these unpleasant emotions, we must acknowledge our own capacity to experience these, sharing our own limit of tolerance with our colleagues. For the patient, once permission has been received, "structure" is the all-important word for the presentation of the feeling. The patient needs the felt assurance that the feeling can be demonstrated in the context of limits and bounds or the process becomes more threatening than relieving. The process of emotion-relieving will require frequent repetition during the convalescent period.

To a large extent, the convalescent period may be seen as a grieving process, a grieving both over what has occurred and over what might have occurred. As such, the process will follow Lindemann's (1944) four stages, beginning with and returning to the shocklike denial phase and progressing through a ventilation of the emotions and the experimenting with different defenses to contain these until some level of coping and adaptation has been attained. In these processes, which will surge forward and slide backward, the role of the attendant therapist is that of assisting the patient in sorting out those defenses that are useful as opposed to those that are maladaptive at the specific time in question. This process will depend on the psychological resources that the individual brings with him to this period in life, the disease process, the external resources available to him in terms of significant others, and real supplies in terms of the social, political, and economic environment. Whereas the grieving process may continue for a considerable time after the convalescent phase and into the rehabilitative one, its significance lies in its requiring the active participation of family, friends, and the attending health workers. Without this, a firm base for the further rehabilitative phase will be lacking, thereby compromising maximal adaptation.

3.14. Rehabilitative Phase of Illness: Coping and Adaptation

Although general principles of adaptation can be identified (Table 1), these will be specific processes for the individual, depending on him, his disease, and his environmental situation (Kimball, 1977b). To a considerable extent, the factors and their interrelationship affecting adaptation have been little more than outlined, based on the intensive study of a limited number of processes. From some of those that have been completed, certain generalizations have been made that are useful in considering other processes. More elusive remain the individual factors that make for successful coping. Certainly, the individual's capacity for new learning is both important and variable. The latter will depend on the individual's innate ability and the affect of age and illness on this. Equally if not more important will be elusive qualities that are identified by such terms as "hope," "determination," and "will power." While most believe that these are essential, a precise identification of them and their relationship to social and physiological factors remain unclear. On the other hand, repeated observations have identified that some emotional states such as high anxiety (Janis, 1958) and depression (Kimball, 1969a), and psychological processes such as absolute denial correlate with poor outcome in terms of optimal rehabilitation and even survival. These are processes that require intensive study and the development of novel hypotheses for testing by new methods.

At the present time, outcome studies of the return to work and social and domestic functioning in many of the chronic and recurring diseases are not encouraging. Explanations for this poor showing suggest a failure to explore the psychosocial determinants of continued morbidity. At the present, the least practitioners can do is to rigorously identify and vigorously pursue the emotional, psychological, and social factors that may be contributing to the less-than-optimal adjustment of the individual to his altered state of functioning, physically, socially, and psychologically. This will demand investigation of family factors, including changes in role and sexual functioning and the responses and attitudes of employers, fellow

Table 1. Tasks of Coping and Adaptation

1. Maintaining a sense of personal worth
2. Keeping distress within manageable limits
3. Maintaining, restoring relationships with significant persons
4. Enhancing the prospects for recovering bodily functions (or alternatives)
5. Identifying the possibility and working toward an acceptable altered life-style
6. Emphasizing an opportunity for growth, the development of new skills
7. Communication and demonstration of these capacities to other

employees, insurance companies, and the population in general and social acquaintances in particular.

4. A Note on Therapy

In the preceding, little has been mentioned about specific therapeutic aspects of the psychosomatic approach. It is to be hoped that the reader has identified that a therapeutic approach is intrinsic to the psychosomatic approach. It is part of the process (Kimball, 1969b). It occurs throughout the interviewing sessions in which data relevant to the person and his illness are collected. Allowing the patient to talk about his illness, to talk about and display his feelings about his illness, to identify his confusions, anxieties, and pains, all will contribute to the evolving diagnostic-therapeutic process. At times, these will indicate specific therapeutic activities, such as the removal or addition of a drug, change of environment, structuring, confrontation, or some other deliberate process. Mostly, however, it will be embodied by the attention of the physician and his staff to the nuances in the behavior of the patient (Kimball, 1977a). At other times, there may be indications for the trial of behavioral methods, a specific drug regimen, or more extended and formalized psychotherapeutic contracts. During specific phases of illness, e.g., the convalescent phase, the grief model lends itself to a therapeutic process (Kimball, 1975).

5. Conclusion

Following a brief review of earlier and present-day concepts regarding the proposed relationships existing among psychologically, biologically, and socially conceptualized events, I have suggested some of the inherent problems presented by these attempts and posed some alternative approaches by which psychosomatic theory may stimulate new empirical research. Also, I have suggested how these changing concepts have influenced our teaching and practice in psychosomatic medicine.

6. References

Alexander, F. *Psychosomatic medicine.* New York: Norton, 1950.
Alexander, F., & French, T. M. *Studies in psychosomatic medicine.* New York: Ronald Press, 1948.
Anthony, E. J. The impact of mental illness on family life. *American Journal of Psychiatry,* 1970, *127,* 138–146.
Bahnson, C. B., & Wardwell, W. I. Parent constellation and psychosexual identification in male patients with myocardial infarction. *Psychological Research,* 1962, *10,* 831–842 (monogr. suppl.).
Bridger, W. H. Sensory discrimination and autonomic function in the newborn. *Journal of the American Academy of Child Psychiatry,* 1962, *1,* 67–82.
Brown, F. Childhood bereavement and subsequent psychiatric disorder. *British Journal of Psychiatry,* 1966, *112,* 1035–1041.
Cannon, W. B. *Bodily changes in pain, hunger, fear and rage.* New York: Appleton, 1920.
Cassell, J., Heyden, S., Bartel, A. G., et al. Incidence of coronary heart disease by ethnic groups, social class and sex. *Archives of Internal Medicine,* 1971, *128,* 901–906.
Cassem, N. H., & Hackett, T. P. Psychiatric consultation in a coronary care unit. *Annals of Intermediate Medicine,* 1971, *75,* 9–14.
Descartes, R. *Les meditations metaphysiques.* D. Mouchet, Paris, 1724.
Deutsche, F., Thompson, D., Pinderhughes, C., et al. *Body, mind and the sensory gateways.* New York: Karger, 1962.

Dunbar, H. F. *Emotions and bodily changes: A survey of literature on psychosomatic interrelationships.* New York: Columbia University Press, 1954.

Engel, G. L. Studies of ulcerative colitis. IV. The significance of headaches. *Psychosomatic Medicine,* 1956, *18,* 334–346.

Engel, G. L. *Psychological development in health and disease.* Philadelphia: Saunders, 1962. (a)

Engel, G. L. Anxiety and depression-withdrawal: The primary affects of unpleasure. *International Journal of Psychoanalysis,* 1962, *43,* 89–97. (b)

Engel, G. L. A reconsideration of the role of conversion in somatic disease. *Comprehensive Psychiatry,* 1968, *9,* 316–326.

Engel, G. L., & Schmale, A. Psychoanalytic theory of somatic disorder: Conversion, specificity and the disease-onset situation. *Journal of the American Psychoanalytic Association,* 1967, *15,* 344.

Erikson, E. *Childhood and society* (2nd ed.). New York: Norton, 1963.

Feinstein, A. R. *Clinical judgment.* Baltimore: Williams & Wilkins, 1967.

Freud, S. The justification for detaching from neurosthenia a particular syndrome: The anxiety neurosis (1894). In E. Jones (Ed.), *Sigmund Freud: Collected papers.* New York: Basic Books, 1959.

Friedman, D. G. *Human infancy: An evolutionary perspective.* Hillsdale, N.J.: Lawrence Erlbaum Assoc., 1974.

Friedman, M., & Rosenman, R. H. Overt behavior pattern in coronary disease: Detection of overt behavior pattern A in patients with coronary disease by a new psychophysiological procedure. *Journal of the American Medical Association,* 1960, *173,* 1320–1325.

Friedman, M., & Rosenman, R. H. Association of specific overt behavior pattern with blood and cardiovascular findings. *Journal of the American Medical Association,* 1969, *169,* 1286–1296.

Gaddini, R. Transitional objects and the process of individuation: A study in three different social groups. *Journal of the American Academy of Child Psychology,* 1970, *9,* 347–365.

Gamow, G. *Expanding universe and the origin of galaxies.* Copenhagen: Munksgaard, 1953.

Gardner, H. *The quest for mind.* New York: Knopf, 1973.

Garma, A. The unconscious images in the genesis of peptic ulcer. *International Journal of Psychoanalysis,* 1960, *41,* 444.

Gellhorn, E. The tuning of the nervous system: Physiological foundations and implications for behavior. *Perspectives in Biology and Medicine,* 1967, *10,* 559–591.

Greene, W. A., Jr. Psychological factors and reticuloendothelial disease. I. Preliminary observations on a group of males with lymphomas and leukemias. *Psychosomatic Medicine,* 1954, *16,* 220–230.

Greene, W. A., Jr., Young, L. E., & Swisher, S. N. Psychological factors and reticuloendothelial disease. II. Observations on a group of women with lymphomas and leukemias. *Psychosomatic Medicine,* 1956, *18,* 284–303.

Grinker, R. R. *Toward a unified theory of human behavior: An introduction to general systems theory* (2nd ed.). New York: Basic Books, 1967.

Groddeck, G. *The book of the it.* New York: New American Library, 1961.

Groen, J. J. Die klinisch-wissenshaftliche Unterschungmethodik in der psychosomatischen Medizin. *Verhandlungen der Deutschen Gesellschaft für Inneres Medizin,* 1967, *73,* 17–27.

Hamburg, D., Hamburg, B., & deGoza, S. Adaptive problems and mechanisms in severely burned patients. *Psychiatry,* 1953, *16,* 1–20.

Harburg, E., Schull, W. J., Erfurt, J. C., et al. Method for estimating heredity and stress. I. A pilot study of blood pressure among Negroes in high and low stress areas, Detroit, 1966–67. *Journal of Chronic Diseases,* 1970, *22,* 69–81.

Hinkle, L. E., Whitney, L. H., Hehman, E. W., et al. Occupation, education, and coronary artery disease. *Science,* 1968, *161,* 238–246.

Holmes, T. H., & Rahe, R. H. The social readjustment rating scale. *Journal of Psychosomatic Research,* 1967, *11,* 213–218.

Jackson, D., Yalom, I. Family research in the problem of ulcerative colitis. *Archives of General Psychiatry,* 1966, *15,* 410–418.

James, W. What is an emotion? *Mind,* 1884.

Janis, I. L. *Psychological stress: Psychoanalytic and behavioral studies of surgical patients.* New York: Wiley, 1958.

Kahn, R. L., Goldfarb, A. I., Pollack, M., & Peck, A. Brief objective measures for the determination of mental status in the aged. *American Journal of Psychiatry,* 1960, *177,* 326–328.

Karush, A., Daniels, G. E., O'Connor, J. F., et al. The response to psychotherapy in chronic ulcerative colitis. II. Factors arising from the therapeutic situation. *Psychosomatic Medicine,* 1969, *31,* 201–226.

Kasl, S. V., Cobb, S. Blood pressure changes in men undergoing job loss. *Psychosomatic Medicine*, 1970, *32*, 19–38.

Kellam, S., Branch, J. D., Agrawal, K. C., & Ensminger, M. *Mental health and going to school*. Chicago: University of Chicago Press, 1975.

Kimball, C. P. Psychological responses to the experience of open-heart surgery. I. *American Journal of Psychiatry*, 1969, *126*, 348–359. (a)

Kimball, C. P. Techniques of interviewing. I. Interviewing and the meaning of the symptom. *Annals of Internal Medicine*, 1969, *71*, 147–153. (b)

Kimball, C. P. Techniques of interviewing. III. The patient's personality and the interview process. *Medical Insight*, 1972, *4*, 26–40.

Kimball, C. P. A liaison department of psychiatry. *Psychotherapy and Psychosomatics*, 1973, *22*, 219–225. (a)

Kimball, C. P. The experience of cardiac surgery. V. Psychological patterns and prediction of outcome. *Psychotherapy and Psychosomatics*, 1973, *22*, 310–319. (b)

Kimball, C. P. Delirium. In Howard F. Conn (Ed.), *Current therapy 1974*, 1974, 833–835.

Kimball, C. P. Medical psychotherapy. *Psychotherapy and Psychosomatics*, 1975, *25*, 193–200.

Kimball, C. P. The ethics of a personal medicine. *Medical Clinics of North America*, 1977, *61*, 867–877. (a)

Kimball, C. P. Psychosomatic theory and its contribution to chronic illness. In G. Usdin (Ed.), *Psychiatric medicine*. New York: Brunner/Mazel, 1977, pp. 259–333.

Kimball, C. P. The languages of psychosomatic medicine. *Psychotherapy and Psychosomatics*. 1977, *28*, 1–12.

Kimball, C. P. Teaching and training of psychosomatic approach: The education of the medical student. Presented at the World Psychiatric Society, Honolulu, Hawaii, August 29, 1977. (d) (in press)

Klein, R. F., Kliner, V. A., Zipes, D. P., et al. Transfer from a coronary care unit. *Archives of Internal Medicine*, 1968, *122*, 104–108.

Koch, R. *Die Aetiologie der tuberkulose physiologischen Gesellschaft Berlin 24 Marz cr gehaltenen Vortrage*. Berlin, A. Hirschwald, 1882.

Kohlberg, L. A cognitive-developmental approach to moral education. *The Humanist*, 1972, Nov./Dec., 13–16.

Kokkedee, J. *The quark model*. New York: Benjamin, 1969.

Kuller, L., & Reisler, D. M. An explanation for variations in distribution of stroke and arteriosclerotic heart disease among populations and racial groups. *American Journal of Epidemiology*, 1971, *93*, 1–9.

LeVine, R. A. *Culture, behavior and personality*. Chicago: Aldine, 1973.

Lindemann, E. Symptomatology and management of acute grief. *American Journal of Psychiatry*, 1944, *101*, 141–148.

Manusco, T. F., Coulter, E. J., & MacDonald, E. J. Migration and cancer mortality experience—a study of native and southern born non-white Ohio residents. In D. D. Hemphill (Ed.), *Trace substances in environmental health. VI. A symposium*. Columbia. University of Missouri, 1973.

Marty, P., & d'Muzan, M. La pensée operatoire. *Revue Francaise de Psychoanalysis*, 1963, Suppl. 1345, Vol. 27.

McGough, J. L. *Psychobiology: Behavior from a biological perspective*. New York: Academic Press, 1971.

McIntyre, J. S. *St. Anselm and his critics: A reinterpretation of the Cur Deus Homo*. Edinburgh: Oliver and Boyd, 1954.

Mechanic, D. The concept of illness behavior. *Journal of Chronic Diseases*, 1962, *15*, 189–194.

Miller, G., & DiCara, L. Learning of visceral and glandular responses. *Science*, 1969, *163*, 434–445.

Minuchin, S., Baker, L., Rosman, B., Liebman, R., Milman, L., & Todd, T. A conceptual model of psychosomatic illness in children. *Archives of General Psychiatry*, 1975, *32*, 1031–1038.

Mirsky, I. A. Physiologic, psychologic and social determinants in the etiology of duodenal ulcer. *American Journal of Digestive Diseases*, 1958, *3*, 285–314.

Nemiah, J., Sifneos, P. *Final report on NIMH Project No. M-262(c)*. A study of the specificity of current psychological factors involved in the production of psychosomatic disease, each suffering from two psychosomatic illnesses, 1964.

Nemiah, J., & Sifneos, P. Affect and fantasy in patients with psychosomatic disorders. In Hill (Ed.), *Modern trends in psychosomatic medicine. II*. London. Butterworth, 1970, pp. 26–34.

Olin, H. S., & Hackett, T. P. The denial of chest pain in 32 patients with acute myocardial infarction. *Journal of the American Medical Association*, 1964, *190*, 977–981.

Parsons, T. The social system. Glencoe, Ill.: Free Press, 1951.

Pavlov, I. P. *Conditioned reflexes* (trans. by G. V. Anrep). London: Oxford University Press, 1927.

Paykel, E. S., Prusoff, B. A., & Uhlenhuth, E. H. Scaling of life events. *Archives of General Psychiatry*, 1971, *25*, 340–347.

Potter, van R. *Bioethics: Bridge to the future.* Englewood Cliffs, N.J.: Prentice-Hall, 1971.

Pratt, J. H. The "home sanatorium" treatment of consumption. *Boston Medical and Surgical Journal*, 1906, *154*, 210–216.

Rahe, R. H. Stress and strain in coronary heart disease. *Journal of the South Carolina Medical Association (Supplement)*, 1976, *72*, 7–14.

Reiser, M. Theoretical considerations of the role of psychological factors in pathogenesis and etiology of essential hypertension. In M. Koster, H. Musaph, & P. Visser (Eds.), Psychosomatics in Essential Hypertension. *Bibliotheca Psychiatrica*, 1970, *144*, 117–124.

Ruesch, J. The infantile personality. *Psychosomatic Medicine*, 1948, *10*, 134–144.

Sapira, J. D., Scheilp, R., Monaity, B., et al. Differences in perception between hypertensive and normotensive populations. *Psychosomatic Medicine*, 1971 *33*, 239–250.

Selye, H. *The stress of life.* New York: McGraw-Hill, 1956, pp. 128–148.

Selzer, H. S., Fajans, S., & Conn, J. W. *Diabetes*, 1956, *5*, 437.

Seubert, K. *Das naturliche System der chemischen Elemente* (Abhandlungen von Lothar Meyer und D. Mendeleev). Leipzig: W. Engelman, 1895.

Shekelle, R. B., Ostfeld, A. M., & Paul, O. Social status and incidence of coronary artery disease. *Journal of Chronic Diseases*, 1969, *22*, 381–394.

Sifneos, P. E. Two different kinds of psychotherapy of short duration. *American Journal of Psychiatry*, 123, 1069–1074, 1967.

Sifneos, P. E. A reconsideration of psychosomatic symptom formations in view of recent clinical observations. *Psychotherapy and Psychosomatics*, 1974, *24*, 151–155.

Skinner, B. F. Operant behavior. *American Journal of Psychology*, 1963, *18*, 503–515.

Thomas, C. B., & Greenstreet, R. L. Psychobiological characteristics in youth as predictors of five disease states: Suicide, mental illness, hypertension, coronary heart disease and tumor. *Johns Hopkins Medical Journal*, 1973, *132*, 16–43.

Uhlenhuth, E. H., & Paykel, E. S. Symptom intensity and life events. *Archives of General Psychiatry*, 1973, *28*, 473–477.

Visotsky, H. M., Hamburg, D. A., Goss, M. E., & Lebovits, B. Coping behavior under extreme stress. *Archives of General Psychiatry*, 1961, *5*, 27–52.

Voth, M. M., Holzman, P. S., Katz, J. B., et al. Thyroid "hot spots": Their relationships to life stress. *Psychosomatic Medicine*, 1970, *32*, 561–568.

Weiner, H., Thaler, M., Reiser, M. F., et al. Etiology of duodenal ulcer. *Psychosomatic Medicine*, 1957, *19*, 1–10.

Williams, R. B., Jr., Kimball, C. P., & Willard, H. N. The influence of interpersonal interaction upon diastolic blood pressure. *Psychosomatic Medicine*, 1972, *32*, 194–198.

Wilson, E. *Sociobiology: The new synthesis.* Cambridge, Mass.: Harvard University Press, 1975.

20

Diagnosing Mental Deficiency

ETTA KARP, MURRY MORGENSTERN, AND
HAROLD MICHAL-SMITH

1. Introduction

Although this chapter is entitled "Diagnosing Mental Deficiency," the word "De-ficiency" is not in current practice in the United States, principally because of its misleading and pejorative implications. In the past, mental deficiency signified moral defect, pervasive deficiencies or defects which were irreversible, biologically fixed and the basis of prediction of future functioning. The basic assumption of deficiency as an unchanging condition is no longer a current notion. "Once a defective, always a defective" was like the old Hindu caste system that kept the individual rooted in a bleak, narrow groove with no prospects, no hope of escape, no expectation of change and/or a happier, more satisfying state.

Contemporary society dismisses the concept of immutability. The retarded can grow, develop, and change under certain conditions. Progress, a vast body of scien-tific, clinical, and medical knowledge, and acceleration of research have discredited old beliefs and recognized their shortcomings and the heavy reliance on a few ques-tionable measurable constructs. Old theories, categorical generalizations, notions of the existence of qualitative and quantitative differences in intellectual factors between the retarded and the average individual have been shown to be fallacious.

The current trend is to remove the lingering "scarlet letter" used to designate, to mark, and to bypass the retarded. Even the less derogatory, misleading term "re-tarded" is considered offensive, stigmatizing, and destructive to this segment of people. Paradoxically, the most prestigious organization interested in mental retardation and organized in 1876 retains the name, American Association on Mental Deficiency (AAMD). Heightened sensitivity to the rights and the privileges of every individual regardless of race, sex, physical well-being, and mental development has focused on the abrogation of any descriptive but discriminatory term likely to label and to affect

ETTA KARP, MURRY MORGENSTERN, and HAROLD MICHAL-SMITH • Mental Retar-dation Institute, New York Medical College, New York, New York 10029.

ETTA KARP, MURRY
MORGENSTERN,
AND HAROLD
MICHAL-SMITH

the equalization process in the individual's pursuit of happiness. However, because another referential term or designation is still lacking, the word "retarded" will be substituted in this chapter for the more demeaning term "deficient."

The retarded individual is viewed today in all his human dimensions, with the same needs, passions, affections, impulses, and feelings as all other people. He cannot be singled out as someone strange or less human than his average contemporaries. The questions that naturally follow are: What is mental retardation? What causes retardation? Can retardation be changed or obliterated? Why are there so many inconsistencies in terminology in this field?

2. The Complexities of Retardation

Some of the questions raised cannot be answered simply, because retardation is a complex, multifaceted condition with no single causal factor that accounts for the diversity of behavioral reactions of the retarded. The lingering effects of some of the old concepts still cling and confuse the picture despite new knowledge and evidence to the contrary.

At the turn of the twentieth century, retardation was viewed as a simple condition based primarily on intellectual capacities. The deficits and intellectual abilities were either inherited or caused by adverse organic factors at a very early time in the individual's life. The factor that differentiated the retarded individual from others was the former's global developmental deficit in his intellectual capacity.

The tests constructed during that time, and proliferating until recently, to measure intelligence or what purported to be intelligence became the only important instrument of intelligence evaluation. Some voices, however, were raised after intelligence testing became widespread, questioning the validity of intelligence tests and expressing concern about the nature of intelligence and what factors could be tapped on a test. Regardless of concern about these controversial issues, intelligence tests were and have been used to influence a wide range of decisions about children and adults, their placement in institutions, special classes, or exclusion from regular elementary schools, labor unions, and employment.

As seen today, retardation may include medical and neurological features such as abnormal brain structure, developmental problems, social maladjustment, social incompetence, and ecological, cultural, intellectual, and behavioral factors that may or may not be present in entirety, yet none can reasonably be considered definitive. Some experts in the field point to social incompetence as the alpha and omega of retardation; others still hang on to the old concept of intelligence, and still others to environmental factors; but no specific has been designated as the nuclear trait. All agree, however, that retardation must be apparent before maturity and that some of the behavioral patterns shown by the retarded can also be seen in many other behavioral disorders commonly found in children and adults.

3. Causes of Retardation

The causes of retardation which interfere with sound development before, during, and after birth are as varied as life itself with its pitfalls, hazards, and seen and unseen dangers. A wide range of recognized but dissimilar factors affect development from the moment of conception to years after birth.

Currently, about 200 causes have been identified, explored, and verified as producing mental retardation. As numerous as this appears, the total represents only about 25% of all the known cases of mental retardation, with the large majority of unknown or questionable origin. Some of the contributing factors occur as the baby develops in the mother's womb, others during the span of the child's physical and neurological development, and many others after birth in the child's world at large—his home and his environment.

Radiation in utero, prematurity, infectious diseases such as congenital syphilis and rubella (German measles) in the mother during the first 3 months of birth, and the Rh factor (blood incompatibility between mother and child) may all produce mental retardation. Rh incompatibility is a recognized cause and is usually known long before a child's birth. If the newborn is immediately given blood transfusions, retardation may be averted.

Genetic factors, e.g., chromosomal abnormalities, result in one type of retardation, Down's syndrome (mongolism) and trisomy 21. Metabolic problems result in another type, e.g., familial amaurotic idiocy (Tay-Sachs) and epiloia (tuberous sclerosis).

Childhood infectious diseases such as scarlet fever, dysentery, erysipelas, and pneumonia accompanied by high fever (above 104°F) may also result in mental retardation.

Toxic agents, e.g., inhalation of noxious fumes given off by the burning of specific types of rubber found in storage batteries and used for fuel among the indigent, affect development. Arsenical fumes, frequently caused by the peeling of moldy wallpaper in very poor homes, affect many growing children. Pica eating, mouthing and swallowing of particles of lead found in the paint on old-fashioned cribs and headboards and in plaster from crumbling walls, jeopardizes wholesome development.

Brain abnormalities originating in prenatal life may directly or indirectly lead to mental retardation. Hydrocephalus (a blocking of ducts) results in the accumulation of fluid in the brain. Craniosynostosis (premature closing of the fontanels of the skull that usually close about the second year of life) causes an elongated head and mental retardation. Severe head injuries caused by falling from high distances, heavy blows, or other accidents to the skull may result in cerebral trauma and brain dysfunction.

As can be seen, causes of conditions associated with mental retardation encompass the developmental, neuropathological, familial, environmental, and social areas. Empirically, it has been found, however, that not all these underlying conditions are demonstrable in all cases, but those identified stand out clearly enough to indicate mental retardation.

4. Definition of Mental Retardation

Mental retardation, a widespread social-behavioral phenomenon, means different things to different societies, subcultures, and people. There is no universal definition despite the universality of the condition. Different definitions have reflected contradictory theoretical views of etiology and prognosis, and have influenced the management and treatment of retarded individuals. A longstanding controversy has been whether the definition should include irreversibility. In Great Britain, for example, emphasis is placed on social incompetency. An individual who manages to be self-supporting, is unobtrusive, and is no outstanding problem to others in his environment regardless of intellectual deficits is not considered retarded. The Soviet Union, on the other hand, considers physical and neurological defects and language, perceptual, and conditioning disorders as the basic characteristics of mental retardation.

Perhaps Clausen's apt summation is far more illuminating. "Mental deficiency does not exist outside the meaning assigned to it." Definitions are arbitrary and reflect the cultural judgment of a particular society at a point in time, so that an individual designated as retarded in one culture may not be considered retarded in another.

The medical model, which is currently our most widely accepted formulation in regard to maladaptive behavior, has had a strong influence on the definition of retardation because of its emphasis on diagnosis. In relation to diagnosis, the accepted definition determines the nature of the disease or abnormality that is identified.

This model has three basic premises as follows:

1. Disturbance in behavior is due to an underlying cause with a resultant emphasis on diagnosis of pathology.
2. This behavior cannot be treated directly, since it is a product or symptom of the cause.
3. Changes in behavior—spontaneous or through various interventions—are not significant unless the core problem has been resolved.

This concern with etiology, diagnosis, and pathology had a restrictive influence on services and programs for the retarded because they were regarded as "sick" and therefore not amenable to habilitation to maximize their limited potential. Paradoxically, as indicated before, some 75% of the mentally retarded give no evidence of a biologically discontinuous defect or exogenous damage to account for the retardation.

This country has taken a more pragmatic approach to the definition of retardation. Clinical concern is far less concerned with causation and diagnosis and more concerned with the possibility of change regardless of intellectual inferiorities and low social competency levels. Practical emphasis, with an eye to what can be achieved, is directed to the plasticity of the individual who is given an environment conducive to change and consequent growth and development.

This is not to deny the value of medical diagnosis and intervention where pathology is indicated in the physiological or organic sense. It is just as important in some cases to understand causes as it is to free other individuals from an assumption of underlying cause.

It should now be apparent that workers in the field of retardation are not all guided by the same philosophy or agree on one definition, and not all communicate on the same level. Too many factors intrude, too many cultural values have changed, too many notions based on conflicting subcultural beliefs exist, too many new attitudes impinge and inevitably lead to confusion and disagreement.

This brief discussion of definition represents the combined thinking of outstanding authorities in the field and was developed under the auspices of the American Association on Mental Deficiency (AAMD). Mental retardation as defined by this committee "refers to significantly subaverage general intellectual functioning existing concurrently with deficits in adaptive behavior and manifested during the developmental period." This definition refers to "subaverage general intellectual func-

tioning." The term "subaverage" stems from a statistical concept of the normal curve
of distribution, an arbitrary assigned average of 100, and the cutoff point or deviation from the number which is considered subaverage intellectual functioning.

Subaverage functioning is based on performance on appropriate objective intelligence tests one standard deviation below the population mean. The developmental period extends to about the age of 16 years.

One of the outstanding features of this definition is the inclusion of adaptive behavior, a recognition of the multifaceted dimensions of retarded behavior. Although
impaired intellectual functioning coexists with impaired adaptability, in the definition the former is still emphasized. Thus, if the clinician finds subaverage intellectual ability without impaired social adaptiveness, intelligence findings are considered doubtful based on the assumption that the "normal" adaptive behavior reflects a higher level of intelligence. On the other hand, if the results of intelligence
testing are above the cutoff of the subaverage level but adaptive behavior is impaired,
it may be assumed that factors other than intellectual ones account for the maladaptive behavior. The clinician, using this definition, excludes etiology and prognosis
when he formulates a diagnosis of retardation.

In accordance with developmental stages, adaptive behavior presents itself in
three basic sequences: maturation, learning, and social adjustment. Maturation is
the important criterion prior to the school years. It refers to the rate of development
of gross and fine motor skills such as crawling, walking, manipulation of buttons,
cutting with scissors. Learning related to the acquisition of academic skills assumes
prime importance during the school years. Social adjustment, important during the
adult years, is manifested by independence, employment, and the ability to take on
personal and social responsibilities. Discussion of evaluation of adaptive behavior
will follow later.

Despite AAMD's definition and the general acceptance of multideterminants of
retardation, it is still not uncommon in clinical practice and administrative procedures to find measured intelligence or the IQ used as the sole criterion of retardation. It seems redundant at this point to enumerate the longstanding criticisms
of intelligence tests. Of greater importance are the more recently expressed concerns of minority group representatives and professionals. These groups have criticized intelligence tests and the resulting IQ as stigmatizing and biased against socially
and economically deprived minority children, excluding them from regular school
settings and denying them opportunities to learn and be trained for competitive
employment.

5. Classification of Mental Retardation

In an attempt to reflect present thinking in regard to the interaction of intelligence and experience and the role of inherited and environmental factors as they
contribute to various forms of retardation, AAMD has developed two classification systems. One is a medical classification based on etiology, in which mental
retardation "is regarded as a manifestation of some underlying disease process or
medical condition." Cause is determined by detection of noxious agents (i.e., chromosomal abnormalities in Down's syndrome) or from symptoms and syndromes typical of the disease (i.e., hydrocephalus). However, inferred etiology based on present
symptoms presents difficulties when a single cause is not present. When this occurs,

etiology is associated with a classification so that the clinician cannot make precise or accurate statements about prognosis.

The other classification system is behavioral based on the definition already discussed: deficits in both measured intelligence and adaptive behavior. Inherent in this system is the assumption that the current abilities measured by standardized individual intelligence tests are normally distributed in the general population. The choice of the appropriate test is the diagnostician's decision. The system uses firm levels of measured intelligence, profound to mild, marked off in terms of standard deviation units. The levels of retardation are translated into IQ values ranges for three commonly used intelligence tests as shown in Table 1.

It should be noted that the borderline category is absent and therefore not a level of retardation. The levels mild, moderate, and severe are reminiscent of educational classification. Mild retardation is much like the category used in schools; it implies "educability." The moderate group pertains to individuals previously referred to as "trainable," the severe group refers to the "dependent retarded," and the profound group refers to those who may require perpetual "life support." With change, an individual classified as moderately retarded may in time move up and function well in the mildly retarded group. An individual classified as moderately retarded may, on the other hand, be more appropriately placed in the severely retarded group.

The classification terms are neither fixed nor static. Mobility up or down is possible and is probably basically helpful in planning programs.

The adaptive levels, like the intellectual ones, depend on the degree of impairment (see Table 2). These levels, unlike intellectual functioning, are scaled from mild negative deviation from the population norms to almost complete lack of adaptation at the extreme lower limit, e.g., a nonambulatory, nonverbal individual who may not be able to feed or dress himself and is cared for in a crib or bed.

The AAMD Adaptive Behavior Scale measures aspects of adaptive and maladaptive behavior. A new edition of the Scale's manual will contain additional procedures for more effective evaluation of the overall behavioral level.

The manual states that valid classification of mental retardation must satisfy the requirements of the definition. Although the adaptive behavioral scale is not yet entirely satisfactory, the determination of mental retardation will still rest on clinical judgment.

The evaluation of adaptive behavior presents less of a problem than that mercurial quality we call intelligence, because behavior, of course, is more clearly observable. If we equate intellectual functioning with the IQ, as discussed earlier, the client is imprisoned within a more or less deliberately limited construct. Moving from the IQ toward a broader perspective of intelligence, validating instruments

Table 1

Level	Obtained intelligence quotient	
	Stanford-Binet and Cattell	Wechsler Scales
Mild	67–52	69–53
Moderate	51–36	54–40
Severe	35–20	39–25 (extrapolated)
Profound	19 and below	24 and below (extrapolated)

Age and level indicated	Illustrations of highest level of adaptive behavior functioning
Age 3 years and above: profound (Note: All behaviors at greater degree of impairment would also indicate profound deficit in adaptive behavior for persons 3 years of age or above.	Independent functioning: Drinks from cup with help; "cooperates" by opening mouth for feeding. Physical: Sits unsupported or pulls self upright momentarily; reaches for objects; has good thumb-finger grasp; manipulates objects (e.g., plays with shoes or feet). Communication: Imitates sounds, laughs or smiles back (says "Da-da," "buh-buh" responsively); no effective speech; may communicate in sounds and/or gestures; responds to gestures and/or signs. Social: Indicates knowing familiar persons and interacts nonverbally with them.
Age 3 years: severe Age 6 years and above: profound	Independent functioning: Attempts finger feeding; "cooperates" with dressing, bathing, and toilet training; may remove clothing (e.g., socks) but not as act of undressing as for bath or bed. Physical: Stands alone or may walk unsteadily or with help; coordinates eye-hand movements. Communication: One or two words (e.g., "Mama," "ball") but predominantly vocalization. Social: May respond to others in predictable fashion; communicates needs by gestures and noises or pointing; plays "pattycake" or plays imitatively with little interaction; or occupies self alone with "toys" few minutes.
Age 3 years: moderate Age 6 years: severe Age 9 years and above: profound	Independent functioning: Tries to feed self with spoon; considerable spilling; removes socks, pants; "cooperates" in bathing; may indicate wet pants; "cooperates" at toilet. Physical: Walks alone steadily; can pass ball or objects to others; may run and climb steps with help. Communication: May use four to six words; may communicate many needs with gestures (e.g., pointing). Social: Plays with others for short periods, often as parallel play or under direction; recognizes others and may show preference for some persons over others.
3 years: mild 6 years: moderate 9 years: severe 12 years and above: profound	Independent functioning: Feeds self with spoon (cereals, soft foods) with considerable spilling or messiness; drinks unassisted; can pull off clothing and put on some (socks, underclothes, boxer pants, dress); tries to help with bath or hand washing but still needs considerable help; indicates toilet accident and may indicate toilet need. Physical: May climb up and down stairs but not alternating feet; may run and jump; may balance briefly on one foot; can pass ball to others; transfers objects; may do simple form-board puzzles without aid. Communication: May speak in two- or three-word sentences ("Daddy go work"); name simple common objects (boy, car, ice cream, hat); understands simple directions (put the shoe on your foot, sit here, get your coat); knows people by name. (If nonverbal, may use many gestures to convey needs or other information.)

(Continued)

Table 2. (*Continued*)

Age and level indicated	Illustrations of highest level of adaptive behavior functioning
	Social: May interact with others in simple play activities, usually with only one or two others unless guided into group activity; has preference for some persons over others.
6 years: mild 9 years: moderate 12 years and above: severe 15 years and above: profound	Independent functioning: Feeds self with spoon or fork, may spill some; puts on clothing but needs help with small buttons and jacket zippers; tries to bathe self but needs help; can wash and dry hands but not very efficiently; partially toilet trained but may have accidents.
	Physical: May hop or skip; may climb steps with alternating feet; rides tricycle (or bicycle over 8 years); may climb trees or jungle gym; play dance games; may throw ball and hit target.
	Communication: May have speaking vocabulary of over 300 words and use gramatically correct sentences. If nonverbal, may use many gestures to communicate needs. Understands simple verbal communications including directions and questions ("Put it on the shelf." "Where do you live?"). (Some speech may be indistinct sometimes.) May recognize advertising words and signs (Ice Cream, Stop, Exit, Men, Ladies). Relates experiences in simple language.
	Social: Participates in group activities and simple group games; interacts with others in simple play ("Store," "House") and expressive activities (art and dance).
9 years: mild 12 years: moderate 15 years and older: severe	Independent functioning: Feeds self adequately with spoon and fork; can butter bread (needs help for cutting meat); can put on clothes and can button and zipper clothes; may tie shoes; bathes self with supervision; is toilet trained; washes face and hands without help.
	Physical: Can run, skip, hop, dance; uses skates or sled or jump rope; can go up and down stairs alternating feet; can throw ball to hit target.
	Communication: May communicate in complex sentences; speech is generally clear and distinct; understands complex verbal communication including words such as "because" and "but." Recognizes signs, words, but does not read with comprehension prose materials.
	Social: May participate in group activities spontaneously; may engage in simple competitive exercise games (dodge ball, tag, races). May have friendship choices which are maintained over weeks or months.
	Economic activity: May be sent on simple errands and make simple purchases with a note; realizes money has value but does not know how to use it (except for coin machines).
	Occupation: May prepare simple foods (sandwiches); can help with simple household tasks (bedmaking, sweeping, vacuuming); can set and clear table.
	Self-direction: May ask if there is "work" for him to do; may pay attention to task for 10 minutes or more; makes efforts to be dependable and carry out responsibility.
12 years: mild 15 years and over: moderate	Independent functioning: Feeds, bathes, dresses self; may select daily clothing; may prepare easy foods (peanut butter sandwiches) for self or others; combs/brushes hair; may shampoo and roll up hair; may wash and/or iron and store own clothes.

Table 2. *(Continued)*

717

DIAGNOSING
MENTAL DEFICIENCY

Age and level indicated	Illustrations of highest level of adaptive behavior functioning

Physical: Good body control; good gross and fine motor coordination.

Communication: May carry on simple conversation; uses complex sentences. Recognizes words, may read sentences, ads, signs, and simple prose material with some comprehension.

Social: May interact cooperatively and/or competitively with others.

Economic activity: May be sent on shopping errand for several items without notes; makes minor purchases; adds coins to dollar with fair accuracy.

Occupation: May do simple routine household chores (dusting, garbage, dishwashing; prepare simple foods which require mixing).

Self-direction: May initiate most of own activities; attend to task 15–20 min (or more); may be conscientious in assuming much responsibility.

15 years and adult: mild

Note: Individuals who routinely perform at higher levels of competence in adaptive behavior than illustrated in this pattern should not be considered as deficient in adaptive behavior. Since by definition an individual is not retarded unless he shows significant deficit in both measured intelligence and in adaptive behavior, those individuals who function at higher levels than illustrated here cannot be considered to be retarded.

Independent functioning: Exercises care for personal grooming, feeding, bathing, toilet, may need health or personal care reminders, may need help in selection of purchase of clothing.

Physical: Goes about hometown (local neighborhood in city, campus at institution) with ease, but cannot go to other towns alone without aid; can use bicycle, skis, ice skates, trampoline or other equipment requiring good coordination.

Communication: Communicates complex verbal concepts and understands them; carries on everyday conversation, but cannot discuss abstract or philosophical concepts; uses telephone and communicates in writing for simple letter writing or orders but does not write about abstractions or important current events.

Social: Interacts cooperatively or competitively with others and initiates some group activities, primarily for social or recreational purposes; may belong to a local recreation group or church group, but not to civic organizations or groups of skilled persons (e.g., photography club, great books club, or kennel club); enjoys recreation (e.g., bowling, dancing, TV, checkers, but either does not enjoy or is not competent at tennis, sailing, bridge, piano playing or other hobbies requiring rapid or involved or complex planning and implementation).

Economic activity: Can be sent or go to several shops to make purchases (without a note to shopkeepers) to purchase several items; can make change correctly, but does not use banking facilities; may earn living but has difficulty handling money without guidance.

Occupation: Can cook simple foods, prepare simple meals; can perform everyday household tasks (cleaning, dusting, dishes, laundry); as adult can engage in semiskilled or simple skilled job.

Self-direction: Initiates most of own activity; will pay attention to task for at least 15–20 min; conscientious about work and assumes much responsibility but needs guidance for tasks with responsibility for major tasks (health care, care of others, complicated occupational activity).

ETTA KARP, MURRY
MORGENSTERN,
AND HAROLD
MICHAL-SMITH

with which to quantify these more elusive qualities are not available. Using the AAMD as our authority, adaptive behavior is defined as "the manner in which the individual copes with the natural and social demands of the environment."

The interesting word here is "demands," the demands of the environment. There are no "demands" when we speak of intelligence. There may be requirements for the purposes of quantification, but even if an impaired individual met those requirements, procedurally speaking, he or she would still be confronted by the "demands" of society for a level of behavior that is consonant with the needs of other human beings who live in a particular community. Mental retardation, per se, does not necessarily affect the mass of normal individuals who constitute society, but deficits in adaptive behavior do.

As the trend toward deinstitutionalization expands and the development of community-based programs for the more severely impaired continues, the question of adaptive behavior becomes more significant. Only in the last 15 years has this behavioral concept become a major factor in the assessment of the mentally retarded—in other words, adaptive behavior has become an additional dimension in assessment and, correspondingly, new problems have arisen in measurement and evaluation.

The simple fact that behavior is now a major factor in evaluation indicates that socialization is an intrinsic consideration, so to speak, of the impaired individual in view of his placement in the larger interpersonal dynamics of school, work, and community. There is, then, an element here that differs from the approach to intelligence, on which we can legitimately ponder a broadening of concept and measurement. Adaptive behavior, however, becomes meaningful in direct relation to existing developmental programs, and a greater degree of pragmatism will be required, as it always is when one is dealing directly with social phenomena. The point is reached pragmatically where an individual's ability to behave appropriately or acceptably in everyday living is a more significant factor than his intellectual functioning. Surely many have observed autistic children who could, on the basis of the psychologist's sensibilities, be considered brilliant, but where the behavior is such as to render that intelligence purely hypothetical and without relation to deinstitutionalized planning.

Adaptive behavior, then, is a community concern, and the evaluation of it is based on standards inherent in the community. The major tenets in the criteria for adaptive behavior were developed in 1961 by the AAMD and were represented by three basic formulations:

1. Independent functioning. This aspect can be best described as the ability of the individual to successfully accomplish, by himself, certain types of activities demanded of him by the general community, in relation to the survival needs of that community and in relation to the typical expectations of the community from others in the same age groups.
2. Personal responsibility. Here it is the willingness—not just the ability but the willingness—of the individual to accomplish, by himself or under some supervision, those critical and basic tasks demanded by the community; the ability, in short, to assume responsibility for his behavior, with its concurrent responsibilities for decision making as reflected in a choice of behaviors.

3. Social responsibility. This can be defined as the ability of the individual to accept responsibility as a member of a group, and to carry out appropriate behaviors in terms of the expectations of the group. This concept is reflected in levels of conformity, socially positive creativity, social adjustment, and emotional maturity. To this, we might add some considerations of civic responsibility, in the sense of the relationship of this to partial or complete socioeconomic independence.

To measure performance according to the criteria thus outlined, there are the Adaptive Behavior Scales, consisting of two parts. The first part assesses performance in the areas of independent functioning, physical development, economic activities, language development, number and time concepts, domestic and general occupation, self-direction, responsibility, and socialization. The second part assesses performance in the areas of violent and destructive behavior, rebellious behavior, antisocial behavior, untrustworthy behavior, withdrawal, stereotyped behavior and odd mannerisms, inappropriate interpersonal manners, inappropriate vocal habits, unacceptable or eccentric habits, self-abuse behavior, hyperactive tendencies, sexually aberrant behavior, psychological disturbances, and the use of medications.

When adaptive behavior is analyzed in the light of the three areas of criteria set for it and the scales designed for its evaluation, one sees a number of underlying realities which do not dovetail all that neatly with the standards reflected by the community at large.

For example, it can be seen that there are age standards and expectations, particularly in relationship to the concept of independent functioning. Generations of normal children have been raised on the societally established parental expectations that a child, at a certain age, should be capable of doing certain things. However, it is known that there may be traditions in the subcultures or in the ethnic minorities where dependence on the mother is fostered beyond the biological/behavioral needs of the child, so that certain capabilities for independent function may be either stunted or postponed. There is also an omnipresent factor, the neurotic overlays possible within a given family structure, in regard to either the premature or the delayed independent functioning of the child; and these parental disturbances may be intensified in the family situation of a retarded child.

Cultural differences between the expectations of one social class and another, in terms of both status and economics, where there are privileges of wealth as well as deprivations of poverty, may exert an other-than-normal effect on the development of a child's independence. Consequently, the priorities set for a child's developmental capabilities at certain points in time can vary to a significant degree, and the measurement of his adaptive behavior may represent deviations that are not necessarily indicative of deficit but may be due to a different or atypical set of determinants.

At another level of reality, one must also consider the inner view of the child in regard to his self-image, his role in the family, and his relationships to his peers. As a child grows, his behavior increasingly reflects the pressures of his peers as well as the values of his adult environment. The demands within the household may well be for scrupulous cleanliness, but a child of a certain status whose play areas are the streets of New York City is going to get dirty if he is to enjoy the street games and play relationships with other children of his own age and status. An impaired child who has an impoverished self-concept and consequently senses an unequal role among his peers may retreat from attempts at independent functioning or he may overcompensate for his sense of inadequacy by conspicuously aberrant behavior.

In short, we have to recognize a number of reality levels: the overall norm; the cultural, social, and economic deviations; the nature of the immediate family constellation; and the reaction formations of the child in terms of his personality and his impairment. Given this conflux of factors, the tolerances of our evaluatory measures must be broadened to encompass the specificities of the child's immediate psychological and circumstantial environment.

The evaluation of the capacity for independent functioning must also relate directly to the second criterion, i.e., personal responsibility. What is at issue here is the matter of individual volition. Does the child wish to perform the functions that are expected of him. Not only is he able to, but is he willing, without a strong degree of coerciveness, to brush his teeth, make his bed, use his eating utensils correctly? If he appears willing to do the things that he is judged capable of doing, we assume that he demonstrates personal responsibility. This construct also involves aspects of trustworthiness as well. Will he undertake certain functions not only willingly but also safely, without constant supervision? Can he be trusted to perform without resultant harm to himself or others? Is he operating at a level which permits others in his environment to conduct their lives without the distraction of constant attention to the child?

Thus the capacity of the child and the willingness of the child to be socialized, to conform to expected routines and established patterns, become the crux of the assessment. Basically, the concern is with the ability of the child to make appropriate decisions, decisions which indicate a basic regard for the self and a basic aptitude for conformance with the requirements of others. Decision making in relation to the intellectually impaired child does have a special significance, because there is a higher degree of suggestibility due to the weakness of the self-image. The concern here is with the ability in the child to reject negative demands as well as to comply with constructive ones.

The third criterion, social responsibility, is, in effect, an outcome of the two preceding conditions. If a child indicates an acceptable level of independent functioning and personal responsibility, then a behavioral role that is acceptable to the community should emerge as he matures. Social responsibility refers to the ability of the impaired individual to maintain a social profile that will enable him to blend into the general mores without distress to the community. This is a very pragmatic concept, because the concern is less with the contributory aspects of social responsibility than with the absence of negative aspects. The goal is a level of adaptive behavior that will permit acceptance of the impaired individual as a member of the community.

The demands of a given community, that is, the social basis on which a community will tolerate an impaired individual, will, of course, vary with geography and with cultural, social, economic, and political pressures, and so on. Modes of language and of dress will certainly vary in regard to specific neighborhoods insofar as neighborhoods do represent, in great part, the various subcultures in our society. Consequently, the very specific ability to conform, without a high degree of visibility as "different," to the particular environment in which the impaired individual is living as a community member is at issue.

In short, the success of the impaired individual depends entirely on his ability to be tolerated by the community. It is sufficient for survival purposes that the personality and functional posture do not create negative reactions—it is not necessary to survival to achieve positive or welcome acceptance. If the latter is achieved, the individual does more than survive; he succeeds.

The real point of this has very little to do, if anything, with the level of the individual's abstract ability, and virtually nothing to do with his academic abilities. The impaired individual does not have to have a concept of time, for example. All he really needs, in this survival context, is to be able to follow a routine which will enable him to be at a job or a class at the appointed hour. If he can do this, he is fulfilling a personal and social responsibility, and the question of his "retardation" is hypothetical. If he can move, in his everyday life, through the routines of community existence without causing alarm, distress, or annoyance to others, then he, for functional purposes, is not retarded, not "stupid."

What is intelligence, functionally speaking, other than a workable method of dealing with the world? In the previous discussion on intelligence and IQ, a broader approach to intelligence was reviewed which can perhaps be comprehended more closely as a mode of approach to people and to life. For practical purposes, intelligence is good adaptive behavior, and perhaps no worldly purpose is served by creating dichotomies in assessment when these dichotomies do not apply realistically to life. What are our assessment objectives, really, in the light of current trends? It is to avoid institutionalization wherever possible, and to provide maximum opportunity for a life that approaches the normal. To classify a child as mentally retarded on the basis of the IQ alone is a disservice to him, provided that the total behavioral aspect augurs well for life in a community.

Conversely, if a child with either more or less intense defects in measured intellectual function fails to indicate the existence of or potential for the assumption of personal and social responsibility to the degree that his nonconformance is conspicuous, in comparison with that of his peers and with the minimum expectations of an open society, then we must provide for him in other ways, such as placement in sheltered workshops, activity centers, or whatever environments or programs are most appropriate for his degree of deviance.

Where nonadaptive behavior exists, we see an individual whom society will regard, without reference to our professional classifications, as "mentally retarded." We can go further and say, in the ultimate realism, that it is society who classifies an individual, not the psychologist. It is the task, then, of psychologists, to accept this view of society as determinant, and to observe and evaluate the total child in the light of his capacity for adaptation to the dynamic interaction of the society in which he is trying to live and to the interpersonal situations in which he must function adequately for his survival. Within the perspective of this goal, relevance must shift from the measurement of intelligence to the comprehension of his total mode. It is in this mode that he expresses himself as a unique human being, and it is in this mode that the members of society will or will not permit him to function.

The Adaptive Behavior Scale can be found in Grossman (1973). In spite of all the thought, effort, and work expended on definition and classification, neither is completely satisfactory. The AAMD proposes to reevaluate and to reformulate shortly and try to arrive at new meaning and a new classificatory system.

6. Diagnosis and Assessment

"Diagnosis," originally introduced by medicine, traditionally means the identification of a disease from its signs and symptoms. Diagnosis serves the physician when he can fit a patient's illness into a classification or find a specific type of treatment that corresponds with the diagnosis. The assumptions basic to this approach are that the somatic causes of illness are regular and predictable in outcome.

In mental retardation, as in many other biosocial conditions, this approach is inadequate, particularly for the psychologist. Research has found no recognizable test patterns to be used by psychologists which can unerringly be diagnostic of any specific condition. The multiplicity of causation and the variety of individuals that fall into this broad category preclude such an approach.

6.1. Multiple Determinants

To the psychologist involved in the individual's total functioning, no one factor can be isolated as primary causation. All factors are in constant interaction with one another, and somatic morbidity or etiology offers little to the understanding of mental retardation.

The growing acceptance of multiple causation has resulted in a new look at diagnosis. For the psychologist, classification does not result in shortcuts to etiological implications. In place of this, accurate descriptions of behaviors are stressed. Following this, the symptoms present are classified into groups which are then compared with empirically established correlates. Theoretically, at least, the clinician can develop probabilities about correlates such as cause or educability which are determined by how an individual's symptoms fit into classification.

Nevertheless, the tendency to use medical terms persists and is often confusing. The term "organicity," for example, frequently appears in psychological evaluation. As Birch points out, "organicity in behavioral functioning is a characteristic manifested by individuals with certain kinds of brain damage and should in no sense be mistaken as the prototype of disturbance which may accompany all instances of injury to the brain."

The psychologist, in recognition of one of his major responsibilities—psychological examination based on functional analysis of behavior, considers this heuristic process assessment. Concentration on new nomenclature is neither euphemistic nor prestige seeking, but is in keeping with the changed emphasis on the behavior of a retarded individual. Assessment as it is used today stresses precise and detailed descriptions of current behavior so that an effective individualized treatment program may be planned and implemented. Assessment also implies procedures used to monitor treatment progress and to evaluate behavior after treatment.

6.2. Testing and Assessment

Testing is done with assessment in mind, but assessment does not necessarily result in a test score. Testing is not equivalent to assessment. Its functions basically are classification and programming, decision making and intervention.

The clinician no longer relies so heavily on test reactions as he did when emphasis was mainly on measured intelligence. Currently, the clinician uses observations in various settings, gathers information about the individual as he was and is, and carefully notes progress, social interactions, and environmental disruptions.

In this approach, the individual is not viewed as a passive recipient in a diagnostic-prescriptive system, but rather as one who responds to his environment and whose response in turn is the consequence of that environment. Its premise is that the individual can change his behavior by acquiring adaptive styles which do not depend on its causes or diagnosis of internal states. Accordingly, it reduces the restrictive results of categorization and stigmatizing.

Certain trends in assessment practices have become evident: (1) an increasing recognition and acceptance of the wide variability which exists in our society with respect to cultural and linguistic patterns, (2) evolving views with regard to education practices and philosophies, and (3) attempts to respond to pressures by organized groups to modify existing practices through litigation, legislation, and actions by professional organizations.

Psychological assessment utilizes a battery of tests yielding information pertinent to an individual's verbal, nonverbal, perceptual, motor, and language skills and personality characteristics. Tests can be useful devices if we acknowledge their strengths and weaknesses. When we use them, we need to recognize that there are basic assumptions underlying their application.

The first assumption is that the clinician is skilled and knowledgeable in test administration, scoring, and analysis, in relating to the client, and in performing other features related to these roles. The clinician must be confident that observed behaviors are sufficient in quantity and representative of the area of function being assessed. Observation is more useful when extended over a period of time in a variety of settings.

Another factor of concern is measurement error. It is assumed that the error magnitude is estimable when a particular measure's reliability and validity are recognized, thus supporting confidence in appropriate statistical interpretations. Standard errors of measurement and estimate can be helpful, but it must be kept in mind that the size of errors in measurement can be only estimated for a particular individual.

Another assumption is that all persons have been exposed to acculturation patterns similar to those of the standardization sample. Of course, the more similar a particular individual is to the sample population, the more confident we are that the selected test is appropriate for our use. In the field of retardation, we often work with persons from physical and sociocultural backgrounds and settings of such difference to warrant questions about a test's appropriateness. This is not to imply that all racial-ethnic minority groups or those from low socioeconomic homes are significantly different from the standardization group. What is needed here is a heightened sensitivity to important differences in child-rearing practices, aspirations, language experiences, and involvement in learning. Such factors may result in acculturation patterns which cannot be directly compared to more typical ones in this country. Whether a particular client's acculturation patterns resemble those reflected in a test's sample can be determined only by a thorough exploration of the person's background. Localized and pluralistic norms may be one way of dealing with problems related to dissimilar acculturation patterns, particularly when group characteristics within a geographical area are significantly different and when results are to be used for programming within a local district. National and local norms may provide greater accuracy and clarity in interpreting test data.

In addition to evaluating behavior in terms of group norms or a standardization sample, assessment may also concentrate on criterion-referenced behaviors of mentally retarded persons. It may be as important to know that a person cannot lace his shoes or draw a horizontal line as it is to know that he is in the tenth percentile of a norm group. Criterion-referenced measures can be useful if they measure specific and relevant behaviors and if they can be interpreted in terms of specific performance standards. Under these conditions, they can provide more precise information on what a child or adult can or cannot do, and can check the rate of progress in acquiring appropriate or important behaviors. The assessor must proceed with caution, however, in their use, because their reliability and validity can be problematic. Furthermore, they may be used to develop standards of performance or desirable goals, thus increasing rather than eliminating cultural biases.

6.3. Assessor-Client Relationship

The assessment process is a complex interaction of the examiner, the client, and situational variables. The assessor himself should be considered a part of the environmental setting in which the assessment occurs. An examiner is not always a facilitator or positive influence on a client's performance. The manner in which rapport is established and maintained, how he responds to the client's attitudes and feelings, and the types of behavior that are reinforced influence performance. Clinicians who are cold and unresponsive and do not enjoy working with disabled clients or who have hidden or overt biases for or against certain kinds of persons may reflect these characteristics in their test interpretations. However, the assessor who recognizes these reactions does not have to feel pressured or threatened by the client's handicap, but rather can begin with the reality of the handicap as part of the client's life problems. Alertness to the sensitivities of the client which is basic in all phases of assessment requires that the assessor see and hear himself as he appears to others.

With the slow or impaired client, one may need a longer initial contact, keener observation of nonverbal cues, and more allowance of time and patience in waiting for a response.

In assessment situations where mental retardation may be a factor, there may be little or no outward manifestation other than behavior. Because of this and the greater social taboo on openly recognizing retardation than other handicapping conditions, there is a greater tendency for overreaction by both the client and assessor. The client may become overly dependent and demanding, and the clinician may be overly guilty, attentive, and concerned. The client's realization that communication of his feelings will be difficult is as important as understanding what others are trying to communicate to him. Nevertheless, the assessor must be an exception to the usual social mores in his approach and manner to these clients, making it possible for them to verbalize their difficulties in understanding things or in people not understanding them.

A point at issue currently is the race of the assessor. It has been suggested that a white examiner engenders feelings of insecurity, self-consciousness, and apprehension among black or other minority group members so that such factors negatively influence performance, particularly in children. Most research does not support this view. There is some evidence that adolescent and adult blacks are more likely to want to work with black psychologists. At times, it may be in the child's or parents' best interests to pair, whether by race or sex. Good clinical judgment can decide when this should occur.

6.4. Language Differences

The assessment of non-English-speaking clients is most valid when it is done in their native language. A translator may be helpful but must be used cautiously since his accent may confuse the client, and differences in meaning presented by translation must be taken into account. It may be helpful also to approach such clients as if they were deaf, using gestures and pictures as well as special instruments which minimize language, to be discussed later.

Assessment procedures with bilingual subjects require different strategies. By definition, the bilingual person has some command of two languages. It is the assessor's responsibility to determine in which language the client feels most comfortable or is most sophisticated. This information can be obtained from the client's teacher or parent and from informal appraisal. In clinical practice, the bilingual psychologist may use both languages depending on responsivity, which may vary from item to item, or test to test. In any event, the basic goal is to use a language style which maximizes the client's opportunity to understand requirements and to be able to respond by using his best language abilities. Testing repertoires have been increased by translating tests into other languages and by developing parallel forms for use with Spanish-speaking clients. However, translation may not necessarily remove language biases unless we are certain that the language used is characteristic of each child or adult we assess. Until such time as we have solved the technical problems in finding ways to minimize language biases of tests, some of the more traditional nonlanguage measures continue to be used but with strong reservations. It becomes patently clear that sound judgment is needed in selection, administration, and interpretation of test results. Familiarity with different linguistic and social-cultural patterns and flexibility and adaptability in using currently available procedures and techniques are intermediate steps before other solutions become available.

7. Assessment Techniques

Assessment is not a goal in itself. It is seen as a major aspect of a process that involves intervention as well. Essential to a comprehensive assessment is information obtained from observational and other available data: language dominance, sensory-motor assessment, adaptive behavior assessment, medical and developmental data, and personality and intellectual assessment.

One of the central aims of assessment follows the Jungian concept of individuation, that is, the development of the individual's resources and potentialities as far and as much as possible. Success to any degree is predicated on the understanding of each individual's unique nature, again as far as it is possible to understand another human being, in order to assist and direct him in his efforts to cope with his world and help him effectively plan for his future in the larger culture.

Understanding of the individual entails a comprehensive study of all the measurable aspects of his life, past and present, with the ultimate goal of knowing him as he copes in his particular world at this particular time in his development. The retarded individual must be prepared to recognize a wider world and the skills it takes to win admission.

Assessment is a continuous process and is involved not only with skills necessary at the time but also with ones needed as the individual grows older. The present needs may emphasize academic programming and socialization—learning to share and a give-and-take relationship to make and hold friends. A later developmental stage may require special training in occupational skills, in understanding and forming heterosexual relationships, and in moving about from community to community.

Psychological assessment is viewed as a fluoroscopic picture of the individual's strengths and weaknesses in all areas of his development—intellectual, emotional, social, perceptual, and vocational—which are constantly reviewed and revised and serve as a baseline for his education, his job training, his social adaptability, his participation in the community, and possibly his function as a marriage partner and a parent.

In the final analysis, assessment is a never-ending process that studies and evaluates an individual's behavior with the intent of measuring objectively and subjectively the areas and skills necessary for learning, adjusting, and coping. The knowledge gleaned from the assessment becomes the foundation of programming and intervention for the materialization of goals.

The test batteries used in diagnostic and in assessment work are basically similar. The content and the structure of the tests highlight strengths and weaknesses of different areas of function and behavior. Areas tapped overlap each other and are not discrete entities. Rather, they are the integral and interactional parts which make up the total configuration or identity of the individual. The areas or domains are cognitive, sensory-motor, perceptual, affective, social, and conative.

It is beyond the scope of this chapter to describe extensively the nature and content of the tests commonly used to sample these behavioral domains. However, it may be useful to understand their place in an assessment battery.

As has been mentioned, the assessment of intellectual development (cognition) has been the core in the study of behavior, not only because intelligence is considered of primary importance for economic and social achievement but also because of the development of IQ tests to measure it precisely. The Stanford-Binet and the Wechsler Scales continue to be the main instruments to measure intellectual functioning despite the never-dormant debates on the nature and definition of intelligence. Current evaluation of intellectual functioning in the field of mental retardation is an essential if not the primary aspect of the battery. Precise and comprehensive assessment of cognitive functioning is needed to delineate the individual's strengths and weaknesses and to understand the deterents to his intellectual growth, whether these be environmental, familial, or physical. Because of the interrelationships of intellectual, social, and emotional development, slowness or retardation in the former can be symptomatic of disturbances in the emotional or neurophysiological spheres. For these as well as other reasons, assessment of intellectual development and function requires the expertise of a trained clinician.

The Binet, designed for children and mainly verbal at the older levels, can be divided into five broad categories: manipulative, language or communicative, discriminative, memory, and reasoning and problem solving. The Wechsler Scales, which are three different tests at different age levels, provide 10–12 subtests arranged in a verbal and nonverbal section. Verbal subtests cover mainly vocabulary, memory, comprehension, numerical reasoning, and concept formation; nonverbal subtests measure visual organization, perceptual-motor integration, and eye-hand coordination.

The size and range of behavior sampled by intelligence tests vary from test to test. The Binet and Wechsler contain many items to cover the abilities to be measured at the various age levels. However, the actual number of items presented to an individual can be quite small. Although both scales have wide content and sample a variety of intellectual behaviors and thought processes, it may not be possible to get an adequate representation of these various aspects for all individuals, especially where retardation may be a factor. An 8-year-old, moderately retarded, administered the WISC may pass only one or two items on a subtest or none at all. In clinical practice, therefore, the Binet may be given at higher age levels when the WISC may be the test of choice.

IQ scales which sample one intellectual activity are sometimes used to replace the Binet and WISC for time convenience. Tests such as the Peabody Picture Vocabulary Test measures receptive language. Even though an IQ is obtained, the assessor must remember that only the single intellectual function is being tapped, whether in the grossly intact individual or in the multiply impaired individual who does not have the verbal or motor ability to respond to the Wechsler. However, the Peabody or the Columbia Mental Maturity Scale may be useful to supplement or verify information obtained from the Binet or Wechsler.

Although intelligence tests have scores standardized on large samples, analysis is not limited to the total IQ score or, in the case of the Wechsler, to the verbal and performance scores or to the scores on various subtests or categories. Analysis of profiles of subtest scores, or patterns within or between subtests, or mental processes is common practice. Comparisons are made between success on one type of task and failure on another or between successes and failures on a similar task, particularly when these occur out of sequence.

These kinds of analyses are necessary to ascertain strengths and weaknesses which may be amenable to remediation or a treatment plan. They can also be useful in relating cognitive function to social or emotional function. One might tentatively hypothesize that a child weak in areas tapping independent judgment and analysis of a situation but adequate in routine learning is too dependent emotionally to make independent intellectual judgments. Variability in patterns of success and failure may suggest lapses in attention, specific disabilities, or physiological handicaps which will need to be corroborated by other elements in the assessment.

However, caution needs to be observed in profile scatter or pattern analysis. There is no evidence, for example, that scatter in and of itself affected behavioral efficiency.

Other qualitative aspects to be considered are the client's approach to test materials, behavioral themes, and associative content. Phrasing, choice of words, and unusual behavior accompanying nonverbal responses provide clues to fears, anxieties, and preoccupations. Inferences drawn from behavior in this structured situation and prediction of behavior in less structured situations must be checked out through other techniques and data. Likewise, inferences from other techniques, history, or school performance may be cross-validated from the analysis of behavior on intelligence tests. As indicated before, information that enhances understanding of the individual and is relevant in modifying behavior is desirable.

In the authors' view, the IQ measures a certain type of functional intelligence but is limited in its ability to explore the full range of possibilities of a particular individual to respond to a wide range of stimuli beyond those offered by our testing instruments. The IQ, therefore, cannot indicate totally an individual's intelligence for effective coping with life's stresses. Other forms of competence exist which can be understood only within a person's concrete personal and environmental experience and the values placed on these experiences in his particular environment. Wide variations in intelligence exist among normal and impaired alike. The restrictions and limitations of the IQ do not necessarily apply only to individuals from ethnic minorities or to children of the white poor. These limitations may apply also to those with normal opportunities for the enrichment of intelligence and experience. If this restrictive condition exists for the children for whom the IQ was originally designed, how much more restrictive is it for those for whom it is not designed?

The direction that clinicians seem to be taking is the loosening of our test schematics, constructs, and tools and the application of our abilities to the individual per se rather than attempts to fit him into some physicalist construct. We need to concentrate on what an individual can do and under what conditions rather than on how much he has.

7.1. Adaptive Behavior

The Vineland Social Maturity Scale is probably the most widely used technique to assess adaptive development. Based on interviews with parents or parent surrogates, activities of daily living divided into areas of self-help, locomotion, occupation, communication, self-direction, and socialization are investigated in this inventory or questionnaire. Most of the skills follow the clinical expectation of normative development over the child's early years to his later status as an adult. Because the scale grouped in age levels like the Binet, with a resulting social age, it is possible to extract from the classification of these items the various kinds of social behavior in which the child seems to be advancing and those in which he has not yet developed. As discussed previously, intellectual performance and social adaptability serve as yardsticks for each other and provide information on their interactive effects on coping and adjustment.

The reliability of the gathered information is often questionable because of parents' anxieties and the wish to make their child seem more like other children. Thus they may give incorrect or exaggerated versions of development or responses colored by their own biases. Sometimes parents are poor observers of their children. Since the Vineland is primarily concerned with developmental skills as they occurred in sequential stages, the questions asked should serve only as guides, and be phrased to lessen anxiety and defensiveness. Rather than confront an anxious mother with the question "Can your child dress himself?" more information can be gained by asking "Tell me how your child dresses himself." It is often possible to verify or spot-check items which can also be evidenced in other parts of the assessment such as drawing, cutting, verbalization, and swallowing nonedibles.

When there are marked discrepancies between parental reports and clinical observations and between social and intellectual functioning in either direction, further investigation is in order. Inferences about parental attitudes of overprotection, stimulation, and encouragement may then be drawn. The Vineland also serves as a convenient device for initiating the parent interview.

7.2. Affective Development

The Rorschach Technique was designed to sample ways of experiencing affect. Originally, it focused on how a person perceives or experiences (*Erlieben*) rather than how he behaves or lives (*Erleben*). The development of the modes of experiencing affect and their representation in the determinants of Rorschach responses are extensively discussed by Ames, Learned, Metranx, and Walker (1952). None of the ten inkblots is representative of everyday objects, although each has a recognizable shape and details. At the very least, each is familiar enough to stimulate the individual's imagination and thoughts which indicate the associative process. The perceptual organization and thought process provide a picture of orientation, fantasy, and ideation. Integration of these elements can lead to an understandable picture of an individual's personality makeup.

The applicability of the Rorschach and other projective techniques to cases where retardation is or may be in the picture has its proponents and critics. The clinician, looking for quantity and variety of responses, may be at a loss when faced with the meager record of a noncommunicative, retarded youngster, resulting in a limited and often negative interpretation. To the clinician familiar with the variety of protocols that may be obtained, more subtle nuances may be accessible for better understanding of the forces influencing adaptive or maladaptive behaviors, support systems, motivational variables, and coping mechanisms. The behaviorist may be more comfortable observing the number of times a child repeats the same activity than considering the child obsessive based on responses to the Rorschach.

Since the Rorschach samples perceptual behavior, the clinician is on uncertain grounds when he attempts to predict broad patterns of social and emotional behavior from patterns of perceptual selection. Research evidence supports this. Users of the Rorschach may be on safer grounds explaining overt behavior than attempting to predict it.

Although the Rorschach is an unstructured technique, the situation may have to be structured for the retarded individual. The instructions given, for example, may be crucial for his understanding of the task. What and how he understands often determines the nature of his responses. If the only instruction given is "Tell me what this looks like" or ". . . what this might be," the tendency may be for him to look for some "right" answer. Adding "Tell me what you see, what kinds of things it makes you think of" may yield idiosyncratic responses rather than merely a popular response. It may be necessary to repeat the directions over several cards or make up a sample blot for the younger child. It is also suggested that for the hyperactive or distractible clients the inquiry is given following the response since they tend to deny their initial impressions or interpret the inquiry as a verification of their responses, which only adds to their self-doubts.

It may be difficult to get the client to specify the determinants so that the inquiry may be rephrased as "Tell me more about it." Care must also be taken not to suggest a response. For example, the response *dog* on Card I may be the usual face, but if the inquiry asks "Show me the parts of the dog," the child may feel that he has to make up a complete dog, giving a confabulated response. Standardized administration and careful inquiry are basic to analysis of responses. There are instances, however, when it may not be possible to stick closely to information obtained in the inquiry. Thus, if a retarded individual gives the appropriate response *flower*, one may have to consider that he is using the color when he adds, "it's pretty" since it cannot be assumed that he is capable of expressing or naming colors.

Paucity of responses is another factor that needs to be considered when using projectives with retarded individuals. A small number of responses may actually reflect limitations in perceptual experiencing so that analysis of the proportion of responses among the various determinants is restricted. One solution has been to transpose them into proportions of the total *R*. Sometimes it may be helpful to administer the cards a second time, asking for an alternate response. If this procedure is used, any additional responses would be interpreted as the percepts the client forms under pressure and suggestion.

Since perceptual development is so very basic in the total development of the individual, the Rorschach, with all its limitations and unknowns, has a place in the assessment of identified or unidentified retarded persons capable of responding to the cards.

7.3. TAT

The stories or themes given in response to the TAT cards are taken to indicate the individual's striving, his attitudes to key figures in his life, and his self attitudes, which stem, it is believed, from his own past experiences. These themes appear to be the conscious part of the individual's experiences, his appraisal of the world around him.

When the client has recognized attentional problems, poor verbal skills, and little patience, a shortened set of cards is advisable.

For males, it has been found satisfactory to use Cards 1, 3BM, 4, 5, 6BM, 7BM, 13MF, and 17BM; for females, Cards 1, 2, 3GF, 4, 5, 9GF, 12F, 13MF, and 18GF. These cards are sufficiently challenging to stimulate imagination and permit idiosyncratic responses.

In many instances, the TAT has advantages over the Rorschach with retarded or developmentally disabled children. Associations on the Rorschach may be meager, providing a limited sampling of ideational content. These associations are partly determined by the nature of the stimuli and the task. In contrast, the TAT is utilized to stimulate fantasy and to project feelings. For the client who has difficulty in structuring stimuli, as on the Rorschach, the content provided by the TAT cards may permit him freer access to his feelings and thoughts. It may be more necessary to prod a child to expand on an initial descriptive or naming response than on a story response. The retarded client giving "Mother and father" may be asked "What are they doing?"

In addition to verbalizations, it is important to be alert to the nonverbal activity and productions of these individuals because they offer clues to emotional interactions. These may represent efforts to communicate feelings for which they may not have the words.

By using combinations of perceptual modes and associative content, the initial step in understanding the child's dynamics can be made. On the Rorschach, the child who sees an aggressive animal and an explosion may be experiencing his reality as hostile and destructive. On the TAT, this content may or may not appear. Whether he projects these experiences outwardly would depend on his defense mechanisms. He may, for example, try to deny or counteract these experiences by expressing wishes for love and affection in his TAT stories.

In using TAT with children, valuable clues are given as to how they are learning to evaluate their social interactions and the types of coping mechanisms they are developing. It can show how they are handling their environment and how they defend themselves against anxiety and stress.

Because of the rich associative material available from the TAT, most clinicians accept its reliability or validity as adequate representation of the child's fantasy and projections. It is generally administered near the end of the test battery, after rapport has been well established. This is important since the retarded child may become particularly anxious or blocked when asked to "reveal his fantasies" to a person whom he may see as a representative of parental authority.

7.4. Figure Drawings (DAP)

Drawings as a means of communication have been known since the day of the cave dwellers. The drawings today in the Draw-A-Person test have become more refined and have more specific meaning since Goodenough's and Harris's use and their revision of this test as a guide to general conceptual development.

Machover introduced the drawing as a projective technique for personality assessment for the young and the old. Most assessment batteries include figure drawing, and in some settings it may be the only projective test given, contrary to all that is known about single test interpretation and its lack of scientific basis.

According to Machover, the body "is the most intimate point of reference in any activity" and as such is both a conscious and unconscious offering that provides a means of expressing body needs and conflicts. In other words, the drawing is a self-projection invested with all one's psychic values and problems. Like the other projective tests, the drawing is only clinically validated, but it does reflect personal problems and emotional adjustment.

Two drawings are required. Queries about size, sex, and other details are answered by "Draw any person you want." If the sex is ambiguous when the drawing is completed, the general question "Give this person a name" should settle the doubt. The opposite sex is then required. "Now draw a man" if the first was a female drawing. It may be necessary to add instructions such as "Make a whole person, not just a stick figure," because this encourages a retarded individual to go beyond stereotypes and to express himself as freely as he chooses. The instructions require an envisioned human body, although there are instances of attempts to use the assessor as the model. As with the Rorschach, a mental image is required before the actual response is produced.

The nature of the inquiry following the completion of the drawings varies widely. With some clinicians, it is extensive and is the basis for many interpretations. The authors limit this inquiry with retarded clients because of nondiscriminatory responses. Although specific signs in the drawings are often interpreted, no single feature per se can carry the weight of the interpretation. If stance in a drawing points toward a rebellious attitude or an overly large hand to aggression, these factors should be verified with other material before including them in the personality picture.

Using Machover's assumption of the meaning of important aspects of the drawings, interpretations are made and used together with the other projective material for an integrated personality picture. Not only is an indication obtained of the extent and nature to which the client has developed his body image, but also clues are provided to the manner to which this image is transmitted into controlled motor activity.

The drawings produced by mentally retarded clients are often identified by their proportion, size, perspective, articulation, points of appendages, and paucity of details. Because of inability to analyze, to conceptualize and relate facts, the drawings can show disproportion, transparency, confused orientation, and incorrect synthesis. Conflict areas and attitudes toward authority figures may also be revealed. Drawings do not appear to be greatly modified by cultural differences, but, in the authors' experience, drawings of retarded adolescent girls of Puerto Rican extraction showed details suggesting greater sexual awareness and interests.

The following discussion is based on representative drawings of clients seen in a clinic for the mentally retarded.

7.4.1. Perspective

Perspective is a difficult concept for even the average child to grasp; it is far more difficult for the retarded child. Spatial relationships such as distance and closeness simply are too abstract for his limited capacities. Poor perception of the spatial relationships involved in his drawings often causes the retarded child to place individual details with little regard to objective reality.

As a rule, the retarded child is at a loss to know where to start when he is confronted with a large white sheet for his drawings. Placement of the drawing is in no specific quadrant, although many use the upper half of the left side. This placement may be attributed not only to spatial difficulties but also to the psychological problems of failure to recognize one's own place in the family or group, with consequent feelings of isolation and withdrawal. Unable to act on his own initiative, the retardate's tendency is to hug the margin as if desperately clinging to a crutch for support. It is not unusual to find the immature retarded child making use of the upper left side placement. Machover maintains that the left side reveals the individual's close ties to, and dependence on, the family. Occasionally, the retarded child's inability to handle space is shown also in the facial features. For example, the facial features may be displaced: the eye may be drawn below the mouth, or the nose may be on the same horizontal plane as the eye.

Body imbalance, which is frequently experienced by the retardate, may show itself graphically in completely skewed figures which look as if they were floating in space. There is no anchorage, nothing to maintain the object in an upright position. Such representations reveal the retardate's feelings of body inferiority.

Symmetry, which indicates balance and control, generally is poor in the drawings of the retarded. This disturbance may be due to confusion in lateral dominance, motor incoordination, and cortical problems, conditions which are found commonly in retardates with central nervous system dysfunctioning. The imbalance may be so extreme that the drawings look as if they are disintegrated.

7.4.2. Proportion

The relative size of objects often is an undeveloped concept in younger or more retarded children, just as the comparative form of adjectives is misunderstood by them. For example, if animals or people are presented in the drawing of a House, either or both may tower above the House.

In disproportionate drawings of the Person, the head most commonly is large, whereas the trunk and the appendages are short and thin or even omitted altogether. Overemphasis of the size of the head frequently is found in the drawings of young "normal" children of from 3 to 6 years of age. For the older retardate, head disproportion seems to be the more usual representation, indicating immaturity and developmental lag, and, according to analytical theory, the oral dependent stage.

It should be remembered that the higher the intelligence level of the retarded child and the better his adjustment, the less striking will be the atypical characteristics of his drawings.

Like the drawings of the "normal" child below the age of 7 years, the retardate's drawings usually are small. Occasionally, however, the other extreme is seen and the page cannot contain the entire graphic production. It is not uncommon to find the retarded child drawing a small Person with overly large, irrelevant details such as a ball or rope drawn close by.

The older retardates, like older "normal" children, come closer to drawing larger figures. Irrelevant details again may be outsized, however, which illustrates graphically the retarded child's poor judgment.

Constricted drawings, whether drawn by the retarded or by the "normal" child, suggest feelings of inferiority and frustration.

7.4.3. Details

Awareness of what happens around one and the recognition of environmental stimuli generally are reflected in drawings by the number and appropriateness of the details. Details are to drawings what colorful description and expressive narrative are to literature. They give life, color, and tone to what is depicted.

The retarded child's drawings, by and large, are bare of details; the Person may be a rigid disproportionate series of circles and a line or lines.

The human figure may lack facial features, appendages, or sexual characteristics. The male and the female figures are drawn alike. A large, round head, eyes that are circles without pupils, perhaps another circle for a nose, short appendages, and large, buttons frequently constitute the Persons portrayed by younger retardates.

The use of circles to represent details suggests the orally arrested development of the retardate who must be buoyed up by the outside and directed step by step to learn to see and regard external stimuli. Dependence on the key figure, usually the mother, is excessive. It is the mother who, figuratively speaking keeps the wheels turning by assisting, guiding, and pointing out the directions.

Facial expression is rarely drawn. Faces drawn by the retardate tend to look alike, are without contour, empty, unseeing, and have little recognizable character. Differentiation may be seen primarily in the mouth. Usually the appendages and the neck are one-dimensional.

Frequently, the retarded child is unable to join the appendages to the body. Disjointed detailing is common among retarded clients with neurological dysfunctioning.

Transparency also is seen frequently in their drawings. A diaphanous skirt or a pair of trousers may be drawn on a figure, but it allows an interior view of the legs, undergarments, etc. Such a transparency usually is drawn by the more retarded child who cannot follow concepts and in general has poor judgment and poor reality testing.

The human figure most likely will reflect feelings of weak basic strength if it is thin, weak, and without many details, and the lines are light in pressure.

7.4.4. Line Quality

Frequently, the line drawn by the retarded child is tremulous, quavering, and/or jerky in quality. Actual breaks in the line where the pencil has wavered because of jerkiness or incoordination are discernible; these all suggest poor motor control and poor motor adaptation. As in the retarded child's reproductions on the Bender, there may be wavering lines instead of clearly defined lines. This incoordination and jerkiness may be related to brain impairment, with associated mental retardation. The lines also may show heavy pressure and appear to have been drawn swiftly and impulsively.

As a technique, drawings stand out because of the short time required to administer, the immediacy of recognition of problems and conflicts, and the constancy of specific aspects such as size, stance, line, and placement. As presently used, drawings often provide dramatic illustrations of the assessor's interpretations, but caution is advised in making generalizations on the basis of drawings alone. The technique attracts many workers who are not versed in psychological principles and dynamics underlying the drawings but feel adequate to analyze them. Too often, such analysis has no clinical validity, although the assumptions made may sound clever.

7.5. Perceptual-Motor Development

The ability to visually discriminate, recognize, organize, and reproduce the world is an essential function of the human organism. It is anticipated that the visual-motor activity involved in copying geometric designs is similar to the functions required in reading and possibly in social interactions. Although neurological difficulties may deter perceptual-motor behavior, they may be only one in a variety of causes responsible for the deficits.

The Bender-Gestalt samples this behavior by having the client reproduce nine figures. The test is short, is easy to give, and yields a mine of information. Bender (1938) and Koppitz (1964) use it for its developmental and clinical values. As a developmental indicator, it can be used only during the maturational period. Children developmentally under 6 years are likely to do so poorly that interpretations would be invalid.

Koppitz's normative studies on children provide some precise scoring. Using the Bender in conjunction with the Seguin Form Board and the Block Designs can provide a broader picture of visual-motor functions. If no gross errors occur on the Bender and if completion of the Seguin Board meets criteria of time and accuracy but the Block Designs cannot be reproduced, then this child may have little difficulty in form perception but considerable difficulty in analyzing and reconstructing more complex stimuli. The manner in which the figures are copied also provides cues about perceptual function: importance to the child of accurate perception; preoccupation with details at the expense of the gestalt; details ignored and a rough sketch satisfactory; shifting the paper and/or the design; errors corrected with elaborating; extraneous additions to the figure.

In using the Bender, age should be taken into account, and additional techniques are required to obtain a wide-enough sampling of behavior. Most importantly, it cannot be assumed that brain damage is the sole cause of deficient performance.

Factors interfering with perceptual-motor function are extensive, and include brain damage, sensory deprivation, and motor weakness; injuries, fatigue, and illnesses; poor motivation; social-cultural deprivation; intellectual retardation; and emotional disturbances. Even when there is a high probability of neurological dysfunctioning, other interfering factors may also be present, such as anxiety and feelings of inadequacy, which may be equally significant in the poor performance.

Distinguishing between receptive and expressive difficulties is important for training purposes, but these distinctions are not always readily observable. If a child draws a figure easily but doesn't recognize errors, this may be a sign of perceptual input difficulty. On the other hand, if the design is copied laboriously, with erasures and corrections, the child may have difficulty in motor reproductions.

Thus far, only visual perception has been mentioned. However, other perceptual modes such as auditory have to be considered, particularly when assessing a suspect child. An auditory perceptual problem may be present if there is frequent misperception of verbal instructions or if instructions have to be repeated. Tests of attention such as Digit Span may also suggest auditory dysfunctioning.

7.6. Educational Achievement

Although school achievement usually cannot be explored extensively by the clinician, a short achievement test is valuable because achievement level is a very common referral problem. Probably the easiest test to interpret is the WRAT. In the light of academic achievement and schooling, it may be one of the most important in the assessment battery.

The WRAT scores indicate the person's current level in the three basic school subjects, word recognition, spelling, and computational arithmetic. More than the level which corresponds to grade placement, the WRAT throws light on the individual's weaknesses in areas which are considered essential as a background for learning academically.

The word recognition score and the verbatim responses to the printed word indicate the approaches to sight reading of words: dependence on phonetics, guessing, substitution of known for unknown words beginning with the same initial sound, configuration, or spelling letter by letter. The sound method, like phonetics, may serve as the best approach to expand the individual's range-of-sight vocabulary, or the configurational method may be reinforced with added attention to initial letter differences, or the left-by-left method may be excluded from the repertoire.

In like manner, scrutiny of the misspelled words leads to clarification of the individual's failures in spelling. These can be attributed to auditory imperception, reversals, unfamiliarity with alphabet, spatial problems, or confusion between letters and their sounds. With the problem recognized, teaching can follow through toward correction of the specific fault.

Close investigation of the arithmetic responses leads to awareness of problems: inability to understand the processes, failure to understand signs, lack of familiarity with combination facts, directional confusion, number reversals, and/or carelessness.

7.7. Dominance and Laterality

All human beings have a right side and a left side, and one or the other may be preferred, as the left hand and the right eye. It has long been recognized that there is some relationship between right- and left-sidedness with certain brain disorders, between dominant hand and cerebral dominance for language. However, currently it is felt that handedness and language are not inevitably and invariably associated.

Right- and left-handedness, however, influence life in innumerable ways, from using eating utensils and mechanical tools to driving a car to orientation in space. Developmentally, in normal growth, one side becomes specialized with the nervous system. If such specialization fails to occur, there is a likelihood of problems, especially in learning. Although researchers and investigators do not always agree, different theories have been advanced to explain the failure to develop clear-cut dominance of one side of the body over the other. Orton in the 1930s stated that interference between the right and left hemispheres of the brain caused problems with reading, writing, and spelling. Dearborn, on the other hand, attributed learning problems to a lack of clear-cut dominance on the left or the right side, especially in people whose preferred or lead eye is on the opposite side from the dominant or lead hand. Most evidence is against both theories.

Understanding of right and left in the spatial world involves one's own body or body image. Ordinarily, understanding of right and left is achieved by the average child by 6–7 years. Distinguishing this on another person comes later, at about 8 years, and understanding laterality difference between right and left in objects develops at about 11 years. Recognition of right and left on one's own body, however, does not ensure recognition of one's right and left facial features and appendages.

Left-handedness is found both in poor and in outstanding readers. Preference for the left eye, however, has been found more frequently in poor than good readers; if dominance is mixed, then hand and eye preference are on different sides of the body; mixed eye–hand dominance may occur more frequently among retarded readers.

Although detailed tests of dominance may not be necessary, informal assessment should be made of laterality and dominance in order to plan programs to help the client, retarded or not, to learn left-right direction in reading. Frequently, it may be sufficient to observe the hand the child uses to write with.

The authors have devised an informal appraisal inventory (Table 3) to tap laterality, dominance, directional orientation, sequencing, auditory discrimination, and memory for meaningful and nonmeaningful material. It is meant to supplement usual test batteries with deeper exploration of deficient areas or functions where findings are ambiguous or nonconfirmatory. Thus not all items need to be given. Many of the items are taken from standardized tests.

Table 3. Neuropsychological Appraisal Inventory

A.

	Confused	Right	Left
Show me your left ear.			
Show me your right eye.			
Show me your right foot.			
Show me your left hand.			
Show me your right thumb.			
Show me your right eyebrow.			
Show me your left cheek.			

B.

	Confused	Right	Left
Show me how you brush your teeth.			
Show me how you brush your hair.			
Show me how you pick up a pencil.			
Show me how you tap a hammer.			
Show me how you wind a watch.			
Show me how you throw a ball.			
Show me how you use a knife.			
Show me how you hold a cup.			
Show me how you shoot a marble.			
Show me how you write your name.			
Place 3 colored pencils on the table.			
Give me the blue pencil.			
Give me the red pencil.			
Give me the lead pencil.			

(Repeat if one hand is not used consistently.)

C.

Directions	Right	Wrong
Turn to the right, then to the left.		
Turn left, right, and left again.		
Turn to left, then left again.		
Show me my right hand.		
Point to my left leg.		
Point to my right ear.		
Point to my left hand.		
Put your left hand on your right ear.		
Put your right hand on your right ear.		

D.

Write the numbers from 1 to 12 (dominant hand).
Write the numbers from 1 to 12 (nondominant hand).

    R—   L—

E.

	Confused	Right	Left
Close one eye and look through the keyhole.			
Do it again.			
Look through this [kaleidoscope] and tell me what you see.			
Put it down.			

(Continued)

Table 3. *(Continued)*

	Confused	Right	Left
Do it again.			
Close one eye and tell me what you see [cone].			
Put it down.			
Do it again.			

Make believe you are going to shoot me right in the middle of my nose. Close one eye, take aim, shoot.

	Shoulder			Eye	
	R___	L___		R___	L___

F. If child fails digits on his age level on Binet, or misses three digits on WISC, try two digits, etc.

Listen to what I say then when I stop, you say what I said.
Digits:

II-6	8-5	3-9	6-3
III	6-4-1	3-5-2	8-3-7
IV-6	4-7-2-9	3-8-5-2	7-2-6-1
VII	3-1-8-5-9	4-8-3-7-2	9-6-1-8-3
IX Reversed	8-4-6-2	3-9-2-1	3-6-2-9
X Forward	4-7-3-8-5-7	5-2-8-6-7-4	7-1-3-8-9-4
XII Reversed	8-1-3-7-9	6-9-5-8-2	5-2-9-4-1
Sup. Ad. Rev.	4-7-1-9-5-2	5-8-3-6-9-4	7-5-2-6-1-8

Nonsense syllables:	Verbatim	Pass	Fail
doy poo			
kah mow			
dee mow pah			
boo dah tay			
bow gah dee tah			
doy boo mow kah			
tah dee gah bow tay			
poo kah dee bah doy			
pah doy poo dee tah bow			
gah tay boo day mow dah			

Words:
Listen to what I say, then when I finish, you say it.

horse–tree
up–house–door
baby–mother–sit–play
around–park–field–seat
went–school–where–was–going

No. correct

G. Sentences:

IV years	We are going to buy candy for mother.
	Jack likes to feed the puppies in the barn.

Table 3. (*Continued*) **739**

V years	Jane wants to build a big castle in her playhouse.
	Tom has lots of fun playing ball with his sister.
VII years	Fred asked his father to take him to see the clown in the circus.
	Billy has made a beautiful boat out of wood with his sharp knife.
XI years	At the summer camp the children get up early in the morning to go swimming.
	Yesterday we went for a ride in our car along the road that crosses the bridge.
A.A.	The redheaded woodpeckers made a terrible fuss as they tried to drive the young away from the nest.
	The early settlers had little idea of the great changes that were to take place in the country.

H. Auditory discrimination:

Letter sounds:

Tell me whether the sounds are the same or different.

	S.	D.			S.	D.
b–p				th–f		
s–t				gr–gl		
d–th				p–p		
e–e				gr–pr		
r–l				pr–tr		
d–d				r–r		
k–s				sl–st		
n–m						

Tell me which words have the

			R.	W.
b	sound	toil–make–baby		
a	sound	bit–back–put		
e	sound	sit–better–sand		
i	sound	boss–dell–pill		
th	sound	think–for–don't		
e	sound	easy–apple–empty		
i	sound	enter–into–on		
p	sound	apple–now–ran		

Words:

Tell me whether the words sound the same or different.

	S.	D.
hit–hut		
bill–bail		
run–run		
set–sat		
art–act		
at–it		
house–house		
friend–fiend		

(Continued)

Table 3. *(Continued)*

	S.	D.
butterfly–butterfly		
scribble–scramble		
grow–grown		
break–break		
dell–dill		
walk–walked		
grand–gland		
light–white		
these–these		
sweater–sled		

I. Rhythm: X   XXX
    Tap: XX   XX
             XX   X   XXX
             X   XX   X   XXX

J. Reversals (words and letters):

no–was–top–how–mat
pat–dog–saw–spilt–raw
boy–on–pot–god–north

K. Divergent thinking:

1. Vocal encoding test (Illinois Test of Psycholinguistic Abilities)

2. "Tell me what sleeps." After child responds, say "Now tell me all the other things that sleep as quickly as you can." Allow 30 sec for a response. If subject stops before expiration of time, ask "What else?" Record all responses. Follow the same procedure with the five scored items as with the warmup item above.

Action–agent

| 1. What swims? |
| 2. What burns?   (wood 2, food 2, toast 1, explosive 2, stick 1) |
| 3. What cuts? |
| 4. What runs? |
| 5. What flies?   (plane 2, birds 2, swan 1, robin 1) |

3. Monroe Language Classification: 1. Name all *animals* you can think of as quickly as you can. 2. *things to eat.* 3. *toys.*
Encourage further responses by saying "Any more?" within the 30-sec period.

L. Block Sort Test (Graham-Ernhart):

M. Tactile Finger Localization (Reitan):

N. Visual Retention Test (Benton; Memory for Designs—S.B.; B.G. from memory):

O. Speech:

    Infantile patterns (letter substitutions)

    Omits letters in words, omits endings.

    Confuses plurals.

    Misuses pronouns.

7.8. Observation

Assessment is neither defined by nor limited to the administration of tests; therefore, it cannot be an evaluation solely in terms of psychometric validity. Assessment also requires conceptual validity or the extent to which hypotheses about a person are confirmed and consistent with observation that follows from the model of the individual constructed in the assessment process.

As mentioned earlier, assessment is a multiphased process in which observation plays an integral role in the understanding of behavior. Observations are made more often in test situations than in everyday situations. The psychological assessment provides opportunities for the first type of observation. As if on stage, the individual is observed from the moment of entrance: his behavior in the waiting room, interaction with the adult or caretaker, interaction with others in the room, behavior on entry into the examination room, approach to the assigned activities, body movements, speech and language, quality of voice and tone, and reactions during the psychometric and personality evaluations. Approaches to problems, attitudes toward test items, energy level, and distractibility fall within the clinician's eye for verbal photography. Appraisal can be made of repeated mannerisms, reactions to external distractions, level of frustration, delaying tactics, defenses used to cover up mistakes, or defenses in general to cope with stress, anxiety, and fatigue.

Observation also enters into the calculation of the person's request for repeated instructions, irrelevant remarks, personal questions asked of the clinician, constant queries about termination of the evaluation. All the above observations focus around the patterns of behavior during the assessment process. These are noted and evaluated in anecdotal style, which obviates the need to employ descriptive language; only the behavior itself is recorded. For more direct behavior in response to certain specific observations, play situations can be set up to cover attitudes to people, represented by dolls, and to violent activities using play weapons and instruments, such as rubber darts, a policeman's stick, a cane, etc.

In other situations, observation can be limited to short periods of behavior that occur at the table, on the playground, in the corridors, during toileting, or in the sheltered workshop. Frequency of an occurrence can be measured within short time periods such as 10 or 15 min, or within short time periods set off during longer periods, such as the first 20 min in the morning and two 20-min periods in the afternoon, one specifically before dismissal or termination of an event.

Observation during an assessment, for example, requires more precision than observation during a working day or a school day. The clinician has to record responses to standardized test material, and yet be alert to every nuance and body movement, and to mood swings, fears, and emotions—in fact, to whatever the individual does, says, or does not say.

Note also must taken of any features that suggest syndromes associated with mental retardation such as physical features: elongated head, low-set ears, wideset eyes, hand flailing, a dwarfed figure, a tiny misshapen head, and drooping eyelids. Appearance, unless characteristic of some defect, is not so important unless it adds to the retardate's burden in living, as the extremely attractive child who is expected, because of stereotypes, to be bright, alert, and socially competent.

Speech is an important facet in mental retardation; it may be infantile, garbled, strange, monosyllabic, echolalic, or dysarthric. Can the individual express himself through words, or does he need gestures and pantomime to communicate ideas? Does he grope for words and generally show dysfluency?

Body movement needs careful attention. Is the individual awkward, jerky with awkward gait? Does he or she seem to cringe or withdraw as if practiced in self-effacement? Are the hands limp, awkward, weak? Which hand is used in writing? Is this hand used consistently?

Other subtle indications of reactions are seen by the individual's attitude toward the assessor, who is viewed as the authority figure. The clinician, of course, may be viewed as benign and friendly, and his smile or nod of encouragement may act as a spur to greater activity and effort. Conversely, the assessor's approval may interfere with the individual's further attempts in the mistaken idea that the goal has been successfully reached.

The presence of the clinician may call out varying emotions. If the individual is not self-conscious, he may hardly notice the clinician's presence; if he is anxious and constricted, the sight of the clinician may further restrict, confuse, or befuddle him. In general, the clinician has to be sensitive and perceptive to nuances and how his personality affects the client.

7.9. Historical Data

A better understanding of a human being requires more than a thumbnail sketch. Everything pertinent to his life should be known and reviewed. These data must comprise familial, physical, and medical status; social history; congenital factors; the individual's birth and medical history; and his developmental, educational, and vocational history if he is old enough to have one. In short, historical data pertain to an individual's genealogy, which includes not only his descent from ancestors and parents but also to his medical and environmental past.

While these data are important in helping to determine the etiology, where possible, of the deficits, they are of equal significance in understanding the impact of these variables on the present behavior and in knowing where and how to begin intervention programs.

8. Problems Related to Assessment

Aside from the lack of refined instruments to assess human behavior in all its dimensions and the controversial issues of the nature and role of intelligence, there are facets that are of concern to many clinicians and other professional workers, for example, the assignment of levels of functioning dependent on quantification and the lack of scientific investigation of behavior relevant to each level.

Although the levels of functioning have been statistically calculated, the limits, whether lower or upper in any of the ranges, are basically only statistical values. The questions raised pertain to behavioral reactions empirically and experimentally known to exist between the function of an individual who obtains an IQ of 51, in the upper limits of the moderate level of retardation, and an IQ of 53, in the lower limits of the mildly retarded level.

The following examples illustrate some problems of assessment. During a parental interview, a mother of six children, employed as a housemaid, explained the division of chores in her own household. Her severely retarded 10-year-old son, a patient in a mental retardation agency, was given the responsibility of the laundry. This boy, mentally 3 years old, succeeded in finding his way to the launderette four blocks distant from his home, separating the colored from the white wash, placing each in a different machine, waiting until the wash was clean and placing each load in different driers; at the same time, he took charge of his 4-year-old sibling. What in the assessment could possibly indicate this boy's potentialities?

A more dramatic example of inadequate assessment due to lack of precise instruments is illustrated by Marty, an 11-year-old boy of moderately retarded intelligence (IQ 50). Uncared for, unschooled because of his mother's alcoholism, Marty spent the greater part of his life on the streets of the city, fending for himself and foraging for food. He eventually attached himself to a neighbor in the same house in which he lived with his alcoholic mother. The neighbor, confused, limited, and overwhelmed by her own children, permitted Marty to tag along, with little concern that he was not her own child. During an agency visit to apply for residential care for her three youngest children, she took Marty with her. Shortly thereafter, Marty appeared alone at the agency, asked for the social worker he had seen, and demanded residential care for himself. He was put off, but after a brief wait he reappeared and requested an emergency meeting with the city officials in charge of such placements. He was permitted to talk to one of the officials by phone, and succeeded in having himself placed. Currently, Marty is a resident of a child care center in the suburbs, in which he is making an adequate adjustment and is showing aptitude for new learning.

Marty's assessment on the intelligence test highlighted his inability to define words and his poor ability to reproduce facts from memory, recognize likenesses and differences, and solve simple arithmetic problems. But what test measures could predict his drive to find a home for himself, his good judgment in turning to a social agency for help, and his ability to convince seasoned professionals of his compelling needs and sincerity?

The nature of the variables responsible for differences in functioning despite closeness of IQ is still obscure, as are the types of various activities (aside from self-help skills) that are subsumed under the four levels of retarded functioning.

Not so pressing but still of lively concern to many clinicians is the concept of mental age, particularly with regard to older retardates. A 20-year-old whose intellectual functioning is assessed at the 3-year-old level is by no means the typical 3-year-old. The difference in life experiences and the presence of defects in areas related to functioning negate such comparison.

Other serious questions relate to differential diagnosis, which in essence means the identification of specific causes accountable for individual behavioral reactions.

ETTA KARP, MURRY
MORGENSTERN,
AND HAROLD
MICHAL-SMITH

In the past, the differential was directed toward amplification of differences between the familial (endogenous) and brain injury (exogenous) types of mental retardation. These distinct types were introduced by Strauss and Werner in 1941 and continued by Lehtenin (1947) and Kephart (1955), who had widespread influence on clinical thinking in the area of mental retardation. Research at the time showed wide differences in perception, performance on the Rorschach, and figure and ground relationship. The studies were often ingenious in construction but technically weak. The criteria for separation of the two groups were critically examined. Other studies, shortly after, did not confirm some of these earlier studies. The importance of Strauss's early work was in the establishment of different behavior patterns in psychological evaluations.

Gallagher (1957) stated that the deficit, as in perception, is more valuable information than the established fact of brain insult. Other investigations have, over the years, tended to go along with this new point.

The feeling has been that organically "damaged" children do not perceive things differently from other children and that all behavior in the final analysis is subject to and determined by the physical activity of the central nervous system. Ego functioning, for example, disrupted by extreme anxiety or by extreme deprivation, can affect perception and resemble organic disease. Simplified, this means that all the behavioral reactions attributed to brain dysfunction, such as poor perception, hyperactivity, perseveration, and other symptoms, cannot be specific to or considered indicative of organic brain disease.

The developmental lags listed in the following outline can occur regardless of the type of retardation.

1. Delayed motor development. Cannot sit up or roll over by the age of 12 months; is unable to walk at the age of 2 years; cannot stand on one foot or hop by the age of 4 years.
2. Delayed speech. Little vocalization by the first year or unable to articulate any words by 18 months; lacks a vocabulary of 100 words by $2\frac{1}{2}$ years; cannot use phrases or construct simple sentences by 3 years; cannot ask questions and emulate adult speech at 6 years.
3. Delayed psychomotor development. Cannot grasp a block and hold it by $2\frac{1}{2}$ years; cannot build a tower of four or more blocks by 3 years; cannot scribble with a pencil by 3 years or draw circles by 4 years.
4. Delayed judgment. Cannot understand hazards such as turning on gas or jumping off heights at home and outdoors by 5 years; cannot find his way in neighborhood by 6 years; greets and follows strangers beyond 5 years.
5. Delayed attention. Cannot listen or attend long enough to follow one simple direction by 4 years; cannot repeat his name by 4 years; cannot recite a nursery rhyme by 6 years.

There is continued concern about psychosis and autism, and the issue raised is whether an individual is retarded, psychotic, or autistic, which some clinicians isolate from childhood psychosis. The relationship between childhood autism and mental retardation is still an unsolved question. Bender (1959) maintains that autistic action and thinking can exist within any number of primary difficulties, such as brain damage, mental retardation, and disordered personal relationships. To her way of thinking, autism is a primitive form of behavior, natural or part of normal development, which lingers on, becomes exacerbated, and signifies a withdrawal defense against intrusion of anxiety in children with many genetic problems, brain disorders, perceptual difficulties, and problems with social relationships. Few clinicians agree with Bender's concept of autism; most consider autism a childhood psychosis of primary disorder.

Pollack, who supplied empirical data on the relationship between schizophrenia and mental retardation based on test performance in schizophrenics, found a strikingly high number of low IQ scores. Approximately 35% scored below IQ 70 and about 44% within the range of 70–89, illustrating the overlap between schizophrenics and the retarded. Scrutiny of the schizophrenic children and other children with different types of disorders showed a higher percentage of low IQs in the former group. Comparison of performance, i.e., in specific areas such as perceptual and motor, showed similar results between the schizophrenics and the retarded.

These findings led Pollack to conclude that childhood schizophrenia and mental retardation are not distinct entities comprising homogeneous groups. A severe behavior disorder with intellectual defect in childhood may reflect behavior consonant to cerebral dysfunction. The primary role, the retardation or the behavior disorder, becomes the function of the clinician's orientation rather than of the child's behavior.

Kessler (1966) states this another way, indicating that differentiation between primary and secondary causes is neither easy to make nor essential, provided that "the diagnosis is an ongoing process combined with a treatment program." Treatment is indicated in both areas regardless of which is primary. In conclusion, there is little evidence to support inferences made regarding the differentiation of psychosis and retardation.

9. Interpretation of Tests

The battery of tests discussed represents a three-sided geometric figure of psychological functions. At the apex are the intelligence tests that tap verbal and nonverbal areas such as memory, reasoning and problem solving, language, concept formation, discrimination, and visual perception organization. Along the sides come the achievement and the perceptual tests, each indicating the effect of impairment on the apex or the intelligence capacities. The baseline represents the traits and characteristics assessed by the projective materials.

Interpretation of test responses requires not only knowledge of the psychological rationale underlying each subtest on the intelligence items as stated by the author of the test, but also the clinician's qualitative point of view on the psychological meaning and significance of test items and content. Wechsler discusses the rationale of each subtest; other clinicians, like Rapaport, Gill, and Schafer have also added their interpretation.

Many clinicians accept Wechsler's underlying psychological rationale of the individual subtests on the WISC but try to relate the concepts to practical behavioral reactions in everyday living. Thus the interpretation of the test item, such as picture arrangement as indicative of anticipation and planning, is extended to mean understanding of the social scene, understanding of sequential acts and their consequences. These responses are not too difficult to translate and interpret because they are part of a structured situation that has a fairly wide range of acceptable responses. Establishing a rationale for responses in unstructured situations such as the Rorschach requires a more definite school of thought.

ETTA KARP, MURRY
MORGENSTERN,
AND HAROLD
MICHAL-SMITH

The philosophy underlying the analysis of the content of the projective materials and the responses on the intelligence tests follows the psychoanalytic belief in projection: everything a person says, every gesture, every facial expression, reflects his inner thoughts. That is, the outside manifestations reflect unexpressed, unconscious inner feelings and attitudes. The notion of projection also implies that an individual's reactions, attitudes, gestures, choice of language, and so forth reflect his personality makeup.

This psychoanalytic rationale is not favored by all clinicians and is one reason that projective techniques are omitted in many test batteries. The behaviorist, for example, or the clinician schooled in "ego psychology" frowns on anything that harks back to analytic psychology or depth psychology. Nevertheless, some clinicians still base their qualitative assessments on this concept. Many clinicians are eclectic in their approach and believe that different schools of psychology have specific values in specific settings and circumstances. Behavior modification has its place, as does analytic theory.

Analysis of all verbal content is based on the projective hypothesis. In addition to analysis of subtest materials that reflect strengths, weaknesses, and areas of severe impairment, all verbal replies on the intelligence tests are analyzed for unconscious, projective meaning. The projective materials, however, offer the most information for psychoanalytic interpretation.

Although scoring in the Rorschach is not standardized, specific elements have been established with regard to determinants, location, color, shading, motion or movement, and category of responses, which are tabulated and interpreted according to empirically established meaning. Many retarded clients capable of giving verbal responses tend to give a limited number of responses, monosyllabic or poor in quality, repetitious, concrete, and on occasion bizarre or absurd. Some of these characteristics such as repetitions, absurdities, and bizarre material lend themselves to interpretation. However, the overall impoverishment of responses minimizes the expectancy of data indicative of personality characteristics. Despite these drawbacks, it is frequently possible to obtain clues to the individual's associative processes and emotional tone which are ordinarily repressed, suppressed, or denied.

Some of the characteristics of the individual usually expected from a projective evaluation pertain to his full image, to that of others, and to his coping mechanisms. For example, how does this individual see himself as a person; in other words, what is his image of himself? How does he view his parents? What are his attitudes to them, particularly to his mother? Does the individual hold others responsible for his failures? Does he focus his complaints around his home or the larger environment? Is there any indication of interest in people, in contact, or in any specific activity? Is there any indication of what triggers off his anxiety, frustration, and/or hostility?

With regard to feeling, does this person withdraw and remove himself, or stay within bounds but fail to participate? Is there any evidence of attitude to authoritarian figures? Is there any inkling of what he feels is their attitude toward him? Is he aware of his sexual role and does this coincide with his behavioral reactions?

What defenses does this person use to cope with the strain and stress of daily living? And, perhaps even more important, what are this individual's strengths? Is there a receptivity to make contact? What are his sensitivities? Can he stay with an idea without digressing or going off into irrelevancies? If there are digressions, do they seem to stem from distractibility or to flight of ideas?

Obviously, not all of these questions can be answered, especially if the protocol is limited and monosyllabic. However, it is the direction interpretation should take.

Interpretation of test data demands not only close scrutiny of items passed or failed but also of the quality of responses. Although vocabulary, for example, is the least vulnerable to deterioration, it does indicate, especially in young age, background and life experiences, as well as an understanding of commonplace words. One's cultural and economical background, ethnic group, and urban or rural setting may be reflected in vocabulary and quality of definitions. Occasionally, an individual of retarded intelligence (mental age 6–0) obtains a vocabulary score at the 8- year level, with weak abstractive and reasoning ability. The inference that immediately comes to mind is a good verbal familial background which the individual has absorbed. Before this can be conclusive, it must be checked out by verbal communication on the Rorschach and the TAT. If the verbal content on these tests is of poor quality, other inferences need to be considered, including the heavy emphasis that has been placed on language at the elementary level which is not readily incorporated in daily communication.

If the item (year VII-#4) "What's the thing for you to do if another boy (or girl) hits you without meaning to do it?" earns the reply "Tell his mother. He'll get no supper," this may or may not be indicative of home training and punishment for misdemeanors.

Item analysis on the Wechsler Intelligence Scale offers a wider interpretive field with regard to knowledge about the individual: the weighted subtest scores that fall below the person's own level indicate the areas of lowest or highest functioning based on the psychological rationale of each, such as attention, abstract thinking, absorption of information, and visual-motor organization.

As emphasized previously, analysis of content and the inferences made must be buttressed by similar hypotheses or inferences from other test material. For example, "In what way are beer and wine alike?" may call out the response "To drink." Further questioning elicits only "My mother." No amount of prodding is more explicatory. The non sequitur to the original response may automatically make one think of an alcoholic female or the possibility of undue drinking in the background. On Card IV on the TAT, the reply given is "He's going away." After much questioning and prodding, a further statement in answer to "Why?" "She's mean, and ugly." "He don't like her no more." And, after continued thought, "Wants a car, hollers a lot." In no response does the idea of alcoholism appear, which does not rule out the possibility of drink as a familial problem, but the original conclusion is not substantiated. What is suggested by the TAT response is the possibility of a hysterical process at work which must also be validated.

Interpretations of the test data, no matter how carefully made, may not always agree from test to test. What then? Occasionally it is possible to integrate contradictory hypotheses and make conflicting facts intelligible. If this is not possible, it may well be that one of the interpretations is wrong, or indeed both may be wrong or both may be right. Differences of this type necessitate other inferences that must be carefully checked out in all the material. It is conceivable that an individual with a schizoid personality can act friendly and warm under certain circumstances, as at the beginning of an assessment, if a good impression is the goal or if superficial friendliness is the gambit in new situations which invariably changes after a longer period of time.

It is inconceivable, however, for an individual to be described as someone who has moved away from reality into a world of his own, and then to expect him to be well aware of the consequences of his social acts. Other adaptive behaviors have to be checked as well as evidence of poor reality testing.

10. The Report

The report is one of the final outcomes of the assessment. The essence or the meat of the report depends on the assessment findings which form the basis of the picture of the individual assessed.

Referrals for assessment come from a variety of different sources—schools, parents, clinics, hospitals, workshops, courts, other social agencies, and prospective employers. The reasons for assessment are usually varied, but each referrent wants to learn something special about the person. For example, the school may want to know why a child has been unable to learn academically, a parent why her son has suddenly become resistant and disobedient, a hospital whether the retarded patient's insistence on severe physical pain is a hysterical outburst or manifestation, the court whether the retarded person understands right from wrong. Other requests may require a specific bit of information as to the intellectual abilities of a child in order to meet legal or administrative requirements for evaluation every 3 years. Another request may ask only for psychological indications of brain dysfunction. Once the referral has been accepted, the report has to address itself to the referrent's needs and the questions raised. Regardless of the agency or person's request, the report has to delineate the individual at the time of assessment and should include the clinician's own interpretation of the findings, his impressions and his observations. The level of intellectual functioning must designate areas of effective and less effective functioning and the relationship of intellectual functioning to the individual's total functioning. Simply stated, the interpretation of his abilities, intellectual, emotional, or nonintellectual, should be related to meaningful aspects of his everyday existence, for example, how poor memory may affect the individual's attention and how this weakness may affect behavior at home, at school, or in other situations.

Although the style of report writing is individual, it must be grammatical, precise, clear, and easily communicative. A dictionary should not be necessary for clarification. Neither should the descriptive terms employed be so stereotypical as to fit any number of other clients.

Because clinical psychology grew out of the assessment of mental disorders, the tendency is to emphasize the pathological. Admittedly, this tendency is becoming less frequently observed in the field of mental retardation, but the word "schizophrenia" must have a special charm if one were to calculate its appearance in the assessment reports of the retarded. Also, mention of weaknesses tends to outnumber mention of strengths. It may well be that professionals in any field focus more attention on shortcomings than on strengths, both of which need mention and explanation.

Psychological assessment reports are often criticized because of their content, lack of content, their language, and paucity of overall information. Some of this criticism is indeed well taken. A referral usually indicates the reason for the assessment; for example, a referral on a 20-year-old retarded adult described him as infantile with child-like behavior, crying, whining, and complaining. The report stressed the same characteristics, finding the young man immature and babyish. Such repetition is not an evaluation in any sense because it does not attempt to explore the ramifications of the behaviors or the setting in which they occurred, nor does it suggest procedures to help overcome this young person's shortcomings. The report merely used synonyms to describe an individual without offering anything worthwhile to understand and to change his behavior.

There is often strong feeling about the language used, and persistent criticism points to the use of unfamiliar professional jargon, references to unknown subtest items, and pompous, pretentious, and erudite-sounding language occasionally used by the inexperienced or insecure clinician.

What must be kept in mind before the report is written is the objective. The written report has to convey a picture of another individual as he behaves, acts, and responds in daily life: what he can manage to do, what he fails to do, his feelings and attitudes, and how he tries to handle anxieties, frustration, anger, rejection, and other problems.

Reports should, as far as possible, answer the questions raised. They should also convey meaning descriptively as well as diagnostically. Clinically, present evaluatory materials are not refined enough to tap at the etiologies of mental retardation, although the neuropsychologist, working with machines, photography, and brain waves, is more likely to evolve behavior patterns indigenous to specific types of mental retardation.

What is a good report? There is no general formula, but a report can be considered good if it is written so that the reader, regardless of his background, understands it, and if the picture presented is of a human being with his faults and his good points, his strengths and his weaknesses, that are recognizable, explicable, and neither condemnatory nor overly accepting. The individual, retarded or nonretarded, should be reflected in word pictures or replicated in words. Suggestions and recommendations, part and parcel of a good report, should be practical, sensible, and appropriate.

11. The Interdisciplinary Team

The formal assessment is not the exclusive concern of the psychological disciplines. Medical practice has, over the years, recognized the need for consultation and examination with specialists to help in patient evaluation of illness. The physician, regardless of his knowledgeability and expertise in a particular area of medicine, cannot be so skilled and experienced in all other branches of medicine as the highly specialized doctors in the related medical disciplines. Similarly, the professional, no matter his area of specialization in the field of mental retardation, is not equipped by training or experience to evaluate each of the varied factors known to have its effect on the individual's functioning.

Realistically, the interdisciplinary team was established as the central source of information and knowledge. This team, in essence, is viewed as a unified body acting as a many-branched assessor capable of evaluating a variety of factors that affect, mold, infringe on, and influence development, growth, and functioning. The team approach to problems by pooled resources, skills, and techniques of the different disciplines offers an integrated picture of the person as he currently functions and, wherever indicated, the reasons for the functioning.

Each discipline's assessment of the recommendations is gathered, discussed in the interdisciplinary group, and, if necessary, changed, reformulated, or revised. These data become the substance of programming and future planning.

Effective and vital as the interdisciplinary team approach is, there are occasional drawbacks, such as the use of similar or the same assessment tools by different disciplines. There is the tendency to report findings to one another for correspondence or agreement, rather than for evaluation of behavioral reactions as seen or interpreted by the individual assessor for greater understanding of the person and his varied dimensions.

12. Conclusion

This chapter on diagnosing mental deficiency, currently called "assessment," aimed not only to cite the negative and positive forces in mental retardation that perplex thinking and confound and complicate the problem of classification, etiology, and differential diagnosis but also to catalogue some of the instruments used.

Trying to differentiate the mentally retarded is like trying to catch and hold the wind. Behaviors, whether erratic, unpredictable, or hypoactive, seen among some may be due to brain injury, to extreme infantilism, or to serious emotional disturbance and/or psychosis. Investigations to establish such differences in children have not been very fruitful, and they inevitably lead to the conclusion that attempts to do so are attempts to stereotype mental retardation. Mentally retarded individuals, whether young or old, are as different and as individual as any of their nondeficient peers.

Standardized tests and the techniques previously discussed are important assessment instruments, but are not the only means of evaluating functioning. Assessment, in the broadest sense, means the study of behavior, which implies knowledge of child development, stages of maturation, and needs and interests of various age groups, as well as familiarity with scientific theories and methodologies.

Such a wide body of knowledge goes hand in hand with direct discriminating observation of behavior patterns and with clinical judgment. Regardless of age of the individual, assessment demands a strong base in psychological theories, concepts, and background. When the variety of developmental disorders in children and their outcomes are considered, it is of paramount importance to assess them early in life. There is no auspicious age to evaluate. Assessment may take place from early infancy and continue until old age. Early assessment, however, is the crux of the detection of problems, and intervention is the brake.

Given the opportunity, the human organism moves toward the life-giving light. Much more has to be explored, researched, and explicated to understand what specific measures can be taken to remediate the problem of retardation as it exists today and to be able to eradicate it tomorrow.

13. Appendix Notes

The authors have included in this chapter a Manual of Operations which has served as a guide for psychologists and psychology trainees at the Mental Retardation Institute. It is used to help staff with limited experience, to ensure administration of a comprehensive, appropriate battery, and to provide consistency and a yardstick for reevaluation and for research purposes.

Department of Psychology—Mental Retardation Institute
New York Medical College

A. Introduction:

This is a guide to assist you in more effective psychological evaluations of your clients. It in no way replaces the test manuals for each specific test, with which, it is assumed, you are completely familiar, or will become so.

Because of the nature of our population, especially children with language difficulties, perceptual problems, cultural differences, etc., special care must be taken to insure the best possible test results.

You have also been given guide sheets for the Rorschach, TAT, Bender, report writing, etc., to assist you in the administration, analysis and interpretation of the test data.

The outlined batteries and test procedures must be followed as stated below. In special instances, changes will have to be made and other tests, rather than the prescribed ones, must be substituted. However, substitutions and changes must be made judiciously and cautiously. Once you have completed the required battery, you are free to add any other tests or to test any dimensions which you consider helpful in further evaluation of the client.

B. Procedures

The prescribed test batteries are to be used regularly except under special circumstances. Any deviations, substitutions, omissions must be accounted for on the psychological report.

I. 2 years of age and below:

1. Gesell, Cattell, or California Mental and Motor Scales. Denver Developmental; Bayley
2. Vineland Social Maturity Scale

II. 2 years through 5 years of age:

1. Stanford-Binet Intelligence Scale (Form L-M)
2. Vineland Social Maturity Scale
3. Human Figure Drawings
4. Basic Geometric Shapes
5. Developmental Test of Visual-Motor Integration (only if basic forms acceptable)

Exceptions:

1. If the subject does not get a basal age on the Binet, the Cattell or the Gesell should be administered.
2. Non-verbal children or those with language difficulties should be given the Merrill-Palmer and the Peabody Picture Vocabulary Test.
3. When there is a significant difference in functioning between the verbal and non-verbal items on the Binet, the following tests should be administered:
    a. WPPSI
    b. Appropriate selected items for the ITPA

Some subjects will not be able to perform on this test battery because of the severity of retardation or uncooperativeness and will need a Developmental Evaluation (inquiry into the chronological course of growth and maturation in all fields: walking, talking, comprehending, etc. plus a Gesell).

III. 6 years to 12 years of age:

1. Stanford Binet, L-M. Between 10–12 years, WISC can be substituted.
2. Wide Range Achievement Test. M.A.—4 and above.
3. Basic Geometric Figures
4. Bender Visual Motor Gestalt Test—if subject can produce a triangle.
5. Vineland Social Maturity Scale (S.Q. is not reported)
6. Rorschach—IQ 40 and above.
7. TAT—IQ 40 and above.
8. Figure Drawings.

Exceptions:

1. For subjects with special disabilities (cerebral palsied, blind, deaf, etc.), extremely difficult or uncooperative subjects, other tests may be used, such as the Leiter, Arthur Point, Pictorial Test of Intelligence, PPVT, Hayes-Binet, Hiskey-Nebraska, Ravens Matrices.

2. If performance on non-verbal tasks is significantly higher on the Binet for older subjects, the WISC Performance Scale and the PPVT must be administered.

3. If the subject does not earn a basal age on the Binet, administer the Cattell or the MP, and the PPVT. Do not report an IQ on MP.

IV. 12 years of age and above:

1. WISC (subjects 16 or over—WAIS)
2. Wide Range Achievement Test
3. Bender Visual-Motor Gestalt Test
4. Vineland Social Maturity Scale (S.Q. not reported). Substitutes or alternates for VSMS: Cain-Levine, Balthazer, Adaptive Behavior Scale
5. Figure Drawings
6. Rorschach Psychodiagnostik, if WISC or WAIS given
7. Thematic Apperception Test (selected cards for Male and Female), if WISC or WAIS given

Exceptions:

1. For severely retarded, regardless of age, who cannot do the WISC or the WAIS, administer either the Binet or the MP, and the PPVT.

C. Administration of Tests:

I. Intelligence Tests

1. Directions for intelligence tests must be followed as given in manuals with one exception only: On the grapho-motor tasks (copying geometric forms):

a. Administer the next geometric form above the passed level. Example: If subject passes circle, *always* give the square.

b. Administer the geometric design preceding the failed level. Example: If subject fails the square, administer the circle.

NOTE: (1) If a form is passed above the ceiling age, *do not* count it in the quantitative score.
(2) If a form is failed below the basal age, *do not* change the basal age.

Developmentally—

age $2\frac{1}{2}$	Scribble circle (demonstrate)
age 3	Circle (no demonstration)—Binet, vertical line (demonstrate)
age 4	Cross (present one already made, do not demonstrate)
age 5	Square (present one already made, do not demonstrate
age 6	Triangle (present one already made, do not demonstrate)
age 7	Diamond (present one already made, do not demonstrate)

2. Be most careful to avoid cuing the patient by gesture, facial expression or verbal hints.

II. Wide Range Achievement Tests (New Form Only):

On the WRAT, use two forms for the reading. The subject reads from one and the examiner records incorrect responses on the other. Write out the actual response given for each word. Use this notated form for the arithmetic and spelling. Always ask subject to write his name on the form.

III. Vineland Social Maturity Scale:

Familiarize yourself with the manual so that you have a clear idea of the criteria in order to score an item plus or minus. Record any pertinent data in regard to the subject's function for each item, as well as impressions of the parent-child relationship.

It is often advisable to ask the informant to describe the subject's performance in the general areas, i.e., toileting, eating, dressing, etc., and then apply this information to the specific items. Avoid asking questions that indicate plus (or minus) answers, i.e., leading questions.

IV. Bender Visual-Motor Gestalt Test:

Be sure to present the plates in their correct position and aligned with the position of the paper. Right-handed subjects generally prefer the cards placed to the left of the paper; left-handed subject to the right. Allow the subject to adjust the plate location as long as they are aligned correctly with the paper. If the subject rotates a plate, return it to its original position. If he repeats this, allow him to proceed but record the rotated position, i.e., Card A, rotated 90 degrees to the right. If the subject rotates the paper, indicate top of paper for the particular design and return paper to the usual position for the next plate. Give one sheet of paper, but be sure the subject understands that he has several plates to copy.

If he turns the sheet over or asks for more paper, allow this. If paper turning continues, indicate top of page; that is, of each design on the sheet.

1. Follow Koppitz criteria for errors in designs.
2. Place extra paper near subject.

V. Drawings

1. Present child with a sheet of paper and ask him to "Draw a person," or "Draw somebody."
2. Do not indicate which sex; if questioned say, "Draw whichever you want."
3. Do not accept a stick figure as the final drawing. When the stick figure is finished, say, "Now draw one with a full body," or "Draw a real person; you know, with a real body and the rest."
4. If sex on the first drawing is undifferentiated, say, "Give this person a first name."
5. Remove drawing and present second sheet and say, "Now draw a boy or a man" (whichever is the opposite sex) "whichever you want."

VI. Thematic Apperception Test:

Record the client's responses verbatim. When you question the subject, please indicate by (Q) before the response. Use the following TAT plates:

TAT (ages 6 through 8)

Boys	Girls
4	4
5	5
6 BM	7 GF
7 BM	8 GF
13 B	13 B

TAT (ages 9 and above)

Boys	Girls
1	1
3 BM	3 GF
4	4
5	5
6 BM	9 GF
7 BM	12 F
13 B	13 MF
13 MF	18 GF
17 BM	

VII. Rorschach

1. Record subject's responses verbatim. A response after questioning should be preceded by (Q).
2. Use location sheets.
3. All responses must be scored and the specified percentages and ratios indicated.
4. Testing the limits should be done with very sparse records and with very negativistic clients.

D. Recording of Data

1. All responses must be recorded verbatim.
2. The correct time must be recorded on all timed tests; i.e., Object Assembly, Block Design, Coding, Picture Arrangement, Bead Stringing, Button Sorting, Seguin Formboards, Wallin, etc.
3. The client's name and date of testing must be written on every sheet and test form.
4. Staple all sheet forms and material together.
5. Description of client's approach, management and performance, particularly on non-verbal tests, should be recorded.
6. If the subject is non-English speaking, a translator can be made available.
7. A summary sheet must be filled out for every client's report.

E. Test Report

1. Follow guide given to you for report writing.
2. Your report should indicate if the test results are considered valid: minimal; if there are indications of higher potentialities, etc.
3. If an IQ was not obtained, state why; report which items were passed or failed and fully describe the child's behavior. A comprehensive descriptive report of an untestable subject should be made.

4. All attempted personality tests should be mentioned and accounted for.

5. Present findings in all areas should be compared to previous results. Try to account for any significant differences between present and previous functioning.

6. The A.A.M.D. Classification of Mental Retardation will be used in your reports as follows:

	IQ
Mild retardation of measured intelligence	67–52
Moderate retardation of measured intelligence	51–36
Severe retardation of measured intelligence	35–20
Profound retardation of measured intelligence	20–below

6a. AAMD—Adaptive Behavior Levels

7. The subject's handedness should be indicated; i.e., hand preference, used right or left hand predominantly, consistently; uses either hand interchangeably, etc.

8. In the observations, keep in mind that the client is a physical being (face, mouth, eyes, unusual muscular movements or postural adjustments) and behavioral manifestations (describe deviant) or stereotyped behavior, etc.).

9. In making recommendations on the report, give a reason for each one.

14. References

Ames, L. B., Learned, J., Metranx, R., & Walker, R. N., *Child Rorschach responses*. New York: Hoeber, 1952.

Bender, L. *A visual motor Gestalt Test and its clinical use*. New York: American Orthopsychiatric Assoc., 1938.

Bender, L. Autism in children with mental deficiency. *American Journal of Mental Deficiency*, 1959, *64*, 81–86.

Birch, H. G. *Brain damage in children: The biological and social aspects*. Baltimore: Williams & Wilkins, 1964, pp. 3–11.

Cronbach, L. J. Assessment of individual differences. In P. Fernsworth & A. McNemar (Eds.), *Annual review of psychology* (Vol. VII). Stanford, Calif.: Annual Reviews, Inc., 1956, pp. 173–196.

Cruickshank, W. M. *Psychology of exceptional children and youth*. Englewood Cliffs, N.J.: Prentice-Hall, 1971.

Freeman, F. A. Intellectual growth of children as indicated by repeated tests. *Psychology monographs*, 1936, *47*, 20–34.

Gallagher, J. J. A comparison of brain-injured and non-brain-injured mentally retarded children on several psychological variables. *Monographs of the Society For Research in Child Development*, 1957, *22*.

Grossman, H. J. (Ed.). *Manual in terminology and classification in mental retardation*. Washington, D.C.: American Association on Mental Deficiency, Spec. Publication Series No. 2, 1973.

Hobbs, N. *The futures of children*. San Francisco: Jossey-Bass, 1975.

Hoffman, L., & Ward Hoffman, M. L. *Review of child development research: Psychological testing of children* (Vol. II). New York: Russell Sage Foundation, 1966, pp. 257–300.

Kagan, J., & Moss, H. A. *Birth to maturity: A study in psychological development*. New York: Wiley, 1962.

Karp, E. The why and the wherefore of intelligence testing of the retarded. *Journal of Clinical Child Psychology*, 1973, 2(1), 35–36.

Kephart, N. C. The slow learner in the classroom. Englewood Cliffs, N.J.: Merrill, 1960.

Kessler, J. W. *Psychopathology of childhood*. Englewood Cliffs, N.J.: Prentice-Hall, 1966.

Klopfer, B., & Kelly, D. *The Rorschach Technique*. New York: World Book Co., 1942.

Koppitz, E. *The Bender Gestalt Test for young children*. New York: Grune & Stratton, 1964.

Ledwith, N. H. *Rorschach responses of elementary school children: A normative study*. Pittsburgh: Unit Press, 1959.

Liverant, S. Intelligence: A concept in need of re-examination. *Journal of Consulting Psychology*, 1960, *24*, 101–110.

Lutey, C. *Individual intelligence testing: A manual*. Greeley, Colo.: Executary Inc., 1966.

Machover, K. *Personality projective in the drawing of the human figure*. New York: 1949.

Mercer, J. Labeling the mentally retarded. Berkeley: University of California Press, 1973.

Michal-Smith, H., & Morgenstern, M. Use of H-T-P with the mentally retarded child on a hospital clinic. In J. Buck and E. Hammer (Eds.), *Advances in the House-Tree-Person Technique: Variations and applications*. Los Angeles: Western Psychological Services, 1970.

Pasamanick, B. Determinants of intelligence. In S. M. Farber & R. H. L. Wilson (Eds.), *Control of the mind: Part 2. Conflict and creativity*. New York: McGraw-Hill, 1963, pp. 3–26.

Pinnean, S. R. *Changes in intelligence quotient: Infancy to maturity*. Boston: Houghton-Mifflin, 1961.

Pollack, M. Brain damage, mental retardation and childhood schizophrenia. *American Journal of Psychiatry*, 1958, *115*, 427–428.

Rapaport, D., Gill, M. N., & Schafer, R. *Diagnostic psychological testing*. London: University of London Press, 1970.

Robb, G. P., Bernardoni, L. C., & Johnson, R. W. *Assessment of individual mental ability*. Scranton, Pa.: Crowell, 1972.

Robinson, H. B., & Robinson, N. M. *The mentally retarded child*. New York: McGraw-Hill, 1965.

Salinger, K. Diagnosis: Who needs it? *Journal of Clinical Issues in Psychology*, 1970, 1(2), 25–27.

Sattler, J. M. Analysis of functions of the 1960 Stanford Binet Intelligence Scale, Form L-M. *Journal of Clinical Psychology*, 1965, *21*, 173–179.

Spiker, C. C., & McCandless, B. R. The concept of intelligence and the philosophy of science. *Psychological Reviews*, 1954, *61*, 255–266.

Spitz, H. H. *Field theory in mental deficiency*. New York: McGraw-Hill, 1963, pp. 11–40.

Steinberg, R. A perspective on the I.Q. *A.P.A. Monitor*, 1977, 8(8).

Stevens, H., & Heber, R. *Mental retardation*. Chicago: University of Chicago Press, 1964.

Strauss, A. A., & Lehtinen, L. E. *Psychopathology and education of the brain-injured child*. New York: Grune & Stratton, 1947.

Strauss, A. A., & Werner, H. The mental organization of the brain-injured mentally defective child. *American Journal of Psychiatry*, 1941, *97*, 1194–1203.

Valett, R. E. *Descriptions of a clinical profile for the Stanford-Binet Intelligence Scale (L-M)*. Palo Alto, Calif.: Consulting Psychologists Press, 1965.

Vernon, M., & Brown, D. A. A guide to psychological tests and testing procedures in the evaluation of deaf and hard of learning children. *Journal of Speech and Hearing disorders*, 1964, *29*, 414–423.

Wesman, A. G.. Intelligence Testing. *American Psychologist*, 1968, *23*, 267–274.

21

Diagnosing Schizophrenia

LEOPOLD BELLAK AND CYNTHIA FIELDING

1. Introduction

The odds against writing something sensible, informed, and useful about the diagnosis of schizophrenia are tremendous. The literature on the subject matter is enormous, as is the diversity of opinions.

Since any diagnosis is predicated on a heuristic hypothesis or concept, we are, by definition, in difficulty, because of the broad range of the concept of schizophrenia. Its scope takes in those on the left who consider it a convenient fiction of the establishment, those in the center who consider it a syndrome of varied etiology and pathogenesis, symptomatology and prognosis, and those on the right who consider it a genetically transmitted metabolic disorder.

Attempts to diagnose schizophrenia are infinite and diverse. Diagnoses have been based on the "feeling" that is induced in the clinician, on the radial pulse, on the leukocyte picture, and on pink spots or mauve spots in electrochromatographic analysis of the urine. Delayed evoked response potentials in the EEG have been studied, as well as a vast number of different signs and symptoms, from Kraepelin and Bleuler to recent attempts including computer diagnosis and the operational criteria proposed for DSM III.

Most clinicians pay very little attention to the tremendous research industry's efforts to delineate and diagnose schizophrenia by these varied means, because so far the payoff for the clinician has been minimal. In essence, if the clinician finds someone with hallucinations, delusions, and a thought disorder in the absence of gross organic findings, and without strong affective features, he is likely to diagnose such a person as schizophrenic. He will then prescribe, by trial and error and his predilection, one of the psychotropic drugs. Perhaps the one major change in the

LEOPOLD BELLAK • Department of Psychiatry, Albert Einstein College of Medicine, Bronx, New York 10461. CYNTHIA FIELDING • Doctoral Program in Clinical Psychology, Florida Institute of Technology, Melbourne, Florida 32901.

past 5 years has been that more American psychiatrists consider the possibility of a manic-depressive disorder if there are any affective features. If the phenothiazines and their relatives do not work, he is likely to give lithium carbonate a chance. If this therapeutic test is successful, the diagnosis will most probably be changed to schizo-affective or affective disorder.

The intent of this chapter is to try to bring a few guidelines from the tremendous research reservoir to the problems of diagnosing schizophrenia in daily chemical work.

A diagnosis is a heuristic hypothesis. Like any hypothesis, its usefulness is measured by its ability to understand, predict, and control. In the case of a diagnosis, it must permit long- and short-range prediction in the form of a prognosis. It must allow inferences concerning a course of action, namely treatment.

A diagnosis as a form of hypothesis must also allow postdiction and hunches concerning preceding events, including etiological and pathogenic ones. Furthermore, it must allow collateral inferences; if A is present, then B and C should also be present. In schizophrenia, some would hold that a thought disorder should be present along with other signs, while some do not consider the presence of thought disorder pathognomonic only of schizophrenia, or its absence as ruling out schizophrenia.

Above all, a diagnosis, like any hypothesis, is of use only if independent judges can agree, with a high degree of statistical reliability and validity, that what is claimed to be present is indeed present. In the field of schizophrenia, very often what one investigator finds cannot be found by others; thus the finding lacks validity.

Looking over the broad field of endeavor, it is possible to speak of two basic trends in the attempts to diagnose schizophrenia. One is primarily concerned with increasing the *reliability* of the diagnosis, and the other one is concerned with establishing the *validity* of the diagnosis. Those familiar with the tenets of scientific methodology may well raise their eyebrows: is it not customary to strive for a combination of reliability and validity in one's findings? That is certainly true in theory, but very often not so in practice. There are a vast number of psychological and psychiatric questionnaires which have great reliability but very questionable validity. That is, if a test is administered to the same person by the same tester a second time, or administered to the same person by a different tester a second time, similar findings are very likely to be made. However, it is regrettable that often the degree to which the test measures what it purports to measure is in question, because construct validity as well as criterion-related validity is poor. Such tests do not correlate well with findings from other measurements or with clinical judgment. There is a whole host of factor analytic data for which the same may be said. They are found again and again with great reliability, but the statistical factors generated by the computer make no sense to the clinician.

The most ambitious attempt to establish reliable criteria for diagnosing schizophrenia can be found in the International Pilot Study of Schizophrenia of the World Health Organization (1976, p. 518). It demonstrated the ability of clinicians to agree on diagnosis, when they were given similar data, within one center. The computer approach by Spitzer, Sheehy, and Endicott (1977), which is now being brought to bear on the definitions in DSM III, is also a challenging enterprise, as are the Present State Examination (PSE) and the associated Catego program of Wing, Cooper, and Sartorius (1974). The PSE is a very sophisticated approach consisting of 140 items, mostly representing familiar psychiatric symptoms, each of which is defined in the glossary. The glossary definitions are necessary to train raters or diagnosticians so that they mean the same thing by a symptom. As Wing (1977, p. 89) says, "A technique such as the PSE is based on the assumption that the examiner knows what he is looking for." That is, of course, the heart of the matter. In order to use this technique, one has to have a certain concept of schizophrenia, and again to quote Wing (1977, p. 91): "Clinicians' decisions are always based upon theory." It is a statement I can heartily agree with. It happens that the PSE is based on, among other things, Schneider's First Rank Symptoms (FRS). Schneider's FRS enjoyed a great deal of popularity, especially among biologically oriented American psychiatrists, actually quite some years after Schneider first formulated these concepts. In the last 2 years, however, systematic studies of FRS have raised serious doubts about their usefulness. Some have found FRS present in nonschizophrenics and not present in schizophrenics (Carpenter, Strauss, & Muleti, 1973). Thus, the PSE may well have reliability: if the users study the glossary, they will show high agreement. However, if the criteria are not valid, it is hard to relate the findings to anything of clinical validity in terms of treatment response and prognosis. As Carpenter, Strauss, and Bartko (1973) mention in the pilot study, diagnostic homogeneity does not relate necessarily or even very likely to etiological and pathogenic communality.

In essence, the position of all those searching for reliability rests on the basic assumption that there is such an entity as "schizophrenia" and that all one needs to do is to agree on the necessary signs and symptoms defining it. If, however, this concept is not valid, then its reliability is worthless.

Curiously enough, the strongest argument against this basic assumption of the groups striving for reliability in the diagnosis of schizophrenia comes from biological research. The most recent research report from NIMH (1976, p. 531) gives increasing evidence that schizophrenics are a heterogeneous group marked by qualitative differences. There seems to be mounting proof that some subgroups may be characterized by neurophysiological abnormalities, others by biochemical ones, and yet others primarily by genetic or experiental ones, with many subgroupings among these major groups. Subdividing schizophrenics clinically by experiental factors also plays a significant role. Goldstein (1970) has suggested that schizophrenics with a good premorbid history and awareness of being ill respond poorly to phenothiazines and well to placebos, minor drugs, or no drugs at all.

To the extent to which these research projects are concerned with criteria that permit diagnoses which postdict a cause or etiology and lead to a testable proposition concerning the treatment of that cause, at least eventually, and a testable specific prognosis or prediction, then to that extent one can say they are concerned with validity.

There are two approaches to the diagnosis of schizophrenia which, in different ways, attempt to cut across the lines of reliability and validity. The first approach by Carpenter, Strauss, and Bartko (1973) relies heavily on the 12 most discriminating signs culled from the PSE, and is a pragmatic one. The diagnosis of schizophrenia is made with a view toward the potential use of the diagnosis and depends on what one wants to accomplish. Different criteria might be found suitable to enlarge on this.

The second approach comes from the authors of the various and collaborative adoptive studies. A most recent and particularly lucid account is one by Wender (1977). He begins with a brief review of the attempts to diagnose schizophrenia, and leads up to a discussion of the scope and validity of the "schizophrenic spectrum" concept, as this group of investigators have come to call it. He reminds us of Kraepelin's classification and of the broader one by Bleuler. He points out that, in European psychiatry, the term "schizophrenia" is still used primarily in the narrower sense that corresponds to Kraepelin's concept of dementia praecox. It coincides to what, in the United States, is called either "chronic schizophrenia," "process schizophrenia,"

LEOPOLD BELLAK
AND
CYNTHIA FIELDING

"true schizophrenia," or "nuclear schizophrenia." This type of schizophrenia can be described by a poor premorbid history, a gradual onset, and all of Bleuler's primary characteristics, as well as his secondary ones. Bleuler's primary characteristics are a loosening of associations, a disturbance of affect, autistic magical thinking, and a profound ambivalence. The secondary symptoms, not considered crucial, are hallucinations, delusions, and motor disturbances such as catatonia.

In the United States, Wender points out, a second form of schizophrenia is referred to as "reactive schizophrenia" or "acute schizophrenic reaction." This group is usually characterized by a good premorbid history, fairly good interpersonal relationships, heterosexual adjustment, and a good work history. The onset tends to be relatively fast, often in relation to some precipitating dynamic factor. This form of schizophrenia is characterized by the presence of secondary characteristics and less evidence of primary ones. Depressive or manic features may play a role. These patients, he says, and the present authors agree, respond well to phenothiazines and ECT and have a good long-term prognosis. However, he feels, as the present authors do, that a certain percentage of these acute schizophrenics will develop into chronic schizophrenics if they are not treated adequately, including therapeutic intervention. Wender further points out that European psychiatrists do not consider acute schizophrenic reactions to be true schizophrenia or even related to it. They call it "schizophreniform psychosis" as Langfeldt does or "psychogenic psychosis."

The third form of schizophrenia in the United States is called "pseudoneurotic schizophrenia" by Hoch and Polantin, and is also sometimes called "ambulatory schizophrenia" or "borderline schizophrenia." Such people usually have a history of chronic poor adjustment, with strangeness to their thinking. Their affective life is characterized by "anhedonia," the inability to feel intense pleasure. Their interpersonal relationships are either absent or excessively dependent. They often have a chaotic sexual life. The psychopathology, as Wender described it, and again the present authors agree, is characterized by its lack of consistency, with various neurotic manifestations ranging over the complete spectrum from phobias, aversions, psychosomatic symptoms, and intense anxiety to feelings of depersonalization and derealization. Again, the present authors agree with Wender that this group of people tends to manifest lifelong disturbances (Bellak & Benedict, 1958), no further deterioration, and no improvement with neuroleptic drugs.

Wender further describes a fourth group most distant from the chronic schizophrenic. He calls this group of people "schizoid," following Kretschmer (1923) and Kallman (1938). This form is characterized by eccentricity, depression, self-centeredness, emotional instability, and a propensity toward fads; these people may thus constitute the "lunatic fringe" of many religious, political, and other movements.

The contribution of the adoptive studies to the understanding of groups with manifestations of psychopathology is Wender's assertion that the studies suggest a genetic relationship among these four disorders. He and his collaborators claim that the comparison of adult groups of adopted schizophrenics with adult groups of adopted nonschizophrenics showed not only a much greater incidence of chronic schizophrenics among the biological relatives of the adopted schizophrenics but also a greater number of reactive schizophrenics, pseudoneurotics, and schizoid personalities among the biological relatives of the adopted schizophrenics. They claim that there is a genetic unity to this group. It is important, in this respect, to keep in mind Rosenthal's (1973) warning that the whole genetic sample is extremely small, and inferences are therefore precarious. In the present authors' opinion, the diagnosis of "schizoid," especially, was made without a basis for any general agreement on the meaning of this term and without adequate studies of interrater reliability. Indeed, the basis of the diagnosis in these adoptive studies, and whether someone belonged or not, relied on the psychiatrist's thumbnail sketch.

2. Ego Function Assessment for the Diagnosis of the "Schizophrenic Spectrum"

Since 1948, and increasingly in 1958 and 1968, the present senior author came to the conclusion that the schizophrenic condition could best be dealt with ration-

Table 1. Ego Functions and Their Components

Ego function	Components
1. Reality testing	Distinction between inner and outer stimuli Accuracy of perception Reflective awareness and inner reality testing
2. Judgment	Anticipation of consequences Manifestation of this anticipation in behavior Emotional appropriateness of this anticipation
3. Sense of reality	Extent of derealization Extent of depersonalization Self-identity and self-esteem Clarity of boundaries between self and world
4. Regulation and control of drives, affects, and impulses	a. Directness of impulse expression b. Effectiveness of delay mechanisms
5. Object relations	a. Degree and kind of relatedness b. Primitivity (narcissistic attachment or symbiotic-object choices) vs. maturity c. Degree to which others are perceived independently of oneself d. Object constancy
6. Thought processes	a. Memory, concentration, and attention b. Ability to conceptualize c. Primary-secondary process
7. Adaptive regression in the service of the ego (ARISE)	a. Regressive relaxation of cognitive acuity b. New configurations
8. Defensive functioning	a. Weakness or obtrusiveness of defenses b. Success and failure of defenses
9. Stimulus barrier	a. Threshold for stimuli b. Effectiveness of management of excessive stimulus input
10. Autonomous functioning	a. Degree of freedom from impairment of primary autonomy apparatuses b. Degree of freedom from impairment of secondary autonomy
11. Synthetic-integrative functioning	a. Degree of reconciliation of incongruities b. Degree of active relating together of events
12. Mastery-competence	a. Competence. How well subject actually performs in relation to his existing capacity to interact with and actively master and affect his environment b. The subjective role, or subject's feeling of competence with respect to actively mastering and affecting his environment c. The degree of discrepancy between component *a* and component *b* (i.e., between actual competence and sense of competence)

ally by thinking of it as a multiple-factor psychosociobiological syndrome of many different etiologies and pathogeneses, which shared as a final common path a serious but variable affliction of the ego functions.

The attempt to assess ego functioning had its origin in the desire to come to grips with the concept of schizophrenia. In the authors' opinion, the crux of the dianosis of schizophrenia for the clinician still lies in the need to give up thinking of schizophrenia as a unitary phenomenon, as one disease. This does not obviate the recognition that there is a clinical condition that shares enough of a common denominator or intragroup similarity to be called the "schizophrenic syndrome." In doing this, one must not forget the individuality of the patient so diagnosed and his need for a highly individual diagnosis, treatment, and prognosis. The senior author has discussed this in a paper on the validity and usefulness of the concept of the schizophrenic syndrome (Bellak, 1970) and in a chapter in *Ego Functions in Schizophrenics, Neurotics, and Normals* (Bellak, Hurvich, & Gediman, 1973).

In view of these propositions, it does not seem worthwhile to engage in a worldwide attempt to find a condition which can be called "schizophrenia," as did the International Pilot Study of Schizophrenia. All that this study established was that observers trained to recognize a number of signs and symptoms, and agreeing to call them schizophrenic at a certain point in their lives, can do so. This was true within a given center, but their ability to do this between centers was not very impressive.

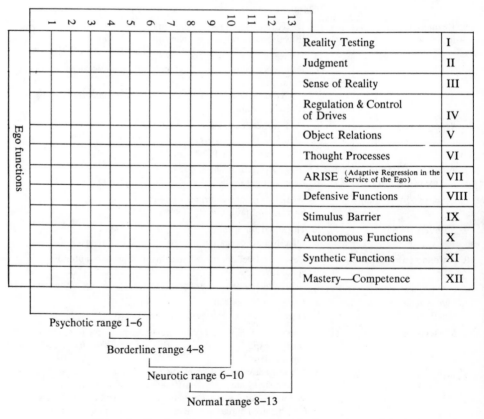

Figure 1. Ego function rating form: schematic diagnostic ranges.

Even if they could have found perfect agreement in centers as well as between centers, the present authors believe it would not mean more than that. Some 100 years ago, well-trained observers could have agreed to call a condition which had certain signs and symptoms such as high temperature, dehydration, fast pulse, fast breathing, and weakness a "fever." Recognizing a fever is not a small or meaningless feat.

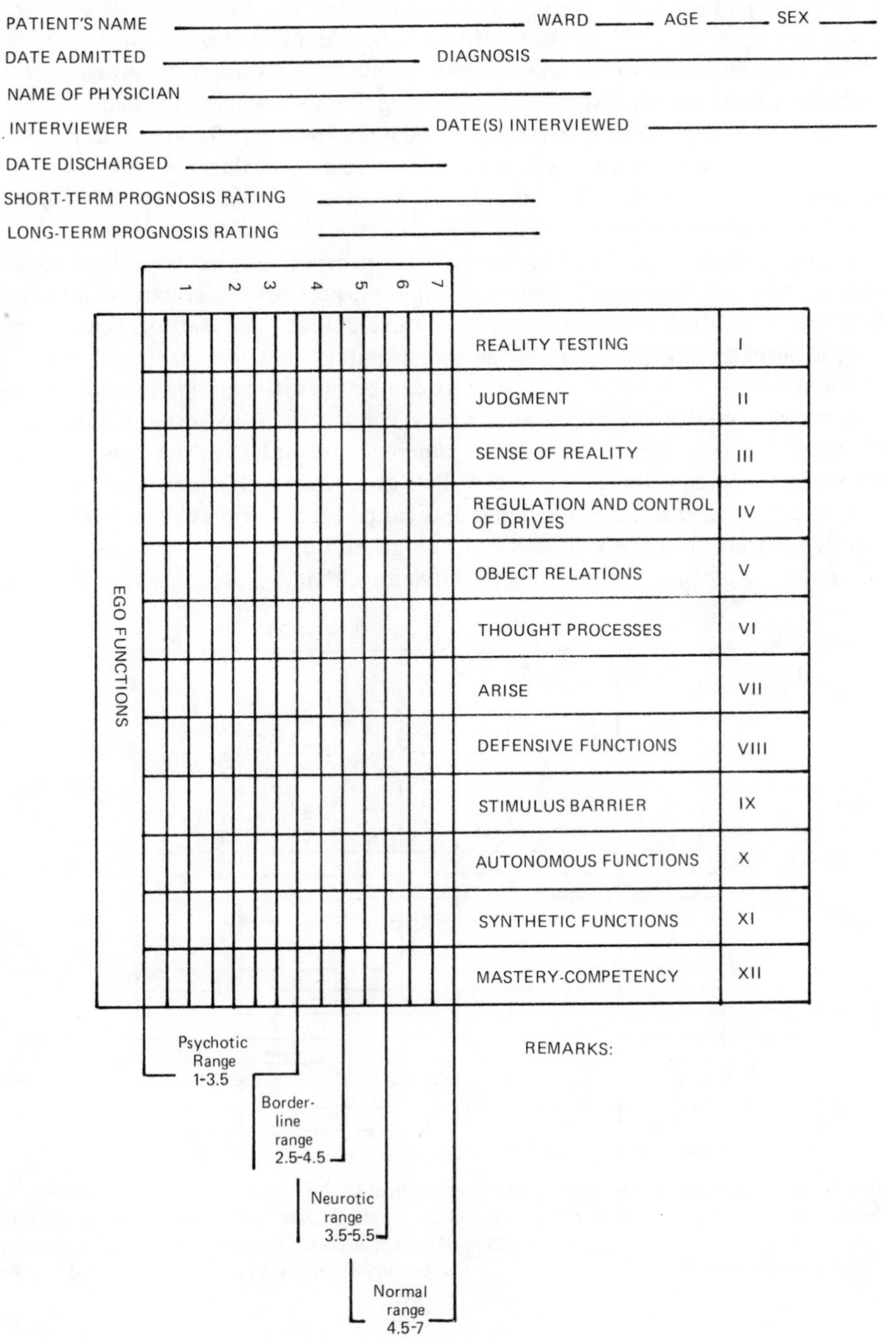

PATIENT'S NAME _____ WARD _____ AGE _____ SEX _____

DATE ADMITTED _____ DIAGNOSIS _____

NAME OF PHYSICIAN _____

INTERVIEWER _____ DATE(S) INTERVIEWED _____

DATE DISCHARGED _____

SHORT-TERM PROGNOSIS RATING _____

LONG-TERM PROGNOSIS RATING _____

EGO FUNCTIONS	1	2	3	4	5	6	7		
								REALITY TESTING	I
								JUDGMENT	II
								SENSE OF REALITY	III
								REGULATION AND CONTROL OF DRIVES	IV
								OBJECT RELATIONS	V
								THOUGHT PROCESSES	VI
								ARISE	VII
								DEFENSIVE FUNCTIONS	VIII
								STIMULUS BARRIER	IX
								AUTONOMOUS FUNCTIONS	X
								SYNTHETIC FUNCTIONS	XI
								MASTERY-COMPETENCY	XII

Psychotic Range 1-3.5

Border-line range 2.5-4.5

Neurotic range 3.5-5.5

Normal range 4.5-7

REMARKS:

Figure 2. Ego functions.

We all agree that generally bed rest is indicated. The random administration of antibiotics to patients with fever would do at least as much good as random administration of phenothiazines to all schizophrenics. However, breaking down the fevers into groups, in which the fever is caused by specific bacteria, viruses, or other etiological factors, makes more specific treatment possible. The reliability of establishing fever with a thermometer needed construct validity for each causal factor. In the absence of such definitive factors, attempts to assess the processes affected by the schizophrenic "fever," and to treat those specific affected ones, must be limited. Although a high temperature may be caused by both pneumonia and cholera, the tremendous fluid loss in cholera is outstanding and its replacement crucial, while in pneumonia the respiratory distress and remedial steps are the main concern.

The present authors' suggestion for a clinical diagnosis that has both nomothetic and ideographic individual validity, as well as providing clinical reliability of diagnosis, is the conceptualization of the schizophrenic syndrome in terms of ego functions. Diagnosis by ego function assessment incorporates the major aspects of a diagnosis already mentioned, that is, prediction, postdiction, collateral inferences, and a treatment. It does not, however, prejudge etiology and pathogenesis.

The psychoanalytic concept of the ego, as part of the tripartite model of the ego, id, and superego, is a useful construct. It can be operationally defined by its functions. If one appraises schizophrenics with regard to the specific ego functions, and with regard to their interaction with the superego and with the drives (as the present authors prefer to call the id), one finds that, as a group, schizophrenics share a low mean of ego functions, but have highly individual ego function patterns, which may possibly separate them into different meaningful groups.

Diagnosis by ego functions has the advantage that it bridges the descriptive and

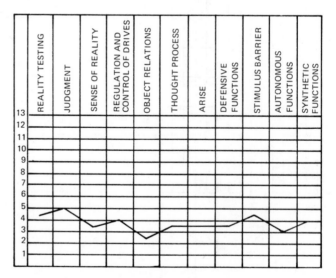

Figure 3.   Ego function assessment profile of a young man in his 20s whose functions nearly all fall around or below 5 with a very poor short-range and long-range prognosis even though the absolute level of functioning is not an extremely low one. From Bellak, Hurvich, & Gediman, *Ego Functions in Schizophrenics, Neurotics and Normals.* Copyright © 1973, by C.P.S., Inc. Reprinted by permission of J. Wiley & Sons, Inc.

the dynamic core. This means that it is possible to arrive at a reliable diagnosis, because independent observers have been shown to agree statistically on their ratings of the ego functions. At the same time, by virtue of the concepts being set within the matrix of psychoanalytic theory and clinical observations, they also have demonstrable predictive powers. As a matter of fact, one way to think of ego function assessment is to see it as a mental status examination in psychoanalytic terms, with quantified ratings and established construct validity.

Although conceptualized decades ago, a 5-year NIMH-supported study resulted, in 1973, in a monograph on *Ego Functions in Schizophrenics, Neurotics, and Normals* (Bellak, et al., 1973). The details of the theoretical nature, and the painful way of arriving at the 12 ego functions that were eventually found both necessary

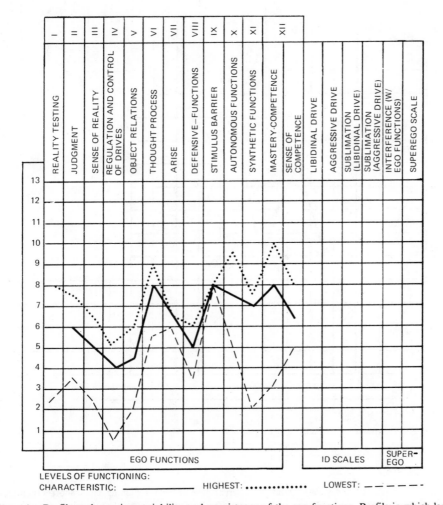

Figure 4. Profile underscoring variability and consistency of the ego functions. Profile in which large differences can be seen between characteristic and lowest level on many functions—regulation and control of drives, synthetic functions, and mastery and competence. Profile highlights areas of vulnerability and strength. From Bellak, Hurvich, & Gediman, *Ego Functions in Schizophrenics, Neurotics and Normals.* Copyright © 1973, by C.P.S., Inc. Reprinted by permission of J. Wiley & Sons, Inc.

and sufficient, are described there. A list of the 12 ego functions and their components is presented in Table 1 and Figures 1–5. Sometimes a 7-point scale is used, and sometimes a 13-point scale. The 7-point scale is easily converted into a 13-point scale by multiplying a scale stop by 2 and subtracting 1. Plotting such curves permits one to assess, at a glance, the amount of discrepancy between ego functioning at times of minimal and maximal intrapsychic and external stress. It also permits the clini-

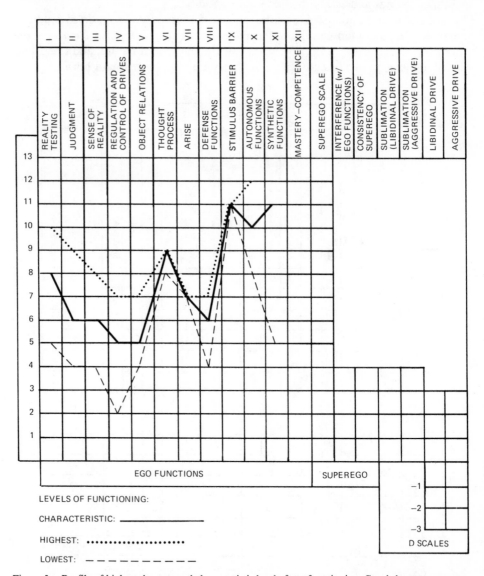

Figure 5. Profile of highest, lowest, and characteristic level of ego functioning. Good short-term prognosis with aid of drugs and good long-term prognosis because of highest level of functioning and because last four ego functions are good. From Bellak, Hurvich, & Gediman, *Ego Functions in Schizophrenics, Neurotics and Normals,* Copyright © 1973, by C.P.S., Inc. Reprinted by permission of J. Wiley & Sons, Inc.

cian to pinpoint the specific ego functions which exhibit the greatest degree of vicissitude, e.g., the relative instability of certain ego functions.

Since the completion of the original work, EFA has been used by others for diverse purposes. Ciompi, Ague, and Danwalder (1976) found it possible to rate progress, using the EFA, in 30 psychoanalytic patients with reliability and validity (Figure 6). Milkman and Frosch (1977) successfully differentiated heroin addicts from amphetamine addicts with EFA profiles (Figure 7).

Recent work in the direction of making EFA simpler and briefer than the original 2-hr interview has been undertaken by Bellak, Conte, and Fielding (1976–1977). Currently, in the status of a pilot study, a 12-page questionnaire, one for each ego function, has been developed, with ten questions for each ego function, each rated

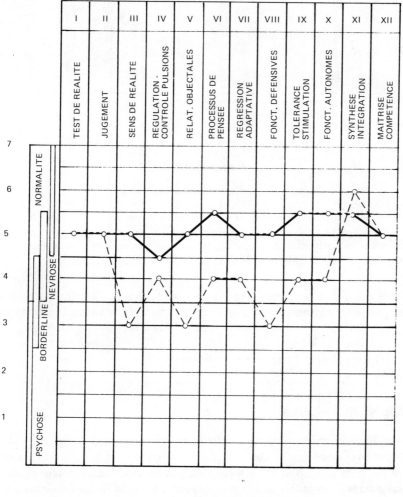

1° évaluation 25.5.1975: moyenne 4.2 points
2° évaluation 16.6.1976: moyenne 5.2 points

Figure 6. An example of an ego function profile of a case in psychoanalysis. Reproduced by permission of the authors.

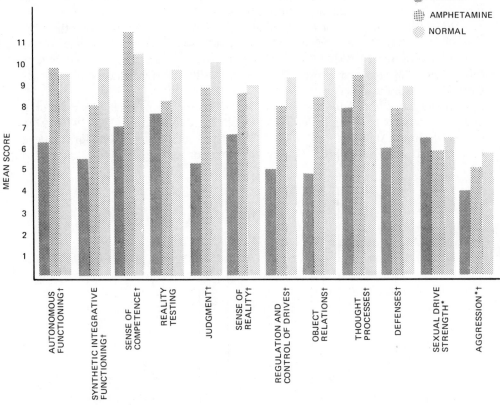

Figure 7. Mean ego function ratings for amphetamine subjects, heroin subjects and normals in the abstinent condition with ratings for sexual and aggressive drive strengths. Reprinted by permission of the *Journal of Psychedelic Drugs*, Madison, Wisconsin.

and combined into a numerical score and a globel score. This should enable any clinician to assess a given patient and to decide graphically which functions are impaired and which are relatively intact. It should also permit him to decide whether crucial functions are impaired enough and the overall ego strength low enough to warrant the diagnosis of "schizophrenic syndrome."

3. Diagnostic Patterns

In addition to making this nomothetic generic diagnosis, a clinician should be encouraged to further qualify this diagnosis with a series of hierarchical statements. For instance, the diagnosis of "schizophrenic syndrome" may be accompanied by "very poor impulse control" and "very poor judgment." This would signal a patient who needs close supervision and drugs to control his impulses. In another patient, inner reality testing might be judged to be very good—i.e., the patient is aware of being ill, recognizing the poor outer reality testing he suffers from. If this is so, it will be useful to keep in mind Goldstein's (1970) findings, that patients with awareness are often further impaired by phenothiazines. The present authors would be especially hesitant to administer phenothiazines if awareness of being ill is accompanied by a poor "sense of self" and some kind of depersonalization, because phenothiazines are likely to lead to a further feeling of being "spaced out."

Any time very poor impulse control and relatively intact thinking are found, possibly combined with a history of asocial behavior, the patient should be carefully examined for evidence of minimal brain damage (MBD) (Bellak, 1976). A careful personal and family history concerning MBD should be taken, and a neurological examination for soft signs administered, as well as a neuropsychological examination.

If the hunch is borne out, then the clinician may well be dealing with a distinct subgroup of the schizophrenic syndrome which warrants certain specific inferences: that this patient has a condition which, at least in part, is caused by the primary factors of MBD—problems in spatial orientation, problems of verbal expression, and a variety of motor and cognitive problems in general. Probably the development of the patient's self-image and body image has been affected, necessitating psychodynamic and remedial work. Furthermore, it is almost a certainty that the patient suffered emotional trauma secondary to the MBD symptoms, such as feeling odd, stupid, and/or clumsy, and that this needs therapeutic attention.

In addition, such patients need extra attention on the ward, because their poor impulse control and rather good reality testing make them the primary group which attempts to run away at the first opportunity or to engage in willful mischief. Therapeutically, such patients usually do not respond well to phenothiazines and may even become worse. However, they may respond well, and almost immediately, to relatively small doses of imipramine (Figure 8). This group responds to imipramine

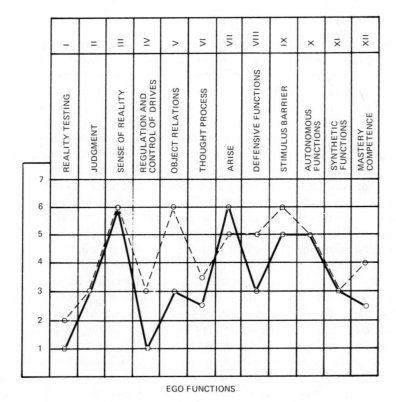

EGO FUNCTIONS

Figure 8. Comparison of average EFA scores of a patient treated with imipramine before and after a 1-week period. From Bellak et al. (1976–1977).

LEOPOLD BELLAK
AND
CYNTHIA FIELDING

very rapidly in comparison with the depressive group's response to the same drug. The reason for this is the immediate amphetaminelike biochemical effect on presynaptic transmission.

One other variable of the schizophrenic syndrome is now under study (Bellak, Meyers, Conti, & Fielding, 1977). It is a clinical hunch that schizophrenics with a reasonably good rating on the last four ego functions and on thought processes are likely to have a good prognosis. Those who have a poor rating on the last four variables and on thought processes may have a good short-range prognosis but are unlikely to have a good long-range prognosis. Some preliminary findings by Ciompi (1977) tentatively bear this out, except that he found that a poor sense of self is a poor prognosticator as well. This, on further consideration, is not surprising if one keeps in mind that crucial role played by success or failure of individuation and the establishment of self-boundaries.

Prognosis should be greatly aided by ego function patterns. A patient with a universally low profile graph can hardly be expected to profit from what we have to offer so far, and is probably best suited for custodial care. A patient in whom reality testing, judgment, and impulse control remain relatively intact even in the acute episode can probably be helped, with rehabilitation, to live constructively in the community, working on some simple job, even if his other functions are relatively poor.

The nature of a patient's object relations needs special scrutiny. It is important for a detailed and sophisticated diagnosis of the primary condition itself, for the kind of therapy suggested, and for the nature of the recovery one can expect.

4. Other Diagnostic Considerations

Following the lead of the research findings for different etiological subgroups of the schizophrenic syndrome, it may be clinically useful to attempt to develop some hunches as to whether a patient's condition is primarily related to experiental factors, to genetic ones, to neurophysiological ones, or possibly to biochemical ones.

The present authors do not see each of these contributing factors as an all-or-none proposition. To the contrary, we feel that, in most people with the "schizophrenic syndrome," there is an interaction of all these and possibly other variables as well, but in different degree. We have, in this context, spoken of a minimax model of schizophrenic etiology," meaning that, in a given patient, some factor—e.g., one of the four mentioned above—plays the maximal role, and one other the minimal role, with the others in second and third place. (We have learned that "minimax" is a term used by mathematicians for a certain type of mathematical model; our use of the term does not relate to the mathematical one.)

The present authors do believe that a careful history might often give some leads along these lines, as will be discussed below, and that such hunches might usefully be taken into consideration in treatment and prognosis. We suggest then that the clinical diagnosis of "schizophrenic syndrome" be accomplished by a description of the ego function profile and, further, by some remark such as "possible neurophysiological factors related to possible encephalitis in childhood" or "related to onset of puberty and conflicts about role within herself and in the family context," etc.

In one group of patients with a strong experiential background, the present authors believe that taking a personal history of such patients within the schizophrenic syndrome will corroborate a hunch that these patients had a relatively good premorbid history, with a significant precipitating situational event causing an acute condition. Furthermore, this type of patient usually responds well to medication and/or psychotherapy, but may well become a chronic patient, especially if he is not helped to work through his dynamic and structural problems. In these cases, delusions and hallucinations can be relatively easily understood by a process akin to dream analysis. If this is accomplished as well by the working through of pre-Oedipal and Oedipal problems, abatement of the acute disorder will most probably ensue. Work with the structural problems of poor internalized objects and an archaic superego, as well as a character analysis, is often necessary for a real basic change and for an excellent prognosis.

The EFA profiles in these patients need to be consistent with what was mentioned earlier on the necessity for relatively good ratings on thought disorder as well as on the last four ego functions. However, a rather severe thought disorder need not be a contraindication, as this is frequently treatable as another defense mechanism. Often, the oversymbolization, the manifest break in relevance, and other manifestations serve as avoidance phenomena of anxiety-loaded thoughts.

Another group, with poor ratings on the last four ego functions, presents features which are generally associated with the chronic or nuclear type of schizophrenia. They also show rather strong evidence of familial occurrence of schizophrenia, suggesting a genetic factor. In the absence of more knowledge about and more treatment capacity for the biological nature of the defects transmitted, prognosis for this group of patients remains rather pessimistic.

However, the picture of chronic psychosis need not necessarily be accompanied by the evidence of genetic factors. In the present authors' opinion, a history of poor object relations, as well as other unfavorable experiential factors from infancy, can produce a similar final common path. In such cases, circumstances permitting, a prolonged psychoanalytic effort may have a better chance of success than in the patients whose restructuring is also interfaced with a disturbed biochemical or neurophysiological substratum.

Yet another subgroup of patients with the schizophrenic syndrome may suffer, as previously mentioned, from various neurophysiological disturbances. We have already discussed one particular subgroup belonging here, namely those suffering from MBD. We do not believe that this is the only group with neurophysiological problems interrelating with the manifest schizophrenic syndrome. A careful personal history, a physical examination, and psychological testing will frequently reveal evidence of a childhood history of high fever, as well as some borderline neurological problems, possibly a somewhat disturbed EEG. As yet, we are not in a position where clinical practice would easily avail itself of hard findings concerning eyetracking (Holzman, Proctor, & Hughes, 1973). Nevertheless, aside from the diagnostic statement of schizophrenic syndrome, frequently in such cases with EFA showing poor ratings for autonomous functioning as well as synthetic integrative functioning, the diagnosis should also mention possible neuropsychological factors. Theoretically, a therapeutic trial on sodium dilantin may be indicated in such cases, in addition to other measures.

Lastly, a group impressed itself on the senior author as long ago as my residency. These patients certainly had to be diagnosed as schizophrenic by all the classical signs and symptoms, including a clear sensorium, but they nevertheless made a toxic impression on me. Their eyes looked feverish, their pupils were dilated, and their skin was shiny smooth, the way I had seen it in patients with rheumatoid arthritis when I worked in a hospital for joint diseases. I do believe that there is a subgroup in which chemical factors play a role. Indeed, it may be that we are only dealing with quantitative variations in dopamine or serum creatine phosphokinase as described by Meltzer (1976).

It has long been the senior author's conviction that etiological research has been so disappointing because the same factors were looked for in all those with the schizophrenic syndrome. To research this, one would try to preselect groups in whom, by history hunches and symptoms, one has to suspect a primary psychological, neurological, biochemical, or genetic factor, and then try to find research evidence of a higher percentage of these factors in each given group than in the other three or four groups. This might be a way of arriving at the quantitatively different contributions of the various factors to the manifest syndrome of the schizophrenic disorders.

Until this time comes, the present authors can only suggest that the clinician incorporate these hunches in his diagnostic formulations and propositions for treatment and prognosis.

5. References

Bellak, L. The validity and usefulness of the concept of the schizophrenic syndrome. In R. Cancro (Ed.), *The schizophrenic reactions* (Menninger Foundation Conference). New York: Brunner/Mazel, 1970.

Bellak, L. A possible subgroup of the schizophrenic syndrome and implications for treatment. *American Journal of Psychotherapy*, 1976, *30*(2), 194–205.

Bellak, L., & Benedict, P. K. (Eds.). *Schizophrenia: A review of the syndrome.* New York: Logos Press, 1958 (now distributed by Grune & Stratton).

Bellak, L., Conte, H., & Fielding, C. Pilot study—Bronx Municipal Hospital, New York, 1976–1977.

Bellak, L., Hurvich, M., & Gediman, H. *Ego functions in schizophrenics, neurotics and normals.* New York: Wiley, 1973.

Bellak, L., Meyers, B., Conte, H., & Fielding, C. Ongoing pilot study, Bronx Municipal Hospital, New York, 1977.

Carpenter, W. T., Jr., Strauss, J. S., & Bartko, J. J. Flexible system for the diagnosis of schizophrenia: Report from WHO international pilot study of schizophrenia. *Science*, 1973, *182*, 1275–1278.

Carpenter, W. T., Jr., Strauss, J. S., & Muleti, S. Are there pathognomic symptoms in schizophrenia? An empiric investigation of Schneider's FRS. *Archives of General Psychiatry*, 1973, *28*, 847–852.

Ciompi, L. Personal communication, University of Lausanne, Switzerland, 1977.

Ciompi, L., Ague, C., & Danwalder, J. P. L'observation de changements psychodynamiques: Experience avec une version simplifiée des "Ego strength rating scales" de Bellak et al. Communication au Xe Congrès International de Psychotherapie, Paris, July 4–10, 1976.

Goldstein, M. J. Premorbid adjustment, paranoid status, and patterns of response to phenothiazines in acute schizophrenia. *Schizophrenia Bulletin*, 1970, *I* (Experimental Issue No. 3), 24–37.

Holzman, P. S., Proctor, L. R., & Hughes, D. W. Eyetracking patterns in schizophrenia. *Science*, 1973, *181*, 179–181.

Kallman, F. J. *The genetics of schizophrenia.* Locust Valley, N.Y.: J. J. Augustin, 1938.

Kretschmer, E. *Physique and character.* New York: Harcourt, Brace & Co., 1923.

Meltzer, H. Y. Neuromuscular dysfunction in schizophrenia. *Schizophrenia Bulletin*, 1976, *2*(1), 106–135.

Milkman, H., & Frosch, W. A. Ego function ratings for amphetamine *S*'s and heroin *S*'s. *Journal of Psychedelic Drugs*, 1977, *9*(1).

Rosenthal, D. Evidence for a spectrum of schizophrenic disorders. Presented at the annual meeting of the American Psychological Association, Montreal, Canada, August 1973.

Schizophrenia Bulletin—NIMH—Special Report: Schizophrenia 1976 (Vol. 2). Washington, D.C.: HEW.

Spitzer, R. L., Sheehy, M., & Endicott, J. DSM-III. Guiding principles. In M. Rakoff, H. C. Stancer, & H. B. Kedward (Eds.), *Psychiatric diagnosis.* New York: Brunner/Mazel, 1977.

Wender, P. H. The scope and validity of the schizophrenic spectrum concept. In M. Rakoff, H. C. Stancer, & H. B. Kedward (Eds.), *Psychiatric Diagnosis.* New York: Brunner/Mazel, 1977, pp. 109–127.

Wing, J. K. The limits of standardization. In M. Rakoff, H. C. Stancer, & H. B. Kedward (Eds.), *Psychiatric Diagnosis.* New York: Brunner/Mazel, 1977.

Wing, J. K., Cooper, J. E., & Sartorius, N. *The measurement and classification of psychiatric syndrome.* New York: Cambridge University Press, 1974.

22

Diagnosis in Old Age

HAROLD WILENSKY

1. Introduction

Disorders of old age cover a broad range and admixture of illnesses and dysfunctions. They range from the relatively universal reactions of mild depression and anxiety to both internal and external loss through the functional psychotic disorders and organic brain syndromes. Other physical diseases typically accompany and contribute to behavioral dysfunction. Prompt, accurate assessment and treatment are crucial at the first signs of disorder. Delay in providing treatment can result in transient dysfunction becoming irreversible regardless of whether the origin of the disorder is found in psychological, biological, and/or sociological stress. Unfortunately, geriatric patients have rarely received the careful evaluation needed (Butler, 1975; Eisdorfer & Stotsky, 1977).

This chapter will first identify problems which contribute to inaccurate assessment and consequent inadequate mental health treatment of the aged and then recommend practical approaches to assessment in accord with the nature of the dysfunction. Foremost among the problems have been the prejudices against the aged which permeate all aspects of our society. Ageism (Butler, 1969) can lead to disastrous consequences, particularly in those aged persons diagnosed or misdiagnosed as suffering from senile dementia. Second, the aged themselves have not been friends and supporters of mental health facilities, rarely seeking help on their own initiative. Third, elderly persons with mental or emotional disorders tend to be multiproblem clients suffering from physical illnesses as well as social, economic, and environmental deprivation. Assessment and treatment call for a cooperative interdisciplinary approach. Team approaches, however, have not had notable success in the history of the treatment of mental and emotional disorders. Finally, the diagnostic practices and techniques psychologists and psychiatrists are most familiar with were developed for use with younger adults. They require considerable modification in administration and interpretation for use with the elderly (Oberleder, 1967; Schaie & Schaie, 1977). Normative data for the frequently used psychological tests are not adequate. Recognition of these obstacles is a prerequisite to the development of a rational, practical approach to clinical assessment.

HAROLD WILENSKY • Psychological Center, City University of New York, New York, New York 10031.

2. Ageism, Stereotyping, and Diagnosis

HAROLD WILENSKY

Ageist prejudices begin to be experienced by the victim sometime during the middle years. Stereotyping had been given legal sanction as soon as a person reached the chronological age of 65. That person was identified by law as a member of a group associated with an expectation of impairment regardless of the individual's functional level (Cain, 1974). In 1978, an act of Congress corrected the inequity of forced retirement at age 65 which was required in some industries. On the other hand, special privileges such as reduced fares, reduced admission fees to museums, theaters, and parks, and special discounts in stores are granted to senior citizens upon request regardless of their financial status.

The negative effects of prejudice are pervasive in our culture (Butler, 1969, 1975). In dealing with mental and emotional disorders, the destructive aspects of prejudice frequently operate in an insidious, disguised manner to delay treatment. Ageism may take the form of the apparently benign acceptance of deviant behavior. Signs and symptoms of disorders that would be cause for elaborate diagnostic study in younger adults tend to be overlooked by friends, family, and community agents such as police, with the explanation "They are only senile" (Butler, 1975). When the signs of disturbance become so compelling that the person must be brought to the attention of a health professional, the professional, all too often subject to similar biases, may also accept the behavior as a sign of senile dementia. The etiology is assumed to be diffuse brain cell loss, a natural correlate of aging. The search for other possible causes of the dysfunction is terminated. The hopeless prognosis of a progressive deteriorative process may set in motion the self-fulfilling prophecy, dooming the patient to a treatment approach that inevitably ensures the accuracy of the prognosis.

Even in cases where the causes may have been transient and self-limiting, the label could lead to the shaping of the patient's behavior in accord with the role expectations of a senile dement held by society and, indeed, by the victim as well. Gruenberg (1967) described this process as a "social breakdown syndrome" which frequently began while the identified patient was still in the community. The patient was relieved of all responsibilities for independent functioning. The identified senile person conformed to the role set, eventually becoming dependent and helpless; institutionalization was necessary, and the deteriorative process continued to the ultimate and predicted conclusion. Admission of elderly patients, particularly those of foreign birth or low socioeconomic status, to state hospitals has been described as the equivalent of a "referral for death" (Markson & Hand, 1970).

The extent of apparently inaccurate diagnosis of chronic brain syndromes in the United States and, by inference, its dire consequences are suggested by the cross-national surveys conducted by Copeland and his associates (1975). They had noted the striking differences in the incidence of organic brain syndromes and functional disorders between those elderly patients hospitalized in the United States and those hospitalized in the United Kingdom. The incidence of organic brain syndrome in the United States (79.8%) was almost 2 times greater than the incidence of the syndrome in England and Wales (42.8%). With regard to functional disorders, the 1967 United States survey revealed a frequency (8.5%) about one-fifth the rate reported in a 1966 survey in England and Wales (46.3%).

Identifying the reasons underlying the differences in admission diagnosis between the two countries was of critical import because of differences in outcome.

Patients with functional disorders have better prognoses than organic brain syndrome patients. Consistent with the differences in the proportion of functional disorders in the two countries, discharge rates within 1 year of admission for the elderly psychiatric patients in England and Wales (61.6%) were 3 times those for the United States patients. In the United States the death rate (43.7%) within 1 year of admission to psychiatric hospitals was about twice that for the elderly patients admitted to the United Kingdom hospitals. (The death rates appeared to be in accord with the incidence of organic brain syndromes in both countries, but rates by diagnostic category were not given.)

When semistructured instruments (The Geriatric Mental Status Schedule and a History Schedule) were employed to obtain objective and comparable diagnostic data, the differences in diagnostic rates all but disappeared, with the United States' rate for organic brain syndrome approaching the much lower incidence of the disorder in the United Kingdom. The apparently great differences in the incidence of these disorders between the countries reflected differences in diagnostic practices rather than in patient populations. Unexplained as yet were the differences in the death rates for elderly psychiatric patients in the United States and in England and Wales. An unresolved issue is the extent to which the higher death rate may be evidence of the dire consequences of the self-fulfilling prophecy associated with the diagnosis of chronic brain syndrome. The hopeless prognosis may well play a role in determining longevity. It remains to be demonstrated whether the death rate for elderly psychiatric patients in the United States would also approach the lower death rate in the United Kingdom should the more objective and presumably more accurate diagnostic procedures be implemented in the United States.

3. Use of Mental Health Facilities

Epidemiological surveys of psychopathology of the aged have typically been employed as evidence for indicting the mental health profession for their neglect of the problems and needs of the elderly. A review of 1970 census data by Kramer, Taube, and Redick (1973) revealed that, while about 10% of the general population was 65 or over, this age group was vastly overrepresented among the patients in mental hospitals, accounting for 30% of the total. In contrast, the elderly group composed only 2% of the patients treated in mental health clinics and 4% of the patients treated in community mental health centers. Estimates of the numbers of older persons seen by private practitioners were also minimal. Butler (1975) concluded that psychiatrists probably spent less than 1 hour per week with older patients; Lawton and Gottesman (1974) indicated that for psychologists the numbers seen were also quite low. Even these figures for outpatients tended to reflect consultations rather than active treatment. Apparently, older individuals have not been making use of mental health professionals until they become so seriously disturbed that they must be hospitalized.

The limited outpatient services for the over-65 group in part have been built into the system of delivery of health services in which it has been the responsibility of the person in need to seek out assistance. With regard to emotional problems, the vast majority of the aged tend not to be psychologically sophisticated. For the current group of aged, the median educational level was about ninth grade, with perhaps one-eighth classifiable as functionally illiterate (Brotman, 1973). For non-whites, the educational level averaged $2\frac{1}{2}$ years less. About 6% were college graduates. Educational level has been shown to be directly related to the readiness to seek out, understand, and remain in psychiatric treatment (Hollingshead & Redlich, 1958). The lower-class, less-educated group rarely sought out therapy but were more likely to be brought to the psychiatrist by authorities in the community. Because of generational and educational differences, the cultural gap between the older person and the mental health professional would tend to be quite large, making for serious problems in communication. The older patient's conception of the need for mental health consultation or treatment may well be that one goes to a head doctor when one is crazy and has to be put away for good. The professionals' biases may well have confirmed the patient's belief as suggested by the low discharge rates for hospitalized elderly psychiatric patients (Copeland et al., 1975).

Up to this point, we have been treating the aged as if they were a homogeneous population. Although large numbers have had less education and are less psychologically sophisticated, it is necessary to begin to differentiate among the individuals. Educational level is increasing; the YAVIS (young, attractive, verbal, intelligent, successful persons) who were preferred as patients by psychotherapists (Schofield, 1964) are also aging, as are their therapists. Add to this the very rapid increase in numbers of gerontological courses being offered in colleges (Lindsey, 1977), and there is hope that the future aged patients and the mental health professionals will begin to view each other in a more objective and more positive manner. Whether there will be sufficient numbers of trained professionals available in the future to provide assistance for the estimated 15% (currently about 3 million persons) who "suffer from significant, substantial, or at least moderate psychopathology" (Pfeiffer, 1977) is doubtful. Accurate diagnosis and sound treatment for emotional and mental disorders have not been attainable for the current generation of elderly (Butler, 1975).

4. The Multiproblem Patient

Stress in a most general sense has been accorded a basic role in the etiology of maladaptive behavior or accelerated decline in psychological functions (Eisdorfer & Wilkie, 1977). In reviewing the diverse situations and conditions that are likely to be classified as stressful events, it becomes apparent that the aged who come to the attention of the clinician are more than likely to have experienced more than a few stressors. No one professional is likely to have the training, knowledge, or time needed to try to alleviate the multitude or situational problems that beset the aged psychiatric patient. Chronic health conditions are most widespread, with national health statistics indicating that about 86% of those 65 and over suffer from one or more chronic conditions. These conditions limited their major activity in 42% of the cases (Busse, 1973). In a survey of mental health programs for the aged, Bourestom (1970) found that about three-fourths of psychiatric patients had physical conditions which limited function, a much higher proportion than found in noninstitutionalized aged.

The aged also are overrepresented in the economically deprived groups. Depending on the criteria used to determine the poverty line, the percentages of elderly persons classified as poor ranged from 15% to 25% (Brotman, 1977; Butler & Lewis, 1973). Brotman (1977) indicated that, for nonwhite aged, the percentage

(32%) falling below the poverty line was more than twice that of the white aged person. Associated with economic deprivation are a host of stressors such as poor diet and substandard housing accommodations. Many of the urban elderly live in deteriorating neighborhoods beset by the constant threat of crime (Clemente & Kleiman, 1976) which curtails mobility, limiting social visiting and such basic activities as shopping for groceries.

Among the multiple problems, social isolation is included as the third major component. The deaths of close friends, family members, and spouses, all rated as severely stressful life events in themselves (Holmes & Rahe, 1967), along with the limitations on mobility already mentioned, contribute to the social isolation and loneliness of the elderly. Social isolation, low socioeconomic status, and poor physical health compose a triad that was associated with devastating low morale in the over-60 population surveyed by Kutner, Fanshel, Togo, and Langner (1956). Although very much in need of community resources, the isolated, poor, sick persons did not make use of available facilities. A similar triad was also included among the factors associated with hospital admission for psychiatric screening (Lowenthal & Berkman, 1967). The mental health professional will readily recognize his impotence in attempting to treat psychiatric disorders in multiproblem patients without concurrent medical, social, and economic assistance. Kutner and his associates (1956) did note that the key variable in the triad was low socioeconomic status. The level of life satisfaction was relatively independent of degree of social isolation and physical condition among the more affluent and better-educated older persons. Perhaps having the means to pay for needed services makes it possible for the individual to obtain the supports to compensate for deficiencies resulting from physical problems and social isolation.

5. Differential Diagnosis: A Misdirected Referral Question

A diagnosis ideally should specify a precise syndrome, an identifiable etiology, an expected course or prognosis, and a treatment plan for the disorder. The current diagnostic classification system (American Psychiatric Association, 1968) has been severely criticized on all counts (Draguns & Phillips, 1971). The labels assigned to patients tend to be unreliable; etiology for most categories is indeterminate; prognoses are unverified; and treatment recommendations are nonspecific. The type of treatment bears little relation to the diagnosis (Stuart, 1970). Frequently, it is determined by the orientation of the therapist rather than by the nature of the disorder. Szasz (1970) is convinced that diagnosis, with its pejorative labels, has done more harm than good. Based on his work with young adults, Rogers (1951) saw little value in assessment and recommended its abandonment.

The criticisms have alerted the clinicians to shortcomings inherent in the system, particularly as it has been applied to functional disorders in younger adults. The model, with its imperfections, is useful with the older patient where immediate determination of etiological factors is essential for the treatment and alleviation of reversible conditions.

Clinicians need first to overcome their negative attitudes toward assessment procedures and diagnostic labels. Second, the process is far more complex with the aged patient. Referral questions which deal with differentiation between organic and functional disorders are not appropriate in practice with older adults. The question implies a dichotomy between psychogenic and biogenic disorders which is overly simplistic at any stage. As has been suggested earlier, with elderly patients the differentiation has been settled with undue frequency in favor of a chronic organic brain syndrome. Unfortunately, such a label tends to terminate the search for remediable causes.

With organic brain syndromes, as with many diseases, the etiological conditions may exist universally within all older adults and yet not be a sufficient explanation for the onset of disordered behavior. Indeed, if the oft-quoted normal loss of brain cells—estimated at a rate of 100,000 per day since childhood—is accurate, after 65 years of losing these irreplaceable cells, a person would have the number of neurons in his brain reduced by about one-fifth of the original 12 billion. Almost every aged person could be presumed to have suffered diffuse loss of brain tissue. Although the diagnostic manual (American Psychiatric Association, 1968) specifies that the syndrome is the result of "diffuse impairment of brain tissue function from whatever cause," the diagnosis itself is based on manifest symptoms: impairment of (1) orientation, (2) memory, (3) intellectual function, and (4) judgment, plus (5) shallow or labile affect. Kay (1972a) stressed the fact that structural damage can be present with or without evidence of intellectual impairment. Autopsies have revealed that as many as one-fourth of nonsenile individuals have senile signs in brain tissue. Generally, a correlation between intellectual impairment and brain disease has been found. The relationship, of course, is far from perfect. Subjects with hypertension, which is associated with arteriosclerosis and cerebrovascular insufficiency, were found to have significantly lower scores on intelligence tests than physically healthy subjects (Wilkie & Eisdorfer, 1971). Corsellis (1962) and Roth, Tomlinson, and Blessed (1966) reported significant correlations between counts of the number of senile plaques in cerebral gray matter and intellectual deterioration.

The excessive numbers of senile diagnoses frequently may have been partial errors in that the diagnoses were incomplete. Butler and Lewis (1973) stressed the fact that patients with multiple problems required the diagnostician to search for multiple causes. The diagnostic process with the elderly called for "a continuing dynamic assessment." During the initial phase of a disorder, the severity of the intellectual and emotional symptoms may obscure the complex etiology. With appropriate treatment and psychological support, the patient may show quite rapid and gratifying change in his condition. The complex interaction of biogenic, psychogenic, and sociogenic causes can then begin to be differentiated.

Geriatric physicians and psychiatrists have warned that any number of physical dysfunctions can produce symptoms which mimic senility (Anderson, 1975; Kay, 1972a; Verwoerdt, 1976). Included are infectious diseases, thyroid malfunction, fecal impaction, anemia, electrolyte disturbance, nutritional deficiencies, toxic conditions, drugs, and a variety of systemic illnesses which result in decreased oxygen or blood supply to the brain. Verwoerdt (1976) referred to this type of differential diagnosis as "primary vs. secondary organic brain syndrome," with the latter "caused by extracerebral-somatic factors" which can be alleviated by treating the physical disorder. Psychological factors can produce symptoms similar to the syndrome associated with severe organic pathology. A depressed person may not put forth the effort needed to attend to even simple questions dealing with orientation. The anxiety associated with admission to a hospital and confrontation with a strange, middle-class, professional authority figure can result in confusion and disorganization of thought processes. Literally any stress can overtax the mental capacity of the aged patient, whereas the same stress would have little effect on a younger person.

Differential diagnosis in the elderly, multiproblem patient should be regarded as the identification of the complex, interacting multiple causes of the disorder and the recommendation of a comprehensive treatment program. Acute reversible brain syndromes may be superimposed on chronic organic brain syndromes; brain syndromes, acute or chronic, may coexist with depression and other functional disorders. Mild senile symptoms may precipitate anxiety and depression, which can further contribute to intellectual disorganization. Senile symptoms may also mask situational factors which might also be contributing to a transient state of confusion. In each case, alleviation of the causes of the acute reversible conditions is urgent, followed by a plan for maintaining or improving the patient's adaptation in a suitable setting.

During the initial phase of a disorder, Kral (1975) and Busse (1973) preferred the adoption of the term "acute confusional state of the aged." This category, suggested by the World Health Organization, would clearly imply that the condition is considered to be a transient consequence of acute stress. The symptoms include clouding of consciousness, disorientation, perceptual distortions, memory difficulties, and, in some cases, hallucinations and delusions. It would have the additional benefit of satisfying administrative pressure for an immediate diagnosis to complete hospital records needed for third-party reimbursement.

In a follow-up of hospitalized patients admitted in this acute state, Kral (1975) reported recovery in 50% of the cases. Of the remaining patients, about half died within a year, and the others developed clinical pictures of senile dementia. The use of "acute confusional state" might also prevent errors resulting from premature diagnosis of chronic organic syndromes in younger patients. Nott and Fleminger (1975) followed 35 middle-aged patients initially referred for admission because of a wide variety of peculiar or bizarre behaviors diagnosed as presenile dementia. In this group, the authors concluded that, because of hasty diagnosis, almost 60% had been erroneously diagnosed. Only 15 cases showed the rapid and progressive deterioration typical of Alzheimer's disease. It should be noted that, although Pfeiffer (1977) pointed out that the deteriorative process does occasionally stop without known reason, a 60% error remains unusually high.

6. Assessment in Acute Disorders

The clinical psychologist relying on traditional diagnostic techniques is likely to discover that most such techniques have been and will continue to be of little value for use with aged patients (Lawton & Gottesman, 1974). The typical battery of clinical tests is far too demanding and time consuming for the older patient, certainly during the initial period of hospitalization when continuous assessment is most urgent. In light of the many and varied medical, psychological, and situational factors contributing to the disturbance, the psychiatrist, too, cannot rely solely on his psychiatric specialties (Pfeiffer, 1977), nor can the psychologist rely solely on his traditional functions. Thorough diagnosis of the patient's problems and the development of a comprehensive treatment plan, of necessity, involve a broad multiprofessional approach. Gurland (1973) has called for an "amalgamation of disciplines" in which one member of the team takes the role of coordinator, organizing the data from the variety of sources relevant to management of the patient. Gaitz and Baer (1970) also have made similar suggestions regarding a role of coordinator.

A position of patient representative, which incorporated part of the role of co-ordinator, has been developed at an inner city hospital (Sydenham Hospital, 1974). The hospital served patients of relatively low educational level and income, many of whom had multiple problems. The patient representative was considered a member of the health team and explained medical and administrative procedures to patients and their relatives, clarifying individual patient's needs and directing their requests to the proper channel. The representative also expedited contacts with outside agencies in obtaining economic assistance, housing, and aftercare following discharge. Except for the department director, during the pilot phase of this program, all positions were filled by college student volunteers.

Patients in an acute state of confusion are not reliable informants. The unfamiliarity of the situation and the strange professionals are likely to enhance the patient's anxiety level and intellectual disorganization. When time is critical in assessing progress of the disorder, it may take several days or more before formal interviews or standardized tests could possibly be administered. Psychologists and psychiatrists have developed very simple, practical systematic scales to chart changes in the patient's mental condition. Among the most widely used scales is the ten-item Mental Status Questionnaire developed by Kahn, Goldfarb, Pollack, and Peck (1960), which includes orientation items and two simple information questions (present and past presidents of the United States). It yields a gross measure of severity of intellectual impairment. The questions can be interspersed within a casual, informal, and nonthreatening conversation. The questionnaire can be repeated as frequently as needed to determine day-to-day changes. It can be administered at different times during the day to identify daily patterns of functioning. Some patients are disorganized on awakening; others may become confused at night. The ease of administration permits its use with minimal training by all levels of staff. Kahn et al. (1960) also employed a simple Face-Hand Test which entailed touching the patient on the cheek and back of the hand simultaneously and having the patient identify the sites of stimulation with eyes closed. The test can be administered to non-English-speaking patients without difficulty. The accuracy of the Mental Status Questionnaire in differentiating between patients manifesting none or mild organic brain syndrome and those with moderate or severe pathology was quite good (approximately 95% accurate). With the Face-Hand Test, there was a sizable proportion of false positives, with about one of four patients with no minimal organic brain syndromes showing positive test results. In the case of false positives, the diagnosis of a chronic organic brain syndrome may have serious consequences in precluding medical treatment. When in doubt, Miller (1977) believes it is less serious to err on the side of depression, if such a differentiation is called for, and to treat the depression rather than make a diagnosis such as senile dementia with its pessimistic prognosis.

Pfeiffer (1975) also developed a Short Portable Mental Status Questionnaire, with norms taking into account level of education. Markson and Levitz (1973) reduced the Kahn et al. (1960) questionnaire to five questions, with scoring that fulfilled Guttman scaling criteria. The score was useful with institutionalized aged to assess extent of memory loss and evaluate changes. In a 14-month follow-up, low scorers were found to have had a higher morbidity than high scorers.

Other extensive scales have been developed which yield more complete assessments of mental and emotional status, as well as competence in activities of daily living. Such scales are useful after the initial screening process has been completed and more time is available. Butler and Lewis (1973) have provided outlines of a longer scorable Mental Status Evaluation, along with a symptom checklist and a thorough Personal Mental Health Data Form. The latter requires a relatively intact informant. Salzman and his associates have provided several reviews of 14 rating scales specifically designed for use with geriatric patients, along with other more general rating scales and tests applicable to aged patients (Salzman, Kochansky, & Shader, 1972; Salzman, Kochansky, Shader, & Cronin, 1972; Salzman, Shader, Kochansky, & Cronin, 1972). The recognition of the contribution of rating scales for use with geriatric patients is evident in the increasing references to new or revised scales in current journals (Fishback, 1977; Lawson, Rodenburg, & Dykes, 1977; Smith, Bright, & McCloskey, 1977).

Despite the invasion of privacy involved for patients living alone, a home visit is often necessary for diagnosis (Pfeiffer, 1977; Group for the Advancement of Psychiatry, 1971). It permits the observer to note the physical condition of the residence, along with the condition in which it has been maintained. The condition of the home may immediately resolve questions concerning placement in a nursing home or other supervised setting when hospitalization is no longer needed. Examination of the kitchen yields information concerning the patient's diet and its nutritional adequacy. Of critical importance are the contents of the medicine cabinet. Many elderly patients ingest quantities of prescribed drugs, over-the-counter medicines, and pills donated by concerned friends. The medicine cabinet may well provide the clue to the acute disorder. Pfeiffer (1977) also suggests talking with neighbors, landlady, or friends to evaluate the support that such persons have provided in the past and can supply after discharge.

6.1. Psychological Tests in the Assessment of Brain Damage

During the period of acute disturbance, the gross evaluation of severity of impairment could best be accomplished with the use of simple mental status questionnaires and behavioral rating scales. The identification of etiological factors depends on procedures which call for minimal or passive cooperation on the part of the patient, such as medical examination, laboratory tests, obtaining historical data from informants, and making home visits regarding drug usage, dietary habits, and psychological or biological stress. For those patients who have recovered from the acute confusional states and for those with mild impairment, more precise measures of functioning can provide baseline scores for evaluation of change. These can also assist in planning treatment programs and, in some cases, contribute to the determination of the presence, location, and nature of the neuropathology.

The relatively new specialty of clinical neuropsychology holds promise of being able to contribute diagnostic techniques which entail no risk to the patient. With younger patients, they have demonstrated validity levels comparable to those of diagnostic medical and neurological procedures. Mattis (1976), employing a WAIS-dominated battery of tests, and Reitan and Davison (1974), using the Halstead-Reitan Neurological Battery, claim good diagnostic accuracy. Utilizing a clinical-actuarial approach with the Halstead-Reitan Battery, Filskov and Goldstein (1974) reported greater accuracy for the psychological tests in determining type and laterality of the neuropathology than for a variety of laboratory procedures. For a sample of 89 patients with known brain damage of various types ranging from diffuse deterioration to focalized, nonprogressive neuropathology, the psychological battery was considerably more accurate than nonintrusive techniques such as the brain scan, EEG, and skull X-rays. Tests even had a somewhat higher number of "hits" than the riskier intrusive procedures such as the pneumoencephalogram and the angiogram. For this impressive study, the mean age of the subjects was about 49 years.

Although the use of neuropsychological diagnostic tests with an older population awaits further standardization, two recent studies suggest that changes due to aging and those due to brain damage can be successfully differentiated. A study by Goldstein and Shelly (1975), using a variety of neuropsychological measures, compared psychological deficits in brain-damaged and non-brain-damaged groups ranging in age from 20 to 62 years. The differences in functioning between young and old, organic and nonorganic, were not systematic. Older non-brain-damaged subjects did better than younger non-brain-damaged subjects on tests of language. With regard to motor performance, the older brain-damaged group functioned at almost identical levels with the older non-brain-damaged group, whereas there were wide discrepancies in motor performance among the younger groups. Although there was some resemblance between aging and brain damage, they concluded that the change in test performance with age is not one of simple decline.

Overall and Gorham (1972) administered the WAIS and the Holtzman Inkblots to over 300 veteran domiciliary members ranging in age from 45 to 84 years. Twenty-eight members (mean age of 67) were diagnosed as suffering from chronic brain syndromes. Older persons did manifest selective performance deficits, but the patterns were clearly distinguishable from the deficits evident in the brain-damaged individuals. With age, Similarities, Digit Symbol, Picture Arrangement, and Object Assembly declined relative to Vocabulary. Information and Vocabulary, where aging effects were minimal, were lower among the brain damaged. More complex differences were found among younger, older, and brain-damaged subjects on Holtzman variables. The authors concluded that normal aging is not simply a road to a chronic brain syndrome.

Wechsler (1958) remained intrigued with pattern analysis despite lack of support for the validity of patterns associated with diagnostic groups. He also adhered to the belief that the Deterioration Index "merits further study." Based on the education-confounded age norms of the Wechsler-Bellevue standardization, Wechsler (1944) selected four subtests that "Hold" with increasing age and four that "Don't Hold" with age. The difference between the weighted subtest scores in the Hold and Don't Hold categories, divided by the sum of the Hold tests, yielded a quotient which it was hoped would reveal the degree of intellectual deterioration and could contribute to the diagnosis of organic pathology. Matarazzo (1972) would strongly disagree with further attempts to find patterns of subtest scores for diagnosis. He sadly concluded: "Alas, hundreds and hundreds of studies on the use of profile, pattern, or scatter analysis with the Wechsler Scales conducted between 1940 and 1970 failed to produce reliable evidence that such a search would be fruitful" (p. 429).

Tests which seek to measure memory specifically have been used clinically in attempts to measure greater-than-normal memory loss presumably indicative of brain damage. The Wechsler Memory Scale (1945), composed of a variety of memory-related tasks and yielding a "Memory Quotient" presumably comparable to the IQ, suffers seriously from a limited standardization sample of 200 adults aged 25–50 years. To obtain MQs beyond age 50 called for extrapolation. In addition, data on reliability were lacking. The Revised Benton Visual Retention Test (Benton, 1963) has normative data up to age 64. Botwinick and Storandt (1974) administered a wide variety of memory tests to a community sample and concluded that the problems involved in developing norms for use with clinical groups were enormous. Not all memory tests are affected equally by age. Furthermore, sex differences appeared to exist. In evaluating memory changes with age, the meaningfulness of the material to the individual and the age at which it was learned determined whether it was recalled. Specific memory tests can provide little information above what can be obtained from more general measures of ability. Factor analytic studies of the WAIS have suggested that, in the aged, the memory factor tends to play a larger role in intelligence measures (Cohen, 1957; Savage & Britton, 1968). In Cohen's analysis, the memory factor in the aged sample loaded on all Verbal subtests except Similarities.

Although still better than informal assessments, the evaluation of the effects of brain disease using tests is particularly difficult with older patients because of the confounding effects of factors unrelated to structural dysfunction. Benton (1967) and Prien (1972) pointed out that impaired functioning could result from hostility or suspicion interfering with cooperation, lack of energy due to depression, communication difficulties, concentration difficulties due to anxiety, an inability to understand the nature of the task because of cultural differences, and limited education. Above all, with many elderly patients, fatigue can make testing with the Halstead-Reitan Battery, which could take 3–7 hr, nearly impossible to complete. A pretest fatiguing condition of 20 min duration has been shown to impair the performance of older persons (mean age 64) more than that of young adults (mean age 38) in the Primary Mental Abilities tests (Furry & Baltes, 1973). Cross-sectional age differences were magnified under the fatigue condition. The interaction of age and fatigue effects would create difficulties in establishing uniform administrative procedures and norms for the lengthy neuropsychological test batteries. At present, the limited normative data and the time and expense of such tests preclude their use in all but the most critical diagnostic problems.

A large number of brief, specialized tests for the diagnosis of organic impairment have been devised, and optimistic studies on limited samples demonstrating the validity of the techniques have been reported. Two recent reviews of diagnostic and assessment techniques with the elderly (Bernal, Brannon, Belar, Lavigne, & Cameron, 1977; Schaie & Schaie, 1977) have surveyed these instruments. In general, validity studies using these techniques were characterized by insufficient sample size, frequently with subjects below age 65. Although diagnostic groups could be differentiated at a statistically significant level, the groups were for the most part clearly identified as brain damaged or nonorganic. These are not typical of the multi-problem patients the geroclinician is likely to assess in practice.

The history of specialized tests for the assessment of brain damage has not shown them to be of value in clinical situations. During the World War II era, Goldstein and Scheerer (1941) developed a series of special tests to measure the loss of the "abstract attitude" as an indicator of brain damage. Clinical psychologists seized on these novel tasks, learned how to administer and how to interpret the general patterns of behavior described in the manual, and after many years discovered that the borderline patients typically referred for differential diagnosis could perform these tasks with relative ease. Skilled clinicians may have been able to make accurate diagnoses based on observation of more subtle cues than were evident in the gross ratings of performance on these concept formation tests. The validity of the Goldstein-Scheerer tests had been demonstrated by differentiating severely brain-damaged patients from nonorganics, diagnoses that could well have been made through observation alone or with a much simpler mental status examination. The Rorschach should be mentioned as a test that has been called on to serve as a diagnostic panacea on the belief that it could contribute to the diagnosis of brain damage above and beyond other techniques. An example of one of the better studies, albeit with younger adults, was conducted by Fisher, Gonda, and Little (1955). The authors tested four sets of Rorschach signs of organic impairment, using as controls subjects who had been seriously considered to be suffering from brain damage and later cleared. Thirty-four of 84 brain-damaged subjects were identified as organic, employing Piotrowski's signs; 94% of these were accurately diagnosed as brain-damaged patients. Although the authors concluded that Piotrowski's signs compared favorably with EEG findings, it should be noted that the Rorschach overlooked 62% of the brain-damaged patients who were classified falsely as nonorganic. Perhaps Rorschach's own reports of two aged persons could serve as examples of the difficulties still being encountered in using inkblots (Rorschach, 1942). In a blind diagnosis of a mentally "well-preserved" 80-year-old woman, "the diagnosis proved to be wrong." Rorschach diagnosed her as a latent or well-preserved schizophrenic and stated that "similar results may be obtained from aged patients otherwise normal." In his report of a 78-year-old male with senile dementia, the severity of impairment was apparently so great that it was necessary to administer the test over several days in order to avoid a completely perseverative record. A test would not be necessary to infer so severe an organic brain syndrome.

6.2. Normal Decline in Abilities

Contributing to the difficulties in diagnosing impairment associated with brain disease are the enormous problems involved in developing norms for older age groups. Until recently, definitions of aging closely resembled the definition of incurable disease in that aging was viewed as a deteriorative process terminating in the death of the organism (Zubin, 1965). This definition reflected the orientation of the scientific and professional community in their expectations in dealing with aged persons. More recent definitions tend to be much more neutral. For example, Birren and Renner (1977), in a review of research, defined aging in terms of "the regular changes that occur in mature genetically representative organisms living under representative environmental conditions as they advance in chronological age." A review of the recent history of the beliefs regarding age and mental ability will provide the background for the clinician to develop a rational approach to the assessment of normal and abnormal aging.

Since the introduction of the Terman revision of the Binet in 1916, a decline in mental ability beyond early adulthood was generally accepted (Matarazzo, 1972). The standardization of the 1939 Wechsler-Bellevue Adult Scale provided norms for adults at different age levels through age 69. Data were available to confirm the long-held hypothesis of a normal decline in intellectual functioning with advancing age (Wechsler, 1944). In standardizing the adult scale, Wechsler was well aware of the correlation between education and IQ (.65–.70) and sought in his sample to obtain educational levels representative of the general population. Apparently, the inverse relationship between age and education which could account in part for the obtained decline in ability in older age groups initially went unnoticed. The fact that the curve for age and brain weight declined in a manner parallel to the decline in intelligence test scores with advancing age past young adulthood was convincing evidence for Wechsler (1944) that the decrements were physiologically based and real. When the longitudinal data collected by Bayley and Bradway and associates began to be analyzed just prior to the publication of the Wechsler Adult Intelligence Scale in 1958, the decline of mental ability with age began to be questioned (Matarazzo, 1972). Nevertheless, Wechsler (1958) adhered to his original position of decline in test scores with age after 25. The inverse correlation of WAIS Full Scale scores with age was impressive (−.42). He tempered his position, however, by summing up the problem as follows: "General intelligence as evaluated by pragmatic criteria appears to maintain itself unimpaired over a much greater portion of adult life, and to decline at a much slower rate than do the mental abilities by which it is inevitably [currently] measured" (p. 142). In accord with his conception of intelligence, there are many nonintellective characteristics which contribute to intelligent behavior other than performance on tests of ability, such as drive, interest, motivation, and general experience.

Recent controversy between psychologists has led to extreme positions with regard to change in mental abilities with age, and the extreme rhetoric is likely to have heuristic value in stimulating the collection of better-controlled normative data. Baltes and Schaie (1976), making use of design techniques to correct for flaws in the cross-sectional studies of intellectual functioning at different age levels, have sought "to debunk the myth of general and universal decline in intellectual performance because it is not supported by data." They accuse theorists (Horn & Donaldson, 1976) who posited a decline in fluid intelligence with age as being "anachronistic" and "reactionary." Acknowledging that crystallized intelligence tended to remain stable with increasing age, Horn and Donaldson (1977) interpret data from identical studies as demonstrating "age decline in many important abilities of intelligence." In a more moderate summation, Botwinick (1977) concludes that decline does take place but that it may not be seen before age 50 or 60 in many functions. For intellectual functions "involving speed of response of non-verbal, perceptual-manipulative skills, decline may be seen before then." There appears to be a general consensus that the age at which decline starts is delayed to later ages with succeeding generations.

The studies of change in intellectual performance with age are of significance to the clinician with regard to the use of age norms in obtaining a measure of IQ and the diagnostic significance of sharp declines in test scores. The age norms that exist for the WAIS were obtained from cross-sectional data and are "strictly cohort specific" (Schaie & Schaie, 1977). Matarazzo (1972) illustrated the problems involved in using obsolescent norms in a clinical situation, positing as an example a case of an executive who was tested at age 35 as part of an industrial appraisal. Twenty years later, he was retested following an accident in which he sustained a brain injury. To use norms for 55-year-olds obtained on the original standardization sample with a lower educational level than the age cohorts of the patient (currently 55-year-olds) would tend to minimize any deficit. The norms for 35-year-olds would probably more appropriately serve as the basis for evaluating change in IQ, making some allowance for possible decrement on speeded motor tasks. In this hypothetical case, a prior test was assumed which permitted direct comparison between earlier and later test scores. In testing a 70-year-old in 1978, greater validity might be obtained by comparing at least his verbal functioning with that of his age cohorts (40-year-olds) when the test was standardized. The 40-year-old standardization group could be presumed to have had greater educational and sociocultural advantages than the then 70-year-old normative group. Again, functioning on the Performance tasks would be expected to show slowed responses, but Verbal tasks would show little or no decrement.

Support for this suggestion can be found in the results of longitudinal studies of mental abilities. In a 20-year longitudinal study, Blum, Jarvik, and Clark (1970) administered the Stanford-Binet Vocabulary and several Wechsler-Bellevue subtests to senescent twins. On retests, stability characterized the performance on all subtests except those with a speeded motor component up through age 73. Between the ages of 73 and 85, they found a more rapid rate of decline on four specific Wechsler subtests: Similarities, Digits Forward, Block Design, and Digit Symbol Substitution. The last subtest in particular showed a decline for all persons in the last test period. In other tasks, individual differences contributed to intratest variations in performance, limiting generalizations regarding longitudinal changes.

Among the more carefully controlled longitudinal studies is the NIMH-sponsored 11-year follow-up of healthy aged men (Granick, 1971). The findings of the initial report (Botwinick & Birren, 1963) contain a wealth of information of importance to the clinician and will be discussed following the description of changes on the repeated psychological tests. The intellectual test performance of 17 survivors of an original sample of 47 healthy aged men held up very well at the last examination when their mean age was 81 (Granick, 1971). Their Full Scale WAIS scores (not converted to IQs) at the three test periods (1956, 1961, and 1967) were 109, 100, and 110, respectively. Performance on the Ravens Progressive Matrices Test was similar to that of the WAIS. The Speed of Copying Digits Test showed a small significant decline from the second to the third testing, consistent with the expected slowing of motor functioning. Draw-a-Person and Speed of Copying Words also revealed statistically significant declines. That these aged subjects were handicapped in comparison with younger persons was evident in the difference between Verbal (mean score of 72) and Performance (mean of 36) Scale scores. The scores obtained on the Performance Scale were considerably below the levels attained by younger persons of similar overall ability. On the other hand, Vocabulary (scaled score of 14.1) and Picture Arrangement (7.7) scores revealed significantly higher functioning on the 11-year retest.

Two points regarding intellectual test performance for this sample are worthy of note. Among the 47 subjects in the 1956 initial testing, 20 men were found to have subclinical or asymptomatic disease states (e.g., high blood pressure and arteriosclerosis). The mean Performance and Full Scale scores for the subclinical disease group were significantly lower than the scores for the healthy group (Botwinick & Birren, 1963). Evidently, even asymptomatic disease resulted in impaired intellectual performance. Second, comparing the scores on the initial testing for the 23 subjects who survived with the 24 men who died revealed significantly higher functioning for the survivors on a majority of the cognitive and perceptual tests. Both Verbal and Performance mean scores were higher for the survivor group (Verbal 70.4, Performance 36.9) than for the nonsurvivors (Verbal 56.0, Performance 29.4) (Granick, 1971). Optimal physical health was also related to survival, with 63% of this group remaining alive at the 11-year follow-up compared with only 30% of the group with mild physical pathology.

6.3. IQ Drop and Death

The intriguing relationship between intellectual decline and death in the elderly was first reported by Kleemeier (1961), who postulated an "imminence-of-death" factor. He indicated that the decline occurred about 2 years prior to death. Jarvik and Falek (1963) reported a longitudinal study with 78 senescent adults, the same population mentioned previously (Blum et al., 1970). The subjects, who were described as ordinary, noninstitutionalized elderly individuals in satisfactory health, were retested with four Wechsler subtests and Stanford-Binet Vocabulary on three occasions over a 12-year follow-up starting at age 60. Subjects who suffered a "critical loss" in two of three subtests had a much higher mortality than those who maintained their level. Vocabulary, Similarities, and Digit Symbol were the sensitive tests and showed decrements as much as 10 years prior to death. Lieberman (1965) and Lieberman and Coplan (1969) employed the Bender-Gestalt, Draw-a-Person, and several projective tests with 25 institutionalized subjects, also seeking to identify psychological changes which predicted death. They reported that changes in test performance began to be apparent about 6–9 months prior to death, with the size of the change rather than the absolute score indicative of a correlation with death. A 7-year follow-up study of 1280 elderly institutionalized subjects by Goldfarb (1969) revealed four characteristics associated with higher mortality. The four variables—(1) diagnosis of severe chronic brain syndrome, (2) nine to ten errors on the Mental Status Questionnaire, (3) impaired ability to care for self, and (4) physical incontinence— suggest very obvious and gross deterioration of functioning and would appear not to be of the same order as studies which deal with apparently healthy subjects.

Reimanis and Green (1971) reported a sharp decline (15.5 Full Scale IQ points on the Wechsler) for ten of 187 veterans in a domiciliary who died within 1 year. Lesser drops were found for those between 1 and 2 years and more than 2 years before death. Hall, Savage, Bolton, Pidwell, and Blessed (1972), using a short form of the WAIS with aged mentally ill patients and normals, found that survivors overall attained higher initial scores than nonsurvivors, but age differences and psychiatric diagnoses limited the generalizability of the findings. The two Performance subtest scaled scores (Object Assembly and Block Design) for the nonsurvivors were significantly lower than the scores of the survivors. A similar difference was not found for the Vocabulary and Comprehension subtests. The two Performance subtests are more novel and are presumed to reflect fluid intelligence, which Hall et al. (1972) believed to be more predictive of imminence of death among schizophrenics and organics than was functioning on the Verbal subtests.

The concepts of "lethal limit" and "terminal drop" were introduced by Riegel and Riegel (1972) in reporting an extensive longitudinal study conducted in Germany. Three hundred and eighty subjects ranging in age from 55 years to over 75 at the start of the study in 1956 were tested initially with the Hamburg Wechsler Intelligence Test for Adults, several personality measures, and five verbal tasks. Much of the authors' report was based on the last five tests. Surviving and cooperative subjects were retested at 5-year intervals in 1961 and 1966. Among the problems in interpreting both cross-sectional and longitudinal results of changes with increasing age were the issues dealing with initial refusers and subjects who later resisted retesting. No data had been obtained on the initial refusers. Cooperation in retesting was associated with survival, with 75% of the subjects who accepted retesting in 1961 surviving until the next period 5 years later. Only 57% of those who refused to be tested in 1961 survived. For those who survived and accepted retesting, intellectual functioning did not decline with age. The authors suggested that the observed decline in performance with age was an artifact due to a "terminal drop" in nonsurviving subjects. The sudden deterioration of intellectual ability occurred within 5 years of death. "At any time during adult life, subjects who perform below average are closer to death than their more able age-mates . . . [they] have already experienced their terminal drop; subjects scoring high retain their abilities and have a good chance for survival" (p. 312). The lower limit of performance was referred to as the "lethal limit," but the authors did not indicate how this limit could be determined for individuals.

Other inferences drawn from these data were that superior subjects showed a faster rate of intellectual growth and a slower rate of decline. Inferior subjects showed slower rates of growth and more rapid decline, particularly in those tasks which relied on novel or unfamiliar material, tasks which could be subsumed within Horn's definition of fluid intelligence (Horn, 1970). Riegel and Riegel (1972) were careful to point out that the growth and decline in intellectual functioning may be due to either intrinsic or extrinsic factors, suggesting that individuals who cope less effectively with their environments may be those who are subject to more rapid decline. Lower-than-average coping ability might be seen in less education, lower income, poorer diets, less than adequate medical care, etc. As has already been indicated, persons from low socioeconomic groups are more vulnerable than higher SES persons to psychiatric illness and more likely to be hospitalized and to die in the institution.

The consensus among these studies of loss of mental abilities prior to death is clear. A sizable deterioration of intellectual ability, one which can be considered a "critical loss" or which reaches a "lethal limit," is a precursor of death. However, the distance from death covered a large period of time. Furthermore, most studies qualified their conclusions by indicating high interindividual variability, which limits the application of this finding in clinical prediction. Jarvik and Falek (1963) noted a decrement as early as 10 years prior to death. Nevertheless, as was pointed out in the discussion of neuropsychological assessment, impaired intellectual functioning in the aged was a most sensitive index of a wide range of stresses, including brain damage. In accord with the position regarding acute disorders, a sudden or large decrement should spur the search for causal factors and their alleviation.

It is improbable that the psychologist would have available prior intelligence test records with which to compare findings to determine whether a sizable decrement in abilities had occurred. The patient's personal history and descriptions by friends or relatives regarding any recent changes in behavior provide data for estimating prior levels of functioning. Patients are sometimes reliable informants regarding changes in abilities, although denial of decline is frequent. The patient's educational attainment, school grades, occupational status, reading habits, hobbies, and cultural pursuits provide bases for estimating prior intellectual ability. An individual whose life-style ranked well above average in intellectual pursuits could be expected to maintain that level on mental tests except for psychomotor slowing well into the 70s or later; a person with a more limited experiential background might be expected to perform at a somewhat lower level. In the latter instance, it would be necessary to attempt to estimate the rapidity of decline which might presage death.

Thus far, the approach to assessment has focused on the diagnosis of acute disorders which would necessitate immediate intervention at a biological level to prevent reversible impairment from becoming chronic. Evaluation of the patient should be continued until it is clear that the condition has improved or stabilized. In acute confusional states or acute organic brain syndromes, the recovery should become evident in a matter of weeks, rarely longer (Kay, 1972a). A treatment program, however, does not end with the alleviation of the medical causes of the acute condition. Typically, the elderly psychiatric patient is a multiproblem patient in whom the etiology of the acute disorder can be traced to situational or behavioral factors which contributed to the physical cause. For example, a fairly common problem among elderly patients admitted for psychiatric screening is alcoholism. Zimberg (1974), reviewing admission rates at Harlem Hospital and San Francisco General Hospital, arrived at estimates in which drinking was a serious problem in at least half of the elderly patients. Men, particularly elderly widowers, were the most vulnerable. The estimated prevalence among widowers living in the community was over 10%, more than twice the estimated rate of alcoholism in the general population. Resorting to drinking provided a means of coping with loneliness and depression. It was also associated with physical disorders, cirrhosis of the liver, seizures, cardiac disease, gastrointestinal disorders, nutritional deficiencies, and organic brain syndromes. Again, attitudes played a role in incorrect diagnoses. Physicians were reluctant to label an elderly patient alcoholic. Only half the actual cases that warranted a diagnosis of alcoholism were so categorized, and accurate diagnosis is a prerequisite to developing an appropriate treatment program.

7. Functional Disorders

Beyond the middle years, aging is inevitably associated with increasing loss. The unique disorders of aging, according to Verwoerdt (1976), are linked to losses. One aspect, loss of mental ability directly resulting from biological decline, has been discussed, with the focus on alleviating or preventing further loss. A secondary aspect deals with the reactions of the person to the losses, both internal and external. From this point of view, the complexities of the interactive network become staggering in their enormity. These are the direct effects of the losses, the patient's ability to recognize the emotional, intellectual, and physical changes that have taken place, the psychological reactions to the changes and losses, and the reactions of others to the changes taking place in the person. Clinical assessment calls for the analysis and understanding of these interacting, interdependent systems, a description of internal and external resources, and the identification of the most practical points of intervention to assist in a new adaptation by the person. There are special points to be covered in history taking (Group for the Advancement of Psychiatry, 1971): the listing of the losses and the patient's present reaction to them, responses to past crises, details concerning retirement experience or changes in social roles, the old-age experiences of significant figures in patient's life, present relationships with spouse, children, and friends, present interests and typical activities, sexual life, attitudes toward death, and personality assets. Information can be obtained from the patient and from relatives and friends. Others who retain an interest in the patient are valuable assets for the patient and can be brought into the treatment program.

While the defensive system of aged persons can run the entire gamut of adaptive or maladaptive mechanisms, Pfeiffer (1977) has found that many elderly patients return to the more primitive types of defense mechanisms. Among the most frequently occurring were unmodified anxiety, depression-withdrawal, projection, somatization, and denial. In these cases, psychological testing may be able to contribute to assessing the person's ability to adapt to changes in his style of life. Individuals with very limited resources may function well in a stable, routinized environment but will lack the flexibility to adapt to changed circumstances without considerable preparation of support systems. More frequently, judgments can be made from direct observation of behavior.

Patients who have been functioning in a varied set of roles and who react with maladaptive behavior following a crisis (retirement, bereavement, or stroke) may benefit particularly from psychological testing as a basis for counseling directed at the development of new interests and roles. Thematic tests can be of value. For the clinician, selected cards from the TAT would probably be most useful in terms of availability of the test and the clinician's familiarity with it. Two other sets of thematic cards depicting scenes which target the specific problems of the aged, the Senior Apperception Technique (Bellak & Bellak, 1973) and the Gerontological Apperception Test (Wolk & Wolk, 1971), have been developed. The SAT tends to be incompletely sketched; the GAT is drawn with more detail. The younger-aged persons may find the persons depicted in the scenes too old in appearance for ready identification. Nevertheless, the cards may be useful for helping some patients who find it difficult to verbalize their problems directly.

The Rorschach meets criteria mentioned by clinicians as being a brief, nonfatiguing, and above all nonthreatening test for most older adults. Nevertheless, the aged did need a good deal of attention and praise. The attempt by Ames, Metraux, Rodell, and Walker (1973) to develop norms for aged persons has been appropriately criticized for its circular, testbound reasoning in that patients were grouped into normal, senile, or presenile according to the "overall adequacy of the record." The Rorschach, however, is used by clinicians more as a semistructured interview rather than a psychometric instrument where it falls far short of the standards a psychological test should meet. The preseniles in the Ames et al. study (1973) were described as defensive, offering excuses and showing fear of being wrong, with somewhat greater numbers of rejections. The "normals" behaved like any adults; the "seniles" were frequently not coherent. Certainly, any inconsistency between what the clinician knows of the patient's behavior in daily living and the level of performance on the Rorschach would call for exploration. A person who appeared to have been functioning adequately prior to the crisis or behavior change which precipitated the mental health referral and who produced a "presenile" record might presumably require greater support in coping with changed circumstances than a person who produced a normal record.

The Holtzman Inkblot Technique and the MMPI come closer to fulfilling the criteria for psychometric instruments, but both tend to be too long to administer to older adults except for research purposes. At the opposite pole in terms of norms, reliability, and validity is the use of drawings with the aged. Wolk (1972) described the use of figure drawings and a chromatic House-Tree-Person test to tap "deeper levels of the personality," but the poor psychomotor control, frequent visual defects, lack of experience in using a pencil, and the childish nature of drawing to many older persons make this technique of questionable value with most patients.

7.1. Depression

The diagnosis of depression in the elderly is for the most part similar to its diagnosis in younger age groups. It is, however, so frequent a symptom in the aged that it can be considered "a characteristic of senescence" (Epstein, 1976). Indeed, it may be difficult to distinguish between complaints due to a normal aging process and those due to a depressive disorder (Gurland, 1976). Obviously, the range for depressive states varies greatly. Although depressions tend to be self-limiting, with potential for fairly rapid favorable outcomes with treatment, the possibility for misdiagnosis does exist (Copeland, et al., 1975). Severely depressed persons can show memory defects and cognitive impairment which may be misdiagnosed as dementia. Such errors are most likely when the depressive disorder occurs in part as a reaction to declining abilities.

Depression may be an early sign of an organic brain syndrome. Further complicating diagnosis are the physical symptoms that frequently accompany depression. These physical symptoms, anorexia and others, can lead to an acute confusional state. Differentiating characteristics are a short history of the symptoms, a family history of depression, and the inconsistent nature of mental impairment. If an error in diagnosis is made, Miller (1977) suggested that it would be preferable to err on the side of depression rather than dementia and to treat the depression. Physical symptoms may also contribute to "mask depressions" in the elderly (Goldfarb, 1974).

In the "depressive equivalents" (Pfeiffer, 1977), patients tended to complain of backaches, headaches, or neckaches and to deny sadness and the losses or deprivations that might precipitate depression. They may resort to self-medication or the use of alcohol to alleviate the pain. Such patients do manifest the fatigue, constipation or diarrhea, weight loss, and sleep disturbances that accompany depression, but they choose to deny feelings of depression. Although it is good practice to follow through on all physical complaints, the physician may devote undue time to the search for medical etiology and overlook the depression, delaying treatment of the emotional disorder. Gurland (1976) reported evidence of greater somatic concern among aged depressives through the use of the semistructured Geriatric Mental Status Interview. He took the position that depressive affect can generally be identified and the disorder can be diagnosed without undue difficulty.

Accurate diagnosis and the rapid alleviating of symptoms are perhaps as critical as in the case of acute brain disorders in that prolonged depressions can have catastrophic social and physical consequences (Epstein, 1976). The loss of energy and the withdrawal that accompany depression lead to isolation, loss of social contacts, and lessened participation in activities. Significant persons in the patient's life tend to develop other contacts, and the void left by the depressed patient may soon be filled. In addition, the reduction in physical activity, lack of concern about personal hygiene, and improper eating habits can contribute to rapid physical decline.

The most common depressive states appear to be reactive to age-related stresses: (1) physical illness, including deafness and blindness, (2) bereavement and loss of significant persons, (3) economic deprivation and poor living conditions, (4) retirement and loss of social roles. Manic-depressive psychoses tend to be less commonly associated with old age; they tend to develop earlier in life. The manicky symptoms of the elderly psychotic also tend to be different from those of the younger patients. The humorous quality and sense of well-being that are common in younger manic patients tend to be replaced by irritability, anger, and grandiosity which bear some similarities to paranoid behavior.

Manic behavior, according to Verwoerdt (1976), occurs less frequently simply because of the high energy expenditure involved in the defensive system. His summation of several studies of outcome in bipolar depressions in later life was pessimistic. His pessimism was not supported by Foster, Gershell, and Goldfarb (1977), who reported that lithium treatment of elderly patients produced the same effects as it did with younger patients. Eisdorfer and Stotsky (1977), reviewing several studies, came to similar conclusions. Antidepressant medication, they indicated, was quite effective in alleviating retarded and mixed depressions, but was less successful in treating agitated depressions or schizoaffective disorders. Electroconvulsive therapy in current practice tended to be used after the failure of patients to respond to drug treatment with frequent success. The choice of treatment depends on the physical condition of the patient. Aged patients are particularly prone to side-effects and require careful supervision.

The treatment program for depressed patients does not end with the alleviation of symptoms. Continued evaluation of mental status is necessary throughout the period of drug treatment because of the possibility of toxic reactions and acute confusional states. The effectiveness of social and psychological interventions to compensate for the losses that may have precipitated the disorder needs to be monitored.

7.2. Suicide

The highest suicide rates are found among the elderly, particularly white males. The vital statistics show a steadily increasing rate of suicide for men with advancing age up to the 80–84 age group, where the rate for white males is 51.4 per 100,000 (Vital Statistics of the United States, 1970). The rates for white females and nonwhite males and females are considerably lower.

Evaluation of suidical risk is a frequent referral question raised by nursing home personnel. The decisions for the clinician regarding action to be taken are difficult ones. Obviously, the professional needs to be alert to signs of suicidal thoughts or plans in patients and to recommend hospitalization (or continue hospitalization) if such ideation is manifest. Ordinarily, Butler and Lewis (1973) point out, older people do not make threats, they "tend simply to kill themselves." The authors provide a long list of diagnostic clues to suicide which are so extensive as to include almost every patient with depressive symptoms. A further complication is the observation that suicidal risk increases with recovery from depression when the patient's energy level has increased to the point where he may be capable of carrying out the act. The difficult choice for the clinician lies with the balance of risks involved in the decision to encourage hospitalization and incur the stress of dislocation from a familiar environment or to attempt to treat the patient in his own setting. Much depends on the evaluation of the support and supervision involved in the setting. Once the patient is hospitalized, the decision arises again in regard to duration of hospitalization—to delay discharge in order to prevent a possible suicide weighed against the effects of continued separation of the patient from his social contacts. The loss of social ties to the community may have as devastating an effect in contributing to the perpetuation of the depression and the concomitant decline in physical as well as psychological functioning. The dilemma cannot be resolved at this stage of our knowledge.

7.3. Grief: Normal and Abnormal

In their review "Psychological Perspectives on Death," Kastenbaum and Costa (1977) noted that studies of bereavement and grief have suggested that they may have a longer and more serious impact on older persons, leaving them more vulnerable to illness and death. These authors attempt to clarify the commonly used terms related to death which many writers have used interchangeably. Frequently "bereavement" is used as synonymous with "grief" and "mourning." Distinguishing these terms can assist clinicians in describing behavior more precisely. Bereavement denotes "survivorship status," whereas grief characterizes "the survivor's distressed state." Mourning is defined in terms of "the culturally patterned manner of expressing the response to death."

In describing mourning reactions, Gorer (1965) divided the pattern into three stages: (1) shock lasting up to a few days after the death of the significant person, (2) intense grief characterized by listlessness, disturbed sleep, lack of appetite, and weight loss for a period of between 6 and 12 weeks, and (3) gradual resumption of interest in life during the year. Our culture tends to define the mourning period as lasting for 1 year. In about one-third of Gorer's sample, the period of grief was extended.

Reviewing several studies on bereavement, Kimmel (1974) pointed out that, for the aged, replacement of a lost love object is more difficult than for the young. The weakened physical condition resulting from the disturbances accompanying grief may contribute to the "higher than expected mortality rates among aged widowed persons." The loss of a confidant may be the most traumatic aspect of the death of a spouse. Visits by friends and family during the entire mourning period may aid in alleviating excessive grief.

Hallucinations in which a "sense of presence" of the dead spouse is felt were reported by almost half of the bereaved persons surveyed by Rees (1975). A smaller percentage reported visual, auditory, or tactile hallucinations. Hallucinations were more frequent in what had been happy marriages. Although only about one-fourth of the persons had revealed their hallucinations to others because of fear of ridicule, Rees interprets the phenomenon as a normal experience which disappears in time.

To sum up, our culture defines mourning as lasting about 1 year, with the period of intense grief enduring for up to 3 months. Ventilation of feelings and contacts with friends and relatives are of benefit in alleviating the distress. Depressive symptoms which persist beyond the normal grief period would call for professional intervention. Anniversaries and holidays are constant reminders which may reinstitute the feelings of sadness and loss experienced during the second stage. Ambivalence and denial complicate the course of grief. Verbalization should be encouraged, and any immediate changes in life-style should be discouraged during the mourning period.

Heyman and Gianturco (1973) reported varying patterns of adaptation to bereavement in a 21-month follow-up study of 41 men and women with an average age of 72. Their findings differed from others regarding sex differences. The lives of the men were less disrupted than those of women because women had to give up their homemaker roles. More typically, men have been found to have higher mortality rates to widowerhood. The individual's prior emotional state contributed to the duration of the depressed state following bereavement. Relatively few persons developed depressions which were evident at follow-up. Indeed, two men who were rated as depressed prior to the death of their spouses experienced a sense of relief after the long-term illnesses of their wives had ended. Perhaps the grieving had taken place prior to death.

7.4. Paranoid Behavior

The development of paranoid ideation occurs with considerable frequency in late life and ranges from relatively brief transitory reactions to persistent persecutory states. Paranoid psychoses without accompanying brain disorder account for about 10% of the admissions of the elderly to mental hospitals (Post, 1966). Delusions also occur in patients with a primary diagnosis of organic brain syndrome. About one-third of the patients Post studied had classical signs of schizophrenia; one-third were deaf; and one-third had a history of suspiciousness, argumentativeness, and undue sensitivity. Post's recommendations for treatment included correction of the sensory losses in hearing or vision and reduction of anxiety. The use of drugs should be limited to supervised administration. Pfeiffer (1977) estimated that "perhaps 60 percent of drug dosages given to paranoid patients in pill form are never taken." The prognosis for schizophrenia beginning in old age, however, tends to be poor (Kay, 1972b).

The schizophrenic psychoses which resemble the disorders of younger persons have poor prognoses. The more frequently occurring paranoid reactions of the aged which deal with issues arising out of everyday life experiences may be alleviated by situational and psychotherapeutic interventions.

Paranoid ideation occurs among those persons who cannot accept decline or loss of functioning within themselves. A paranoid solution may be the most comfortable way of explaining ordinary events for which the person cannot accept responsibility. The delusions take the form of accusing someone in the immediate environment of harming them or their property. In a fairly typical case, a widow living alone accused the building superintendent of entering her apartment, breaking a vase, stealing food from her refrigerator, and pouring chocolate syrup on her clothing. Apparently a meticulous housekeeper in the past, she could not accept her declining motor control, which may have accounted for the broken vase and stained clothing or memory lapses concerning foods she had probably consumed or never purchased. Although the police listened patiently to her complaints, the superintendent found it difficult to overlook her accusations, particularly since they were accompanied by ethnic slurs. The patient, referred to a community mental health center by the police, had been a social isolate, suspicious of others, and quarreled regularly with her daughter for not being more attentive. Although she refused to become involved in a senior citizens' center, she accepted several appointments at the center for therapy which she used to voice her complaints. Her daughter was encouraged to visit more frequently and assist in housecleaning and shopping. The daughter also encouraged the superintendent to call her should the problem recur, which provided him with an opportunity to take action and defend himself. The accusations diminished.

In a nursing home consultation, a woman began to accuse the nursing aides of beating her at night so that she awakened in severe pain. She denied that her arthritic condition could account for the discomfort she experienced. The nursing home personnel were advised to accept her delusional beliefs. Her verbal abuse of residents, however, necessitated psychiatric hospitalization.

A sizable portion of the aged population in mental hospitals consists of schizophrenics who have grown old in the hospital. With advancing age, the symptomatology of schizophrenia tends to ameliorate (Verwoerdt, 1976). Psychomotor activity tends to be reduced; hallucinations become less troublesome and may diminish in frequency; delusions sometimes disappear. Although many old schizophrenics have been deinstitutionalized by placement in foster homes or health-related facilities, the traumatic effects of transfers should be carefully considered. Such placements have resulted in increased withdrawal from activities to the detriment of the former patient.

The assessment of paranoid behavior calls for a comprehensive evaluation of the patient in his environment. Frequently, the individual will be prepared to describe the situation quite fully, including personal experiences, but will become suspicious or fearful of formal psychological tests. Evaluation of cognitive functioning, however, can contribute to understanding the role decline in mental abilities may play in the disorder. The pervasiveness or specificity of the delusional system can probably be more readily assessed through interviews with the patient and other persons involved with him.

7.5. Psychoneuroses, Personality Disorders, Transient Situational Disturbances

Admissions to outpatient psychiatric services and public mental hospitals in the United States indicate that different disorders tend to occur during specific age periods. Organic, affective, and paranoid disorders have been identified as occurring with high frequency in the aged population. Grouped with the depressive and paranoid disorders were conditions that could formally be classified as depressive neurosis, transient situational disturbance (i.e., adjustment reaction of late life), or personality disorders (paranoid personality). Alcoholism, which frequently accompanied acute organic brain syndromes, was rarely diagnosed as such (Zimberg, 1974). Anxiety is frequently a symptom in transient disorders, reactions to physical illness or decline, and as a part of a depressive syndrome.

In reviewing biometric surveys by the National Institute of Mental Health, Meyer (1974) noted that, for persons over 65, first admissions to public mental hospitals for psychoneuroses, personality disorders, and transient situational disorders dropped precipitously. For the 45–64 year age group, these psychogenic disorders accounted for about 60% of all first admissions; for the over-65 year group, they accounted for only 6%. The very small numbers of aged persons seen in outpatient clinics suggest that relatively few diagnoses of these types are made for the older adult.

Meyer (1974) speculated that chronic psychoneuroses that developed early in life were mitigated by aging, or patients suffering from the more severe nonpsychotic disorders may have decompensated into psychoses or have died so that only those with the milder disorders, which did not require treatment, have survived. Verwoerdt (1976) also attempted to account for the drop in the numbers of aged in the psychogenic diagnostic categories. He suggested changes in intensity of drive levels and conflicts as possible explanations. Dependent persons may no longer be threatened by the competitive aspects of our society, particularly after retirement, when there is less need to maintain an independent façade. Sexual drives diminish, although in the hysterical personality the lack of narcissistic gratification may lead to depression or hypochondriasis. The obsessive-compulsive personality may be able to compensate for declining memory through his orderly behavior patterns, but increasing stress may precipitate depression. The schizoid personality, with his preference for solitude, may adapt quite well to the social isolation that occurs in old age. When isolates are required through institutionalization to live in close contact with others, serious interpersonal conflicts develop. They continue to function as they did when living at home, not dressing completely, unaware of their impact on others, and, particularly in the dining hall, reacting with anger to restrictions. If they are forced to share a room, their roommates bear the brunt of their asocial behavior.

These explanations are, of course, speculative. Longitudinal studies of neurotic patients do not exist. The more plausible hypothesis is that old persons simply do not seek out psychiatric treatment. Anxiety symptoms which may accompany short-lived transient disorders may be treated successfully with minor tranquilizers by physicians without referral to a mental health professional. Hence elderly patients do not receive such diagnoses until they are so severely incapacitated that they receive more severe diagnoses.

7.6. Hypochondriacal Neurosis

Because hypochondriacal individuals may never have contact with a mental health clinic, this disorder also is likely not to be included in statistical surveys. Pfeiffer (1977) believes it to be "the next most frequent functional psychiatric disorder in the later years behind depressive and paranoid reactions." The well-known symptoms entail a "preoccupation with the body and with fear of presumed diseases of various organs" (American Psychiatric Association, 1968). Perhaps the derogatory reference of some medical personnel to older patients with many physical complaints as "old crocks" is an informal classification of hypochondriasis or the closely related syndrome, neurasthenic neurosis. Both Verwoerdt (1976) and Pfeiffer (1977) vividly portray the frustrations experienced by physicians who treat such patients. Somatic complaints must be taken seriously, yet to find nothing wrong physically will result in the patient's seeking out a "better doctor." Curing the original complaint leads to the development of a new set of symptoms; failing to cure leads to being labeled incompetent. Psychological interpretations tend to be totally rejected. The patients' anxieties are clearly tied to tangible physical symptoms, and they apparently obtain considerable gratification from contacts with doctors and reports about their illnesses to others who will listen and sympathize. Pfeiffer (1977) suggests making use of the MMPI to confirm the diagnosis, which can reassure the physician and help in the development of a treatment plan. Verwoerdt (1976) recommends that the patient's need to be cared for should be respected and offers a detailed procedure for the physician to follow which permits the patient to retain his defenses and the physician to make efficient use of his time.

The psychophysiological disorders are presumed to have their origin in the response of the individual to stressful events. Steinbach (1975) indicated that the onset of the more common psychosomatic disorders (ulcers, colitis, asthma) tended to occur well before age 60. Even rheumatoid arthritis, essential hypertension, and cardiovascular disorders, which have unusually high prevalence rates among the aged, begin earlier in life. Regardless of age at onset, stress is recognized as contributing to the development and exacerbation of physical disease and to the acceleration of the aging process, although it is recognized that stress may also have its positive aspects in leading to new and improved adaptation (Eisdorfer & Wilkie, 1977). A link is strongly suggested between anxiety and behavior patterns which invite excessive stress and the development of coronary heart disease. As mentioned previously, cardiovascular disease has been associated with lowered intellectual functions and lowered rates of survival. Steinbach (1975) emphasized the "vicious interaction circle" that is created in such patients in which the somatic disease causes psychiatric disorder which in turn leads to further somatic deterioration and on. The identification of personality characteristics, behavior patterns, and situational events which contribute to stress, and particularly maladaptive reactions to stress, would be of benefit to the clinician in developing a therapeutic program aimed at altering the patient's life-style to ameliorate the exposure to stress and its negative effects.

9. A Rational Approach to Assessment

Diagnostic procedures with the aged can never be routinized. The selection of techniques to be used depends on the nature of the referral, physical condition, age, background, stage of life, and situational variables such as available external resources for providing treatment and support. The initial focus has been on the patient with an acute confusional disorder, where prompt identification and treatment of etiological factors are essential in order to prevent irreversible damage. The complexities of the diagnostic problem are enormous in that typically there are a multitude of interacting biological, psychological, and social factors contributing to the acute condition. Certainly, medical examination and treatment are of primary importance. Even with the identification of physical causal conditions, depression, cognitive impairment, or loss of supporting persons may have contributed to the acute disorder directly or to the underlying physical condition.

During this initial diagnostic phase, the more formal psychological tests frequently are impractical. An instrument of choice would be one of the relatively simple, brief mental status questionnaires which can be administered by any member of the multidisciplinary team working with the patient. The questionnaire can be repeated several times during the day, and from day to day, to chart changes that may occur regularly and to monitor any changes as treatment progresses. Whenever possible, the same member of the team should conduct the interviews and brief evaluations of the patient to reduce the stress of adapting to the unfamiliar and threatening strangers.

Aged persons in acute distress are also frequently seen in emergency rooms of hospitals. Ideally, a geroclinical consultant should be available at the emergency room to determine whether or not the elderly patient understands the prescription or instructions offered by the overworked personnel and to determine what additional problems may contribute to the patient's current complaint. Too often, older individuals are given what Butler (1975) labeled "the emergency-room hustle," in which the patient is treated and given instructions to return or obtain medication. Because of cognitive impairment due to the immediate stress or a chronic deficit, the patient may not comprehend the instructions, remember when to take medication, or return for a follow-up. A consultant, possibly a patient representative, could determine what additional help the patient may need in order to carry out the physician's instructions.

During the initial phase, assessment of the home situation and interviews with relatives or friends are needed to determine the patient's level of functioning prior to the current crisis. On occasion, severely impaired individuals have been able to function at home, with children, spouse, or siblings, providing the basic necessities of life and satisfying social contacts. Such a patient may have been unable to do more than recognize his relatives, even occasionally forgetting his name. These patients would obtain the maximum number of errors on the Kahn et al. (1960) questionnaire when examined. The relatives' reports of either gradual or precipitous decline prior to the current episode would provide a crude baseline for estimating level of recovery following the acute episode. It is important to note that, even with clearly diagnosable severe dementia, the patient may be able to return home when hospitalization is no longer needed.

When the patient's condition has stabilized, it may be possible to administer formal tests of intellectual ability. The available norms are not likely to be of value in estimating the degree of change from the patient's level of functioning prior to the episode. The expected level would have to be inferred from the individual's experiential background, the types of activities engaged in previously, his age, and physical condition. The precise scores provide baseline measures for future comparison. Observations of performance yield data for estimating the degree of independence and adaptibility and permit judgment regarding the ability of the person to adapt to a changed life situation where there has been a loss of a significant supporting person or a forced move to a new location. Test scores should never be used to determine the capacity of a person to function effectively in his environment. Fisher (1973) urged the use of Robert White's concept of competence as a more appropriate measure. Competence could be rated through using a number of cognitive and social accessibility scales.

Clinicians are aware of the limitations of the validity of samples of test behavior administered in a strange situation by persons who are of a different cultural background in predicting adaptation to the real-life situation of the patient. Toward this end, Lawton (1970) has focused on procedures for making a favorable placement for the patient after a contact with a clinician. The patient's well-being depends on not being challenged beyond his resources, on minimizing environmental stress. Lawton has conceptualized "sublevels of individual organization." These are arranged in a hierarchy of groups of functions in which persons engage in different types of environmental settings. The lowest level of organization would call for the provision of basic life maintenance supports provided in a hospital setting, ranging through various levels of support in institutional settings up to self-maintenance in the community. He suggested a test battery to match the individual's level of functioning to that required by the particular environmental setting. Lawton and Brody (1969) devised an Instrumental Activities of Daily Living Scale which rates eight skills:

"telephoning, shopping, food preparation, housekeeping, laundry, use of public transportation, self-medication, and handling of finances." The scale covers areas on which the clinician can attempt to evaluate competence and make a rough match to the environment suited to the individual's well-being.

In the context of assessing the person's competence to function in the community, Bloom and Blenkner (1970) focused on "contentment," appraising this variable through interviews with the elderly person and with observers, supplemented by the use of brief standardized tests to attempt to predict outcome. To minimize the threat of a test situation, they introduced the test with the comment that it was like questions on a quiz program. Tissue (1971) developed a simple five-item scale of psychological readiness for withdrawal. For those persons in good health, morale was high when activity level matched disengagement style. For those in poor health, morale was low.

It is apparent that a multiplicity of methods exist and can be used as guides for the geroclinician. Regarding the choice of specific standardized test material, in all likelihood the tests with which the clinician is most familiar would be the ones to employ, with his judgment providing for the adaptation of whatever norms exist. Cautions regarding sensory deficits, the need for patience and gentleness, and the fact that the patient's behavior in the strange office may yield a strikingly different picture from behavior at home must be reiterated. In those cases where a severe chronic brain syndrome does exist, treatment programs can be developed to maximize the ability of the patient for self-care (Barns, Sack, & Shore, 1973; Rebok & Hoyer, 1977). Day hospital rehabilitation programs have been developed to train both the brain-damaged patient and his relative or caretaker to adapt to continued living at home. Even a few months at home is of great importance and can enhance the life satisfaction of elderly persons. Assessment in such cases includes appraisal of the supporting persons' abilities as well as those of the patient. Repeated evaluations of the patient's progress in the treatment program will permit revisions in goals. The follow-up examinations need not be extensive unless there is unaccountable change in the patient's level of functioning.

The crises that lead to referral to mental health professionals do include adjustment problems created by retirement, physical disease, and bereavement, which call for changes in the life-style of the individual or the family. To the extent that the patients are motivated to accept therapy or counseling on an individual, family, or group basis, the approach to assessment would be quite similar to that with younger adults. One or more intake interviews may be called for, with or without formal psychological tests. While this group of psychologically sophisticated persons is growing, there remain sizable numbers of persons with serious problems in adaptation who will not seek assistance. Occasionally, guidance can be provided through contact with their middle-aged children.

While there is still much evidence of the tragic consequences of growing old in America, the decade of the 1970s has witnessed highly positive changes which bode well for the future aged. Most striking has been the dramatic growth in interest in the field of gerontology. Courses and programs are now being offered at well over 1200 colleges in the United States; this is 3 times the number offered 5 years earlier (Lindsey, 1977). The increase in the numbers of persons systematically studying the aging process, the increase in the numbers and political power of aged persons, and the increase in federal and local community aid for programs for the elderly suggest that we have passed the nadir in our treatment of the older American. We can expect funds to become more available to provide services and to train the additional professionals to supply the needed services. Above all, the demoralizing pessimism that has plagued the field is being replaced by a readiness on the part of mental health professionals to take action.

10. References

American Psychiatric Association. *Diagnostic and statistical manual of mental disorders* (2nd ed.) DSM-II. Washington, D.C.: American Psychiatric Association, 1968.

Ames, L. G., Metraux. R. W., Rodell, J. L., & Walker, R. M. *Rorschach responses in old age.* New York: Brunner/Mazel, 1973.

Anderson, W. F. Concomitant physical states. In J. G. Howells (Ed.), *Modern perspectives in the psychiatry of old age.* New York: Brunner/Mazel, 1975.

Baltes, P. B., & Schaie, K. W. On the plasticity of intelligence in adulthood and old age: Where Horn and Donaldson fail. *American Psychologist*, 1976, *31*, 720–725.

Barns, E. K., Sack, A, & Shore, H. Guidelines to treatment approaches: Modalities and methods for use with the aged. *The Gerontologist*, 1973, *13*, 513–527.

Bellak, L., & Bellak, S. S. *Senior Apperception Technique.* Larchmont, N.Y.: C.P.S., 1973.

Benton, A. L. *Revised Visual Retention Test: Manual.* New York: Psychological Corporation, 1963.

Benton, A. L. Psychological tests for brain damage. In A. M. Freedman & I. H. Kaplan (Eds.), *Comprehensive textbook of psychiatry.* Baltimore: Williams & Wilkins, 1967.

Bernal, B. A. A., Brannon, L. G., Belar, C., Lavigne, J., & Cameron, R. Psychodiagnostics of the elderly. In W. D. Gentry (Ed.), *Geropsychology: A model of training and clinical service.* Cambridge, Mass.: Ballinger, 1977.

Birren, J. E., & Renner, V. J. Research on the psychology of aging: Principles and experimentation. In J. E. Birren & K. W. Schaie (Eds.), *Handbook of the psychology of aging.* New York: Van Nostrand Reinhold, 1977.

Bloom, M., & Blenkner, M. Assessing functioning of older persons living in the community. *The Gerontologist*, 1970, *10*, 31–37.

Blum, J. E., Jarvik, L. F., & Clark, E. T. Rate of change on selective tests of intelligence: A twenty-year longitudinal study of aging. *Journal of Gerontology*, 1970, *25*, 171–176.

Botwinick, J. Intellectual abilities. In J. E. Birren & K. W. Schaie (Eds.), *Handbook of the psychology of aging*, New York: Van Nostrand Reinhold, 1977.

Botwinick, J., & Birren, J. E. Mental abilities and psychomotor responses in healthy aged men. In J. E. Birren, R. N. Butler, S. W. Greenhouse, L. Sokoloff, & M. R. Yarrow (Eds.), *Human aging: A biological and behavioral study.* PHS No. 986, Washington, D.C.: U.S. Government Printing Office, 1963.

Botwinick, J., & Storandt, M. *Memory, related functions and age.* Springfield, Ill.: Thomas, 1974.

Bourestom, N. C. Evaluation of mental health programs for the aged. *Aging and Human Development*, 1970, *1*(3), 187–198.

Brotman, H. B. Who are the aging? In E. W. Busse & E. Pfeiffer (Eds.), *Mental illness in later life.* Washington, D.C.: American Psychiatric Association, 1973.

Brotman, H. B. Income and poverty in the older population in 1975. *The Gerontologist*, 1977, *17*, 23–26.

Busse, E. W. Mental disorders in later life-organic brain syndromes. In E. W. Busse & E. Pfeiffer, (Eds.), *Mental illenss in later life.* Washington, D.C.: American Psychiatric Association, 1973.

Butler, R. N. Age-ism: Another form of bigotry. *The Gerontologist*, 1969, *9*, 243–246.

Butler, R. N. *Why survive? Being old in America.* New York: Harper & Row, 1975.

Butler, R. N. & Lewis, M. I. *Aging and mental health.* St. Louis, Mo.: Mosby, 1973.

Cain, L. D. The growing importance of legal age in determining the status of the elderly. *The Gerontologist*, 1974, *14*, 167–174.

Clemente, F., & Kleiman, M. B. Fear of crime among the aged. *The Gerontologist*, 1976, *16*, 207–210.

Cohen, J. The factorial structure of the WAIS between early adulthood and old age. *Journal of Consulting Psychology*, 1957, *21*, 283–290.

Copeland, J. R. M., and associates. Cross-national study of diagnosis of mental disorders: A comparison of the diagnoses of elderly psychiatric patient admitted to mental hospitals serving Queens Co., N.Y., and the former Borough of Camberwell, London, *British Journal of Psychiatry*, 1975, *126*, 11–20.

Corsellis, J. A. N. *Mental illness and the ageing brain*. London: Oxford University Press, 1962.

Draguns, J. G., & Phillips, L. *Psychiatric classification and diagnosis: An overview and critique*. New York: General Learning Press, 1971.

Eisdorfer, C., & Stotsky, B. A. Intervention, treatment, and rehabilitation of psychiatric disorders. In J. E. Birren & K. W. Schaie (Eds.), *Handbook of the psychology of aging*. New York: Van Nostrand Reinhold, 1977.

Eisdorfer, C., & Wilkie, F. Stress, disease, aging and behavior. In J. E. Birren & K. W. Schaie (Eds.), *Handbook of the psychology of aging*. New York: Van Nostrand Reinhold, 1977.

Epstein, L. J. Depression in the elderly. *Journal of Gerontology*, 1976, *31*, 278–282.

Filskov, S. B., & Goldstein, S. G. Diagnostic validity of the Halstead-Reitan Neuropsychological Battery. *Journal of Consulting and Clinical Psychology*, 1974, *42*, 382–388.

Fishback, D. B. Mental status questionnaire for organic brain syndrome, with a new visual counting test. *Journal of American Geriatric Society*, 1977, *25*, 167–170.

Fisher, J. Competence, effectiveness, intellectual functioning, and aging. *The Gerontologist*, 1973, *13*, 62–68.

Fisher, J., Gonda, T. A., & Little, K. B. The Rorschach and central nervous system pathology: A cross validation study. *American Journal of Psychiatry*, 1955, *111*, 487–492.

Foster, J. R., Gershell, W. J., & Goldfarb, A. I. Lithium treatment in the elderly. I. Clinical usage. *Journal of Gerontology*, 1977, *32*, 299–302.

Furry, C. A. & Baltes, P. B. The effect of age differences in ability-extraneous performance variables on the assessment of intelligence in children, adults, and the elderly. *Journal of Gerontology*, 1973, *28*, 73–80.

Gaitz, C. M., & Baer, P. E. Diagnostic assessment of the elderly: A multifunctional model. *The Gerontologist*, 1970, *10*, 47–52.

Goldfarb, A. I. Predicting mortality in the institutionalized aged. *Archives of General Psychiatry*, 1969, *21*, 172–176.

Goldfarb, A. I. Masked depression in the elderly. In S. Lessee (Ed.), *Masked depression*, New York: Jason Aronson, 1974.

Goldstein, G., & Shelly, C. H. Similarities and differences between psychological deficit in aging and brain damage. *Journal of Gerontology*, 1975, *30*, 448–455.

Goldstein, K., & Scheerer, M. Abstract and concrete behavior, an experimental study with special tests. *Psychological Monographs*, 1941, *53*, No. 2.

Gorer, G. *Death, grief and mourning in contemporary Britain*. London: Cresset Press, 1965.

Granick, S. Psychological test functioning. In S. Granick & R. D. Patterson (Eds.), *Human aging II: An eleven-year follow-up biomedical and behavioral study*. DHEW Publication No. (HSM) 71-9037. Washington, D.C.: U.S. Government Printing Office, 1971.

Group for the Advancement of Psychiatry. *The aged and community mental health: A guide to program development* (Vol. 8). Report No. 81, November 1971.

Gruenberg, E. M. The social breakdown syndrome—some origins. *American Journal of Psychiatry*, 1967, *123*, 1481–1489.

Gurland, B. J. A broad clinical assessment of psychopathology in the aged. In C. Eisdorfer & M. P. Lawton (Eds.), *The psychology of adult development and aging*. Washington, D.C.: American Psychological Association, 1973.

Gurland, B. J. The comparative frequency of depression in various adult age groups. *Journal of Gerontology*, 1976, *31*, 283–292.

Hall, E. H., Savage, R. D., Bolton, J., Pidwell, D. M., & Blessed, G. Intellect, mental illness, and survival in the aged. *Journal of Gerontology*, 1972, *27*, 237–244.

Heyman, D. K., & Gianturco, D. T. Long-term adaptation by the elderly to bereavement. *Journal of Gerontology*, 1973, *28*, 359–362.

Hollingshead, A. B., & Redlich, F. C. *Social class and mental illness*. New York: Wiley, 1958.

Holmes, T. H., & Rahe, R. H. The social readjustment rating scale. *Journal of Psychosomatic Research*, 1967, *11*, 213–218.

Horn, J. L. Organization of data on life span development of human abilities. In L. R. Goulet & P. B. Baltes (Eds.), *Life span developmental psychology*. New York: Academic Press, 1970.

Horn, J. L., & Donaldson, G. On the myth of intellectual decline in adulthood. *American Psychologist*, 1976, *31*, 701–719.

Horn, J. L., & Donaldson, G. Faith is not enough: A response to the Baltes-Schaie claim that intelligence does not wane. *American Psychologist*, 1977, *32*, 369–373.

Jarvik, L. F., & Falek, A. Intellectual stability and survival in the aged. *Journal of Gerontology*, 1963, *18*, 173–176.

Kahn, R. L., Goldfarb, A. T., Pollack, M., & Peck, A. Brief objective measures for the determination of mental status in the aged. *American Journal of Psychiatry*, 1960, *117*, 326–328.

Kastenbaum, R., & Costa, P. T. Psychological perspectives on death. *Annual Review of Psychology*, 1977, *28*, 225–250.

Kay, D. W. K. Epidemiological aspects of organic brain disease in the aged. In C. M. Gaitz (Ed.), *Aging and the brain*. New York: Plenum, 1972 (a).

Kay, D. W. K. Schizophrenia and schizophrenia-like states in the elderly. *British Journal of Hospital Medicine*, October 1972, 369–376 (b).

Kimmel, D. C. *Adulthood and aging*. New York: Wiley, 1974.

Kleemeier, R. W. Intellectual changes in the senium or death and the I.Q. Paper presented at the meeting of the American Psychological Association, New York, 1961.

Kral, V. A. Confusional states. In J. G. Howells (Ed.), *Modern perspectives in the psychiatry of old age*. New York: Brunner/ Mazel, 1975.

Kramer, M., Taube, C. A., & Redick, R. W. Patterns of use of psychiatric facilities by the aged: Past, present, and future. In C. Eisdorfer & M. P. Lawton (Eds.), *The psychology of adult development*. Washington, D.C.: American Psychological Association, 1973.

Kutner, B., Fanshel, D., Togo, A. M., & Langner, T. S. *Five hundred over sixty*. New York: Russel Sage Foundation, 1956.

Lawson, J. S., Rodenburg, M., & Dykes, J. A. A dementia rating scale for use with psychogeriatric patients. *Journal of Gerontology*, 1977, *32*, 153–159.

Lawton, M. P. Assessment, integration, and environments for older people. *The Gerontologist*, 1970, *10*, 38–46.

Lawton, M. P., & Brody, E. M. Assessment of older people: Self-maintaining and instrumental activities of daily living. *The Gerontologist*, 1969, *9*, 179–186.

Lawton, M. P., & Gottesman, L. E. Psychological services to the elderly. *American Psychologist*, 1974, *29*, 687–693.

Lieberman, M. A. Psychological correlates of impending death: Some preliminary observations. *Journal of Gerontology*, 1965, *20*, 181–190.

Lieberman, M. A., & Coplan, A. S. Distance from death as a variable in the study of aging. *Developmental Psychology*, 1969, *2*, 71–84.

Lindsey, R. Gerontology is still a very young science. *The New York Times*, June 19, 1977, p. 9E.

Lowenthal, M. F., & Berkman, P. *Aging and mental disorder in San Francisco*. San Francisco: Jossey-Bass, 1967.

Markson, E. W., & Hand, J. Referral for death: Low status of the aged and referral for psychiatric hospitalization. *Aging and Human Development*, 1970, *1*, 261–272.

Markson, E. W., & Levitz, G. A Guttman scale to assess memory loss among the elderly. *The Gerontologist*, 1973, *13*, 337–340.

Matarazzo, J. D. *Wechsler's measurement and appraisal of adult intelligence*. Baltimore: Williams & Wilkins, 1972.

Mattis, S. Mental status examination for organic mental syndrome in the elderly patient. In L. Bellak & T. B. Karasu (Eds.), *Geriatric psychiatry: A handbook for psychiatrists and primary care physicians*. New York: Grune & Stratton, 1976.

Meyer, J. E. Psychoneuroses and neurotic reactions in old age. *Journal of the American Geriatric Society*, 1974, *22*, 254–257.

Miller, E. *Abnormal ageing: The psychology of senile and presenile dementia*. London: Wiley, 1977.

Nott, R. N., & Fleminger, J. J. Presenile dementia: The difficulties of early diagnosis. *Acta Psychiatrika Scandinavia*, 1975, *51*, 188–191.

Oberleder, M. Adapting current psychological techniques for use in testing the aged. *The Gerontologist*, 1967, *7*, 188–191.

Overall, J. E., & Gorham, D. R. Organicity versus old age in objective and projective test performance. *Journal of Consulting and Clinical Psychology*, 1972, *39*, 98–105.

Pfeiffer, E. Successful aging. In L. E. Brown & E. O. Ellis (Eds.), *Quality of life: The later years*. Acton, Mass.: Publishing Science Group, 1975.

Pfeiffer, E. Psychopathology and social pathology. In J. E. Birren & K. W. Schaie (Eds.), *Handbook of the psychology of aging*. New York: Van Nostrand Reinhold, 1977.

Post, F. *Persistent persecutory states of the elderly*. London: Pergamon Press, 1966.

Prien, R. F. *Chronic organic brain syndrome.* Washington, D.C.: Veterans Administration, Department of Medicine and Surgery, 1972.

Rebok, G. W., & Hoyer, W. J. The functional context of elderly behavior. *The Gerontologist*, 1977, *17*, 27–34.

Rees, W. D. The bereaved and their hallucinations. In B. Schoenberg, I. Gerber, A. Weiner, A. H. Kutscher, D. Peretz, & A. Carr (Eds.), *Bereavement, its psychosocial aspects.* New York: Columbia University Press, 1975.

Reimanis, G., & Green, R. F. Imminence of death and intellectual decrement in the aging. *Developmental Psychology*, 1971, *5*, 270–272.

Reitan, R. M., & Davidson, L. A. (Eds.). *Clinical neuropsychology.* Washington, D.C.: Winston & Sons, 1974.

Riegel, K. F., & Riegel, R. M. Development, drop and death. *Developmental Psychology*, 1972, *6*, 306–319.

Rogers, C. R. *Client-centered therapy: Its current practice, implications and theory.* Boston: Houghton, 1951.

Rorschach, H. *Psychodiagnostics.* New York: Grune & Stratton, 1942.

Roth, M., Tomlinson, B. E., & Blessed, G. Correlation between scores for dementia and counts of senile plaques in cerebral grey matter of elderly subjects. *Nature*, 1966, *209*, 109–110.

Salzman, C., Kochansky, G. E., & Shader, R. T. Rating scales for geriatric psychopharmacology—A review. *Psychopharmacology Bulletin*, 1972, *8*(3), 3–50.

Salzman, C., Kochansky, G. E., Shader, R. T., & Cronin, D. M. Rating scales for psychotropic drug research with geriatric patients. II. Mood ratings. *Journal of the American Geriatric Society*, 1972, *20*, 215–221.

Salzman, C., Shader, R. T., Kochansky, G. E., & Cronin, D. M. Rating scales for psychotropic drug research with geriatric patients. I. Behavior ratings. *Journal of the American Geriatric Society*, 1972, *20*, 209–214.

Savage, R. D., & Britton, P. G. The factorial structure of the WAIS on an aged sample. *Journal of Gerontology*, 1968, *32*, 183–186.

Schaie, K. W., & Schaie, J. P. Clinical assessment and aging. In J. E. Birren & K. W. Schaie (Eds.), *Handbook of the psychology of aging.* New York: Van Nostrand Reinhold, 1977.

Schofield, W. *Psychotherapy: The purchase of friendship.* Englewood Cliffs, N.J.: Prentice-Hall, 1964.

Smith, J. M., Bright, B., & McCloskey, J. Factor analytic composition of the Geriatric Rating Scale (GRS). *Journal of Gerontology*, 1977, *32*, 58–62.

Steinbach, A. Psychosomatic states. In J. G. Howells (Ed.), *Modern perspective in the psychiatry of old age.* New York: Brunner/Mazel, 1975.

Stuart, R. B. *Trick or treatment.* Champaign, Ill.: Research Press, 1970.

Sydenham Hospital. *Patient representative.* Mimeographed job description. Sydenham Hosptial, New York, August 2, 1974.

Szasz, T. *The manufacture of madness.* New York: Harper & Row, 1970.

Tissue, T. Disengagement potential: Replication and use as an explanatory variable. *Journal of Gerontology*, 1971, *26*, 76–80.

Verwoerdt, A. *Clinical geropsychiatry.* Baltimore: Williams & Wilkins, 1976.

Wechsler, D. *Measurement of adult intelligence* (3rd ed.). Baltimore: Williams & Wilkins, 1944.

Wechsler, D. A standardized memory scale for clinical use. *Journal of Psychology*, 1945, *19*, 87–95.

Wechsler, D. *The measurement and appraisal of adult intelligence* (4th ed.). Baltimore: Williams & Wilkins, 1958.

Wilkie, F., & Eisdorfer, C. Intelligence and blood pressure in the aged. *Science*, 1971, *172*, 959–962.

Wolk, R. L. Refined projective techniques with the aged. In D. P. Kent, R. Kastenbaum, & S. Sherwood (Eds.), *Research planning and action for the elderly: the power and potential of social science.* New York: Behavioral Publications, 1972.

Wolk, R. L., & Wolk, R. B. *The Gerontological Apperception Test.* New York: Behavioral Publications, 1971.

Zimberg, S. The elderly alcoholic. *The Gerontologist*, 1974, *14*, 221–224.

Zubin, J. Perspectives on the conference. In M. M. Katz, J. O. Cole, & W. E. Barton (Eds.), *The roles and methodology of classification in psychiatry and psychopathology.* PHS No. 1584, Washington, D.C.: U.S. Government Printing Office, 1965.

23

Diagnosing Personality States

FREDERICK C. THORNE and VLADIMIR PISHKIN

1. History and Theory of Modern Integrative (State) Psychology

1.1. Introduction

Although much has been written about specific psychological states such as anxiety, anger, and sex, Thorne (1967a, 1970) has presented the only comprehensive system of integrative psychology capable of explicating the general theory, nature, diagnosis, and case-handling implications of *state* psychology. It is emphasized that the theory, methodology, and applications of a thoroughgoing state psychology are basically different from psychological trait and personality structure theory. All raw behavior occurs only in the form of psychological states, defined as momentary cross-sections of the stream of psychic life. State psychology is molar and global in studying the dynamics of ongoing mental life. Methodologically, it represents an expansion of the psychiatric concept of mental status enlarged to include all the aspects of the stream of consciousness across time as the person runs critical episodes of life management.

Action behavior patterns may be regarded as molar units for the study of underlying psychological states. Diagnostically, there are the dual problems of discriminating what psychological states it is clinically important to study and then of differentiating the etiology and psychological significance of the critical states. All of this implies that the clinician understands the concept and nature of psychological states and is familiar with methods for their study. Pilot studies indicate that, as of 1977, few psychologists understand the concept or how to deal with state phenomena clinically. Hence this chapter deals with theory, methods, research findings, and clinical implications of the diagnosis of psychological states, but translated into the terminology and study of real-life action units rather than that of underlying structures and functions.

Thorne (1955) published a book called *Principles of Psychological Examining,*

FREDERICK C. THORNE • Clinical Psychology Publishing Co., Inc., Brandon, Vermont 05733.
VLADIMIR PISHKIN • Veterans Administration Hospital, Oklahoma City, Oklahoma 73104.

Part Two of which dealt comprehensively with the study of factors organizing the integration of behavior. This book contains a large number of diagnostic outlines which tremendously enlarge clinical psychological space as follows:

Outline for Constitutional Analysis (pp. 206–207)
Outlines of Maturational Factors and Rates (pp. 222–223)
Diagnosis of Disorders of Consciousness (pp. 235–239)
Attributes of Feelings and Emotions (pp. 247–250)
Biological Classification of Feelings and Emotions (pp. 250–255)
Outline of Psychosexual Development (pp. 266–267)
The Principal Factors of Ability (pp. 285–298)
Outline of Cognitive Thinking (pp. 308–309)
A Classification of Ideologies (pp. 368–369)
Control Factors (pp. 354–359)
Outline for Appraisal of Control (pp. 369–372)
Outline of Habit Formations (pp. 381–387)
Attitudes and Interests (pp. 393–401)
A Classification of the Principal Types of Situational Problems (pp. 409–420)
Outline of Role-Playing Behaviors (pp. 424–427)
Outlines of Life-Style Factors (pp. 434–435, 436–437, 444)
Outline of Ego Functioning (pp. 449–451)

This list of outlines is not considered to be complete, because advancing knowledge continuously adds new information. However, it was based on factor analytic studies up to 1955, much of which information still has factorial validity even though being continuously expanded by new factorial studies.

Thorne (1964) devised a diagnostic classification system and nomenclature for psychological states. This system was based on a multitrait, multilevel, multifactor, empirical analysis of the factors organizing integrated states. A standard three-part formula was devised, consisting of (1) a statement of behavioral (in)adaptability, (2) symptom/syndromal descriptions, and (3) a statement of psychodynamic etiological determination. The diagnostic classification was derived partially by surveying the dictionary for common terms describing unusual behavior types not included in official classifications but nevertheless readily recognizable by empirical observations. The classification refers primarily to pathological and eccentric types but could be readily expanded to include superior or charismatic types. In 1964, no factorial investigations were available to validate the factors described empirically; however, the introduction of the Integration Level Test Series (described later) began to provide a research bundle of evidence supporting the hierarchical level hypothesis.

Thorne's early interests in expanding diagnostic systems stemmed partially from an attempt to apply medical diagnostic methods to psychology, and partially as a reaction to Carl R. Rogers's dictum that diagnostic procedures were contraindicated in nondirective counseling and psychotherapy. However, the reader should note that Rogerian reflection of feelings deals with, and emphasizes the importance of, the psychological state of the moment as the principle problem of case handling.

Thorne (1967a) published another book, entitled *Integrative Psychology*, which provides the systematic theory of the nature of psychological states in terms of the basic concepts of unification and integration. This book includes expanded outlines as follows:

Outline of Symptomatic-Syndromal Descriptive Classifications (pp. 91–92)
Outline of the Differential Diagnosis of Psychological States (pp. 93–97)

Chapters 11 and 12 deal at length with fear, anger, and sex excitement states.

This book, taken as a whole, provides a global molar view of the basic foundations of state psychology. Practical applications to psychological case handling are dealt with in Thorne (1968a, 1968b).

Finally, Thorne (1970) provided a diagnostic classification and nomenclature for existential state reactions together with factor analytic studies of the Existential Study, which provides research evidence for the validity of such factors (Thorne & Pishkin, 1973).

This new system of integrative psychology may appear very complex and cumbersome to the novice, but it is absolutely necessary for understanding of the diagnostic and case-handling implications of integrative (state) psychology.

1.2. Types and Purposes of Diagnosis

It has not been generally understood that there are many types of diagnosis suited to specific types of problems. Psychodiagnosis does not exist in a vacuum in the sense that it has no purposes or usages. Psychodiagnosis always is referential to clinical and/or applied questions related to specific psychological problems in specific institutions or agencies. Historically, different institutions and agencies such as schools, police, courts, social work and rehabilitation agencies, business and industry, medicine, marriage and sex counseling, the military have each utilized psychodiagnosis for different purposes in different ways to answer specific questions.

Operationally, it is useful to differentiate between clinical diagnosis and applied process diagnosis. Clinical diagnosis as utilized classically in medicine and psychiatry was concerned with the identification of the causes and symptomatology of diseases, disorders, defects, deficits, and pathological processes. Clinical diagnosis typically utilized deductive methods to identify pathological conditions using standard diagnostic classifications and nomenclatures. Clinical diagnosis came to serve the dual purpose of (1) identifying the nature of clinical conditions for purposes of treatment and (2) serving as the basis for statistical classifications of disease. Classical clinical diagnosis in psychiatry broke down in the last half of the twentieth century when the official classification system and nomenclature were questioned as to validity. The "myth of mental disease" controversy questioned the existence of "schizophrenia" and "psychoneuroses" as diseases in the medical sense as the underlying clinical phenomena were reinterpreted as interpersonal reaction disorders. In any case, clinical diagnosis is just one type of diagnostic process.

Differential diagnosis involves the differentiation and identification of various classes of etiological factors. The purpose is to discriminate among the various types of diseases, disorders, defects, deficits, and pathological conditions included in official classification and nomenclature systems.

Clinical process diagnosis involves the moment-to-moment diagnosis developments in the case-handling process.

Clinical pathological diagnosis involves the study of disorders in the various organ systems and functions. In clinical psychology and psychiatry, it involves the study of traits, personality structures, psychological states, dynamic processes, drives, needs, temperament, intelligence, control mechanisms, attitudes, interests, ideologies, role playing, social strivings, life-styles, and existential status.

Clinical classification diagnosis involves the differentiation of conditions for statistical record purposes according to some standard system.

Prognostic diagnosis involves making predictions of future outcomes.

In medicine, clinical diagnosis has been primarily concerned with the condition of the organism with respect to disease, disorders, illness, defects, and incapacitation. This works well with organic medicine involving physical pathology. It works less well in psychiatry where, with the exception of a few organic psychoses classifiable as disease processes, most of the disorders are functional in nature, often with unknown etiology and involving purely psychic processes.

Applied psychology as practiced in schools, child guidance clinics, welfare agencies, business and industry, the military, etc., has had very different purposes and methods. Applied psychology has been more particularly concerned with human efficiency and life management problems in practical life situations involving coping and adaptation. Applied efficiency and life management diagnoses are more concerned with the specific psychological states of the person performing in specific life situations. Since most life problems involve integrative disorders, the concept of integrative diagnosis is useful.

Human efficiency engineering as developed in applied psychology involves applied diagnosis to specific work situations in which the person must adapt to more or less fixed environmental conditions, i.e., to do specific jobs.

Life management diagnosis involves the analysis and evaluation of behavior to determine personal-social-situational adequacy of ongoing self-actualization, productivity, and achievement. Here the diagnostic problem is to determine why the person is not doing well in specific coping behaviors. The judgment as to whether the person is doing well may be purely relative. The judgment as to what is considered "doing well" can be made either by the person himself or by others, preferably competent experts.

The difference in methods between clinical and applied psychology should be well understood. Clinical practice has been more concerned with abnormality, disease, disorder, defects, and pathogenicity in the psychobiological organism. Applied psychology has been concerned more with the efficiency and achievements of the person in action in all life situations. State psychology is particularly relevant to the purposes of applied psychology. However, both clinical and applied psychology must depend on psychodiagnosis.

1.3. Toward a Breakthrough in Basic and Applied Psychology*

Postulate I.   Many of the invalidities and shortcomings of the whole field of psychology up to 1975 stem from failure to differentiate the purposes and methods of basic science psychology and applied psychology.

*On the evening of August 25, 1977, while in a light sleep, I (F.C.T.) started dreaming about psychology. With intense feelings of intellectual excitement, I suddenly developed a succession of global, molar insights bringing together and unifying a large number of molecular problems on which I had been thinking for many years. Although most of these molecular problems had been worked over and thought out previously, I had never before had a global insight into how they all fit together. Introspectively, all elements of this dream were exceptionally realistic and apparently rational and logical. The basic insights of the dream are listed in the text in the form of simple postulates which fit together systematically.

Basic science psychology primarily deals with the nature and functions of the psychobiological organism, incorporating the specific contributions of a multi-disciplinary approach, including genetic, constitutional, anatomical, biochemical, physiological, pathological, biological, behavioral, and sociological sciences. Psycho-biology deals with the nature of man, studying the interactions of heredity and environment in the functioning of organisms.

Applied science deals with real-life conditions and situations in the global unit of the-person-running-the-business-of-his-own-life-in-the-world. Applied science utilizes the contributions of basic science in diagnosing, evaluating, assessing, modifying, and treating practical life management coping problems, but translated into the terminology and study of real-life action units rather than in terms of underlying structures and functions.

> Postulate II.   Real-life phenomena may be identified, recognized, described, and manipulated without necessarily understanding their nature.

In physics, the characteristics of gravity and electricity are known, even though their causes and nature are not understood.

In psychology, consciousness is subjectively experienced even though its nature and causes are not understood. Psychology should not overlook, ignore, or deny those phenomena of subjective experience simply because it is not known how to deal with and measure them objectively. Basic science deals with the nature of behavior. Applied science deals with real-life behavior and its meanings. The purposes and contents of basic and applied sciences are different, i.e., one investigates and the other applies, so that perception, memory, and learning can be dealt with phenomenally without knowing their underlying processes.

Historically, the development of psychological science has been heavily influenced by the need to be scientific. Since the scientific method requires a rigorously objective and materialistic experimental-statistical approach, the field has become too method-centered in the sense that basic science tends to exclude all subjective phenomena which it cannot objectify.

> Postulate III.   The subject of psychology has become bogged down by preoccupation with theory, models, concepts, and other abstractions which are unproven and/or unprovable.

Psychology as an academic subject has become bogged down by a mass of invalid, irrelevant, and obsolete approaches by deductive methods of questionable applicability. When it is asked "What is truly known in psychology which has valuable practical applicability?" much of basic science knowledge turns out to be inapplicable, trivial, incomplete, irrelevant, and invalid. In fact, theorizing and conceptual model building may not be as important as finding out what actually works.

Psychology as applied science has turned out to be largely invalid (the failure of diagnosis), useless (the failure of psychotherapies), erroneous (prediction failures), or inapplicable (unsuitable for field purposes). Underlying all these failures is the invalidity of theories and methods. Too often, this has been due to the attempt of psychology to borrow from other fields rather than develop its own relevant methods and findings.

> Postulate IV.   The general failure of basic science psychology to come up with sound foundations for applied psychology has led to much professional disillusionment and some nihilism. However, instead of abandoning the field

because of the failures of classical approaches, we should start out from the beginning in applied psychology and develop more valid theory and methods. An eclectic approach is necessary.

The history of psychology is replete with a large variety of schools, systems, theories, and approaches, most of them unvalidated, and depending on a whole spectrum of operational methods. The primary need is to identify, analyze, and classify all possible operational approaches, determine their indications and contraindications, and discover their validity for different purposes. A thoroughgoing eclectic approach is necessary to accomplish this.

The place to start is to reintroduce the topics of consciousness, subjective experience, introspection, phenomenology, and existentialism into the field of psychology, because, without them, psychology is not psychology but only behavior physiology. The map of psychological space must be enlarged to encompass all relevant phenomena. Unfortunately, American psychology has been dominated by behaviorism and objectivism to the extent that its most important topics have been excluded or even denied. This must stop. Psychology's business is the psyche.

With particular reference to the field of psychodiagnosis, the disillusionment and nihilism stemming from the gradual recognition that traditional classifications and nomenclatures of mental disease (disorders) were invalid and obsolete, that classical diagnostic methods were invalid or irrelevant for predictive purposes, and that many of the schools and systems of classical psychology were incomplete—all of this led to the rejection of diagnosis as a necessary part of clinical case handling. Psychodiagnosis was dealt a further body blow by Carl R. Rogers's pronouncement that diagnosis was not necessary, and was even contraindicated in nondirective case handling, and also George Albee's statement that clinical psychology was dead.

The new breakthrough consists in diagnosing actual raw behaviors in the form of clinically significant psychological states and their integration. Traits and personality structures are conceptual abstractions often many levels removed from important raw behaviors. Trait and personality structure measurements largely have turned out to be invalid and/or irrelevant for predictive and behavior modification purposes.

> Postulate IVa.   Psychological states are the proper elements for valid and relevant psychodiagnosis.

The diagnosis of psychological states necessarily involves the study of changing internal and external conditions. If it is still desired to study the commonalities of behavior formerly dealt with by trait and structure theory, such constancies can be regarded as the central tendencies of states which persist across time and which give the impression of being constancies if so classified and studied by self-fulfilling methods directed toward constancy rather than change.

> Postulate IVb.   Traits are the central tendencies of psychological states persisting across time.

> Postulate V.   Raw behaviors occur only in the form of psychological states.

This is the rationale for a new state psychology. The limits of objective methodology directed primarily toward study of commonalities and central tendencies has resulted in the formulation of trait and structural psychologies which turn out to be invalid, irrelevant, and obsolete. The concept of personality has the same validity as the concept of mind. Unfortunately, preoccupation with common traits and structures has resulted in overlooking the changes which are the primary characteristic of fluctuating states.

Trait and structure concepts are theoretical abstractions many levels removed from raw behavior data. Trait and structural psychologies require the interpretation of changing scores on any measure as due to error variance. State psychology regards changing scores as reflecting changing states. Indeed, traits can be regarded as only the central tendencies of states; i.e., behavior constancies occur because etiological factors and equations remain unchanged over longer or shorter periods. State psychology is a breakthrough to the future. It deals primarily with real-life, momentary behavior (action) units.

> Postulate VI.   Recognition of the primacy of raw behaviors occurring in the form of a stream of life involving a succession of states reflective of constantly changing conditions requires explanations of what organizes psychological states.

State theory requires an entirely different and new approach to behavior study than trait or structural theories. When it is recognized that such phenomena as suicidal tendencies always involve states rather than traits (there is no trait of suicidal tendencies), it is necessary to determine the etiological equations which organize all states. The general clinical finding that trait formulations do not predict much requires clinicians to study the critical episodes involving either conspicuously successful adaptation or, conversely, poor adaptation and failure. This requires the intensive study of clinically significant states.

> Postulate VII.   Integration resulting from the unification of experience is the central and most important psychic process. Integrative psychology is the foundation necessary to explain and work clinically with psychological states.

The greatest psychological need is to integrate and unify experience self-consistently. Environmental stimulation, either internal or external, is chaotic unless organized, unified, and integrated experientially. Adaptive integrations underlie all normal, healthy, productive, and creative behaviors. Conversely, lack of integration, disintegration, or negative integrations underlie all psychopathology. Level of integration is the central cardinal factor both in health and in illness.

The principles of integration have been skipped lightly over or ignored in American psychology, which has not formally recognized their importance. Psychiatry, in contrast, regards integration as reflected in the mental status concept as fundamentally important. In fact, a person cannot stay oriented, "on the ball," "with it," "functioning on all eight cylinders," unless integration is maintained across time. No other function is as important as integration. Therefore, psychodiagnosis must deal with integrative status—with the status of integration vs. disintegration vs. negative integrations across time in the clinically critical episodes of life.

> Postulate VIIa.   A primary objective of psychodiagnosis is to study integrative status.

> Postulate VIII.   Consciousness is the locus of waking states, i.e., it is the locus of experiencing.

No study of real-life behavior can be complete without considering the state and contents of consciousness. This fact is so experientially self-evident that it is incomprehensible how any theory of psychology can ignore or deny it. The impact of behaviorism on American psychology has been so great that few texts even mention the topic, so that objective psychologies completely exclude experiencing in which the state and contents of consciousness are an important factor. Obviously, no person claims to be completely functional unless fully conscious, and no experimenter works with subjects who are asleep. No other science has so completely ignored its birthright as has objective positivism and its variants.

All volitional behaviors involve conscious choice, decision making, and controls. Peak behaviors and experiences always are mediated in consciousness. Preoccupation with methodological concerns resulting in animal experimentation, highly controlled laboratory experiments, and behavioristic theory has led to the ignoral in American psychology of many of the most highly human behaviors studied by the phenomenologists such as Husserl, Heidegger, and Boss. Finally, the very conscious experiencing which makes life livable, e.g., happiness, esthetics, sex play, entertainment, is totally excluded from psychologies which ignore or deny subjective experience and introspection as a basic method of study. It is interesting that bright, well-educated laymen often can make sophisticated psychological judgments as valid as or even more valid than those of psychological professionals preoccupied with unvalidated theories (Thorne, 1961b).

> Postulate IX.   The contents of consciousness are critical for understanding the meanings of behavior. They may be critically important for diagnosing psychological states.

The contents of meanings of any behavior may be more significant than the raw behavior itself. For example, take the act of holding up a cup in the hand in the air. The significant thing is not the motor pattern of holding the cup, but the contents of the cup. The psychological meaning of the act is what the cup holds, i.e., water, alcohol, medicine, or poison. For example, inviting a little girl to enter a car is not as significant as what the driver intends to do to her. For example, the act of kissing has meaning only as regards how it is done. In other words, the motive and the manner in which an act is performed are more important than the motor pattern. People say one thing and do another. Diagnosing the meaning may be critically important clinically.

> Postulate X.   Only clinically significant episodes require analysis.

Most behavior has no particular dynamic significance in terms of critical outcomes. The important principle is to deal clinically only with the psychological states in which the person committed clinically significant acts. It is not necessary to investigate psychological states involving trivial or noncontributory actions. Clinical intervention is indicated only with behavior which is critical for producing healthy states or modifying unhealthy states.

> Postulate XI.   Life management is the crux of all applied (clinical) psychology practice.

The real issue in all applied practice is how to improve practical performance. To the degree that any person can control performance, the critical issue is life management, i.e., how well the person is coping with important problems. Adaptability is the important criterion. Only the hermit can live completely unto himself, and even a solitary existence requires many adaptive responses. Social living requires adaptation to many situations, particularly ones involving social adjustment.

Postulate XII.   Integration is the basis for all adaptive controls. Therefore, the diagnosis of integrative status may be critically important.

The higher the number of relevant factors integrated in responding to complicated life problems, the more adaptable levels of control are achieved. Controls are based on unifying self-consistently all the inputs necessary for integrated behaviors. Psychic life involves a continuous stream of integrative processes, attempting to unify every relevant factor necessary for problem solutions. Therefore, the integrative milieu must be studied diagnostically.

Postulate XIII.   All the traditional basic science concepts of sensation, perception, learning, memory, concept formation, etc., should be reevaluated in terms of integrative theory.

Perception, learning, association, concept formation, etc., may be regarded as different integrative subfunctions involving different types of unifying process. It is not necessary to refer to the basic science psychology of perception and learning which dealt more with the conditions and processes of perception and learning rather than with integrated contents. Clinically, the important question is what a person perceives and learns rather than how. The fact that humans can perceive, learn, form concepts, etc., is in the same category that a person can walk. The significant feature is not that one can walk but where one walks.

Postulate XIV.   Underlying and determining every psychological state is an integrative milieu which is defined as the global product of the unification of the psychological field of forces of the moment.

Underlying every integrated state is a field of dynamic forces called the integrative milieu, which can be represented by an etiological equation. In coping behavior, it is necessary to represent all the factors which must be unified and made internally consistent to produce the psychological state of the moment. Unfortunately, utilizing current invalid and/or inadequate clinical methods, it is not always possible to identify, diagnose, and modify all factors which are actually organizing behavior.

Postulate XV.   A clear distinction should be made between concepts and terminology suitable for basic science psychology and those suitable for applied psychology.

Confusion has been introduced in the past by failure to differentiate concepts and terms appropriate for basic and applied science. Basic science has tended to define concepts in terms of the operations underlying them. Applied science has developed terms suited to phenomenal appearances and empiric experience.

For example, consider such terms as "mind," "personality," "intelligence," "motivation." "Mind" is a lay term for any conscious state or mental activity; however, this concept has been rejected scientifically as not being materially objectifiable. "Personality" is an abstraction, defined in at least 30 ways, but referring particularly to the social impact of behavior; it has no more objectivity than the concept of mind. "Motivation" has been defined in psychology as anything which stimulates action; it is a semantic abstraction, often used uncritically by both basic science and applied psychologists. Let us now consider the importance of dealing with phenomenal acts rather than theoretical concepts.

Psychology simply accepts the empirical fact that motivational processes phenomenally exist, and then proceeds to discover their practical applications in getting people motivated. While it may be desirable to understand the nature of basic processes, such information is not absolutely necessary for case handling. Historically, the concept of motivation probably was an attempt by the behaviorists to rationalize the role of organismic factors when the S-R formula was changed to S-O-R.

Postulate XVI.   Only a comprehensive state psychology based on integration theory is capable of explaining the most complicated human behaviors.

The episodes of events such as the Watergate scandal cannot be understood except in terms of the mental states of those involved. No trait or personality structure theory is capable of explaining the behavior complexities of all those involved.

The concept of full humanness implies that man at his highest levels of creativeness, rationality, adaptability, aesthetic sensibility, affective sensitivity, awareness, nobleness, altruism, courage, bravery, and general life management is largely the cause of his own effects, because nothing else can program and control such behaviors. Skinnerian psychology is totally unable to explicate such behavior.

Only a systematic eclecticism is capable of encompassing the incredibly complex organismic and situational factors involved in real-life situations involving such complex people as Presidents Nixon and Carter, for example. The classical methods of psychodiagnostics were too simplistic and narrow to deal with all pertinent integrational factors in explicating complicated behaviors.

The concept of "intelligence" has been defined both in basic science and in applied terms. This differentiation should be clearly understood, because the two types of definitions have greatly different implications. Basic science concepts have defined intelligence in terms of the operational methods whereby it is measured, e.g., tests of abilities, memory, vocabulary, comprehension, perceptual discriminations, concept formation. In applied practice, none of these involves what is commonly known by laymen as intelligence. In terms of applied psychology, intelligence refers to life management involving the appropriateness and effectiveness of all management actions, i.e., the person who manages well is intelligent. Intelligence is what a person can do, and how he adapts and competes.

This postulate applies to all the principal concepts of psychology, including perceptions, learning, memory, concept formation, affective life, and volition, which can be defined in either basic science or applied terms. To demonstrate how important it is to clearly differentiate concepts and terms suitable for basic science psychology and applied psychology, consider the whole area of volition and controls. Basic science objective psychology has rejected and/or ignored the whole topic referred to as will(power) because it has no methods capable of objectifying such a concept, and, therefore, denies its material reality. Applied psychology, however, empirically observes phenomena of control and therefore develops the concepts of will(power), volition, and self-control which are used in formulating dynamics for case-handling.

Similar comments apply to the concepts of needs, drives, intents, desires, wishes, and motivation in general. Basic science psychology attempts to discover the biological, biochemical, physiological, and psychological processes underlying motivational phenomena. Applied psychology deals with presumably purposeful action sequences attempting to analyze, identify, uncondition, or recondition the underlying integrative dynamics. Applied psychology is concerned primarily with the content and meanings of behavioral action units, i.e., what the person is doing. To accomplish this, the applied psychologist must analyze and understand life management operations. Basic science psychology studies the structures, processes, and mechanisms which make integrated behaviors possible. Applied clinical science studies their meanings, contents, and management.

The fact is that no theory or psychological system extant is capable of adequately explicating man at his highest levels of perceptiveness, learning ability, rationality, affective sensitivity, productivity, creativity, character development, and overall full humanness.

Most of psychological research to date has been performed on special groups such as children or the abnormal in very limited laboratory situations and has utilized a variety of objective methods unsuitable for dealing with man at highest levels of integration. Behaviorism applies best to captive audiences of animals and young children. Gestalt research started primarily on animals. Freudian psychology was based on studies of pathological cases. With the advent of objectivism, introspectionism and self-psychologies went into disrepute. Phenomenological, personalistic, and existential psychologies have only recently been widely considered. None of these psychologies gets very far in explicating complicated people whose inner lives are very rarely comprehensively explored. State psychology promises to come closer because it deals with the very essence of a person, namely, the states underlying raw behaviors at any temporal cross-section of life and its situations.

2. The Clinical System: Critical Psychological States

2.1. Definitions

Critical psychological states involve behavior which has important personal and/or social consequences. Not all behaviors are clinically significant in that critical episodes stem therefrom. It is manifestly impossible to investigate the whole stream of psychic life, waking and sleeping, from birth to death. The clinician must select samples of behavior judged to be dynamically important in explaining significant behaviors.

A large percentage of behavior under normal conditions has little or no clinical significance and hence does not warrant clinical investigation. Usually, when a person is referred for assessment and clinical evaluation, the referral is accompanied by a list of presenting problems and/or chief complaints which outline the objective and subjective problems and serve as a convenient starting point for clinical investigations.

A principal aim of clinical study is to ascertain the psychological state of the person at the time significant acts were committed. Because every psychological state reflects the status of underlying integrative processes, the study of the critical events of a person's life record requires the study of integrative (mal)functioning to discover how well the person succeeded in unifying that particular episode of experience.

Clinical psychiatry recognizes the importance of studying critical psychological states in its emphasis on the study of mental status. Psychiatrically, it is considered very important to study the mental status of the person at the time when clinically significant acts were committed. Mental status examinations, one type of diagnostics, essentially involve the study of psychological states.

2.2. Introspective Methods for Studying Psychological States

In contrast to objective psychology, which studies only objectively measurable behaviors (the "nothing-buts"), the central data of state psychology consist of subjective experience mostly studied by introspective methods reporting the state and contents of consciousness. Ideally, the subject should have had some training in studying his own subjective experiencing and then communicating its contents in reasonably adequate terms. Further diagnostic information can be obtained by supplemental objective methods, which, however, rarely reproduce subjective experiencing as exactly or as richly.

The easiest approach is to ask a person what he is conscious of, thinking about, feeling, planning, etc. From time immemorial, people wanting to understand another person have said "A penny for your thoughts." A second method is to ask direct questions concerning inner mental life, including specific feelings and thoughts. Finally, a person may reveal much about subjective inner experience in the form of writings, musical compositions, art works, and other productions.

In spite of the notorious unreliability of introspective and subjective reporting due to deliberate concealment, malingering, psychopathology, etc., it must not be assumed that all introspective data are valid. Many persons are very truthful and faithful about reporting inner mental life. In our opinion, subjective reports should be accepted as honest and valid until their unreliability or invalidity is proven. Projective psychology has resulted in much waste and invalidity because of the assumption that unconscious factors underlie all behaviors, with the result that subjective reports are discounted and only projective test results are considered valid. If a person is richly communicative, the resulting productions may be taken at face value, particularly when self-damaging admissions are made.

Perhaps more significant is the factor of conscious, deliberated, meditated concealment of inner mental life. The word "personality" is derived from the Greek word *persona*, meaning "mask." Outward behavior cannot be assumed to be truly or completely reflective of inner mental life. Nevertheless, it should be given diagnostic weight and utilized, particularly for screening purposes, to uncover indications of a person's life problems. This applies to all comparable methods of subjective reporting, including fiction and nonfiction writing, playwriting and acting, art work, music, and other forms of expression which are self-revealing or even projective.

What is clinically important is that all subjective experiencing and introspective reporting refer to specific psychological states which may be diagnostically important. Although some unconscious repression, censoring, and distortion may occur, or the person may deliberately malinger, most expressive behavior may be interpreted as directly reflecting an underlying psychological state. Where professed intentions and actions are inconsistent, further diagnostic investigation is indicated to discover what actually lies behind overt behaviors.

2.3. Direct Observations of Psychological States and Interactions

Intelligent laymen may empathize very competently with the psychological states of another in terms of what the other person is doing, looking at, hearing, feeling, thinking, and acting out expressively. Observation reveals whether the person is asleep, waking up, fully awake, enjoying, rejecting, loving, hating, etc. Often simply observing what another person is attending to is very clinically important.

> Postulate XVII. Empathy may reveal much information about another person's psychological state.

Rogerian nondirectivism places high emphasis on empathically "getting with" the client so as to understand feeling states. Further data are elicited by nondirectively reflecting the client's feelings, such as by saying, "You feel . . ."

It is preferable for the clinician to actually observe the client in the situations where he gets into trouble and does not cope well. If the problem involves interpersonal difficulties, the person should be observed interacting with the key persons in the problems. The clinician should observe the whole situation to gather clues as to the psychological states involved in all parties to the problem. The sensitive observer often can gather clues as to the nature of underlying psychological states and can diagnose the dynamics of maladjustment.

Miniature situations also can be devised to discover how the person reacts to factors which are considered potentially important. Once maladaptive behavior has been identified, it can be manipulated clinically to obtain more effective coping.

> Postulate XVIII. Psychological states can be directly observed in actual or contrived problem situations.

In general, field observations of what actually goes on are most important in obtaining unbiased judgments as to significance.

2.4. Life Record Sources of Diagnostic Data

The life record can provide very pertinent information about the psychological states underlying clinically significant behavior episodes. The diagnostician must develop skills in interpreting life record data for information relating to significant psychological states. Many significant events may be one of a kind, as where a person commits suicide, commits homicide, becomes impotent, or commits other actions having profound existential significance. It is not the act itself which may be clinically important but rather the nature of the psychological state at the moment when the act was committed.

> Postulate XIX. Life record data should be interpreted diagnostically in terms of their implications for clinically significant psychological states.

The person must have been in a specific psychological state at the time of significant recorded actions, so the problem becomes one of discovering the particular conditions, situations, and states when important actions occurred. Consider, for examples, changes in psychological states existing immediately before and after a person discovers he has cancer, the marriage partner or relative has just died, the wife or husband has been unfaithful, a job has been lost, war has been declared, and innumerable other events have occurred which may be presumed as basically changing the conditions of life. Particularly dramatic as an example of how drastically states can change quickly is a male's contents of consciousness just prior to and after sexual orgasm. Before orgasm, he feels the sex act is paramount; just after he may feel totally disgusted with himself and the woman, with sex appetite completely gone.

In all history taking, it is desirable to obtain verbatim accounts of exactly what the person said and did rather than interpretive statements by others who may not be competent observers. It is particularly important to obtain evidence concerning conspicuous changes in the subject's behaviors which may indicate major changes in inner psychological states. Critical actions usually are preceded by forewarning signs and symptoms that something is changing for better or worse.

Clinical judgment studies (Thorne, 1961b)* indicate that past history is the best predictor of future behavior, assuming that no basic changes in existential status have occurred. The dynamics of behavior change may be either very slow or very rapid, so that as much continuity as possible should be obtained in history taking.

There are many developmental periods in which change is quite predictable, such as adolescence, the onset of menstruation in females, pregnancy, menopause, and old age.

Attention should be directed particularly to the relation of critical life episodes to behavior changes. Stream-of-life charts are intended to graphically depict the relation between temporal events and behavior changes. It may be invaluable to chronicle past events subjectively, as in a diary, so that a continuing record is available concerning just how the person experiences reality. Subjective reactions constitute just as important a source of evidence as objective observations, and an attempt should be made to correlate subjective and objective aspects of experience. What the person feels and experiences may be very important data to the clinician if not to the objectivist experimenter.

2.5. Other Methods of Studying Psychological States

Literally any expressive behavior may yield clues as to the psychological state underlying such behaviors. Life charts may be constructed to indicate the relationships between various events and situations in life and psychological reactions. Time investment studies or self-report diaries can provide very important information concerning circadian rhythms, mood states, demoralization states, and other reactions which may persist across time. Psychophysical methods such as paired comparisons may be used to compare the intensity or extensity of state reactions.

The important consideration in all objective measurement methods is that the methods and the data should be interpreted from the "state" orientation rather than in terms of more abstract traits or personality structures. Because state factors can vary widely across time, it may be necessary to repeat measures across time as long as significant changes might be expected. Our own factor analytic results reported in later sections of this chapter indicate that factors may vary widely between testings, with the same items showing different loadings, or with factors appearing in different orders—all across time. In highly variable attitudinal or ideological factors which are known to show high cultural change, such as attitudes toward sex or femininity, it may be expected that rapidly changing states will produce markedly different behaviors. Thorne (1967a) gives many examples of action tendencies which may vary through 180° due to sudden alterations of underlying states. Such changes are particularly characteristic of feeling-emotional behaviors which occur only as states.

---

*The book *Personality* presents the first definitive statement of the necessity for differentiating the phenomena of psychological states diagnostically and therapeutically.

Clinical experience indicates that many of the traditional trait or personality structure tests are invalid, are irrelevant, and/or have low predictive significance. Projective tests, in particular, have generally either proven invalid for the investigation of underlying dynamics because Freudian theories are invalid or proven inapplicable because critical behaviors may have non-Freudian etiology.

It is possible that trait and factor tests have been considered invalid because they are not interpreted in terms of "state" theory and would prove more effective if so interpreted. Also, trait and projective test results may have been disregarded in the past because unreliability was treated as error variance or invalidity rather than as measuring actual change in the etiology of behavior. Another difficulty with indirect, subtle projective items is that they may stimulate mental set responding, e.g., social desirability or aquiescence sets, when the subject tries to answer ambiguous, unstructured items.

In any case, Thorne (1965) developed the Integration Level Test Series, consisting of eight 200-item questionnaires sampling eight hierarchical levels of factors potentially organizing integrated states which are considered as clinically significant. The items consist largely of obvious, direct questions specifically referring to important psychological states which deserve further investigation. The purpose is to identify levels at which integrative difficulties may be occurring, either in the present or past. If the subject responds significantly, it is assumed that at some time (not necessarily in the present) the subject may have had adaptive difficulties in that area of coping.

2.7. Psychodiagnostic Orientation and Employment Status

The applied/clinical orientation of psychological specialists is influenced largely by this employment status and purpose of the psychodiagnostic examination. Specialists tend to be hired for special purposes so that employment status determines what they do operationally, either experimentally or clinically. Clinical psychologists and industrial psychologists may operate as differently as day from night in spite of what theoretical influences they may have been exposed to during training.

Child psychologists study growth and development, utilizing various indices of maturation.

Educational psychologists tend to concentrate on learning disabilities and school behavior problems.

Vocational advisors assess talents and do job counseling.

Marriage and sex counselors deal with interpersonal relations and sex adjustment.

Business and financial counselors deal with the management of money, property, and debts.

Industrial counselors deal with human efficiency and personnel management.

Clinical psychologists deal with psychopathology as reflected in maladaptation or maladjustment.

Community psychologists deal with social action problems.

Other applied psychologists, such as military psychologists, deal with very specific problems.

FREDERICK C.
THORNE AND
VLADIMIR PISHKIN

In all of these applications, the study of the psychological states of the persons involved may be critically important in understanding the causation of critical actions. All this requires that the specialists have intimate experience and competency in dealing with special situations and their dynamics.

Postulate XXI. Employment requirements tend to determine how various types of specialists operate.

3. ILTS

The Integration Level Test Series (ILTS) consists of a series of objective questionnaires constructed to measure different levels of factors which may organize behavior integration. The concept of personality integration long has been utilized in clinical psychology and psychiatry without any systematic efforts for objective measurement. It is postulated that all normal psychological states reflect the operation of various hierarchical levels of factors organizing integration.

A prime need of the organism is to organize experience into psychologically meaningful integrates or wholes. Integration reflects the operations or processes whereby lower and more discrete elements of experience are integrated into self-consistent meaningful wholes. During the course of a day, different psychological states, ranging from sleeping to the highest cognitive behaviors, reflect increasingly more complex "integrations of integrates," with successive hierarchies of functions providing the necessary psychophysiological substates in support of the highest level integrations.

The concept of hierarchies of integration presupposes that various levels of complexity of behavior organization may be observed and measured. Psychologically, it is important to measure all the levels of factors which may organize the integration of psychological states. Where such levels of organizing factors show temporal constancy so as to constitute enduring predispositions to behave in certain ways, these commonalities may be referred to as personality (traits). Clinically, it is important to measure both isolated psychological states and relatively enduring personality traits (commonalities).

The Integration Level Test Series was constructed to sample several important levels of factors potentially organizing psychological integration. Accordingly, eight scales were developed to tap certain critical domains of state integration.

The Personal Health Survey is a 200-item objective questionnaire measuring the psychosomatic foundations of psychological states including general health, general development, gastrointestinal system, cardiovascular system, miscellaneous systems, central nervous system, neuromuscular system, anxiety-fear states, anger-frustration states, schizophrenia, affective psychoses, and character disorders.

The Sex Inventory (Male Forms) consists of 200-item objective questionnaires evaluating sexuality in adults.

The Femininity Study consists of 200 items designed to tap female sexuality.

The Personal Development Study consists of a 200-item questionnaire dealing with the utilization in personality of the classical Freudian mechanisms.

The Ideological Survey consists of a 200-item objective questionnaire sampling ideological factors contributing to *Weltanschauung*.

The Social Status Survey is a 200-item objective questionnaire measuring important role-playing and social status factors contributing to important adjustment skills.

The Life-Style Analysis consists of 200 items divided into two groups measuring Adlerian life styles and Murray's need systems.

The Existential Study consists of 200 items reflecting a person's feelings concerning how well he has been running the business of his life in the world.

In order to accomplish standardization and establish factorial structure of these scales, a total of 2716 subjects were tested from nine different clinical groups. These groups were identified as follows:

Diagnostic Code Group 1.   Incarcerated felons at the Central Prison, Raleigh, North Carolina. Mean age 26.4 years (range 13–57); mean education 8.9 years (range 3–20); 95.3% Protestant, 4.7% Roman Catholic; 44% married, 37% single, 19.4% divorced.

Diagnostic Code Group 2.   Incarcerated felons at Colorado State Penitentiary, Canon City. Mean age 31.8 years (range 21–52); mean education 9.6 years (range 6–21 years); 86.2% Protestant, 12.3% Roman Catholic; 51% married, 32% single, 17% divorced.

Diagnostic Code Group 3.   Alcoholics committed to the Willmar Minnesota State Hospital. There were 58 males, mean age 43.2 years (range 29–58); mean education 11.4 years (range 7–15); 45% Protestant, 55% Roman Catholic; 47% married, 24% single, and 29% divorced. There were 31 females, mean age 44.6 (range 25–64); mean education 12.1 years (range 8–16); 60% Protestant, 40% Roman Catholic; 60% married and 40% single.

Diagnostic Code Group 4.   Sixty-two female psychology students at Skidmore College, Saratoga Springs, New York.

Diagnostic Code Group 5.   Students of the objectivist philosophy of Ayn Rand from the Nathaniel Branden Institute, New York City. There were 80 males, mean age 29.0 years (range 19–56); mean education 15.2 years (range 6–20); 1.6% Protestant, 1.6% Roman Catholic, 3.2% Jewish, 93.6% "none" or "atheist"; 33% married, 60% single, 7% divorced. There were 75 females, mean age 28.2 years (range 17–54), mean education 14.3 years (range 9–18), 4% Protestant, 1.4% Catholic, 2.7% Jewish, 91.9% "none" or "atheist"; 47.7% married, 43% single, and 15.3% divorced.

Diagnostic Code Group 6.   Unmarried mothers who were participating in a research project at the Florence Crittenton Home in Chicago, Illinois, where they were residents. Mean age 17.1 years (range 15–20); mean education 9.8 years (range 7–12); 88% Protestant, 12% Catholic; 100% single.

Diagnostic Code Group 7.   College students, University of Alberta, 75 males, 84 females. No demographic data are available because all subjects were instructed to answer the test anonymously and did not give any identifying data.

Diagnostic Code Group 8.   Psychiatric patients with a primary diagnosis of chronic undifferentiated schizophrenia from Central State Hospital, Norman, Oklahoma. There were 236 males, mean age 41.8 years (range 22–53); mean education 10.43 years (range 7–16); 69% Protestant, 31% Roman Catholic; 52% married, 21% single, and 27% divorced; mean length of psychiatric hospitalization 11.6 years (range 3–16). There were 152 females, mean age 42.6 years (range 22–59); mean education 11.8 years (range 8–17); 71% Protestant, 29% Roman Catholic; 68% married, 18% single, and 14% divorced; mean length of hospitalization 10.9 years (range 3–15).

Diagnostic Code Group 9. A total of 278 adults obtained through the cooperation of Walter V. Clarke and Associates, management consultants of Fort Lauderdale, Florida. The subjects were all gainfully employed executives of client companies serviced by the Walter V. Clarke organization who were taking seminars in business leadership and management problems. The vocational status of the subjects ranged from supervisory foremen through high-level executives, with the average being in the middle-executive range. The group ranged between 25 and 60 in age, averaged better than 12 years of education, and included only males. By virtue of their vocational status and being selected for further leadership training by their employer companies, this group may be described as consisting of vocationally adaptable, highly self-actualized people.

3.1. Life-Style Analysis

Perhaps of all the major schools of psychology, there have been fewer objective studies of Adlerian analytic psychology than any other major system. For many reasons, Adlerian theories have not received the research validation which they deserve in spite of growing empirical and clinical evidence concerning their value. At a time when Freudian psychoanalysis has been whittled down to size, Adlerian theories are receiving more universal acceptance because of their broader applicability. For reasons not fully explicated, Alfred Adler never attracted many scientifically oriented followers, and it was not until the Ansbachers (1956) expanded on his theories in detail that Adler began to receive much professional attention in America.

Adlerian psychology may be regarded as one of the first state-oriented systems. Adler's emphasis on the outward thrust of life in the direction of movements toward expansion and overcoming difficulties, and his insistence that human destiny is largely social, that most life problems are social problems, that human interrelatedness and social embeddedness are important—all these emphasize movement and change as the person runs the business of life in a changing world.

One of the most important Adlerian concepts is that of life-style, the more or less characteristic schema (offensive-defensive strategy and tactics) implicit in the person's attack on his problems. In short, the life-style concept easily can be operationalized and should be amenable to objective study. According to Adler, life-styles are conditioned very early in life and tend to continue throughout life as high-level organizers of complex behaviors.

During the first half of the twentieth century, motivation theory achieved high status in theoretical psychology, with motivation finally emerging as a key concept and perhaps the major determiner of behavior. Murray (1938) was one of the first to operationalize a scientific approach to the study of motivations with his Thematic Apperception Test (TAT) and need theories. The TAT was widely used between 1940 and 1960, when its lack of predictive validity was demonstrated. Nevertheless, need theory continued to be widely accepted and had many projective applications.

One important issue concerns the relation of needs to life-styles. It has been postulated that needs organize life-styles, but to date there have been no factorial studies correlating measures of needs in relation to life-styles.

In 1965, Thorne devised the Life-Style Analysis, a 200-item objective questionnaire intended to measure Adlerian life-styles in relation to the Murray (1938) need system. It was hypothesized that each person develops typical need systems which are worked out by the development of distinctive life-styles (schemas) involving specific uses of strategies and tactics for gaining ends.

3.1.1. Factored Scales

Five main factors emerged from the total group data. This general finding indicates that no large general or secondary factors could be extracted from the data, which were determined very complexly (Pishkin & Thorne, 1975).

Factor I. Aggressive-Domineering Life-Style. This scale reflects a domineering, aggressive life-style of competing against other people when the items are answered positively. The items all reflected power needs, with specific items that elicited as many as 76% of the subjects who admitted various expressions of power needs. Although social desirability factors undoubtedly moderated the open expression of such needs, the overall content of the items relates to power needs.

Factor II. Conforming Life-Style. This factor consists of items all of which express (at least on verbal levels) awareness of social desirability and/or a conforming life-style. The differential percentages of responding by the various groups indicate a variety of factors that underlie the same responses in different groups. In general, the groups known to be immature, unadjusted, or delinquent are utilizing conforming attitudes defensively, as by "going along" with people. In contrast, the Branden Institute (Ayn Rand) students and the college students appear to be rejecting conformism by expressing rebellious individualism.

Factor III. Defensive Withdrawal. Strong vs. weak ego strength appears to underlie realistic coping vs. defensive rationalizations and withdrawal. Interpretation of the dynamic patterns among the various groups must depend on comparison of the base rates of responding to each item in relation to the factorial structure of each group. The most unadjusted groups (1, 2, 3, 6, 8) tend to show defense by denial or rationalizations, while the more normal groups (5, 7) are more able to admit error and fallibility.

Factor IV. Amoral Sociopathy. Two items express indifference to helping wounded animals and bullying people. Another item, "What other people think does not concern me," characterizes the unsocialized egocentric who gets his own way and does not conform to authority. This may be referred to as "irrational" self-interest, as differentiated from a more altruistic "rational" self-interest.

3.1.2. Findings

The factorial results are more consistent with Adlerian self-psychology and style-of-life theory. Factor I (Aggressive-Domineering), Factor II (Conforming), and

Factor V (Resistive-Defiant) have high face and construct validity as life-style factors. These factors also are consistent with Karen Horney's types of going with and against people.

Factors III (Weak Ego Strength) and IV (Amoral Sociopathy) both relate to immature, unsocialized self-functioning. Factor III implies more ego defensiveness, while Factor IV is interpreted as an immature selfishness. On the whole, pathological states are represented by the schizophrenic group in Factors III, IV, and V.

Murray's need factors did not appear in the present analysis, either because they were not represented strongly enough to contribute much to the variance or because the items did not turn out to be valid indices of needs.

Item analysis across diagnostic groups indicates a large number of causal (etiological) relationships consistent with the expected and observed differences between normal and clinical groups. No claims are made for standard structures or traits that underlie observed pattern similarities that can be interpreted only in terms of studying group patterns across all the tests and factors of the Integration Level Test Series. The results are more consistent with psychological state theory, which postulates very complex and variable determinations that must be investigated individually across all groups and scales. Relatively low reliabilities of item responding across time also support the state hypothesis rather than personality structure and trait theories.

The factorial results also are more consistent with state theory in that traits did not show up consistently. Where constancy appears, it is interpreted according to state theory as reflecting a constant etiological equation in which the same integrative milieu continues across time.

3.2. The Existential Study

Existential psychology and psychiatry have received increasing attention during the past 20 years, but little has been accomplished in the development of objective measures of existential concepts. Normative and validational studies are almost completely lacking because most existential concepts have had philosophical, metaphysical, or anecdotal origins. From its origins in the works of Kierkegaard and Sartre, European existential psychology, in particular, has involved highly speculative and abstruse theorizing, with often obscure implications. Viktor Frankl, after World War II, did most to relate highly speculative theoretical concepts to empirical clinical data in his concepts of noogenic neuroses and clinical symptomatology.

In 1961, Thorne made an operational analysis of the methods and contributions of all schools of psychology and demonstrated that existential psychology dealt with important areas of high-level integrative phenomena related to self-functioning and the state of being in the world. Thorne's (1967a) integrative psychology related the study of psychological states to all the hierarchical levels at which behavior can be organized, including existential factors at the level of self-functioning.

The Existential Study is a 200-item objective questionnaire designed to measure self-concepts, self-status, self-esteem, self-actualization, existential morale and demoralization, meanings of life, attitudes toward the human condition, and destiny, suicide, and existential success-failure. It contains items intended to objectify Frankl's existential neuroses, if in fact such do exist.

3.2.1. Definitions

existentialism: The study of states of being, of the conditions of existing as a conscious person in the world.

existential anxiety: Anxiety specifically reactive to existential concerns. Actually, this may involve all anxiety viewed as a reaction to the insecurities of life.

existential examination: The preoccupation of the conscious self with the meanings of life, with the worth of any life, and with the general conditions of self-actualization.

existential neurosis: After Frankl, noogenic neuroses involve existential demoralization, existential vacuum, and a general loss of the meanings of values of life

existential problem: A more limited concern with a specific life question, such as whether to commit suicide.

existential status: The momentary status of self-actualization achieved by a person—literally, his or her existential "batting average" based on the individual success-failure ratio that reflects levels of accomplishment achieved.

existential vacuum: A symptom of Frankl's noogenic neurosis that involves a loss or emptiness of meaning in life—having no goals, interests, or purposes.

self-actualization: The degree to which a person actualizes potentialities and opportunities, implying that full existence depends on maintaining the highest levels of integration across time.

state of being: A momentary cross-section of the stream of psychic life, particularly subjective (conscious) awareness of the state of existence.

human condition: The condition of the person in the world, with particular reference to the limiting conditions of humanness and social situation. Literally, being "stuck" with one's self, sex, race, age, soma, psyche, etc.

3.2.2. Procedure

The items of the Existential Study were constructed from actual patient communications collected over years of psychiatric practice, and often consist of verbatim statements from patients that concern their existential concerns. An empirical analysis of a collection of patient statements that reflect existential problems yielded three major areas of concerns that relate to (1) preoccupations with the meanings and worth of the self, (2) difficulties in getting along with other people, and (3) more generalized concerns over the status of Man in the world, i.e., with the human condition in general, with particular reference to societal conditions at time and place. It became apparent that man is stuck with himself, with the human nature of others with whom he must cope, and with the human condition in general (what it means to be a human at any point in history). The test was constructed to consist of 200 items roughly divided into three sections related to reaction to the self, to others, and to the human condition.

Since the Existential Study originally was conceived as one of a series of psychological state-measuring instruments, it first was necessary to resolve technical issues of the validity and reliability of subjective reporting. Because this instrument deals with high-level conscious integrations that deal with the subjective meanings of

FREDERICK C.
THORNE AND
VLADIMIR PISHKIN
life, it was decided to use direct, obvious items, on the assumption that subjective reportings of item responses were both reliable and valid. Pilot studies had shown that, in spite of the operation of response sets such as social desirability, acquiescence, and ulterior motivations, the subjects on the whole appeared to be responding truthfully and consistently. When the subject makes a direct admission of socially undesirable reactions, it may be assumed that he is responding realistically. We accept the tenet that direct questions often are the most economical sources of reliable and valid information.

Based on an empirical analysis of primarily existential complaints of patients observed in clinical practice, Thorne (1970) devised a diagnostic classification and nomenclature for existential state reactions that introduced a new dimension in psychopathology. It remains for future research to study the interrelationships of empirically observed clinical existential reactions and the objective existential factor scales derived from the Existential Study.

Since existential state factors obviously derive only from the contents of states of consciousness and can be reported only subjectively, we have found it to be clinically useful to examine the Existential Study item responses of each subject qualitatively to gain an impression of his existential problems and reactions. Healthy subjects report little difficulty in integrating existential problems, and they evidence high existential morale. Unhealthy subjects report that they have been crushed by life, are experiencing severe existential anxiety, and display chronic existential demoralization states reflected both in objective behavior manifestations and in test responses.

It is postulated that existential concerns involve some of the highest-level integrations of which man is capable, the subjective nadirs and peaks of being as well as some of the most human types of experiencing. No system of psychology may be regarded as comprehensive that does not recognize and deal with the purely subjective contents of conscious experiencing that often are the only cues to an understanding of what the person is doing and what he is experiencing in real life. Therefore, the Existential Study opens up an entirely new domain on the highest integrative levels for psychological study.

Testing was conducted in groups of different sizes, depending on the installation, according to standard instructions. Usually the test was included as part of a routine battery except with students, when it was given during classes as part of the assignment. All subjects were advised that the results in no way would affect their status.

The statistical procedure utilized to analyze the Existential Study data consisted of principal component factor analyses with varimax rotation; the rotated factors were orthogonal (Pishkin & Thorne, 1973).

3.2.3. Results

Factored Scales. Five main factors were extracted from the overall group data from nonschizophrenic subjects, whereby Diagnostic Group 8 served as the pathological, nonintegrated control group and became the basis for five scales that consisted of ten most highly loaded items, plus other items that usually load .40 or higher and are included for informational purposes to clarify the nature of the factor.

Factor I. Demoralization State/Existential Neurosis. This scale contains six items that reflect self-actualization failures, four items that indicate lack of existential morale, three items that indicate such symptoms of existential vacuum as boredom, loneliness, and purposelessness, three items that indicate negative self-esteem, and four items that indicate suicidal impulses. This pattern of low self-esteem, existential failure, existential vacuum, and desires to "end it all" may be considered to define existential demoralization states and/or neuroses. Literally, the self is sick about itself, and most of the items can be interpreted alternatively as self-inconsistencies.

Factor II. Religious Dependency Defenses.   This factor had not been predicted as such when the ES was constructed empirically, even though items related to religious beliefs had been included on the basis of the clinical observation that religious beliefs seem to protect against depression. This factor consists of ten items that load .60 or better and ten items that load .40 or better, all of which endorse belief in God and hope of Heaven, thankfulness for the Lord's blessings, expression of trust that He will take care of His children, and denial of the right to choose suicide. This is regarded as a defense against existential anxiety and demoralization.

Factor III. Existential Confidence/Morale.   This factor includes eight items that express high self-esteem and confidence, four items that express high morale, and three items that deny suicidal ideas. The remainder generally deny the existential vacuum. The factor is defined as an existential morale factor that expresses the confidence that stems from self-actualization.

Factor IV. Self-Actualization Esteem.   This factor has ten items that express high self-actualization, four items that express high morale, two items that express high fortitude (guts), and three high self-esteem items. On the grounds that competent performance always depends on high internal controls, this may be regarded as a high internal control factor that results in high self-actualization and esteem.

Factor V. Concern over the Human Condition.   This factor includes 20 items related to destiny, fate, and the human condition. The world is regarded as a hazardous, dangerous, and hostile place that threatens security. Most of these items reflect existential anxiety; indeed, concern over the human condition is a basic source of anxiety. An alternative explanation is that many items reflect beliefs in the external control of behavior, i.e., life is overpowering and individual controls are failing.

Factor Interpretation.   In terms of general existential theory, these factors are interpreted as consistent with and supporting the construct and factorial validity of the roles of self-actualization and esteem, faith and hope, and high morale as positively influencing self-executive functioning. A clear existential neurosis factor emerged, in addition to existential anxiety related to the insecurities of the human condition. Two factors may be interpreted alternatively as internal control and external control.

It should be emphasized that we regard all the factors (except perhaps Factor II) as true "states" subject to constant change and fluctuation as the attitudinal status of the person changes in reaction to changes of intrapersonal, interpersonal, and general situational factors. Literally, the state of affairs is changing constantly so that constant change of existential attitudes is postulated. Developmental studies are necessary to trace the causal interrelationships that result in basic attitudinal shifts.

Based on the five factors measured by the Existential Study, but not denying the possibility of the discovery of additional factors if other items are included, it appears that general existential attitudes have affective (Factor III), cognitive (Factors II, IV, and V), and conative (Factor I) components, if classical models are to be followed. More consistent with psychological state theory, however, is the interpretation that all five factors simply represent different attitudinal reactions that reflect different modes of attempting to integrate disparate aspects of experience into unified self-functioning.

To be clinically significant, test scores must reveal statistically significant and clinically meaningful differences among diagnostic groups. In general, the different diagnostic groups did reveal clinically significant differences in relation to level of self-concept, existential demoralization, and concern over the human condition consistent with what might be expected from general group characteristics. Based on item-response differences and different factor profiles, the Existential Study scores differentiated the various diagnostic groups on the basis of general existential morale and satisfaction with the way life was going.

On all factor scales, the group of Ayn Rand students scored most normally on all factors—they denied demoralization and rejected religious dependency, while at the same time they reported cynical attitudes toward human nature, expressed high expectations of life, reported high self-concepts, and generally were optimistic about the human condition. The Ayn Rand students obviously were reflecting intellectual commitment to Rand's objectivist philosophy by endorsing its view of the meanings of existence. The Rand students scored a mean rank order on all five factor scales of 4.5, where 5.0 is rated most existentially healthy. It remains for other research to discover whether rational existential insights have been translated into actual self-actualization in real life.

The college student group showed a much different profile, with above-average ratings on concern over the human condition, dependent religiosity, and high morale, and the lowest ratings of self-concept and philosophical optimism. While they rated (on an average ranking of 2.8) next highest to the Rand students, they apparently did not have any strengthening philosophy such as objectivism and, consequently, expressed confusion and cynicism about the human condition.

The incarcerated prisoner group rated slightly above average in rankings on Factors I, II, III, and IV, but below average on concern over the human condition. The prisoners expressed the views that things rapidly are going to hell in the world, life is getting very dangerous, a person can take only so much in life, they have just about had it, and now only want to exist in peace. The prison group also expressed high demoralization, as manifested by "don't know what to do with myself," life is unbearable, shame over their records, self-hate, being a failure, and feeling passed by in life.

The group of unmarried mothers revealed a pattern of low self-concept, high existential demoralization and feelings of being overwhelmed by the human condition and their problems. This group had the lowest ranking of any on Factor V, and perceived the world as a very threatening place over which they feel little control, with no one really caring. On the self-concept Factor IV, they deny being happy, lack fortitude, are dissatisfied with themselves for not breaking even, and feel vulnerable to the bad in life.

The alcoholic population from Willmar State Hospital showed the highest existential demoralization and reported not knowing what to do with themselves, feeling that life is unbearable, being ashamed, hating themselves for failure, and feeling that life has been pretty tough and is passing them by. They show low confidence in life (Factor III), are afraid of ending up in an institution, of being unable to control their destiny, and consider themselves dull and uninteresting.

The schizophrenic group, which empirically represents those who have been unsuccessful in their attempts at self-actualization and are unable to exist within the socioeconomic structure of the society, has been chronically institutionalized. These subjects showed a completely different profile characterized by a great deal of dissatisfaction with oneself, depression, and worthlessness, as well as dissatisfaction with life in general. There is insecurity—"vague fears and anxieties." One does not get much out of life—"something is missing." Depression is the dominant feature present, in addition to some confusion. There is much dissatisfaction with the self, and it is felt that there has been little accomplishment in life. Insecurity, free-floating anxieties, and lack of direction are present.

The schizophrenics were especially low on Factors III and IV, and demonstrated low self-esteem and lack of internal controls. However, their above-range loading on Factor V reflects an orientation toward external control of behavior and a breakdown of individual controls.

The item composition of comparable factors in different groups was different, the order of emergence of the various factors differed slightly, there were different loadings of identical items between groups, there were group differences in response sets, and, finally, there were differential base rates of responding to highly loaded items between groups. The psychotic group clearly revealed a unique factor structure that reflects existential disintegration.

These patterns of factorial results are interpreted as validating the central hypotheses that psychological states are being measured, that mental status patterns vary and change among different groups, and that repeated factor analyses must be performed within and between groups to follow changing patterns of psychological states. It has been established that general patterns of existential factors can be replicated across clinical groups, which must, however, be studied separately in order to comprehend their integrative dynamics.

3.3. The Ideological Survey

The Ideological Survey (IS) is a 200-item self-report questionnaire for the study of ideas and attitudes relating to the role of the individual in society, with specific reference to factors relating to the self-concept and morale.

Ideological composition (defined as the unique constellations of ideational and attitudinal systems specific to each individual) is a relatively ignored area in both psychiatric mental status examinations and objective psychological measurement. As of this date, no standardized objective measuring devices are available for sampling clinically important ideological areas. Historical reasons for ignoring ideological composition include behavioristic denial and ignoral of the importance of subjective mental life and psychoanalytic preoccupation with affective, impulsive, and repressed unconscious factors in "depth" psychology.

The system of integrative psychology developed by the senior author (Thorne, 1967a) postulates that cognitive factors importantly organize rational-intellectual levels of integration. Clinically, it is important to measure not only the quantitative aspects of cortical integrative quality (intelligence) but also the existential meanings of ideological contents. Ideological factors must be weighted properly in determining the etiological equations underlying the organization of important integrations.

A most important existential concern relates to the meanings of man in relation to society. Conflicting political philosophies of the extreme left and right place diametrically opposed interpretations on the relationship of the individual to society. Leftist philosophies view the state as all-important, with individual men existing only for the service of society as reflected by collectivist and state welfare positions. Rightist philosophies view the individual as the prime value, with the state existing only for the protection and potentiation of the individual. Proponents of opposing philosophies have argued vociferously in support of their positions, but little has been done scientifically to assess the actuarial outcomes in mental health of adhering to different ideological positions.

The literary works of Ayn Rand deal compellingly with the issue of man and society. Her first novel, *The Fountainhead* (1943), is a fictional clinical case history describing the struggle of a rugged individualist confronting contemporary social-trending society. Her major novel, *Atlas Shrugged* (1957), allegorically describes the fate of a society in which individualism is being destroyed by collectivism, depicting in its characters the case histories and outcomes of persons adopting individualistic vs. collectivist styles.

To discuss the fundamentals and application of her objectivist philosophy, Rand, together with her colleague, the psychologist Nathaniel Branden, in 1961 founded a special publication first called the *Objectivist Newsletter* and later *The Objectivist,* which was dedicated to the systematic communication of her ideas. The objectivist position stresses reason as man's most important resource and is particularly concerned with the epistemological implications of ideological composition.

Since Rand's objectivist philosophy is sharply at variance with the prevailing views in our culture, her ideas often encounter sharp opposition. In our opinion, this dispute cannot be resolved by debate or logic but only by the scientific assessment of the outcomes of adhering to any particular ideological opinion. The Ideological Survey was devised to make possible objective measurement and evaluation of the outcomes of holding conflicting ideological positions as they may be related to mental illness.

In order to obtain a representative sampling of core ideas reflecting the extreme positions of capitalism vs. socialism, an ideological survey was made of public literature representing both philosophies. In particular, the authors made an ideological analysis of all the published writings of Ayn Rand and Nathaniel Branden, including *The Fountainhead, Atlas Shrugged, We the Living, For the New Intellectual, The Virtue of Selfishness,* and the complete back files of *The Objectivist* magazine through 1966.

Every sentence communicating an objectivist or socialist idea was transcribed on a separate card and filed until the search was completed. The cards were then classified and categorized as to the content and meaning communicated by each idea. Inventory items were constructed, utilizing Rand's words wherever possible or condensing the meaning to a form suitable for a true-false questionnaire item.

The collection of items was then evaluated in collaboration by both authors to include not only the most significant meanings but also all ideas having psychological or mental hygiene importance. In this way, the collection was cut down to the 200 potentially most significant ideas which became the basis for the IS.

The preliminary empirical classification of the discrete items into logical categories immediately resulted in the identification of clusters of ideas stemming from a core concept. The entire collection of ideas was thus classified into "core," "central," and "corollary" ideational units according to their primary (irreducible) or secondary (collateral) significance in an ideational constellation or cluster.

The basic concepts of the objectivist ideology were classified by us into the basic concepts of Nature, Reality, Life, Existence, Man, Feelings and Emotions, Mind, Reason, Concept Formations, Epistemology, Productivity, Economic Systems, Morality, and Mental Health. In each category, the objectivist viewpoint supported individualism, while the socialistic position reflected collectivism and state welfare philosophy. A brief summary of the core ideas of Rand's objectivist position as we selected them follows:

Nature and Reality: Reality is that which exists. Existence exists.
>   Law of Identity: *A* is *A*. A thing is itself.
>   Objective reality is the criterion of truth.
>   When faced by an apparent contradiction: Check your premises.

Existence and Life: Only one fundamental alternative in the universe: existence or nonexistence.
>   Full living must be earned by maximal effort.
>   The maintenance of life is not unconditional.
>   Life is a process of self-sustaining and self-generated action.
>   Full life is a value to be bought—thinking is the only coin noble enough to buy it.

Man: Man is a rational being, but rationality is a matter of choice.
>   Man has no automatic code of survival.
>   Man has to be man, hold his life as a value, learn to sustain it, to discover the values it requires, and to practice his virtues—by choice.

Mind and Reason: Mind exists. Consciousness exists.
>   Man is a being of volitional consciousness.
>   The more man develops his mind, the greater is the range of choices open to him.
>   Reason is the faculty that identifies and integrates the material provided by man's senses.
>   Rationality rests on the recognition of the fact that existence exists.
>   Rationality is a matter of choice: To think or not to think.
>   Reason is man's basic means of survival. Rationality is man's basic virtue from which all the others proceed.
>   Man's foremost moral obligation: The constant, clearest, fullest use of his rational faculty.
>   Reason is an absolute which permits no compromise.

Feelings and Emotions: Emotions are the automatic consequences and expressions of a man's estimate of that which furthers or threatens his life. The capacity for emotions is innate, but their content is determined by a man's values.
>   Happiness: The state of consciousness proceeding from the achievement of one's values: the successful state of life.
>   Anxiety is man's hidden dread of inability to deal with existence.
>   Neurotic fear stems from the knowledge and fact of a man's basic default, of suspending reason, of refusing to think. Guilt stems from knowing he has done it volitionally.

Morality: Code of basic values accepted by choice.
>   There is a morality of reason, proper to man; man's life is its standard of value.

FREDERICK C.
THORNE AND
VLADIMIR PISHKIN

All that is proper to the life of a rational being is good—all that destroys it is evil. A moral code must be defined for and not against man.

Highest moral purpose: The achievement of one's own happiness in accordance with a rational standard of value.

Self: The self-concept is the nucleus of ego functioning.

Self-esteem is man's highest value and basic psychological need. Self-esteem is the conviction that one is competent to live and worthy of living.

Man must strive to acquire values of character which make all his other achievements possible.

An individualist is a man who lives for his own sake and by his own mind, sacrificing neither himself to others nor others to himself.

Motivation: The achievement of one's happiness in accordance with one's *rational* self-interest is man's proper motive.

Sacrifice of the self or self-immolation is immoral.

Man is an end in himself and not the means to the ends of others.

Work and Property: Every man is the owner of his mind, his life, and his effort. Productivity creates wealth.

Rights are conditions of existence required by man's nature for his proper survival. There is only one fundamental right (all the others are its consequences or corollaries): A man's right to his own life. Rights cannot exist without the right to translate them into reality: The right of property.

Money is the material shape of the principle that men who wish to deal with one another must deal by trade and give value for value.

Trade is a moral symbol of respect for human beings: The trader is a man of justice who earns what he gets and does not give or take the undeserved.

If one renounces the material world, one surrenders it to evil.

Mental Health: Man's survival and mental health demand that he place nothing above his own rational judgment. The requirements of man's survival establish this need.

Mental health, depending on biologically appropriate mental functioning, requires unbreached cognitive contact with reality.

Mental health depends on a reality-oriented use of one's consciousness—unobstructed, integrated, fully utilized.

Irrationality involves a reversal of the cause-effect relationship of cognition and evaluation (reason and emotion), allowing emotions to determine thinking, action, and judgment.

No man can survive the moment of pronouncing himself irretrievably evil or a total failure—should he do it, his next moment is insanity or suicide.

Lack of self-esteem results in a neurotic state, with anxiety and guilt stemming from incompetence to deal with existence.

Valuing the opinions of others higher than objective reality results in a psychological syndrome in which a person holds the consciousness of other men as his ultimate epistemological frame of reference; desire for approval or popularity replaces objective appraisal of reality.

Incorrect premises are the basis for irrational actions.

Altruism holds the promise of that which is every neurotic's dream: A way to bypass reality.

Pseudo-self-esteem is a neurotic mechanism for evading reality and faking a self-value one does not possess. Pseudo-self-esteem is maintained by two means: Evading and repressing feelings and ideas that could affect self-appraisal adversely, and seeking to derive a sense of efficacy from something other than rationality.

Concessions to irrationality turn consciousnss from accurate perceptions of reality to the act of faking reality.

If you hold the irrational as your standard of value and the impossible as your concept of the good—if you long for rewards you have not earned, for a fortune or love you don't deserve—if you search for loopholes in the laws of causality and identity, for an *A* that becomes a non-*A* at your whim —then nothing but frustration and failure can result.

3.3.1. Sources of Illogical Thinking

The fallacy of the frozen abstraction: Substituting some one particular concrete for the wider abstract class to which it belongs.

The fallacy of the stolen concept: Using a concept, while ignoring, denying, or contradicting the antecedent concepts on which it logically depends. All knowledge and concepts have a hierarchical structure. When using concepts, one must recognize their genetic roots—what they logically depend on and presuppose.

The fallacy of self-exclusion: A theory whose claim to truth is incompatible with its own content.

The fallacy of hominem: Attempting to refute an argument by impeaching the character of an opponent.

3.3.2. Hypothetical Model Formulations

The ideological dichotomy represented by the Rand-Branden objectivist philosophy at one extreme and the collectivist position at the opposite extreme involves

Table 1

Objectivist (A)	Antithesis (B)
Firm knowledge and contact with reality.	Out of contact with reality.
Understands and applies the laws of identity and causality.	Ignores identity and causality or misinterprets them.
Dedicated to full living and getting the most out of existence.	Content with the status quo and following roads of least resistance.
Struggling for self-actualization; aggressively pursuing success.	Has largely given up on things.
Maximal use of reason and rational thinking; long-term goals.	Depending on wish fulfillments; short-term pleasures.
Fully focused consciousness; faces all problems directly.	Deliberately turns consciousness away from problems.
Dedicated to the truth and the highest effort at self-improvement	Evades the truth, which is often too painful; substitutes ulterior motives.
High self-esteem and self-concept.	Low self-esteem; low self-concept.
Motivated by rational self-interest.	Motivated by submission to others and altruism.
Productive and achieving.	Nonproductive and failing.
Recognizes property rights and respects the rights of others.	Expects something for nothing; unrealistic entitlements.
Check his premises to correct error.	Tries to overlook contradictions.
Authentic.	Phony.
The individualist.	The mindless follower.

some intriguing implications which can be incorporated in hypothetical models predicting the outcomes from basing actions on one ideological position or another. The hypothetical characterizations outlined in Table 1 stem from the dichotomy of ideological-attitudinal systems stemming from the objectivist position *(A)* and its antithesis *(B)*.

Rand's book *Atlas Shrugged* contains predictions concerning the personal and social consequences of actions based on the antithetical ideological positions of objectivist vs. collectivist philosophies. In our opinion, the scientific proof of the validity of either position depends on the actuarial outcomes of holding any particular ideological position in relation to mental health. The IS should provide an objective instrument for discovering who holds what ideological position, and for identifying relationships with important criterion variables of mental health and disorder.

3.3.3. Findings

The Ideological Survey (IS) was administered informally as opportunity presented by members of the Walter V. Clarke organization to seminar participants consisting of employees of client companies. The purposes of the test were not explained, and it was generally well accepted by the subjects, who regarded it as part of their training experiences. None of the subjects had received any familiarization with the Rand-Branden objectivist position, and, as far as the authors knew, none of the subjects knew anything about the purpose of this investigation.

The IS consists of 200 items sampling key ideas derived from the objectivist philosophy (individualism) vs. collectivism. The subjects were instructed to mark each item "true" if they agreed with it or "false" if they disagreed with it, or to omit the item if they could not answer. Participation was voluntary and no adverse reactions to the test were reported.

Varimax rotation was carried out until 50 factors were identified, including all with an eigenvalue of 1.0 or over. Five factors had a sufficient number of items loading over .30 to be meaningful. The remaining factors consisted of single items or small clusters reflecting more or less specific attitudes or ideas more characteristic of the normal group than of psychiatric patients. These will be reported later (Pishkin & Thorne, 1968).

Factor I. Fifty-one items on the IS loaded higher than .30 on this factor. Of the 20 items loading higher than .40, there is an almost equal division between purely ideological responses supporting rugged individualism and responses indicating high self-regard and morale. Although it might be argued that business executives are indoctrinated with capitalistic philosophical positions and tend to identify with management, the association of individualism with high self-sentiment and morale argues for both these factors as contributing to a positive mental health, high self-actualization factor. Depending on the semantic level of categorization. Factor I is defined as "Secure Individualism." It also reflects self-determinism and tendency for independent action.

Factor II. Twenty-four items load over .30 on this factor. Here again we note a cluster of purely ideological items of moralistic implication in association with a small cluster expressing concern over personal inadaptability. Thirteen of the items with the highest loadings endorse self-interest as a prime motive and reject what might be characterized as collectivist ideology. The remaining 11 items express concern over personal inefficiency. This factor is defined as "Egocentrism" and may also be seen as a factor representing high self-esteem.

Factor III.   Of the 15 items loading over .30, seven are concerned with personal adequacy and the remaining eight relate to ethics and morality. The underlying factor appears to be "Doing Right." The self-concern items express ethical concern conforming with conventional morality and equitable relationships with others.

Factor IV.   Of the nine items loading over .30, three clearly state concern about rational thinking and personal responsibility and the remaining items express a positivistic attitude toward the possibilities for self-determination. This is a "Self-Determination" factor characterized by self-assurance and confidence.

Factor V.   Eight items load over .30. These items relate to "Independent Self-Assertion" and reject "conforming to the powers that be for the sake of being popular and accepted." This factor specifically rejects the idea that collective good is the highest value, and places emphasis on objective evaluation of what is "good."

Taken together, the five significant factors extracted from our population of highly self-actualized business executives fall into a highly consistent picture of a person who (1) shows rugged individualism with high morale, (2) is motivated by rational self-interest, (3) is concerned about doing right, (4) is controlled by rational self-determination, and (5) is characterized by independent self-assertion. If the reader will refer back to an earlier paper describing the rationale of the construction of the IS (Thorne & Pishkin, 1968), a remarkable agreement will be noted between the theoretical postulations and the actual statistical factor analytic evidence. These findings may be regarded as providing an objective characterization of factors related to self-actualization, positive mental health, and high morale.

3.3.4. Follow-Up Study

A follow-up study investigated ideological composition in institutionalized psychiatric patients characterized by vocational inadaptability and general existential failure. Empirical experience indicates that inadaptable people tend to subscribe to defensive ideologies rationalizing their failures. In particular, the Rand-Branden objectivist position postulates an ideological characteristic of "The Disabled Man" as cited in an earlier paper describing the rationale of construction of the IS.

The subjects were 408 male white psychiatric patients from three Veterans Administration hospitals (Tuskegee, Alabama; Little Rock, Arkansas; and Oklahoma City, Oklahoma). The range in education was from eighth grade to 4 years of college, mean 11.34 years. The subjects were between 28 and 52 years of age, mean 38.6 years. All were volunteers and were instructed that the IS was administered as a part of the overall testing procedure. All were diagnosed as having schizophrenic reactions of different types.

Five meaningful patient factors were extracted composed of items with loadings higher than .30. In addition, a large number of single items and small clusters appeared on which the patient group responded significantly differently from normals.

FREDERICK C.
THORNE AND
VLADIMIR PISHKIN

Patient Factor I.   This factor may be characterized as the "Dependency" factor. This is a very general factor, with 104 items out of 200 loading higher than .30; of these, 21 items loaded higher than .50. Of the 104 items, 45 are identical in content but opposite in sign with the items composing Normals Factor I reported in the companion study of ideological responses in business executives. Patient Factor I clearly is the bipolar opposite of Normals Factor I. Once again, this factor comprises two groups of items expressing existential failure and demoralization and a defeatist ideology. It should be noted that where both groups react to Factor I items the loadings of the patients tend to be slightly higher but not significantly so. Analyzing the additional items with patient loadings on Factor I greater than .30, and which are not represented in Normals Factor I, the patients show a very broad deterioration of morale. Paradóxically, many patients still express individualistic sentiments (ego ideals) in juxtaposition with many expressions of defeat and inadequacy. The additional elements shown by the patients included a wider ideological position, more dependence on religion ("My life belongs to God" and "Religion is the highest authority"), more expressions of conformity to gain acceptance and popularity, more expressions of feelings of personal inadequacy, more expressions of vocational inadaptability (work boring, behind in work, loses too much time off, and thinks work rut bad), and cynical toward life (others have all the luck, what people don't know won't hurt them, every man has his price, never had a chance in life, recommends "buck-passing," some are licked before they start, you have to be a good "operator," the little man hasn't got a chance). Patient Factor I also appears to reflect the frustrated demoralization leading to dependency. The overwhelming emphasis is on failure and disillusionment. The patients perceive capitalism and management as exploiting the workers, who must band together for protection and mutual support. There are strong indications by this group of endorsing good as what is right for society, altruism as the highest principle, and guaranteed social security for all.

Patient Factor II.   This factor has the characteristics of "Low Self-Esteem." Nine of 26 items loading higher than .30 on Patient Factor II are also found on Normals Factor II. All of these nine items refer to self-critical attitudes. Of the remaining items of Normals Factor II not found on Patient Factor II, the majority relate to altruism, including rejection of "My life belongs to God," religion the highest authority, altruism the highest value, blessed are the meek and humble. This indicates the strongly individualistic factor running through the items of Normals Factor II, with rejection of the collectivist ideology. Of the items on Patient Factor II not identical with Normals Factor II, almost all relate to feelings of personal inefficiency which must reflect low self-concept. Patients Factor II may also be interpreted as an inferiority complex factor.

Patient Factor III.   Only two items (126 and 196) are found also on Normals Factor III. This factor is difficult to interpret except that three of the four items with the highest positive loadings reflect the "Desire to be of Service" by the psychiatric patients, while most of the remainder reflect regret over not having done better.

Patient Factor IV.   This factor is related to Normals Factor IV, which involves rational self-determination. Patient Factor IV involves expression of some of the same ideals of self-determination and is considered a "Self-Serving Expediency" factor. Items 83 and 185 justify the need for stretching the truth, while item 46 endorses the idea that moral perfection is impossible to man.

Patient Factor V.   Patient Factor V appears to be essentially comparable to Normals Factor V, and represents "Social Compromise." With patients, this factor seems to represent character disorder aspects of psychopathology, while for normals it taps assessment of one's role in society.

Comparing Normals Factor I with Patients Factor I as to item composition, it is obvious that we are dealing largely with a bipolar factor involving secure individualism (morale) vs. frustrated demoralization (dependency) at the extremes; however, Patient Factor I is much more generalized and diffuse in its contribution and may be regarded as a superfactor. It is significant that the first 21 items with loading over .50 on Patient Factor I all express ideological contents reflecting defensive demoralization. This ideology not only might have been predicted from the Rand-Branden model but also reflects the frustrated complaints commonly heard from lower laboring classes.

In contrast, Normals Factor I shows not only a smaller number of items and lower loadings but also a less solid ideological composition, with six out of the first 20 items reflecting attitudes toward the self rather than an ideological system. Apparently, normal secure individualism is a much more limited and narrow factor than frustrated demoralization leading to dependency.

Patient Factor II, which we have labeled "Low Self-Esteem," consists of many items which alternatively might be interpreted as reflecting poor self-control in many areas. Twenty-four of the 26 items reflect ineffectuality and failure in managing the business of life with reasonable prudence; i.e., the person is out of control and recognizes it.

It will require further developmental research to determine whether the defensive collectivist ideology expressed by this frustrated and dependent schizophrenic population is a primary cause of, or a secondary reaction to, the pervasive existential failure which characterizes the group.

3.4. The Femininity Study

The Femininity Study (FS) was constructed in 1968 after pilot studies with the Sex Inventory (Female Form) had indicated that the latter test was not measuring sexuality in females with the same reliability and validity as the Sex Inventory (Male Form) has measured sexuality in males. Not only were females markedly more reluctant to answer obvious-direct items that concerned sexuality than were males, but it also became apparent that female sexuality is much more complexly determined psychosocially than is male sexuality.

It also became apparent that women had special problems related to the self-concept, feelings of personal worth, inadequacies in role playing, and other existential problems. The Women's Lib movement not only succeeded in uncovering the special predicament of women in a male world but also began to exert strong influences on changing women's attitudes toward femininity and problems of sex discrimination. Large differences in the stereotyped patterns of male vs. female roles in life, as well as the biological implications of reproductive functions in females, rendered it necessary to adopt a much more complicated strategy for the measurement of typically feminine behaviors. Therefore, The FS was developed to measure more than simply female sexuality and to measure important domains of femininity in many other areas.

Accordingly, the FS was constructed to measure objectively many aspects of the feminine self-concept, female role playing, and attitudes not systematically sampled in earlier tests. Wide sex differences appear not only culturally but also individually at different temporal periods. It is postulated that the state of evolution of the feminine role components of the self-concept develops progressively from rudimentary levels in early life.

It may be assumed that sexuality is primarily a state phenomenon, with change and individual differences as the main attributes. It is necessary to study changes in the status of femininity in special clinical groups successively and separately across time. It cannot be assumed that any special group inevitably will reflect overall statistical factors across time. The status of femininity in any special group can be followed only by repeated measurements of its development across time. Within the biological trait limits of maleness and femaleness, femininity actually exists primarily as states.

3.4.1. The Issue of Masculinity vs. Femininity

The concept of femininity as unipolar rather than bipolar automatically rules out many of the theoretical issues that have beclouded bipolar theory. The Femininity Study was constructed as a unipolar measuring instrument that is not concerned primarily with the differentiation of masculine vs. feminine response tendencies but rather with differences across time between females with different demographic characteristics. The research literature generally has demonstrated the difficulty in constructing items that differentiate between males and females except those in the areas of interests and motivations. Where such differentiating items exist, clinical significance attaches to males with female interests and females with male interests, and related problems of sexual differentiation and inversion.

Rather than becoming concerned with male vs. female differences, our preliminary studies with the FS had been directed primarily toward the normative data and base rates for different groups of females. This objective can be approached by different methods. Sannito, Walker, Foley, and Posavec (1972) attempted to arrive at typically feminine response tendencies by having a group of ten clinical psychologists judge each test item as to feminine response directions, disregarding items that could not be so classified as typically feminine responses. This approach involves the dangers of forcing the data into preconceived categories and disregards natural base rates. Another difficulty with having judges evaluate the femininity of individual items is that different groups of judges may rate items differently.

Of ten judges who rated the direction of responses to each item as typically feminine or unfeminine in the Sannito et al. study (1972), ten of ten judges agreed on the most feminine scoring for 75 (37.5%) items, nine of ten judges agreed on the scoring of 42 (21%) items, eight of ten judges agreed on the scoring of 32 (16%) items, seven of ten judges agreed on the scoring of 24 items (12%), six of ten judges agreed on the scoring of 15 (7.5%) items, while on the remaining 12 (6%) items only five of ten judges agreed on the scoring. The amount of agreement on the most "feminine" scoring direction is considered remarkably high in view of the fact that many items referred to clinically significant although sexually nonspecific behaviors that could be shown by either sex.

3.4.2. Item Construction

In accordance with the strategy (Thorne, 1976a) developed in the construction of other state tests, obvious-direct items were used throughout the FS on the theory that subjects tend to perceive less ambiguity in items with clear manifest content. Younger, "enlightened" generations appear to be much less inhibited in responding in sensitive areas and tend to respond very frankly to items that might appear to have derogatory content. The internal consistency of item responding, particularly in sensitive areas in which subjects may be admitting negative characteristics, tends to confirm the validity of accepting the item responses at face value in most cases.

Obvious-direct items also appear to be indicated when one is dealing with state phenomena, where it is necessary to make specific references in order to obtain specific answers. Preliminary studies indicated that subtle-indirect items tend to be more ambiguous; when the subject does not perceive supposed meanings clearly, there is a tendency to respond with response sets such as social desirability or acquiescence. The intention is to state items unambiguously enough so that the subject easily understands their intended meanings and can respond validly either in terms of present states or in memories of past states experienced.

The FS items were constructed without any preconceptions with regard to normative feminine response tendencies. It was intended that normative rates would be established empirically by the actual base rates of different clinical groups with differing demographic characteristics. Whether any item would be retained in factored scales would be a function of base rate differentiating power among different groups.

The test items were constructed from actual verbatim comments or responses made by women who were being studied for sex-role adjustment problems. The major consideration was to construct items that sampled clinically significant behaviors. Even though some behaviors may be nonspecific sexually, it is assumed that different male vs. female sex-role requirements may place different clinical weightings on the same responses at different times and places. For example, item 124, "Occasionally, children frustrate me so much I could scream," was not rated by ten judges as typically "feminine." However, such a response from a female was judged clinically significant in relation to the female parent role because women normally associate more closely with children than do males.

It was postulated that female sexuality states could be measured on the basis of face validity items designed to tap 11 areas of female adjustment: social role, parent role, career role, homemaker role, role confidence, sex identification, development and maturation, sex drive and interests, promiscuity, homosexuality, and health and neurotic conflict. One of the basic issues was to determine whether factor analyses could demonstrate validity in relation to feminine states of specific groups of female populations. The findings are reported for research purposes only and are not intended as measures of predictable traits or personality structures, because psychological states are in constant change across groups.

Five main factors were extracted, and interpretations are based operationally on the content of the highest-loaded items and the finding of clusters of items with common obvious meanings (Pishkin & Thorne, 1977b).

Factor I. Heterosexual Social Role Inadaptability. Nine of the ten highest-loaded items refer specifically to difficulties in attracting and holding the attentions of men, too few dates, inability to compete for men with other females, etc. These women feel lonely and socially uneasy.

Factor II. Parental Role Inadaptability.   The highest-loaded items reflect lack of confidence and success in child management. These women also express anxiety over all social relationships. Insecurity in heterosexual contacts also is reported.

Factor III. Homemaker Role Inadaptability.   The four highest-loaded items all express dislike for homemaking roles and for household dirty work. A career is preferred over marriage, and severe menstrual cramps are experienced.

Factor IV. General Affective Instability.   The highest-loaded items indicate emotional instability and/or psychosomatic symptoms.

Factor V. Maternal Role Inadaptability.   Items express frustration and conflict over children and their management as well as homosexual tendencies and conflicts.

Perhaps the most significant findings derived from the factoring of item responses from all the diagnostic groups combined as a general population are the high base rates of felt inadequacy and inadaptability across all groups. In general, the base rates suggest a continuum from the presumably most normal college females through the alcoholic women to the institutionalized schizophrenic group. Although the institutionalized women consistently show much great inadaptability in all domains, as many as 50% of the college females report affective instability secondary to heterosexual, maternal, parental, and homemaker inadaptability. The methodology of this study does not permit the analysis of hen-egg problems related to whether the affective instability or the role inadaptabilities are primary or secondary. It may be assumed that all kinds of psychodynamics are operating in such varied populations.

Interpreted according to the theory of integrative psychology that underlies the organization of various clinically significant psychological states, it appears that patterns of defective integration and/or disintegration occur in many combinations and permutations in constant change across time. Integration theory postulates an almost infinite variety of integration deficits, and our data tend to confirm the universalities of such inadaptabilities.

Disregarding the fact that Diagnostic Code 8 consisted of institutionalized women diagnosed as schizophrenic, and instead simply classifying them as cases of most global disintegration, whereas the alcholic women may be considered as more integrated, and the college females as most integrated, the factorial results do succeed in identifying various patterns of inadaptability that occur against a more general background of imperfect integrations.

The base rate results seem to indicate that American women have extensive "hangups" in the areas of heterosexual social roles, maternal roles, parental roles, and homemaker roles, together with general affective instability and psychosomatic symptoms that exist as secondary reactions. In other words, the average female in our culture has important interpersonal relationship problems, particularly with the opposite sex and with children. Sex is the great problem, either because an adjustment has not been achieved yet or because it has failed. There are large problems in role-playing adaptability, particularly as sex partner, mother, parent, and homemaker. In the terms of integrative psychology, large numbers of females either are failing or have failed in "putting it all together," in "getting on the ball," or in integrating all necessary factors required for competent functioning in many aspects of managing the business of life.

Why such inadaptabilities have developed is a matter for study in subsequent research on developmental and etiological relationships. What we have demonstrated here is that such problems do exist in large sectors across populations.

3.5. Sexuality in Adult Males

The objective measurement of sexuality presents difficult technical problems due to the delicate nature of the issues involved and the question of obtaining truthful answers as far as the subject can consciously report his sexual feelings. Because of the influence of Freudian theories of the repression of sexuality, most measurement attempts have utilized indirect projective approaches. However, long clinical experience with instruments such as the MMPI indicates the difficulty of constructing projective items which can be established as valid measures of sexuality.

3.5.1. Study

Because pilot studies conducted by us had indicated the relative invalidity and unproductivity of subtle-indirect, projective-type items in the study of adult male sexuality, and also because the Kinsey studies had indicated the feasibility of using obvious-direct questions, this study utilized a very obvious-direct approach in proposing questions concerning the most intimate aspects of sexuality. It is hypothesized that, in the 1960s in the United States, taboos against the frank discussion of sexuality in all classes of the population lessened to the point where truthful replies may be obtained using direct methods.

The subject consisted of adult males, including students at the University of Miami, inmates of the California Rehabilitation Center at Corona with addiction problems, and convicted felons of all types from the North Carolina State Hospital.

The Sex Inventory was administered by the group method, using the standard instructions printed at the top of the answer sheet by clinical psychologists at each of the cooperating institutions. The subjects were advised that they could give or omit their names as they saw fit and that in no case would any of the results be used against them. Records which were obviously invalid because of large numbers of incomplete items or inability to complete the test were discarded.

The Sex Inventory (Thorne, 1966) consists of 40 subtle-indirect and 160 obvious-direct items relating to all aspects of sexuality. Pilot studies performed with large samples of comparable subjects using earlier forms of the inventory indicated that the items were largely intelligible to subjects with 8 years of education and that most subjects were responding frankly and with internal consistency of answers. The items are stated in basic English, and few subjects required help in completing the records.

3.5.2. Statistical Analysis

A special program for factoring a 190×190 item matrix was written by Dean Clyde and Richard J. Sherin of the Biometric Laboratory, University of Miami, and run on the IBM 7040. This program involved computing product moment coefficients equivalent to ϕ coefficients and allowing for missing data, computing principal components with unities in the diagonals, and using a normalized varimax rotation.

Varimax rotation was carried out until 50 factors were identified, of which eight factors had a sufficient number of items with loadings over .30 to be meaningful. Analysis of the percentages of variance contributed the various factors indicated the great heterogeneity of factors sampled by the Sex Inventory.

Factor I. Sex Drive and Interest.   The largest single factor extracted was labeled "Sex Drive and Interest" (Factor I) because of the breadth of positive interests and attitudes expressed toward a wide variety of expressions of sexuality. Thirty items of the Sex Inventory showed loadings over .25 on this factor. Analysis of the content of these items reveals that sex drive manifests itself in a wide variety of interests and forms of expression. The high internal consistency of the items making up this factor indicates the validity of obvious-direct items sampling an area as delicate as sexuality.

Factor II. Sexual Frustration and Maladjustment.   Factor II, representing 3.37% of the variance, was labeled "Sex Frustration and Maladjustment" because the items are consistent in reflecting dissatisfaction with sex life, feelings of deprivation, difficulties with the opposite sex, guilt and worry over sex, and fears about sex impulse control. It is interesting that 36% of the entire group expressed a desire to see a psychiatrist in this connection. Close to 40% of the entire group ($N = 545$) admit to serious problems in securing outlets for sexuality or in expressing it. These findings in general support Kinsey's results concerning the incidence of sexual frustration and maladjustment among males.

Factor III. Neurotic Conflict Associated with Sex.   Factor III contributed the third highest percentage of variance (3.42%) represented by a large number of symptoms of anxiety, guilt, depression, nervousness, irritability, psychosomatic conditions, impulsiveness, and paranoid projections. In contrast to Factor II, where all the items were more or less directly connected with sex problems and involved direct references to sexuality, the items reflecting Factor III are characterized by more generalized neurotic conflict and symptomatology. Perhaps Factor II represents a condition in which disturbance is exactly represented in consciousness with no repression of causes, while Factor III reflects typical psychoanalytic repression mechanisms resulting in neurosis. Again, attention should be drawn to the high percentages of subjects admitting problem behaviors and the resulting conflicts.

Factor IV. Sexual Fixations and Cathexes.   An attempt was made during construction of the Sex Inventory to include items sampling a wide variety of sex cathexes. The percentages of variance contributed by all of these items was low, and no items were highly correlated enough to justify any kind of a scale. It appears that sexual conditioning and cathexes are highly specific and must be treated individually. We have not attempted to construct any kind of a scale representing these items, and it is suggested that positive responses to the more deviant items constitute indications for more intensive clinical investigations.

Factor V. Repression of Sexuality.   Factor V, contributing 1.05% of variance, consists of two clusters of items. The first cluster has been identified as a factor of repression because it involves items expressing difficulties of expressing sexuality, disapproval of sex activities, repressive attitudes, and regression desires. The second cluster involves conservative and reactionary attitudes toward sex, including approval of chastity, disapproval of uncontrolled sexuality, and suppression of socializing with outgroups. It is interesting that this latter cluster includes an item, denying ever having had a sex climax, indicating that the conservative-repressive attitudes have been carried out in action.

Factor VI. Loss of Sex Controls.   The Sex Inventory was deliberately constructed to include a number of obvious-direct items referring specifically to symptoms related to poor impulse control and tendencies to act out dangerously. The first nine items had loadings over .20 and, together, reflect a syndrome of imminent breakdown of sex controls. It is significant that the incidences of significant responses to these items in the total sample of 545 cases ranged from 5% expressing a need to be institutionalized for protection against sex impulses to 36% expressing a need to see a psychiatrist. Although our population is admittedly skewed, including an atypical number of confirmed sex deviants, it speaks well for the validity of the Sex Inventory that these trends show up on an objective questionnaire. Incidentally, a sufficient number of normal college students also admitted problems of sex control to indicate the generality of the factor in the general population. The items in the second group did not load highly on Factor VI but did load highly on other scales and are included because clinical judgment indicates their importance as indices of lowered impulse control. These items include three (8, 120, and 196) loading highly on sex frustration and maladjustment, two (7 and 65) loading highly on neurotic conflict, and two (24 and 139) representing the socially dangerous cathexes of child molestation and indecent exposure. The items of Factor VI are all designated as "Stop" items, potentially indicative or pathognomonic of breakdown of impulse controls. It is intended that these Stop items should serve as a positive indication that the person is potentially dangerous sexually and should be subjected to further intensive clinical investigation. Persons admitting one or more of these signs should be committed for further observation or should be retained in an institution until such signs clear up.

Factor VII. Homosexuality.   Factor VII involves 1.86% of the variance and includes two clusters of items whose existence and relationships had not been predicted during construction of the Sex Inventory but which logically enough represent inverse facets of the condition. The first cluster consists of a number of homosexual signs expressing preference for the same sex and unease with the opposite sex. This combination of preference for one's own sex and nervousness with the opposite sex is probably to be regarded as pathognomonic of homosexuality. It is again significant that obvious-direct items are the most highly loaded on this factor, with only one projective item (23) being loaded highly enough to be included. The second cluster of items, involving denial of homosexuality, may be regarded as eliminating homosexuality by exclusion. This cluster of items reflects the claim of normality in that being a "queer" or attracted to one's own sex is denied as well as preference for the same sex or perverted thoughts. These people do not understand homosexuality and deny that it is normal. It may well be that the failure to claim normality is by implication a sign of homosexuality.

Factor IX. Promiscuity and Sociopathy. Factor IX includes four clusters of items which are interpreted clinically as reflecting a range of amoral and sociopathic tendencies. The first cluster reflects liberal-radical attitudes toward sexuality which may lead to promiscuity or amoral behavior. The second cluster of items reflects three clusters involving extreme degrees of illegitimacy and promiscuity. Here again these items are internally consistent and probably reflect low superego functioning.

The implications of this study are somewhat curtailed by the unrepresentative nature of the population studied. When study of the Sex Inventory first began in 1961, it was planned to obtain a representative population sample and clinical groups of various types of sex delinquents equated on the demographic variables of age, education, socioeconomic level, race, and religion. Unfortunately, within the limits of the private resources with which this investigation was conducted during the first 5 years, it proved impossible to locate and secure the cooperation of all segments of the population. Strong biases against the overt study of sexuality still exist, and the only institutions where large-scale cooperation was obtained were prisons and corrective institutions.

The research design was adopted of using general prisoners (felons convicted of property crimes such as breaking and entering, burglary, forgery, and auto theft) as controls for sex criminals (aggravated sex, rape, indecent exposure, and homosexuality). There is evidence that the general prison population is comparable in many demographic variables with the special groups of sex offenders. A third prison group, differentiated on the basis of earlier unpublished studies which showed atypical patterns of sexuality, consisted of felons convicted of crimes involving physical violence against persons including assault and battery, manslaughter, and homicide. To represent high levels of intelligence and socioeconomic status, the college group was added to the various prison groups. Finally, the group of convicted drug addicts was included as partially representative of adolescents in rebellion against conventional society.

The very heterogeneous composition of the population under study provided an extremely rigorous test for the factorial research design. Pilot studies showed that different clinical groups were answering most of the items of the Sex Inventory in opposite ways depending on their different backgrounds and ideological-attitudinal composition. The fact that such a large amount of contradictory responding existed among the widely heterogeneous groups undoubtedly lowered the level of correlations and loadings of items and factors. However, because such a large number of clear-cut factors were extracted and in view of the relatively low percentage of variance contributed by the principal factors, it may be concluded that factorial validity has been established.

The general reliability and validity of the use of obvious-direct items for the study of sexuality are supported by the general consistency of individual responding on the inventory and the logical consistency of the factors extracted. Test-retest reliability studies showed satisfactory intraclass correlations. A much more severe test is provided by factoring a 190×190 item matrix with consistent results.

3.6. The Personal Development Study

The Personal Development Study (PDS) is one of the eight subtests of the Integration Level Test Series which objectively measures different hierarchical levels of factors organizing the integration of psychological states. One of the original purposes of the ILTS was to investigate the contributions of the major systems of psychology in the causations of behavior. The Freudian metapsychology postulates the operation of various mechanisms in the unconscious determination of mental life. The PDS consists of a 200-item questionnaire involving ten scales of 20 items, each constructed empirically to measure ten Freudian mechanisms. It was hypothesized that if unconscious mechanisms actually do organize all psychological states, then statistical factor analyses should identify important mechanisms underlying a wide variety of items.

Perhaps the most thoroughgoing application of Freudian theory has been in projective psychology, which postulates the operation of Freudian mechanisms both in the dynamics of everyday life and in psychopathology. Projective psychology plays down the significance of the manifest contents of behavior and instead seeks to discover the latent operations of Freudian mechanisms.

In the grand research design (Thorne, 1976a,) which proposed a series of objective measurements covering a wide spectrum of possible etiological factors as represented by the major schools of psychology, a battery of eight tests called Integration Level Test Series was constructed which would include the classical Freudian mechanisms. Accordingly, a 200-item questionnaire was devised entitled the Personal Development Study (Thorne, 1965) to discover whether Freudian mechanisms were operating across a wide variety of behaviors and could be measured validly. The purpose was to discover what mechanisms are operating and in what patterns in different clinical groups. Additionally, Rosenzweig's (1947) mechanisms of extrapunitiveness, intropunitiveness, and impunitiveness also were included as a further test of the projective principle.

Factorial structure of the PDS was accomplished in a 200-item questionnaire empirically constructed of ten scales purportedly measuring classical Freudian mechanisms, together with Rosenzweig's (1947) extrapunitive, intropunitive, and impunitive modes of obstacle dominance. The basic issue is whether such constructs have factorial validity and can be measured objectively using self-ratings.

Subjects were administered the PDS in groups of different sizes, depending on the installation, using standard instructions as printed on the sheets as part of the ILTS battery. All subjects were advised that the tests would in no way affect their status and that participation was completely voluntary.

The statistical analysis consisted of making an item analysis across all groups, followed by a principal component factor analysis of the overall data of all groups combined and of each group separately with varimax rotation.

3.6.1. Factored Scales

Five factors were extracted from the total group data. This general finding indicates that only a small amount of the variance was accounted for by the five factors (Pishkin & Thorne, 1977b).

Factor I. Projection.   Twelve of the 20 items came from PDS Empirical Scale III labeled "Projection," and the content of these items is consistent with the generally understood intepretation of this label. Psychiatrically, it is important to differentiate reality-based feelings of being treated poorly from paranoid projections of persecution which have no reality basis. In this connection, items express existential anxiety over not having been too successful in life, which may have some reality basis. Our interpretation is that the main cluster reflects paranoid projections, and the smaller cluster may reflect realistic feelings of being rejected and treated poorly.

Factor II. Optimism-Responsibility.   This factor was difficult to interpret. Nine items came from Empirical Scale X (Impunitiveness), six items came from Empirical Scale VIII (Extrapunitiveness), and three items came from Scale IX (Intropunitiveness). On the other hand, the content of 11 items expresses an optimistic, almost Pollyannaish, world view that good always triumphs. Eight items express ideas that right is right, that there are proper ways to do things, that people make their own problems, and that deserved punishments should be meted out. These two clusters caused the factor to be labeled "Optimism-Responsibility." However, the larger cluster could also be interpreted as "Repression-Suppression" and the smaller cluster as "Extrapunitiveness." This factor is also seen as having pronounced superego qualities.

Factor III. Reaction and Symptom Formation.   This factor also is difficult to interpret. Four items each came from the Empirical Extrapunitive, Intropunitive, and Reaction Formation Scales, and three items from the Symptom Formation Scale. However, interpreted in terms of item content, four items reflect Jungle Rule aggressiveness, four items suggest withdrawal, four items reflect sensitive criticality, and three items suggest sublimation. In general, this appears to be a defensiveness factor, but wide base rate differences between groups indicate that different groups are using different defenses. The college students tend to be least defensive and the institutionalized schizophrenics most defensive. This factor appears to be measuring different things in different groups, as evidenced by wide differences in endorsement rates across groups.

Factor IV. Repressive-Compulsive.   This is another factor difficult to interpret. Six items came from the Empirical Reaction Formation Scale, five items from Empirical Scale I (Repression), four items from Scale VIII (Extrapunitiveness), and three items from Scale IV (Identification). Examining loadings and item contents, five items refer to repression/suppression, along with three items referring to religious beliefs. Three small clusters refer to bringing out the best in people, doing what's correct or right, and neatness. This apparently is a repression/suppression factor which might also be labeled "high superego" in Freudian terms but which also reflects high social desirability acquired by training as an alternative explanation.

Factor V. Intropunitiveness-Guilt.   Nine items came from Empirical Scale IX (Intropunitiveness), four items came from Scale II (Regression) expressing fixation and dependency, and three items came from Scale VI (Symptom Formation). Content analyses supported these interpretations. Since all 20 items have negative loadings indicating an overall group denial of these tendencies, large intergroup differences in base rate responding indicate different existential connotations of such responding. Because the college students have done better in life, they can afford to deny self-blame and guilt. Conversely, the alcoholics and schizophrenics have failed more and have more to feel guilty about. Low percentage of "true" responses implies healthy ways of responding, because the factor loadings are negative.

3.6.2.   Group Differences in Base Rate Responding

Comparison of the percentages of each diagnostic group responding "true" to each item reveals marked differences between groups. In general, the college students of Group 7 set base rates for normal responding. The alcoholics and the unmarried mothers reveal more pathological reactions, both qualitatively and quantitatively, than the college students, but still must be regarded as within the normal range. The institutionalized schizophrenics of Group 8 lie at the opposite end of the continuum, consistently showing more and greater pathological responding.

Although the base rate data were collected primarily to reflect important group differences, they also provide important information concerning pathological trends in the overall population. Examination of results indicate that, with the exception of Factor I, on which the college group often rates very low, most items reflect relatively high pathological tendencies across the whole population. Rather than dichotomous splits, the results indicate a continuum of levels of integration across groups.

It is evident that the different populations reflect many permutations and combinations of strong and weak factors, in changing patterns across time and with various mixtures of clusters (factors). Hence we do not regard the factors as representing fixed psychological traits or personality structures but only as reflecting psychological states in constant change, and not necessarily occurring at any particular time. The relationships are so complex, and hen-egg problems so common, that it is not possible to make definitive statements which have any wide applicability. On the whole, extensive use of scatter diagrams failed to reveal any consistent trends representing Freudian standard mechanisms, as postulated in the first PDS paper (Pishkin & Thorne, 1977c).

In reporting the five main overall factors in this study, we have mentioned the difficulties in interpreting and naming several factors. Instead of making inferences concerning the nature of the factors, we have rejected theorizing in favor of an operational statement of the item contents in relation to generally accepted clinical meanings. This approach avoids getting mired in purely theoretical speculations and semantic morasses in attempting to translate or equate concepts from many different theoretical positions. It became obvious from surveying the raw item data that the same factor could have many item expressions and that the same items could refer to several factors. Also, the same item responses often could be given different theoretical interpretations and might even vary in significance in different contexts. Therefore, it seems safer to eschew all theorizing and simply present the data.

In our opinion, integration theory can simplify the interpretive problem greatly. Since all raw behaviors can be considered to be more or less unified (self-consistent) integrates, the clinical problem becomes one of trying to discover what factors organize any particular integrative pattern. Instead of becoming entangled in all sorts of theoretical abstractions such as the concepts of learning, perception, concept formation, and Freudian mechanisms, it is much simpler and more valid to regard all factors as involving various integrational dynamics. In brief, large differences between the empirical and the factored scales were found in this study, suggesting that Freudian interpretations are too simplistic. Cluster analyses of items across scales indicated various permutations and combinations of items highly loaded on factors. The factors are interpreted in terms of integration theory.

3.7. The Personal Health Survey

The Personal Health Survey (PHS) (Thorne & Pishkin, 1978) is a 200-item objective questionnaire sampling the psychosomatic supports of psychological states, including general health, general development, gastrointestinal system, cardio-vascular system, miscellaneous (genitourinary, respiratory, endocrine, skin) systems,

FREDERICK C.
THORNE AND
VLADIMIR PISHKIN

central nervous system, neuromuscular system, anxiety-fear states, anger-frustration states, schizophrenia, affective psychoses, and character disorders.

Positive mental health depends on general physical health and development, normal functionings of psychophysiological supporting systems, healthy psychosomatic relationships, and the absence of psychoses, neuroses, and character disorders. The 200 PHS items are divided into 12 scales constructed to measure conditions potentially disintegrating normal functionings.

The PHS originally was constructed of 12 scales consisting of characteristic symptoms of physiological supporting organ systems, together with affective, cognitive, and conative mental syndromes. Theoretically, at least, there should be high convergent/construct validity between empirically and statistically derived factors relating to health syndromes. It is important to ascertain the base rates of incidence of various types of disorders in different age, sex, socioeconomic, educational, and clinical groups, because it is first necessary to demonstrate the actual existence of disease and disorder in any particular group before attempting to study its factorial structure.

There is also the issue of attempting to differentiate between nonspecific symptoms and signs and those which are specific or pathognomonic. Symptom patterns may vary widely across time and conditions (states).

Subjects were administered the PHS using standard written instructions in groups of different sizes depending on local conditions. Usually, the test was given as a part of the ILTS battery except in isolated cases where the test was administered singly. All subjects were advised that the testing would in no way affect their status, and that it was completely voluntary.

The statistical procedure consisted of an item analysis of the percentages of diagnostic groups answering each item false, followed by a principal component factor analysis of the overall data of all groups combined with varimax rotation. The rotated factors were orthogonal (Thorne & Pishkin, 1978).

3.7.1. Factored Scales

Five main factors were extracted from the total group data. The relatively small percentage of variance accounted for implies that no large general or secondary factors could be extracted from the data, which were complexly determined.

Factor I. Autonomic Instability. The most highly loaded items, all with loadings higher than .40, relate to psychosomatic symptoms and/or hypochondriasis with underlying autonomic instability. In the relatively young diagnostic groups under study here, the incidence of such symptoms was relatively low because of their general good health. Nevertheless, as high as 50% of the various groups reported such complaints. When the diagnostic groups were arranged as to incidence of complaints, the unmarried mothers and alcoholics had most complaints and the felons and college students least.

Factor II. Sociopathic Exploitive Life-Style. This factor showed the highest congruent/construct validity, with ten out of 12 items with loadings above .30 having been included in the original empirically constructed character disorder scale. Referring to the comparative percentages of the various diagnostic groups responding "true" to the items of this scale, two distinct types emerge. The felons have the highest incidence of admission of such symptoms, followed by the alcoholics. In contrast, the unmarried mothers and college students deny such symptoms. The emergence of this factor is considered to validate Thorne's concept of the sociopath as involving an exploitive life-style disorder.

Factor III. Normal Mental Status. Most of the items in this scale involve denials of mental symptoms of affective and cognitive disorders. In rank order of admission of having such symptoms, the schizophrenics rate highest, followed by the unmarried mothers and alcoholics, with the felons and college students claiming relative mental normality.

Factor IV. Stress Pattern. This factor was relatively difficult to interpret because of (1) the relatively uniform patterns of responding across groups, (2) the general denial of such complaints in the clinical diagnostic groups, and (3) the relatively high incidence of admission of such complaints in the college students. Most of the items can be interpreted as referring to the symptoms of pressure and stress. The alcoholics show the highest incidences of such symptoms, followed by the college students and unmarried mothers, with the felon group largely denying such symptoms.

Factor V. Denial of Psychosis. The relatively high and uniform denial of psychotic symptoms across Groups 2, 7, 6, and 3 indicates very low base rates of psychosis for these populations. About 20% of the alcoholics fear a mental breakdown.

The PHS samples physical and mental symptoms having probable relationships to positive mental health, which is presumed to depend on general physical health and development, normal functionings of supporting organ systems, healthy psychosomatic relationships, and the absence of global psychic disintegrations (psychoses), partial disintegrations (psychoneuroses), or negative integrations (character disorders). Actually, it requires relatively aged populations who have lived long enough to develop physical and mental disabilities to provide a proper test for this type of inventory. Where a disease (disorder) has a relatively low incidence even within the most susceptible age groups, it may show basically negative findings in younger age groups currently under study.

Nevertheless, it should be instructive to discover what patterns appear with items which are basically not relevant to the age group. The first finding is that, in relation to the overall factor structure, the factoring of special groups shows much lower comparability of factors across groups and the appearance of many more subfactors specific to special groups. A scatter diagram was constructed with the overall factors on the Y axis, and the 20 factors of Diagnostic Groups 2, 3, 6, and 7 on the X axis, with the following results:

Overall Factor I, Autonomic Instability, had four items identical with Factor II, Group 2; four items identical with Factor II, Group 3; five items identical with Factor II, Group 6; and four items identical with Factor I, Group 7. These findings indicate a weak or low comparability of a psychosomatic factor across all groups, usually involving gastrointestinal or cardiovascular instability.

Overall Factor II, Sociopathic Exploitiveness, has representation only in four items in Factor III, Group 3 (alcoholics). Although sociopathic symptoms were admitted by all groups, they never appeared in the full-blown syndrome of Overall Factor II.

Overall Factor III, Normal Mental Status, reappeared in five identical items with Factor I, Group 3; seven identical symptoms in Factor I, Group 6; and six identical symptoms with Factor V, Group 7. All these items consisted of denials of symptoms.

Overall Factor IV, Stress, had no clear matches with the group factors, although Factor II, Group 3, had four identical items. Nevertheless, all groups had stress items represented, although not in syndromes representing factors.

Overall Factor V, Denial of Psychosis, had a clear match only with six identical items of Factor IV, Group 3, and four identical items with Factor III, Group 7, although all groups had many single items denying psychotic disintegration.

3.7.2. Other Findings

Perhaps the most significant findings from the overall and group factor analyses was the failure of clear-cut syndromes of organ system symptoms to appear as factors. Although the PHS had been constructed with 20 items representing each of the principal organ systems, less than 20% of such items ever appeared in one of the overall factors or in the group factors. When such clusters did appear, they were always in association with other psychosomatic clusters (principally GI and CV clusters) or with clusters of anxiety-tension symptoms. The general picture thus is one of mixed psychosomatic patterns indicating general autonomic instability when it did appear in these age groups. The general conclusion is that mixed psychosomatic patterns were common across all groups but that pure organ system factors did not appear.

3.8. Social Status Study

The Social Status Study is a 200-item objective questionnaire measuring role-playing and social status factors in personal adjustment. It consists of ten scales of 20 items, each sampling adaptibility in role-playing and social status areas:

Scale I. Citizen Role. Twenty items measuring citizenship and effort to make the world a better place to live in. Scale II. Social Person Role. Twenty items sampling sociability and social skills. Scale III. Social Class Roles. Twenty items measuring ego involvement with social class and status factors. Scale IV. Parent and Family Roles. Twenty items measuring role playing as parent and family member. Scale V. Financial Manager Role. Twenty items measuring role-playing success in handling money and property. Scale VI. Sex Partner Role. Twenty items sampling adjustment as sex partner. Scale VII. Worker Role. Twenty items measuring adjustment as a worker. Scale VIII. Marriage Partner Role. Twenty items sampling marital attitudes. Scale IX. Leader-Follower Roles. Twenty items sampling leadership. Scale X. Political Role. Twenty items measuring attitudes on political issues.

Factor analysis, based on the eight clinical populations of the items, is currently in progress.

4. The Clinical Implications of Integrative (State) Psychology

4.1. Expanding Psychological Space

Behavior changes constantly. State psychology deals with the continuously changing behavior states which constitute the stream of psychic life. Both psychological theory and its practice change completely when integration theory reorients psychological thinking to the real phenomena of behavior change. Instead of deductive methods attempting to project structural systems and theories on raw behavior data, the clinician substitutes inductive approaches to interpreting the data derived from clinically significant states and episodes. The clinician will find his thinking revolutionized when he starts thinking in terms of change rather than constancies of behavior in the form of classical trait and personality structure formations.

It is too much to expect that psychologists who have been educated and trained in the classical schools and systems of psychology can reorient their theory and practice in terms of newer integrative (state) psychology overnight. Indeed, the history of clinical medicine indicates that older, indoctrinated generations may have to die off before younger generations can be taught and learn to practice newer viewpoints.

Modern clinical training programs may even operate to perpetuate obsolete methods, because the designers and administrators of such programs are so committed to classical theory and methods that they fear their training programs will not be approved by official accrediting bodies unless such obsolete approaches are included.

In a series of unpublished investigative studies, Thorne (1970–1977) has systematically questioned leading psychological scientists concerning their information and attitudes toward state phenomena. Even though many publications on state psychology have appeared since 1950, few of the authorities appeared cognizant of this literature and most could not define or understand the terms "state" and "integration." We are indeed dealing with entirely new dimensions better known by psychiatrists than psychologists.

The apparent reason why psychiatrists are more understanding and sensitive to psychological state phenomena than clinical psychologists is their training in making mental status examinations, which are not usually part of the training of clinical psychologists. The concept of mental status implies the existence not only of psychological states but also of changing status. It is commonly recognized in psychiatry that every examination should include an appraisal of mental status and that such mental status examinations should be repeated at frequent intervals to follow changing status faithfully.

Clinical psychologists have been trained largely as measurement technicians who may or may not make mental status observations during testing and case handling. In the standard psychiatric team pattern, the psychiatrist was supposed to diagnose and treat the patient, psychologists were supposed to do supplementary tests, and social workers were supposed to monitor postdischarge or preadmission case handling. Thus psychologists have not systematically evaluated mental status in their practice, certainly not while performing experiments.

4.2. New Concepts of Psychopathology

Thorne (1976b) developed a new system of psychopathology based on the implications of state psychology and defects or disorders of disintegration. This approach postulates that the cyclic, changing nature of psychological states inevitably produces integrational deficits and disorders during all life periods as the person is involved in a continuous struggle to maintain integration under all the changing conditions and situations of life. The clinical problem exists in diagnosing what integrative mechanisms are breaking down, when and where. The clinical problem consists in differentiating the behavior units (episodes) which are clinically significant, because so much of behavior is nonconsequential and noncritical for the most important adaptive coping behaviors in life.

The concept of adaptability is clinically important in order to establish criteria for determining clinical investments in diagnosis and treatment. The central fact is that every person must "get on the ball" and "put it all together," i.e., stay integrated across time at the highest possible levels. In terms of the well-known humanistic rights to run one's own life as one sees fit and not to be coercively interfered with by others (society), the concept of adaptation is preferred as being more neutral than the concept of adjustment, which is too relative to factors of time and place.

Clinically, the important consideration with state factors is that they are usually transient, momentary, and ever-changing. A person may be coping well 99% of the time but may enter transient states for shorter or longer periods where he may be violently dangerous to himself or others, or may be transiently incapacitated and unproductive or inefficient.

Conversely, a person who is basically mentally unhealthy or about average may show transient states in which he is supernormal, creative, productive, loving, and altruistic. State psychology can explain the underlying dynamics of both the peak and nadir experiences of life better than any other psychological system can.

4.3. Decompensation States

The concept of psychological decompensation is very descriptive of what happens with temporary deficits of integration or disintegration. In the diagnostic outlines referred to above, many conditions are described and classified as involving integrative disorders of transient or momentary duration. Unusual conditions cause the decompensation state, which disappears when normal conditions are reestablished.

4.4. Temporary Insanity

Psychiatry and the legal profession have had difficulties in understanding, describing, categorizing, naming, and disposing with cases showing temporary aberrations, often with dangerous manifestations, which are of only temporary duration, and which cannot be classed as mental diseases although the person is obviously transiently disordered. These conditions are well explained in terms of psychological state theory; i.e., the person is transiently lacking integration or is disintegrated psychologically. The transient state may be personally or socially dangerous, but the person can be expected to return to normality when the underlying etiological equation changes and becomes more normal, producing a more normal psychological state.

4.5. Wide Behavioral Variability

In classical psychometrics, unreliability of measures has been regarded as due to error variance. State psychology regards much of behavioral variance as due to normal changes in psychological states. In many studies of the factorial composition of the subtests of the Integration Level Test Series, Thorne and Pishkin (1968–1977) found that factorial composition tends to change markedly from one study to another, between and within groups, and individually, across time. Change is to be predicted by state psychology, and the clinician must deal with change validly.

4.6. Developmental Changes

Wide fluctuations of all psychological processes may be expected between all developmental periods as predicted by psychological state theory. Rather than speaking of personality as constant because the person either looks or acts the same, it is more valid to look for change, identify it, describe it, and work with it.

4.7. Drastic Personality Reorganizations

The central tendencies of behavior (personality) can change remarkably with drastic changes in conditions. Consider, for example, what happens when a person learns that he has cancer or that his wife (husband) is unfaithful, or when a clergyman loses his religion. The concept that the world was round rather than flat instantly changed our entire cosmology. Similar changes of feelings, emotions, ideas, plans, successes or failures, etc., can drastically alter state reactions.

4.8. Medical and Legal Competence and Responsibility

Although basic science psychology largely ignored problems of mental competency and voluntary intent because it did not have objective methods to study them, laymen understand the phenomena involved and utilize the concepts of competence and deliberate intent in settling medical and legal issues. Psychologists and psychiatrists are called on to render judgments as to mental competence. The McNaughten legal decision rules that a person is not guilty if (1) he did not know of the consequences of his actions, or (2) if he did know the consequences of his actions (knowing what he or she was doing) but was unable to control his actions because of an irresistible impulse. Although the law is constantly being liberalized, whether or not a person is competent and responsible is an important psychological issue.

It is obvious that a person's psychological state at the time of committing a significant action is critical to disposition of the case. Many kinds of psychological evidence concerning mental status are relevant to the issues. Unfortunately, there are so many schools and theories in psychology and psychiatry without definite evidence as to which is relevant in any particular case that the courts are treated to the spectacle of expert witnesses testifying literally on opposite sides concerning the same data. Cyclic changes of expert opinion have ranged from extreme repression/suppression to extreme permissiveness and tolerance.

Such concepts as temporary insanity, transient decompensation, character disorders, personality reactions, and even the psychoses and psychoneuroses need to be better understood and objectively measured. In this connection, the concepts of integrative state psychology are very relevant diagnostically as long as decisions of disposition or case handling are involved.

4.9. Statistical Implications

State psychology, which involves change, has entirely different statistical implications from trait psychology, which supposedly involves commonalities. Large variability in most psychological measurements usually is interpreted as unreliability due to error variance. Tests which are found to be unreliable usually are discarded as not providing valid, stable measures. Only relatively recently have repeated testings with the same tests been used to follow changes in "personality" structures.

Since life itself and persons in particular are never exactly the same from moment to moment, and because each succeeding moment brings greater or lesser observable change, it follows that psychological states are in constant flux, changing constantly through life from birth to death. Therefore, because change is to be expected in inner psychological states, it follows that changing outer behaviors and test results may be truly reflecting normal changes which are not necessarily due to error variance.

Predictions of an unknown future are, by definition, impossible unless it can be demonstrated that the same etiological formulas produce unchanging psychological states across time. Some psychological states such as sleep, hunger, thirst, menstruation, and sexual excitement occur with such regular cycles that they can be predicted. However, life in the world is much more chaotic unless well organized socially, so that many developments and problems are unpredictable. Also, many life events are one of a kind, which may be unpredictable and unpreventable.

This means that psychological state data usually apply only to the moment obtained, and cannot necessarily be used for predictive purposes. All the clinician can conclude is that the person was in a specific psychological state at the time of testing, or had had previous experience with such a state, or had somehow learned about it from outside sources. In state tests such as the Integration Level Test Series, the test results will not necessarily be reliable since bona fide state changes may be occurring, and will have only suggestive predictive value because the future itself and all it brings cannot be predicted.

The results of state tests should be used primarily as screening devices to indicate factors which may have been operative in the past or at the time of testing but which may not necessarily operate in the future. Supplementary investigations should be conducted to discover the temporal source, frequency, duration, intensity, and dynamic significance in relation to critical behavior episodes.

The most important use of psychological state data is probably to monitor integrative status including the nature or patterning of the integrative milieu, integrative stability, integration levels, positive and negative integrations, and disintegration. The problem is to diagnose integrative status across time. To objectify integrative changes, we need a statistics of change to show which organizing factors are operating, how, and when.

4.10. Research Design for Psychological States

Thorne (1976a) has outlined a grand research design for the investigation of psychological states with reference to their nature, duration, and change, utilizing both subjective and objective methods. The measurement of change requires entirely new experimental-statistical methods capable of measuring change in factors organizing integration, and particularly states and contents of consciousness. Particularly important is the development of methods capable of clarifying cause-effect relationships among many hierarchical levels of factors.

4.11. The Nature of Clinical Practice

It is to be expected that the whole nature of clinical practice will change when psychologists recognize the significance of integrative state psychology. State measurements will replace trait measurements. New types of state measurements case-handling methods will have to be devised. Diagnosis will return to a position of prime importance because all clinical case-handling should be based on a complete understanding of causation and how causal factors can be handled. The number of types of diagnoses will be expanded greatly, particularly clinical process diagnosis. Eclecticism will become universally adopted because increasing realization of behavior complexity will require an increasing complexity of valid diagnostic and treatment methods.

In the past, too many clinicians have been searching for universal short-cuts and panaceas to deal with all conditions. It was once claimed that Rogerian counseling and therapy could be learned in 3 weeks. Many with only master's-level training are labeling themselves as psychologists when actually such training currently is largely invalid, irrelevant, and obsolete. There is no substitute for long clinical experience leading to wisdom, and there are no simple methods which will solve everything.

Clinical and applied practice in the future will be based more solidly on many kinds of diagnosis, dealing with a wide spectrum of psychological domains of which many today are still unexplored. Improved psychodiagnosis is the foundation of necessary breakthroughs to more valid practices. In the future, comprehensive diagnostic workups will take days or months rather than minutes or hours.

ACKNOWLEDGMENT

The authors are indebted to Dr. T. S. Knawiec for criticizing the manuscript of this chapter.

5. References

Ansbacher, H., & Ansbacher, R. *The individual psychology of Alfred Adler*. New York: Basic Books, 1956.

Murray, H. A., & The Harvard Psychological Clinic. *Explorations in personality*. New York: Oxford University Press, 1938.

Pishkin, V., & Thorne, F. C. A factorial study of ideological composition in institutionalized psychiatric patients. *Journal of Clinical Psychology*, 1968, *24*, 273–277.

Pishkin, V., & Thorne, F. C. A factorial study of existential state reactions. *Journal of Clinical Psychology*, 1973, *29*, 392–402.

Pishkin, V., & Thorne, F. C. A comparative study of the factorial composition of responses on the life style analysis across clinical groups. *Journal of Clinical Psychology*, 1977, *33*, 249–255. (a)

Pishkin, V., & Thorne, F. C. A factorial structure of the dimensions of femininity in alcoholic, schizophrenic and normal populations. *Journal of Clinical Psychology*, 1977, *33*, 10–17. (b)

Pishkin, V., & Thorne, F. C. A factorial study of personal development of unmarried mothers, college, alcoholic, and schizophrenic populations. *Journal of Clinical Psychology*, 1977, *33*, 609–617. (c)

Rand, A. *The fountainhead*. New York: Bobbs, 1943.

Rand, A. *Atlas shrugged*. New York: Random House, 1957.

Rand, A., & Branden, N. (Eds.). *The objectivist*. New York, 1961.

Rosenzweig, S. *Rosenzweig Picture Frustration Study: Revised Form for Adults manual*. St. Louis: Author, 1947.

Sannito, T., Walker, R. E., Foley, J. M., & Posavec, E. J. A test of female sex identification: The Thorne Femininity Study. *Journal of Clinical Psychology*, 1972, *28*, 531–539.

Thorne, F. C. *Principles of psychological examining*. Brandon, Vt.: Clinical Psychology Publishing Company, Inc., 1955.

Thorne, F. C. *Personality*. Brandon, Vt.: Clinical Psychology Publishing Company, Inc., 1961. (a)

Thorne, F. C. *Clinical judgment*. Brandon, Vt.: Clinical Psychology Publishing Company, Inc., 1961. (b)

Thorne, F. C. Diagnostic classification and nomenclature of psychological states. *Journal of Clinical Psychology*, 1964, Monogr. Suppl., No. 17.

FREDERICK C.
THORNE AND
VLADIMIR PISHKIN

Thorne, F. C. *Integration Level Test Series*. Brandon, Vt.: Clinical Psychology Publishing Company, Inc., 1965.

Thorne, F. C. The Sex Inventory. *Journal of Clinical Psychology*, 1966, *22*, 367–374.

Thorne, F. C. *Integrative psychology*. Brandon, Vt.: Clinical Psychology Publishing Company, Inc., 1967. (a)

Thorne, F. C. Classification of etiological equations. In *Integrative psychology*. Brandon, Vt.: Clinical Psychology Publishing Company, Inc., 1967. (b)

Thorne, F. C. Diagnostic classification and nomenclature for existential state reactions. *Journal of Clinical Psychology*, 1970, *26*, 403–420.

Thorne, F. C. A grand research design for the investigation of psychological states. *Journal of Clinical Psychology*, 1976, *32*, 209–224. (a)

Thorne, F. C. Towards a new system of psychopathology. *Journal of Clinical Psychology*, 1976, *32*, 751–761. (*b*)

Thorne, F. C., & Pishkin, V. The Ideological Survey. *Journal of Clinical Psychology*, 1968, Monogr. Suppl., No. 25, 1968.

Thorne, F. C., & Pishkin, V. The Existential Study. *Journal of Clinical Psychology*, 1973, Monogr. Suppl., No. 42.

Thorne, F. C., & Pishkin, F. V. The Life Style Analysis. *Archives of the Behavioral Sciences*, 1975, Monogr. Suppl., No. 45.

Thorne. F. C., & Pishkin, V. The objective measurement of femininity. *Archives of the Behavioral Sciences*, 1977, Monogr. Suppl., No. 50 (a)

Thorne, F. C., & Pishkin, V. The Personal Developmental Study, *Archives of the Behavioral Sciences*, 1977, Monogr. Suppl., No. 51 (b)

Thorne, F. C. & Pishkin, The Personal Health Survey, *Archives of the Behavioral Sciences*, 1978, Monogr. Suppl., in press.

Thorne, F. C., Haupt, T. D., & Allen, R. M. Objective studies of adult male sexuality utilizing the Sex Inventory. *Journal of Clinical Psychology*, 1966, Monogr. Suppl. No. 21.

24

Diagnosing Neurotic Disorders

MARTIN MAYMAN AND JENNIFER COLE

1. Introduction

Among mental health practitioners, it is generally assumed that sound clinical work rests squarely on sound diagnostic assessment. This has long been a truism in all medical specialties. It was virtually the be-all and end-all of psychiatry during the last century and the beginning of this century. More recently, especially among non-medical practitioners, the art of differential diagnosis is no longer so highly revered. Attaching a diagnostic label to a set of presenting symptoms or to a prevailing character style which a patient manifests initially in his work with a therapist has been reduced in many clinical settings to the status of an annoying bureaucratic requirement. There are some clinicians, most notably Karl Menninger (Menninger, Mayman, & Pruyser, 1963), who have spoken out forcefully and eloquently against the dangers inherent in diagnostic labeling, which too often becomes a subtle form of pejorative, dehumanizing rejection of the patient because of his illness.

Diagnosis, if it is of any value today—and it is our belief that it is—is a process which has evolved from the art of pigeonholing to a functional analysis of a patient's current ego state. The soundest conception of its purpose is well stated by Wallerstein (1975), who, although he is speaking about the diagnostic process in psychoanalysis, expresses a point of view applicable to diagnosis in all of psychiatry:

> I regard prediction . . . as central to the *clinical analytic* enterprise and to the ways in which analysts habitually think, though its crucial role here is usually implicit and can therefore remain unacknowledged. Actually, though, every responsible action in analytic diagnosis and treatment involves predictions derived empirically from the observable data or deductively from analytic theoretical propositions. If a patient is assigned to a diagnostic category, reactions, symptoms, and special characteristics belonging to the designated pathological entity are implied. Diagnosis in fact is of little meaning unless prediction-oriented, unless the application of the label carries some connotations as to what may be expected in the development of the illness and in the projected treatment course.

MARTIN MAYMAN and JENNIFER COLE • Department of Psychology, University of Michigan, Ann Arbor, Michigan 48104.

In its broadest sense, a diagnostic assessment includes any and all judgments one makes about a particular patient in comparison with other patients. This need not be limited to the act of assigning a diagnostic label from the classical psychiatric nomenclature. We are being equally diagnostic when we make a judgment of "how sick" a particular patient may be, or when we decide that a particular patient's defenses are of such a nature as to justify one course of treatment rather than another.

Perhaps before going further we should outline the point of view from which this chapter is written. We will be discussing in the last two sections the most familiar neurotic patterns encountered in the course of diagnostic or therapeutic work with patients. However, people are far more complex than any nosological system we can use to classify them. So, too, with respect to personality patterns. While we may be able to identify an individual's primary, salient neurotic pattern, it is important to keep in mind that there exist for him other adaptive potentialities which he may have sacrificed or foregone in order to achieve whatever equilibrium he now maintains. In the course of intensive psychotherapy, one commonly finds that a person emerges as a multifaceted being who can turn a very different face to the world than that which he initially presented. He may gain (or regain) access to other personality styles, perhaps only abortively, but occasionally more permanently. The more one knows a person, the more one comes to discover the complex coalescence of multiple neurotic and normal patterns which make up that personality.

It should be clear by now that we make the major assumption that neurotic conditions, while traditionally carrying identifying labels, are by no means disease entities clearly distinguishable one from the other. Neuroses are responses to a series of internal and external stresses which render a person more or less dysfunctional, uncomfortable, unhappy, and unfulfilled. We shall present several major "syndromes," with the caveat that this medical label is misleading. We are referring rather to common configurations of inner pressures, resultant symptoms, and coping styles of varying utility, which together compose "character structures" or "personality styles."

We shall attempt to present a survey of the contemporary ways of looking diagnostically at the major psychoneurotic disorders currently encountered in diagnostic consultations and treatment clinics. Our approach is a clinical one, descriptive in what we hope is a clinically useful fashion. For a classical exposition of diagnostic nomenclature, the reader is referred to several sources. The *Diagnostic and Statistical Manual of Mental Disorders* (DSM II) first took the form we see it in today when, during World War II, the Surgeon-General's office set about reorganizing the standard psychiatric nosology according to more functional principles of psychodynamic classification. A major revision of that manual is being prepared and may soon be published. Of value in briefer form is the introductory section of Rapaport, Gill, and Schafer's *Diagnostic Psychological Testing* (1968), in which the authors describe those diagnostic groupings on which their research was based. Other works of more specific revelance will be referred to where applicable.

2. Global Assessment of Mental Illness or Health

The most pragmatic approaches to diagnosis are those which attempt a comprehensive assessment of ego strengths and weaknesses, concentrating on those ego functions which are most relevant to the clinical work at hand. One such diagnostic profile, defined carefully and applied systematically to the predictive process in clinical work, was developed by the Menninger Foundation's Psychotherapy Research Project (Wallerstein, Robbins, Sargent, & Luborsky, 1956). A closely related diagnostic profile is that used at the Hampstead Clinic, which like the Menninger Clinic is a psychoanalytically oriented clinical setting (Anna Freud, 1965). A more intensive cross-sectional profile of ego functions, presented in the form of a manual to aid in their assessment for diagnostic purposes, is that developed recently by Bellak and his co-workers (Bellak, Hurvich, & Gediman, 1973). A wisely used schema for diagnosing degree of psychopathology is the Luborsky Health-Sickness Rating Scale (1962), a highly differentiated calibration of the degree of life disruption effected by a patient's neurotic or psychotic disorder. This instrument is unique in that it includes at the upper end of the scale the degree of a person's healthy intactness and effectiveness. This diagnostic instrument is a far simpler one to use than the Wallerstein, Bellak, or A. Freud profiles. Like them, it was developed for use in psychoanalytic practice, although it is equally applicable in nonpsychoanalytic settings. Other, more narrowly focused measuring instruments for assessing the degree of psychopathology are suggested in the NIMH publication *Psychotherapy Change Measures* (Waskow & Parloff, 1975). Several measures of variables included in the Menninger or Hampstead profiles (level and quality of object relationship, quality of reality testing, level of drive development) are described in Chapter 13 (Mayman & Krohn) of *Psychotherapy Change Measures*.

The comprehensive diagnostic system which grew out of the Menninger Foundation Psychotherapy Research Project was based on certain assumptions derived from psychoanalytic theory, from which predictions could be made about the process of change and cure. A static, descriptive approach is explicitly avoided. Rather, the balance of interpersonal forces is assessed in an attempt to describe each unique individual and to enable researchers to evaluate that fluid movement toward and away from greater "health." The interested reader is referred to literature published on this project over the past 20 years. The profile rests on these six assumptions:

1. Mental illness derives from otherwise insoluble intrapsychic conflicts.
2. These conflicts are in part unconscious.
3. Intrapsychic conflicts are related to early childhood experiences and represent inadequately resolved infantile conflicts.
4. Prior to the onset of clinical illness, the intrapsychic conflicts are handled through the idiosyncratic patterning of impulse-defense configurations, character traits, and perhaps more or less ego-syntonic symptoms, which together make up the personality structure of the individual.
5. Through varying combinations of inner and outer stresses (sometimes clearly discernible as "precipitating events"), the previously utilized methods of maintaining homeostatic equilibrium fail and symptoms or ego-dystonic character traits, or both, appear.
6. The patterning of the symptoms and associated ego-dystonic character traits reveals important elements of the inner conflicts, the ways the ego tries to cope with them, as well as important aspects of the fundamental character organization of the individual (Wallerstein, 1956).

Given these assumptions, the following "patient variables" were identified and defined. A full definition of each is presented by Wallerstein et al. in their paper.

2.1. Assessment of Relevant Patient Variables

MARTIN MAYMAN
AND JENNIFER COLE

I. Sex and age
II. Anxiety and symptoms
   1. Anxiety
   2. Symptoms
   3. Somatization
   4. Depression and guilt feelings
      a. Depression
      b. Conscious guilt
      c. Unconscious guilt
   5. Alloplasticity
III. Nature of conflicts
   1. Core neurotic problem
   2. Current life problem
IV. Ego factors (and defenses)
   1. Self-concept
   2. Patterning of defenses
   3. Anxiety tolerance
   4. Insight
   5. Externalization
   6. Ego strength
V. Capacities factors
   1. Intelligence
   2. Psychological mindedness
   3. Constitutionally endowed aspects of ego strength
   4. Capacity for sublimations
VI. Motivational factors
   1. Honesty
   2. Fee
   3. Extent of desired change
   4. Secondary gain
VII. Relationship factors
   1. Quality of interpersonal relationship
   2. Transference paradigms
VIII. Reality factors
   1. Presence of "neurotic life circumstance"
   2. Adequacy of finances to the treatment requirements
   3. Attitudes of significant relatives
   4. Physical health

Bellak et al. turn a more high-powered lens on the ego factors in psychopathology. They isolate 12 major ego variables and break each of these down further into two or more component variables. These 12 ego variables, extensively defined in their book, are

1. Reality testing
2. Judgment
3. Sense of reality of the world and of the self

4. Regulation and control of drives, affects, and impulses
5. Object relations
6. Thought processes
7. Adaptive regression in the service of the ego
8. Defensive functioning
9. Stimulus barrier
10. Autonomous functioning
11. Synthetic-integrative functioning
12. Mastery-competence

The Hampstead profile overlaps in many respects the Menninger profile and that developed by Bellak and his co-workers. But, as do each of the others, it places somewhat different emphases on the component variables of the profile. Again, the bare bones of the outline are cited (and occasionally paraphrased) here. Each of the variables is defined in considerably greater detail by Anna Freud.

2.2. Diagnostic Profile

   I. Reason for referral (arrests in development, behavior problems, anxieties, inhibitions, symptoms, etc.)
  II. Description of child (personal appearance, moods, manner, etc.)
 III. Family background and personal history
  IV. Possibly significant environmental influences
   V. Assessments of development
   A. Drive development
      1. Libido—Examine and state
         a. with regard to phase development:
            whether the child has proceeded to his age-adequate stage and whether this highest level is being maintained or has been abandoned regressively for an earlier one.
         b. with regard to libido distribution:
            whether self-regard, self-esteem, a sense of well-being are achieved without undue dependence on the object world
         c. with regard to object libido:
            level and quality of object relationships
      2. Aggression—Examine the aggressive expressions at the disposal of the child
         a. according to their quantity
         b. according to their quality
         c. according to their direction
   B. Ego and superego development
      a. intactness or defects of ego apparatus
      b. intactness or otherwise of ego functions
      c. the defense organization:
         whether employed against individual drives; whether defenses are age adequate, balanced, and effective, and overly dependent on the object world or independent of it (superego development)

VI. Genetic assessments: regression and fixation points manifest in
   a. overt behavior
   b. fantasy activity
   c. symptomatology
VII. Dynamic and structural assessments (conflicts)
   a. external conflicts between the id-ego agencies and the object world (arousing fear of the object world)
   b. internalized conflicts between ego-superego and id after the ego agencies have taken over and represent to the id the demands of the object world (arousing guilt)
   c. internal conflicts between insufficiently fused or incompatible drive representatives (such as unsolved ambivalence, activity vs. passivity, masculinity vs. feminity)
VIII. Assessment of some general characteristics
   a. the child's frustration tolerance
   b. the child's sublimation potential
   c. the child's overall attitude to anxiety
   d. progressive developmental forces vs. regressive tendencies
IX. Diagnosis

From these data and inferences, the diagnostician should reach one of six conclusions:

1. that, in spite of current manifest behavior disturbances, the personality growth of the child is essentially healthy and falls within the wide range of "variations of normality"
2. that existent pathological formations (symptoms) are of a transitory nature and can be classed as by-products of developmental strain
3. that there is permanent drive regression to previously established fixation points which leads to conflicts of a neurotic type and gives rise to infantile neuroses and character disorders
4. that there is drive regression as above plus simultaneous ego and superego regressions which lead to infantilisms, borderline, delinquent, or psychotic disturbances
5. that there are primary deficiencies of an organic nature or early deprivations which distort development and structuralization and produce retarded, defective, and atypical personalities.
6. that there are destructive processes at work (of organic, toxic, or psychic, known or unknown origin) which have effected, or are on the point of effecting, a disruption of mental growth

One of the products of the Menninger Psychotherapy Research Project was the Health-Sickness Rating Scale (Luborsky, 1962), which was devised to measure the outcome of psychotherapy. The scale employs seven criteria which should be weighed in arriving at an estimation of the patient's degree of disturbance:

1. The patient's need to be protected and/or supported vs. the ability to function autonomously.
2. The seriousness of the symptoms (the degree to which they reflect personality disorganization).
3. The degree of the patient's subjective discomfort and stress.

4. The patient's effect on his environment (danger, discomfort, etc.).
5. The degree to which he can utilize his abilities.
6. The quality of his interpersonal relationships (warmth, intimacy, genuineness, distortion of perception of relationships, impulse control in relationships).
7. The breadth and depth of his interests.

Persons can be assigned a scalar ranking from a hypothetical 100, indicating optimal "normality," to 10, for one who would quickly die without closed-ward care. One of the strengths of this system is its utility in assessing and reflecting progression and regression during illness and recovery and in highlighting those areas among the seven aforementioned in which progress or regression is occurring. Most neurotic patients fall between 50 and 75 on the Luborsky scale. At the upper reaches of this range, symptoms, inhibitions, and character problems cause more than everyday discomfort and may motivate the person to seek treatment. As a patient approaches the "50" mark, instability and difficulty in maintaining himself in his life situation become increasingly characteristic; stability is achieved by such patients only as a result of great and costly effort.

We stated earlier that this chapter would not attempt to present a summary of the standard psychiatric nomenclature but rather some useful references and orienting points regarding the diagnostic process. Toward this end, what follows is a characterization of two modal types which, in a number of diagnostic systems, define two polar opposites of defensive style, character structure, sense of reality, affect organization, and interpersonal relatedness. Shapiro (1965) has dichotomized the continuum of character styles into those which are primarily hysteriform and those which are primarily obsessional. In this, he follows closely the position taken by Rapaport, Gill, and Schafer (1968). In what follows, we shall attempt a comprehensive summary from a number of sources of the essentially hysteriform neurotic condition and the essentially obsessional neurotic condition.

3. Hysterical Neurotic Conditions

The term "hysteria" in its present-day usage refers to a "character neurosis" as much as it does to a "symptom neurosis." The hysterical personality is generally characterized by repressive inhibitions in specific areas or involving specific cognitive or motor functions, particularly when these involve sexual or competitive feelings. Hysterical persons also engage in a great deal of "acting out," that is, symptomatic, preprogrammed repetition of certain life patterns in love, work, or play. This represents an unconscious seeking out of similar situations (doomed love affairs, older men, a tyrannical boss, etc.) which represent an unwitting recapitulation of an early object relationship and its coordinate ego state. Both acting out and inhibition may, and frequently do, appear in one person at different times and around specific issues. They have in common their role in representing an unconscious conflict and a repetitive, maladaptive attempt at working it through or attempting to find compromise neurotic gratification in place of unconsciously forbidden normal gratification.

The neurotic symptoms most often associated with hysterical neuroses are phobias and conversion symptoms. As with character styles, they may tap into conflicts and relationship paradigms deriving from an Oedipal developmental level, or, in more disturbed patients, the symptoms appear more regressive in character and indicate a primary pregenital neurosis.

The phobia serves to bind anxiety associated with particular unconscious conflicts and utilizes the mechanism of avoidance typical of hysteria. The phobic object or situation generally symbolizes a feared object or the person's own forbidden impulses—sexual and/or aggressive. The symbol is a displacement, then, from one object onto another and also serves to disguise the original conflict. Mild phobias or phobias of specific places, objects, situations, etc., are common in hysteria; phobias which border on the bizarre or which have a primitive or consuming nature are probably not. Common developmental phobias of childhood do not imply later hysterical psychopathology. Agoraphobia, like the school phobias of childhood, is now believed to relate to separation problems and suggests a pre-Oedipal source. The nature, prevalence, and importance of phobic symptoms are very well presented and documented by Weekes (1977).

The conversion symptom, when it appears in hysteria (see Chodoff, 1954, for a discussion of this subject), also utilizes symbolization and displacement. This symptom, when unraveled, proves to represent a conflict over some sexual or aggressive impulse and the action of a conscience or superego to suppress and disguise this impulse. The result frequently includes the inhibition of some normal function, e.g., a paralysis of the hand or a loss of sexual potency. The anxiety which one would expect to see in response to the conversion symptom may be largely or wholly denied by the hysteric, a phenomenon which has been termed "belle indifference." Actually, anxiety is present and can usually be elicited or its effect observed in the patient's daily functioning. The symptom also serves to punish the individual for his forbidden wishes and may elicit the kind of attention and help one seeks from the environment.

But such symptoms are embedded in a character structure defined by typical personality traits and cognitive styles. We must again stress the limits of the inclusiveness of any set of descriptions of this sort, because there are always other sides to the personality which may become evident in time or under different circumstances.

The hysteriform character structure is often as diagnostic of hysteria as are the traditional hysterical symptoms. Overall, the individual's reality testing is good, except for specific blind spots or areas of selective repression or denial around conflicted impulses, both internal and external, and situations which provoke or elicit those impulses. The capacity to disown and deny conflictful aspects of reality may sometimes give the hysteric an air of naiveté which at times approaches a form of pseudostupidity. A surprising amount of native intelligence may exist behind this defensive façade.

The hysteric's attention is largely oriented toward outer events. The ego tends to be perception bound at the expense of an adequate awareness of more subjective events like fantasy, impulses, and feelings. Externalization becomes a preferred mode of defense. (See Shapiro, 1965, and Voth & Mayman, 1966, for a fuller explication.) There can be a certain banality, a proneness to take things at face value, which gives hysterics a somewhat shallow or superficial air. Nonetheless, they are highly attuned to interpersonal cues and situations.

Affectively, the hysteric has a surface warmth and sparkle, emotional lability, and widespread deployment of affect as part of a distinctive defensive system. The use of affects can border on histrionics (Seton, 1965). The manifest feelings, which at first are thrown up as a defensive screen as if to ward off covert or repressed feelings, may prove eventually to be "real" feelings, but are used in such a way as to be obstacles during major portions of therapeutic work. Seton makes the point that the very affect which is used defensively by the hysteric as a smoke screen must itself come under therapeutic scrutiny eventually for its repressed content.

Behaviorally, the hysteric is action oriented, hence the tendency to act out conflicts rather than be cognizant of them. In selected areas, the hysteric will appear impulsive or incapable of exercising self-discipline. This is an integral part of the defensive system, allowing the hysteric to remain unaware of these impulses and even to achieve a certain gratification which would otherwise be impossible because of the forbidden nature of the repressed impulses and fantasies. If action were impossible, the likelihood of these conflicts becoming conscious would increase, posing a threat to the defenses. This fact is utilized in the analytic treatment of hysterics, in that the suppression of acting out encourages remembering rather than repeating.

While hysterical behavior may be inappropriate at times, the conscience or superego is generally well developed. There is an awareness of social propriety and a strong sense of what a good person "should do" under particular circumstances. This strict conscience may frequently be externalized onto others, particularly authority or parent figures. The hysteric anticipates criticism, disapproval, or censure for attitudes or actions of which he himself disapproves, and may try to avoid the now-externalized punishment. He has restricted access to his inner feelings, but prefers to perceive in the outer world those attitudes and judgments which are his own. The readiness to form transferences is part of this process; important people from the past, or aspects of them, are externalized onto current persons to whom the hysteric responds as though they are in fact his past objects.

The hysteric's heavy reliance on the defenses of displacement, externalization, avoidance, and denial have been mentioned. Repression is still considered a cornerstone of hysterical defensive functioning, that is, the repression of fantasies and impulses which are forbidden. The reemergence of repressed sexual impulses can be observed in the sexualization which frequently permeates even mundane events in the hysteric's life. This may be obvious only to others, because the hysteric is generally unaware of his sexual feelings at that moment and would be taken aback if this were suggested. There is a fear of mature, genital sexuality, and conflict over pregenital libidinal and aggressive wishes toward opposite- and same-sex persons.

One important and debated aspect of hysteria which we can only address superficially here concerns the sex differences noted in diagnosis. That is, more than 3 times as many women are diagnosed hysterical as men, and the reverse holds true as regards the diagnosis of obsessive-compulsive personality (see Chodoff & Lyons, 1958). There is nothing implicit in our current theories of psychosexual development which would dictate a predominance of hysterical (phallic-Oedipal) conflicts in females as opposed to males. Earlier theories, including Freud's, which undertook to explain this phenomenon, are largely superseded now. Chodoff and Lyons suggest that derogatory descriptions of hysteria were made exclusively of women by male psychiatrists: emotional lability, seductiveness, frigidity, naiveté, a global diffuse cognitive style, and lack of attention to precision are all traits traditionally considered "feminine."

We suggest that hysterical conflicts are actually as common in men as they are in women, although the manifest behavior will differ along culturally determined lines. Men certainly have phobic symptoms, are fearful about all kinds of disturbances in bodily functions, can be hypochondriacally anxious in rather phobic ways, and have other phobic symptoms like fear of injections, fear of flying, claustrophobia, and agoraphobia. We do not have adequate surveys of neurotic symptoms in the general population to enable us to determine their relative frequency in men and women, but in clinical practice one commonly observes the aforementioned symptoms in one's male patients.

Not only in symptom formation but also in character structure we find as many men as women hysterics. Often, this does not seem to be true, but this is only because we fail to recognize that male hysterics do not manifest the same traits as do female hysterics. Generally, hysteria in male character structures appears in one of two forms. The first is a phallic-assertive, counterphobic, hypermasculine male. The other is an essentially shy, proper, mannerly man who is sexually inhibited but in other respects is masculinely competent. We find strong defenses against the free expression of sexuality, coexistent with a well-developed capacity for forming close, well-differentiated, warm, and stable object relationships. The type marked by more massive inhibitions is associated with fairly clear indications of extensive castration anxiety. Still a third type, which most nearly approaches the so-called typical female hysterical character, is the expansive, effusive, impetuous, egocentric, emotionally labile male who is currently considered one form of narcissistic personality.

In both sexes, the prototypical hysterical configuration shows distinctive features which bear the earmark of phallic-level sexuality (Mayman, 1968, 1974). This includes phallic-urethral issues of pride or shame, and fears of loss of control pertaining originally to bladder control itself but displaced during development onto fear of loss of control of feelings. The phallic-intrusive modality is typically more evident in male development, but will be manifest among females as well. It concerns the intense interest in and pursuit of intrusive aims originally toward the body of the parent. Curiosity and adventuresomeness are derivatives of intrusiveness but are usually inhibited or repressed. Phallic-locomotor drives, on the other hand, are easily sublimated into athletic pursuits, and concern pleasure in one's own body, in moving powerfully, gracefully, and rapidly. Often the association is made between speed and sexual excitement, with loss of control in this area representing loss of sexual control. Thus the path is laid for motor inhibitions and defensively restricted pleasure in physical activity. Competitiveness is also a phallic character trait which can appear in any arena which becomes invested with symbolic phallic prowess, be it sports, money making, intellectual achievement, etc.

It is important to consider separately the infantile personality as one form of pregenital hysterical character which falls on the more disturbed end of the hysteriform spectrum, and with whom the hysteric is often confused. They differ both qualitatively and in matter of degree, sometimes shading into one another, particularly in the initial clinical picture (Kernberg, 1975).

In the quality of reality contact, the infantile personality demonstrates a hysteriform involvement in outer events, but with greater scotomization of unpleasant and undesirable aspects of reality and more conspicuous reliance on primitive defenses such as denial and flight. The emotional shallowness observed in the hysteric is exaggerated in the infantile personality. He is suggestible but less consistently pliant, because of the greater charge of aggressive affects and more blatant ambivalence. Behavior is more willful, erratic, and unpredictable.

Affectively, the infantile personality may be engaging, but this surface responsiveness is strongly colored with less modulated narcissistic features. Their self-centeredness, egocentricity, and demandingness may quickly turn into retaliatory anger on slight frustration. Affects are even more labile, with a correspondingly heightened capacity for histrionic display of an inappropriate sort. Because of the heavy reliance on denial and dissociation, the infantile personality is prone to depressive mood swings.

Behaviorally, the impulsivity of an infantile personality greatly exceeds the action orientation typical of the hysteric. Thoughtlessness may border on the impetuous, tension and anxiety are poorly tolerated, and drive discharge is more imperative, less discriminate, and less modulated by conscious intention. Effective, sustained effort in the pursuit of goals is correspondingly more difficult for the infantile personality; thus there are fewer areas of relatively adaptive, conflict-free functioning. Quite blatant or crude symptomatic acts or acting out may appear in their behavior.

Some of the reasons for these differences become clearer when we understand the more primitive aspects of the ego and superego in the infantile personality. The superego is more archaic, rigid, and demanding in a less realistic way. Thus the predominant anxiety concerns are archaic retaliation rather than the more mature loss of love which threatens the hysteric. Compliance with superego injunctions is necessarily of a more extreme form, with erratic swings between manipulative compliance and the acting out of defiance; identification with the harsh superego alternates with the throwing over of moral constraints. Projection of superego demands onto external figures spurred by guilt which is consciously denied results in quite distorted perceptions of others' motives and attitudes. Id content or impulses may likewise be projected onto others, making accurate reality testing and steady relationships quite difficult.

Rather than being primarily bound up in triadic conflicts from the phallic-Oedipal period, the infantile personality is greatly involved with the maternal introject, with dyadic relations to his objects. Less shaded images of idealized good and bad objects and self prevail, with images of mother as ungiving, cold, destructive, engulfing, and frustrating. A corresponding amount of primitive rage will accompany these perceptions. The fears which permeate relationships derive from these threatening images of the object: the infantile character longs for symbiotic union but fears engulfment, abandonment, injury, and loss of self. Ambivalence is acted out in wide swings from one extreme to the other; opposing views of self and object world are maintained by defensive "splitting" (Kernberg, 1975, Kohut, 1971). The hysteric generally experiences one or another side of the ambivalence as ego-dystonic; this is generally kept under repression. The infantile personality retains the capacity to experience and alternate between both sides of his ambivalence consciously, because of his heavy reliance on the mechanisms of dissociation, splitting, and denial. The infantile personality will have less well-differentiated reactions to members of each sex. Both may be reacted to as seductively need-gratifying objects. The infantile personality is more likely to be sexually promiscuous than is the hysteric. The capacity for stable, enduring relationships is handicapped by the abovementioned regressive features; life overall is a more chaotic and less maturely involved affair. Primitive sadistic and masochistic fantasies and behavior may break through, because of superego pathology and the primitive state of the drives and object images.

4. Obsessional Neurotic Conditions

MARTIN MAYMAN
AND JENNIFER COLE

The term "obsessional" typically refers to a proliferation of ideational defenses and symptomatology in an overmeticulous, doubt-ridden personality, all of which have a paralyzing effect on the capacity to act freely (Rapaport, Gill, & Schafer, 1968). The obsessive-compulsive character style, which we will present here, is a rather well-delineated one (Shapiro, 1965; Salzman, 1968). Shapiro chooses to highlight four aspects of obsessive-compulsive functioning: (1) rigidity, (2) compulsive activity, (3) the dominant sense of "should," and (4) the compelling need to perform activities which are in some way realized to be absurd.

Rigidity may refer to the individual's "character armor," sometimes manifest almost literally in the tightness of the musculature, sometimes figuratively as in the tenacity with which one adheres to schedules, etc. On the cognitive level, dogmatism and the tendency to be opinionated and inflexible in one's views are common characteristics of obsessional functioning. The obsessive is not easily able to adapt his mental set flexibly to suit the nature of the incoming information or situation. The obsessive-compulsive person abhors looseness and is incapable of planless spontaneity. He does not easily experience the surprise of discovery or novelty in his encounters with the world. Obsessional persons are generally fact oriented, capable of and inclined to amass a great deal of "objective" knowledge, liking order which pulls all these discrete bits of information together.

The obsessive-compulsive individual's need to control his experience of reality and accomplish certain specific tasks often gives him a driven appearance and a subjective sense of being driven. He feels this impulsion as somewhat external to himself, but does not know its source. The sense of self-awareness is almost never lost; detached self-examination may even be omnipresent. He is aware of himself and how he is functioning, and frequently of the role which he is filling.

The pervasive sense of doubt and inability to decide, derivatives of the ambivalence which plagues his developmental history, make it difficult for the obsessive-compulsive person to experience free will. He may ruminate endlessly, and then rapidly decide on the basis of an arbitrary or extraneous feature of the issue at hand, without the sense of freedom to move among various options to a firmly felt, satisfying decision. The obsessional person characteristically feels anxious when this mode of cognition is interfered with or when confronted with situations which do not lend themselves to this style of mastery.

Nonetheless, the obsessive-compulsive individual substitutes will power for genuine, autonomous, immediate experience (Shapiro, 1962). Will power is not very functional in decision-making; thus the decision may actually be made in a rather abrupt fashion which results from the winning out of one or the other side of the ambivalence that the obsessive person feels in virtually every decision he makes or every act he performs.

A great deal of worry and rumination typically accompanies major decisions. The obsessive-compulsive personality prefers to have policies or rules which he can follow, experiencing adherence to them as adherence to some objective code which is real and absolute and which exists somehow apart from himself, even if these policies or rules were originally chosen or arranged by him. The sense that one had to do as one did seems to be comforting to the obsessional neurotic and affords him a sense of purpose in his actions, a reassuring sense of himself as the agent of some supraindividual authority.

The dual features of dogmatism and doubt which pervade the obsessional's style stem from his apparent inability to experience a subjective sense of conviction about any decision he makes. He cannot just feel the truth or rightness of some idea, action, choice, or whatever. Dogmatism, being stubbornly opinionated, eliminates the need to consider and decide between alternatives and provides the illusion of correctness, even though important aspects of an issue may be ignored. All of this represents the effort to bypass the sticky ambivalence which plagues the obsessional person.

The obsessional person knows that for him to change his routine will not injure anyone, will not really trigger the catastrophe he fears, but he will go to desperate ends to preserve it, as though unconscious intentions and fantasies represented the real truth for him. The critical distinction between intrusive thoughts or preoccupations and outright delusions lies in the obsessional's capacity to retain his self-critical ego functions, to take intellectual distance from these convictions. He may present himself for treatment because he is, for example, plagued by the conviction that he will kill someone, even though he knows he will never do so.

Certain defense mechanisms are characteristic of the obsessional neurotic in his struggle against ambivalence toward others and against his own rather sadistic superego. The obsessional conflict is generally manifested in terms of thinking or ideational symptomatology. Intellectualizing defenses are predominant, and this neurosis, in fact, seldom occurs in those of less than strong intellectual endowment (Rapaport et al., 1968). Thinking itself has been intimately implicated in drive discharge. Thus the defenses against instinctual impulses are represented in the defenses against certain types of thinking and certain thought contents. However, when the neurosis involves a heavy reliance on compulsive behavior rather than on obsessional thought functioning, intellectualizing as a defense may be largely or wholly absent.

Isolation of affect and of the thought content related to that affect is one of the primary defensive maneuvers typical of this neurosis. Certain fantasies may exist in consciousness with no conscious guilt feelings, while overpowering feelings of guilt may be attached to apparently meaningless or trivial actions or ideas. Particularly aggressive affects may be manifest in symptomatic behavior which appears to have no meaning to the patient, i.e., he may calmly leave an analytic hour, but then fiercely kick a stone which he inadvertently trips over.

Compulsive behavior serves to ward off acute outbreaks of anxiety through the ostensibly nonsensical but unconsciously efficacious magic ritual. Magical "undoing" has the purpose of negating unconscious hostile impulses. Obsessions and compulsions may represent a magical talisman against the danger associated with these impulses or magical assurance of the protection of an important love object. There are any number of ways in which one action may be employed to nullify another. The handwashing compulsion is the classical example of a mechanism of undoing, of washing away the dirty or aggressive impulses or fantasies. Usually, some of the aggressive content, particularly the aggression directed at objects, will appear in more subtle form in the symptom and be gratified indirectly. The handwashing ritual, especially if repeated 30 or 40 times a day, injures both the person who does it and anyone else inconvenienced by these acts, thereby satisfying sadistic and masochistic impulses which have to be warded off. Some mothers, to take another example, are compulsively cautious with their children, consciously wishing to protect them from harm, but in fact imposing painful restrictions and stirring unnecessary anxiety in their children.

MARTIN MAYMAN
AND JENNIFER COLE

Reaction formations against unacceptable impulses are also typically seen in the obsessive-compulsive personality. Cloying sweetness which lacks genuine warmth may be superimposed on a wish to be hostile, derogatory, or attacking. Overt solicitousness (sometimes annoying in the extreme) may defend against its opposite wish to cause harm or to wish ill to a loved one.

Psychoanalytic theory relates the ambivalence of the obsessive character to object-relational issues which are most salient in the anal phase. This becomes especially apparent in the obsessive's characteristic preoccupations with derivative forms of the wish to hoard, control, expel, or withhold, be messy, or be free of any or all imperfections. There may be a reluctance to part with possessions, particularly anything which was once close to the body or identified with the self. A preoccupation with money, savings, and miserliness represents this conflict displaced onto money. Reaction formations against a soiling instinct may be represented in scrupulous cleanliness, fastidiousness, and orderly behavior, with occasional breakthrough of the original instinct in secret pockets of filthiness. Rigid punctuality and compulsive lateness represent derivatives of the conflict over making it to the toilet in time, and are commonly observed displacements in the obsessional neurotic. One readily observes in all of these symptoms the important role of ambivalence and an infantile assertion of autonomy which is typical in the pre-Oedipal anal phase which persists in heightened form in the obsessional neurotic. The struggle between love and hate, the wish to control or be controlled by the object, to withhold and preserve or expel and destroy will appear and reappear in multiple forms in the psychotherapeutic exploration of this symptomatology.

The ambivalence originally experienced toward one's childhood objects is now experienced toward one's own thoughts or ideas. The negativism typical of the anal phase becomes manifest in the obsessional thought style. There is obviously great potential here for interference with intellectual functions. A special kind of work inhibition is common among this group, although the obsessional thinking style can be advantageous in certain areas of intellectual endeavor. The intellectual obstinacy so typical of the obsessional personality is easily seen as a derivative of early battles over control of the sphincter, of the feces during toilet training, and of the toilet training schedule itself. In some obsessive personalities, the conflict between the wish to withhold and the wish to expel, or even to injure the object with one's fecal product, may be observed in the alternation between clamming up and "verbal diarrhea." Speech or ideas may be experienced as a bombardment or an aggressive attack on others and therefore may be a secondary cause for superego retribution, requiring further defensive operations.

Typical of the obsessive-compulsive neurosis is the continual struggle between expression of the impulse and identification with the superego prohibition against the impulse, with a partial return of the repressed instincts. The defensive operation may become increasingly intricate and tiresome, generalizing to many areas of thinking and living, frequently impinging on the comfort and lives of the obsessional neurotic and those around him. The superego itself has regressed to an anal-sadistic position and the talion principle, i.e., an eye for an eye, is frequently observed in the construction of obsessional symptomatology. "Sphincter morality" is often evident, that is, a guilt over being caught in the forbidden deed rather than a more appropriate and balanced sense of guilt about really hurting others or violating inner standards with which one has fairly unambivalently identified onself. Atonement for an impulse may allow the individual to express the impulse again. In this sense, the superego is, to a greater or lesser degree, corruptible; it can be manipulated by certain magical acts.

We indicated above that it is commonly assumed that hysteria is far more prevalent among women than among men. Similarly, the assumption is widely held that obsessive-compulsive neurosis is far more commonly encountered in men than it is in women. Once again, it is our impression that this conclusion is reached only if one takes a narrowly circumscribed view of this condition. If one allows for culturally imposed sex differences to affect some of the manifest forms by which women are likely to express obsessive or compulsive tendencies, one will find that the condition is as prevalent among women as among men. There have, however, been a number of studies recently which suggest that the culture itself exerts a heavy pressure on men to isolate themselves from, and dampen their feelings, which would have them behave in a manner characteristic of the obsessional neurotic (Goldstine, 1974). It is widely believed that women are more in touch with their own feelings than are men. Whether these sex differences do, in fact, exist and whether or not the culture does foist a sex-based choice of defense on people is something which we need to learn much more about before it can be taken as a truism of clinical practice.

5. References

American Psychiatric Association, Committee on Nomenclature and Statistics. *Diagnostic and statistical manual of mental disorders*. Washington, D.C.: American Psychiatric Association, 1968.

Bellak, L., Hurvich, M., & Gediman, H. *Ego functions in schizophrenics, neurotics and normals*. New York: Wiley, 1973.

Chodoff, P. A reexamination of some aspects of conversion hysteria. *Psychiatry*, 1954, *17*, 75–81.

Chodoff, P., & Lyons, H. Hysteria, the hysterical personality and "hysterical" conversion. *American Journal of Psychiatry*, 1958, *114*, 734–740.

Freud, A. *The writings of Anna Freud*, Vol. 6. New York: International Universities Press, 1965, 108–147.

Goldstine, T. *Impersonal and interpersonal orientations in the conception of autonomy: A study of sex differences*. Unpublished Ph.D. dissertation. Ann Arbor: University of Michigan, 1974.

Kernbert, O. *Borderline conditions and pathological narcissism*. New York: Jason Aronson, 1975.

Kohut, H. *The analysis of the self*. New York: International Universities Press, 1971.

Luborsky, L. Clinicians' judgments of mental health. *Archives of General Psychiatry*. 1962, *7*, 407–417.

Mayman, M. Early memories and character structure. *Journal of Projective Techniques and Personality Assessment*, 1968, *32*, 303–316.

Mayman, M. The shame experience, the shame dynamic, and shame personalities in psychotherapy. Paper presented to the American Psychological Association, September, 1974.

Menninger, K., Mayman, M., & Pruyser, P. *The vital balance*. New York: Viking, 1963.

Rapaport, D., Gill, M., & Schafer, R. *Diagnostic psychological testing*. Edited by R. Holt. New York: International Universities Press, 1968.

Salzman, L. *The obsessive personality*. New York: Science House, 1968.

Seton, P. Uses of affect observed in a histrionic patient. *International Journal of Psychoanalysis*. 1965, *46*, 226–236.

Shapiro, D. Aspects of the obsessive-compulsive style. *Psychiatry*, 1962, *25*, 46–55.

Shapiro D. *Neurotic styles*. New York: Basic Books, 1965.

Voth, H., & Mayman, M. The psychotherapy process: Its relation to ego-closeness—ego-distance. Part I. *Journal of Nervous and Mental Disease*, 1966, *143*, 324–337.

Voth, H., & Mayman, M. Diagnostic and treatment implications of ego-closeness/ego-distance: Auto-kinesis as a diagnostic instrument. *Comprehensive Psychiatry*, 1967, *8*, 203–216.

Wallerstein, R. *Psychotherapy and psychoanalysis*. New York: International Universities Press, 1975.

Wallerstein, R., Robbins, L., Sargent, H., & Luborsky, L. The psychotherapy research project of the Menninger Foundation. *Bulletin of the Menninger Clinic*, 1956, *20*, 221–280.

Waskow, I., & Parloff, M. *Psychotherapy change measures*. Rockville, Maryland: National Institute of Mental Health, 1975.

Weekes, C. *Simple, effective treatment of agoraphobia*, New York: Hawthorn, 1977.

25

Diagnostic Procedures in the Criminal Justice System

FRED J. PESETSKY AND ALBERT I. RABIN

1. Introduction

Discretion exists in determining whether an individual will be entered into the criminal justice system. Victims may refuse to file complaints or swear out arrest warrants, the police may fail to make arrests, or prosecutors may drop a case for one reason or another. However, once an individual has been entered into the criminal justice proceedings by criminal charges being brought against him, he is subject to a process in which there is a considerable amount of discretion that is used in the application of legal sanctions. Legal decisions to which an accused may be subjected include not only the enforcement of those sanctions defined by law but also the determination of whether the individual should be excused from the application of those sanctions. Legal determinations that are exclusionary in function are predominantly concerned with the mental or emotional makeup of the individual. When the defendant's condition is such as to indicate the presence of a mental illness, an initial consideration for exclusion from the criminal proceedings is that of determining his competency to stand trial. Our legal system is designed to exclude those mentally ill individuals who are unable to understand the nature of the proceedings against them or to assist in their own defense. Mental illness may also be a determinant that excludes the application of legal sanctions as an excusing factor implied in the verdict of "not guilty by reason of insanity." These decisions require the input of medical and psychological data on which the legal decisions may be based.

Psychological data also influence discretionary decisions that are made after determination of the legal facts in applying sanctions such as placing an individual on probation or sentencing him to an institution. If sentenced to an institution, the type of institutionalization, the conditions of imprisonment, the treatment and programming

FRED J. PESETSKY • 1905 Grovedale, Jackson, Michigan 49203. ALBERT I. RABIN • Department of Psychology, Michigan State University, East Lansing, Michigan 48824.

FRED J. PESETSKY
AND ALBERT I. RABIN

to which an individual is exposed, and an individual's subsequent release are all broad discretionary tactics which are based on both behavioral and impressionistic data which may or may not be relevant to the decision that is made. Input from psychologists and psychiatrists is heavily relied on for making many of these decisions.

Friedman (1975) attempts to describe legal systems in behavioral terms and views the delivery of sanctions as providing reward or punishment. The major focus is on sanctions being a form of deterrence in that punishment will produce more deterrence and less forbidden behavior. He views the deterrent effect of sanctions as either general, in that there is a greater likelihood that the population or part of it when hearing about a sanction or seeing it in operation would modify its behavior accordingly, or special, in which the application of punishment is to reduce or eliminate the commission of future crime by the person being punished.

The difficulty of the type of sanction, positive or negative, or its impact on various types of offenders is viewed by Friedman as being determined by the characteristics of the threat or promise and the characteristics of the behavior to be controlled. Input from the behavioral scientists in determining sanctions to be applied may allow for greater specific deterrence, while laws indicating formal sanctions to be applied may provide for more general deterrence.

Once the sanction of imprisonment is imposed, correctional approaches and programming are employed in an attempt to alter the individual. This correctional approach is based on the general impression that simple delivery of sanctions is insufficient in providing specific deterrence. If the deterrent value of legal sanctions were indeed effective, there would be little need for correctional treatment or programming designed to alter the individual to whom the sanctions have been applied.

The type of treatment to which an individual would be exposed during the course of his "punishment" may depend on three factors. The first consideration of some criminologists is that enforced treatment is a continuation of punishment. A second consideration may be that correctional programming and treatment during incarceration make the punishment more benevolent by providing the opportunity for change. The third determination may be that our own benevolence is directed toward reducing the negative impact of the applied sanctions.

The rationale by which decisions are made in the criminal justice system and their actual operation may be viewed through the paradigm utilized by Chronbach and Gleser (1957). These authors applied decision theory to psychological testing and personnel decisions. They presented the characteristics of decision processes as having an individual about whom a decision is required, having available two or more treatments which may be applied, and rendering the decision on the basis of information possessed about the individual. That information becomes processed by means of an established principle of interpretation or strategy, which produces either a terminal decision or an investigatory decision calling for additional information. If the decision is investigatory, it indicates what tools or procedures may be used to gather that information and subsequently lead to a further decision. This cycle would continue until eventually a terminal decision is made by assigning an individual to a treatment option. The outcome of that decision would be the individual's performance under the assigned treatment.

Diagnostic procedures, the gathering of information and classification of data, are significant processes influencing both the terminal decision and its outcome. Once an individual is accused of the commission of a crime and formally entered into the criminal justice system, he becomes subject to the sequential series of decisions. This includes pretrial decisions, those decisions made during courtroom proceedings, postconviction decisions by the court, and decisions during the application of prescribed sanctions.

In all of these decisions, there is a continued reliance on receiving information about the individual. Much of that information concerns an individual's personal adjustment, interpersonal relationships, and specific behavior patterns. Psychologists and psychiatrists are generally recognized by our society as experts who possess definitive knowledge and skills in obtaining information about an individual, who match that information to the decision to be made, and who predict the outcome of the decision. Understandably, the validity of this assumption is highly questionable if not erroneous. The major contribution that may be made by any diagnostician in this system is that of providing information to the legal and judicial experts who carry the responsibility as decision makers. When the behaviorial scientist avoids his assumption of that responsibility, he is free to use his expertise in making his appraisal of an individual. This enhances objectivity by not allowing the decision to influence information gathering. Independence of diagnostic assessment may then occur without the intrusion of personal or philosophical biases that are inherent in decisions and their outcomes.

It is also of interest that many of the decisions that are made are not mutually exclusive, although frequently they should be. For instance, there is a tendency to regard an individual found incompetent to stand trial as not guilty by reason of insanity, because the mental illness related to the former is viewed as intrinsic to the latter. However, an individual may become mentally ill after the commission of a crime because of the impact of having committed the act or because of the stress of being involved in criminal proceedings. If not considered exculpable, the finding of incompetency and subsequent restoration to competency may materially affect subsequent decisions without regard to the individual's present condition and needs. Initial decisions may also preclude calling for further investigatory decisions at later phases in the criminal justice procedure, or they may prevent a diagnostician from more fully using the tools, skills, or other resources at his disposal. Because an individual may be exposed to a variety of terminal decisions, it may be fruitful to evaluate those decisions as they occur in the criminal justice process and review those factors that should be included in information-gathering procedures.

The paradigm of Chronbach and Gleser clearly demonstrates the relationship between the techniques and instrument of assessment and the outcome of decisions in terms of cost factors. When applied to personnel selection, the cost factors provide an indication of the effectiveness of the decisions in terms of economic considerations and efficiency of operations to business management. The impact may be measured in terms of the effect on the organization as well as on the individual involved, inasmuch as personnel decisions do have an effect on the life-style of the individual concerned. More significant intrinsic factors are found in criminal justice decisions, because the cost factors may be secondary to intangibles of greater significance. The outcome of decisions, for instance, influences an individual's life and life-style and the lives and well-being of others.

In view of the resurgence of interest in the death penalty, the outcome of a treatment decision is clearly significant. Length of imprisonment and conditions of

FRED J. PESETSKY
AND ALBERT I. RABIN

confinement are additional treatment options of major consequence to both the individual and other members of society. The outcome of decisions is highly influenced by considerations of an individual's "dangerousness" to others in an effort to protect society from further criminal transgressions. While the philosophy of protection of the public dictates the application of criminal sanctions, the same philosophy has an impact on the assessment process which may dictate what information is entered into the decision-making. The cost factors of protection of the public, along with protection of an individual and his civil liberties, requires that the assessment process be as objective as possible. The reliance on input of information from mental health practitioners requires the use of comprehensive and sophisticated diagnostic procedures which may be far removed from the current state of the science and the art of psychological assessment and prediction. Because decisions have to be made from the current state of diagnostic assessment, use should be made of available resources, including both actuarial data and clinical impressions, which are based on information-gathering procedures oriented toward independent decisions at various stages of the criminal justice process.

2. Pretrial Decisions

Diagnostic procedures most often initiated for pretrial decisions center on the determination of ability to stand trial. The competency decisions clearly refer to the defendant's comprehension skills. The competency decision may be based on definitions which vary from one jurisdiction to another, but the basic ingredients are the same. Legal competency is determined when an individual is found capable of understanding the nature of the proceedings against him and is able to assist in his defense. The question of competency is raised to the court prior to trial to determine whether the defendant is capable of assuming the role of a defendant. While this remains a legal determination, the information on which the decision is based is predominantly medical and psychological. How and why the competency of the defendant is questioned are clearly not objectively determined with any degree of consistency.

One of the authors (F. P.) had the opportunity to participate in the evaluation of a convicted offender to determine whether the individual could be regarded as mentally ill by any criterion, including his history. He acknowledged deliberately deceiving his attorney and refusing to openly communicate with him because he was not cleared by the CIA to handle top-secret information. Obviously, if that impression was communicated to his attorney, his competency to stand trial would have been questioned and the appropriate proceedings initiated. Whether this allegation is fact or fiction would be immaterial, because the presentation of the statement would have indicated the possibility of the individual's being mentally ill—the concept on which the determination of competency is grounded.

Limited intelligence, restricted abstraction capacity, social or educational deprivation, or other factors are less likely, if at all, related to the concept of competency when mental illness is not indicated. Individuals are allegedly restored to competency in mental hospitals, not educational institutions or institutions for the mentally retarded. A retardate may have charges against him dropped if committed to an institution, but that will depend on whether the stringent criteria for admission are met, not on the basis of the legal definition of competency.

Although the matter of competency may be an issue of degree of impaired functioning, it is viewed as a discrete entity which is either absent or present. Very often, the particular crime is the significant factor in raising the question. The use of violence or the presence of typical or bizarre features may indicate the possibility of mental illness. Thomas and Hess (1963) studied patients committed to a state hospital as "incompetent to stand trial," with interesting and embarrassing results. They found that in many of the records there was no indication of mental illness or insanity. They also found that the psychiatrist would frequently assume the role of a judicial expert by directing the decision makers into prescriptive programming rather than answering the question of competency. The investigators also found that the majority of psychiatric reports were empty and meaningless but accepted and used by the courts as "evidence." It was also discovered that courts often granted permission for "incompetent" persons to have a hospital parole to their homes in society for as long as 3 years before there was any conclusion to the legal process.

There have since been changes in the procedures followed in some jurisdictions in making the determination of competency task oriented. However, the lack of objective criteria of competency may militate against objective determinations. Robey (1965) and Lipsitt and McGarry (1971) have attempted to provide more standardized criteria to be applied in determining the competency question. The more systematized approach is presented in a checklist format by Robey (1965) in directing diagnostic attention to three areas of "competency." Comprehension of court proceedings is the first segment for review and is regarded as a relatively simple cognitive task. The second determination is that of the individual's ability to assist counsel and is likely to be more difficult. The facts of the case and legal strategy are influenced by more factors than the presence of a mental illness. The final area of concern is addressed toward an evaluation of the defendant's "susceptibility to decompensation" while awaiting or standing trial to estimate the "potential" for becoming incompetent after the evaluation.

The checklist may direct diagnostic attention in an attempt to standardize the evaluation process. However, no operational criteria of competency to stand trial are offered or available in psychological or legal definitions.

Without a consensually validated set of criteria for the determination of competency, the assertions of Robey provide a beneficial beginning for a task-oriented evaluation. However, concepts of mental illness may reduce the effectiveness of such evaluations because they may bias a task which calls for what Szasz (1963) views essentially as a determination of a defendant's ability to perform cognitively the role of being a defendant. Moving the focus from mental illness to an evaluation of cognitive functioning will prevent the evaluator from making a diversion into unrelated issues. The matter of competency should remain independent of findings of mental illness because the presence of such disorders need not materially effect the functions being evaluated.

While the clinical diagnosis of mental illness may intrude on the independent determination of competency to stand trial, further intrusions may occur when subsequent responsibilities are added to the functions of the evaluator by responsible social agents or by the diagnostician's own perceptions. This may easily occur when the determination of "incompetency" may be preparatory to determination of diminished responsibility or exculpability, which are themselves independent legal determinations. The implications of a future outcome of being found "not guilty by reason

FRED J. PESETSKY
AND ALBERT I. RABIN

of insanity" are inherent in initial evaluations of competency to stand trial. When an agent or agency is charged with simultaneously making both determinations, each determination contaminates the other. The processes may be separate, but they are not independent.

An illustration of a threefold contaminatory effect may be found in the operation of the Center for Forensic Psychiatry in Michigan. This unit was originally established to perform evaluations of competency and to provide required treatment to restore those so adjudicated to a state where they were able to assume the defendant's role and to stand trial. Additional responsibilities were subsequently assigned as the Center extended its evaluations to include questions of insanity for subsequent pleas of findings of diminished responsibility or exculpability. Competency and insanity are distinct legal findings and can remain discrete tasks only when evaluators address the questions independently. With both considerations being made simultaneously, the finding of competency can materially affect the findings and testimony of insanity, and the anticipation of questions of insanity will affect the determination of competency. The third contamination occurred when the state of Michigan passed legislation establishing a plea of "guilty but mentally ill." This is a legal judgment in addition to "not guilty by reason of insanity." An individual found not guilty by reason of insanity would be sent to a mental hospital, with his subsequent release from incarceration being determined by his recuperation from a "mental illness." The finding of "guilty but mentally ill" differs little from the "guilty" verdict because the individuals so adjudicated are institutionalized in the prison. The "guilty but mentally ill" allegedly differ from those found "guilty" by receiving treatment during their confinement. However, if they do "recuperate" from a mental illness, they continue to serve their criminal sentence. The "insane" are excused from criminal sanctions and hospitalized, and are released when they are considered no longer mentally ill. The "guilty but mentally ill" go to prison and continue to remain in prison until paroled or discharged.

The matter of competency refers solely to the cognitive ability of an individual to assume the role of the defendant. The exculpability in a finding of insanity is determined by a mental illness ostensibly influencing the commission of the act, and "guilty but mentally ill" is a finding that an individual is mentally ill but that the criminal actions are not directly or necessarily the product of that illness.

It is clear that the diagnostic agents charged with the three determinations will find it exceedingly difficult if not impossible to simultaneously address the three tasks independently.

3. Trial Decisions

Excluding unique verdicts such as Michigan's "guilty but mentally ill," the preponderance of trial decisions address themselves to the problem of exculpability or diminished responsibility. The typical trial procedure evaluates evidence for the determination of guilt. A plea of "not guilty by reason of insanity" is essentially a plea of guilty. The difference between this plea and the guilty plea stresses that the individual lacked criminal intent due to being mentally ill, so as to fit the legal criteria that excuse these actions.

While the legal tests, definitions, or criteria vary across jurisdictions, Rappeport (1975) reports that most jurisdictions in the United States use essentially the Mc-Naughten Rule or the American Law Institute's Model Penal Code Test. Rappeport is quick to note that many authors imply that a person must be psychotic in order to be considered not guilty by reason of "insanity." The concept of insanity has no objective criteria, however, and diagnostic procedures are directed toward labeling an individual as mentally ill. Diagnostic procedures stop with the affixing of the psychiatric label, and speculation then begins.

It is easy to understand the difficulties in extrapolating from a label of mental illness to an estimate of insanity if we view the sematics of the legal rules. Rappeport (1975) cites these rules: McNaughten: "At the time of committing of the act, the party accused was laboring under such a defect of reason, from a disease of the mind, as not to know the nature and quality of the act he was doing; or, if he did know it, that he did not know what he was doing was wrong" (p. 289). American Law Institute: "A person is not responsible for criminal conduct if, at the time of such conduct as a *result of Mental Disease* or *Defect* he lacks *substantial* capacity to either *appreciate* the criminality (wrongfulness) of his conduct, or to *conform* his conduct to the requirements of the law" (pp. 292–293).

The Durham Rule from the 1954 decision by Judge Bazelon, Chief Justice of the United States Court of Appeals in the District of Columbia, is cited by Halleck (1971): "The Rule we now hold is simply that an accused is not criminally responsible if his unlawful act was the product of mental disease or defect" (p. 213). "Disease" referred to a condition considered capable of improving or deteriorating, while "defect" was viewed as capable of neither.

These rules seem relatively simple until the semantics is considered. What is meant by "nature of the act" and by "quality of the act"? How do they differ? If a subject knew both, whatever they mean, by what standard will it be determined that he knew it was "wrong"? What criteria of wrongness are to be imposed? Regardless of experts who assume they know the meanings, those meanings are not inherent in the law. Smith and Musk (1976) report the impression of others that the testifying psychiatrists (and other expert witnesses) are rarely asked about what words such as "substantial capacity" and "appreciate" mean to them. The meaning of the words may vary both denotatively and connotatively from one expert to another.

The reliability and validity of psychiatric diagnosis have been challenged for years. The labeling process has been well influenced by factors other than symptomatology, such as economic status, political ideology of the subject, and even the presence of an attorney for the client. These factors are well reviewed and demonstrated by the research of Braginsky and Braginsky (1974). These authors view the identification and classification of deviants as part of the process of "social sanitation," of removing those deviants from the "mainstream of society."

This social sanitation, however, is not the function of the identification and classification of offenders in the decision of insanity. Greater benevolence is ostensibly involved in this process, because the effort is to extricate a "sick" individual from harm by the exposure to criminal sanctions. The imposition of punitive sanctions serves to protect society, while the finding of insanity provides an alternative of treating the individual.

In essence, we stigmatize an individual as mentally ill to avoid stigmatizing him as being criminal. Burt (1976) analyzes the legal reform movement in the mental health area to show that our benevolence lies behind the conceptual (labeling) and spatial (institutionalizing) segregation of the mentally ill. This same phenomenon occurs in decision-making regarding insanity.

The basis of this segregation continues to be the diagnosis of a mental illness despite our changing concept of abnormal behavior. Rabin (1974) reviews the changes in the concept of mental abnormality and explains part of the unreliability of diagnosis as a function of the varied conceptions. He considers the adversary situation of insanity hearings as illustrative of the lack of reliability of the judgment of abnormality and its determination by the "personal predilection of the expert."

Diagnosticians who become so involved would well heed the comments of Morris (1968), who asks whether it would be appropriate or valid to make a diagnosis on the basis of an examination which takes place months to years after the criminal act, particularly when it would be based on the report of the only observer present, one who is allegedly irrational and mentally ill—the defendant.

If this paradox is clearly recognized in the examination of the offender and if the limitations are recognized, not only should diagnostic considerations be relied on with caution but also the court should be clearly informed of the limitations of the examinations and the speculations of the examiner. The basis of the speculations, derived from diagnostic appraisal, is the most meaningful datum to be communicated to the court as an informational source rather than the expert's assuming the decision-making role. Increased reliability may be obtained when the diagnostic examination is maintained as distinct from the legal decision in spite of court efforts to have the experts make that decision.

In a 1976 trial in Detroit, an individual accused of a capital crime was evaluated by experts after the crime had occurred. The experts disagreed both on diagnosis and on their conclusions regarding the individual's "sanity." An additional expert was subpoenaed for testimony in view of his having treated the individual in the past. While he was originally subpoenaed by the defense, his testimony was clearly favorable to the prosecution. In the course of the trial, very little was made of the fact that testifying experts had evaluated the defendant many months after his apprehension until the defense attempted to discredit the testimony of the expert who had seen the individual for evaluation and treatment over a year prior to the offense. It was only with this witness that the defense attorney focused on the basis for the witness's conclusions and the fact that the data submitted were a result of contacts a long time before the criminal offense occurred. When the witness openly admitted that his testimony might not be appropriate or valid, the defense attorney raised the issue of whether the impressions might be more valid if the witness had evaluated the defendant in greater proximity to the offense or even during the enactment of the offense. The response was clearly positive, much to the delight of the prosecuting attorney and to the subsequent chagrin of the defense. The prosecutor had planned to present still another expert witness, a clinical psychologist who was directly present and fully witnessed the enactment of the crime. In this one case, a strong legal consideration of the basis from which the diagnostician gained his impressions was used to establish credibility. It did resolve Morris's paradox and emphasized the data on which speculations were based.

4. Posttrial Decisions

Criminal justice is viewed by Kittrie (1971) primarily as an instrument of crime control which proscribes acts designated as crimes and establishes penal sanctions for the purpose of deterrence. Society, however, has shifted to a more aggressive stance of crime prevention by adopting the role, functions, and operations of a "therapeutic state" which protects itself by isolating and controlling socially dangerous persons. The benevolent treatment trend is readily apparent in the decisions which exclude the mentally ill from the application of punitive sanctions, but the therapeutic state model is also inherent in postconviction decisions in the determination of dispositions and sentences.

The philosophy leads to the utilization of behavioral scientists and practitioners in providing input into sentencing decisions which may lead to imprisonment, placement on probations, or assignment to alternative programming as part of, or in lieu of, punishment. Alternatives to imprisonment became increasingly popular following Menninger's (1968) critical analysis of the negative influences of punitive sanctions. The current (as of 1978) emphasis of court decisions is to maximize the protection of society, but little attention is being paid to humanistic aspects of the resultant processes to which the convicted offender is subjected. This had led to an increased reliance on incarceration as decision makers overemphasize the possible dangerousness of the offender in order to reduce potential hazards to society.

Diagnostic processes are being used to apply the principle of the least restrictive alternative, an approach recently analyzed by Rubin (1975) in decisions of probation or imprisonment. Gilman (1975) advocates sentencing procedures that distinguish between two groups of criminals. Imprisonment would be reserved for those with a past pattern of repetitive violence, but all others would be considered ineligible for imprisonment. He would eliminate all psychiatric predictions or diagnostic evaluations for sentencing. Nevertheless, diagnostic evaluations continue to be elicited as information on which the judge may base his decisions.

This continuing reliance on diagnostic procedures may be partly based on the orientation that there are essentially two ways of maintaining social control over deviants. Goldstein (1975) provides a review of research and theory on human aggression which presents a framework of those methods. His "short-term" measure is that of preventing those individuals who behaviorally demonstrate their propensity for engaging in violence from doing so. This would be in line with the concept of maintaining public safety by incarceration. The short-term qualification is appropriate, because eventually the institutionalized person must be released. The longer-range function would be that of preventing the ability and desire to aggress from arising by removing rewards for violence and correcting or modifying those factors leading to the aggressive acts. Recognition of both short- and long-term measures may allow diagnostic work to address means of maintaining public safety as well as increase the significance of the informational input into the sentencing process.

This input may assist in preventing extraneous variables from entering the diagnostic process. Reynolds and Sanders (1975) discuss a study by Landy and Aronson as evidence that a defendant's social attractiveness can influence severity of sentence given by simulated jurors. The authors point out that the most salient factor was the social attractiveness of the defendant, but that age was also a consideration if that attractiveness was ambiguous. These same factors may operate to influence the diagnostic information of allegedly objective diagnosticians. Friedman and Mann (1976) found that the staff members of a correctional institution who had considerable contact with a youth in a rehabilitation program could not predict recidivism better than chance. Their decisions did influence discharge processes of the youth. The key influence on the staff was the level of seriousness and degree of violence of the youth's most serious offense. The other significant, but less powerful, influence was the degree to which the youth was liked. The greater the liking, the less criminal behavior was predicted. It is likely that the same variables may enter the diagnostic process and distract from its objectivity and goal.

The long- and short-term goals of public protection are based on information designed to have predictive value concerning future violence. While the above studies indicate that extraneous factors influence predictions and judgments, the state of the art or science is such that the ability of anyone to predict criminal behavior from diagnostic processes is highly questionable. Steadman (1976) reports on a study of 967 patients transferred from two New York hospitals for the "criminally insane" to civil hospitals. Psychiatric determinations of dangerousness were vastly overpredicted. The number of false positives was double the number of accurate predictions on which offenders would exhibit assaultive, nondefensive behavior toward others. Kozol, Boucher, and Garogalo (1972) asserted that dangerousness can be reliably diagnosed and effectively treated, because only 6.1% (5 of 82) of sex offenders who underwent treatment at their facility and were discharged on recommendation of their clinical staff subsequently committed serious assaultive crimes. This was in contrast to those released by court order against the advice of the clinical staff where 34.7% (17 of 49) committed serious assaultive crimes subsequent to discharge. The authors, however, failed to control for length of time at risk in the community. Wenk, Robinson, and Smith (1972) applied Kozol's indicators of dangerousness to 4146 California Youth Authority wards and found that the most efficient variable for prediction was the individual's history of actual violence. This accounted for half the subjects who later became violent. Their violent recidivism rate was 3 times that of the remainder of the group. The authors also found, in agreement with Steadman (1976), that the greatest difficulty with the predictions was the excessive number of false positives. While violence predictions were made by Wenk et al. for 1006 youths, only 52 had their past pattern of violence repeated.

Diagnostic input into the sentencing process by psychiatrists and others, in spite of lack of accurate predictability, is persistently used. Bohmer (1975) attempted to analyze the use and influence of psychiatric reports on judicial sentencing over a 5-year period in Philadelphia. Her interviews with judges revealed that they cannot understand the reports written for them by psychiatrists, but they increasingly view sex offenders in a psychiatric light. Bohmer's research revealed a low rate of acceptance of psychiatric recommendations. The judges followed those recommendations by giving a prison sentence in only 42% of the time. Interestingly, they also sentenced to imprisonment much more frequently than the psychiatrist recommended it. Recommendation for probation was followed only 37% of the time. During the 5-year research period, the psychiatrists began to recommend prison sentences more often. The summary impression of this research project is that the psychiatric report was found to have little influence on sentencing decisions.

More positive light on the contribution of diagnostic information to posttrial decisions is shed by Dana, Hannifin, Lancaster, Lore, and Nelson (1963), who studied routine psychological diagnostic and treatment planning reports in a juvenile probation department. Predictions of prognosis from psychological reports were found to have an overall accuracy rate of 80.5%. When recommendations in the report were followed, the accuracy rate was mildly increased to 82.5%.

What is apparent is that courts stress the acquisition of psychological, sociological, and other diagnostic information to contribute to the decision making after conviction. The need is perceived and acted on regardless of a lack of empirical validity of predictions and the failure of the court to act on the specific recommendations. The greatest need is for using diagnostic processes for obtaining more information about the defendant, with the goal of public safety being paramount. It is that goal that also leads to overprediction of criminal behavior and sacrifices civil liberties needlessly. Philosophically, one may ask whether the payoff in public protection is worth the sacrifice to individuals. The base rate of repetitive violence is small, but the false positives are altogether too high. Recognizing the base rate and avoiding prediction may assist the diagnostician in this segment of the decision-making process in providing only information germane to the task assigned: that of determining an appraisal of the needs of the offender and how to service those needs under the least restrictive conditions possible. This will allow the examiner to responsibly take into account the rights of the offender and the rights of society.

5. Correctional Program Decisions

Entry into the correctional system initiates diagnostic procedures designed for the purpose of classification of the offender on the basis of his program and security needs. The 1973 report of the National Advisory Commission on Criminal Justice sets forth rather exemplary views in its section on standards and goals in corrections. Classification is considered a process for determining needs and requirements of the institutionalized offender and for assigning him to programs according to his needs and existing resources. The Commission comments that too often the purpose for which a classification system might serve has not been specified, although most systems are designed for "treatment" purposes. The Commission also notes that its cursory analysis of existing systems reveals that they may be more properly called classification systems for management.

Maier (1976) reports that the classification generally occurs in a reception center where the diagnostic procedures have the intent of classifying the offender for assignment to a program designed to modify his characteristics and/or aspects of his environment which are responsible for his involvement in deviant activity. He further states that the problem with this system is that the "treaters" do not seem to know how to bring about changes in individuals by way of a treatment process. He stresses this impression by his consideration that the intervention strategies which follow from the offender typologies consist of old alternatives. Most of the offender categories tend to be based on subjective impressions of the diagnostic agents rather than being empirically determined. Warren (1971) cross-tabulated some 16 typological systems to find six subtypes of offenders; these systems were considered as leading to effective management and treatment. Decision-making was regarded as being facilitated by classification of offenders as Asocial, Conformist, Antisocial-Manipulator, Neurotic, Subcultural-Identifier, or Situational.

Using a factor analytic approach, Peterson, Quay, and Cameron (1959) were able to establish dimensions of delinquency which have classification potential. That potential was made operational by Quay and Parsons (1970) in a federal center for juvenile offenders. The authors utilized the factor-analytically developed dimensions to classify delinquents as inadequate, neurotic, psychopathic, or subcultural. Comparable objective studies have not been accomplished for the adult criminal, although such classification dimensions might assist the diagnostic process involved in both institutional management and treatment programming for the offender.

The effectiveness of assigned treatment is accurately challenged by Martinson (1974), whose poignant review of treatment programs of all varieties in corrections indicates that nothing seems to affect the recidivism rate. Palmer (1975) takes issue with Martinson by his conclusions that some of the cited studies have demonstrated at least partial success. The issue may be one of reliability and validity of the diagnostic/classification procedures on which assignment to treatment is based. Appropriate assignment to psychological, vocational, educational, and other treatment programs is required before effectiveness of programs is determined. Program assignment is a decision based on information which must be salient to the issue at hand. The discrediting of treatment programs, the popular current correctional view, assumes that diagnosis was related to decisional outcome.

Bazelon (1972) indicted psychologists for failing to change the majority of offenders but assumed that their contribution was significant in determining correctional programming. Too often the impact of psychological recommendations has been ignored or has been minimally effective because of overriding concern for "custody" and "security" which affects the classification process. Silber (1974) finds mental health workers few and far between, and treatment the exception rather than the rule. He cites reasons for most prisoners receiving little or no systematic treatment. In 1976, the ratio of professional staff to prisoners was 1:179 nationally.

Psychological treatment agents were just not available. Using available survey data, Silber concludes that most prisoners do not demonstrate the traditional psychotic and neurotic symptomatology ordinarily in the province of the mental health worker. Character disorders composed the preponderance of diagnostic labels among prisoners. Finally, Silber notes that the custodial staffs of prisons usually viewed the professionals with both hostility and ambivalence.

He does recommend diagnosis at reception centers becoming a two-way process which provides feedback to the offender and allows him to participate in the decisions made. Informing the offender of the results of his evaluation and reasons for recommended options may well assist in motivating the offender into changing his behavioral patterns. The feedback process may also provide for the correction of data on which diagnosis is based. This is far from standard procedure, however, and would in all likelihood meet with resistance from many professionals unsure of their skills and tasks.

Shover (1974) attempted to determine the process by which practitioners learned techniques and diagnostic semantics of institutions, interviewed and diagnosed inmates, and trained their successors. He found novices placed in their responsibilities in corrections without agreed-on and empirically reliable techniques for analyzing the possible causes of the criminality of offenders. There is no body of theory endorsed by those in corrections. Diagnostic categories applied in corrections were considered arbitrary, ambiguous, and ad hoc. Agency diagnostic procedures were self-serving and directed toward "lubricating the work flow and minimizing disruptions to routine." Cynical attitudes were developed by the novices as competency in classification grew, and the disillusioned left, while those who remained appeared to accept the disillusionment and personal dissatisfaction in exchange for job security.

Another interesting commentary on the system's socialization process is illustrated in Moynihan's (1976) dissertation on the socialization of volunteer and professional correctional workers. He found them "getting burned," from their perspective, as they view themselves as systematically deceived by the tacit assumptions and procedural operations of the correctional enterprise. Being ideologically cheated is a resounding self-perception due to conceptualizations of rehabilitation being superficial and antiquated so that rehabilitative goals are not achieved. Correctional administration emphasized procedural activity and operations to the degree that the workers found themselves required to acquiesce to the primary correctional system function of public safety.

There is no doubt that this socialization within the system profoundly affects diagnostic and information-gathering procedures; it also provides the diagnosticians and data gatherers with a myopic screen that subjects the data to distortions and selectivity. This affects the establishment of classification systems by varied correctional departments. The operations of the classificatory system are additionally a function of the degree of sophistication of the diagnostic personnel, the instruments used, the available institutional resources, and bureaucratic pressures to complete routine administrative processes. The general task of classification may be the institutional assignment of an individual based on sex, length of sentence, age, and other objective factors. The more significant contributions of the diagnostic process are related to the following, not all-inclusive, areas:

1. Level of security or custodial restriction. Assignment to an institution based on security needs is frequently depicted in terms of maximum, medium, and minimum custodial control. Diversion into community programs may also be accomplished within this framework. The contributing factors may include objective criteria such as length of sentence, escape history, type of crime, or legal specification. Intangible influences may include an estimate of the individual's need for protection because of the possibility of homosexual assault or victim potential in a predatory population. Either of these factors may lead to either an increase or a decrease of security restrictions. Assessments of violence-prone prisoners and estimates of "impulse control" are other factors affecting security-level determinations. How these determinations are made varies across systems and among diagnostic experts.

2. Educational and vocational programming. Achievement and vocational interest and aptitude tests frequently are used to assign individuals to programs which may range from special education programs through college courses. Vocational training and speech correction may be offered if the resources are available. Routine work assignments may be esoteric outcomes of this area of assessment.

3. Intellectual functioning. Both group and individually administered intelligence tests may be used to establish an estimate of current functioning to determine program classification, and may also serve as a source of data for "understanding" the individual criminal behavior. Programs for the mentally retarded are few, but this information may shed light on institutional management problems as well as possible placements when the individual leaves the system. The severely retarded never make it into

FRED J. PESETSKY
AND ALBERT I. RABIN

the criminal system because they qualify for alternative programming, but a larger number of the mildly retarded may find themselves in a correctional system which may recommend specialized handling at the institutional level. However, unless specific programs are available, the special management just does not get provided.

4. Institutional counseling. Personality tests may be administered and, along with clinical interviewing and social histories, may indicate a need for an individual to receive counseling to assist in achieving a gamut of goals ranging from assisting in prison adjustment to rehabilitation. Goals are generally excluded from the recommendation for counseling, and counselors in the correctional system frequently lack any professional or formal training in "counseling." While goals are left vague or unspecified, recommendations for individual or group counseling are almost a general requirement.

5. Mental health needs and services. Psychiatric and psychological services may be available within a correctional system, or resources from that state's department of mental health may be used to provide needed care for the mentally ill. Functional neuroses and psychoses as well as neurological problems require assessment, and care in a residential mental health program or while an individual matriculates within a prison population may be necessary. Hospital or community mental health services may be provided as a function of the classification process if those resources exist. Generally, the resources that exist are corrective rather than preventive. The mental health professional may also be imposed on to provide treatment services for acting-out disciplinary problems and assume the goal of social control under the aegis of treatment. This is particularly the case when there is a clear acceptance of the stereotypes that the mentally ill are dangerous and that the dangerous are mentally ill.

6. Medical needs. The involvement of physicians in the classification process provides for the assessment of physical illnesses, problems, and disabilities which may require placement in institutions possessing the required resources for both acute and chronic care. This includes medical demands which may temporarily or permanently override other program determinations. Diabetes, epilepsy, physical handicaps, and specialized conditions may exert a powerful influence over program recommendations. Medical practices may also become involved as part of the process of correction or treatment of the offender; plastic surgery, for example, may be a valuable tool in producing psychological and behavioral change.

7. Special treatment programs. Correctional systems may have a variety of treatment programs which cater to distinctive offenders. These programs may be at the disposal of the offender, or he may be directly or tacitly coerced into participating in them.

Programs to deal with chemical abuse are dichotomized into those for alcoholics and those for other drug abusers. The programs are determined by either educational or therapeutic orientations, with little assignment to the groups so organized on the basis of diagnosis. This provides little consideration of differential treatment as dictated by individual needs.

The major goal for the assigned treatment method is independence from chemicals, but this is a symptomatic approach. Krystal and Raskin (1970) explored three areas of drug-personality interactions: affect, object representation, and modification of consciousness. It would appear that a more sophisticated assignment to treatment programs based on diagnostic procedures assessing these factors may provide for more rapid and effective treatment. In achieving a prescription of differential treatment, motivation for drug use may consider factors such as Wikler and Rasor's (1953) finding that addicts have chief sources of anxiety related to pain, sexuality, and expression of aggression. Heller and Mordkoff (1972) postulate two types of abusers on the basis of choice of drug, with heroin addicts being considered as psychopathic personalities with little evidence of overt reports of anxiety, guilt, insecurity, or depression and with dominating antisocial personalities. Other or multiple drug abusers are highlighted as possessing antisocial personalities along with anxiety and depression. A similar typology is evident in the writings of Ausubel (1958), indicating that drugs are used to cope with emotional difficulties. Anxiety is self-treated by the neurotic through the drug choice; the psychotic uses the drug to alleviate depression or suppress delusions, and the thrill of drug use and its effects, being an ego-enhancing experience, is reinforcing for the psychopath.

It would appear that increased diagnostic attention in the reinforcements of the drug, motivations for the drugs, and the selection of the drug of choice may produce information to dictate the treatment needs of drug abusers and the orientations or goals that should be inherent in treatment alternatives.

With the repeal (in Michigan and other states) of criminal sexual psychopath laws, the sex offender has been diverted into the correctional system rather than being institutionalized in mental health facilities. This has led to a proliferation of treatment programs for the sex offender in the correctional setting. Diagnosis of individual needs, values, motivations, and emotional and mental states has given way to a more popularly accepted approach based on assignment due to the nature of the crime. Specialized treatment may be indicated, for example, for sex offenders, but rarely is there a differential set of programs established on the basis of individual diagnostic considerations.

Kozol (1971) attempts to describe a number of myths about the sex offender, and, in particular, the belief that all sex offenders are dangerous. This may be one of the factors that leads to sex offenders receiving global treatment, because the major goal is that of public safety. Receiving treatment to achieve that goal is commendable if it indeed does succeed in diminishing the dangerous potential of repetitive behavior. However, this behavior is not that repetitive, and the belief on which it is based appears erroneous.

Diagnostic procedures employed with sex offenders may follow for the identification of the "dangerous" or "repeaters" in order to reduce the number of false positives. Individual diagnosis of sex offenders may also allow the sex offense to be viewed as symptomatic, habitual, accidental, or part of an individual's life-style. Differential treatment may then be recommended.

A final group of specialized treatment programs is made available for the violent or psychopathic offender. Violence and psychopathy may not necessarily go together, but if violence is one of the symptoms of the psychopathic individual then he is

FRED J. PESETSKY
AND ALBERT I. RABIN

included in the violent group. Likewise, some groups in correctional settings are ambiguously referred to as "low-impulse-control groups" and are in treatment programs to which the psychopathic and/or violent offender is assigned. Management and treatment on the basis of the crime containing assaultive behavior fail to acknowledge the psychological, situational, and physiological factors which may contribute to the behavior, independently or in combination and interaction. Psychopathic, low-impulse-control, and violent classifications of individuals are overinclusive and subject to misdiagnosis, mismanagement, and mistreatment to the degree that the safety and well-being of the offender, the institution, and society are endangered.

Psychopathic individuals have had a successful response to treatment using the medication imipramine hydrochloride (Foster, 1975). Violent offenders whose behavior was a function of temporal lobe epilepsy or another organic brain condition may be treated by a combination of medication and psychotherapy (Mark & Ervin, 1970; Small, 1973; Blumer, 1975; Walker, 1961).

Rader (1977) found the extent of psychopathology to differ among exposers, rapists, and assaulters, with the rapist being the most psychologically disturbed of the group and the assaulter being more of a "garden variety" type of psychopath. The research produced results essentially similar to that on code types of the MMPI found in the prison population (Persons & Marks, 1971).

The violent offender classified as such by his behavior may be mistreated when accurate diagnosis of causal factors is not made. One of the authors (F. P.) had been personally involved in the diagnosis and treatment of three offenders with existing patterns of violence. Two offenders were diagnosed as paranoid schizophrenic and one was diagnosed as psychopathic. Psychotherapy and chemotherapy (tranquilizers) were prescribed but to little avail, as violent behaviors continued. In the course of therapy, clues appeared to warrant diagnostic evaluation whereupon the diagnosis of temporal lobe epilepsy was supported. The use of anticonvulsant medication produced immediate effects. The psychological disequilibrium of the patients was replaced by feelings of well-being and the violent behavior disappeared.

The fact that most correctional treatment programs are not based on diagnosis or extensive psychological and behavioral assessment does little to check recidivism or otherwise protect the public and the individual. Klopfer's (1964) article, "Psychotherapy without Diagnosis, Blind Lead the Blind," is poignant as an indictment of the correctional system whose diagnostic procedures are minimal and superficial, at best. Recognition of limitations of current procedures and attempts toward improvement by attempting to assess individual needs and influences in producing criminal behavior are found in the concept of parole contracts (Gettinger, 1975). The concept refers to matching individual needs, as diagnostically assessed, with correctional programs. The parole contract or "Mutual Agreement Program" (MAP) is an agreement between the offender and the correctional and releasing authorities so that definite parole dates are established. The offender must be released on the fulfillment of those conditions which call for an inmate to complete correctional activities such as counseling, educational courses, group therapy, or vocational training and to maintain a specified level of adjustment. Nine states and the District of Columbia are presently using such contracts with approximately 4000 inmates.

Such performance and service contracts are probably most feasible when based on objective and accurate assessment. Finckenauer and Rauh (1976) view the disadvantages of the MAP as overshadowing any advantages. Contracts are viewed as operating under the untested assumption that positive changes in the repertoire of the inmates are going to occur. Given the established attitudes of diagnosticians in the correctional system, the concern for mechanical processing, the restrictive diagnostic procedures, the current level of resources, and the state of the art and science of prediction and rehabilitation, the operation of MAP may mislead correctional administrators, the offender, and the general public. Finckenauer and Rauh anticipate that the MAP may encourage manipulation by inmates, prison staff, and parole boards. This would have the effect of rewarding deviant behavior or those attitudes and inclinations producing it.

The conclusion of Martinson (1974) that nothing works in corrections, if accurate, indicates that the MAP is or will become an innocuous bureaucratic procedure whose only impact is to indicate that "something is being done." Sommer (1976) criticizes prison systems for adopting the approach to do something, anything, if something is amiss or goes astray. It gives the impression that corrective action has been taken, but the conclusion is not necessarily valid. It would appear that a more corrective process would be involved in directing attention to the decision-making in the system and the reliability and validity of the diagnostic procedures and other information-gathering techniques. The assignment of programs and establishment of contracts may be entirely based on factors immaterial to an individual's needs. The well-known YAVIS syndrome was an effective constellation indicating the characteristics of the patient who would receive preferential psychotherapy because he was young, attractive, verbal, intelligent, and successful. It may be that this same syndrome operates to determine correctional classification and program assignment rather than the determination based on relevant factors that contribute to the commission of the crime, or on the individual needs of the offender.

6. Base Level and Exit Assessment

If we are indeed to improve the state of the art and the knowledge of treating offenders, the proper starting point would be the identification of offenders. Offender typologies used in classification systems in the correctional process are based on subjective speculation, and they lack the sophisticated objectivity that is reflected in the typologies or dimensions of delinquency of Quay (1970). An attempt to determine the dimensions of criminality should begin with a diagnostic assessment of all criminals at the correctional entry stage. This could be initiated at some stage of the trial process. However, the individual is not criminal until he has been so adjudicated by the court. The time of presentence following adjudication would be another possibility. But qualified diagnosticians are not readily available to all courts. Correction reception information systems usually provide diagnostic personnel and programs for all but probationers. Ideally, it would be the court that would be able to provide the base level determination (BLD) for each convicted offender. This would be a diagnostic assessment of the individual and his crime as a standard to determine the makeup of the offender for the development of typologies. The base level determination would also be the control or comparison standard against which changes are measured. The BLD could serve to provide an understanding of criminal behavior and to assist in determining how existing community or prison programs may be utilized in protecting the public by restrictions and/or treatment. It would additionally indicate the type of programs that should be developed on a community or institutional level. The use of actuarial data may provide an estimate of the potential hazard, i.e., maintaining an individual in the community. These data from nature of crime studies will direct the diagnostician toward recommending programs in restrictive or institutional settings. An actual pattern of continued criminal involvement or repetitive episodic criminality also indicates increased need for treatment under conditions of confinement or restriction.

The degree of control required would indicate whether appropriate community alternatives exist or whether confinement is necessary. Should evaluations indicate that institutionalization is an option used because of the lack of community resources, the extent to which this is happening will document the need for community program development. The lack of programs, community or institutional, to meet the needs of the offender and to protect the public, on both short-term and long-term bases, may also be documented when diagnosticians specify what is necessary for public safety and offender needs. Compromise recommendations should be clearly noted, as well as recommendations for management and treatment using only existing resources. The BLD would also provide the opportunity for both individual diagnosis and for evaluating those programs to which individuals have been assigned. Individual diagnosis through the BLD would be instrumental in obtaining estimates of current needs of current offenders. This would allow for the elimination of costly and ineffective programs which do not service current needs. Replacement by programs developed for the greatest need may occur when the finances of outmoded programs are redirected.

Diagnostic procedures at the point of criminal justice entry may provide a standardized diagnostic service that could intensively gather information to be used at a decision-making point in the system, culminating in comparison diagnostics at the point of exit. Continued dangerousness or hazard to society may be estimated by viewing changes in the individual as a result of, or in spite of, efforts at rehabilitation or treatment. Exit testing or diagnostic assessment prior to release has no comparison criteria and provides little more than a global predictive effort based on little knowledge of the offender and pure speculation of change. These assessments are, nonetheless, required by procedure or law in a number of jurisdictions. The BLD should be structured so as to provide an assessment of the dimensions of an individual's current level of psychological adjustment and state of integration. This includes personality factors and states of organization that are unique for the individual, as well as stresses and cognitive and emotional functioning. The presence of social, emotional, or organic disorders and their level of significance are included in this assessment.

Since the evaluation was required as the result of deviant behavior, emphasis should be placed on those factors which appear to bear a causal relationship to the criminal action. This relationship should be clearly specified. The individual meaning of the criminal act to the subject and its relationship to his "life-style" can be ascertained by its patterned, episodic, or accidental nature.

The significance of the act to the individual and determination of whether it is syntonic or dystonic is to be assessed in exploring the motivations for the act, including the "psychodynamics" or highly individualistic purpose it serves.

Because situational and interpersonal components may be present, their level of significance should be included in the total evaluation. These components serve to provide motivational insights and may be of direct causal consequence.

Once clinical impressions are gained, it is necessary to include the actuarial data determined by the nature of the offense. The inclusion and integration of these data in the assessment process provide a predictive base in determining the likelihood of repetition. This serves to assess the type of management required for public safety and determines the conditions under which a treatment program may be required.

The final assessment direction would focus on the individual's motivation for change and should follow a feedback of recommendations and the information on which they are based. This allows the entry of the individual into the diagnostic process when his perceptions and involvement may provide additional information to support or change management and treatment specifications.

While the above information may allow for the use of psychiatric or other nosological labels, the true diagnosis would be the total evaluation. This would prevent the confusion that appears from the use of labels, because dimensions of criminality would be stressed for more complete informational input into the decision makers. Diagnostic emphasis on the dimensions which contribute to criminal behavior also serves to provide a more complete evaluation which may be used for a variety of decisions as well as permit further evaluations to have a resource for comparison to evaluate changes. The BLD thus allows for the use of the individual as his "own control."

If the recommendations of Silber (1974) to criminal justice workers are heeded, attention may be initiated at the initial decision of classification, that is, the diagnostic process which would be able to be modified from its adequate state to a more sophisticated level.

7. Models and Diagnostic Procedures

The orientation from which diagnosticians operate not only determines the procedures that are used but also influences the information elicited and the ensuing findings and actions. The fads and fashions of model construction and utilization in the behavioral sciences have done little to reduce or eliminate the lack of connection between diagnosis and intervention. In application of behavioral models in the criminal setting, there is no standardized acceptable approach which relates existing models to the philosophy or goals of correctional agents (correctional models).

Rabin (1974) emphasizes the lack of a demonstrable relationship between specifically diagnosed conditions and intervention as prescribed. Diagnostic procedures are established by those systems and organizations which perceive their applicability to the system's need. In the correction of criminally deviant patterns of behavior, the purposes of the prevalent model for correction cannot be eliminated from the way in which diagnostic procedures are established or used. Sommer (1976) suggests that correctional systems suffer a condition he diagnoses as the "model muddle." The variety of correctional systems influences what can be expected of the process of imprisonment. Deterrence, rehabilitation, reform, vengeance, restitution, incapacitation, reeducation, and integration in the community are some of his designated correctional models. There is always some degree of overlap between models, and their governing of day-to-day correctional operations includes the governing of diagnostic models in the information-gathering process.

The influence of these correctional models on the diagnostic process may be found in the social interaction between diagnostician and subject (Rabin, 1974). It is perhaps this interaction that has led to research findings which demonstrate the influence of social economic level (Hollingshead & Redlich, 1958; Lee, 1968; Efron, 1970), political ideology (Braginski & Braginski, 1974), and ego-reinforcing compliments (Braginski & Braginski, 1974) on the diagnosis of mental disorders. Influences of YAVIS and physical attractiveness affected judgments of mental health (Katz & Zimbardo, 1977) and harshness of sentencing by simulated jurors (Reynolds & Sanders, 1975).

What is needed is not the acceptance of a particular model, be it medical, correctional, social-behavioral, humanistic, or otherwise, because our knowledge and understanding of criminal behavior and ways to correct it are grossly limited. There is rather a need to establish diagnostic procedures which will produce information at the decision level, a diagnostic process which will be devoid of theoretical bias and based on operational concepts.

Perhaps the tendencies for excursion into theoretical abstractions can be curtailed in considering the purposes that diagnostic assessments serve. Klopfer (1968) states that, from the viewpoint of the three parties (examiner, patient, and reader of the report), diagnostic studies serve three purposes:

1. The understanding of the patient
2. The prediction of future behavior
3. Establishment of a record of the patient's psychological state at a given time, place, and under a given set of circumstances

It would seem that all three functions are pertinent to diagnostic assessment at any given point in the decision-making processes in the criminal justice system. Too frequently, however, diagnosticians fall prey to what Klopfer calls a basic fallacy in clinical evaluation and clinical research: that there is only "such a thing as a 'basic' or 'true' personality" (p. 257).

Klopfer suggests that diagnostic procedures become attuned to three levels: public communication and public image, level of conscious self-concept, and level of "private symbolization." Diagnostic techniques and psychological objective and projective testing would obtain information from one or more of the three levels. Report of findings would then specify the levels from which the data is obtained.

Implicit in Klopfer's levels of assessment is a diversion from theoretical, philosophical, and moral models concerning the criminal into a model for assessment designed specifically for the purposes of understanding, prediction, and establishment of a specified base level of behavioral functioning. Recognition of different levels of assessment will, however, not be sufficient to prevent moral values from entering into the prescriptive and predictive action phase of the assessment, because this is where the greater amount of bias is introjected. This is particularly the case as most evaluations occur on the first level of assessment.

A well-known psychiatric authority on murders was requested to conduct an evaluation of a 55-year-old white male who shot and killed a work supervisor. The psychiatrist indicated that, on the basis of the patient's history and his clinical impressions, "Mr. S. has always been a hard-working, law-abiding individual. He was highly dependent upon his wife. In the fall of 1975, Mr. S. suffered a depressive illness as a reaction to his wife's hospitalization, surgery and prolonged separation. On September 18, 1975, there was an additional stress of having been fired from his job as a security guard. This was apparently precipitated by his poor work performance, which in turn was secondary to his depressive illness. He focused his anger on his supervisor, proceeded to the plant, and killed him instantly. After the act he behaved in a way designed to insure his immediate apprehension. While incarcerated, he developed a severe psychotic depression characterized by delusions, hallucinations and bizarre suicidal attempts by lacerating his eyes with broken glass from his own eye glasses. He was hospitalized in a mental hospital and I reviewed that report. In the interview, he was a profoundly depressed emaciated individual who is desperately in need of psychiatric care. If he is sent to prison, such action will constitute, in my opinion, cruel and unusual punishment of this severely ill individual and would amount to a death sentence."

The individual was found guilty of first-degree murder and remanded to a prison. Trial occurred after he had been restored to "competency." Placement in prison on a life sentence was mandatory for the crime of first-degree murder. The assessment of the quoted psychiatrist did not address the question of either competency or insanity but was an attempt to gain conviction under Michigan's new verdict of "guilty but mentally ill," which would not provide differential handling in spite of implications of the law for treatment. The evaluation may have been based on history, but was also based on clinical impressions. It is misleading because it is a recounting of facts from history. That history or self-presentation may have been the basis for statements concerning the crime, but the only clinical impression is that of recording depression in an emaciated individual in need of psychiatric care. The entry of values is clear in the prescription provided, being that of avoiding imprisonment, but not specifying what alternatives may be considered other than the judicial expert judgment of "cruel and unusual punishment" and imprisonment constituting a "death penalty."

It may be of interest to note that, when the individual was received in corrections, part of the classification process provided an additional psychiatric evaluation which stated: "The depressive psychotic episode was the aftermath of his killing. I have seen this in hundreds of murderers and it is reflective of his guilt. Placement in prison should provide the punishment that he psychologically needs and would probably offset any tendency for a repetition of his acute depressive psychosis."

Both examiners had access to the same data, but their conclusions are quite different, whether based on experience with murders, moralistic values or philosophical inclinations, or knowledge of the psychological impact of incarceration on prisoners. Or was there a game of oneupmanship being played as both are considered by experience and publication to be "experts" on "murderers"? Case history did reveal that the patient had been diagnosed as epileptic and had been on neuroleptic medication, in addition to tranquilizers which readied him for trial. It would appear that the experts involved addressed themselves to different problems at hand. The first psychiatrist was assigned the task of restoring the patient to competency, the second psychiatrist was hired to help the offender avoid the sanction of imprisonment, and the third psychiatrist was to determine alternatives or resources to be used during imprisonment. However, there are no evaluations which clearly provide an understanding of the patient, provide a basis for prediction of future behavior, or establish a record of the patient's state other than his depressed condition, which could be reliably diagnosed by anyone.

While most diagnostic assessment procedures should encompass these goals, superficial problem assessments are undertaken cursorily without regard to the fact that even initial evaluations will serve as a basis for future assessments and decisions. Recognizing the Klopferian levels may aid in producing more intensive diagnostic

FRED J. PESETSKY
AND ALBERT I. RABIN

assessment and in gathering information to provide data to contribute to the reliability and validity of both prescriptive and predictive arguments.

Because clinical judgments have been considered unreliable and of questionable validity, there has been an emphasis on actuarial predictions (Meehl, 1954). Kime (1976) reports early findings on the risk of violent behavior of individuals paroled from the Michigan Department of Corrections. Using a sample of 2033 offenders, he found the base rate of violent behavior for the total sample at 10.5%. He attempted to determine those combinations of factors which might best predict violent behavior and to identify any groups with unusually high or low potential for violence. Significant variables, in combination with two or three others, were type of crime, marital status at the time of the crime, juvenile history, age at first arrest, being raised by the mother alone, and prison adjustment. Group A, which constituted 18% of the sample and exceeded the violence base rate with a rate of 24%, was characterized as having served time for an assaultive crime and being single. Other high-risk groups were identified with violence rates of 34%, 38%, 37%, and 44%, far in excess of the base rate for the population. The same factors were used to identify low-risk groups utilizing the same process as with the high-risk groups, which is familiar to insurance companies in developing their actuarial tables. However, while these factors may categorize the offenders in high and low groups, Johnson and Kime (1975) accept the unreliability of clinical judgments of continued dangerousness but do rely on them to possibly modify the risk categories of some individuals, particularly if treatment has indicated significant change which may alter the classification of an offender's risk group. Perhaps the combination of clinical and actuarial data in the diagnostic process may improve predictive validity of classifications and judgments.

There are studies which have shown superiority of clinical judgments over actuarial procedures (Lindzey, 1965; Reitan, 1964), but the use of actuarial data in the diagnostic process may be a way to maximize the validity of the decisional process. A blending rather than an either/or function is recommended.

Reitan (1964), in using the battery of psychological tests developed by Halstead (1947) to determine brain damage, was able to identify etiology and locale of brain lesions with fairly high accuracy. He also found that the diagnoses were more accurate using clinical intuition rather than statistical methods. There was a problem of objectifying clinical inference in order to duplicate results obtained by the clinical method. Russell, Neuringer, and Goldstein (1970), in resolving this problem, described the development of "neuropsychological keys" which were based on rules of inference used by neuropsychologists. A similar approach may be useful in diagnosis and classification in the criminal justice system if the actuarial and clinical ingredients are known. Knowing the ingredients may provide novices and others with a wide recognition of the features that should be assessed in applying diagnostic procedures in order to prevent the diagnostic process from being myopic.

Whatever ingredients are proposed for the evaluative process, the tripartite conceptual model for the evaluation of mental health (social deviance, pathology, criminality) and psychotherapy (institutionalization, alternative treatments) may indicate that biases would continue. Strupp and Hadley (1977) suggest that goals and values of diagnostic and treatment activities may be judged differently depending on whether society, the individual, or the mental health professional makes the judgment.

In summary, it is essential for diagnosticians within the criminal justice system to view their procedures and findings from the vantage point of themselves as individuals and professionals, from the standpoint of the client or patient, and from the frame of reference of the system and society. Recognition of salient features in the following section on a paradigm for such an evaluation may assist the diagnostician in this task.

8. Paradigm for the Evaluation of Criminal Offenders

8.1. The Act

Deviant behavior is often subjectively defined and culturally relative. However, there are some criminal behaviors that are more universally codified., Friedman (1975) distinguishes between criminal acts as mala in se and mala prohibita. The former refers to legally proscribed activities that are viewed as inherently "bad," "criminal," or "wrong," such as murder, rape, assault. The latter refers to legally proscribed acts that are deviant, criminal, or "bad" simply because they are prohibited by law.

In coping with the deviant and his conduct, it is necessary to determine precisely what the individual is attempting to communicate through that conduct (Smith & Pollack, 1976). It is well recognized that deviants continue with their criminal pattern of behavior in spite of recognizing that their actions may well be personally destructive as well as socially harmful. Smith and Pollack view that criminal conduct as a response to stress and suggest providing other ways to relieve the stress to persuade the deviant to conform. While these authors are simplistic in their views, the focus on the "meaning" of criminal conduct is the initial stage of the diagnostic process.

That conduct, as a form of acting out, varies according to its form, place, direction, and duration (Chwast, 1965). The forms of the acting out are listed by Chwast as by the individual, by dyads, by groups, and by the family (pp. 102–103). The location of the acting out may be in the family, in the peer group, against authority, and within the community. The direction of criminal acting out can occur with a person, place, or object being the target. Finally, the duration may be episodic in pattern, or transitory or continuous.

The criminal style from awkward to sophisticated reflects how embedded an individual's life-style is in the commission of that crime and reflects the meaning of the act to the actor. The style also reveals properties important to the predictive process; those acts which are highly meaningful or reinforcing emotionally or cognitively may be high in the hierarchy of responses in the behavioral repertoire of the individual.

The situation or circumstances of the act are reflected in the strategy leading to its commission and contribute to an understanding of the expressive, instrumental, or accidental nature of the action. Other factors to be reviewed are also considered as aspects of the situation or circumstances of the crime. Whether the situation appears by chance, is sought out by the perpetrator, or is created by the actor is more understandable when the criminal style is analyzed.

The style of the crime may indicate more significant individual variables influencing the behavior. Those individuals whose crime is structured for easy apprehension may indicate the consequences of conviction as more significant than the act itself. A 19-year-old who broke into a neighborhood home and stole a number of articles including the ever-popular television set, portable record player, and sporting equipment did so after a freshly fallen snow. Not only did the police follow the tracks, but also, when they rang the offender's doorbell, the offender opened the door with all the stolen merchandise in radiant view behind him. His evaluation by a corrections diagnostician revealed intense hatred for his mother; it appeared that, dynamically, his crime served the function of self-protection. Struggling to control his impulse to kill his mother and feeling he was losing that control, he found security in being imprisoned. The criminal label and incarceration served not only to protect him from his impulses but also simultaneously to punish him for them.

8.2. The Strategy

The adaptive value of crime is paramount in the theoretical formulations of Halleck (1971). Crime is a way in which individuals experience "biological, psychological and sociologically determined situations of their existence." Crime is regarded by Halleck as a solution the offender chooses to adapt to life stress. The act itself involves motoric action or behavioral responses and, on occasion, the refusal to perform motoric acts, as may be the case in crimes of negligence. The adaptive function of behavioral consequences culminating in a criminal activity can be viewed as positive, purposive, and directed.

As in the typology of aggression (Buss, 1971), criminal behavior may be expressive or instrumental in the adaptive sequence. Expressive acts may be more emotionally motivated in behavior expressing psychological problems and conflicts, symptomatic of pathological personality structure, or providing a cathartic value to the individual. When instrumental, the behavioral sequence is one which provides a more tangible reinforcer to the individual due to cognitive rather than emotional functioning.

The expressive or instrumental qualities of the act may be reflected in the sophistication and skills required for its commission. The nature of the criminal behavior expressed also aids in determining the extent of emotional or cognitive factors involved, as in criminal behavior committed for "fun" rather than for more pathological or criminalistic motives. Even features of "job satisfaction" are found in a view of crime as adaptation and should not be overlooked by diagnosticians. Plate (1975) provides information concerning career criminal activities which clearly indicates the instrumental value that may be involved in the commission of a crime. High profit, tax exempt, with reasonably short "office hours" suggests that only minimal efforts may be required, with high "payoff" being an inducement.

8.3. The Actor

Most diagnostic evaluations are based primarily on the psychological state or personality structure of the offender. This diagnostic process is a two-way street, because the diagnostician and offender are in interaction with one another while under the guide and direction of social expectancies of action infringing on the liberties of the client. Such infringement occurs through something being done "to" (although the benevolent diagnosticians and decision makers would prefer the word "for") the subject of the diagnostic procedure.

Qualities of the interaction and philosophy of the diagnostician have already been discussed. There is no doubt that the interaction will be more cooperative and responsive with the YAVIS individual, and this will ultimately reflect on the evaluation, recommendations, and action. Aside from these factors, there are other ways of influencing the evaluation process. Rosenhan (1973) and his associates obtained admission to psychiatric hospitals through informing a doctor that they heard voices saying "hollow," "empty," and "thud." Regardless of the normal behavior evidenced on the ward, the pseudopatients were unable to convince the staff that they were not "schizophrenic." It would appear that once a diagnostician is attuned to the possible presence of pathology and so labels it, continuation of his label, and indeed his perceptions of the patient, becomes a self-fulfilling prophecy. The prophecy becomes evidenced in criminal justice evaluations, because being "mentally ill" may excuse one from sanctions of the crime, provide special treatment, or enable the offender to view himself as "sick" rather than "bad." This was reflected in a television documentary on individuals found not guilty by reason of insanity. An overwhelming number of those persons acknowledged playing the "insanity game." There are some diagnosticians who will refute such a notion by reporting that there is a double stigma attached to being both "mad" and "bad" by virtue of being a mentally ill offender. The only problem is that the stigma may be in the mind of the diagnostician, but not in the view of the offender.

A 26-year-old college graduate student killed his wife and went to attend an esoteric lecture following the action. On his return home, he called the police and reported that his wife was shot. The investigating officers were unable to find an indication that his wife was shot. When the offender was asked how he knew his wife was shot, he pointed to a rifle in the corner, stating that that was not where it was kept. The police officers found the subject's wife lying on the bed and found no blood. They did determine that perhaps she was shot, after they turned the body over, lifted the victim's hair, and used a flashlight to see a bullet hole in the base of the victim's skull. The offender was indeed YAVIS. He was examined and treated, although not found incompetent, and was recommended for return to the community for treatment. Because this recommendation was alien to the judicial system, the individual was convicted, but psychiatric evaluations were as instrumental as YAVIS in changing the first-degree murder charge to manslaughter. The focus on the attractiveness of the defendant and his glib use of psychiatric jargon indicating that he was emotionally disturbed overruled the diagnostic impression of the style of the crime, which was convincingly cool, calculated, and well integrated. This was reflected in the investigating officers' report, which also detailed the emotional state of the defendant. However, professional diagnosis was not their strong suit. Their observations were astute and of diagnostic importance because they reflected the style of the crime, which the diagnosticians chose to ignore with their benevolent emphasis on the individual professing to need professional help. Their interaction with the offender was equally ignored as they failed to realize the value to the offender, who played the role of an emotionally disturbed young man being evaluated by benevolent diagnosticians who control sanctions by their recommendations.

Responding to Klopher's first level of assessment was sufficient, albeit selective, because diagnoses based only on conscious statements in an adversary situation were viewed as truthful and accurate. Our attempts to find pathology and provide an "indepth" evaluation also allow for a tendency to avoid the acceptance of the subject's statements at the first level. When an offender claims the criminal activity was "fun," that may not be regarded as sufficiently complete. One examiner in a correctional center was taken aback because the offender told him he did not want the money from the armed robberies he pulled, but was more interested in the fun, excitement, and thrill of it. The style of the crimes would have lent credence to his view, but that was not sufficient. Said the examiner: "The patient offers numerous rationalizations for his criminal conduct in an effort to have others view his crimes as being thrill-seeking. This avoids the real recognition that his unresolved homosexual feelings for his father are the main motivation for his crimes. He does receive 'thrills' but only because he holds a phallic symbol on a father figure (men are generally in his stickups). This is just one example of how his sexual perversion insidiously manifests itself." The major difficulty is that the examiner's statement is based on attempting to fit the style of the crime into a theoretical framework of preconceived assumptions.

In our efforts to apply diagnostic evaluations and make predictions, our attempts at understanding the individual become restricted because of our failure to apply the knowledge we already have. Most of our diagnostic energies are invested in crimes which have a bizarre quality or involve violence producing physical destruction or abuse of a victim. This tends to keep diagnosticians in the mold of mental health workers by the unpredicated assumption that mental illness and such crimes are related. But even mental health workers fail to use existing knowledge and classifications or typologies which might be useful in the diagnostic enterprise.

Toch's (1969) typology of violence-prone strategies could be of assistance in viewing the patterns of violence-prone individuals which could produce insight into their activities. If Toch called these strategies symptoms of mental illness, their impact would be long recognized. All three of Klopher's levels would be pertinent in understanding these strategies, as well as in providing some subjective estimate of the probability of recurrence. When included in the total diagnostic assessment, the tendency to use violent actions and their significance to the individual may lead to greater understanding.

Diagnosticians also may inadvertently ignore individual aspects of episodic behavior disorders. Monroe (1974) defines such disorders as generally recurrent and intermittent, disrupting the life-style of the individual. Episodic dyscontrol is seen as a subgroup, where an abrupt single act or short series of acts is carried through to achieve at least partial relief of tension or immediate gratification of a specific need. He distinguishes between primary dyscontrol as an immediate reaction to an external stimulus, seeking need gratification, and seizure dyscontrol as the result of brain dysfunction. We often fail to recognize that organic brain disorders are the greatest mimickers of the functional disorders. Small (1973) offers a variety of findings that suggest neurological implications from case history data, psychological testing, clinical interview impressions, and patient complaints. Unless the neurological impairment is obvious, little significance is placed on the data. One patient who killed an individual in the process of an attack of temporal lobe epilepsy was viewed by a number of clinicians as dangerous but not mentally ill. This was predicated on their notion that epileptics do not kill in the course of seizures. There is still conflict regarding the temporal lobe phenomenon in spite of the work of Mark and Ervin (1970), who also considered the possibility of controlled, skillfully executed acts of violence as a function of the phenomenon. Because medical reviews indicated a consensus that epileptics were not dangerous, that bias may well be distorting the diagnostic evaluations and decisions on individuals who may have the syndrome described in Mark and Ervin and Honigfeld and Howard (1973). The diagnosis and possible use of the condition as a determinant of diminished responsibility are relatively rare even when a full syndrome is displayed in accordance with the characteristics described by Mark and Ervin. Abnormal EEG patterns may also be ignored because a criminal behavior may not fit the consensus. However, that consensus appears more based on those patients in epileptic clinics, while the temporal lobe patients who do act out violently, erratically, or skillfully may end in prison without the least suspicion of organic involvement. Possession of the syndrome may well end up diagnosed as schizophrenia (latent type is preferable because the symptoms may wax and wane) or dissociative neurosis. If the recommended treatment of medication and/or psychotherapy is for those conditions, the diagnosis is apt to be changed to psychopathy, and secure incarceration will result because treatment does not produce change. A program of psychotherapy along with dilantin or mysoline may have produced greater change in behavior and been more appropriate to the temporal lobe phenomenon if it were diagnosed.

It may be that diagnosticians are more impressed with level of pathology (extent), which serves to guide decision makers more than the refined definition of type of pathology. Rader (1977) investigated the level of pathology in sex offenders, finding the rapists the most psychologically disturbed of the groups, assaulters next, and exposers the least disturbed. The extent of pathology did affect sanction decision because the least psychologically disturbed tended to be placed on probation while the most disturbed were inclined to be sent to prison or committed. This may appear to be inconsistent with the philosophy inherent in the concept of diminished responsibility and may reflect a tendency to view the level of pathology as indicative of "dangerousness" or need for control rather than treatment.

Most of these results, however, were achieved by scores on the Minnesota Multiphasic Personality Inventory (MMPI). Being reflective of Level I, which involves self-perceptions, level of pathology may reflect an attempt by the subject to adopt the "sick role." That role appears to be inconsistent with probation placement. More comprehensive assessment appears indicated to define the "pathology" of an individual.

The diagnostic instruments currently in vogue for individual assessment are of the paper-and-pencil variety, particularly in the correctional diagnostic and classification process, as time and ease of administration are main considerations. The application of diagnostic procedures, at the three levels suggested by Klopfer, would yield a more comprehensive view of personality structure.

Self-presentation through consciously controlled tests or interview responses may indicate that an individual either is assuming that sick role or is indeed sustaining psychological dysfunction. The sick role would reflect Level I data concerned with public communication and public image. Further evaluation is necessary to determine the consistency of that image with self-perceptions. This would allow the examiner to become more aware of pathology and how it intrudes on the individual's life-style. Level III, private symbolization, affords an estimate of the extent of any pathology and its influence on the personality structure.

Consistency of pathology in all three levels would indicate a more psychologically disturbed individual whose behavior (criminal and otherwise) is a function of that disorder. Need for control and treatment options can be highly specified, and predictions are more inclined to be of greater accuracy as an individual's defenses and means of coping are identified.

Focus on one level does not permit the full determination of the nature and extent of the pathology and the identification of the means of coping, or provide an understanding of how the pathology is related to the actual criminal behavior.

8.4. The Victim

A comprehensive diagnostic process cannot be achieved without an understanding of the role of the victim, particularly in those cases involving sexual attack or other interpersonal violence. Aggression may be a displacement on an innocuous target or one who symbolically represents a significant figure. Symbolic representations are more prone to be discovered in repeaters because the resolution of conflict by the destruction or injury of the offending target tends to be incomplete. A murderer or assaulter whose victim matches characteristics of his mother or father or who otherwise displaces anger on the victim has only a substitute with a substitute target. The act itself may not gratify or satisfy the need to express the anger. The symbol is destroyed, but the real target continues to exist and serves to keep the feelings stimulated. Symbolic representation may not succeed as a complete activity because the original offending stimulus continues to exist and to offend.

Research on murders (Wille, 1974; Tanay, 1969) indicates that the victim received signals from the perpetrator regarding the action that would be forthcoming. However, the signals were either ignored or led to an intensification or facilitation of the act. Some murders have been regarded as the victim's suicide, with the perpetrator being the tool for the victim's demise (Wille, 1974). It is difficult to validate this impression, which may be accurate for a very small proportion of murders, because the victim is unable to provide any data. Victimology studies of assaults or would-be murders where prompt medical attention prevented victim death may provide more information on victim characteristics and interaction with the offender. Some individuals persist in consistently, and almost constantly, being victimized in interpersonal relationships, and the same could apply to being victims of property and interpersonal crimes.

The importance of shifting attention to the role of the victim as well as the perpetrator of a violent act is also emphasized by Bard (1971) in his study of police intervention in intrafamilial violence. He estimates that approximately 10% of injuries sustained by police occur on their becoming involved in handling of family disputes. Support is offered by Sarbin (1967), who presents his thesis that humiliating or degrading transformation of an individual's identity into a "nonperson" in interpersonal encounters evokes violent behavior. The medical concept of "iatrogenesis" is useful in understanding interpersonal violence and the role of the victim. Bard states that "the term refers simply to a disorder resulting from the actions of the physician during his ministrations" (p. 158). Iatrogenesis may be viewed as referring to the treatment of one condition creating another. Bard's notion of iatrogenic violence indicates that the manner with which a seemingly aggressive act is handled may lead to the eruption of violence. This interaction is of diagnostic importance because the criminally assaultive behavior of an offender may be iatrogenic in nature. The basic cause may lie in the interaction pattern between victim and perpetrator. The perpetrator may indeed have been victimized.

Since the victim's role in the interaction may have been instrumental to the crime, diagnosis of the offender must include an assessment of the interaction between that offender and the victim.

This interaction may also reveal properties of the offender in view of how he may select victims who have characteristics meaningful to him. Craik (1971) discusses the systematic assessment of "places," using concepts and techniques from the field of personality assessment. The assessment of places directs attention to their physical-spatial properties, the organization of components within them, their traits, and their behavioral and institutional attributes. All these features are also inducements for an individual to frequent certain types of places. Personality and individual needs and conflicts are reflected in the places that are chosen with high frequency and over a long time. One offender could not accept the interpretation that he was attempting to resolve his homosexual desires. He denied any feelings for other men, sexually and otherwise, but was able in his conversations with other offenders to demonstrate his knowledge of all the "swinging" bars in Detroit. However, all the bars he cited were "gay" bars.

Places also contain people; people who may become victims. The place in which the victims are found may indicate characteristics which motivate the individual because of the behavioral drawing attributes and the functional nature of the place or because the place makes the victim into a target.

Similarities exist with frequenting of places, selectivity of victims, and drug choice which occurs after the drug abuser has "shopped around"; all reflect selective needs of the offender. Their effect on the offender psychologically and his need for them are a crucial part of the diagnostic procedure.

On less pathological terms, the meaning of the criminal sequence may reflect the individual's sustaining a "flow experience" which may defy explanation. Csikszent-mihalyi (1975) studied chess masters, dancers, mountain climbers, composers, and others, and found a commonality. What they shared was "flow," which was a satisfying "high," an exhilarating feeling of creative accomplishment and heightened functioning. There was almost a oneness with the doing of the activity and oneself. The intrinsic motivation was in the "doing." One of the authors (F. P.), working with dangerous offenders, found this to be the major motivation for such activities as armed robbery, taking heroin, and assaulting. While this appeared in a few individuals, it is not a generalized or typical finding. It has occurred with sufficient frequency to be considered in a diagnostic process, and is of sufficient import as it maximizes the violence potential of the individual. Future behaviors are likely to be repetitions of the past, attempts to enjoy that flow experience which resists alteration, because no reasonable substitute can readily be provided. Like the artist who loses interest in a painting when it is completed, or the dancer who loses interest after performing, and the mountain climber after reaching the peak, the criminal with the flow experience from his behavior looks to the next process of doing. Satisfaction and gratification come from the doing and not from the accomplishment.

This flow experience may initially occur accidentally, but later some violence-prone individuals may keep their destructive urges in a "holding pattern" by searching for or creating appropriate targets to rationally permit themselves the privilege of experiencing the process. This may be a consistent or intermittent pattern.

The "privilege of experience" refers not only to the flow experience but also to intermittent indulgence that may be tension relieving, pleasurable, or erotic, or which may break boredom. Expression of emotional or psychological conflicts or a multitude of other reinforcements may be provided by the victim and the process. This tendency is supported by the findings on stimulus seekers and stimulus reducers, with the seekers immersed in the process and the reducers directed by the goal or effect of that process.

9. Techniques and Tools

The accomplishment of a complete assessment of the criminal offender using an interactional approach is a formidable task. It requires the examination of multilevel aspects of the individual, the situation, and the victim at the same time. It is far simpler to conduct a superficial evaluation relative to the initial decision and to ignore major decision making that will occur at various points of the criminal justice process.

The matter of pretrial decisions is the simplest, because the basis for the evaluations is generally the assessment of extent of pathology from which impressions of competency and insanity are obtained. Regardless of diagnostic procedures utilized, the orientation of the examiner outweighs the data collected.

An interactional analysis may produce some improvement by virtue of increasing diagnostic sensitivity and providing behavioral specifically as the basis of the decisions. The actual techniques and instruments will vary according to the preferences and biases of the individual diagnosticians or dictates of the agency which provides the service.

Current diagnostic procedures involve the use of MMPI as the predominant personality inventory, along with a mixture of interest and aptitude tests. Intelligence estimates are a general "must," although their relationship to programming is as questionable as the other devices. Perhaps the lack of relevancy of diagnostic studies to correctional programming is due to the diagnosticians performing the service. As behavioral experts, they are responsible not only for the use of diagnostic instruments and establishing procedures but also for selecting the devices. Incorporating the various methods of personality assessment attuned to the levels of personality may well improve the strategies of decision-making. The adjective checklists, inventories, and projective techniques summarized by Megargee and Menzies (1971) as assessing aggression can be incorporated into a multilevel assessment of criminal behavior.

Current techniques at the disposal of the diagnostician are abundant, but many of the professionals involved lack the necessary knowledge of the techniques and training in their application.

1. Case history. In the correctional system, case workers are typically assigned at the early stage. While there is an emphasis on attempting to obtain a social history by diagnosticians in the pretrial stage, some of the information is already present in reports prepared for correctional authorities. The presentence investigator's report is designed to provide descriptive material of the criminal act from the frame of reference of the complainant or victim, witnesses, police investigators, and the offender himself. Social history data are also required, but court workers performing this task have usually had no professional training in obtaining case histories. Nevertheless, some of them are remarkably perceptive and complete in their reports. Information presented may indicate the need for additional diagnostic resources to be recommended.

2. Objective personality tests. As screening devices, the objective personality tests are invaluable, particularly the popular MMPI with its indices of pathology. However, subject to conscious distortion by the respondent, information is still presented without considering his involvement and role in the assessment process. Skilled clinicians are able to gain psycho-dynamic impressions from the MMPI, using a clinical rather than a sign approach. The California Personality Inventory (CPI) has been referred to as the MMPI for normals. It is somewhat useful in providing information to the prison staff and prison counselor which may facilitate the individual's adjustment. It also permits the incompetent clinician to provide impressions which sound professional. The Sentence Completion Test will yield data as a function of the sentence stems, generally providing Level I information, although Levels II and III may appear. Other inventories may be used, but their nosological net is not as extensive as the ones mentioned.

3. Interests, aptitudes, and achievement. Since correctional systems attempt to provide remedial programs in academic and vocational preparation, a variety of tests are used contingent on the preferences of the classification units. For the simplistic programs available for female offenders (Velimesis, 1975), testing or other appraisals serve no purpose. The Kuder is used for general areas of vocational interest because of its ease of administration and interpretation.

4. Intellectual functions. Intelligence tests are typically the paper-and-pencil variety which is included in routine batteries. The WAIS may be given when the results on the routine tests are low, indicating a question of adequacy of intellectual functioning, or for additional specific diagnostic information. Disturbances of intellectual functioning and neurological complaints or symptoms may require the refined estimates provided by the WAIS.

5. Neurological screening. The EEG is a frequent asset to diagnostic assessment where the possibility of brain dysfunction is suspected. Other tests such as the Bender-Gestalt and the Halstead-Reitan may be useful. The Halstead-Reitan can be used only when diagnosis is worth the expense of the test and the salary of the trained diagnostician to use it. It is used to localize brain damage, and its use is limited to those diagnostic centers servicing neurological problems. There is little need for the criminal justice agencies to incorporate its use in classification procedures. Referral may be made to an agency which provides such testing if indicated.

6. Projective testing. The use of the Thematic Apperception Test (TAT) and the Rorschach has fallen in frequency because of the emphasis most universities and students place on objective procedures. Lindzey (1965) had shown clinical judgments from the TAT to be more successful than objective testing, but the test is time-consuming and many clinicians are too busy or too bored with the test to bother with it. The Rorschach provides information at Level III concerning personality structure and reality testing that can make a significant impact on the diagnostic process. The projective techniques may also be used to provide a standardized interpersonal situation to an individual (provided that it is

properly administered), because nowhere else does the offender get a standardized situation to which he can respond. The major difficulty with its use is that specialized training is required. The Hand Test shows promise in evaluating extent and direction of hostile and aggressive responses. (Bricklin, Piotrowski, & Wagner, 1962).

7. The clinical interview. A free-floating interaction, the interview is rarely standardized and is limited by the interaction between the diagnostician and interviewee. That interaction is rarely assessed, because all effort is generally directed toward the patient's responses. Diagnosticians, as a result of their academic and field training, or its lack, will demonstrate varied individual competency. In addition, the interview is often centered on the purpose of evaluation. Clinicians who are experienced in mental health settings are oriented toward people who voluntarily seek help. In the criminal justice system, this is not the case, and fear, defensiveness, and suspiciousness prevail on the part of the client. The system dictates how the diagnostician will be perceived by the offender, who is often remarkably perceptive of the "psychology game" and the role that would be most advantageous to assume. As the offender's perceptions of the process, person, and purpose of the examiner influence his responses, the examiner's perceptions of the offender influence his interaction. That interaction is rarely analyzed, although it is a most significant part of the diagnostic procedure.

8. Nonverbal behavior. Any clinician will tell of the importance of non-verbal behavior and acknowledge that he always uses this source of information concerning the client. The truth is that skilled clinicians respond to nonverbal behavior consciously and unconsciously, but both the sophisticated and naive diagnosticians rarely note it unless it is strikingly dramatic. North (1972) and Argyle (1975) provide a plethora of research and information concerning personality assessment through movement and bodily communications. Gilbert, Kirkland, and Rappeport (1977) provide a test technique for evaluating personality and social behavior with children, but clinicians and other diagnosticians do not formalize inquiries into or impressions of the subject's nonverbal behavior. Willis (1975) presents a fascinating analysis and assessment of the expressive style of the motorbike culture in England, where nonverbal and movement assessment receives considerable research and clinical attention. Concepts of places and situations, of flow feelings, of personal meaning to dress activity and interaction, and of peers are derived from the nonverbal communications and movements. The body as a medium of expression is generally ignored by American diagnosticians in favor of verbal communication patterns, although body responses and actions could be evaluated on all three personality levels.

The literature on personality assessment is relatively lacking in descriptions of the instruments used in assessment or classification of criminal offenders. Test batteries, routine and otherwise, vary from one agency to another, with most being created or changed ad hoc. Processing people rather than goal-oriented diagnosis seems to be the major function of diagnosticians. Tests appear to be chosen for their speed and efficiency of administration rather than for their effectiveness in providing information or establishing a base level for future comparisons. Regardless of the battery of instruments used by the diagnostician, the effectiveness of clinical diagnosis will be determined by the ability of the diagnostician to apply himself and his skills as an artist and scientist. Integrating actuarial and clinical data presupposes a recognition by the diagnostician of the relevant factors in criminal behavior, a training in the use of clinical tools, and a recognition that personality level is to be incorporated into the assessment. Awareness of system and personal biases and of his interaction with an offender within those biases may assist the diagnostician to adhere to his data and provide specified support for his conclusions or recommendations. By doing so, the diagnostician will find himself providing a significant service to the offender, to the criminal justice system, and, indeed, to the society he serves.

10. References

Argyle, M. *Bodily communication.* New York: International Universities Press, 1975.

Ausubel, D. P. *Drug addiction: Physiological, psychological and sociological aspects.* New York: Random House, 1958.

Bard, M. The study and modification of intra-familial violence. In J. Singer (Ed.), *The control of aggression and violence.* New York: Academic Press, 1971.

Bazelon, D. L. Psychologists in corrections. Are they doing good for the offender or well for themselves? In S.L. Brodsky (Ed.), *Psychologists in the criminal justice system.* Marysville, Ohio: American Association of Correctional Psychologists, 1972.

Blumer, D. Temporal lobe epilepsy and its psychiatric significance. In F. Benson, & D. Blumer (Eds.), *Psychiatric aspects of neurological disorders.* New York: Grune & Stratton, 1975.

Bohmer, C. Judicial use of psychiatric reports in the sentencing of sex offenders. Ann Arbor, Mich.: Xerox University Microfilms, 1975, 169 pp. (dissertation, University of Pennsylvania).

Braginsky & Braginsky. *Mainstream psychology: A critique.* New York: Holt, Rinehart and Winston, 1974.

Bricklin, B., Piotrowski, Z., & Wagner, E. *The Hand Test: A new projective test with special reference to the prediction of overt aggressive behavior.* Springfield, Ill.: Thomas, 1962.

Burt, R. A. Helping suspect groups to disappear. In G. Bermant, C. Nemeth, & N. Vidar, (Eds.), *Psychology and the law.* Lexington, Mass.: Lexington Books, 1976.

Buss, A. H. Aggression pays. In J. Singer (Ed.), *The control of aggression and violence.* New York: Academic Press, 1971.

Chronbach, L. J. & Gleser, G. C. *Psychological tests and personnel decisions.* Urbana: University of Illinois Press, 1957.

Chwast, J. Delinquency and criminality: An acting out phenomenon. In L. E. Abt, & S. L. Weissman, (Eds.), *Acting out.* New York: Grune & Stratton, 1965.

Craik, K. H. The assessment of places. In P. McReynolds (Ed.), *Advances in psychological assessment* (Vol. II). Palo Alto, Calif.: Science and Behavior Books, 1971.

Csikszentmihalyi, M. *Beyond boredom and anxiety.* San Francisco: Jossey-Bass, 1975.

Dana, H., Hannifin, P., Lancaster, C., Lore, W., & Nelson, D. Psychological reports and juvenile probation counseling, *Journal of Clinical Psychology*, 1963, *19*, 352–355.

Efron, C. Psychiatric bias: An experimental study of the effects of social class membership on diagnostic outcome. Unpublished master's thesis, Wesleyan University, 1970.

Finckenauer, J. O., Rauh, C. Contract parole: Some legal and rehabilitative issues of mutual agreement programming for parole release. *Capital University Law Review*, 1976, *5*, 175–195.

Foster, T. W. Drug therapy for sociopathic offenders: An experimental treatment program utilizing imipramine hydrochloride. Ann Arbor, Mich.: Xerox University Microfilms, 1975, 319 pp. (dissertation, Ohio State University).

Friedman, C. J., & Mann, F. Recidivism; the fallacy of prediction. *International Journal of Offender Therapy and Comparative Criminology*, 1976, *20*, 153–164.

Friedman, L. M. *The legal system: A social science perspective.* New York: Russel Sage Foundation, 1975.

Gettinger, S. Parole contracts: A new way out. *Corrections Magazine*, 1975, *2*, 3–8, 45–52.

Gilbert, G. S., Kirkland, D. D., & Rappeport, L. Nonverbal assessment of interpersonal affect *Journal of Personality Assessment*, 1977, *41*, 13–18.

Gilman, D. The sanction of imprisonment: For whom, for what, and how. *Crime and Delinquency*, 1975, *21*, 337–347.

Goldstein, J. H. *Aggression and crimes of violence*. New York: Oxford University Press, 1975.

Halleck, S. *Psychiatry and the dilemmas of crime*. Berkeley: University of California Press, 1971.

Halstead, W. C. *Brain and intelligence*. Chicago: University of Chicago Press, 1947.

Heller, M. E., & Mordkoff, A. M. Personality attributes of the young, non-addicted drug user. *International Journal of Addiction*, 1972, *7*, 65–72.

Hollingshead, A. B., & Redlich, F. C. *Social class and mental illness: A community study*. New York: Wiley, 1958.

Honigfeld, G., & Howard, A. *Psychiatric drugs: A desk reference*. New York: Academic Press, 1973.

Johnson, P. M., & Kime, W. L. *Performance screening—A new correctional synthesis*. Lansing, Mich.: Department of Corrections (mimeo), 1975.

Katz, M., & Zimbardo, P. Making it as a mental patient. *Psychology Today*, April 1977, 122–126.

Kime, W. L. *Early findings: Risk of violent behavior on parole*. Lansing, Mich.: Corrections Department (mimeo), 1976.

Kittrie, N. N. *The right to be different: Deviance and enforced therapy*. Baltimore: The Johns Hopkins Press, 1971.

Klopfer, W. G. The blind leading the blind: Psychotherapy without assessment. *Journal of Projective Techniques and Personality Assessment*, 1964, *28*, 87–392.

Klopfer, W. G. Interation of projective techniques in the clinical case study. In A. I. Rabin (Ed.), *Projective techniques in personality assessment*. New York: Springer, 1968.

Kozol, H. W. Myths about the sex offender. *Medical Aspects of Human Sexuality*, June 1971.

Kozol, H. W., Boucher, R. J. & Garogalo, R. F. The diagnosis and treatment of dangerousness. *Crime and Delinquency*, 1972, *18*, 371–392.

Krystal, H., & Raskin, H. A. *Drug dependence: Aspects of ego functions*. Detroit: Wayne State University Press, 1970.

Lee, S. Social class bias in the diagnosis of Mental Illness. Ann Arbor, Mich.: University Microfilms, 1968.

Lindzey, G. Seer versus sign. *Journal of Experimental Research in Personality*, 1965, *1*, 17–26.

Lipsitt, P. O., & McGarry, A. L. Competency for trial: A screening instrument. *American Journal of Psychiatry*, 1971, *1*, 128.

Maier, G. J. Therapy in prisons. In D. J. Madden & J. R. Lion (Ed.), *Rage, hate, assault and other forms of violence*. New York: Spectrum Publications, 1976.

Mark, V., & Ervin, F. *Violence and the brain*. New York: Harper & Row, 1970.

Martinson, R. What works? Questions and answers about prison reform. *The Public Interest*, Spring 1974. 22–54.

Meehl, P. E. *Clinical versus statistical prediction: A theoretical analysis and a review of the evidence*. Minneapolis: University of Minnesota Press, 1954.

Megargee, E. I., & Menzies, E. S. The assessment and dynamics of aggression. In P. McReynolds (Ed.), *Advances in psychological assessment* (Vol. II). Palo Alto, Calif.: Science and Behavior Books, 1971.

Menninger, K. *The crime of punishment*. New York: Viking Press, 1968.

Monroe, R. R. The problem of impulsivity in personality disturbances. In J. R. Lion, (Ed.), *Personality disorders: Diagnosis and management*. Baltimore: Williams & Wilkins, Co. 1974.

Morris, N. Psychiatry and the dangerous criminal. *Southern California Law Review*, 1968. *41*, 514–547.

Moynihan, M. H. Getting burned: A study in the socialization of correctional workers. Ann Arbor, Mich.: Xerox University Microfilms, 1976, 192 pp. (dissertation, University of Colorado).

North, M. *Personality assessment through movement*. London: Macdonald & Evans, 1972.

Palmer, T. Martinson's revisited. *Journal of Research in Crime and Delinquency*, 1975, *12*, 133–252.

Persons, R. W., & Marks, P. A. The violent 4-3 MMPI personality type. *Journal of Counsulting and Clinical Psychology*, 1971, *35*, 189–196.

Peterson, D. R., Quay, H. C., & Cameron, G. R. Personality and background factors in juvenile delinquency as inferred from questionnaire responses. *Journal of Consulting Psychology*, 1959, *23*, 395–399.

Plate, T. *Crime pays*. New York; Simon & Schuster, 1975.

Quay, H., & Parsons, L. *The differential classification of the juvenile offender*. Morgantown, W. Va.: Robert F. Kennedy Youth Center, 1970.

Rabin, A. I. Changing concepts of mental abnormality. *The Centennial Review*, Spring 1974, *18*.

Rader, C. M. MMPI profile types of exposers, rapists, and assaulters in a court services population. *Journal of Consulting and Clinical Psychology*, 1977, *45*, 61–69.

Rappeport, J. R. Personality disorders in the court. In J. R. Lion (Ed.), *Personality disorders: Diagnosis and management*. Baltimore: Williams & Wilkins, 1975.

Reitan, R. M. Psychological deficits resulting from cerebral lesions in man. In J. M. Warren & K. Akert (Eds.), *The frontal granual cortex and behavior*. New York; McGraw-Hill, 1964.

Reynolds, D. C., & Sanders, M. S. Effect of defendant attractiveness, age, and injury on severity of sentence given by simulated jurors. *Journal of Social Psychology*, 1975, *96*, 149–150.

Robey, A. Criteria for competency to stand trial: A checklist for psychiatrists. *American Journal of Psychiatry*, 1965, *122*, 616–623.

Rosenham, D. L. On being sane in insane places. *Science*, 1973, *179*, 250–257.

Rubin, S. Probation or prison; applying the principle of the least restrictive alternative. *Crime and Delinquency*, 1975, *21*, 331–336.

Russell, E. W., Neuringer, C., & Goldstein, G. *Assessment of brain damage: Neuropsychological key approach*, New York: Wiley-Interscience, 1970.

Sarbin, T. The dangerous individual, an outcome of social identity transformation. *British Journal of Criminology*, July 1967, 285–295.

Shover, N. Experts and diagnosis in correctional agencies. *Crime and Delinquency*, 1974, *20*, 248–358.

Silber, D. E. Controversy concerning the criminal justice system and its implications for the role of mental health workers. *American Psychologist*, 1974, *29*, 239–244.

Small, L. *Neuropsychodiagnosis in psychotherapy*. New York: Bruner/Mazel, 1973.

Smith, A., & Pollack, H. Deviance as a method of copying. *Crime and Delinquency*, 1976, *22*, 3–16.

Smith, B. D. & Musk, H. The violent offender in the court. In D. J. Madden & J. R. Lion (Eds.), *Rage, hate, assault and other forms of violence*. New York: Spectrum Publications, 1976.

Sommer, R. *The end of imprisonment*. New York: Oxford University Press, 1976.

Steadman, H. J. Predicting dangerousness. In D. J. Madden & J. R. Lion (Eds.), *Rage, hate, assault, and other forms of violence*. New York: Spectrum Publications, 1976.

Strupp, H. H., & Hadley, S. W. A tripartite model of mental health and therapeutic outcomes: With special reference to negative effects in psychotherapy. *American Psychologist*, 1977, *32*, 187–196.

Szasz, T. *Law, liberty and psychiatry*. New York: Macmillan, 1963.

Tanay, E. Psychiatric study of homocide. *American Journal of Psychiatry*, 1969, *125*, 1252–1258.

Thomas, M., & Hess, J. H., Jr. Incompetency to stand trial: Procedures, results, and problems. *American Journal of Psychiatry*, 1963, *119*, 713–720.

Toch, H. *Violent men: An inquiry into the psychology of violence*. Chicago: Aldine, 1969.

Velimesis, M. The female offender. *Crime and Delinquency Literature*, 1975, *7*, 94–112.

Walker, A. E. Murder or epilepsy? *Journal of Nervous and Mental Disorder*, 1961, *133*, 430–437.

Warren, M. Q. Classification of offenders as an aid to efficient management and effective treatment. *Journal of Criminal Law, Criminology, and Political Science*, 1971, *62*, 239–258.

Wenk, E., Robinson, J. O., & Smith, G. W. Can violence be predicted? *Crime and Delinquency*, 1972, *18*, 393–402.

Wikler, A., & Rasor, R. W. Psychiatric aspects of drug addiction. *American Journal of Medicine*, 1953, *14*, 566–570.

Wille, W. S. *Citizens who commit murder*. St. Louis, Mo.: Warren Green Inc., 1974.

Willis, P. E. The expressive style of the motor-bike culture. In J. Bentall & T. Polhemus (Eds.), *The body as a medium of expression*. New York: Dutton, 1975.

Index

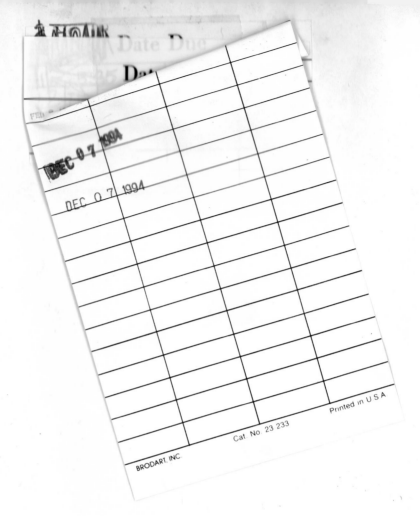